AF694983

Thieme

Oral Cancer

Evaluation, Therapy, and Rehabilitation

Carole Fakhry, MD, MPH, FACS
Professor
Department of Otolaryngology–Head and Neck Surgery and Oncology
Director
Johns Hopkins Head and Neck Cancer Center
The Johns Hopkins University School of Medicine
Baltimore, Maryland, USA

Karen T. Pitman, MD, FACS
Associate Professor
Department of Otolaryngology–Head and Neck Surgery
The Johns Hopkins University School of Medicine
Baltimore, Maryland, USA

Ana P. Kiess, MD, PhD
Assistant Professor
Department of Radiation Oncology and Molecular Radiation Sciences
The Johns Hopkins University School of Medicine
Baltimore, Maryland, USA

David W. Eisele, MD, FACS
Andelot Professor and Director
Department of Otolaryngology–Head and Neck Surgery
The Johns Hopkins University School of Medicine
Baltimore, Maryland, USA

384 illustrations

Thieme
New York • Stuttgart • Delhi • Rio de Janeiro

Library of Congress Cataloging-in-Publication Data is available from the publisher.

Important note: Medicine is an ever-changing science undergoing continual development. Research and clinical experience are continually expanding our knowledge, in particular our knowledge of proper treatment and drug therapy. Insofar as this book mentions any dosage or application, readers may rest assured that the authors, editors, and publishers have made every effort to ensure that such references are in accordance with **the state of knowledge at the time of production of the book.**

Nevertheless, this does not involve, imply, or express any guarantee or responsibility on the part of the publishers in respect to any dosage instructions and forms of applications stated in the book. **Every user is requested to examine carefully** the manufacturers' leaflets accompanying each drug and to check, if necessary in consultation with a physician or specialist, whether the dosage schedules mentioned therein or the contraindications stated by the manufacturers differ from the statements made in the present book. Such examination is particularly important with drugs that are either rarely used or have been newly released on the market. Every dosage schedule or every form of application used is entirely at the user's own risk and responsibility. The authors and publishers request every user to report to the publishers any discrepancies or inaccuracies noticed. If errors in this work are found after publication, errata will be posted at www.thieme.com on the product description page.

Some of the product names, patents, and registered designs referred to in this book are in fact registered trademarks or proprietary names even though specific reference to this fact is not always made in the text. Therefore, the appearance of a name without designation as proprietary is not to be construed as a representation by the publisher that it is in the public domain.

© 2020. Thieme. All rights reserved.

Thieme Medical Publishers New York
333 Seventh Avenue
New York, New York 10001 USA
+1 800 782 3488
customerservice@thieme.com

Georg Thieme Verlag KG
Rüdigerstrasse 14, 70469 Stuttgart, Germany
+49 [0]711 8931 421, customerservice@thieme.de

Thieme Publishers Delhi
A-12, Second Floor, Sector-2, Noida-201301
Uttar Pradesh, India
+91 120 45 566 00, customerservice@thieme.in

Thieme Publishers Rio de Janeiro,
Thieme Publicações Ltda.
Edifício Rodolpho de Paoli, 25º andar
Av. Nilo Peçanha, 50–Sala 2508,
Rio de Janeiro 20020-906 Brasil
+55 21 3172-2297

FSC www.fsc.org 100% Paper from well-managed forests FSC® C103101

Cover design: Thieme Publishing Group
Typesetting by Thomson Digital, India

Printed in USA by King Printing Company, Inc. 5 4 3 2 1

ISBN 978-1-62623-968-5

Also available as an e-book:
eISBN 978-1-62623-969-2

This book, including all parts thereof, is legally protected by copyright. Any use, exploitation, or commercialization outside the narrow limits set by copyright legislation, without the publisher's consent, is illegal and liable to prosecution. This applies in particular to photostat reproduction, copying, mimeographing, preparation of microfilms, and electronic data processing and storage.

We dedicate this book to our patients who have faced oral cancer, and to our mentors, colleagues, and trainees who have helped us do our best in caring for them.

Carole Fakhry, Karen T. Pitman, Ana P. Kiess, and David W. Eisele

Contents

Videos

Video 11.1 Speech samples following subtotal glossectomy.

Video 22.1 Ulnar artery perforator flap.

Video 24.1 Radial forearm fasciocutaneous transfer for retromolar trigone reconstruction.

Video 44.1 Postoperative fiberoptic endoscopic evaluation of swallowing.

Video 44.2 Subtotal glossectomy.

Foreword

The management of squamous cell carcinoma of the upper aerodigestive tract has evolved significantly in recent decades. For patients with carcinoma of the oropharynx, hypopharynx or larynx, functional organ preservation through the application of new surgical and nonsurgical modalities has become the overarching principle of treatment, as the quest for therapies that provide significant survival benefit continues. In contrast, primary surgery remains the preferred treatment for patients with cancers of the oral cavity and has been demonstrated to provide better disease control and functional outcome than nonsurgical methods. Nearly 40 years ago, it was established that definitive radiation therapy for squamous cell carcinoma of the oral cavity was associated with an unacceptable incidence of severe fibrosis, xerostomia, and osteoradionecrosis of the jaws. Contemporary methods of reconstruction introduced in the late 1980s permitted transfer of vascularized soft tissue and bone to reconstruct the tongue, floor of the mouth, and mandible with a high degree of success and acceptable functional outcome. Reliable free tissue transfer now provides the head and neck oncologic surgeon with the latitude to resect tumors with adequate margins, knowing that advanced reconstruction would provide restoration of form and function and well-vascularized tissues that could better withstand postoperative radiotherapy. It is likely that the combination of more complete surgical resection, guided by contemporary imaging to assess the local extension of oral cavity tumors more accurately, and advanced reconstruction have contributed to the improved survival observed in these patients.

Oral Cancer: Evaluation, Therapy, and Rehabilitation is an important addition to the existing textbooks devoted to head and neck oncology. The editors are internationally recognized leaders with extensive experience in treating head and neck cancer. In this book, they have provided the most current evidence-based management principles available. Each chapter covering oncologic evaluation and treatment is paired with a companion chapter on state-of-the-art reconstruction particular to each site. A key element in the treatment of patients with oral cancer is contemporary surgical reconstruction, and leaders in the field have contributed site-specific chapters covering the reconstructive options that are time tested and effective for restoring form and function. The contributing authors stress the importance of multidisciplinary evaluation and management by a team of experts, which is a fundamental concept throughout this book.

The book starts with a discussion of epidemiology and the molecular events that are precursors to invasive cancer, providing an understanding of the molecular biology of oral cancer progression that is critical to developing risk assessment models and identifying targets for new therapies. On this broad foundation, subsequent chapters provide an in-depth discussion of patterns of disease progression and a comprehensive management approach for each of the oral cavity subsites. Appropriately, prosthetic rehabilitation, implantology, and speech and swallowing rehabilitation are covered in detail and serve as an adjunct to the chapters on therapy and surgical reconstruction. The textbook appropriately concludes with a discussion on the management of early and late treatment sequelae and strategies to mitigate these untoward events. These are followed by discussions on the future directions in cancer therapy that are unfolding and include the hope for immunotherapy and targeted therapy to improve treatment outcomes and lower morbidity. The scientific basis for these new modalities is addressed as well. This textbook is an important state-of-the-art resource for those who seek to become educated in managing patients with tumors of the oral cavity. Its comprehensive scope will be an invaluable resource for the multidisciplinary team whose responsibility is to comprehensively care for these patients with common goals of achieving a cure and providing a meaningful quality of life.

Randal S. Weber MD, FACS
Professor
Chief Patient Experience Officer
John Brooks Williams and Elizabeth Williams Distinguished University Chair in Cancer Medicine
Department of Head and Neck Surgery
University of Texas M. D. Anderson Cancer Center
Houston, Texas, USA

Preface

Oral cancer comprises a significant proportion of head and neck malignant neoplasms worldwide and carries the potential to considerably disrupt form and function. Surgery, the primary treatment modality, can impair appearance, speech, mastication and swallowing, each of which may be further exacerbated by adjuvant treatments. Successful prevention and early detection of oral cancer remain elusive to date, yet it can be the best opportunity to reduce the suffering and mortality from oral cancer. Recent advances in the understanding of the underpinnings of oral cancer at the molecular level and in the immunological interface between tumor and patient have enabled progress towards more effective treatment strategies, which may also inform future prevention or early detection.

This textbook provides a comprehensive in-depth review of each phase of the survivorship trajectory for oral cancer patients. Oral cancer is a heterogeneous entity that can arise from divergent exposures and premalignant entities. At the diagnostic stage, the biopsy that is initially performed by a head and neck specialist is interpreted by a pathologist. While much of the diagnostic and therapeutic pathway hinges upon accurate pathologic evaluation, it also relies upon further assessment by neuroradiology, speech-language pathology, radiation oncology, medical oncology, nutrition, dentistry, psychology, social work, and nursing. The input of the multidisciplinary team is synthesized at each stage of care and this theme is carried through all stages of the survivorship trajectory.

In this book, the issues relevant to oral cancer in each phase are examined in-depth. For example, dental issues are examined separately from the vantage point of pre-treatment, postsurgical rehabilitation, postradiotherapy, dental complications of oral cancer treatment, and sequelae such as trismus. Swallowing and speech assessments before and after therapy are considered separately and include video illustrations. Strategies for radiation therapy as primary, adjuvant, and salvage therapy are explored as well as the sequelae and complications of radiation therapy. Given that surgery serves as the main treatment modality for the majority of histopathologic entities of oral cancer, surgical considerations for each subsite of the oral cavity are considered, not only from an ablative but also from a reconstructive perspective. For each chapter, epidemiology, typical clinical presentations, diagnostic methods, anatomic and treatment considerations, and sequelae of therapy are reviewed. With each chapter key considerations or pearls are highlighted. Lastly, recurrent and metastatic oral cancer management is discussed in a similar focused manner.

This book provides the present state-of-the-art diagnostic, therapeutic, and rehabilitative strategies for oral cancers with a consistent emphasis on the theme of multidisciplinary care. Due to the complexity of management of patients with oral cancer, their care must be carefully coordinated to allow access to a comprehensive team of experts who work collaboratively to ensure optimal treatment outcomes.

We are grateful to the experts who have contributed their insights, perspectives, and expertise to the content of this book. We hope that this book will assist practitioners at all levels of experience. We are optimistic that the future holds with it many advances and improvements in oral cancer care and outcomes.

Carole Fakhry, MD, MPH, FACS
Karen T. Pitman, MD, FACS
Ana P. Kiess, MD, PhD
David W. Eisele, MD, FACS

Contributors

Rina Abrams, MS, CCC-SLP
Speech Language Pathologist
Assistant Professor of Otolaryngology–Head and Neck Surgery
The Johns Hopkins University School of Medicine
Baltimore, Maryland, USA

Hassan Arshad, MD, FACS
Associate Professor of Oncology
Department of Head and Neck/Plastic and Reconstructive Surgery
Roswell Park Comprehensive Cancer Center
Buffalo, New York, USA

Nafi Aygun, MD
Professor
Russell H. Morgan Department of Radiology and Radiological Sciences
Division of Neuroradiology
Johns Hopkins University
Baltimore, Maryland, USA

H. Michael Baddour, MD
Assistant Professor
Department of Otolaryngology
Emory University School of Medicine
Atlanta, Georgia, USA

Brittany R. Barber, MD
Assistant Professor
Department of Otolaryngology–Head and Neck Surgery
University of Washington
Seattle, Washington, USA

Justin A. Bishop, MD
Director of Anatomic Pathology
Associate Professor
Department of Pathology
University of Texas Southwestern Medical Center
Dallas, Texas, USA

Kofi Boahene, MD, FACS
Professor
Department of Otolaryngology–Head and Neck Surgery
The Johns Hopkins University School of Medicine
Baltimore, Maryland, USA

Lauren M. Bolding, DDS, MS, FACP
Clinical Associate
Department of Otolaryngology–Head and Neck Surgery
The Johns Hopkins University School of Medicine
Baltimore, Maryland, USA

Karim Boudadi, MD
Assistant Professor
Department of Oncology
The Johns Hopkins University School of Medicine
Baltimore, Maryland, USA

Christopher Britt, MD
Assistant Professor
Department of Otolaryngology
Loyola University Medical Center
Maywood, Illinois, USA

Patrick J. Byrne, MD, FACS, MBA
Director
Division of Facial Plastic and Reconstructive Surgery
Professor
Department of Otolaryngology–Head and Neck Surgery
Department of Dermatology
Department of Biomedical Engineering
Member of Miller Coulson Academy of Clinical Excellence
The Johns Hopkins University School of Medicine
Baltimore, Maryland, USA

Amy Cao, DDS
Dentist
Woodinville Family Dental
Woodinville, Washington, USA

Jason Y.K. Chan, FRCSEd (ORL)
Assistant Professor
Department of Otorhinolaryngology–Head and Neck Surgery
The Chinese University of Hong Kong
Hong Kong SAR, China

Steven S. Chang, MD FACS
Director
Head and Neck Cancer Program
Henry Ford Cancer Institute
Detroit, Michigan, USA

David Chen, MD
Chief Resident
Department of Otolaryngology–Head and Neck Surgery
The Johns Hopkins University School of Medicine
Baltimore, Maryland, USA

Jennifer Christenson, DO
Clinical Instructor
Department of Otolaryngology–Head and Neck Surgery
Oregon Health and Science University
Portland, Oregon, USA

Yee Seul Chun, DDS
Dentist
The Johns Hopkins Hospital
Baltimore, Maryland, USA

James H. Clark, MD
Assistant Professor
Department of Otolaryngology–Head and Neck Surgery
The Johns Hopkins University School of Medicine
Baltimore, Maryland, USA

Natasha Cohen, MD, MSc, FRCSC
Adjunct Professor
Division of Otolaryngology
Queen's University
Kingston, Ontario, Canada

Catherine M. Concert, RN, DNP, FNP-BC, AOCNP, NE-BC, CNL,CGRN, FNAP, FNYAM
Nurse Practitioner
Department of Radiation Oncology
NYU Langone Health
New York City, New York, USA

Ruth J. Davis, MD
Resident
Department of Otolaryngology–Head and Neck Surgery
The Johns Hopkins University School of Medicine
Baltimore, Maryland, USA

Matthew P. Deek, MD
Resident
Department of Radiation Oncology and Molecular Radiation Sciences
The Johns Hopkins University School of Medicine
Baltimore, Maryland, USA

Shaun C. Desai, MD, FACS
Assistant Professor
Facial Plastic and Reconstructive Surgery
Department of Otolaryngology–Head and Neck Surgery
The Johns Hopkins University School of Medicine
Baltimore, Maryland, USA

Anil D'Cruz, MS, DNB, FRCS (Hon)
Director
Department of Oncology
Apollo Hospitals
Mumbai, Maharashtra, India

David W. Eisele, MD, FACS
Andelot Professor and Director
Department of Otolaryngology–Head and Neck Surgery
The Johns Hopkins University School of Medicine
Baltimore, Maryland, USA

Mark El-Deiry, MD, FACS
Associate Professor
Department of Otolaryngology
Chief
Division of Head and Neck Surgery
Director
Head and Neck Oncology Surgery Center
Emory University School of Medicine
Atlanta, Georgia, USA

Joel B. Epstein, DMD, MSD, FRCD(C)
Professor
Cedars-Sinai Medical Center
Los Angeles, California, USA
City of Hope National Medical Center
Duarte, California, USA

Carole Fakhry, MD, MPH, FACS
Professor
Department of Otolaryngology–Head and Neck Surgery and Oncology
Director
Johns Hopkins Head and Neck Cancer Center
The Johns Hopkins University School of Medicine
Baltimore, Maryland, USA

Christine G. Gourin, MD, MPH, FACS
Professor
Department of Otolaryngology–Head and Neck Surgery
Head and Neck Surgical Oncology
The Johns Hopkins University School of Medicine
Baltimore, Maryland, USA

Jennifer H. Gross, MD
Head and Neck Surgery Fellow
Department of Otolaryngology
University of Miami
Miami, Florida, USA

Theresa Guo, MD
Resident
Department of Otolaryngology - Head and Neck Surgery
The Johns Hopkins University School of Medicine
Baltimore, Maryland, USA

Vishal Gupta, MD
Assistant Professor of Oncology and Otolaryngology
Department of Head and Neck/Plastic and Reconstructive Surgery
Roswell Park Comprehensive Cancer Center
Buffalo, New York, USA

Pelin Güneri, PhD, DDS
Professor
School of Dentistry
Ege University
Izmir, Turkey

Andrea L. Hanick, MD
Physician
Head and Neck Institute
Cleveland Clinic
Cleveland, Ohio, USA

Wesley L. Hicks Jr., MD, FACS
Professor and Chairman
Department of Head and Neck/Plastic and Reconstructive Surgery
Roswell Park Comprehensive Cancer Center
Buffalo, New York, USA

Susan Hill, MAPS, RD, CSO
Supportive Oncology Services
Henry Ford Cancer Institute
Detroit, Michigan, USA

Allen S. Ho, MD
Director
Head and Neck Cancer Program
Associate Professor of Surgery
Cedars-Sinai Medical Center
Los Angeles, California, USA

Won Jin Ho, MD
Hematology Oncology Fellow
The Sidney Kimmel Comprehensive Cancer Center
The Johns Hopkins University School of Medicine
Baltimore, Maryland, USA

Kenneth S. Hu, MD, FASTRO
Associate Professor
Department of Radiation Oncology
Department of Otolaryngology–Head and Neck Surgery
NYU Langone Health
New York City, New York, USA

Erik Interval, MD
Fellow
Head and Neck Surgical Oncology
Estabrook Cancer Center
The Nebraska Methodist Hospital
Omaha, Nebraska, USA

Glenn T. Jennings, MS, DABR
Medical Physicist
Department of Radiation Oncology
NYU Langone Health
New York City, New York, USA

Ashok Jethwa, MD
Clinical Fellow
Department of Otolaryngology–Head and Neck Surgery
University of Toronto
Toronto, Ontario, Canada

Gerard J. Ondrey
Medical Student
University of Minnesota Medical School
Minneapolis, Minnesota, USA

Maie A. St. John, MD, PhD, FACS
Professor and Thomas C. Calcaterra Chair
Department of Head and Neck Surgery
Co-Director
UCLA Head and Neck Cancer Program
Jonsson Comprehensive Cancer Center
David Geffen School of Medicine at UCLA
Los Angeles, California, USA

Andrew W. Joseph, MD, MPH
Assistant Professor
Facial Plastic and Reconstructive Surgery
Department of Otolaryngology–Head and Neck Surgery
University of Michigan Health System
Ann Arbor, Michigan, USA

Hyunseok Kang, MD
Associate Professor
School of Medicine
University of California San Francisco
San Francisco, California, USA

Arij Kazmi, DMD
Dentist
McGill University
Montreal, Quebec, Canada

Majid Khan, MD
Associate Professor of Radiology
Director
Non-Vascular Spine Intervention
Russell H. Morgan Department of Radiology and Radiological Science
The Johns Hopkins Hospital
Division of Neuroradiology and Neuro-interventional Radiology
Baltimore, Maryland, USA

Ana P. Kiess, MD, PhD
Assistant Professor
Department of Radiation Oncology and Molecular Radiation Sciences
The Johns Hopkins University School of Medicine
Baltimore, Maryland, USA

Wayne Koch, MD
Professor
Department of Otolaryngology–Head and Neck Surgery
The Johns Hopkins University School of Medicine
Baltimore, Maryland, USA

Jamie A. Ku, MD
Otolaryngology–Head and Neck Surgeon
Sections of Head and Neck Surgery and Oncology and Facial Plastic and Reconstructive Surgery
Cleveland Clinic Foundation
Cleveland, Ohio, USA

Elizabeth M. Kurian, MD
Associate Professor
Department of Pathology
University of Texas Southwestern Medical Center
Dallas, Texas, USA

Stephen Y. Lai, MD, PhD, FACS
Professor
Department of Head and Neck Surgery
Division of Surgery
The University of Texas MD Anderson Cancer Center
Houston, Texas, USA

Leah I. Leinbach, DMD, MPH
Assistant Professor
Department of Otolaryngology–Head and Neck Surgery
Director
General Practice Residency
Division of Oral Maxillofacial Surgery-Dentistry
The Johns Hopkins University School of Medicine
Baltimore, Maryland, USA

Lauren Levi, DMD
Dental Oncology Attending and Clinical Instructor
Icahn School of Medicine at Mount Sinai
New York City, New York, USA

Ryan J. Li, MD
Assistant Professor
Department of Otolaryngology–Head and Neck Surgery
Oregon Health and Science University
Portland, Oregon, USA

Kershena Liao, MD
Resident
Department of Otolaryngology–Head and Neck Surgery
UT Southwestern Medical Center
Dallas, Texas, USA

Diana J. Lu, MD
Radiation Oncologist
Samuel Oschin Comprehensive Cancer Institute
Cedars-Sinai Medical Center
Los Angeles, California, USA

G. Nina Lu, MD
Assistant Professor
Department of Otolaryngology–Head and Neck Surgery
Division of Facial Plastic and Reconstructive Surgery
University of Washington School of Medicine
Seattle, Washington, USA

William Lydiatt, MD, EMBA
Chief Medical Officer
Vice President of Medical Affairs
Methodist and Women's Hospitals
Omaha, Nebraska, USA

Rajarsi Mandal, MD
Assistant Professor
Department of Otolaryngology–Head and Neck Surgery
The Johns Hopkins University School of Medicine
Baltimore, Maryland, USA

Angela L. Mazul, PhD, MPH
Assistant Professor
Department of Otolaryngology/Head and Neck Surgery
Division of Public Health Sciences
Department of Surgery
Washington University School of Medicine
St. Louis, Missouri, USA

Ranee Mehra, MD
Director
Head and Neck Medical Oncology
Professor of Medicine
Marlene and Stewart Greenebaum Comprehensive Cancer Center
Baltimore, Maryland, USA

Vikas Mehta, MD, MPH, FACS
Associate Professor
Department of Otorhinolaryngology–Head and Neck Surgery
Montefiore Medical Center/Albert Einstein College of Medicine
Bronx, New York, USA

Brett A. Miles, MD, DDS, FACS
Professor
Department of Otolaryngology–Head and Neck Surgery
Co-Chief
Division of Head and Neck Cancer Surgery
Director
Head and Neck Oncologic and Microvascular Reconstructive Surgery Fellowship Program
Icahn School of Medicine at Mount Sinai
New York City, New York, USA

Michael G. Moore, MD, FACS
Associate Professor
Director of Head and Neck Surgery
Co-Director of Skull Base Surgery
Department of Otolaryngology–Head and Neck Surgery
UC Davis Medical Center
Sacramento, California, USA

Kevin M. Motz, MD
Resident Physician
Department of Otolaryngology–Head and Neck Surgery
The Johns Hopkins University School of Medicine
Baltimore, Maryland, USA

Wojciech K. Mydlarz, MD
Director
Head and Neck Surgery–National Capitol Region
Assistant Professor
Department of Otolaryngology–Head and Neck Surgery
The Johns Hopkins University School of Medicine
Baltimore, Maryland, USA

Frank Ondrey, MD, PhD, FACS
Associate Professor
Department of Otolaryngology–Head and Neck Surgery
Co-Leader
Carcinogenesis and Chemoprevention Program
Masonic Cancer Center
University of Minnesota Medical School
Minneapolis, Minnesota, USA

Brandi R. Page, MD
Associate Residency Program Director
Radiation Oncology Residency Program
Assistant Professor
Radiation Oncology and Molecular Radiation Sciences
The Johns Hopkins University School of Medicine
Baltimore, Maryland, USA

Aru Panwar, MD, FACS
Surgeon
Head and Neck Surgical Oncology
Methodist Estabrook Cancer Center
The Nebraska Methodist Hospital
Omaha, Nebraska, USA

Mihir R. Patel, MD
Associate Professor
Department of Otolaryngology/Head and Neck Surgery
Emory University School of Medicine
Atlanta, Georgia, USA

Alexander E. Pazoki, MD, DDS, FACS
Assitant Professor
Department of Otolarygology–Head and Neck Surgery
Director
Division of Oral and Maxillofacial Surgery–Dentistry
The Johns Hopkins University School of Medicine
Baltimore, Maryland, USA

Tim J. Phillips, MD
Clinical Instructor
Department of Otolaryngology–Head and Neck Surgery
UC Davis Medical Center
Sacramento, California, USA

Karen T. Pitman, MD, FACS
Associate Professor
Department of Otolaryngology–Head and Neck Surgery
The Johns Hopkins University School of Medicine
Baltimore, Maryland, USA

Harry Quon, MD, MS
Co-Director
Johns Hopkins Head and Neck Cancer Multidisciplinary Clinic
Associate Professor
Radiation Oncology and Molecular Radiation Sciences
The Johns Hopkins University School of Medicine
Baltimore, Maryland, USA

Saudur Rahman, MD
Radiologist
Health System Clinician
Feinberg School of Medicine
Northwestern Lake Forest Hospital
Northwestern Medicine
Lake Forest, Illinois, USA

Eleni M. Rettig, MD
Instructor
Department of Otolaryngology-Head and Neck Surgery
Associate Surgeon
Brigham and Women's Hospital & Dana-Farber Cancer Institute
Harvard Medical School
Boston, Massachusetts, USA

Jeremy D. Richmon, MD
Associate Professor
Department of Otolaryngology–Head and Neck Surgery
Massachusetts Eye and Ear
Harvard Medical School
Boston, Massachusetts, USA

Zain Rizvi, MD
Assistant Professor
Department of Otolaryngology–Head and Neck Surgery
University of Washington School of Medicine
Seattle, Washington, USA

Lisa M. Rooper, MD
Assistant Professor of Pathology
Departments of Pathology and Oncology
The Johns Hopkins University School of Medicine
Baltimore, Maryland, USA

Michael G. Roskies, MD
Fellow
Department of Otolaryngology–Head and Neck Surgery
University of Toronto
Toronto, Ontario, Canada

William R. Ryan, MD, FACS
Associate Professor
Head and Neck Oncologic/Endocrine/Salivary Surgery
Department of Otolaryngology–Head and Neck Surgery
University of California
San Francisco, California, USA

Zachary Saltman, DMD
Oral and Maxillofacial Surgeon
Germantown Oral and Facial Surgery Center
Germantown, Maryland, USA
Columbia oral and Facial surgery Center
Columbia, Maryland, USA

Nicole C. Schmitt, MD
Assistant Professor
Division of Head and Neck Surgery
Department of Otolaryngology–Head and Neck Surgery
The Johns Hopkins University School of Medicine
Baltimore, Maryland, USA

James J. Sciubba, DMD, PhD
Professor (Retired)
The Johns Hopkins School of Medicine
Consultant
The Milton J. Dance Head and Neck Center
The Greater Baltimore Medical Center
Baltimore, Maryland, USA

Rosh K.V. Sethi, MD, MPH
Instructor in Surgery
Department of Otolaryngology–Head and Neck Surgery
Harvard Medical School
Boston, Massachusetts, USA

Andrew G. Sikora, MD, PhD
Vice Chair for Research
Co-Director
Head and Neck Cancer Program
Bobby R. Alford Department of Otolaryngology–Head and Neck Surgery
Baylor College of Medicine
Houston, Texas, USA

Ghassan G. Sinada, DDS
Maxillofacial Prosthodontist
Milton J. Dance Head and Neck Center
Greater Baltimore Medical Center
Towson, Maryland, USA

Ryan M. Smith, MD
Assistant Professor
Facial Plastic and Reconstructive Surgery
Department of Otorhinolaryngology–Head and Neck Surgery
Rush University Medical Center
Chicago, Illinois, USA

Gregory Stachelek, MD, PhD
Resident
Department of Radiation Oncology
The Johns Hopkins University School of Medicine
Baltimore, Maryland, USA

Heather M. Starmer, MA CCC-SLP, BCS-S
Clinical Associate Professor
Department of Otolaryngology, Head and Neck Surgery
Director
Head and Neck Cancer Speech and Swallowing Rehabilitation
Stanford Cancer Center
Stanford, California, USA

Marietta Tan, MD
Assistant Professor
Department of Otolaryngology–Head and Neck Surgery
The Johns Hopkins University School of Medicine
Baltimore, Maryland, USA

Theresa Tharakan, MD
Resident Physician
Department of Otolaryngology–Head and Neck Surgery
Washington University School of Medicine
St. Louis, Missouri, USA

Carl M. Truesdale, MD
Resident Surgeon
Department of Otolaryngology–Head and Neck Surgery
University of Michigan Health System
Ann Arbor, Michigan, USA

Anthony P. Tufaro, MD, DDS, FACS
Professor of Surgery
Chief of Plastic Surgery
University of Oklahoma Health Sciences Center
Oklahoma City, Oklahoma, USA

Richa Vaish, MS, MCh
Assistant Professor
Department of Head and Neck Services
Tata Memorial Hospital
Mumbai, Maharashtra, India

Peter S. Vosler, MD, PhD
Assistant Professor
Department of Otolaryngology–Head and Neck Surgery
Head and Neck Surgical Oncology and Microvascular Reconstruction
The Johns Hopkins University School of Medicine
Baltimore, Maryland, USA

Kimberly Webster, MA, MS, CCC-SLP
Speech Language Pathologist
Assistant Professor of Otolaryngology–Head and Neck Surgery
The Johns Hopkins University School of Medicine
Baltimore, Maryland, USA

John W. Werning, MD, DMD
Otolaryngologist
ProMedica Physicians Group
Toledo, Ohio, USA

Amy Williams, PhD, LP
Director
Psychology Practicum Program
Division of Health Psychology
Vice Chair
Complex Case Review Committee
Henry Ford Cancer Institute
Director of Research and Senior Staff Psychologist
Department of Otolaryngology–Head and Neck Surgery
Henry Ford Health System
Detroit, Michigan, USA

Eddy W.Y. Wong, FRCSEd (ORL)
Chief
Division of Head and Neck Surgery
Clinical Associate Professor
Department of Otorhinolaryngology–Head and Neck Surgery
The Chinese University of Hong Kong
Consultant
Department of Ear, Nose, and Throat
Prince of Wales Hospital
Shatin, Hong Kong SAR, China

Kimberly E. Wooten, MD
Assistant Professor of Oncology
Department of Head and Neck/Plastic and Reconstructive Surgery
Roswell Park Comprehensive Cancer Center
Buffalo, New York, USA

Mary Jue Xu, MD
Resident Physician
Department of Otolaryngology–Head and Neck Surgery
University of California San Francisco
San Francisco, California, USA

Sherry X. Yan, MD
Resident Physician
Department of Radiation Oncology
NYU Langone Health
New York City, New York, USA

Zenon Yeung, FRCSEd (ORL)
Deputy Chief
Division of Head and Neck Surgery
Clinical Assistant Professor
Department of Otorhinolaryngology–Head and Neck Surgery
The Chinese University of Hong Kong
Hong Kong SAR, China

Jose P. Zevallos, MD, MPH, FACS
Chief
Division of Head and Neck Surgery
Joseph B. Kimbrough Professor of Head and Neck Surgery
Department of Otolaryngology/Head and Neck Surgery
Washington University School of Medicine
St. Louis, Missouri, USA

Zachary S. Zumsteg, MD
Assistant Professor
Department of Radiation Oncology
Samuel Oschin Comprehensive Cancer Institute
Cedars-Sinai Medical Center
Los Angeles, California, USA

Section I

Background

1 Epidemiology of Oral Cavity Cancer

Jennifer H. Gross, Angela L. Mazul, and Jose P. Zevallos

Summary

Oral cavity cancer is one of the most common cancers worldwide. The leading risk factors include the use of tobacco, alcohol, and betel quid, which is predominantly used in Asia. Fortunately, the overall incidence and survival in the United States have improved with the decrease in tobacco use. Recommended treatment generally includes definitive surgery, with adjuvant therapy in indicated cases. The most important prognostic factor is the presence of nodal metastasis, and overall survival decreases dramatically as overall stage increases. Therefore, early detection of premalignant or malignant lesions could lead to improved survival. Resection and reconstruction of oral cavity malignancies are uniquely challenging, as they require consideration of both structure and function and can lead to significant posttreatment changes in quality of life. This chapter will provide an overview of the epidemiology, risk factors, clinical presentation, anatomy, and treatment considerations of this complex disease.

Keywords: epidemiology, risk factor, clinical presentation, anatomy, treatment

1.1 Introduction

Oral cavity cancer is among the most common cancers worldwide and is often associated with significant patient morbidity and poor survival. Patients may have advanced disease at presentation and therefore require treatment with surgery, radiation therapy, and chemotherapy. While surgical advances over the last 40 years have resulted in better functional outcomes, oncologic outcomes for oral cavity cancer are largely unchanged.[1] Over the last several decades, there has been an increased understanding of etiologic factors associated with oral cancer that extends beyond traditional carcinogenic factors. Investigators have focused on the impact of diet and dental health as potential etiologic factors and have explored the increasing incidence of oral cavity cancer among younger patients. In this chapter, we review the epidemiology of oral cavity cancer, with an emphasis on highlighting established and emerging risk factors associated with this disease. A complete understanding of oral cancer epidemiology is essential towards targeting interventions and improving primary and secondary prevention for oral cavity cancer.

1.2 Epidemiology

1.2.1 Histology

Squamous cell carcinomas constitute more than 90% of all oral cavity cancer and will be the focus of this chapter. However, other malignant tumors can arise from the epithelium, connective tissue, minor salivary glands, lymphoid tissue, and melanocytes. Minor salivary gland carcinomas represent less than 5% of the oral cavity cancers. Most arise in the hard palate (60%), lips (25%), and buccal mucosa (15%). Mucoepidermoid carcinoma is the most common type (54%), followed by low-grade adenocarcinoma (17%), and adenoid cystic carcinoma (15%). Other tumors are mucosal melanomas, osteosarcoma of the mandible or maxilla, and odontogenic tumors such as ameloblastoma.[2]

1.2.2 Incidence/Burden of Disease

Oral cavity squamous cell carcinoma (OCSCC) is one of the most common head and neck cancers, accounting for approximately 30% of all cases. In the United States, from 2000 to 2010, the incidence of oral cavity cancer was 4.3 per 100,000. Globally, the age-standardized rate was 2.7 per 100,000 with substantial differences by region, race, and sex. In general, rates of oral cavity cancer are higher in southern Asian counties with Papua New Guinea, Maldives, Sri Lanka, and Pakistan with the highest rates.[3]

Race and Gender Distribution

In the United States, from 2000 to 2010, the incidence of OCSCC was much higher among non-Hispanic white males (6.4 per 100,000 population, age-standardized to the 2000 population) compared to non-Hispanic black males (4.2 per 100,000 population). This racial difference is also reflected in females (3.4 per 100,000 population), where non-Hispanic white women have higher rates than non-Hispanic black women (2.1 per 100,000 population). Hispanic males (3.4 per 100,000) also have higher rates compared to Hispanic women (2.1 per 100,000 population).[4]

Even globally, the incidence of oral cavity is consistently greater among men than among women. The male:female rate is 2:1 overall, and it is the highest for central and eastern Europe (5:2) and lowest for northern Africa, western Asia, and Oceania (1:4).[3]

Recently, there has been a dramatic increase in the incidence of oral tongue squamous cell carcinoma of young females, and to a lesser extent young males.[5,6] Studies of the prognosis of this subgroup are mixed with no clear consensus.[7–9] The genomic profile of older smokers with tongue cancer is shown to be the same as younger nonsmokers.[10] This subgroup was determined with epidemiologic methods, and since these tumors are not human papillomavirus (HPV) associated or smoking and alcohol related, the etiology remains uncertain.[11]

1.2.3 Survival

Survival for OCSCC has improved over the past decade.[4] In the Surveillance, Epidemiology, and End Results (SEER) Program, the 5-year overall survival is 57.1%.[12] There are some differences by race, with non-Hispanic blacks having the lowest 5-year survival at 42.7%, and non-Hispanic whites with a 58.0% 5-year survival. However, there is tremendous heterogeneity by stage. As stage increases, 5-year survival decreases dramatically. Five-year survival by stage I is 78.1%, stage II is 60.3%, stage III is 48.7%, stage IVA is 33.2%, stage IVB is 23.8%; and stage IVC is 12.3%.[12]

1.2.4 Risk Factors

Tobacco

Tobacco is the leading risk factor for OCSCC, accounting for over a quarter of OCSCC cases.[13,14] However, the association between OCSCC and tobacco is smaller than when compared to other subsites of head and neck cancer.[15–17] Previous epidemiologic studies have demonstrated that cigarette smokers have almost three times the risk of OCSCC when compared with noncigarette smokers.[18] Even low-frequency smokers (one to two cigarettes a day) have a 50% increased risk of OCSCC.[19]

Duration of smoking also plays an important role in OCSCC. A study found that at a low level of consumption (≤ 15 cigarettes per day), smoking more cigarettes per day for a shorter duration was more deleterious than smoking fewer cigarettes per day for a longer duration.[20] However, this relationship changes for heavier smokers (> 15 cigarettes per day). Among heavy smokers, smoking more cigarettes per day for a shorter duration was less deleterious than fewer cigarettes per day for a longer duration. The excess risk of OCSCC due to tobacco virtually disappears 20 years after smoking cessation and independently of the quantity previously consumed.[20]

Studies evaluating smokeless tobacco and OCSCC have been inconsistent. The relationship is complex due to the concurrent use of cigarettes or other fillers such as betel leaves, areca nuts, quicklime, condiments, spices, or sweeteners depending on the region. Animal models of smokeless tobacco have been largely negative. However, in the United States, smokeless tobacco (non-cigarette-smoking) users have demonstrated an approximately twofold increase in the risk of OCSCC.[21] Ultimately, the International Agency for Research on Cancer has concluded that there is sufficient evidence of carcinogenicity in smokeless tobacco.[22]

Alcohol Use

Although not as strongly correlated as tobacco use, high alcohol consumption is also a major risk factor for OCSCC. Alcohol accounts for an 18% increased risk of OCSCC.[15] The risk increases with daily consumption, duration of consumption, and lifetime cumulative consumption.[23,24] Heavy beer and liquor drinkers (30 + drinks per week) were about five times more likely than nondrinkers to develop OCSCC.[25] Heavy wine drinking was associated with an increased risk of OCSCC (odds ratio [OR] = 3.2), but there was an attenuated association most likely attributed to differences in socioeconomic status.[25]

Interaction between Tobacco and Alcohol Use

Smoking and alcohol consumption have a synergistic interaction that results in an exponentially increased risk in OCSCC and other head and neck cancers. Among never drinkers, heavy smokers had almost 13 times the risk of OCSCC compared with never smokers/never drinkers. However, among those who consume over two alcoholic beverages a day, heavy smokers had almost 31 times the risk of OCSCC compared with never smokers.[26] This same study suggests that 23.5% of OCSCC are attributed to both alcohol and cigarette smoking.[26,27]

Betel Quid

Betel quid contains betel leaf, areca nut, and slaked lime, and it may contain tobacco. It is used by 600 million people worldwide, predominantly in Asia.[28] Betel quid has been classified as an oral carcinogen in humans by the International Agency for Research on Cancer, with evidence for a dose–response relationship (i.e., risk increases in a step-wise fashion with increased exposure).[28] In Asian studies, betel quid chewing appeared to be a stronger risk factor for cancer than either smoking or alcohol consumption.[29] In a recent review, betel quid without tobacco was associated with a sevenfold increase in the risk of OCSCC and a 15-fold increased risk when betel was combined with tobacco.[30]

Diet

The most consistent finding between diet and OCSCC risk is the association between consumption of fruit and vegetables with decreased risk.[31] In a large prospective cohort study, high consumption of fruits and vegetables was associated with a decreased risk of OCSCC (OR = 0.6; 95% confidence interval [CI]: 0.4–0.9) when compared with low consumption of fruit and vegetables.[31] Since fruits and vegetables do not have a high source of protein or fat, carbohydrates, fiber, and vitamins and minerals likely contribute to this association. Other types of food have been studied less frequently and with inconsistent results. In a meta-analysis, high consumption of processed meat (i.e., meat preserved by smoking, curing, salting, or by addition of chemical preservatives) was associated with an increased risk (OR = 1.91; 95% CI: 1.19–3.06) of OCSCC. However, total meat (white and red meat) consumption was not significantly associated with OCSCC.[32]

To further strengthen the association between diet and OCSCC, studies have suggested a link between combined dietary indexes and OCSCC. In a case-control study, OCSCC was associated with a "western" diet, or a diet with high consumption of fried foods, fat, and processed meats.[33] In the same study, more pro-inflammatory diets were also associated with an increased risk.[34]

The association between tea and OCSCC is inconsistent and depends largely on the temperature of tea and location. Maté—an herbal tea commonly consumed in South America—was associated with an increased risk of oral cavity (and oropharynx) cancer.[35,36] Yet, a meta-analysis found a decreased risk of OCSCC with overall tea consumption. When the meta-analysis considered type of tea, green tea was significantly associated with decreased risk of OCSCC, while black tea was not associated. However, most of the green tea studies were in Asian countries, making them less generalizable.[37]

Similarly, coffee consumption is likely also associated with a decreased risk of OCSCC. A pooled analysis found an inverse relationship between OCSCC and coffee consumption (OR: 0.5; 95% CI: 0.3–0.7 for coffee drinkers of more than four cups of coffee per day vs. nondrinkers).[38] This association was also reflected in a French case-control study.[39] In a meta-analysis, coffee was associated with a decreased risk of OCSCC and pharyngeal cancer.[40]

Oral Human Papillomavirus Infection

Although HPV infection has been linked definitively to oropharyngeal cancer, its role in OCSCC etiology is controversial. In a meta-analysis that included 5,478 cases worldwide, HPV deoxyribonucleic acid (DNA) was found in 24.5%.[41] Another study of 1,264 cases found 7.4% of OCSCC tumors had HPV DNA.[42] Both studies demonstrate large heterogeneity by region and sex, potentially leading to the difference in prevalence. To date, there is no clear molecular evidence that OCSCC is driven by HPV infection. Unlike oropharyngeal cancer, there does not appear to be a survival advantage for HPV-positive OCSCC.[43–47] Additionally, for OCSCC as a whole, no significant relationship was observed between high-risk sexual behaviors and the risk of cancer.[48]

Oral Health

Various measures of oral health, such as the number of missing teeth, number of dental checkups, and tooth mobility, have been associated with OCSCC.[49–52] Although these results could be confounded by low socioeconomic status and education level as well as the consumption of tobacco and alcohol, poor oral and dental health is a significant risk factor for OCSCC. In a pooled analysis, having the worst oral hygiene score was associated with three times greater risk of OCSCC when compared to having an optimal oral hygiene score.[50]

1.3 Clinical Presentation

Patients with oral cavity lesions (benign, premalignant, or malignant) often present initially to a primary care provider or dentist. Due to the wide variety of presentations and pathology in oral cavity lesions, they are often ambiguous and referred to an otolaryngologist or head and neck surgeon in order to rule out malignancy.

1.3.1 Benign Lesions

There are a variety of anatomic variants occurring in the oral cavity that can be confused with pathologic findings, including dental tori, Fordyce granules, and geographic tongue. Dental tori are bony outgrowths most commonly arising from the lingual surface of the mandible or the hard palate. They can be caused or exacerbated by trauma and generally do not require removal. Fordyce granules are small, papular sebaceous glands found in clusters, usually on labial or buccal mucosa. Again, these lesions are safe to leave alone. Geographic tongue, or benign migratory glossitis, presents with erythematous patches that migrate over the surface of the tongue. It is present in 3% of Americans and can often be confused with more concerning lesions such as leukoplakia.[53] Another lesion that sometimes causes concern among primary care providers or dentists is the iatrogenic dental amalgam tattoo. These lesions are found in approximately 1% of the U.S. adult population and can be mistaken for a nonbenign lesion. An amalgam tattoo presents most commonly as a dark-colored macule on mucosa adjacent to a restored tooth.[54]

Multiple categories of systemic illness can present with oral manifestations, including immunologic disorders (e.g., lupus, scleroderma, inflammatory bowel disease, human immunodeficiency virus [HIV]/acquired immunodeficiency syndrome [AIDS]), vitamin deficiencies (e.g., vitamin B12 deficiency), colonization or infection (e.g., candidiasis, herpes simplex virus), hematologic disorders (e.g., hereditary hemorrhagic telangiectasia), and endocrinopathies (e.g., hypothyroidism).

1.3.2 Premalignant Lesions

Premalignant oral cavity lesions can resemble benign lesions, but differ in that they have a risk of malignant transformation. Recognition and early detection are important in the prevention of OCSCC. Risk factors of both premalignant and malignant lesion development are similar and are discussed in the "epidemiology" section of this chapter. The most common premalignant oral cavity lesions are leukoplakia, erythroplakia, oral submucous fibrosis, and lichen planus.[55] Leukoplakia is a painless, white plaque determined by diagnosis of exclusion. Histologically, these lesions are comprised of hyperkeratosis with alteration in epithelial thickness. The risk of malignant transformation associated with leukoplakia is as high as 18% within 5 years.[56] Erythroplakia is overall less common, but it has a greater than 90% chance of transforming into a dysplastic or malignant lesion.[57] It presents as a red, flat macule with a velvety appearance. Oral submucous fibrosis is primarily found in southeast Asian countries where chewing betel quid is more common. It appears as a fibrotic, blanching oral mucosal lesion that can later lead to significant trismus. The risk of malignant transformation is 7.6% within 10 years.[58] Oral lichen planus (OLP) is characterized by inflammation of the stratified squamous epithelium, possibly from autoimmune activation of CD8 + T cells. There are six types of OLP, the most common of which is the reticular pattern. This subtype presents as asymptomatic, often bilateral, and symmetric "fine white striae."[55] A 2010 review reported a risk of malignant transformation of up to 10%.[59]

1.3.3 Malignant Lesions

Malignant oral cavity lesions can be variable in appearance, presenting signs and symptoms, and location. Nonhealing ulcers, mucosal irregularities, and exophytic masses are common presentations of oral cavity malignancies (▸ Fig. 1.1, ▸ Fig. 1.2, ▸ Fig. 1.3). A complete history and physical examination is essential, with a focus on assessing risk factors and a complete head and neck examination. Symptoms can range from severe pain to hypoesthesia or anesthesia due to adjacent sensory nerve invasion. Trismus and bleeding are signs potentially concerning for malignant pterygoid invasion and tumor necrosis, respectively. A firm neck mass in a patient with an oral cavity lesion should increase suspicion for malignancy.

1.4 Diagnosis and Evaluation

1.4.1 Physical Examination

The first step on initial presentation is a comprehensive history and physical examination. A physical examination of the oral cavity should include visualization and palpation of all oral cavity subsites (oral tongue, floor or mouth, alveolar ridge, hard palate, buccal mucosa, retromolar trigone). The dentition should be evaluated, and dentures should be removed for better visualization. A full cranial nerve examination is a necessary component, with emphasis on tongue mobility (cranial nerve

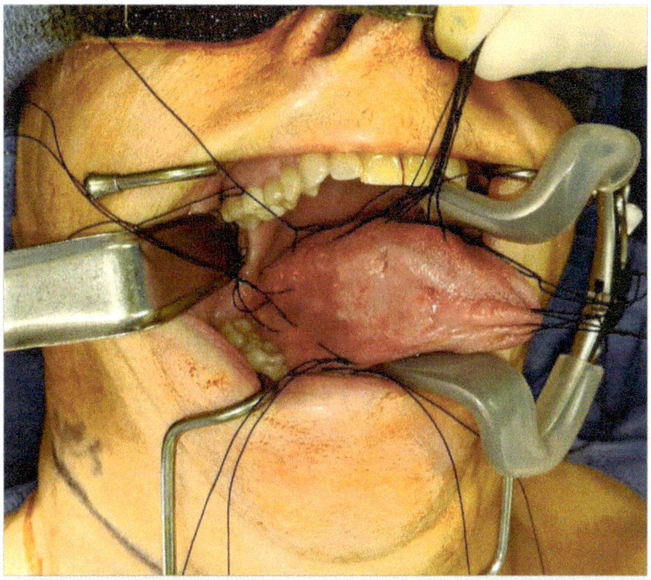

Fig. 1.1 Lateral tongue squamous cell carcinoma.

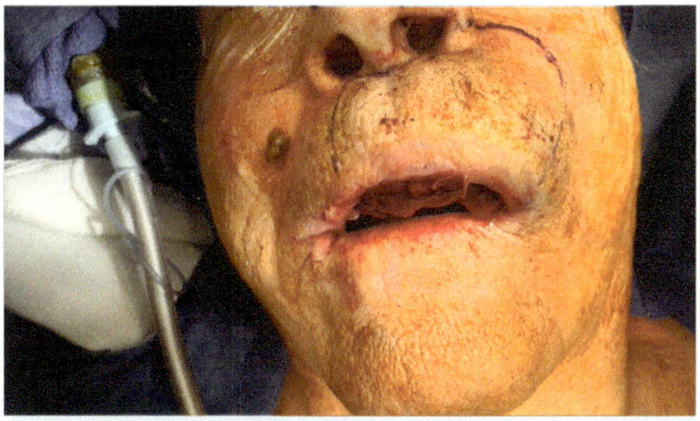

Fig. 1.2 Alveolar ridge squamous cell carcinoma.

XII) and sensation in the distribution of the inferior alveolar and mental nerves (cranial nerve V). The complete examination should also include either an indirect mirror or a direct fiberoptic view of the oropharynx and larynx. Understanding the extent or invasiveness of the tumor is essential when planning therapy, and clinicians should assess the potential for invasion into the deep muscles of the tongue, floor or mouth, mandibular or maxillary bone, or pterygoid musculature.

Imaging

Imaging is a critical tool in assessing tumor invasion of soft tissue and muscle, bone, or neural structures, as well as to evaluate for regional or distant metastases. The National Comprehensive Cancer Network (NCCN) recommends a computed tomography (CT) scan and/or a magnetic resonance imaging (MRI) with chest imaging as indicated and to consider a positron emission tomography (PET/CT) for advanced-stage disease. A CT scan with contrast is generally the mode of imaging performed during initial evaluation. It is very useful in assessing tumor

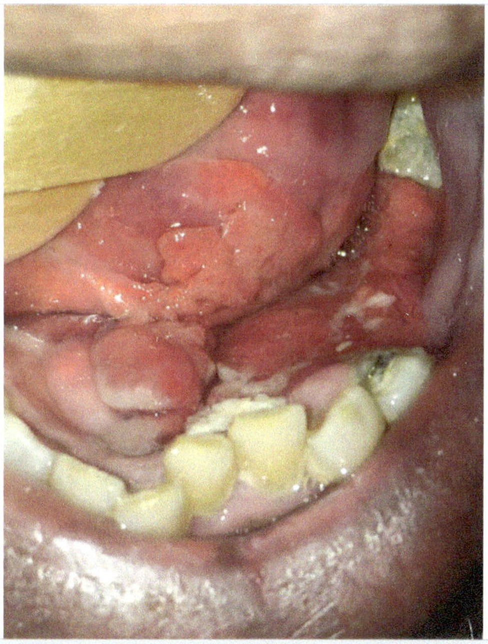

Fig. 1.3 Ventral tongue and floor of mouth squamous cell carcinoma.

mucosal and bony extent, is relatively cost-effective, and often readily available. An MRI is a useful adjunct in tumors with concern for perineural spread. PET alone has been shown to be more sensitive and specific than other imaging modalities in detecting primary and locally recurrent head and neck cancers.[60] PET/CT has the added benefit of improved localization and correlation with anatomic findings, and it can be useful in the detection of unknown or synchronous primaries or in diagnosing distant metastases. PET/CT has been shown to be extremely useful in the staging and management of advanced head and neck cancer, and its use continues to become more prevalent.[61]

Biopsy

A tissue sample is essential for the diagnosis of an oral cavity lesion. Surgical biopsies can be taken in the clinic under local anesthesia or in the operating room for select patients. Any ambiguous regional or distant lesions will also need histopathologic diagnosis, more commonly obtained by either fine needle aspiration (FNA) or core biopsy. The most common histologic diagnosis is squamous cell carcinoma, representing 90% of oral cavity cancers.[62] Other variants include adenocarcinoma, mucoepidermoid of a salivary gland, cutaneous basal cell carcinoma or melanoma of the lip, or primary tumors of the mandible.

Staging

Oral cavity cancer survival depends largely on stage at presentation, and the American Joint Committee on Cancer (AJCC) tumor node and metastasis (TNM) staging system is the gold standard. In January 2018, the AJCC 8th edition was enacted with significant alterations in both T and N staging for oral cavity cancer (▶ Table 1.1). T1 through T3 staging is still primarily dependent on tumor size, and T4a and T4b tumors are now described as "moderately advanced" and "very advanced," as opposed to "resectable" and "unresectable." Depth of invasion

Table 1.1 AJCC 8th edition T stage

Tx	Cannot assess
Tis	Carcinoma in situ
T1	≤ 2 cm, depth of invasion (DOI) ≤ 5 mm
T2	≤ 2 cm, DOI: 5–10 mm OR: 2–4 cm, DOI ≤ 10 mm
T3	Tumor > 4 cm OR DOI > 10 mm (and not T4)
T4a	Moderately advanced: (lip) invades bone, involves floor of mouth, inferior alveolar nerve, or skin (oral cavity) invades adjacent structures only (mandible or maxilla, maxillary sinus, facial skin)
T4b	Very advanced: invades masticator space, pterygoid plates, or skull base, or encases carotid

Table 1.2 AJCC 8th edition N stage

pNx	Cannot assess
pN0	No nodes
pN1	1 node ≤ 3 cm, extranodal extension (ENE) negative
pN2a	1 node ≤ 3 cm, ENE positive, OR 1 node 3–6 cm, ENE negative
pN2b	Multiple nodes ≤ 6 cm, ENE negative
pN2c	Bilateral or contralateral nodes ≤ 6 cm, ENE negative
pN3a	Node > 6 cm, ENE negative
pN3b	1 node > 3 cm, ENE positive, OR multiple nodes (ipsilateral, bilateral, or contralateral) with any ENE positive

(DOI) has also been added for its prognostic value. Regardless of its size, a tumor with DOI of 5 to 10 mm is automatically staged as a T2, and DOI greater than 10 mm changes the stage to a T3. Additionally, N staging continues to rely on lymph node number and size. However, both the clinical staging and pathological N staging now include assessment of extranodal extension (ENE). As demonstrated in ▶ Table 1.2, ENE positivity upstages a lymph node less than 3 cm from N1 to N2a and all other nodal stages to N3c.[63]

1.5 Anatomic Considerations/ Relevant Anatomy

The oral cavity primarily serves as the entrance to the aerodigestive tract. Eating and digestion begin in the oral cavity, with emphasis on mastication, salivation, and bolus propulsion to the pharynx. It also serves as the key site for speech modification, a respiratory conduit for inspiration, and a chemosensory organ for taste.

1.5.1 Anatomic Subsites

The oral cavity includes the following eight anatomic subsites: the lips, the upper and lower alveolar ridges and gingiva, the hard palate, the floor of mouth, the buccal mucosa, the oral tongue (the anterior two-thirds), and the retromolar trigone.[64] Having an intimate knowledge of adjacent anatomical structures is extremely important in order to perform a safe, negative margin resection and to be able to counsel the patients appropriately before treatment. The oral cavity is bounded by the vermillion border anteriorly, the buccal mucosa laterally, the hard and soft palate junction superiorly, the anterior tonsillar pillar and circumvallate papillae posteriorly, and the floor of mouth inferiorly.

Oral cavity mucosa is lined with stratified squamous epithelium, which consists of multiple layers of adherent epithelial cells. Due to their close proximity, they are well adapted to resist daily mechanical and chemical insults, and the outer layer frequently sloughs off and is replaced by the deeper layer. Frequent replacement of cells and associated proliferation and turnover increases the likelihood of development of cellular anomalies and subsequent carcinogenesis in the setting of endogenous or exogenous insults.[65] In general, thinner nonkeratinized mucosa within the oral cavity undergoes higher rates of proliferation and mitosis, which correlates with a higher incidence of carcinoma. Specifically, the floor of mouth, ventral tongue, and buccal mucosa subsites have the longest S phase of mitosis, in contrast with the palate and dorsal tongue.[66] As expected, these areas have been found to correlate with a higher incidence of malignant transformation/carcinoma.[67]

1.5.2 Muscular Anatomy

There are four bilateral pairs of muscles of mastication: the masseter, temporalis, medial pterygoid, and lateral pterygoid muscles. The masseter is the workhouse of the muscles of mastication, acting to elevate and protrude the mandible. It originates and inserts at the zygomatic arch and mandibular ramus, respectively. The temporalis muscle is a large, fan-shaped muscle that originates at the temporal fossa, extends under the zygomatic arch, and inserts on the coronoid process of the mandible. It serves to elevate and retract the mandible. The bulk of the medial pterygoid muscle originates from the medial surface of the lateral pterygoid plate and inserts onto the medial mandibular ramus and angle, joining the masseter to form the pterygomasseteric sling. It functions to elevate and weakly protrude the mandible and assist with excursion. The lateral pterygoid muscle has two heads: the superior runs from the greater wing of the sphenoid to the temporomandibular joint capsule and the inferior runs from the lateral surface of the lateral pterygoid plate to the condylar surface of the mandible. It primarily protrudes the mandible, assists with excursion, and is the only muscle of mastication to depress (or open) the jaw. Tumor invasion of the lateral pterygoid can lead to significant trismus.

The paired extrinsic tongue muscles are anchored to bone and act to protrude, retract, and allow horizontal movement of the tongue. The genioglossus, hyoglossus, and styloglossus function within the oral cavity, while the palatoglossus contributes to movement of the base of the tongue. The genioglossus extends from the mandibular mental spine to the hyoid and ventral tongue and is the major contribution to tongue protrusion. The hyoglossus originates from the greater cornu and side of the body of the hyoid, inserting onto the lateral tongue and acting to depress and retracting the tongue. The styloglossus arises from the styloid process and the stylomandibular ligament and inserts on the anterolateral and anterior tongue surface. This muscle depresses and elevates the tongue.

The paired intrinsic tongue muscles include the superior and inferior longitudinal, transverse, and vertical muscles and are generally thought to control the tongue's shape and displacement. They form a "meshlike structure" without clear demarcation of tissue planes between them.[68] As a result, a tongue malignancy can easily spread within the intrinsic tongue musculature. It is important to keep this anatomy in mind when performing a margin-negative tumor resection.

The four paired suprahyoid muscles (digastric, stylohyoid, geniohyoid, and mylohyoid) generally act to elevate the hyoid bone and assist with swallowing. The mylohyoid is an important landmark as the inferior border of the oral cavity, separating the sublingual and submandibular spaces. These two spaces communicate via the posterior free border of the mylohyoid, allowing potential spread of infection or malignancy from the floor of mouth to the neck.

1.5.3 Dentition

Teeth are composed of enamel, pulp, dentin, and cementum. The cementum covers the dental root and is bound to the alveolar bone by specialized connective tissue called periodontal ligaments (PDLs). Periodontal disease from poor oral hygiene is very common and can lead to chronic inflammation, a major risk factor in development of oral cavity cancer.[69] Mucosal tumors can spread to the alveolus and mandible by direct extension through exposed PDLs.

1.5.4 Innervation and Taste

The mandibular nerve is the third branch of the trigeminal nerve and itself branches into the lingual nerve and the inferior alveolar nerve, terminating in the mental nerve. The mandibular nerve and its branches provide general sensation to the lower half of the oral cavity, including the mandibular dentition and PDLs, oral tongue, floor of mouth, buccal mucosa, lower lip, and all four pairs of masticator muscles. The second branch of the trigeminal nerve, the maxillary nerve, provides general sensation to the upper half of the oral cavity. Motor function of the paired extrinsic (excluding the palatoglossus) and intrinsic tongue muscles is supplied by the hypoglossal nerve.

The dorsal tongue is covered with three types of lingual papillae: circumvallate, fungiform, and filiform. They each contain hundreds of taste buds that supply afferent taste sensation to the chorda tympani branch of the facial nerve.

1.5.5 Salivary Glands

Saliva is a very important part of oral hygiene and barrier protection and is secreted from the six major salivary glands bilaterally as well as the hundreds of minor salivary glands. Salivary mucin is known to bind to the surface of oral mucosa in order to hydrate, lubricate, and protect against microorganisms, along with antimicrobial peptides.[70,71] The paired parotid glands secrete mainly serous, stimulated saliva through ducts that pierce the buccinator and open into the mouth adjacent to the maxillary second molar. The paired submandibular glands secrete the majority of mucous, unstimulated saliva through bilateral ducts at the anterior floor of mouth. They are divided into superficial and deep lobes by the mylohyoid muscle. The two smallest named salivary glands are the sublingual glands. They secrete mixed serous and mucous saliva and are located in the lateral superficial floor of mouth, adjacent to the mandibular canines.

1.6 Treatment Considerations and Approaches

Primary surgical resection is the preferred treatment for oral cavity cancer, followed by adjuvant radiation therapy and/or chemotherapy in indicated cases and based on pathologic features.[72] Definitive doses of radiation therapy have been shown to lead to an unacceptable rate of mandibular osteoradionecrosis (ORN).[73] As a result, definitive chemoradiation therapy (CRT) is generally reserved for poor surgical candidates due to unresectable tumor burden or underlying comorbidities.

1.6.1 Surgical Options and Approaches

Primary Tumor

The primary surgical objective for treatment of a head and neck cancer with curative intent is a margin-negative resection. The extent of resection depends on the location of the primary tumor, which often involves vital structures within the head and neck. No strict definitions exist for recommended surgical margins in oral cavity tumors, but multiple studies have shown a significant difference in locoregional recurrence and survival (disease free or overall) with a margin greater than 5 mm.[74–76] Intraoperatively, the surgeon often makes this assessment tactilely and sends surgical margins for frozen histologic confirmation. In advanced-stage tumors, a composite resection involving soft tissue and adjacent bone is often indicated. The bony maxilla and mandible form the framework of the oral cavity, so any oral cavity malignancy will eventually involve bone if left untreated. Bony margins are more difficult to ascertain, as the technology to rapidly decalcify bone for frozen histologic analysis is not currently available. Various methods of obtaining bony margins have been described, including bone marrow scrapings and thin cortical bone margins by osteotome, but none have yet been widely adopted.[77,78] Composite extirpation of an oral cavity cancer may require partial maxillectomy or a rim versus segmental mandibulectomy for clear margins.

Neck Treatment

The most important prognostic factor in oral cavity cancer is the presence of nodal metastasis. Surgical treatment of a clinically N0 neck relies on the probability of occult nodal metastasis, while treatment of an N+neck is absolutely indicated. Selective neck dissection (or modified radical) is now considered the standard of care, in comparison with the more historical radical neck dissection. In a lateralized oral cavity cancer, the nodal basins most at risk are the ipsilateral levels I through III.[79,80] Per the decision tree analysis performed by Weiss et al in 1994, risk of occult nodal metastasis greater than 20% in any head and neck cancer warrants elective treatment of the neck.[81] This threshold continues to be the prevailing opinion today.

Advanced tumor stage, aggressive pathologic features, and immunocompromised status are among the major indicators for performing an elective neck dissection. For those patients with lower risk of occult nodal disease, surgical treatment of the neck is helpful for both prognostic value and guiding the decision for adjuvant therapy. Multiple retrospective studies have illustrated that primary tumor thickness of at least 3 to 4 mm is correlated with increased risk of cervical nodal metastasis.[82–84] More recently, a randomized control trial by D'Cruz et al., demonstrated a significantly increased rate of overall and disease-free survival in those patients with greater than 3.0 mm tumor depth who had elective neck dissections. The results demonstrated a 3-year 13% overall survival advantage in early-stage oral cancer patients with tumor depth greater than 3 mm who underwent elective versus therapeutic neck dissection.[85] Primary tumors of the floor of mouth tend to exhibit more frequent regional spread due to their proximity to neurovascular structures. Therefore, T1 lesions or greater warrant an elective neck dissection.[86]

Sentinel lymph node (SLN) biopsy is an effective, minimally invasive option for identifying occult nodal metastasis in early oral cavity cancers (cT1–T2). It can detect aberrant nodal drainage from the primary tumor while reducing the need for a potentially unnecessary elective neck dissection. It can also be used in patients with lower but not negligible risk of occult nodal disease, as in primary lip cancers.[87] According to a recent review and meta-analysis of over 3,500 cT1–T2 patients, SLN biopsy had a pooled identification rate of 96.3%, sensitivity of 87%, and negative predictive value of 94%.[88] With the appropriate surgical technique and experience, the head and neck cancer surgeon should consider SLN biopsy as an alternative to elective neck dissection in selective early oral cavity cancers.

Reconstructive Options

Head and neck ablative defects require consideration of both structure and function and are therefore uniquely challenging for the head and neck reconstructive surgeon. General principles adhere to the reconstructive ladder, with use of secondary intention, primary closure, skin grafts, local flaps, regional flaps, or free flaps. Unlike other anatomic areas, the head and neck often require a combination of reconstructive techniques to appropriately address the needs of a specific ablative defect. It is important to address concerns with oral intake, speech, breathing, aesthetics, and tissue coverage of vital structures (i.e., carotid artery or dura). Goals of reconstruction are a critical component of discussion with patients, and planning should be coordinated with appropriate multidisciplinary care providers. Development of free tissue transfer has markedly improved the functional and cosmetic outcomes for head and neck cancer patients with large, composite defects, and they should be considered in the appropriate patients[89] (► Fig. 1.4, ► Fig. 1.5, ► Fig. 1.6).

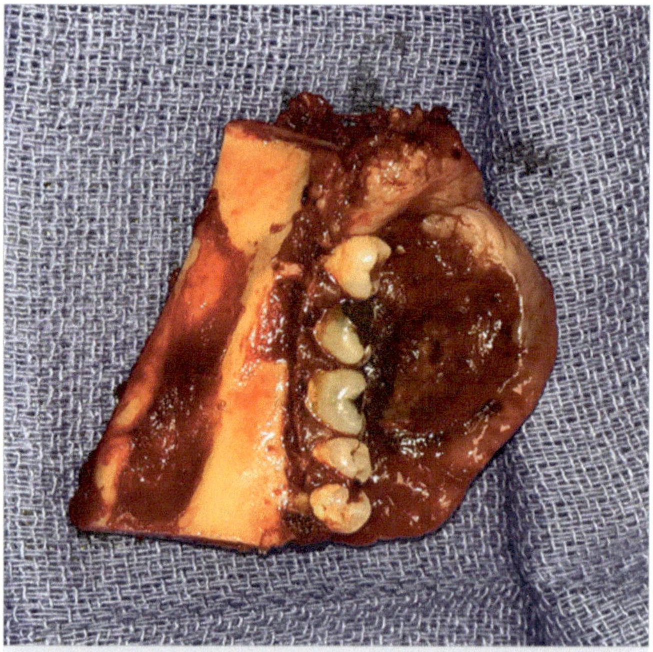

Fig. 1.5 Composite resection.

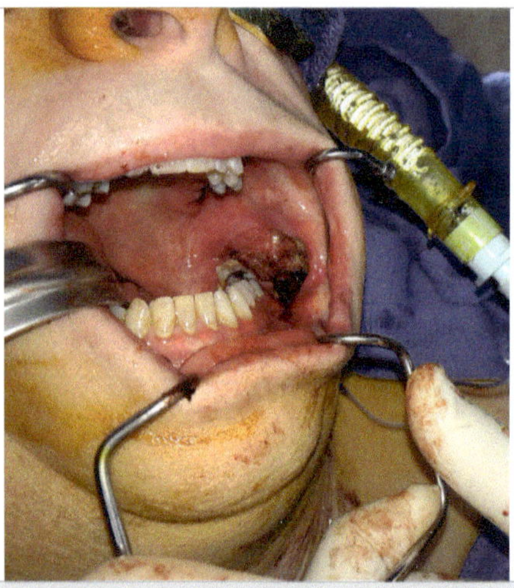

Fig. 1.4 Buccal mucosa squamous cell carcinoma invading the mandibular gingiva and alveolar ridge cortex.

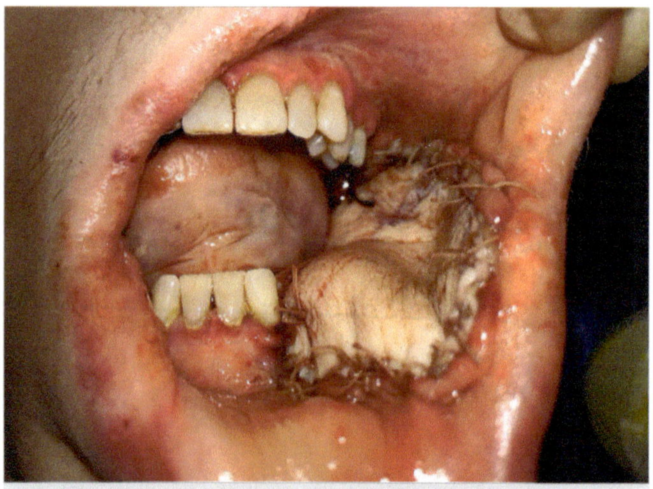

Fig. 1.6 After reconstruction with a fibular free flap.

1.6.2 Medical Options

Radiation and Chemotherapy

Surgery is the preferred treatment for oral cavity cancer; thus, radiation therapy and/or chemotherapy are generally utilized in the postoperative adjuvant setting. Postoperative radiotherapy (PORT) is recommended for advanced tumor stage III–IV and positive nodal disease.[72] The addition of concurrent chemotherapy is reserved for positive tumor margins or ENE, as adjuvant CRT has shown to significantly improve disease-free survival and locoregional control in those patients when compared to PORT alone.[90,91] Appropriate adjuvant dosage for optimizing locoregional control while minimizing toxicity is generally 60 Gy, and it should be administered within 6 weeks postoperatively.[92,93]

Radiation and chemotherapy primarily target and damage proliferating and differentiating cells, causing oral mucosa to become thin or ulcerated.[65] These effects can be seen especially in those thinner nonkeratinized areas, namely, the floor of mouth, buccal mucosa, and ventral tongue, causing mucositis and ulceration. These lesions can lead to pain, dehydration, and poor nutritional status that occasionally requires enteral feeding. Radiation permanently decreases proliferation in all affected tissues and degrades their normal matrices, endothelial cells, and fibroblasts. As a result, radiated tissues have increased fibrosis and ischemia, presenting clinically with trismus, fistula formation, tissue necrosis, and infection. Toxicity effects are exponentially related to the total dose of radiation.[92] Adding concurrent chemotherapy augments the rate of acute adverse toxicity and has even led to death.[94] When counseling patients on the risks and benefits of adjuvant therapy, it is important to have an honest discussion about the survival advantages as well as the tissue toxicities.

Multimodality, Multidisciplinary Therapy

Multimodality therapy is often the treatment of choice for advanced-stage oral cavity cancer. Multidisciplinary treatment refers to the coordination of multiple specialists for the care of a patient. Addressing the oncologic and quality-of-life needs of a head and neck cancer patient is complex. Effective care requires the input of head and neck surgery, medical oncology, radiation oncology, radiology, pathology, audiology, oral surgery, prosthodontic dentistry, speech pathology, and nutrition. Multiple tertiary academic centers now have multidisciplinary clinics to streamline the patients' numerous clinic visits, ultimately aiming to decrease time to treatment and improve overall completeness of care.[95] A recent study even showed an increase in oropharyngeal disease-specific survival with implementation of a multidisciplinary clinic for patients treated with definitive CRT.[96] For definitive surgical patients, one of the most pressing time constraints is to initiation of adjuvant therapy within the recommended postoperative 6 weeks. Expediting postoperative care is crucial, as delay to adjuvant treatment is associated with decreased survival.[97]

1.7 Surgical Sequelae

Surgical sequelae fundamentally include the outcomes after completion of ablation, reconstruction, and possible adjuvant therapy. It is challenging to delineate independent effects of each step of treatment, as they rarely occur in isolation. Patients with lip tumors develop concerns with oral competence and microstomia. Tongue defects impair speech articulation and bolus propulsion necessary for swallowing. Buccal tumors can lead to considerable trismus. Tumors involving the mandible have a significant impact on mastication and occlusion. Hard palate tumor resection and reconstruction may result in velopharyngeal insufficiency or oronasal fistula formation. Immediate postoperative edema often necessitates tracheostomy tube placement at the time of surgery to prevent airway compromise. All subsites of oral cavity cancer can lead to significant changes in physical appearance.

1.7.1 Long-Term Sequelae/ Rehabilitation

Survivors of head and neck cancer often live with long-term sequelae of radiation and/or chemotherapy in addition to surgery. Postradiation dental caries or periapical abscesses sometimes necessitate dental extraction, and development of mandibular or maxillary osteoradionecrosis is a known complication. These patients can benefit from pre- and post-extraction hyperbaric oxygen and should be treated by dentists or oral surgeons familiar with head and neck cancer patients.[98] Xerostomia and trismus are exceedingly common and lead to dysgeusia, dysphagia, malnutrition, and poor overall quality of life. As a result, patients sometimes require placement of an enteral feeding tube. Treatment of trismus includes jaw exercises and rehabilitation or mechanical stretching in the operating room. Persistent oronasal or oroantral fistulas can be managed surgically or with a prosthodontic palatal obturator. Speech concerns can be addressed by a specialized speech and language pathologist during individualized speech therapy sessions. Development of neck lymphedema is a very common complication due to impaired lymphatic drainage. It can cause stiffness and even swallowing difficulties, with significant improvements after physical therapy and manual lymphedema massage.[99] An often overlooked sequela is a strong association between head and neck cancer survivors and depressive mood.[100] Dysfunctions in eating and salivating are almost universal after oral cavity cancer treatment, and they are major risk factors for development of depression.[101] These patients may benefit from seeking counseling or attending survivorship meetings. Again, utilizing multidisciplinary care is paramount to your patient's overall functional status and can significantly impact both quality of life and survival.[102]

Key Points

- Oral cavity lesions are heterogeneous in appearance and symptomatology.
- Workup includes a histologic tissue diagnosis and appropriate imaging (CT or MRI with possible PET/CT).
- Definitive surgery ± adjuvant therapy is the mainstay of treatment.
- Primary tumor depth greater than 3 mm or floor of mouth tumors T1 or greater necessitates an elective neck dissection in the N0 neck.

- Consider an SLN biopsy in early-stage tumors.
- Head and neck reconstruction is very challenging and sometimes requires more than one reconstructive technique to optimize functional and aesthetic outcomes.
- Multidisciplinary care increases survival.

References

[1] van Dijk BAC, Brands MT, Geurts SME, Merkx MAW, Roodenburg JLN. Trends in oral cavity cancer incidence, mortality, survival and treatment in the Netherlands. Int J Cancer. 2016; 139(3):574–583

[2] Montero PH, Patel SG. Cancer of the oral cavity. Surg Oncol Clin N Am. 2015; 24(3):491–508

[3] Shield KD, Ferlay J, Jemal A, et al. The global incidence of lip, oral cavity, and pharyngeal cancers by subsite in 2012. CA Cancer J Clin. 2017; 67(1):51–64

[4] Weatherspoon DJ, Chattopadhyay A, Boroumand S, Garcia I. Oral cavity and oropharyngeal cancer incidence trends and disparities in the United States: 2000–2010. Cancer Epidemiol. 2015; 39(4):497–504

[5] Muller K, Kazimiroff J, Fatahzadeh M, et al. Oral Human Papillomavirus Infection and Oral Lesions in HIV-Positive and HIV-Negative Dental Patients. J Infect Dis. 2015; 212(5):760–768

[6] Li R, Koch WM, Fakhry C, Gourin CG. Distinct epidemiologic characteristics of oral tongue cancer patients. Otolaryngol Head Neck Surg. 2013; 148(5): 792–796

[7] Udeabor SE, Rana M, Wegener G, Gellrich N-C, Eckardt AM. Squamous cell carcinoma of the oral cavity and the oropharynx in patients less than 40 years of age: a 20-year analysis. Head Neck Oncol. 2012; 4:28

[8] Brägelmann J, Dagogo-Jack I, El Dinali M, et al. Oral cavity tumors in younger patients show a poor prognosis and do not contain viral RNA. Oral Oncol. 2013; 49(6):525–533

[9] Siegelmann-Danieli N, Hanlon A, Ridge JA, Padmore R, Fein DA, Langer CJ. Oral tongue cancer in patients less than 45 years old: institutional experience and comparison with older patients. J Clin Oncol. 1998; 16(2):745–753

[10] Pickering CR, Zhang J, Neskey DM, et al. Squamous cell carcinoma of the oral tongue in young non-smokers is genomically similar to tumors in older smokers. Clin Cancer Res. 2014; 20(14):3842–3848

[11] Patel SC, Carpenter WR, Tyree S, et al. Increasing incidence of oral tongue squamous cell carcinoma in young white women, age 18 to 44 years. J Clin Oncol. 2011; 29(11):1488–1494

[12] SEER Program. SEER* Stat Database: Incidence-SEER 18 Regs Research Data + Hurricane Katrina Impacted Louisiana Cases, Nov 2017 Sub (2000–2015) < Katrina/Rita Population Adjustment > - Linked To County Attributes - Total U.S., 1969–2016 Counties, National Cancer Institute, DCCPS, Surveillance Research Program, released April 2018, based on the November 2017 submission. Available at: www.seer.cancer.gov

[13] World Health Organization, International Agency for Research on Cancer. Tobacco smoke and involuntary smoking. Vol. 83.Lyon, France: International Agency for Research on Cancer; 2004

[14] Hashibe M, Brennan P, Benhamou S, et al. Alcohol drinking in never users of tobacco, cigarette smoking in never drinkers, and the risk of head and neck cancer: pooled analysis in the International Head and Neck Cancer Epidemiology Consortium. J Natl Cancer Inst. 2007; 99(10):777–789

[15] Hashibe M, Brennan P, Chuang SC, et al. Interaction between tobacco and alcohol use and the risk of head and neck cancer: pooled analysis in the International Head and Neck Cancer Epidemiology Consortium. Cancer Epidemiol Biomarkers Prev. 2009; 18(2):541–550

[16] Hashibe M, Sturgis EM. Epidemiology of oral-cavity and oropharyngeal carcinomas: controlling a tobacco epidemic while a human papillomavirus epidemic emerges. Otolaryngol Clin North Am. 2013; 46(4):507–520

[17] Lubin JH, Muscat J, Gaudet MM, et al. An examination of male and female odds ratios by BMI, cigarette smoking, and alcohol consumption for cancers of the oral cavity, pharynx, and larynx in pooled data from 15 case-control studies. Cancer Causes Control. 2011; 22(9):1217–1231

[18] Wyss A, Hashibe M, Chuang SC, et al. Cigarette, cigar, and pipe smoking and the risk of head and neck cancers: pooled analysis in the International Head and Neck Cancer Epidemiology Consortium. Am J Epidemiol. 2013; 178(5): 679–690

[19] Berthiller J, Straif K, Agudo A, et al. Low frequency of cigarette smoking and the risk of head and neck cancer in the INHANCE consortium pooled analysis. Int J Epidemiol. 2016; 45(3):835–845

[20] Lubin JH, Purdue M, Kelsey K, et al. Total exposure and exposure rate effects for alcohol and smoking and risk of head and neck cancer: a pooled analysis of case-control studies. Am J Epidemiol. 2009; 170(8):937–947

[21] Wyss AB, Hashibe M, Lee YA, et al. Smokeless tobacco use and the risk of head and neck cancer: pooled analysis of US studies in the INHANCE Consortium. Am J Epidemiol. 2016; 184(10):703–716

[22] Cogliano V, Straif K, Baan R, Grosse Y, Secretan B, El Ghissassi F, WHO International Agency for Research on Cancer. Smokeless tobacco and tobacco-related nitrosamines. Lancet Oncol. 2004; 5(12):708

[23] Goldstein BY, Chang S-C, Hashibe M, La Vecchia C, Zhang Z-F. Alcohol consumption and cancers of the oral cavity and pharynx from 1988 to 2009: an update. Eur J Cancer Prev. 2010; 19(6):431–465

[24] Baan R, Straif K, Grosse Y, et al. WHO International Agency for Research on Cancer Monograph Working Group. Carcinogenicity of alcoholic beverages. Lancet Oncol. 2007; 8(4):292–293

[25] Purdue MP, Hashibe M, Berthiller J, et al. Type of alcoholic beverage and risk of head and neck cancer: a pooled analysis within the INHANCE Consortium. Am J Epidemiol. 2009; 169(2):132–142

[26] Radoï L, Paget-Bailly S, Cyr D, et al. Tobacco smoking, alcohol drinking and risk of oral cavity cancer by subsite: results of a French population-based case-control study, the ICARE study. Eur J Cancer Prev. 2013; 22(3):268–276

[27] Radoï L, Menvielle G, Cyr D, Lapôtre-Ledoux B, Stücker I, Luce D, ICARE Study Group. Population attributable risks of oral cavity cancer to behavioral and medical risk factors in France: results of a large population-based case-control study, the ICARE study. BMC Cancer. 2015; 15:827

[28] IARC Working Group on the Evaluation of Carcinogenic Risks to Humans. Betel-quid and areca-nut chewing and some areca-nut derived nitrosamines. IARC Monogr Eval Carcinog Risks Hum. 2004; 85:1–334

[29] Radoï L, Luce D.. A review of risk factors for oral cavity cancer: the importance of a standardized case definition. Community Dent Oral Epidemiol. 2013; 41:97–109,–e78–91

[30] Merchant AT, Pitiphat W. Total, direct, and indirect effects of paan on oral cancer. Cancer Causes Control. 2015; 26(3):487–491

[31] Freedman ND, Park Y, Subar AF, et al. Fruit and vegetable intake and head and neck cancer risk in a large United States prospective cohort study. Int J Cancer. 2008; 122(10):2330–2336

[32] Xu J, Yang XX, Wu YG, Li XY, Bai B. Meat consumption and risk of oral cavity and oropharynx cancer: a meta-analysis of observational studies. PLoS One. 2014; 9(4):e95048

[33] Bradshaw PT, Siega-Riz AM, Campbell M, Weissler MC, Funkhouser WK, Olshan AF. Associations between dietary patterns and head and neck cancer: the Carolina head and neck cancer epidemiology study. Am J Epidemiol. 2012; 175(12):1225–1233

[34] Mazul AL, Shivappa N, Hébert JR, et al. Proinflammatory diet is associated with increased risk of squamous cell head and neck cancer. Int J Cancer. 2018:(e-pub ahead of print)

[35] Dasanayake AP, Silverman AJ, Warnakulasuriya S. Maté drinking and oral and oro-pharyngeal cancer: a systematic review and meta-analysis. Oral Oncol. 2010; 46(2):82–86

[36] Deneo-Pellegrini H, De Stefani E, Boffetta P, et al. Maté consumption and risk of oral cancer: case-control study in Uruguay. Head Neck. 2013; 35(8):1091–1095

[37] Wang W, Yang Y, Zhang W, Wu W. Association of tea consumption and the risk of oral cancer: a meta-analysis. Oral Oncol. 2014; 50(4):276–281

[38] Galeone C, Tavani A, Pelucchi C, et al. Coffee and tea intake and risk of head and neck cancer: pooled analysis in the international head and neck cancer epidemiology consortium. Cancer Epidemiol Biomarkers Prev. 2010; 19(7): 1723–1736

[39] Radoï L, Paget-Bailly S, Menvielle G, et al. Tea and coffee consumption and risk of oral cavity cancer: results of a large population-based case-control study, the ICARE study. Cancer Epidemiol. 2013; 37(3): 284–289

[40] Turati F, Galeone C, La Vecchia C, Garavello W, Tavani A. Coffee and cancers of the upper digestive and respiratory tracts: meta-analyses of observational studies. Ann Oncol. 2011; 22(3):536–544

[41] Ndiaye C, Mena M, Alemany L, et al. HPV DNA, E6/E7 mRNA, and p16INK4a detection in head and neck cancers: a systematic review and meta-analysis. Lancet Oncol. 2014; 15(12):1319–1331

[42] Castellsagué X, Alemany L, Quer M, et al. ICO International HPV in Head and Neck Cancer Study Group. HPV involvement in head and neck cancers: comprehensive assessment of biomarkers in 3680 patients. J Natl Cancer Inst. 2016; 108(6):djv403

[43] Syrjänen S, Lodi G, von Bültzingslöwen I, et al. Human papillomaviruses in oral carcinoma and oral potentially malignant disorders: a systematic review. Oral Dis. 2011; 17 Suppl 1:58–72
[44] Isayeva T, Li Y, Maswahu D, Brandwein-Gensler M. Human papillomavirus in non-oropharyngeal head and neck cancers: a systematic literature review. Head Neck Pathol. 2012; 6 Suppl 1:S104–S120
[45] Schwartz SR, Yueh B, McDougall JK, Daling JR, Schwartz SM. Human papillomavirus infection and survival in oral squamous cell cancer: a population-based study. Otolaryngol Head Neck Surg. 2001; 125(1):1–9
[46] Elango KJ, Suresh A, Erode EM, et al. Role of human papilloma virus in oral tongue squamous cell carcinoma. Asian Pac J Cancer Prev. 2011; 12(4):889–896
[47] Duray A, Descamps G, Decaestecker C, et al. Human papillomavirus DNA strongly correlates with a poorer prognosis in oral cavity carcinoma. Laryngoscope. 2012; 122(7):1558–1565
[48] Heck JE, Berthiller J, Vaccarella S, et al. Sexual behaviours and the risk of head and neck cancers: a pooled analysis in the International Head and Neck Cancer Epidemiology (INHANCE) consortium. Int J Epidemiol. 2010; 39(1): 166–181
[49] Ahrens W, Pohlabeln H, Foraita R, et al. Oral health, dental care and mouthwash associated with upper aerodigestive tract cancer risk in Europe: the ARCAGE study. Oral Oncol. 2014; 50(6):616–625
[50] Hashim D, Sartori S, Brennan P, et al. The role of oral hygiene in head and neck cancer: results from International Head and Neck Cancer Epidemiology (INHANCE) consortium. Ann Oncol. 2016; 27(8):1619–1625
[51] Guha N, Boffetta P, Wünsch Filho V, et al. Oral health and risk of squamous cell carcinoma of the head and neck and esophagus: results of two multicentric case-control studies. Am J Epidemiol. 2007; 166(10):1159–1173
[52] Mazul AL, Taylor JM, Divaris K, et al. Oral health and human papillomavirus-associated head and neck squamous cell carcinoma. Cancer. 2017; 123(1): 71–80
[53] Chaubal T, Bapat R. Geographic tongue. Am J Med. 2017; 130(12):e533–e534
[54] Buchner A. Amalgam tattoo (amalgam pigmentation) of the oral mucosa: clinical manifestations, diagnosis and treatment. Refuat Hapeh Vehashinayim (1993). 2004; 21(3):25–28, 92
[55] Yardimci G, Kutlubay Z, Engin B, Tuzun Y. Precancerous lesions of oral mucosa. World J Clin Cases. 2014; 2(12):866–872
[56] Liu W, Wang YF, Zhou HW, Shi P, Zhou ZT, Tang GY. Malignant transformation of oral leukoplakia: a retrospective cohort study of 218 Chinese patients. BMC Cancer. 2010; 10:685
[57] Shafer WG, Waldron CA. Erythroplakia of the oral cavity. Cancer. 1975; 36 (3):1021–1028
[58] Cox SC, Walker DM. Oral submucous fibrosis. A review. Aust Dent J. 1996; 41 (5):294–299
[59] Farhi D, Dupin N. Pathophysiology, etiologic factors, and clinical management of oral lichen planus, part I: facts and controversies. Clin Dermatol. 2010; 28(1):100–108
[60] Di Martino E, Nowak B, Hassan HA, et al. Diagnosis and staging of head and neck cancer: a comparison of modern imaging modalities (positron emission tomography, computed tomography, color-coded duplex sonography) with panendoscopic and histopathologic findings. Arch Otolaryngol Head Neck Surg. 2000; 126(12):1457–1461
[61] Ha PK, Hdeib A, Goldenberg D, et al. The role of positron emission tomography and computed tomography fusion in the management of early-stage and advanced-stage primary head and neck squamous cell carcinoma. Arch Otolaryngol Head Neck Surg. 2006; 132(1):12–16
[62] Walker DM, Boey G, McDonald LA. The pathology of oral cancer. Pathology. 2003; 35(5):376–383
[63] Amin M, Edge S, Greene F, et al. AJCC cancer staging manual. 8th ed. New York, NY: Springer; 2017
[64] Li R, Agrawal N, Fakhry C. Anatomical sites and subsites of head and neck cancer. In: Fakhry C, D'Souza G, eds. HPV and Head and Neck Cancers. Head and Neck Cancer Clinics. New Delhi: Springer; 2015:1–11
[65] Squier CA, Kremer MJ. Biology of oral mucosa and esophagus. JNCI Monographs. 2001; 2001(29):7–15
[66] Thomson PJ, Potten CS, Appleton DR. Mapping dynamic epithelial cell proliferative activity within the oral cavity of man: a new insight into carcinogenesis? Br J Oral Maxillofac Surg. 1999; 37(5):377–383
[67] Mashberg A, Meyers H. Anatomical site and size of 222 early asymptomatic oral squamous cell carcinomas: a continuing prospective study of oral cancer. II. Cancer. 1976; 37(5):2149–2157
[68] Saito H, Itoh I. Three-dimensional architecture of the intrinsic tongue muscles, particularly the longitudinal muscle, by the chemical-maceration method. Anat Sci Int. 2003; 78(3):168–176
[69] Sahingur SE, Yeudall WA. Chemokine function in periodontal disease and oral cavity cancer. Front Immunol. 2015; 6:214
[70] Schenkels L, Gururaja TL, Levine MJ. Salivary mucins: their role in oral mucosal barrier function and delivery. In: Rathbone MJ, ed. Oral Mucosal Drug Delivery. New York, NY: Marcel Dekker; 1996:191–220
[71] Weinberg A, Krisanaprakornkit S, Dale BA. Epithelial antimicrobial peptides: review and significance for oral applications. Crit Rev Oral Biol Med. 1998; 9 (4):399–414
[72] Iyer NG, Tan DS, Tan VK, et al. Randomized trial comparing surgery and adjuvant radiotherapy versus concurrent chemoradiotherapy in patients with advanced, nonmetastatic squamous cell carcinoma of the head and neck: 10-year update and subset analysis. Cancer. 2015; 121(10):1599–1607
[73] Reuther T, Schuster T, Mende U, Kübler A. Osteoradionecrosis of the jaws as a side effect of radiotherapy of head and neck tumour patients–a report of a thirty year retrospective review. Int J Oral Maxillofac Surg. 2003; 32(3):289–295
[74] Loree TR, Strong EW. Significance of positive margins in oral cavity squamous carcinoma. Am J Surg. 1990; 160(4):410–414
[75] Chen TY, Emrich LJ, Driscoll DL. The clinical significance of pathological findings in surgically resected margins of the primary tumor in head and neck carcinoma. Int J Radiat Oncol Biol Phys. 1987; 13(6):833–837
[76] Sutton DN, Brown JS, Rogers SN, Vaughan ED, Woolgar JA. The prognostic implications of the surgical margin in oral squamous cell carcinoma. Int J Oral Maxillofac Surg. 2003; 32(1):30–34
[77] Mahmood S, Conway D, Ramesar KC. Use of intraoperative cytologic assessment of mandibular marrow scrapings to predict resection margin status in patients with squamous cell carcinoma. J Oral Maxillofac Surg. 2001; 59 (10):1138–1141
[78] Oxford LE, Ducic Y. Intraoperative evaluation of cortical bony margins with frozen-section analysis. Otolaryngol Head Neck Surg. 2006; 134(1): 138–141
[79] Huang S-F, Kang CJ, Lin CY, et al. Neck treatment of patients with early stage oral tongue cancer: comparison between observation, supraomohyoid dissection, and extended dissection. Cancer. 2008; 112(5):1066–1075
[80] Lim YC, Lee JS, Koo BS, Kim SH, Kim YH, Choi EC. Treatment of contralateral N0 neck in early squamous cell carcinoma of the oral tongue: elective neck dissection versus observation. Laryngoscope. 2006; 116(3):461–465
[81] Weiss MH, Harrison LB, Isaacs RS. Use of decision analysis in planning a management strategy for the stage N0 neck. Arch Otolaryngol Head Neck Surg. 1994; 120(7):699–702
[82] Yuen AP, Lam KY, Wei WI, et al. A comparison of the prognostic significance of tumor diameter, length, width, thickness, area, volume, and clinicopathological features of oral tongue carcinoma. Am J Surg. 2000; 180(2):139–143
[83] Asakage T, Yokose T, Mukai K, et al. Tumor thickness predicts cervical metastasis in patients with stage I/II carcinoma of the tongue. Cancer. 1998; 82 (8):1443–1448
[84] Huang SH, Hwang D, Lockwood G, Goldstein DP, O'Sullivan B. Predictive value of tumor thickness for cervical lymph-node involvement in squamous cell carcinoma of the oral cavity: a meta-analysis of reported studies. Cancer. 2009; 115(7):1489–1497
[85] D'Cruz AK, Vaish R, Kapre N, et al. Head and Neck Disease Management Group. Elective versus therapeutic neck dissection in node-negative oral cancer. N Engl J Med. 2015; 373(6):521–529
[86] Hicks WL, Jr, Loree TR, Garcia RI, et al. Squamous cell carcinoma of the floor of mouth: a 20-year review. Head Neck. 1997; 19(5):400–405
[87] Civantos FJ, Stoeckli SJ, Takes RP, et al. What is the role of sentinel lymph node biopsy in the management of oral cancer in 2010? Eur Arch Oto-Rhino-Laryngol. 2010; 267:839–844
[88] Liu M, Wang SJ, Yang X, Peng H. Diagnostic efficacy of sentinel lymph node biopsy in early oral squamous cell carcinoma: a meta-analysis of 66 studies. PLoS One. 2017; 12(1):e0170322
[89] Chim H, Salgado CJ, Seselgyte R, Wei F-C, Mardini S. Principles of head and neck reconstruction: an algorithm to guide flap selection. Semin Plast Surg. 2010; 24(2):148–154
[90] Peters LJ, Goepfert H, Ang KK, et al. Evaluation of the dose for postoperative radiation therapy of head and neck cancer: first report of a prospective randomized trial. Int J Radiat Oncol Biol Phys. 1993; 26(1):3–11
[91] Bachaud JM, David JM, Boussin G, Daly N. Combined postoperative radiotherapy and weekly cisplatin infusion for locally advanced squamous cell carcinoma of the head and neck: preliminary report of a randomized trial. Int J Radiat Oncol Biol Phys. 1991; 20(2):243–246

[92] Ang KK, Trotti A, Brown BW, et al. Randomized trial addressing risk features and time factors of surgery plus radiotherapy in advanced head-and-neck cancer. Int J Radiat Oncol Biol Phys. 2001; 51(3):571–578
[93] Awwad HK, Lotayef M, Shouman T, et al. Accelerated hyperfractionation (AHF) compared to conventional fractionation (CF) in the postoperative radiotherapy of locally advanced head and neck cancer: influence of proliferation. Br J Cancer. 2002; 86(4):517–523
[94] Cooper JS, Pajak TF, Forastiere AA, et al. Radiation Therapy Oncology Group 9501/Intergroup. Postoperative concurrent radiotherapy and chemotherapy for high-risk squamous-cell carcinoma of the head and neck. N Engl J Med. 2004; 350(19):1937–1944
[95] Townsend M, Kallogjeri D, Scott-Wittenborn N, Gerull K, Jansen S, Nussenbaum B. Multidisciplinary clinic management of head and neck cancer. JAMA Otolaryngol Head Neck Surg. 2017; 143(12):1213–1219
[96] Light T, Rassi EE, Maggiore RJ, et al. Improving outcomes in veterans with oropharyngeal squamous cell carcinoma through implementation of a multidisciplinary clinic. Head Neck. 2017; 39(6):1106–1112
[97] Graboyes EM, Garrett-Mayer E, Ellis MA, et al. Effect of time to initiation of postoperative radiation therapy on survival in surgically managed head and neck cancer. Cancer. 2017; 123(24):4841–4850
[98] Chavez JA, Adkinson CD. Adjunctive hyperbaric oxygen in irradiated patients requiring dental extractions: outcomes and complications. J Oral Maxillofac Surg. 2001; 59:518–522; discussion 523–524
[99] Piso DU, Eckardt A, Liebermann A, Gutenbrunner C, Schäfer P, Gehrke A. Early rehabilitation of head-neck edema after curative surgery for orofacial tumors. Am J Phys Med Rehabil. 2001; 80(4):261–269
[100] Barber B, Dergousoff J, Slater L, et al. Depression and survival in patients with head and neck cancer: a systematic review. JAMA Otolaryngol Head Neck Surg. 2016; 142(3):284–288
[101] Wu Y-S, Lin PY, Chien CY, et al. Anxiety and depression in patients with head and neck cancer: 6-month follow-up study. Neuropsychiatr Dis Treat. 2016; 12:1029–1036
[102] Karvonen-Gutierrez CA, Ronis DL, Fowler KE, Terrell JE, Gruber SB, Duffy SA. Quality of life scores predict survival among patients with head and neck cancer. J Clin Oncol. 2008; 26(16):2754–2760

2 Patient Populations at Increased Risk for Oral Cavity Cancer

Kevin M. Motz and Marietta Tan

Summary
Oral cavity cancer occurs more frequently in certain geographic areas and patient populations. In some regions of the world, higher rates of oral cancer are attributable to frequent usage of tobacco, alcohol, and betel quid. Furthermore, patients with either specific genetic predispositions or acquired immunosuppression are also at increased risk for the development of oral cancer. This chapter will review those populations at greater risk for oral cavity cancer.

Keywords: betel quid, fanconi anemia, dyskeratosis congenita, xeroderma pigmentosum, epiderma bullosis, immunosuppression

2.1 Introduction

Oral cavity cancer (OCC) comprises the group of neoplasms that present within the confines of the vermillion border of the lips anteriorly and the circumvallate papillae and the junction of the hard and soft palates posteriorly. OCC is a significant problem worldwide, with peaks in its incidence occurring both in specific geographic regions and in individual patient populations. The most common type of OCC is squamous cell carcinoma (SCC), but other malignant tumors arising from epithelial or mesenchymal tissues can occur. While the overall incidence of OCC is relatively low, areas such as France, Brazil, and South Asia have increased rates of the disease. In addition, OCC is more common in specific at-risk patient populations that have either genetic predispositions or underlying chronic acquired or iatrogenic immunosuppression. The geographic locations and populations at increased risk for OCC will be discussed in this chapter.

2.2 Geographic Variation in OCC Incidence

OCC has a global incidence ranging from 0.4 to 23.1 cases per 100,000 individuals, with an estimated 275,000 new cases of OCC diagnosed each year.[1,2] OCC is more common in men, and the risk of malignancy increases with age.[2] SCC accounts for up to 95% of oral cavity malignancies, while sarcomas, lymphomas, salivary gland tumors, and melanomas account for the remainder of cases.[3–6]

The incidence of OCC varies considerably by geographic region, a phenomenon attributed to disparate rates of exposure to tobacco, alcohol, and other modifiable risk factors.[7] In most industrialized nations, the overall incidence of OCC is declining, secondary to a decrease in the use of tobacco products, a major risk factor for SCC.[8,9] For example, in much of North America, Australia, and Western Europe with the exception of France, the incidence of OCC is relatively low, ranging from 0.4 to 4 cases per 100,000 individuals. However, the incidence of OCC in France is exceedingly high, with 42.3 cases per 100,000 male individuals.[2] The increased incidence of OCC in France is related to the increased use of tobacco and alcohol, which can increase risk of OCC by up to 3,800%.[10] In Brazil, which is commonly cited as having a high incidence of OCC, the majority of cases are clustered in the southern and southeastern regions of the country. The concentration of cases in those regions is attributed to higher rates of tobacco use, as well as lower socioeconomic status and reduced access to health care services.[11] Finally, the developing countries of India, Pakistan, Sri Lanka, and Bangladesh have some of the highest rates of OCC in the world, with incidences of up to 9 to 11 cases per 100,000 individuals.[9] In these countries, OCC accounts for up to 25% of new cancer diagnoses[2] and is associated with high rates of tobacco, alcohol, and betel quid usage.

2.2.1 Betel Quid Chewing

Betel quid chewing represents a modifiable risk factor that increases the risks of both oral premalignant lesions and OCC. "Betel quid" refers to combinations of betel leaf, areca nut, and slaked lime, with or without the addition of tobacco leaf, which is then chewed or packed into the gingivobuccal sulcus of the mouth. Various combinations of these ingredients can be made into betel quid, or each ingredient can be consumed individually.[12] Sweeteners and essences, such as menthol, are also commonly added to betel quid. Betel quid formulations are highly variable by region and may have different designations based on composition. Mass-produced betel quid substitutes, known as pan masala (which does not contain tobacco) and gutka (which contains tobacco), are also widely available.[13] Given the variability in content, when the term "betel quid" is used, it is important to determine the formulation's specific components. In particular, the addition of tobacco further increases the risks of betel quid. For example, a meta-analysis of 25 studies from the Indian subcontinent showed a relative risk of OCC of 8.47 for betel quid with tobacco, compared to 2.41 for betel quid without tobacco.[14] It is also important to note that the concomitant use of alcohol or cigarette smoking with betel quid chewing increases the risks of oral premalignancy and OCC in a synergistic manner.[15,16]

Global estimates of betel quid use indicate that there are currently nearly 700 million consumers worldwide.[12] The chewing of betel quid in different forms, a custom which dates back thousands of years, has become deeply ingrained in a number of sociocultural traditions. The earliest use of betel quid as a masticatory object dates back to 430 BC. Indian scripts dating back to the 4th century indicate that betel quid was originally thought to be a therapeutic agent and was used to treat a wide range of human disease. It was also recognized for its euphoric and stimulant effects.[17] The highest rates of betel quid use are clustered in the countries of India, Pakistan, Bangladesh,

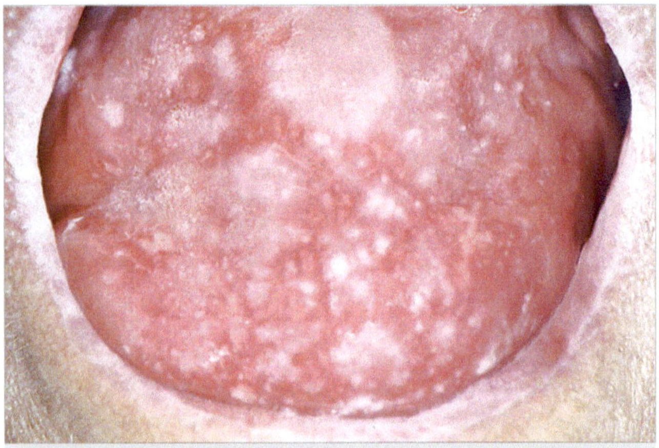

Fig. 2.1 Oral submucous fibrosis affecting the tongue. (Source: Laskaris G, ed. Color Atlas of Oral Diseases. Diagnosis and Treatment. 4th ed. New York, NY: Thieme; 2017.)

Sri Lanka, and Taiwan. In these areas, up to 40% of the population use betel quid in various forms.[18]

Premalignant oral lesions associated with the use of betel quid include leukoplakia, erythroplakia, oral submucous fibrosis, and lichen planus.[12,19,20] The presence of leukoplakia or erythroplakia secondary to betel quid use is common and has been associated with an increased risk of oral malignancy. Betel quid use can also lead to oral submucous fibrosis, a premalignant condition characterized by subepithelial inflammation and fibrosis (▶ Fig. 2.1). The rate of malignant transformation of oral submucous fibrosis to carcinoma has been estimated at 8% over a 17-year period. Moreover, patients with oral submucous fibrosis may be up to 400 times more likely to progress to malignancy compared to tobacco users without premalignant lesions.[12] Nonmalignant consequences of oral submucous fibrosis also exist and contribute to morbidity. Depending on the degree of fibrosis, oral submucous fibrosis can result in trismus, dysarthria, limited ability to provide oral hygiene, and limited food consumption leading to malnourishment. In particular, trismus may complicate surveillance and surgical resection of dysplastic or malignant lesions. These considerations should be taken into account when initiating treatment plans for patients with OCC secondary to betel quid use.[12,21]

In addition to increasing the risk of OCC, betel quid use also increases the risk of malignancies of the esophagus, larynx, lung, liver, and pancreas.[22] A dose-dependent relationship exists between the duration and amount of betel quid use and the risk of malignancy. Given these risks, patients who utilize betel quid should undergo increased surveillance of oral lesions, and clinicians should maintain a heightened suspicion for carcinoma. Furthermore, patients should receive counseling on the risks of use and the benefits of cessation, as the cessation of betel quid use reduces the risk of malignancy by up to half.[14]

2.3 Inherited Syndromes

The incidence of OCC is increased in patients with certain inherited syndromes. The predisposition to malignancy in these individuals can be explained by the "two-hit" hypothesis, in which the first "hit" is the inherited mutant allele, while the second "hit" is an acquired somatic mutation leading to malignant transformation.[23] Genomic instability in some patient populations may also lead to earlier and more frequent development of malignant lesions.[24] Individuals with these syndromes therefore require close surveillance to monitor for the development of premalignant or malignant oral cavity lesions. These patients should also be counseled on smoking and alcohol cessation, in order to mitigate their risk of malignancy.

2.3.1 Fanconi Anemia

Fanconi anemia (FA) is a rare, autosomal recessive disorder caused by mutations in any of at least 15 known genes, each involved in deoxyribonucleic acid (DNA) repair and stabilization pathways. Defects in these pathways lead to chromosomal instability and thereby increase the risk of malignancy, including lymphocytic and myelocytic cancers, as well as solid organ tumors.[25] FA is also characterized by bone marrow failure and sensitivity to DNA cross-linking agents. Acute myeloid leukemia is the most common malignancy associated with FA. However, as the life expectancy of FA patients has improved due to advances in leukemia management, the incidence of solid organ tumors has risen to as high as 28% by 40 years of age.[26] Solid tumors in FA patients occur most commonly in the head and neck, the majority of which arise in the oral cavity. The incidence of head and neck SCC is 240- to 700-fold greater in FA than in the general population,[27–29] and OCC comprises over two-thirds of head and neck cancers diagnosed in FA.[30]

In individuals with FA, OCC and other head and neck cancers are known to be aggressive and carry a poor prognosis.[26] The propensity of FA patients to develop OCC, coupled with poor tolerance of radiation therapy and chemotherapy, underscores the need for careful and frequent screening, starting as early as late childhood, in this population.[26,30]

2.3.2 Dyskeratosis Congenita

Dyskeratosis congenita (DC) is a rare inherited disorder caused by defects in telomere maintenance. The most common form of DC is X-linked recessive, but autosomal dominant and autosomal recessive forms have been observed.[31] Clinically, it is characterized by bone marrow failure, premature aging, and increased risk of malignancy. Patients with DC present with a triad of mucocutaneous findings: oral leukoplakia, reticulated hyperpigmentation of the skin, and nail dystrophy. Leukoplakia affects up to 80% of patients with DC and most commonly affects the oral mucosa (▶ Fig. 2.2).[32] The leukoplakia associated with DC can affect any mucosal subsite within the oral cavity and is considered a premalignant condition.[31] Secondary to the increased propensity for oral leukoplakia, the risk of OCC is significantly increased in DC, with an incidence of tongue cancer 1,154-fold greater in patients with DC than in the general population.[33] Given the increased frequency and early onset of premalignant mucosal changes in DC, up to 35% of oral cancer malignancies arise in the third to fifth decades of life in these patients. Individuals with DC therefore require close surveillance of leukoplakic lesions, to ensure early detection and treatment of malignancy.[34]

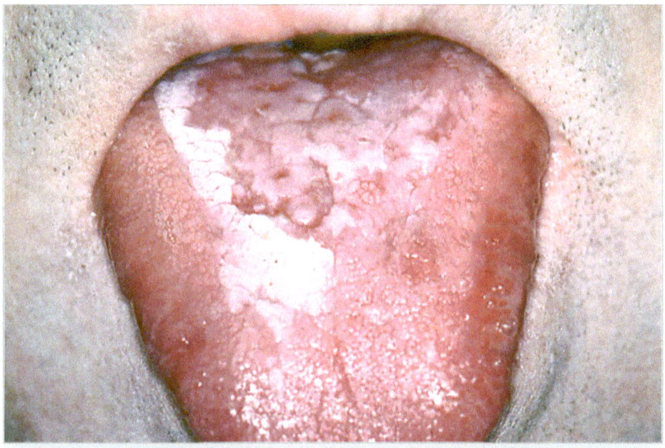

Fig. 2.2 Leukoplakia on the dorsum of the tongue in a patient with dyskeratosis congenita. (Source: Laskaris G, ed. Color Atlas of Oral Diseases. Diagnosis and Treatment. 4th ed. New York, NY: Thieme; 2017.)

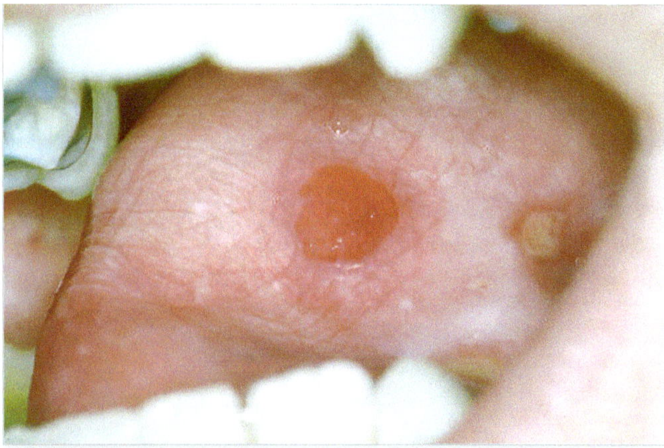

Fig. 2.3 Bulla formation on the tongue in a patient with epidermolysis bullosa. (Source: Laskaris G, ed. Color Atlas of Oral Diseases. Diagnosis and Treatment. 4th ed. New York, NY: Thieme; 2017.)

2.3.3 Xeroderma Pigmentosum

Xeroderma pigmentosum (XP) is a rare, autosomal recessive disorder characterized by hypersensitivity to ultraviolet radiation, secondary to defective nucleotide excision repair mechanisms.[23] Individuals with XP are at increased risk of developing skin cancers, with 50% of patients developing cutaneous malignancies between the ages of 10 and 14 years. The majority of malignancies associated with XP occur on the face, scalp, lips, and eyelids. However, other sites, such as the oral tongue or gingiva, can be affected. SCC affecting the anterior tongue, presumably resulting from sun exposure to the tip of the tongue, is estimated to occur over 20,000-fold more frequently in XP patients under the age of 20 compared to the general population. In addition, malignant neoplasms arising from oral cavity sites other than the tongue occur 400 times more frequently in young XP patients than in the general population.[35,36] Patients with XP therefore require close surveillance with frequent and thorough examination of the skin, lips, and oral cavity. Early identification and treatment of premalignant or malignant lesions are imperative.

2.3.4 Epidermolysis Bullosa Spectrum

Epidermolysis bullosa (EB) is a spectrum of diseases hallmarked by blistering and mechanical fragility of the skin. There are four main types of EB: intraepidermal, junctional, dermolytic, and mixed. In addition, there are over 30 subtypes of EB.[37] The clinical presentation of EB can be highly variable and reflects the marked genetic heterogeneity among subtypes in this disease spectrum. The presentation and severity of oral manifestations in EB differ by type or subtype of disease, but patients commonly present with multiple intraoral bullae that rupture, leading to ulceration and erosion (▶ Fig. 2.3). Multiple cases of OCC, most commonly affecting the tongue, have been reported in individuals with EB who survive the second and third decades of life. Patients with generalized recessive dystrophic EB therefore need close monitoring of oral lesions.[38–41]

2.4 Acquired Immunosuppression and Immune Dysregulation

A functional immune system is thought to play a protective role in preventing tumor development. The theory of immune surveillance, first proposed by Burnet in 1970, states that thymic-dependent effector lymphocytes play a role in the elimination of developing cancers.[42] This process may be diminished in patients with acquired immunosuppression, thereby allowing the development of certain malignancies. These malignancies include lymphomas, Kaposi's sarcoma, renal cell cancer, hepatobiliary cancers, and SCC of the skin, cervix, and anogenital region.[42–44] In OCC, a similar immunologic etiology has been observed. Immunosuppressed patients have a reported 2- to 15.7-fold increased risk of developing an oral malignancy.[45] Increased incidences of OCC have been reported in patients that are immunosuppressed secondary to human immunodeficiency virus (HIV)/acquired immunodeficiency syndrome (AIDS), solid organ transplantation (SOT), hematopoietic stem cell transplantation (HSCT), and graft-versus-host disease (GVHD). However, the risk of specific associated malignancies varies based on the etiology of immunosuppression.

2.4.1 Human Immunodeficiency Virus

HIV is a lentivirus that can lead to AIDS. HIV infects $CD4^+$ T lymphocytes and other immune cells, resulting in the eventual depletion of $CD4^+$ T cells and the loss of cell-mediated immunity.[46] Immunosuppression secondary to HIV leads to an increased propensity for disease-specific infections, as well as an increased risk of specific malignancies, including OCC. There is a 2.3-fold increased incidence of cancers of the oral cavity and pharynx in patients with HIV/AIDS compared to the general population.[47] The relative risk of developing OCC in HIV/AIDS increases as $CD4^+$ T-cell counts decline, and evidence suggests that restoration or maintenance of immune competence with antiretroviral therapy can reduce the risk of malignancy.[48] HIV/AIDS patients who develop premalignant oral lesions should be closely monitored. In addition, patients should be counseled on cessation of modifiable risk factors such as tobacco and alcohol use, in order to mitigate the risk of oral malignancy.

2.4.2 Solid Organ Transplantation

Suppression of the immune system to prevent rejection is a critical component in the management of SOT. However, immunosuppression is known to increase the risk of de novo malignancies, including OCC,[49] by weakening immune surveillance and worsening susceptibility to oncogenic viral infections. In patients with SOT, there is a 5.5-fold increased risk of OCC, with a 10.7-fold increased risk for malignancy specifically of the tongue.[50] The risk of developing cancer at different primary sites also varies depending on the transplanted organ. For example, the incidence of OCC is up to 10-fold higher in liver transplant recipients compared to the general population, but only fourfold to fivefold higher in kidney, heart, or lung transplant recipients.[49,51]

The specific risk of malignancy in patients with SOT appears to be related to the duration and degree of immune suppression and does not appear to be agent specific.[52,53] SOT patients who develop OCC have worse survival rates at 1 year compared to nontransplanted patients with OCC.[54] Furthermore, treatment of head and neck malignancies in this population may be complicated by the need for ongoing immunosuppression to ensure transplant viability. Due to the propensity for worsened survival and locoregional control in SOT patients with head and neck cancer, identification and treatment of oral cavity malignancies at an early stage is critical.[51,55] These outcomes highlight the importance of continued surveillance in patients who have undergone SOT.

2.4.3 Hematopoietic Stem Cell Transplantation/Chronic Graft-versus-Host Disease

HSCT is a curative therapy for the management of multiple malignant and nonmalignant hematological disorders. The frequency of HSCT has steadily increased over the past 30 years.[56,57] It is now well recognized that patients who have undergone HSCT have an increased risk for the development of secondary solid organ tumors, with a 2.7-fold increased incidence of all solid tumor types when compared to the general population. The risk is significantly higher for oral cavity malignancies, with a 19.5-fold increased risk of tongue cancers and a 12.5-fold increased risk of cancers of the gum or other sites in the oral cavity. In addition, the risk of developing OCC after HSCT increases over time, thereby placing younger HSCT patients in a higher risk category.[58]

The increased risk of OCC in this patient population has been attributed to chronic graft-versus-host disease (cGVHD), a sequela of HSCT that occurs in 60 to 80% of long-term survivors. Chronic GVHD results when transplanted donor T lymphocytes mount an immune response against recipient tissue, due to differences in histocompatibility antigens. Oral manifestations of cGVHD result from chronic submucosal inflammation and can lead to leukoplakia, fibrosis, and lichen planus (▸ Fig. 2.4). The increased risk of OCC in patients who have undergone HSCT is attributed to the chronic inflammation associated with cGVHD; it is thought that the repeated immunologic injury predisposes the oral mucosa to malignant transformation.[59,60] In addition, patients requiring HSCT are likely to have previously undergone cytotoxic therapy with radiation or chemotherapy, thus further increasing their risk of secondary malignancy. Given the increased risk of OCC in patients with cGVHD, increased surveillance is necessary, albeit not always straightforward. Oral manifestations of cGVHD include hyperkeratosis, ulceration, erythema, and pain, all of which can make detection of secondary oral cavity malignancies more challenging.

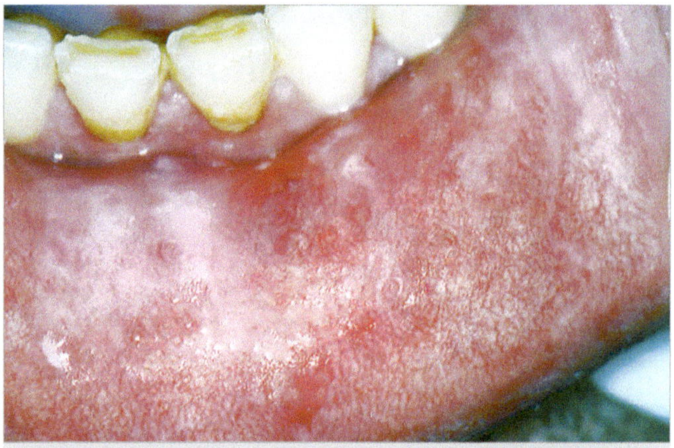

Fig. 2.4 Oral manifestation of chronic graft-versus-host disease. (Source: Laskaris G, ed. Color Atlas of Oral Diseases. Diagnosis and Treatment. 4th ed. New York, NY: Thieme; 2017.)

2.5 Clinical Presentation

Patients with the inherited syndromes described above often present with OCC at younger ages and in the setting of other mucosal disease. In particular, individuals with XP develop OCC at very young ages compared to the general population, with most patients presenting before 20 years of age.[35,36] Individuals with FA and DC also develop OCC at young ages. One study found that FA patients developed OCC at a mean age of 32 years, compared to 63 years in the general population.[26] Similarly, patients with DC developed SCC of the head and neck at a median age of 32 years.[33] Furthermore, in patients with inherited syndromes such as FA, OCC often develops in the absence of a history of tobacco and alcohol use, which are common risk factors for oral cancer in the general population.[26] These individuals may present with more advanced cancers at initial diagnosis compared to the general population.[28]

Patients with acquired immunosuppression due to either SOT or HSCT may also develop OCC at younger ages than the general population and without exposure to other risk factors like tobacco or alcohol.[51,60] After SOT, the mean time to diagnosis of noncutaneous head and neck cancer is 7.8 years, though the mean interval is shortest in liver transplantation (27 months) and as long as 14 years in kidney transplantation.[51,61] The time to diagnosis of OCC after the development of cGVHD in HSCT likewise ranges from 2 to more than 10 years.[60]

2.6 Treatment Considerations

Individuals who develop OCC in the setting of inherited syndromes or acquired immunosuppression must be given special consideration when planning treatment. These patients should be managed within a multidisciplinary setting. The underlying etiology of the disease process, the patient's functional and immune status, and the use of previous cytotoxic therapies should be considered.

In general, the primary treatment modality in OCC is surgical resection with or without adjuvant radiation and chemotherapy. Given that complete surgical resection can often produce large oral cavity defects, reconstructive options and potential wound-healing issues must be given careful consideration. A history of previous radiation, underlying immunosuppression, and hematologic dyscrasias can lead to secondary complications of surgery and should be investigated preoperatively and managed aggressively when possible.

Underlying genetic anomalies can lead to increased rates of complications from radiation or chemotherapy. In particular, the underlying DNA repair defects in FA make these patients extremely sensitive to both radiation and cytotoxic chemotherapy. Radiation therapy results in high rates of severe mucositis, dysphagia, and pancytopenia in patients with FA, and several deaths have been reported due to severe systemic complications resulting from radiation.[30] Over 40% of patients are not able to complete radiation therapy.[62] In addition, FA patients are exquisitely sensitive to cisplatin, a DNA cross-linking agent and the mainstay of current head and neck SCC chemotherapeutic regimens. Conventional chemotherapy can therefore result in significant toxicity and should be avoided in FA.[30,63] Consequently, surgery is the mainstay of treatment of OCC and other head and neck cancers in patients with FA. Surgery can be well tolerated in these patients, but preoperative assessment of bone marrow function and potential need for platelet or blood transfusion is critical.[30]

The use of chemotherapy for the management of OCC in patients who have undergone renal transplantation should also be given careful thought, due to the concern for worsening graft function. Surgical resection and radiation therapy are therefore the preferred treatment modalities for most early-stage cancers in patients who have undergone renal transplantation. However, one study of head and neck cancer after SOT found that even cisplatin-based chemotherapy was safe in kidney transplant patients, with no reported major renal toxicities.[64] In some patients, there may also be a role for judicious reduction in immunosuppression, provided there is close monitoring of graft function.[65]

2.7 Conclusion

OCC is a relatively rare malignancy, but its incidence is increased in specific at-risk populations. Individuals exposed to modifiable risk factors, such as tobacco, alcohol, or betel quid use, have increased incidences of OCC. Variable rates of exposure to these modifiable risk factors explain many of the geographic differences in OCC disease burden. In patients with significant exposure to products such as betel quid, a higher index of suspicion should be present when evaluating oral lesions. In addition, patients with specific underlying genetic abnormalities or acquired immunosuppression are at particular risk for the development of OCC. Increased screening for and surveillance of premalignant lesions is imperative in these patients.

Key Points

- While the overall incidence of OCC is low, it is elevated in specific geographic areas with increased exposure to modifiable risk factors and in specific populations with certain underlying inherited or acquired conditions.
- Increased incidences of OCC have been identified in France, Brazil, and South Asia, secondary to the increased use of tobacco, alcohol, and betel quid.
- Betel quid is the combination of betel leaf, areca nut, slaked lime, and possibly tobacco; its use has been shown to increase the risk of OCC.
- The risk of OCC is increased in patients with specific inherited conditions, including FA, DC, XP, and EB spectrum.
- Immunosuppression increases the risk of OCC in patients with HIV/AIDS, SOT, and HSCT.
- cGVHD increases the risk of OCC in patients who have undergone HSCT.

References

[1] Moore SR, Johnson NW, Pierce AM, Wilson DF. The epidemiology of mouth cancer: a review of global incidence. Oral Dis. 2000; 6(2):65–74

[2] Warnakulasuriya S. Global epidemiology of oral and oropharyngeal cancer. Oral Oncol. 2009; 45(4-5):309–316

[3] Chen JK, Eisenberg E, Krutchkoff DJ, Katz RV. Changing trends in oral cancer in the United States, 1935 to 1985: a Connecticut study. J Oral Maxillofac Surg. 1991; 49(11):1152–1158

[4] Roder D, Wilson D. Oral cancer in South Australia: incidence and case survival. Aust Dent J. 1983; 28(5):312–315

[5] Ostman J, Anneroth G, Gustafsson H, Tavelin B. Malignant oral tumours in Sweden 1960–1989: an epidemiological study. Eur J Cancer B Oral Oncol. 1995; 31B(2):106–112

[6] Ernani V, Saba NF. Oral cavity cancer: risk factors, pathology, and management. Oncology. 2015; 89(4):187–195

[7] de Camargo Cancela M, Voti L, Guerra-Yi M, Chapuis F, Mazuir M, Curado MP. Oral cavity cancer in developed and in developing countries: population-based incidence. Head Neck. 2010; 32(3):357–367

[8] Franceschi S, Bidoli E, Herrero R, Muñoz N. Comparison of cancers of the oral cavity and pharynx worldwide: etiological clues. Oral Oncol. 2000; 36(1): 106–115

[9] Chaturvedi AK, Anderson WF, Lortet-Tieulent J, et al. Worldwide trends in incidence rates for oral cavity and oropharyngeal cancers. J Clin Oncol. 2013; 31(36):4550–4559

[10] Radoï L, Menvielle G, Cyr D, Lapôtre-Ledoux B, Stücker I, Luce D, ICARE Study Group. Population attributable risks of oral cavity cancer to behavioral and medical risk factors in France: results of a large population-based case-control study, the ICARE study. BMC Cancer. 2015; 15(1):827

[11] Antunes J, Toporcov TN, Biazevic MGH, Boing AF, Bastos JL. Gender and racial inequalities in trends of oral cancer mortality in Sao Paulo, Brazil. Rev Saude Publica. 2013; 47(3):470–478

[12] Sharan RN, Mehrotra R, Choudhury Y, Asotra K. Association of betel nut with carcinogenesis: revisit with a clinical perspective. PLoS ONE. 2012; 7(8): e42759

[13] Nair U, Bartsch H, Nair J. Alert for an epidemic of oral cancer due to use of the betel quid substitutes gutkha and pan masala: a review of agents and causative mechanisms. Mutagenesis. 2004; 19(4):251–262

[14] Guha N, Warnakulasuriya S, Vlaanderen J, Straif K. Betel quid chewing and the risk of oral and oropharyngeal cancers: a meta-analysis with implications for cancer control. Int J Cancer. 2014; 135(6):1433–1443

[15] Amarasinghe HK, Usgodaarachchi US, Johnson NW, Lalloo R, Warnakulasuriya S. Betel-quid chewing with or without tobacco is a major risk factor for

oral potentially malignant disorders in Sri Lanka: a case-control study. Oral Oncol. 2010; 46(4):297–301
[16] Liu B, Shen M, Xiong J, et al. Synergistic effects of betel quid chewing, tobacco use (in the form of cigarette smoking), and alcohol consumption on the risk of malignant transformation of oral submucous fibrosis (OSF): a case-control study in Hunan Province, China. Oral Surg Oral Med Oral Pathol Oral Radiol. 2015; 120(3):337–345
[17] Sharan RN. Association of betel nut with carcinogenesis: a review. Cancer J. 1996; 9(1):13–19
[18] Nelson BS, Heischober B. Betel nut: a common drug used by naturalized citizens from India, Far East Asia, and the South Pacific Islands. Ann Emerg Med. 1999; 34(2):238–243
[19] Lee C-H, Ko AM-S, Warnakulasuriya S, et al. Population burden of betel quid abuse and its relation to oral premalignant disorders in South, Southeast, and East Asia: an Asian Betel-quid Consortium Study. Am J Public Health. 2012; 102(3):e17–e24
[20] Solanki J, Gupta S. Prevalence of quid-induced lichenoid reactions among western Indian population. J Exp Ther Oncol. 2015; 11(1):63–66
[21] Arakeri G, Rai KK, Boraks G, et al. Current protocols in the management of oral submucous fibrosis: An update. J Oral Pathol Med. 2017; 46(6):418–423
[22] Chen P-H, Mahmood Q, Mariottini GL, Chiang T-A, Lee K-W. Adverse health effects of betel quid and the risk of oral and pharyngeal cancers. BioMed Res Int. 2017; 2017:3904098
[23] Prime SS, Thakker NS, Pring M, Guest PG, Paterson IC. A review of inherited cancer syndromes and their relevance to oral squamous cell carcinoma. Oral Oncol. 2001; 37(1):1–16
[24] Lengauer C, Kinzler KW, Vogelstein B. Genetic instabilities in human cancers. Nature. 1998; 396(6712):643–649
[25] Knipscheer P, Räschle M, Smogorzewska A, et al. The Fanconi anemia pathway promotes replication-dependent DNA interstrand cross-link repair. Science. 2009; 326(5960):1698–1701
[26] Kutler DI, Patel KR, Auerbach AD, et al. Natural history and management of Fanconi anemia patients with head and neck cancer: a 10-year follow-up. Laryngoscope. 2016; 126(4):870–879
[27] Rosenberg PS, Alter BP, Ebell W. Cancer risks in Fanconi anemia: findings from the German Fanconi Anemia Registry. Haematologica. 2008; 93(4):511–517
[28] Kutler DI, Auerbach AD, Satagopan J, et al. High incidence of head and neck squamous cell carcinoma in patients with Fanconi anemia. Arch Otolaryngol Head Neck Surg. 2003; 129(1):106–112
[29] Rosenberg PS, Greene MH, Alter BP. Cancer incidence in persons with Fanconi anemia. Blood. 2003; 101(3):822–826
[30] Lin J, Kutler DI. Why otolaryngologists need to be aware of Fanconi anemia. Otolaryngol Clin North Am. 2013; 46(4):567–577
[31] Handley TPB, McCaul JA, Ogden GR. Dyskeratosis congenita. Oral Oncol. 2006; 42(4):331–336
[32] Dokal I. Dyskeratosis congenita in all its forms. Br J Haematol. 2000; 110(4): 768–779
[33] Alter BP, Giri N, Savage SA, Rosenberg PS. Cancer in dyskeratosis congenita. Blood. 2009; 113(26):6549–6557
[34] Sirinavin C, Trowbridge AA. Dyskeratosis congenita: clinical features and genetic aspects. Report of a family and review of the literature. J Med Genet. 1975; 12(4):339–354
[35] Kraemer KH, Lee MM, Scotto J. DNA repair protects against cutaneous and internal neoplasia: evidence from xeroderma pigmentosum. Carcinogenesis. 1984; 5(4):511–514
[36] Kraemer KH, Lee MM, Scotto J. Xeroderma pigmentosum. Cutaneous, ocular, and neurologic abnormalities in 830 published cases. Arch Dermatol. 1987; 123(2):241–250
[37] Fine J-D, Eady RAJ, Bauer EA, et al. The classification of inherited epidermolysis bullosa (EB): report of the Third International Consensus Meeting on Diagnosis and Classification of EB. J Am Acad Dermatol. 2008; 58(6):931–950
[38] Wright JT. Oral manifestations in the epidermolysis bullosa spectrum. Dermatol Clin. 2010; 28(1):159–164
[39] Reed WB, College J, Jr, Francis MJ, et al. Epidermolysis bullosa dystrophica with epidermal neoplasms. Arch Dermatol. 1974; 110(6):894–902
[40] Fine J-D, Johnson LB, Weiner M, Li K-P, Suchindran C. Epidermolysis bullosa and the risk of life-threatening cancers: the National EB Registry experience, 1986–2006. J Am Acad Dermatol. 2009; 60(2):203–211
[41] Wright JT, Fine J-D, Johnson LB. Oral soft tissues in hereditary epidermolysis bullosa. Oral Surg Oral Med Oral Pathol. 1991; 71(4):440–446
[42] Burnet FM. The concept of immunological surveillance. Prog Exp Tumor Res. 1970; 13:1–27
[43] Frisch M, Biggar RJ, Engels EA, Goedert JJ, AIDS-Cancer Match Registry Study Group. Association of cancer with AIDS-related immunosuppression in adults. JAMA. 2001; 285(13):1736–1745
[44] Biggar RJ, Chaturvedi AK, Goedert JJ, Engels EA, HIV/AIDS Cancer Match Study. AIDS-related cancer and severity of immunosuppression in persons with AIDS. J Natl Cancer Inst. 2007; 99(12):962–972
[45] Atsuta Y, Suzuki R, Yamashita T, et al. Japan Society for Hematopoietic Cell Transplantation. Continuing increased risk of oral/esophageal cancer after allogeneic hematopoietic stem cell transplantation in adults in association with chronic graft-versus-host disease. Ann Oncol. 2014; 25(2):435–441
[46] Maartens G, Celum C, Lewin SR. HIV infection: epidemiology, pathogenesis, treatment, and prevention. Lancet. 2014; 384(9939):258–271
[47] Grulich AE, van Leeuwen MT, Falster MO, Vajdic CM. Incidence of cancers in people with HIV/AIDS compared with immunosuppressed transplant recipients: a meta-analysis. Lancet. 2007; 370(9581):59–67
[48] Silverberg MJ, Chao C, Leyden WA, et al. HIV infection, immunodeficiency, viral replication, and the risk of cancer. Cancer Epidemiol Biomarkers Prev. 2011; 20(12):2551–2559
[49] Collett D, Mumford L, Banner NR, Neuberger J, Watson C. Comparison of the incidence of malignancy in recipients of different types of organ: a UK Registry audit. Am J Transplant. 2010; 10(8):1889–1896
[50] Adami J, Gäbel H, Lindelöf B, et al. Cancer risk following organ transplantation: a nationwide cohort study in Sweden. Br J Cancer. 2003; 89(7):1221–1227
[51] Nelissen C, Lambrecht M, Nevens F, et al. Noncutaneous head and neck cancer in solid organ transplant patients: single center experience. Oral Oncol. 2014; 50(4):263–268
[52] Dantal J, Hourmant M, Cantarovich D, et al. Effect of long-term immunosuppression in kidney-graft recipients on cancer incidence: randomised comparison of two cyclosporin regimens. Lancet. 1998; 351(9103):623–628
[53] Rama I, Grinyó JM. Malignancy after renal transplantation: the role of immunosuppression. Nat Rev Nephrol. 2010; 6(9):511–519
[54] Deeb R, Sharma S, Mahan M, et al. Head and neck cancer in transplant recipients. Laryngoscope. 2012; 122(7):1566–1569
[55] Alsidawi S, Price KA, Chintakuntlawar AV, et al. Characteristics and long-term outcomes of head and neck squamous cell carcinoma after solid organ transplantation. Oral Oncol. 2017; 72:104–109
[56] Passweg JR, Baldomero H, Gratwohl A, et al. European Group for Blood and Marrow Transplantation (EBMT). The EBMT activity survey: 1990–2010. Bone Marrow Transplant. 2012; 47(7):906–923
[57] Gratwohl A, Baldomero H, Aljurf M, et al. Worldwide Network of Blood and Marrow Transplantation. Hematopoietic stem cell transplantation: a global perspective. JAMA. 2010; 303(16):1617–1624
[58] Curtis RE, Rowlings PA, Deeg HJ, et al. Solid cancers after bone marrow transplantation. N Engl J Med. 1997; 336(13):897–904
[59] Margaix-Muñoz M, Bagán JV, Jiménez Y, Sarrión MG, Poveda-Roda R. Graft-versus-host disease affecting oral cavity. A review. J Clin Exp Dent. 2015; 7(1):e138–e145
[60] Demarosi F, Lodi G, Carrassi A, Soligo D, Sardella A. Oral malignancies following HSCT: graft versus host disease and other risk factors. Oral Oncol. 2005; 41(9):865–877
[61] Vajdic CM, McDonald SP, McCredie MR, et al. Cancer incidence before and after kidney transplantation. JAMA. 2006; 296(23):2823–2831
[62] Birkeland AC, Auerbach AD, Sanborn E, et al. Postoperative clinical radiosensitivity in patients with fanconi anemia and head and neck squamous cell carcinoma. Arch Otolaryngol Head Neck Surg. 2011; 137(9):930–934
[63] Scheckenbach K, Wagenmann M, Freund M, Schipper J, Hanenberg H. Squamous cell carcinomas of the head and neck in Fanconi anemia: risk, prevention, therapy, and the need for guidelines. Klin Padiatr. 2012; 224(3):132–138
[64] Rabinovics N, Hadar T, Mizrachi A, Bachar G, Purim O, Popovtzer A. Adjuvant treatment for head and neck cancer in solid organ transplant recipients. Oral Oncol. 2015; 51(5):e23–e25
[65] Chapman JR, Webster AC, Wong G. Cancer in the transplant recipient. Cold Spring Harb Perspect Med. 2013; 3(7):a015677

Section II

Premalignancies of the Oral Cavity

3 Premalignant Oral Lesions

Joel B. Epstein and Pelin Güneri

Summary

Oral premalignant lesions/oral premalignant disease/oral premalignant conditions are referred as "oral potentially malignant disorders" since they are defined as "a morphologically altered tissue in which cancer is more likely to occur than its normal counterpart" by the World Health Organization (WHO). The histological indicator of increased risk of oral cancer progression is the oral epithelial dysplasia, which is explained as "the histopathologic changes seen in a chronic, progressive, and premalignant disorder of the oral mucosa which may present itself clinically as leukoplakia, erythroplakia, or leukoerythroplakia, or may also be seen in verrucous or papillary leukoplakias, in the margins of a chronic mucosal ulcer, or in the adjacent mucosa of invasive squamous cell carcinoma." In addition to leukoplakia and erythroplakia, oral lichen planus and submucous fibrosis which is mostly observed in certain geographical areas have been included in the clinical definition of oral potentially malignant epithelial lesions (OPMEL). In this chapter, the epidemiology, incidence, major causes comprising tobacco, alcohol, age and gender, molecular alterations/chromosome instability/genetics, human papillomavirus (HPV), inflammation, infections of oral microbiota, socioeconomic status, immunosuppression, and the clinical characteristics of OPMEL are presented. The most common adjunct methods and devices utilized for assistance to the clinical practitioner for detection and evaluation of OPMEL are also discussed.

Keywords: oral leukoplakia, erythroplakia, oral lichen planus, submucous fibrosis, dysplasia, toluidine blue, cytology

3.1 Introduction

WHO has advocated the term "oral potentially malignant disorders" (OPMD) for "a morphologically altered tissue in which cancer is more likely to occur than its normal counterpart" rather than "premalignant lesions," "premalignant disease," or "premalignant conditions," since only some of those lesions may transform into oral malignancies.[1] Oral epithelial neoplasia is initiated with a focal clonal overgrowth of altered cells near the oral basement membrane, which expands both upward and laterally, and replaces the healthy oral mucosal epithelium.[2,3] This pathobiology of a neoplastic process begins with normal tissue progressing through various stages of alteration and finally leading to invasive carcinoma.[4,5] Thus, it is considered that carcinogenesis most often occurs as a multistep process through the continuum from normal mucosa to oral carcinoma.[5,6] Continuous exposure to potentially carcinogenic factors eventually leads to cellular alterations in a localized area or within the region exposed to the potential carcinogen,[5,7–9] leading to risk of oral premalignant lesions/conditions/OPMD.[4,8–11] This regional exposure hypothesis has been referred as "the field cancerization" first described in 1851 after increased risk of oral cancer in the oral mucosa of pipe smokers had been established.[12] It has been supported by the lateral expansion of oral malignant areas rather than infiltration in depth,[7] observation of multiple second primary tumors with higher prevalence than primary oral cancers,[5,8] and the development of synchronous distant tumors within the upper aerodigestive tract.[2,7,8,13] A definition for field cancerization is "the presence of one or more areas of oral mucosa consisting of epithelial cells with genetic alterations with a monoclonal origin, without invasive growth and metastatic behavior."[4] High incidence of local recurrences and second primary tumors are considered to be the result of a process where a single cell is transformed to produce a premalignant field by clonal expansion.[2] In this field of various subclones, two separate tumors with the same clonal origin may develop, and may be erroneously referred to as local recurrences.[2] Also, histological evaluation of the margins may appear cancer free, but tumor-associated genetic alterations may be retained within the adjacent tissue to the operation area, leading to more than 25% of head and neck cancers following surgical removal of the cancer lesions.[4]

Oral epithelial dysplasia is considered a histological indicator of premalignancy that carries an increased risk of oral cancer development.[14–16] It is defined as "the histopathologic changes seen in a chronic, progressive, and premalignant disorder of the oral mucosa which may present itself clinically as leukoplakia, erythroplakia, or leukoerythroplakia, or may also be seen in verrucous or papillary leukoplakias, in the margins of a chronic mucosal ulcer, or in the adjacent mucosa of invasive squamous cell carcinoma."[14]

Generally, a premalignant lesion may contain cytological features similar to that of oral malignant ones,[10] may be present prior to the diagnosis of malignant changes at the same location,[17–19] and may be observed within the whole epithelial layers.[10] Hyperplastic basal cells, enlarged and hyperchromatic nuclei, and drop-shaped rete ridges have been considered the elementary criteria for diagnosis of an epithelial dysplasia.[14] The structural and cellular alterations that are considered the indicators of dysplasia have been reported elsewhere in detail.[12,16,20,21]

The grading of oral epithelial dysplasia has been controversial in the literature, with the most commonly used histological grading system for oral epithelial dysplasia including four steps with increasing severity of histological transformation:[10,12,14,20] (1) mild epithelial dysplasia, with minimal dysplastic alterations showing immature basal cell proliferation confined to the lower third of the epithelium; (2) moderate epithelial dysplasia, demonstrating dysplastic changes extending into the middle one-third of the epithelium; (3) severe epithelial dysplasia, with abnormal proliferation of dysplastic cells from the basal layer to the upper third of the epithelium; and (4) carcinoma in situ, with dysplastic cells with enlarged, hyperchromatic nuclei and various typical and atypical mitotic activities through the entire thickness of the epithelium but without evidence of connective tissue invasion.

Hyperplasia was included in the most initial stage of dysplasia in some reports,[20] but was later excluded since it was not an indicator of malignant risk.[15,22] Also, carcinoma in situ has not been included in dysplasia staging and was not considered as dysplasia, but an actual preinvasive malignancy due to the presence of undifferentiated, primitive cells from the basal to the top layer of the epithelium[12,15] because connective invasion cannot be ruled out.

The subjectivity of grading of dysplasia, low agreement among and between observers because of the subjective nature of the assessment, lack of established objective criteria, the inability to define the exact criteria to predict the malignant risk on histologic grounds, and arbitrary classification of dysplasia have been reported.[12,15,21,23–25] To overcome the shortcomings of conventional grading system advocated by the WHO, a binary system that combines the mild and moderate dysplasia as low risk and severe dysplasia and carcinoma in situ as high-risk lesions has been proposed.[10,15,21,24] Similarly, the Ljubljana grading system, which has focused on the clinical decision points to classify the oral hyperplastic lesions as simple and abnormal hyperplasia (no need for close follow-up), atypical hyperplasia (needs close follow-up), and carcinoma in situ (requires treatment), has been presented.[22,26]

Even though the presence of dysplasia has been associated with a risk of progression to cancer,[12,14,24,27] other reports describe an independent nature of oral oncogenesis from the degree of dysplasia.[13,15] Continuing research suggests that in future, various markers of the genetic and molecular changes of the cells involved in malignant transformation should be included in any lesion classification for accurate evaluation.[15,26]

3.2 Epidemiology

Considering that oral cancer represents the end stage of a continuum of oral epithelial alterations and provided that oral premalignant lesions may precede oral cancer,[3,17–19] the etiological factors for development of oral premalignant lesions are thought to be those recorded for oral cancer.[16] Thus, the well-known effects of tobacco and alcohol have been considered the major causes of oral premalignant lesions.[28–34] However, it should be noted that both internal and external factors including betel quid use, aging, gender, UV radiation, infections (candida and the human papilloma virus),[31,32,35] decreased immune response,[36–38] genetic susceptibility,[3] and chronic oral trauma[39,40] may play a role in oral carcinogenesis.

3.2.1 Incidence, Causes, Clinical Characteristics

Tobacco

Tobacco has been accepted as a primary etiologic factor in oral cavity and oropharyngeal cancers.[30] Heavy use of smokeless tobacco in the form of nass, naswar, khaini, pan masala, gutkha, and betel quid (a combination of betel leaf, slaked lime, areca nut, and catechu) or smoking in the form of cigarette, bidi, chutta, reverse type of smoking, and hookah have been associated with higher risk of upper respiratory tract carcinogenesis.[3,33] Even though the exact interactive mechanism is not clearly defined, the carcinogenic action of tobacco and alcohol is synergistic[30] and the risk of developing oral cancer is 38 times higher among heavy drinkers and smokers when compared to nonusers.[32] A dose–response relationship for smoking frequency, duration, and cumulative consumption has been documented.[29] Estimated risk of 1.4-fold for oral cavity cancers for "ever users" versus "never smokers" among "never drinkers" of alcohol has been reported, supporting a causal relationship.[29]

Tobacco chewing has been considered a risk factor for oral premalignant lesions probably being a potential cause of field cancerization of oral mucosa.[28,41] The odds ratio for ever tobacco chewers was 37.8 when adjusted for other confounding etiological factors,[28] with a linear dose–response association between oral cancer and chewing tobacco in terms of age at initiation, duration, and frequency of chewing per day.[41] Tobacco chewing has also been associated with the risk of multiple OPMD and alcohol was linked with the risk of multiple oral premalignant lesions.[28]

Electronic cigarettes (EC) present aerosol toxicants and carcinogens, which are present in cigarette smoke, such as carcinogenic tobacco-specific nitrosamines, aldehydes, volatile organic compounds, phenolic compounds, polycyclic aromatic hydrocarbons, tobacco alkaloids, heavy metals, flavors, nicotine,[42] and radionuclides.[43] The levels of potentially toxic compounds in their aerosol have been controversial: some suggest that EC aerosols expose users to carcinogenic substances that induce deoxyribonucleic acid (DNA) damage and reactive oxygen species, decrease the cellular total antioxidant capacity, and increase cancer risk,[42,44] whereas others provide comparable results with EC to tobacco.[43,45,46]

Alcohol

Although making a distinct assessment of the etiological impact of individual alcoholic beverages on oral cavity cancer development has been difficult because of combined consumption of alcohol and tobacco,[29] an increased risk for oral cancer with alcoholic beverage consumption increased the odds ratios from 3.0 to 14.8 with heavy consumption even after controlling for smoking.[47,48] All studies from the United States, Europe, and Asia have shown that alcohol abuse was significantly associated with oropharyngeal cancer.[47] The adjusted relative risks were between 6.2 and 9.22 for more than four drinks a day and 3.9 for consumption of four to seven times per week. When only oral cancer is taken into account, a positive and dose-related association with alcoholic beverage consumption has been reported in various regions of the world.[47,49] The ethanol content of the alcoholic beverages has been attributed as the cause of carcinogenic effect, mostly because of its activity as a solvent for other carcinogens and the potential to damage DNA.[29]

Age and Gender

Oral squamous cell carcinoma (OSCC) is mostly observed in older patients,[39,50–54] and especially noticed in males.[50,52] However, more recent studies are identifying OSCC at earlier ages and without known risk factors. Others stated either equal incidence of OSCC in females and males[55] or higher incidence of OSCC in female patients,[54] especially in those younger than 40 years.[56]

Generally, oral cancer risk increases with age,[32] with the highest incidence (26.8%) observed between 55 and 64 years in the United States from 2003 to 2007,[53] which has been attributed to immunosenescence-related changes in cellular and serological immune responses affecting the process of generating specific responses,[57] and cumulative risk factor exposure. More recently, possibly due to the changes in etiological factors, the number of patients younger than 40 years and in their 40s and 50s has been increasing,[32,58] with a prevalence of 11.3% of oral cancer among patients younger than 45 years.[59]

Similar to OSCC, oral dysplasia is observed more commonly in patients between the age of 50 and 69 years, with a mean age of 59.3 years.[14] Mild, moderate dysplasia and carcinoma in situ were identified at 57 to 58 years of age, whereas severe dysplasia and verrucous hyperplasia with dysplasia were observed in older patients, around 65 years of age.[14]

Molecular Alterations/Chromosome Instability/Genetics

Oral cancer development is initiated with autonomous proliferation of cells harboring DNA damage, which are not controlled by cell-growth regulation mechanisms.[3] Clinically healthy-appearing oral mucosa may contain insidious early dysplastic changes with chromosomal aberrations that precede the malignant transformation.[10,60–62] Risk of the genomic alterations has been associated with increased probability of oral cancer development,[3,24,63] and a genetic progression model involving microsatellite markers at 10 commonly altered chromosomal loci has been proposed for oral premalignant lesions.[60]

Loss of heterozygosity (LOH), microsatellite instability (MSI), and loss of regions at chromosome arms 1p, 2q, 3q, 5q21–22, 8p21–23, 9p21–22, 11q13, 11q23, 13q, 14q, 17p, 18q, and 22q have been observed in oral cancer tissues.[3,31,63,64] The lack of protective effects of tumor suppressor genes p16 (9p21), APC (5q21–22), and p53 (17p13) due to mutations has also been related to oral cancerogenesis.[3,63] Invasive tumors presented chromosomal changes mostly within arms 5p, 9q, 11q, and 19p, suggesting that the genetic mutation may be different during the initial phases and invasion.[63] As the severity of histopathologic findings increases, the allelic loss also increases showing that oral carcinogenesis is a dynamic process[8] in which a single mutated cell could progress to cancer, whereas other daughter cells could wait to develop cumulative molecular changes to become malignant.[60]

Additionally, second primary tumors in oral cancer patients have been considered to originate from one clonal population, sharing a common genotype.[2,4] Histologically normal mucosa of tumor adjacent areas of the patients with multiple oral mucosal primary tumors may indeed contain TP53 mutated cells, which may be present within more than 200-cell diameter area.[4]

Human Papillomavirus

HPV is a nonenveloped, double-stranded, circular DNA virus with a double-stranded DNA molecule.[65,66]

Oral mucosa may be a site of HPV infections and recurring HPV-associated lesions, and a prevalence of HPV (from 0.6–81%) has been reported.[65] HPV transmission to the oral cavity may be associated with sexual contacts, perinatal transmission of the neonate during birth,[65,67] and autoinfection via anogenital HPV infection.[68]

In recent decades, infection by high-risk genotypes of HPV has been presented as a risk factor for oral cancer,[66,69–72] although more specifically for the malignant lesions in the oropharynx, including the base of the tongue, soft palate, tonsils, and pharyngeal wall.[65,68,73,74] The prevalence of HPV infection in oropharyngeal squamous cell carcinoma (OPSCC) has been reported to be up to 90%,[69,72–74] and associated with increasing prevalence of HPV-associated head and neck squamous cell carcinoma (HNSCC) in the United States, Western Europe, Canada, and Australia.[68,71,74] Patients with HPV-related OSCC are generally younger, more commonly male, have a higher socioeconomic status,[67,68,71,72] a higher lifetime number of sex partners,[66,72] and mostly present as smaller lesions,[66,67] at a higher stage and with large metastatic lymph nodes.[65–67]

The type and oncogenic phenotype of HPV are determined by differences in the DNA base sequences of E6 and E7, and high- and low-risk HPV subtypes have been defined. The most common high-risk subtypes include HPV-16 and HPV-18,[66,72,74,75] whereas low-risk subtypes include HPV-6 and HPV-11.[65,76] HPV-positive tumors are associated with a better prognosis compared to HPV-negative SCC.[65–67,73,74,77]

The role of HPV in oral cancer has been investigated using polymerase chain reaction that showed the presence of HPV DNA in 0 to 80% of OSCC cases;[65,71] mostly, HPV-16 or HPV-18 were observed among 16 to 73% of the patients.[75,78,79] HPV-16 and HPV-18 were three times more common in oral dysplastic lesions and invasive cancers than benign mucosal lesions. In a study of oral dysplasia, HPV-16 and HPV-18 rates were not associated with the severity of oral dysplastic lesions.[75] Other studies suggest variable presence of high-risk HPV subtypes associated with the severity of dysplasia, with the highest proportion in severe dysplasia or greatest risk for malignancy reported.[78,80–82]

Malignant transformation of oral mucosal cells is associated with high-risk HPV subtypes, including HPV-16 and HPV-18.[67] HPV-6, HPV-16, and HPV-18 were noted in oral leukoplakia (OL), whereas HPV-6, HPV-11, and HPV-18 were reported in oral erythroplakia (OE) lesions.[67] HPV-16 and HPV-18 were also observed in 9.2% of oral lichen planus (OLP) lesions, suggesting a possible impact of HPV upon the transformation of OLP to OSCC.[81] HPV-18 was the most frequently detected genotype among OLP and OL patients, followed by HPV-16, HPV-33, HPV-31, and HPV-6.[83]

Inflammation/Infection

In addition to molecular epithelial change, the effect of chronic inflammation in tumor initiation, promotion, and progression by altering the local environment has been reported.[35,84–86] It is suggested that an environment that incubates the components of a persistent reactive response such as the chronic inflammatory cells, cytokines, growth factors, and DNA-damaging elements in the tissues surrounding the foci with malignant challenges may contribute to the development of neoplasia via stimulation of cell division stimulated by a continuous repair process despite antitumor responses of the host.[11,84,86–89] In addition to chronic inflammatory conditions of the epithelium, further accumulation of acquired immune response to cancerous development may also intervene with the whole process.[86,87] The malignant transformation of OPMD has been attributed to a cascade of molecular stimuli originating with chronic inflammatory infiltrate.[89,90] Expression of hypoxia-related proteins,[6] regulatory T cells, and tumor-associated macrophages, and expression of anti-inflammatory cytokines, proinflammatory cytokines, and inflammatory-induced endogenous oncogenic alterations containing micro-RNAs (miRNAs) or transcriptional changes may play a role in progression of oral premalignant lesions to OSCC.[89–91]

Oral Hygiene

In the literature, poor oral hygiene,[31,35,40,49] periodontal disease,[35,49,92] significant tooth loss (over 6–20 teeth),[40,48,49,92–94] five or more defective teeth,[40] trauma associated with improper complete dentures,[40] and infrequent dental controls[94] have been noted as risk factors for oral cancer after adjusting for tobacco and alcohol consumption, whereas regular dental checkups and tooth brushing were associated with decreased risk.[40,92–95] The risk is higher for alcohol consumers, and may be due to oral microflora and mucosal cell conversion of ethanol within saliva to carcinogenic acetaldehyde.[35,92,94]

Repetitive dental ulcers were found to be associated with HNSCC,[96] and denture-related mucosal traumas have been associated with increased risk for oral cancer.[39,40]

Socioeconomic Status

Individuals from low socioeconomic populations have been reported to be at increased risk of oral cancer because of less awareness about preventable risk factors of oral cancer like tobacco and alcohol use,[59,97,98] poor nutrition,[39,97,99] and less access to health care.[48] Both the incidence and survival rates of cancer have been associated with socioeconomic factors.[30,48] People with low income had a higher prevalence of tobacco and alcohol use and poorer diet lacking fruits and vegetables.[39,97] However, even in nonsmoking alcohol-consuming groups and in both high- and low-income countries, the odds of developing oral cancer was high when associated with low income, low occupational social class, and low education level.[39,48,49,97]

The world-standardized incidence rate for oral cancer among males is higher in more developed countries, whereas the mortality rates is almost the same.[48] On the other hand, for females, both the world-standardized incidence rate and the mortality rate for oral cavity cancer are higher in less developed countries,[48] possibly due to delayed diagnosis and limited health care access for treatment in those areas,[48,97] in addition to prevalence and duration of exposure to known risk factors for cancer.

Immunosuppression

Long-term immunodeficiency observed in patients with solid organ or hematologic cell transplants or chronic autoimmune diseases has been attributed as a contributing factor in carcinogenesis due to the lack of protective activity against oncoviruses including Epstein–Barr virus (EBV), human herpes virus 8 (HHV-8), and HPV, compromised immune surveillance of malignant cells, and pro-oncogenic properties of some immunosuppressive agents.[37] Because of the decrease in T and natural killer (NK) cells, which are vital for cellular immunity and management of cancerogenesis, malignant transformations may be increased in patients receiving immunosuppressive therapy.[36–38]

Commonly administered immunosuppressants including tacrolimus, cyclosporine, methotrexate, monoclonal antibodies, and steroids have been associated with increased risk of carcinogenesis.[36–38]

3.3 Clinical Presentation

OPMD and OSCC patients may infrequently complain of bleeding of the mouth and throat, unilateral pain/numbness/discomfort, ear pain, trismus, limited movement of involved tissue, teeth mobility, neck mass, sore throat, difficulty in speaking, chewing, and swallowing, weight loss, and malodor.[51,100–103] These symptoms are associated with advanced stage of cancer and are related to the location of the lesion.[103] However, as OPMD and initial OSCC lesions are commonly asymptomatic or minimally symptomatic until the advanced stages of the disease, which then leads to diagnosis,[51,102–104] the presence of symptoms that are not indicative of malignancy might mislead clinicians.[18,105] Increased[106] or similar levels of physical pain between patients with oral premalignant conditions and OSCC[107] have also been reported. The significant challenge is detection and differentiation of OPMD and OSCC from variations of normal mucosa and from more common benign/inflammatory mucosal lesions.[18,102]

The list of oral premalignant lesions varies in the literature. The broadest list includes proliferative verrucous leukoplakia,[12,19] erythroplakia,[12,19,25] reverse smokers palate,[12] oral submucous fibrosis (OSMF),[12,19] speckled/granular/nonhomogeneous leukoplakia,[12,25] tobacco pouch keratosis,[19] leukoplakia tobacco keratosis/nicotine stomatitis,[12,19] and OLP.[12,19]

Clinically, these lesions induce oral mucosal changes in surface texture, color, and size; cause loss of surface integrity and contour deviations; and may also influence the mobility of intraoral or extraoral structures.[31,108] Even though over 30% of patients with OSCC and OPSCC receive oral cancer screening within 3 years before a diagnosis of OSCC,[109] the unpredictable nature of potential progression of OPMD can lead to occurrence of malignant lesions at any time.

Mixed color of OPMD has been reported as a potential indicator of increased risk of malignant nature.[103,110–112] Similarly, irregular/mixed texture of the lesion is also an indicator of malignant nature and smooth texture was a sign of benign nature.[111,113]

Chronic oral mucosal ulcers with nonelevated borders have been suggested as a clinical feature of oral malignancy.[50,111–115] The confined nature of the lesion, which was depicted with defined and regular margins, was suggestive of benign lesions, while irregular and undetectable margins were reported as indicators of malignant potential.[111,113]

3.3.1 Oral Leukoplakia

OL is the most common form of OPMD,[19,32,116] which is observed clinically in up to 4.9% of the world population.[11,19,24,32,117,118] It is defined by the WHO as "a white patch or plaque that cannot be characterized clinically or histologically as any other disease"[118] or "white plaques of questionable risk having excluded (other) known diseases or disorders that carry no increased risk for cancer."[24,119,120] Smoking, alcohol, HPV infection, candidiasis, and reduced concentrations of serum vitamin A and C, beta-carotene, and folic acid[24,117,118] are etiological factors of OL.

A provisional diagnosis is made when a lesion at clinical examination cannot be clearly diagnosed as any other disease of the oral mucosa with a white appearance; a definitive diagnosis of OL is made as a result of the identification and elimination of suspected etiological factors and, in the case of persistent lesions following a period of 2 to 4 weeks, histopathological examination.[116,117]

Clinically, OL is broadly classified into homogeneous and nonhomogeneous subtypes.[24,117,119,120] Homogeneous plaques are predominantly white, of uniform flat, thin appearance with shallow cracks of surface keratin, and have a smooth, wrinkled, or corrugated surface with a consistent texture throughout[24,119] (▶ Fig. 3.1). This clinical pattern shows a low risk of malignant transformation (5%).[118,119,121] Nonhomogeneous variants include mixed, white and red, but retaining predominantly white character (speckled), small polypoid outgrowths, rounded red or white excrescences (nodular), and wrinkled or corrugated surface appearance (verrucous).[24,116,119] Malignant transformation is reported as 25% of nonhomogenous OLs, revealing a higher risk than homogenous lesions.[118] Proliferative verrucous OL is an independent entity from the set of leukoplakias, more often observed in elderly women, usually in the gingival region that may affect large areas of mucosa, as whitish verrucous lesions, or in a less keratinized polypoid form with well-defined borders.[118] These lesions are characterized by a multifocal presentation, resistance to treatment,[24] and high rate of malignant transformation of up to 80%.[24,118]

The majority of OL represent benign conditions, and should be differentiated from candidiasis, lupus erythematosus, lichen planus, traumatic/irritative lesions, chemical burns, syphilis, papilloma, hereditary white lesions, and geographic tongue,[13] because long-standing OL lesions may be potential precursors of oral cancer.[11,117,120] The reported malignant transformation rate ranges from 0.13 to 36.4%, depending upon the study design,[11,24,110,118,120,122,123] within a period of 1 to 30 years.[12,123] Histological analysis of the lesions is the current standard to examine their biological potential.[24,116,117]

Having nonhomogenous nature,[24,117,120,124] being larger than 200 mm,[117,120,124] location on the tongue or floor of the mouth,[117,125] female gender,[117,125] age older than 60 years,[24] presence of dysplasia,[117] previous history of SCC,[118] regular consumption of alcohol or cigarettes,[118] and occurrence in nonsmokers[117,125] are correlated with higher risk of transformation. Nonhomogeneous OL on tongue/floor of the mouth had a 43.10-fold higher risk compared to homogeneous lesions located on the other sites,[125] but histological analysis of the lesions is mandatory to discover their biological potential.[24,117,124]

3.3.2 Oral Lichen Planus

OLP is a chronic inflammatory mucocutaneous disorder that is characterized by periods of exacerbation and remission.[119,126,127] It commonly involves the mucosa of the oral cavity, but can involve the skin, the vulvar and vaginal mucosa, the glans penis, the scalp (resulting in alopecia), and the nails.[128] OLP occurs in 70 to 77% of patients with cutaneous LP,[126] but 15% of patients with predominantly OLP may develop cutaneous lesions.[129]

The age of onset is generally between the fourth and sixth decades of life with females affected 1.5 to 3 times more than males.[126,128,130] The estimated prevalence of OLP is between 0.5 and 3%.[126,128,129,131,132]

The typical oral manifestations of OLP are reticular, papular, atrophic and/or erosive, plaquelike, and bullous forms.[126,127,130,133] Some authors simplified the clinical grouping describing three types of lesions: reticular (Wickham's striae, plaques, and papules); atrophic (erythematous); and erosive (ulcerative and bullous), with the posterior buccal mucosa the most frequently affected site[129,134] (▶ Fig. 3.2, ▶ Fig. 3.3).

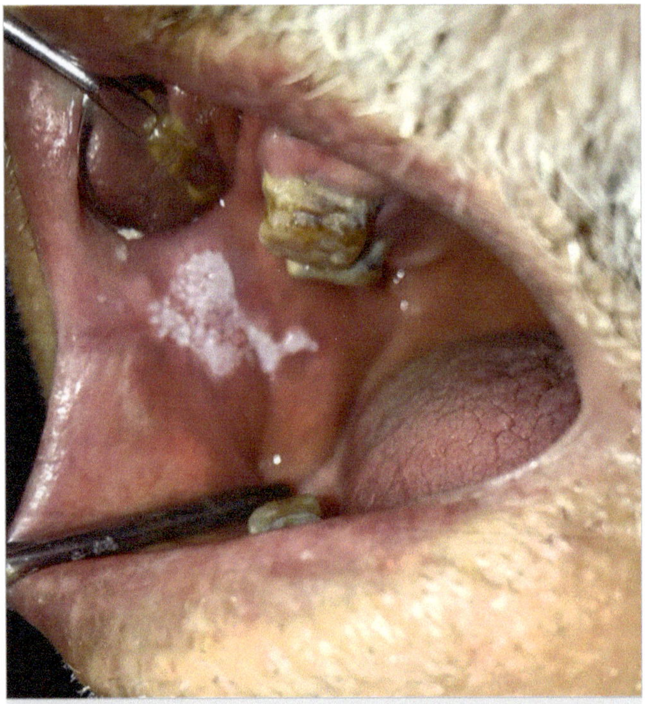

Fig. 3.1 Leukoplakia lesion on the right buccal mucosa with histological diagnosis of SIN1.

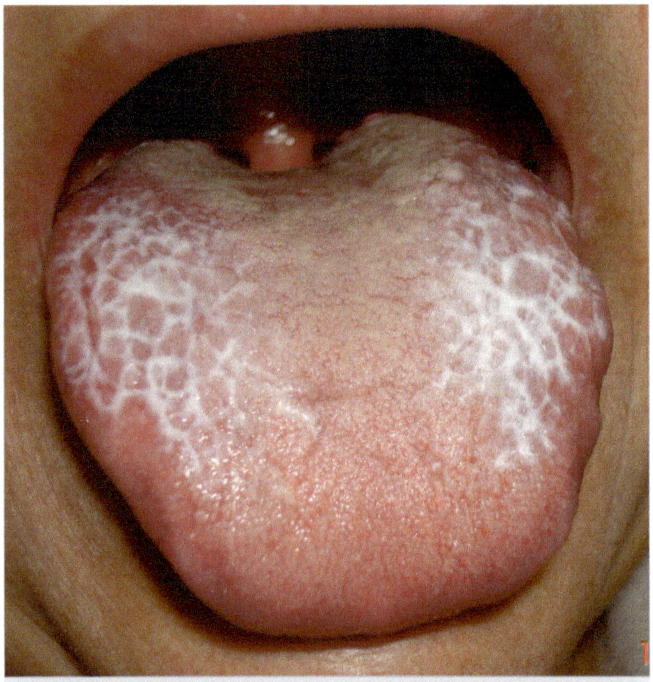

Fig. 3.2 Reticular oral lichen planus on the tongue.

Each of these clinical forms of OLP may occur as the only form of OLP seen in a patient, or concurrently with one or more of the other forms of OLP.[130] Mucosal lesions are usually multiple and commonly present with bilateral distribution.[128] In some OLP patients, gingival location presenting as white papules or plaques may resemble homogeneous and nonhomogeneous leukoplakia.[127,128]

Clinical symptoms may be absent or minimal and is most commonly observed in the classic reticular form, while erythema, erosions, and ulceration are generally painful manifestations.[132]

An exogenous or an endogenous antigen presentation by the oral keratinocytes initiates the pathogenesis of OLP, followed by a complex inflammatory response containing mainly $CD4^+$ and $CD8^+$ T cells, macrophages, mast cells, and the associated cytokines and cytotoxic molecules.[132] The histological picture of OLP lesions present with dense inflammatory infiltrate in the upper lamina propria, liquefaction degeneration of basal keratinocytes, and basal membrane hyperkeratosis or atrophy of the keratin layer.[132]

Etiological or initiating factors include hepatitis C virus; psychological stress (high levels of anxiety or depression); contact hypersensitivity to dental materials, especially to amalgam; herpes viruses (HSV1, EBV, and HHV-6); HIV; HPV; and hepatitis B virus.[129,135] Medications or dental materials may induce lesions similar to OLP, termed "oral lichenoid reactions,"[126,128] which are difficult to distinguish from OLP.[119] Drug-induced oral lichenoid reactions have been reported with nonsteroidal anti-inflammatory agents, angiotensin-converting enzyme inhibitors, β-blockers, methyldopa, and penicillamine.[126] In addition to amalgam, oral lichenoid reactions can result from contact hypersensitivity to dental materials such amalgam, gold alloy, composite, and dental acrylics, and they can resolve after replacement of the causative dental material.[126] Oral lichenoid lesions may occur in patients with acute or chronic graft-versus-host disease.[128]

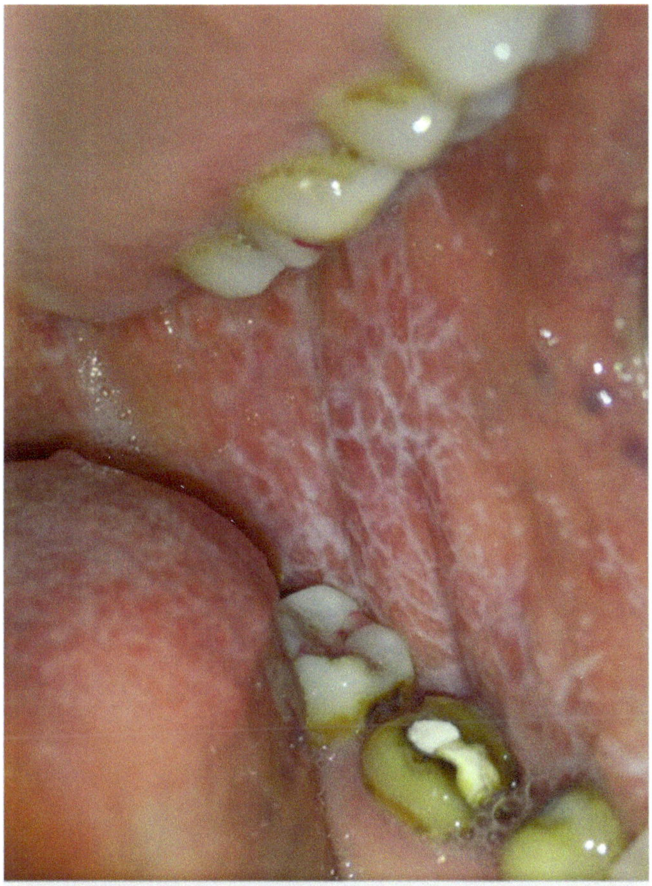

Fig. 3.3 Reticular oral lichen planus on the left buccal mucosa.

The premalignant potential of OLP is still debated,[119,126,136] but it is generally accepted that lichen planus/lichenoid lesions can be OPMD[119,137] and lichenoid lesions may have a higher malignant transformation rate than OLP.[138] In order to assess the malignancy potential of OLP, follow-up for a minimum of 6 years has been advised.[139] The exact mechanisms that drive lichen planus/lichenoid lesions to cancer is not known, but it is suggested that the chronic inflammatory microenvironment might lead to altered growth control of epithelial cells, and when combined with oxidative stress from oxidative and nitrative products might provoke DNA damage over time, which results in cancer development.[132,138] Furthermore, the changes in the lesion microenvironment and altered host immune response may be of importance.

The rate of transformation ranges from 0 to 10%, according to the study population and study design, after mean follow-up of 1.5 to 10 years.[126–128,132,136] The literature suggests that there may be a higher frequency of OLP transforming into SCC in some locations, such as tongue, followed by buccal mucosa and gingiva. Even though results are inconclusive regarding the clinical form,[127] malignant transformations may be observed more in atrophic, erosive, and ulcerative lesions.[136] When intraepithelial neoplasia with squamous intraepithelial neoplasia (SIN) II and SIN III is present in the biopsy, the risk of malignancy is increased by 9%.[138] Long-term monitoring may be problematic, but at a minimum, annual monitoring is recommended for asymptomatic white reticular OLP,[128,131] whereas atrophic/erosive/ulcerative forms shall be monitored from 1 to 3 months depending on the extensiveness and severity of their lesions.[131]

3.3.3 Erythroplakia

OE has been described as "a fiery red patch that cannot be characterized clinically or pathologically as any other definable lesion."[16,124,140] OE occurs most commonly in middle-aged and elderly adults;[97,124,140,141] alcohol and tobacco have been reported to be risk factors.[97,124,140] The prevalence of OE has a range of between 0.004 and 0.83%.[16,140]

OE may have a smooth and velvety surface or an irregular, red granular surface interspersed with white or yellow foci.[140,141] If the redness is dominant, then the lesion may be described as granular erythroplakia, but when there are numerous, small irregular foci of leukoplakia dispersed in the erythroplakic patch, it is described as speckled leukoplakia.[140] Clinically, OE is unicentric, may be adjacent to leukoplakia, and remains soft and not indurated until the development of carcinoma.[140] Lesions are clearly demarcated from the surrounding oral mucosa,[140] and are mostly located at the floor of the mouth, ventrolateral tongue, and soft palate.[141,142] Presence of granular, elevated, or speckled surface in an erythroplastic area suggests an increased risk of an invasive nature of the lesion.[141] Application of adjuncts such as toluidine blue (TB) may increase the diagnostic accuracy of clinical evaluation,[99] but considering that majority of OE lesions present with severe dysplasia, carcinoma in situ or carcinoma,[12,25,124,140] any persistent red lesion in suspicious sites requires follow-up.[142]

3.3.4 Submucous Fibrosis

The WHO has defined OSMF as a "slowly progressive disease in which the fibrous bands form in the oral mucosa, ultimately leading to severe restriction of movement of the mouth, including the tongue."[143] It is a chronic, progressive, debilitating, and potentially malignant disorder characterized by fibrosis of the lining mucosa of the upper digestive tract involving the oral cavity, oropharynx, and the oesophagus.[119,144–146] OSMF presents with juxtaepithelial inflammation and progressive fibrosis of submucosa. The fibrosis may lead to reduced jaw opening and limited oral opening due to rigid lips and cheeks. Dysphagia may occur due to involvement of the pharynx and the upper third of the esophagus. Oral burning sensation may be due to sclerosing stomatitis.[16,119,143,146,147] Limited movement of the tongue may occur.

OSMF is mostly observed in males involving the buccal mucosa.[143,144] The main etiological factor has been defined as areca nut use,[143,148] either alone or in combination with tobacco or as betel quid.[143,146,149] However, only a small portion of areca nut users develop the disease, suggesting that genetic predisposing factors are also involved.[146,148,150] Additionally, capsaicin in chilies, copper in areca nut or water, micronutrient deficiencies of iron, zinc, and essential vitamins, a possible autoimmune basis to the disease with demonstration of various autoantibodies, and an association with specific human leukocyte antigens (HLA) have been proposed.[144,150,151]

Even though OSMF was previously confined to geographical areas such as South East Asia and India,[143,145,146,148] it is observed among the Asian immigrants throughout the world.[145,150]

Clinical characteristics of OSMF are the results of fibrosis and hyalinization of subepithelial tissues, either due to increased collagen synthesis or reduced collagen degradation.[150,151] With the changes in the cell cycle, DNA, keratinocytes and keratin, tumor-cell proliferation and survival, angiogenesis, fibrosis through epithelial–mesenchymal transitions, and tissue hypoxia, malignant transformation in OSMF may occur.[143,149,152] The rate of transformation of OSMF to OSCC ranges from 3 to 19%,[144,146,147,149,150] even up to 30% over years.[145,151]

Severely atrophic oral mucous membrane of OSMF patients may be at increased risk to development of other potentially malignant lesions such as leukoplakia and erythroplakia because of the acanthosis and proliferation of epithelial lining, indicating a transition from fibrosis to SCC.[144] The risk of malignant transformation of OSMF increases with the presence of epithelial dysplasia and leukoplakia.[144,148,149]

Stage, nodal involvement, and disease-free survival have been better in OSCC patients with OSMF and it has been suggested that OSCC associated with OSMF is histopathologically a diverse cancer.[143,148,149]

3.4 Diagnosis and Evaluation

Technical developments may contribute to the efficacy of detection and diagnostic evaluation for OSCC. Adjuncts to the clinical evaluation must be simple and inexpensive and assist in distinguishing benign, inflammatory, and reactive mucosal lesions from dysplastic and neoplastic change.[115] Imaging with computed tomography, magnetic resonance imaging, positron emission tomography, ultrasonography, and nuclear medicine may contribute to diagnosis and staging.[153]

Several adjunctive visualization aids have been introduced.[154–156,157,158] These products and devices include oral exfoliative cytology/oral brush cytology, v staining, and in vivo imaging devices (e.g., fluorescent light).[154,159,160]

3.4.1 Exfoliative Cytology

Oral exfoliative cytology is used to obtain epithelial cells from all layers of oral mucosa with a bristle brush to examine the cell morphology under a light microscope.[161] It is promoted as rapid, inexpensive, and well-tolerated method to assess the need for scalpel biopsies in clinically benign-appearing lesions.[157,162] However, the results of the studies that have assessed the sensitivity and specificity of brush cytology in detecting dysplasia or OSCC are controversial.[163] While a number of reports have shown the value of brush cytology,[159,164] others reported large numbers of false-positive and false-negative results,[165–167] ranging between 30 to 84%[168] and 63% for dysplastic lesions.[169] Mehrotra et al performed a study where immediate scalpel biopsies were obtained after brush biopsies from oral lesions, and they reported 96.3% sensitivity and 100% specificity for dysplasia or carcinoma.[170] Potential limitations, such as the inability to acquire transepithelial collections in necrosis and/or mucosal infection, which are frequently observed with carcinomas, have been reported.[162,163] Also, mucosal sites and lesions with a high degree of keratinization may prevent collection of enough basal cells in leukoplakia, and inflammatory conditions frequently may lead to atypical results.[162,163,171]

Oral brush cytology (OralCDx BrushTest system) was developed to investigate mucosal abnormalities with low-risk clinical features.[156,172–174] A specially designed brush is utilized to obtain a transepithelial sample of cells from a mucosal lesion.[156,172–174] The cell material obtained is transferred to the slide and fixed[172] and computer program is used to evaluate the cellular material, which is reported as "positive," "atypical," or "negative."[156,170] The sensitivity of Oral CDx ranged from 71 to 100%, specificity from 25 to 94%, and PPV from 33 to 86%;[161,175] however, the challenge remains in differentiating inflammatory/reactive change from dysplastic change. Other evaluation of exfoliative cells including assessing molecular changes may enhance the utility of cytologic evaluation.

3.4.2 Toluidine Blue Staining

TB, which is also known as tolonium chloride, is a metachromatic vital dye that binds to tissues undergoing rapid cell division such as inflammatory, regenerative, and neoplastic tissue, and sites of DNA change.[155,161] It has been used in detection of potentially malignant abnormalities of the uterine cervix and the oral cavity[165] (► Fig. 3.4). TB may be applied as a mouth rinse or topical, resulting in the royal blue staining of abnormal tissue.[167,176] Since traumatic/inflammatory mucosal changes and ulcerations have high cellular metabolic rate, they also stain and may lead to false-positive findings.[176,177] The relevance of TB in identification of OPMD and early diagnosis of OSCC[167,176,

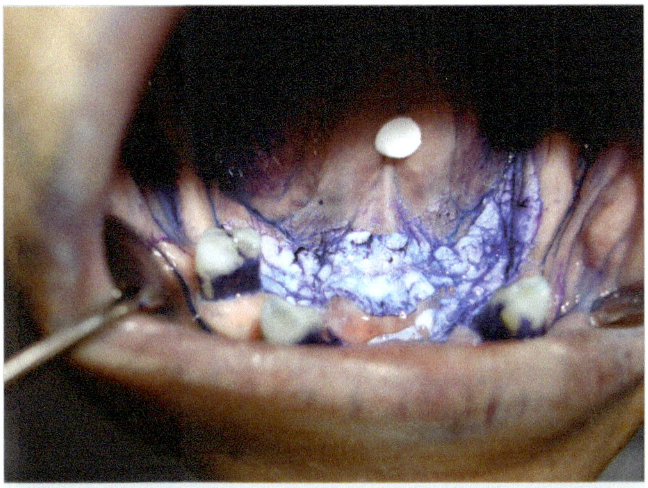

Fig. 3.4 Royal blue staining observed after application of toluidine blue, which is used to define the margins and the areas that require biopsy.

[178,179] to assess margins and biopsy site of the lesions before biopsy[180–183] and follow-up of patients with previous oral cancer have been reported.[178] The ranges of sensitivity/specificity and positive predictive value (PPV)/negative predictive value (NPV) of TB staining are as follows: sensitivity changed between 38 and 98%, specificity between 9 and 93%, PPV between 33 and 93%, and NPV between 22 and 92%.[158,165,166,176,179,184–188] The sensitivity and specificity of TB are reported to be higher for malignant lesions, but the sensitivity was lower for potentially malignant lesions.[164] On the other hand, molecular abnormalities may be present at margins of lesions and at oral sites, which may be histologically benign.[168,176,189] Considering that positive TB staining presents lesions with LOH and may precede histological transformation[179,190] due to binding to sites of molecular change, "false-positive" TB results based upon histomorphology may actually represent molecularly "true-positive" lesions with risk of progression to OSCC.[191]

3.4.3 Optical Systems

The development of oral neoplasia is associated with abnormal metabolic and structural changes in tissue optical properties.[192–194] Fluorescence diagnostics and light-based detection systems are grounded on the assumption that suspicious mucosal tissues might reveal different absorbance and reflectance profiles when exposed to various forms of light or energy.[176,195] Supporting this concept, some authors report progressive reduction in blue-green intensity of light in dysplastic and cancerous tissues.[196,197] Tissue fluorescence loss has been associated with LOH in oral mucosa.[196,197] However, its ability to distinguish the dysplastic nature of the lesions remains controversial.[192,193] In identified SCC at the time of surgery, loss of fluorescence has been shown to predict lesion margins and has been shown to improve surgical outcomes.[196]

Several devices that utilize light for assisting clinical oral cancer diagnosis have been presented to the dental market. Among these, ViziLite system (Zila Pharmaceuticals, Phoenix, AZ) has a capsule that emits light when activated.[166,198] Normal cells absorb the light and have a bluish color, whereas the light is reflected by abnormal cells with a higher nucleus-to-cytoplasm ratio, leading to acetowhite appearance with marked and distinguishable borders.[166,199–203] Some authors reported increased ability to detect mainly white and white-red oral lesions,[162,199,200] whereas others stated its low potential for discrimination between malignant, benign, and inflammatory oral lesions.[162,166,176,195,198,202,203] Microlux Diagnostic Light (Microlux/DL, AdDent, Danbury, CT) is another device that uses refractive light technology and enhances visibility of oral white lesions, but could not discriminate between inflammatory, benign, and malignant nature of lesions.[204] OraScoptic DK (Orascoptic, Kerr Co., Middleton, WI) is a similar device to Microlux, producing light of similar wavelength to ViziLite, but the supporting literature about its efficacy rare.[176]

The visually enhanced lesion scope (VELscope; LED Dental, White Rock, BC, Canada) uses the fluorescence properties of oral mucosa and aids in diagnosing mucosal abnormalities before they become visible.[162,196,197] Advanced detectability of oral mucosal abnormalities with VELscope has been shown,[205] but its specificity was low.[206,207] Others reported no additional benefit with the use of optical diagnostic systems.[157,208,209] The role of adjuncts has limited study in general practice and in lower risk populations, making recommendations for use in the primary care setting challenging, as PPV and NPV are not known and all are faced with the challenge of differentiating inflammatory from dysplastic change. Molecular markers hold promise for future application.

Key Points

Potential characteristics suggesting oral dysplastic/neoplastic conditions:

- More common in older patients.
- With red and white mixed color.
- Having irregular texture.
- Defined and irregular margins or with undetectable margins.
- Associated with firm and fixed lymphadenopathy.
- Causing pain and loss of function should increase suspicion of malignancy potential of the lesion.
- Adjuncts supporting the clinical examination may include cytology and visual adjuncts; and future molecular analyses may also assist the tissue examination.

References

[1] Goyal D, Goyal P, Singh HP, Verma C. An update on precancerous lesions of oral cavity. Int J Med Dent Sci. 2013; 2:70–75

[2] Tabor MP, Brakenhoff RH, van Houten VM, et al. Persistence of genetically altered fields in head and neck cancer patients: biological and clinical implications. Clin Cancer Res. 2001; 7(6):1523–1532

[3] Nagpal JK, Das BR. Oral cancer: reviewing the present understanding of its molecular mechanism and exploring the future directions for its effective management. Oral Oncol. 2003; 39(3):213–221

[4] Braakhuis BJ, Tabor MP, Kummer JA, Leemans CR, Brakenhoff RH. A genetic explanation of Slaughter's concept of field cancerization: evidence and clinical implications. Cancer Res. 2003; 63(8):1727–1730

[5] Liao CT, Wallace CG, Lee LY, et al. Clinical evidence of field cancerization in patients with oral cavity cancer in a betel quid chewing area. Oral Oncol. 2014; 50(8):721–731

[6] Zhang X, Han S, Han HY, et al. Risk prediction for malignant conversion of oral epithelial dysplasia by hypoxia related protein expression. Pathology. 2013; 45(5):478–483

[7] Slaughter DP, Southwick HW, Smejkal W. Field cancerization in oral stratified squamous epithelium; clinical implications of multicentric origin. Cancer. 1953; 6(5):963–968

[8] Ha PK, Califano JA. The molecular biology of mucosal field cancerization of the head and neck. Crit Rev Oral Biol Med. 2003; 14(5):363–369

[9] Angadi PV, Savitha JK, Rao SS, Sivaranjini Y. Oral field cancerization: current evidence and future perspectives. Oral Maxillofac Surg. 2012; 16(2):171–180

[10] Ai H, Barrera JE, Meyers AD, Shroyer KR, Varella-Garcia M. Chromosomal aneuploidy precedes morphological changes and supports multifocality in head and neck lesions. Laryngoscope. 2001; 111(10):1853–1858

[11] Güneri P, Epstein JB. Why are we still unable to accurately determine the malignant potential or the behavior of oral mucosal lesions? Oral Oncol. 2017; 71:177–179

[12] Bouquot JE, Speight PM, Farthing PM. Epithelial dysplasia of the oral mucosa-diagnostic problems and prognostic features. Curr Diagn Pathol. 2006; 12:11–21

[13] Mogedas-Vegara A, Hueto-Madrid JA, Chimenos-Küstner E, Bescós-Atín C. The treatment of oral leukoplakia with the CO2 laser: a retrospective study of 65 patients. J Craniomaxillofac Surg. 2015; 43(5):677–681

[14] Lumerman H, Freedman P, Kerpel S. Oral epithelial dysplasia and the development of invasive squamous cell carcinoma. Oral Surg Oral Med Oral Pathol Oral Radiol Endod. 1995; 79(3):321–329

[15] Warnakulasuriya S, Reibel J, Bouquot J, Dabelsteen E. Oral epithelial dysplasia classification systems: predictive value, utility, weaknesses and scope for improvement. J Oral Pathol Med. 2008; 37(3):127–133

[16] Dionne KR, Warnakulasuriya S, Zain RB, Cheong SC. Potentially malignant disorders of the oral cavity: current practice and future directions in the clinic and laboratory. Int J Cancer. 2015; 136(3):503–515

[17] van der Waal I. Potentially malignant disorders of the oral and oropharyngeal mucosa; terminology, classification and present concepts of management. Oral Oncol. 2009; 45(4–5):317–323

[18] Güneri P, Epstein JB. Late stage diagnosis of oral cancer: components and possible solutions. Oral Oncol. 2014; 50(12):1131–1136

[19] Carreras-Torras C, Gay-Escoda C. Techniques for early diagnosis of oral squamous cell carcinoma: systematic review. Med Oral Patol Oral Cir Bucal. 2015; 20(3):e305–e315

[20] Barnes L, Eveson JW, Reichart P, Sidransky D, eds. World Health Organization Classification of Tumours. Pathology & Genetics: Head and Neck Tumours. IARC Press: Lyon, France; 2005:179–183

[21] Kujan O, Oliver RJ, Khattab A, Roberts SA, Thakker N, Sloan P. Evaluation of a new binary system of grading oral epithelial dysplasia for prediction of malignant transformation. Oral Oncol. 2006; 42(10):987–993

[22] Zerdoner D. The Ljubljana classification: its application to grading oral epithelial hyperplasia. J Craniomaxillofac Surg. 2003; 31(2):75–79

[23] Hellquist H, Cardesa A, Gale N, Kambic V, Michaels L. Criteria for grading in the Ljubljana classification of epithelial hyperplastic laryngeal lesions. A study by members of the Working Group on Epithelial Hyperplastic Laryngeal Lesions of the European Society of Pathology. Histopathology. 1999; 34 (3):226–233

[24] Kumar A, Cascarini L, McCaul JA, et al. How should we manage oral leukoplakia? Br J Oral Maxillofac Surg. 2013; 51(5):377–383

[25] Scully C. Challenges in predicting which oral mucosal potentially malignant disease will progress to neoplasia. Oral Dis. 2014; 20(1):1–5

[26] Sengiz S, Pabuççuoğlu U, Sarioğlu S. Immunohistological comparison of the World Health Organization (WHO) and Ljubljana classifications on the grading of preneoplastic lesions of the larynx. Pathol Res Pract. 2004; 200(3): 181–188

[27] Chandu A, Smith AC. The use of CO2 laser in the treatment of oral white patches: outcomes and factors affecting recurrence. Int J Oral Maxillofac Surg. 2005; 34(4):396–400

[28] Thomas G, Hashibe M, Jacob BJ, et al. Risk factors for multiple oral premalignant lesions. Int J Cancer. 2003; 107(2):285–291

[29] Hashibe M, Brennan P, Benhamou S, et al. Alcohol drinking in never users of tobacco, cigarette smoking in never drinkers, and the risk of head and neck cancer: pooled analysis in the International Head and Neck Cancer Epidemiology Consortium. J Natl Cancer Inst. 2007; 99(10):777–789

[30] Petersen PE. Oral cancer prevention and control: the approach of the World Health Organization. Oral Oncol. 2009; 45(4–5):454–460

[31] Scully C, Bagan J. Oral squamous cell carcinoma overview. Oral Oncol. 2009; 45(4–5):301–308

[32] Brocklehurst P, Kujan O, Glenny AM, et al. Screening programmes for the early detection and prevention of oral cancer. Cochrane Database Syst Rev. 2010(11):CD004150

[33] Gupta S, Shah JS, Parikh S, Limbdiwala P, Goel S. Clinical correlative study on early detection of oral cancer and precancerous lesions by modified oral brush biopsy and cytology followed by histopathology. J Cancer Res Ther. 2014; 10(2):232–238

[34] Zygogianni AG, Kyrgias G, Karakitsos P, et al. Oral squamous cell cancer: early detection and the role of alcohol and smoking. Head Neck Oncol. 2011; 3:2

[35] Meurman JH. Infectious and dietary risk factors of oral cancer. Oral Oncol. 2010; 46(6):411–413

[36] Alsidawi S, Price KA, Chintakuntlawar AV, et al. Characteristics and long-term outcomes of head and neck squamous cell carcinoma after solid organ transplantation. Oral Oncol. 2017; 72:104–109

[37] Hirai H, Tomioka H, Mochizuki Y, Oikawa Y, Tsushima F, Harada H. Clinical course of oral squamous cell carcinoma in patients on immunosuppressant and glucocorticoid therapy. J Oral Maxillofac Surg. 2017; 75(9):1980–1986

[38] Zamoiski RD, Yanik E, Gibson TM, et al. Risk of second malignancies in solid organ transplant recipients who develop keratinocyte cancers. Cancer Res. 2017; 77(15):4196–4203

[39] Güneri P, Cankaya H, Yavuzer A, et al. Primary oral cancer in a Turkish population sample: association with sociodemographic features, smoking, alcohol, diet and dentition. Oral Oncol. 2005; 41(10):1005–1012

[40] Rosenquist K, Wennerberg J, Schildt EB, Bladström A, Göran Hansson B, Andersson G. Oral status, oral infections and some lifestyle factors as risk factors for oral and oropharyngeal squamous cell carcinoma. A population-based case-control study in southern Sweden. Acta Otolaryngol. 2005; 125 (12):1327–1336

[41] Gupta B, Bray F, Kumar N, Johnson NW. Associations between oral hygiene habits, diet, tobacco and alcohol and risk of oral cancer: a case-control study from India. Cancer Epidemiol. 2017; 51:7–14

[42] Ganapathy V, Manyanga J, Brame L, et al. Electronic cigarette aerosols suppress cellular antioxidant defenses and induce significant oxidative DNA damage. PLoS One. 2017; 12(5):e0177780

[43] McAdam K, Kimpton H, Porter A, et al. Comprehensive survey of radionuclides in contemporary smokeless tobacco products. Chem Cent J. 2017; 11 (1):131

[44] Yu V, Rahimy M, Korrapati A, et al. Electronic cigarettes induce DNA strand breaks and cell death independently of nicotine in cell lines. Oral Oncol. 2016; 52:58–65

[45] Goniewicz ML, Knysak J, Gawron M, et al. Levels of selected carcinogens and toxicants in vapour from electronic cigarettes. Tob Control. 2014; 23(2): 133–139

[46] Franco T, Trapasso S, Puzzo L, Allegra E. Electronic cigarette: role in the primary prevention of oral cavity cancer. Clin Med Insights Ear Nose Throat. 2016; 9:7–12

[47] International Agency for Research on Cancer; World Health Organization. IARC Monographs on the Evaluation of Carcinogenic Risks to Humans. Vol. 96. Alcohol Consumption and Ethyl Carbamate. Lyon, France: IARC; 2010:279–329

[48] Curado MP, Hashibe M. Recent changes in the epidemiology of head and neck cancer. Curr Opin Oncol. 2009; 21(3):194–200

[49] Balaram P, Sridhar H, Rajkumar T, et al. Oral cancer in southern India: the influence of smoking, drinking, paan-chewing and oral hygiene. Int J Cancer. 2002; 98(3):440–445

[50] Al-Rawi NH, Talabani NG. Squamous cell carcinoma of the oral cavity: a case series analysis of clinical presentation and histological grading of 1,425 cases from Iraq. Clin Oral Investig. 2008; 12(1):15–18

[51] Bagan J, Sarrion G, Jimenez Y. Oral cancer: clinical features. Oral Oncol. 2010; 46(6):414–417

[52] Gorsky M, Epstein JB, Oakley C, Le ND, Hay J, Stevenson-Moore P. Carcinoma of the tongue: a case series analysis of clinical presentation, risk factors, staging, and outcome. Oral Surg Oral Med Oral Pathol Oral Radiol Endod. 2004; 98(5):546–552

[53] Brocklehurst P, Kujan O, O'Malley LA, Ogden G, Shepherd S, Glenny AM. Screening programmes for the early detection and prevention of oral cancer. Cochrane Database Syst Rev. 2013(11):CD004150

[54] Nowosielska-Grygiel J, Owczarek K, Bielińska M, Wacławek M, Olszewski J. Analysis of risk factors for oral cavity and oropharynx cancer in the authors' own material. Otolaryngol Pol. 2017; 71(2):23–28

[55] Jainkittivong A, Swasdison S, Thangpisityotin M, Langlais RP. Oral squamous cell carcinoma: a clinicopathological study of 342 Thai cases. J Contemp Dent Pract. 2009; 10(5):E033–E040

[56] Ribeiro AC, Silva AR, Simonato LE, Salzedas LM, Sundefeld ML, Soubhia AM. Clinical and histopathological analysis of oral squamous cell carcinoma in

young people: a descriptive study in Brazilians. Br J Oral Maxillofac Surg. 2009; 47(2):95–98

[57] Castelo-Branco C, Soveral I. The immune system and aging: a review. Gynecol Endocrinol. 2014; 30(1):16–22

[58] Warnakulasuriya S. Global epidemiology of oral and oropharyngeal cancer. Oral Oncol. 2009; 45(4–5):309–316

[59] Gupta N, Gupta R, Acharya AK, et al. Changing trends in oral cancer: a global scenario. Nepal J Epidemiol. 2016; 6(4):613–619

[60] Califano J, van der Riet P, Westra W, et al. Genetic progression model for head and neck cancer: implications for field cancerization. Cancer Res. 1996; 56(11):2488–2492

[61] Sarode SC, Sarode GS, Karmarkar S, Tupkari JV. A new classification for potentially malignant disorders of the oral cavity. Oral Oncol. 2011; 47(9): 920–921

[62] Zhang L, Poh CF, Williams M, et al. Loss of heterozygosity (LOH) profiles: validated risk predictors for progression to oral cancer. Cancer Prev Res (Phila). 2012; 5(9):1081–1089

[63] Garnis C, Chari R, Buys TP, et al. Genomic imbalances in precancerous tissues signal oral cancer risk. Mol Cancer. 2009; 8:50

[64] Li X, Lee NK, Ye YW, et al. Allelic loss at chromosomes 3p, 8p, 13q, and 17p associated with poor prognosis in head and neck cancer. J Natl Cancer Inst. 1994; 86(20):1524–1529

[65] Gupta S, Gupta S. Role of human papillomavirus in oral squamous cell carcinoma and oral potentially malignant disorders: a review of the literature. Indian J Dent. 2015; 6(2):91–98

[66] Maxwell JH, Grandis JR, Ferris RL. HPV-associated head and neck cancer: unique features of epidemiology and clinical management. Annu Rev Med. 2016; 67:91–101

[67] Khot KP, Deshmane S, Choudhari S. Human papilloma virus in oral squamous cell carcinoma: the enigma unravelled. Chin J Dent Res. 2016; 19(1):17–23

[68] Gooi Z, Chan JY, Fakhry C. The epidemiology of the human papillomavirus related to oropharyngeal head and neck cancer. Laryngoscope. 2016; 126 (4):894–900

[69] Kreimer AR, Clifford GM, Boyle P, Franceschi S. Human papillomavirus types in head and neck squamous cell carcinomas worldwide: a systematic review. Cancer Epidemiol Biomarkers Prev. 2005; 14(2):467–475

[70] Gillison ML, Alemany L, Snijders PJ, et al. Human papillomavirus and diseases of the upper airway: head and neck cancer and respiratory papillomatosis. Vaccine. 2012; 30 Suppl 5:F34–F54

[71] Gillison ML, Chaturvedi AK, Anderson WF, Fakhry C. Epidemiology of human papillomavirus-positive head and neck squamous cell carcinoma. J Clin Oncol. 2015; 33(29):3235–3242

[72] D'Souza G, McNeel TS, Fakhry C. Understanding personal risk of oropharyngeal cancer: risk-groups for oncogenic oral HPV infection and oropharyngeal cancer. Ann Oncol. 2017; 28(12):3065–3069

[73] Nichols AC, Dhaliwal SS, Palma DA, et al. Does HPV type affect outcome in oropharyngeal cancer? J Otolaryngol Head Neck Surg. 2013; 42:9

[74] Mallen-St Clair J, Alani M, Wang MB, Srivatsan ES. Human papillomavirus in oropharyngeal cancer: the changing face of a disease. Biochim Biophys Acta. 2016; 1866:141–50

[75] Jayaprakash V, Reid M, Hatton E, et al. Human papillomavirus types 16 and 18 in epithelial dysplasia of oral cavity and oropharynx: a meta-analysis, 1985–2010. Oral Oncol. 2011; 47(11):1048–1054

[76] Farsi NJ, Rousseau MC, Schlecht N, et al. Aetiological heterogeneity of head and neck squamous cell carcinomas: the role of human papillomavirus infections, smoking and alcohol. Carcinogenesis. 2017; 38(12):1188–1195

[77] Chaturvedi AK, D'Souza G, Gillison ML, Katki HA. Burden of HPV-positive oropharynx cancers among ever and never smokers in the U.S. population. Oral Oncol. 2016; 60:61–67

[78] Mathew A, Mody RN, Patait MR, Razooki AA, Varghese NT, Saraf K. Prevalence and relationship of human papilloma virus type 16 and type 18 with oral squamous cell carcinoma and oral leukoplakia in fresh scrappings: a PCR study. Indian J Med Sci. 2011; 65(5):212–221

[79] Oliveira MC, Conceição Andrade M, Santos Menezes F. Epidemiology of HPV in head and neck cancer. In: Broeck DV, ed. Human Papillomavirus and Related Diseases: From Bench to Bedside—A Clinical Perspective. Rijeka, Croatia: InTech; 2012:197–207

[80] Szarka K, Tar I, Fehér E, et al. Progressive increase of human papillomavirus carriage rates in potentially malignant and malignant oral disorders with increasing malignant potential. Oral Microbiol Immunol. 2009; 24(4):314–318

[81] Gorsky M, Epstein JB. Oral lichen planus: malignant transformation and human papilloma virus: a review of potential clinical implications. Oral Surg Oral Med Oral Pathol Oral Radiol Endod. 2011; 111(4):461–464

[82] Reed SG, Wahlquist AE. Adults with oral high-risk human papillomavirus (hpv) and/or smoking history have a higher risk for clinically diagnosed oral premalignant lesions. J Evid Based Dent Pract. 2015; 15(3):134–136

[83] Campisi G, Giovannelli L, Aricò P, et al. HPV DNA in clinically different variants of oral leukoplakia and lichen planus. Oral Surg Oral Med Oral Pathol Oral Radiol Endod. 2004; 98(6):705–711

[84] Lin WW, Karin M. A cytokine-mediated link between innate immunity, inflammation, and cancer. J Clin Invest. 2007; 117(5):1175–1183

[85] Balkwill FR, Mantovani A. Cancer-related inflammation: common themes and therapeutic opportunities. Semin Cancer Biol. 2012; 22(1):33–40

[86] Sano Y, Kogashiwa Y, Araki R, et al. Correlation of inflammatory markers, survival, and COX2 expression in oral cancer and implications for prognosis. Otolaryngol Head Neck Surg. 2018; 158(4):667–676

[87] Coussens LM, Werb Z. Inflammation and cancer. Nature. 2002; 420(6917): 860–867

[88] Ghallab NA, Shaker OG. Serum and salivary levels of chemerin and MMP-9 in oral squamous cell carcinoma and oral premalignant lesions. Clin Oral Investig. 2017; 21(3):937–947

[89] Sun Y, Liu N, Guan X, Wu H, Sun Z, Zeng H. Immunosuppression induced by chronic inflammation and the progression to oral squamous cell carcinoma. Mediators Inflamm. 2016; 2016:5715719

[90] Shi W, Yang J, Li S, et al. Potential involvement of miR-375 in the premalignant progression of oral squamous cell carcinoma mediated via transcription factor KLF5. Oncotarget. 2015; 6(37):40172–40185

[91] Kamperos G, Nikitakis N, Sfakianou A, Avgoustidis D, Sklavounou-Andrikopoulou A. Expression of NF-κB and IL-6 in oral precancerous and cancerous lesions: an immunohistochemical study. Med Oral Patol Oral Cir Bucal. 2016; 21(1):e6–e13

[92] Divaris K, Olshan AF, Smith J, et al. Oral health and risk for head and neck squamous cell carcinoma: the Carolina Head and Neck Cancer Study. Cancer Causes Control. 2010; 21(4):567–575

[93] Zheng TZ, Boyle P, Hu HF, et al. Dentition, oral hygiene, and risk of oral cancer: a case-control study in Beijing, People's Republic of China. Cancer Causes Control. 1990; 1(3):235–241

[94] Chang JS, Lo HI, Wong TY, et al. Investigating the association between oral hygiene and head and neck cancer. Oral Oncol. 2013; 49(10):1010–1017

[95] Moreno-López LA, Esparza-Gómez GC, González-Navarro A, Cerero-Lapiedra R, González-Hernández MJ, Domínguez-Rojas V. Risk of oral cancer associated with tobacco smoking, alcohol consumption and oral hygiene: a case-control study in Madrid, Spain. Oral Oncol. 2000; 36(2):170–174

[96] Li S, Lee YC, Li Q, et al. Oral lesions, chronic diseases and the risk of head and neck cancer. Oral Oncol. 2015; 51(12):1082–1087

[97] Hashibe M, Jacob BJ, Thomas G, et al. Socioeconomic status, lifestyle factors and oral premalignant lesions. Oral Oncol. 2003; 39(7):664–671

[98] Zhang J, Gao F, Yang AK, et al. Epidemiologic characteristics of oral cancer: single-center analysis of 4097 patients from the Sun Yat-sen University Cancer Center. Chin J Cancer. 2016; 35:24–29

[99] Chainani-Wu N, Epstein J, Touger-Decker R. Diet and prevention of oral cancer: strategies for clinical practice. J Am Dent Assoc. 2011; 142(2):166–169

[100] Haya-Fernández MC, Bagán JV, Murillo-Cortés J, Poveda-Roda R, Calabuig C. The prevalence of oral leukoplakia in 138 patients with oral squamous cell carcinoma. Oral Dis. 2004; 10(6):346–348

[101] Epstein JB. Screening for oral potentially malignant epithelial lesions and squamous cell carcinoma: a discussion of benefit and risk. J Can Dent Assoc. 2014; 80:e47

[102] Messadi DV, Wilder-Smith P, Wolinsky L. Improving oral cancer survival: the role of dental providers. J Calif Dent Assoc. 2009; 37(11):789–798

[103] Barnes L, Eveson JW, Reichart P, Sidransky D, eds. World Health Organization Classification of Tumours. Pathology and Genetics: Head and Neck Tumours. Lyon, France: IARC Press; 2005:170

[104] Remmerbach TW, Meyer-Ebrecht D, Aach T, et al. Toward a multimodal cell analysis of brush biopsies for the early detection of oral cancer. Cancer. 2009; 117(3):228–235

[105] Pentenero M, Navone R, Motta F, et al. Clinical features of microinvasive stage I oral carcinoma. Oral Dis. 2011; 17(3):298–303

[106] Karbach J, Al-Nawas B, Moergel M, Daubländer M. Oral health-related quality of life of patients with oral lichen planus, oral leukoplakia, or oral squamous cell carcinoma. J Oral Maxillofac Surg. 2014; 72(8):1517–1522

[107] Yang Y, Zhang P, Li W. Comparison of orofacial pain of patients with different stages of precancer and oral cancer. Sci Rep. 2017; 7(1):203

[108] Lee JJ, Hong WK, Hittelman WN, et al. Predicting cancer development in oral leukoplakia: ten years of translational research. Clin Cancer Res. 2000; 6(5): 1702–1710

[109] Scully C, Field JK, Tanzawa H. Genetic aberrations in oral or head and neck squamous cell carcinoma 2: chromosomal aberrations. Oral Oncol. 2000; 36 (4):311–327

[110] Reibel J. Prognosis of oral pre-malignant lesions: significance of clinical, histopathological, and molecular biological characteristics. Crit Rev Oral Biol Med. 2003; 14(1):47–62

[111] Epstein JB, Gorsky M, Cabay RJ, Day T, Gonsalves W. Screening for and diagnosis of oral premalignant lesions and oropharyngeal squamous cell carcinoma: role of primary care physicians. Can Fam Physician. 2008; 54(6):870–875

[112] Epstein JB, Güneri P, Boyacioglu H, Abt E. The limitations of the clinical oral examination in detecting dysplastic oral lesions and oral squamous cell carcinoma. J Am Dent Assoc. 2012; 143(12):1332–1342

[113] Epstein JB, Zhang L, Rosin M. Advances in the diagnosis of oral premalignant and malignant lesions. J Can Dent Assoc. 2002; 68(10):617–621

[114] Zakrzewska JM, Downer C, Lopes V. The oral medicine clinic: what is its role? J R Soc Med. 1994; 87(7):390–392

[115] Poh CF, MacAulay CE, Laronde DM, Williams PM, Zhang L, Rosin MP. Squamous cell carcinoma and precursor lesions: diagnosis and screening in a technical era. Periodontol 2000. 2011; 57(1):73–88

[116] van der Waal I, Axéll T. Oral leukoplakia: a proposal for uniform reporting. Oral Oncol. 2002; 38(6):521–526

[117] van der Waal I, Schepman KP, van der Meij EH, Smeele LE. Oral leukoplakia: a clinicopathological review. Oral Oncol. 1997; 33(5):291–301

[118] Martorell-Calatayud A, Botella-Estrada R, Bagán-Sebastián JV, Sanmartín-Jiménez O, Guillén-Barona C. Oral leukoplakia: clinical, histopathologic, and molecular features and therapeutic approach. Actas Dermosifiliogr. 2009; 100(8):669–684

[119] Warnakulasuriya S, Johnson NW, van der Waal I. Nomenclature and classification of potentially malignant disorders of the oral mucosa. J Oral Pathol Med. 2007; 36(10):575–580

[120] Lodi G, Franchini R, Warnakulasuriya S, et al. Interventions for treating oral leukoplakia to prevent oral cancer. Cochrane Database Syst Rev. 2016; 7: CD001829

[121] Silverman S, Jr, Gorsky M, Lozada F. Oral leukoplakia and malignant transformation. A follow-up study of 257 patients. Cancer. 1984; 53(3):563–568

[122] Holmstrup P, Vedtofte P, Reibel J, Stoltze K. Long-term treatment outcome of oral premalignant lesions. Oral Oncol. 2006; 42(5):461–474

[123] Foy JP, Bertolus C, William WN, Jr, Saintigny P. Oral premalignancy: the roles of early detection and chemoprevention. Otolaryngol Clin North Am. 2013; 46(4):579–597

[124] van der Waal I. Potentially malignant disorders of the oral and oropharyngeal mucosa; present concepts of management. Oral Oncol. 2010; 46(6):423–425

[125] Lee JJ, Hung HC, Cheng SJ, et al. Carcinoma and dysplasia in oral leukoplakias in Taiwan: prevalence and risk factors. Oral Surg Oral Med Oral Pathol Oral Radiol Endod. 2006; 101(4):472–480

[126] Farhi D, Dupin N. Pathophysiology, etiologic factors, and clinical management of oral lichen planus, part I: facts and controversies. Clin Dermatol. 2010; 28(1):100–108

[127] Garcia-Pola MJ, Llorente-Pendás S, González-Garcia M, García-Martín JM. The development of proliferative verrucous leukoplakia in oral lichen planus. A preliminary study. Med Oral Patol Oral Cir Bucal. 2016; 21(3):e328–e334

[128] Al-Hashimi I, Schifter M, Lockhart PB, et al. Oral lichen planus and oral lichenoid lesions: diagnostic and therapeutic considerations. Oral Surg Oral Med Oral Pathol Oral Radiol Endod. 2007; 103 Suppl:25.e1–25.e12

[129] Malik U, Gupta S, Malik SD, Vashishth S, Zaheeruddin, Raju MS. Treatment of symptomatic oral lichen planus (OLP) with 0.1% tacrolimus powder in Oraguard-B: a pilot prospective study. Saudi Dent J. 2012; 24(3–4):143–148

[130] Shen ZY, Liu W, Feng JQ, Zhou HW, Zhou ZT. Squamous cell carcinoma development in previously diagnosed oral lichen planus: de novo or transformation? Oral Surg Oral Med Oral Pathol Oral Radiol Endod. 2011; 112(5):592–596

[131] Siar CH, Mah MC, Gill PP. Prevalence of bilateral "mirror-image" lesions in patients with oral potentially malignant epithelial lesions. Eur Arch Otorhinolaryngol. 2012; 269(3):999–1004

[132] Georgakopoulou EA, Achtari MD, Achtaris M, Foukas PG, Kotsinas A. Oral lichen planus as a preneoplastic inflammatory model. J Biomed Biotechnol. 2012; 2012:759626

[133] Hietanen J, Paasonen MR, Kuhlefelt M, Malmström M. A retrospective study of oral lichen planus patients with concurrent or subsequent development of malignancy. Oral Oncol. 1999; 35(3):278–282

[134] Munde AD, Karle RR, Wankhede PK, Shaikh SS, Kulkurni M. Demographic and clinical profile of oral lichen planus: a retrospective study. Contemp Clin Dent. 2013; 4(2):181–185

[135] Thornhill MH. Immune mechanisms in oral lichen planus. Acta Odontol Scand. 2001; 59(3):174–177

[136] van der Meij EH, Schepman KP, van der Waal I. The possible premalignant character of oral lichen planus and oral lichenoid lesions: a prospective study. Oral Surg Oral Med Oral Pathol Oral Radiol Endod. 2003; 96(2):164–171

[137] van der Waal I. Oral potentially malignant disorders: is malignant transformation predictable and preventable? Med Oral Patol Oral Cir Bucal. 2014; 19 (4):e386–e390

[138] Casparis S, Borm JM, Tektas S, et al. Oral lichen planus (OLP), oral lichenoid lesions (OLL), oral dysplasia, and oral cancer: retrospective analysis of clinicopathological data from 2002–2011. Oral Maxillofac Surg. 2015; 19(2): 149–156

[139] Rajentheran R, McLean NR, Kelly CG, Reed MF, Nolan A. Malignant transformation of oral lichen planus. Eur J Surg Oncol. 1999; 25(5):520–523

[140] Reichart PA, Philipsen HP. Oral erythroplakia: a review. Oral Oncol. 2005; 41 (6):551–561

[141] Mashberg A, Garfinkel L. Early diagnosis of oral cancer: the erythroplastic lesion in high risk sites. CA Cancer J Clin. 1978; 28(5):297–303

[142] Hassona Y, Scully C, Almangush A, Baqain Z, Sawair F. Oral potentially malignant disorders among dental patients: a pilot study in Jordan. Asian Pac J Cancer Prev. 2014; 15(23):10427–10431

[143] Chaturvedi P, Malik A, Nair D, et al. Oral squamous cell carcinoma associated with oral submucous fibrosis have better oncologic outcome than those without. Oral Surg Oral Med Oral Pathol Oral Radiol. 2017; 124(3):225–230

[144] Chourasia NR, Borle RM, Vastani A. Concomitant association of oral submucous fibrosis and oral squamous cell carcinoma and incidence of malignant transformation of oral submucous fibrosis in a population of Central India: a retrospective study. J Maxillofac Oral Surg. 2015; 14(4):902–906

[145] Brennan PA, Arakeri G. Oral submucous fibrosis-an increasing global healthcare problem. J Oral Pathol Med. 2017; 46(6):405

[146] Tekade SA, Chaudhary MS, Tekade SS, et al. Early stage oral submucous fibrosis is characterized by increased vascularity as opposed to advanced stages. J Clin Diagn Res. 2017; 11(5):ZC92–ZC96

[147] Rai V, Mukherjee R, Routray A, et al. Serum-based diagnostic prediction of oral submucous fibrosis using FTIR spectrometry. Spectrochim Acta A Mol Biomol Spectrosc. 2018; 189:322–329

[148] Speight PM, Khurram SA, Kujan O. Oral potentially malignant disorders: risk of progression to malignancy. Oral Surg Oral Med Oral Pathol Oral Radiol. 2018; 125(6):612–627

[149] Arakeri G, Patil SG, Aljabab AS, et al. Oral submucous fibrosis: an update on pathophysiology of malignant transformation. J Oral Pathol Med. 2017; 46 (6):413–417

[150] Tilakaratne WM, Klinikowski MF, Saku T, Peters TJ, Warnakulasuriya S. Oral submucous fibrosis: review on aetiology and pathogenesis. Oral Oncol. 2006; 42(6):561–568

[151] Bari S, Metgud R, Vyas Z, Tak A. An update on studies on etiological factors, disease progression, and malignant transformation in oral submucous fibrosis. J Cancer Res Ther. 2017; 13(3):399–405

[152] Gadbail AR, Chaudhary MS, Sarode SC, et al. Ki67, CD105, and a-SMA expressions better relate the binary oral epithelial dysplasia grading system of World Health Organization. J Oral Pathol Med. 2017; 46(10):921–927

[153] Rapidis AD, Gullane P, Langdon JD, Lefebvre JL, Scully C, Shah JP. Major advances in the knowledge and understanding of the epidemiology, aetiopathogenesis, diagnosis, management and prognosis of oral cancer. Oral Oncol. 2009; 45(4–5):299–300

[154] Epstein JB, Gorsky M, Fischer D, Gupta A, Epstein M, Elad S. A survey of the current approaches to diagnosis and management of oral premalignant lesions. J Am Dent Assoc. 2007; 138(12):1555–1562, quiz 1614

[155] Allegra E, Lombardo N, Puzzo L, Garozzo A. The usefulness of toluidine staining as a diagnostic tool for precancerous and cancerous oropharyngeal and oral cavity lesions. Acta Otorhinolaryngol Ital. 2009; 29(4):187–190

[156] Fedele S. Diagnostic aids in the screening of oral cancer. Head Neck Oncol. 2009; 1:5

[157] Mehrotra R, Singh M, Thomas S, et al. A cross-sectional study evaluating chemiluminescence and autofluorescence in the detection of clinically innocuous precancerous and cancerous oral lesions. J Am Dent Assoc. 2010; 141(2):151–156

[158] Giovannacci I, Vescovi P, Manfredi M, Meleti M. Non-invasive visual tools for diagnosis of oral cancer and dysplasia: a systematic review. Med Oral Patol Oral Cir Bucal. 2016; 21(3):e305–e315

[159] Mehrotra R, Gupta DK. Exciting new advances in oral cancer diagnosis: avenues to early detection. Head Neck Oncol. 2011; 3:33

[160] Laronde DM, Williams PM, Hislop TG, et al. Influence of fluorescence on screening decisions for oral mucosal lesions in community dental practices. J Oral Pathol Med. 2014; 43(1):7–13

[161] Güneri P, Epstein JB, Kaya A, Veral A, Kazandı A, Boyacioglu H. The utility of toluidine blue staining and brush cytology as adjuncts in clinical examination of suspicious oral mucosal lesions. Int J Oral Maxillofac Surg. 2011; 40 (2):155–161

[162] Trullenque-Eriksson A, Muñoz-Corcuera M, Campo-Trapero J, Cano-Sánchez J, Bascones-Martínez A. Analysis of new diagnostic methods in suspicious lesions of the oral mucosa. Med Oral Patol Oral Cir Bucal. 2009; 14(5):E210–E216

[163] Rethman MP, Carpenter W, Cohen EE, et al. American Dental Association Council on Scientific Affairs Expert Panel on Screening for Oral Squamous Cell Carcinomas. Evidence-based clinical recommendations regarding screening for oral squamous cell carcinomas. J Am Dent Assoc. 2010; 141(5):509–520

[164] Gupta A, Singh M, Ibrahim R, Mehrotra R. Utility of toluidine blue staining and brush biopsy in precancerous and cancerous oral lesions. Acta Cytol. 2007; 51(5):788–794

[165] Onofre MA, Sposto MR, Navarro CM. Reliability of toluidine blue application in the detection of oral epithelial dysplasia and in situ and invasive squamous cell carcinomas. Oral Surg Oral Med Oral Pathol Oral Radiol Endod. 2001; 91(5):535–540

[166] Ram S, Siar CH. Chemiluminescence as a diagnostic aid in the detection of oral cancer and potentially malignant epithelial lesions. Int J Oral Maxillofac Surg. 2005; 34(5):521–527

[167] Gandolfo S, Pentenero M, Broccoletti R, Pagano M, Carrozzo M, Scully C. Toluidine blue uptake in potentially malignant oral lesions in vivo: clinical and histological assessment. Oral Oncol. 2006; 42(1):89–95

[168] Hodgson DR, Foy CA, Partridge M, Pateromichelakis S, Gibson NJ. Development of a facile fluorescent assay for the detection of 80 mutations within the p53 gene. Mol Med. 2002; 8(5):227–237

[169] Oral Cancer Foundation. http://oralcancerfoundation.org. Accessed on September 23, 2011

[170] Mehrotra R, Mishra S, Singh M, Singh M. The efficacy of oral brush biopsy with computer-assisted analysis in identifying precancerous and cancerous lesions. Head Neck Oncol. 2011; 3:39

[171] Mehrotra R. The role of cytology in oral lesions: a review of recent improvements. Diagn Cytopathol. 2012; 40(1):73–83

[172] Sciubba JJ. Improving detection of precancerous and cancerous oral lesions. Computer-assisted analysis of the oral brush biopsy. U.S. Collaborative OralCDx Study Group. J Am Dent Assoc. 1999; 130(10):1445–1457

[173] Eisen D. The clinical features, malignant potential, and systemic associations of oral lichen planus: a study of 723 patients. J Am Acad Dermatol. 2002; 46 (2):207–214

[174] Frist S. The oral brush biopsy: separating fact from fiction. Oral Surg Oral Med Oral Pathol Oral Radiol Endod. 2003; 96(6):654–655

[175] Casparis S, Borm JM, Tomic MA, Burkhardt A, Locher MC. Transepithelial brush biopsy: oral CDx®—a noninvasive method for the early detection of precancerous and cancerous lesions. J Clin Diagn Res. 2014; 8(2):222–226

[176] Patton LL, Epstein JB, Kerr AR. Adjunctive techniques for oral cancer examination and lesion diagnosis: a systematic review of the literature. J Am Dent Assoc. 2008; 139(7):896–905, quiz 993–994

[177] Cancela-Rodríguez P, Cerero-Lapiedra R, Esparza-Gómez G, Llamas-Martínez S, Warnakulasuriya S. The use of toluidine blue in the detection of premalignant and malignant oral lesions. J Oral Pathol Med. 2011; 40(4):300–304

[178] Epstein JB, Feldman R, Dolor RJ, Porter SR. The utility of tolonium chloride rinse in the diagnosis of recurrent or second primary cancers in patients with prior upper aerodigestive tract cancer. Head Neck. 2003; 25(11):911–921

[179] Zhang L, Williams M, Poh CF, et al. Toluidine blue staining identifies high-risk primary oral premalignant lesions with poor outcome. Cancer Res. 2005; 65(17):8017–8021

[180] Kerawala CJ, Beale V, Reed M, Martin IC. The role of vital tissue staining in the marginal control of oral squamous cell carcinoma. Int J Oral Maxillofac Surg. 2000; 29(1):32–35

[181] Missmann M, Jank S, Laimer K, Gassner R. A reason for the use of toluidine blue staining in the presurgical management of patients with oral squamous cell carcinomas. Oral Surg Oral Med Oral Pathol Oral Radiol Endod. 2006; 102(6):741–743

[182] Siddiqui IA, Farooq MU, Siddiqui RA, Rafi SMT. Role of toluidine blue in early detection of oral cancer. Pak J Med Sci. 2006; 22:184–187

[183] Driemel O, Kunkel M, Hullmann M, et al. Diagnosis of oral squamous cell carcinoma and its precursor lesions. J Dtsch Dermatol Ges. 2007; 5(12):1095–1100

[184] Mashberg A. Final evaluation of tolonium chloride rinse for screening of high-risk patients with asymptomatic squamous carcinoma. J Am Dent Assoc. 1983; 106(3):319–323

[185] Mashberg A. Reevaluation of toluidine blue application as a diagnostic adjunct in the detection of asymptomatic oral squamous carcinoma: a continuing prospective study of oral cancer III. Cancer. 1980; 46(4): 758–763

[186] Silverman S, Jr, Migliorati C, Barbosa J. Toluidine blue staining in the detection of oral precancerous and malignant lesions. Oral Surg Oral Med Oral Pathol. 1984; 57(4):379–382

[187] Warnakulasuriya KA, Johnson NW. Sensitivity and specificity of OraScan (R) toluidine blue mouthrinse in the detection of oral cancer and precancer. J Oral Pathol Med. 1996; 25(3):97–103

[188] Epstein JB, Oakley C, Millner A, Emerton S, van der Meij E, Le N. The utility of toluidine blue application as a diagnostic aid in patients previously treated for upper oropharyngeal carcinoma. Oral Surg Oral Med Oral Pathol Oral Radiol Endod. 1997; 83(5):537–547

[189] Partridge M, Li SR, Pateromichelakis S, et al. Detection of minimal residual cancer to investigate why oral tumors recur despite seemingly adequate treatment. Clin Cancer Res. 2000; 6(7):2718–2725

[190] Epstein JB, Zhang L, Poh C, Nakamura H, Berean K, Rosin M. Increased allelic loss in toluidine blue-positive oral premalignant lesions. Oral Surg Oral Med Oral Pathol Oral Radiol Endod. 2003; 95(1):45–50

[191] Güneri P, Epstein JB. The need to reassess studies on detection of potentially premalignant and malignant oral lesions. Oral Oncol. 2010; 46(1):e2–e3

[192] Pavlova I, Williams M, El-Naggar A, Richards-Kortum R, Gillenwater A. Understanding the biological basis of autofluorescence imaging for oral cancer detection: high-resolution fluorescence microscopy in viable tissue. Clin Cancer Res. 2008; 14(8):2396–2404

[193] Schwarz RA, Gao W, Redden Weber C, et al. Noninvasive evaluation of oral lesions using depth-sensitive optical spectroscopy. Cancer. 2009; 115(8): 1669–1679

[194] Rashid A, Warnakulasuriya S. The use of light-based (optical) detection systems as adjuncts in the detection of oral cancer and oral potentially malignant disorders: a systematic review. J Oral Pathol Med. 2015; 44(5):307–328

[195] Seoane Lestón J, Diz Dios P. Diagnostic clinical aids in oral cancer. Oral Oncol. 2010; 46(6):418–422

[196] Poh CF, Zhang L, Anderson DW, et al. Fluorescence visualization detection of field alterations in tumor margins of oral cancer patients. Clin Cancer Res. 2006; 12(22):6716–6722

[197] Poh CF, Ng SP, Williams PM, et al. Direct fluorescence visualization of clinically occult high-risk oral premalignant disease using a simple hand-held device. Head Neck. 2007; 29(1):71–76

[198] Ujaoney S, Motwani MB, Degwekar S, et al. Evaluation of chemiluminescence, toluidine blue and histopathology for detection of high risk oral precancerous lesions: a cross-sectional study. BMC Clin Pathol. 2012; 12:6

[199] Huber MA, Bsoul SA, Terezhalmy GT. Acetic acid wash and chemiluminescent illumination as an adjunct to conventional oral soft tissue examination for the detection of dysplasia: a pilot study. Quintessence Int. 2004; 35(5): 378–384

[200] Epstein JB, Gorsky M, Lonky S, Silverman S, Jr, Epstein JD, Bride M. The efficacy of oral lumenoscopy (ViziLite) in visualizing oral mucosal lesions. Spec Care Dentist. 2006; 26(4):171–174

[201] Kerr AR, Sirois DA, Epstein JB. Clinical evaluation of chemiluminescent lighting: an adjunct for oral mucosal examinations. J Clin Dent. 2006; 17(3): 59–63

[202] Farah CS, McCullough MJ. A pilot case control study on the efficacy of acetic acid wash and chemiluminescent illumination (ViziLite) in the visualisation of oral mucosal white lesions. Oral Oncol. 2007; 43(8):820–824

[203] Oh ES, Laskin DM. Efficacy of the ViziLite system in the identification of oral lesions. J Oral Maxillofac Surg. 2007; 65(3):424–426

[204] McIntosh L, McCullough MJ, Farah CS. The assessment of diffused light illumination and acetic acid rinse (Microlux/DL) in the visualisation of oral mucosal lesions. Oral Oncol. 2009; 45(12):e227–e231

[205] Scheer M, Neugebauer J, Derman A, Fuss J, Drebber U, Zoeller JE. Autofluorescence imaging of potentially malignant mucosa lesions. Oral Surg Oral Med Oral Pathol Oral Radiol Endod. 2011; 111(5):568–577

[206] Awan KH, Morgan PR, Warnakulasuriya S. Evaluation of an autofluorescence based imaging system (VELscope™) in the detection of oral potentially malignant disorders and benign keratoses. Oral Oncol. 2011; 47(4):274–277

[207] Rana M, Zapf A, Kuehle M, Gellrich NC, Eckardt AM. Clinical evaluation of an autofluorescence diagnostic device for oral cancer detection: a prospective randomized diagnostic study. Eur J Cancer Prev. 2012; 21(5):460–466

[208] Balevi B. Assessing the usefulness of three adjunctive diagnostic devices for oral cancer screening: a probabilistic approach. Community Dent Oral Epidemiol. 2011; 39(2):171–176

[209] McNamara KK, Martin BD, Evans EW, Kalmar JR. The role of direct visual fluorescent examination (VELscope) in routine screening for potentially malignant oral mucosal lesions. Oral Surg Oral Med Oral Pathol Oral Radiol. 2012; 114(5):636–643

4 Management of Oral Premalignant Lesions

James J. Sciubba

Summary

Oral mucosal epithelial transformation through a series of genetic and structural changes is known to occur in several mucosal diseases, with these changes ultimately producing clinical phenotypic alterations ranging from purely erythematous, smooth lesions (erythroplakia) to predominantly white patterns, or a mixed pattern of each. Lesions with altered surface qualities where papillary to verrucous features are present, proliferative verrucous leukoplakia, offers behavioral differences marked by significantly elevated risk of carcinoma development versus typical leukoplakia. Additionally, the relatively more common immune driven condition, oral lichen planus, also possesses transformation behavior in a relatively small percentage of cases. Submucous fibrosis, a common condition geographically distributed over Southeast Asia and India, forms the basis of very large numbers of oral squamous carcinoma cases within this region. Recognition of these mucosal diseases clinically and characterized by tissue biopsy can allow intervention along with long-term posttreatment follow-up.

Keywords: transformation, biopsy, dysplasia, immune dysfunction

4.1 Introduction

Management of oral premalignant mucosal diseases (OPMDs) and conditions remains a clinical challenge. The goal for management of oral premalignant diseases is prevention of progression to invasive malignant disease. Possible approaches include reducing exposure to carcinogens ("environmental") or risk of progression among exposed individuals by means of employing medical, nonsurgical means to terminate or reverse carcinogenic events.[1] The spectrum of clinically encountered oral potentially malignant epithelial disorders, often without an obvious cause, represent, over time, a range of risk of becoming malignant. Progressive accrual of genetic alterations with recognized patterns and timing have been described along a biologic pathway to malignant transformation.[2]

4.2 Diagnosis

The first step in clinical management, of course, is identifying a clinical abnormality as premalignant with a properly performed mucosal biopsy with subsequent histopathologic evaluation as the recognized standard of care. Numerous adjunctive diagnostic techniques are available to clinicians; however, most of these modalities for clinical evaluation to date lack precision, are difficult to interpret, and do not allow prediction or anticipation of clinical behavior.[3] Thus, classic pathologic analysis must be considered the most accurate and predictable diagnostic modality, although submitted tissue specimens represent a single-spot analysis at a specific time point in what represents an evolutionary biologic process that may lead to true malignant transformation, with levels and degrees of epithelial dysplasia being the morphologic hallmarks of such an evolution in most cases.

4.3 Epidemiology

Conditions defined as potentially malignant, therefore having an increased risk of developing into squamous cell carcinoma, include leukoplakia, and a variant, proliferative verrucous leukoplakia (PVL), erythroplakia, combined leukoplakia–erythroplakia (erythtroleukoplakia or speckled leukoplakia), submucous fibrosis, oral lichen planus/oral lichenoid lesions, and possibly chronic candidiasis. The current World Health Organization (WHO) definition of leukoplakia is "a white plaque of questionable risk having excluded other (causes) known diseases or disorders that carry no increased risk for cancer," which will serve as the benchmark for this chapter.[4] Conditions that appear clinically abnormal such as frictionally induced or traumatic keratosis, surface keratosis secondary to a chronic biting habit (morsicatio), and acute candidiasis will thus, by definition, be excluded. The global prevalence of OPMDs has been reported to range from 1 to 5%.[5,6] Aside from erythroplakia, the overall risk of OPMDs evolving to squamous cell carcinoma is low, with the clinical problem being that of defining or characterizing which of the individually expressed lesions will progress to dysplasia and transform to invasive cancer. The estimated rate of malignant transformation ranges from 0.13 to 36.4% at a yearly rate of 1.36%.[7] The mechanisms of transformation from a benign state to one of premalignancy and finally invasive carcinoma involve a series of genetic alterations that are cumulative, but not always reversible. These gene-based alterations may be based on hereditary susceptibility, environmental factors, or random deoxyribonucleic acid (DNA) replication errors/mutations.[8]

4.3.1 Oral Premalignant Diseases

Premalignant oral mucosal disease is characterized by a biologically altered epithelium that is at risk for progression to squamous cell carcinoma that presents as several clinical phenotypes. Levels of risk for malignant transformation vary among members within this group of conditions, which include leukoplakia and its variant, PVL, erythroplakia, submucous fibrosis, and lichen planus. A more inclusive, useful but nonspecific, term, keratosis of unknown significance, includes cases that do not demonstrate reactive histologic features as well as absence of dysplasia, and thus will not be presented here.[9] Driving management considerations of OPMDs is the presence of and degree of oral epithelial dysplasia (OED), with most studies relating to leukoplakia. The spectrum of OED, regardless of which specific premalignant condition is being evaluated, is generally in keeping with the subjective grading criteria of the WHO according to which epithelial alterations range along a continuum from mild to moderate, severe, and carcinoma in situ.[10] As with pathology of the uterine cervix, useful parallels exist within this context as to the notion of intraepithelial neoplasia of the oral mucosa as well as the grading of such, although the OED grading schemes are less rigid.

The specific oral premalignant diseases discussed will include leukoplakia (idiopathic and tobacco related), the leukoplakia variant, proliferative leukoplakia, erythroplakia, submucous fibrosis, and oral lichen planus and oral lichenoid lesions. Each condition relates to variable degrees of risk in progressing to carcinoma with varying forms of management.

4.4 Management Considerations

4.4.1 Oral Leukoplakia

A broad spectrum of treatment philosophies and preferences has been published concerning the spectrum of oral mucosal conditions deemed premalignant, yet overall there is no single modality that has been studied in a carefully designed randomized clinical trial. The wide range of treatment options in the literature range from surgical to medical with widely disseminated studies analyzed in an evidence-based manner reporting limited evidence where active treatments offer no better results than placebo in reducing the risk of developing oral cancer.[11,12] Crucial in helping understand the entire concept of management of any oral premalignant disease is the presence or absence of epithelial dysplasia and the degree of dysplasia if present, based on biopsy analysis. The clinical relevance and importance of OED being present resides with understanding that a percentage of these lesions carry a risk of progression to invasive cancer with the risk of this progression ranging from 6 to 36%.[13] The transformation risk of oral leukoplakia ranges from 0.13 to 17.5% over a period ranging from 0.5 to 30 years.[14,15] What seems to be clear in most studies is the relationship between an increasingly greater risk of dysplasia transforming to invasive cancer as the degree of epithelial dysplasia increases. A reduction of risk to malignant transformation by surgical excision has been stated to be favored over active surveillance, with lesions not excised showing a significantly higher rate of transformation versus those instances where excision was accomplished.[16] Recent studies also have emphasized the role of active treatment in the form of wide local excision and/or laser ablation in substantially reducing or preventing recurrence of oral premalignant disease and cancer progression, including cases of mild epithelial dysplasia.[17,18]

Following establishment of a diagnosis of an oral mucosal premalignant disease or condition, management, and further risk reduction, the elimination of environmental carcinogens (tobacco and alcohol consumption) may be helpful, despite an absence of proven treatment approaches to confidently prevent the development of cancer within the context of treated epithelial dysplasia.[19] Management philosophies vary widely across a spectrum of treatment modalities ranging from habit and risk factor control to medical interventions, including chemoprevention and dietary considerations, surgical removal or ablation, close surveillance and observation, and more often a combination of these strategies. It seems clear, however, that the worst possible outcome for not treating this class of conditions simply allows worsening of the disease.

For leukoplakia with proven dysplasia present, the most common treatment or interventional modality is surgical excision, with many alternative treatments published. The most predictable results are achieved within the context of lesions that are localized, discrete, and show clinically evident margins. Mehanna and colleagues noted a significant reduction in the rate of malignant transformation of dysplastic leukoplakia treated surgically versus those not having surgery, though the risk for malignant transformation was not entirely eliminated.[16]

Alternative forms of surgery for treatment of oral premalignant lesions include laser ablation (CO_2, most commonly), with recurrence rates ranging widely from 3 to 41% and subsequent malignant transformation rates from 0 to 15%.[20] In the cases of homogeneous leukoplakia treated with CO_2 laser ablation, highest success rates were achieved with margins of 3- and 1-mm depth.[21] Unfortunately, little pooled data exist regarding predicting or documenting malignant transformation rates in higher risk leukoplakia types. Additionally, there is evidence regarding higher recurrence rates in the cases of multifocal dysplastic leukoplakia.[22]

PVL was defined as a specific form of leukoplakia in 1985 by Hansen and colleagues.[23] It is separated from typical oral leukoplakia by its more aggressive biologic profile with a high recurrence rate and high risk of transformation to invasive squamous cell carcinoma. It begins as a smooth homogeneous leukoplakia plaque that advances over a wider surface area to involve multiple sites, either as a contiguous process or as a discontinuous one, assuming a multifocal distribution. Of note, affected individuals often do not carry the same risk profile as those associated with oral leukoplakia and squamous cell carcinoma.[24] Additionally, the demographic profile of PVL versus typical oral leukoplakia differs in that nonsmokers and older women dominate in published series overall, with the pathologic qualities of PVL characterized by variation within each region ranging from benign hyperkeratosis to carcinoma, with other pathologic variations including verrucous hyperplasia, verrucous carcinoma, and, less frequently, verrucous carcinoma.[25]

Management options must consider the specific histopathologic features present. Often, multiple biopsies are generally performed, with an average of nine biopsies performed during the lifetime of a person with PVL.[26] The degree of dysplasia present will determine the level of management. Some treatments may relate to observation alone if dysplasia is absent, while premalignancy beyond mild dysplasia will require complete removal, by scalpel excision, laser ablation, photodynamic therapy, systemic retinoids, each with equivocal results, with surgical excision being the most commonly employed modality.[27] Some advocate the use of surgery combined with methisoprinol in the cases where papilloma virus was present in an effort to add an antiviral modality and an immunostimulant effect.[28] As recurrence and progression are very frequent, with 71% of patients recurring or progressing to carcinoma in the light of multiple treatment interventions, long-term vigilance and multiple biopsies over a lifetime are needed.

Prevention strategies, including chemoprevention, have included use of retinoids, antioxidants, cyclooxygenase-2 (COX-2) inhibitors, and vitamin A and derivatives, all without clear success in halting or reducing progression and malignant progression. Overall prognosis is poor given the recurrence rate and frequency of transformation to invasive carcinoma.[29]

4.4.2 Oral Lichen Planus

Oral lichen planus, a T-lymphocyte-mediated condition, and oral lichenoid lesions fall within the spectrum of oral premalignant diseases/conditions, with a generally considered range of malignant transformation from 0 to 3.5% of cases, with a greater rate consistently noted for oral lichenoid lesions at 3.2%, and that for all combined forms or subsets or variants of lichen planus being 1.09%.[30] A recent publication has suggested that oral cancer incidence rates in those with oral lichen planus/oral lichenoid lesions are underestimated because of the usual exclusionary criteria imposed as far as how carcinomas may arise in areas of the oral cavity beyond the immediate region where lichen planus/lichenoid lesions are present and where carcinogenic events are present.[31] Alterations of gene expression at the posttranscriptional level mediated in part by microRNA activity are considered, among the precarcinogenic events, critical.[32] Importantly, and as anticipated, an increased risk of transformation has been noted in those with risk factors, which include smoking, alcohol abuse, and hepatitis C infection.[33] Also to be considered is which form or subtype of oral lichen planus is present and the specific rate of malignant transformation associated with that form.[34] Some investigators emphasize the greater risk of malignant transformation relative to oral lichenoid lesions over more classic cases of oral lichen planus.[35]

While no specific treatment strategy exists to prevent dysplastic or neoplastic transformation of oral lichen planus, active treatment, in addition to eliminating risk behaviors, must be employed in addition to ongoing follow-up evaluations on a regular basis. Given the immune dysfunction as the initiating event, and subsequent inflammatory process, clinicians have employed a battery of approaches to address both aspects of this disease and associated symptoms. In the cases of biopsy-proven, minimally evident, lower risk reticular oral lichen planus, routine annual to semiannual observation is acceptable, with monitoring to assure either clearance or complete regression or transition to erosive and atrophic lesions, which have a higher risk of evolving to dysplastic transformation or carcinoma in a small percentage of cases, as noted above.

The mainstay of first-line active management has been the judicious use of corticosteroids in a topical and/or systemic fashion in the majority of cases, and to a lesser degree, intralesionally in focally unresponsive or recalcitrant instances. Commonly, the use of potent to ultrapotent corticosteroids in the form of clobetasol propionate or other less potent fluocinonide is employed. In the cases of severe disease or cases refractory to topical management, a short course of oral prednisone (0.5–1.0 mg/kg) for up to 6 weeks may be appropriate.[36] Steroid administration in the form of intraorally placed fluticasone spray has been used with effectiveness greater than betamethasone oral rinses.[37]

Nonsteroidal approaches are also helpful and efficacious and are often employed in instances where steroid treatment is contraindicated. Such steroid-sparing approaches in the cases of non-erosive diseases, which include the use of retinoic acid or isotretinoin gel, are an alternative. Nonsteroidal systemic immunosuppression in the form of methotrexate, azathioprine, or mycophenolate mofetil may be a consideration, as well as hydroxychloroquine and dapsone. Additionally, the use of topically applied calcineurin inhibitors, including tacrolimus and pimecrolimus, has been advocated in studies noting safety and efficacy in recalcitrant cases of erosive variant oral lichen planus.[38]

The recent introduction of superficial and higher energy types of treatment including low-level laser use has been noted with stated encouraging results.[39] Managing refractory cases of erosive-atrophic lesions has involved removal of lesions with the use of higher energy CO_2 laser treatment. In these instances, 10,600-nm continuous wave, 5-W energy levels in a slightly defocused fashion has been used, with over 75% of patients demonstrating variable degrees of improvement in clinical score.[40]

Additional nonpharmacologic approaches to management of oral lichen planus involve several recently published options including the use of photodynamic therapy. This technique involves administration of a photosensitizer or photosensitive agent, including a newly described chlorine 6–derived photosensitizer, Photolon, followed by use of a specific wave length excitatory light source.[41] Light exposure allows excitation of the photosensitizer, followed by generation of reactive oxygen species including singlet oxygen and free radicals. As a result, cell destruction follows by way of plasma membrane lysis and intracellular protein dysfunction and inactivation.[42] Superficial treatment in the form of irradiation ranging from 630 to 980 nm, 20 to 300 mW, and 10 seconds to 15 minutes has been effective in management of symptomatic oral lichen planus by attacking infiltrating lymphocytes.[43] An additional sensitizer in the form of methylene blue and a diode laser at 660-nm wavelength has shown superiority over topically placed corticosteroids with minimal side effects.[44]

4.4.3 Oral Submucous Fibrosis

Oral submucous fibrosis (OSMF) represents a well-recognized oral premalignant disorder with clustering of cases in India, Southern Asia, and Southeast Asia. A progressive and chronic course is characteristic with chiefly oral mucosal location, with a lesser degree of involvement of the pharynx and superior portion of the esophagus. Symptoms range from persistent burning of the oral mucosa, intolerance to spicy foods, and, most importantly, compromise of oral function and trismus. Etiologic factors chiefly involve use of and consumption of areca nut products including betel quid, pan masala, and gutka, with the major areca-derived components driving the premalignant behavior of OSMF being arecoline, alkaloids, and polyphenols, with a likely contributing relationship to a genetic predisposition in affected individuals, with little evidence to support development of OSMF in those without areca nut use.

Studies have revealed arecoline-reducing production of metalloproteinase inhibitors (TIMP-1). Increasing fibroblast contracture, reduced vascularity by way of reduction of endothelial cell proliferation, contributes to the pathogenesis, as do structural changes of collagen mediated by copper-dependent lysyl oxidase. Major fibrosis-inducing factors also include growth factors and inflammatory cytokines.[45]

Approaches to management include conservative medical treatment and surgical alternatives with possible prosthetic rehabilitation. If cessation of areca use precedes development of trismus, symptoms will often resolve. As with most oral premalignant conditions, there is no reliable evidence for the clinical efficacy of any specific management plan or protocol.

Medical management of OSMF beyond physical therapy is varied, with variable levels of effectiveness. More directed medical treatment modalities include modulation of inflammation and the immune process with steroids, interferon-γ, placental extracts, levamisole, colchicine, and, recently, administration of thioctic acid (alpha lipoic acid). The latter agent may reduce symptoms of OSMF by virtue of its stated antioxidant role and inhibition of free radical formation.[46] Use of pentoxifylline as a blood flow promoter, tissue oxygenation augmentation, and fibrinolysis promoter has been utilized with modest success. Beta-adrenergic agonists have shown promise as reversing fibrosis in OSMF.[47] Carotenoids, in particular lycopene, have been used in managing early-phase OSMF as have tea-derived pigments, vitamins, and zinc, as they help control the effects of copper-associated lysyl oxidase upregulation.[48] Fibrinolytic therapy, including the use of hyaluronidase, collagenase, and chymotrypsin, is also a treatment option in selected cases.[49]

Surgical management of OSMF in those with established fibrosis and trismus with reduction of interincisal opening less than 25 mm becomes a valid option. The goal of treatment is directed toward division of the fibrotic tissue with resurfacing of the surgical gap with a nasolabial flap or buccal fat pad.[50] A standard protocol independent of the extent of fibrosis includes appropriate imaging and biopsy confirmation of an absence of a malignant infiltrate possibly mimicking OSMF. Muscle release following incision of fibrous bands, followed by myotomy of masticatory muscles with possible coronoidectomy, is often employed, depending on the degree of oral opening following the release procedure. Additionally, for small and medium-sized defects of the buccal mucosa, a superiorly based platysma myocutaneous flap has been shown to be a valid surgical reconstructive alternative.[51] Following resurfacing of the surgical defect, postoperative physical therapy is mandatory, beginning 3 days postoperatively.[52]

4.4.4 Erythroplakia

As defined, erythroplakia represents a red, homogeneous, often velvety patch on the oral mucosa that cannot be accounted for by any other specific disease entity. Sites of predilection include the alveolar mucosa including the sulcus area, retromolar trigone region, and floor of the mouth. It is usually found in adults older than 50 years and is associated with a significantly higher risk of dysplasia or carcinoma at the time of the clinical diagnosis. In Shafer and Waldron's classic study of 58 cases of erythroplakia, 91%, at initial presentation, were biopsy proven to represent at least severe epithelial dysplasia, in situ carcinoma, or squamous carcinoma.[53] Management is complete excision subsequent to obtaining a tissue biopsy where a level of dysplasia is likely identified. Recurrence is common with mandatory careful periodic follow-up care.[54]

Key Points

- The goal of management of oral premalignant lesions is prevention of progression to malignant lesions, which is a potential outcome of their natural history.
- The gold standard for identification and categorization of premalignant lesion remains pathologic evaluation. Management is dependent on type of oral premalignant lesion.
- Management alternatives and approaches for typical oral leukoplakia vary widely with levels of dysplasia guiding the level and intensity of treatment.
- Risk reduction of dysplastic forms of leukoplakia evolving to invasive cancer by way of ablation or excision is favored over surveillance alone.
- PVL versus typical oral leukoplakia with noted differences in transformation risk to invasive cancer mandates a more aggressive approach to treatment.
- Oral lichen planus and oral lichenoid lesion management relates primarily to use of anti-inflammatory agents and monitoring in association with elimination of known risk factors.
- The medical and surgical treatment challenges posed by OSMF relative to malignant transformation and management in advance of malignant transformation are formidable with prevention a key strategy.

References

[1] Hong WK, Sporn MB. Recent advances in chemoprevention of cancer. Science. 1997; 278(5340):1073–1077

[2] Califano J, Westra WH, Meininger G, Corio R, Koch WM, Sidransky D. Genetic progression and clonal relationship of recurrent premalignant head and neck lesions. Clin Cancer Res. 2000; 6(2):347–352

[3] Huber MA. Adjunctive diagnostic techniques for oral and oropharyngeal cancer discovery. Dent Clin North Am. 2018; 62(1):59–75

[4] Warnakulasuriya S, Johnson NW, van der Waal I. Nomenclature and classification of potentially malignant disorders of the oral mucosa. J Oral Pathol Med. 2007; 36(10):575–580

[5] Petti S. Pooled estimate of world leukoplakia prevalence: a systematic review. Oral Oncol. 2003; 39(8):770–780

[6] Smith LW, Bhargava K, Mani NJ, Malaowalla AM, Silverman S, Jr. Oral cancer and precancerous lesions in 57,518 industrial workers of Gujarat, India. Indian J Cancer. 1975; 12(2):118–123

[7] Napier SS, Speight PM. Natural history of potentially malignant oral lesions and conditions: an overview of the literature. J Oral Pathol Med. 2008; 37(1): 1–10

[8] Tomasetti C, Li L, Vogelstein B. Stem cell divisions, somatic mutations, cancer etiology, and cancer prevention. Science. 2017; 355(6331):1330–1334

[9] Woo SB, Grammer RL, Lerman MA. Keratosis of unknown significance and leukoplakia: a preliminary study. Oral Surg Oral Med Oral Pathol Oral Radiol. 2014; 118(6):713–724

[10] Barnes L, Eveson J, Reichart P, Sidransky D, eds. World Health Organization of Classification of Tumours. Pathology and genetics of tumours of the head and neck. Lyon, France: IARC Press; 2005

[11] Lodi G, Franchini R, Warnakulasuriya S, et al. Interventions for treating oral leukoplakia to prevent oral cancer. Cochrane Database Syst Rev. 2016; 7: CD0901829

[12] Warnakulasuriya S, Ariyawardana A. Malignant transformation of oral leukoplakia: a systematic review of observational studies. J Oral Pathol Med. 2016; 45(3):155–166

[13] Reibel J. Prognosis of oral pre-malignant lesions: significance of clinical, histopathological, and molecular biological characteristics. Crit Rev Oral Biol Med. 2003; 14:47–62

[14] Silverman S, Jr, Gorsky M, Lozada F. Oral leukoplakia and malignant transformation. A follow-up study of 257 patients. Cancer. 1984; 53(3): 563–568

[15] Schepman KP, van der Meij EH, Smeele LE, van der Waal I. Malignant transformation of oral leukoplakia: a follow-up study of a hospital-based population of 166 patients with oral leukoplakia from The Netherlands. Oral Oncol. 1998; 34(4):270–275

[16] Mehanna HM, Rattay T, Smith J, McConkey CC. Treatment and follow-up of oral dysplasia: a systematic review and meta-analysis. Head Neck. 2009; 31 (12):1600–1609

[17] Zhang L, Lubpairee T, Laronde DM, Rosin MP. Should severe epithelial dysplasia be treated? Oral Oncol. 2016; 60:125–129

[18] Arnaoutakis D, Bishop J, Westra W, Califano JA. Recurrence patterns and management of oral cavity premalignant lesions. Oral Oncol. 2013; 49(8): 814–817

[19] Field EA, McCarthy CE, Ho MW, et al. The management of oral epithelial dysplasia: the Liverpool algorithm. Oral Oncol. 2015; 51(10):883–887

[20] Mogedas-Vegara A, Hueto-Madrid JA, Chimenos-Küstner E, Bescós-Atín C. Oral leukoplakia treatment with the carbon dioxide laser: A systematic review of the literature. J Craniomaxillofac Surg. 2016; 44(4):331–336

[21] Nammour S, Zeinoun T, Namour A, Vanheusden A, Vescovi P. Evaluation of different laser-supported protocols for the treatment of oral leukoplakia: a long-term follow-up. Photomed Laser Surg. 2017; 35(11):629–638

[22] Yang SW, Tsai CN, Lee YS, Chen TA. Treatment outcome of dysplastic oral leukoplakia with carbon dioxide laser: emphasis on the factors affecting recurrence. J Oral Maxillofac Surg. 2011; 69(6):e78–e87

[23] Hansen LS, Olson JA, Silverman S, Jr. Proliferative verrucous leukoplakia. A long-term study of thirty patients. Oral Surg Oral Med Oral Pathol. 1985; 60 (3):285–298

[24] Onofre MA, Sposto MR, Navarro CM, Motta ME, Turatti E, Almeida RT. Potentially malignant epithelial oral lesions: discrepancies between clinical and histological diagnosis. Oral Dis. 1997; 3(3):148–152

[25] Sciubba JJ, Helman JI. Current management strategies for verrucous hyperkeratosis and verrucous carcinoma. Oral Maxillofac Surg Clin North Am. 2013; 25(1):77–82, vi

[26] Abadie WM, Partington EJ, Fowler CB, Schmalbach CE. Optimal management of proliferative verrucous leukoplakia: a systematic review of the literature. Otolaryngol Head Neck Surg. 2015; 153(4):504–511

[27] Poveda-Roda R, Bagan JV, Jiménez-Soriano Y, Díaz-Fernández JM, Gavaldá-Esteve C. Retinoids and proliferative verrucous leukoplakia (PVL). A preliminary study. Med Oral Patol Oral Cir Bucal. 2010; 15(1):e3–e9

[28] Femiano F, Gombos F, Scully C. Oral proliferative verrucous leukoplakia (PVL); open trial of surgery compared with combined therapy using surgery and methisoprinol in papillomavirus-related PVL. Int J Oral Maxillofac Surg. 2001; 30(4):318–322

[29] Munde A, Karle R. Proliferative verrucous leukoplakia: an update. J Cancer Res Ther. 2016; 12(2):469–473

[30] Fitzpatrick SG, Hirsch SA, Gordon SC. The malignant transformation of oral lichen planus and oral lichenoid lesions: a systematic review. J Am Dent Assoc. 2014; 145(1):45–56

[31] Gonzalez-Moles MA, Gil-Montoya JA, Ruiz-Avila I, Bravo M. Is oral cancer incidence among patients with oral lichen planus/oral lichenoid lesions underestimated? J Oral Pathol Med. 2017; 46(2):148–153

[32] Aghbari SMH, Gaafar SM, Shaker OG, Ashiry SE, Zayed SO. Evaluating the accuracy of microRNA27b and microRNA137 as biomarkers of activity and potential malignant transformation in oral lichen planus patients. Arch Dermatol Res. 2018; 310(3):209–220

[33] Aghbari SMH, Abushouk AI, Attia A, et al. Malignant transformation of oral lichen planus and oral lichenoid lesions: A meta-analysis of 20095 patient data. Oral Oncol. 2017; 68:92–102

[34] Eisen D. The clinical features, malignant potential, and systemic associations of oral lichen planus: a study of 723 patients. J Am Acad Dermatol. 2002; 46 (2):207–214

[35] Reed SG. Oral lichenoid lesions and not oral lichen planus have the character for malignant transformation to oral squamous cell carcinoma. J Evid Based Dent Pract. 2008; 8(4):238–239

[36] Voûte AB, Schulten EA, Langendijk PN, Kostense PJ, van der Waal I. Fluocinonide in an adhesive base for treatment of oral lichen planus. A double-blind, placebo-controlled clinical study. Oral Surg Oral Med Oral Pathol. 1993; 75 (2):181–185

[37] Hegarty AM, Hodgson TA, Lewsey JD, Porter SR. Fluticasone propionate spray and betamethasone sodium phosphate mouthrinse: a randomized crossover study for the treatment of symptomatic oral lichen planus. J Am Acad Dermatol. 2002; 47(2):271–279

[38] Eisen D, Carrozzo M, Bagan Sebastian JV, Thongprasom K. Number V Oral lichen planus: clinical features and management. Oral Dis. 2005; 11(6): 338–349

[39] Al-Maweri SA, Kalakonda B, Al-Soneidar WA, Al-Shamiri HM, Alakhali MS, Alaizari N. Efficacy of low-level laser therapy in management of symptomatic oral lichen planus: a systematic review. Lasers Med Sci. 2017; 32(6):1429–1437

[40] Pakfetrat A, Falaki F, Ahrari F, Bidad S. Removal of refractory erosive-atrophic lichen planus by the CO2 laser. Oral Health Dent Manag. 2014; 13(3):595–599

[41] Sobaniec S, Bernaczyk P, Pietruski J, et al. Clinical assessment of the efficacy of photodynamic therapy in the treatment of oral lichen planus. Lasers Med Sci. 2013; 28(1):311–316

[42] Trehan M, Taylor CR. Low-dose excimer 308-nm laser for the treatment of oral lichen planus. Arch Dermatol. 2004; 140(4):415–420

[43] Mostafa D, Tarakji B. Photodynamic therapy in treatment of oral lichen planus. J Clin Med Res. 2015; 7(6):393–399

[44] Mostafa D, Moussa E, Alnouaem M. Evaluation of photodynamic therapy in treatment of oral erosive lichen planus in comparison with topically applied corticosteroids. Photodiagn Photodyn Ther. 2017; 19:56–66

[45] Tilakaratne WM, Ekanayaka RP, Warnakulasuriya S. Oral submucous fibrosis: a historical perspective and a review on etiology and pathogenesis. Oral Surg Oral Med Oral Pathol Oral Radiol. 2016; 122(2):178–191

[46] Bhandarkar GP, Shetty KV, Kulkarni K. Thioctic acid in oral submucous fibrosis (India's disease): a better tomorrow. J Stomatol Oral Maxillofac Surg. 2018; 119(2):129–134

[47] Sharma JK, Gupta AK, Mukhija RD, Nigam P. Clinical experience with the use of peripheral vasodilator in oral disorders. Int J Oral Maxillofac Surg. 1987; 16 (6):695–699

[48] Warnakulasuriya S, Kerr AR. Oral submucous fibrosis: a review of the current management and possible directions for novel therapies. Oral Surg Oral Med Oral Pathol Oral Radiol. 2016; 122(2):232–241

[49] Chole RH, Gondivkar SM, Gadbail AR, et al. Review of drug treatment of oral submucous fibrosis. Oral Oncol. 2012; 48(5):393–398

[50] Arakeri G, Brennan PA. Oral submucous fibrosis: an overview of the aetiology, pathogenesis, classification, and principles of management. Br J Oral Maxillofac Surg. 2013; 51(7):587–593

[51] Bande C, Joshi A, Gawande M, et al. Utility of superiorly based platysma myocutaneous flap for reconstruction of intraoral surgical defects: our experience. Oral Maxillofac Surg. 2018; 22(1):45–51

[52] Arakeri G, Rai KK, Boraks G, et al. Current protocols in the management of oral submucous fibrosis: an update. J Oral Pathol Med. 2017; 46(6):418–423

[53] Shafer WG, Waldron CA. Erythroplakia of the oral cavity. Cancer. 1975; 36(3): 1021–1028

[54] Sciubba J, Scully C. Oral leukoplakia. BMJ Best Practice. Available at: http://bestpractice.bmj.com/bestpractice/monograph/621/highlights/summary.html

Section III

Diagnostic Evaluation of Oral Cavity Cancers

5 Evaluation and Staging for Cancers of the Oral Cavity

Erik Interval, William Lydiatt, and Aru Panwar

Summary
High-quality care for patients with oral cavity cancer requires comprehensive evaluation by a health care team experienced in the management of complex head and neck cancers. Assignment of disease stage must accurately reflect prognosis, guide management strategies, and allow comparison of like populations. The eighth edition of the American Joint Committee on Cancer (AJCC) staging system introduces major changes that incorporate emerging evidence in support of the prognostic value of depth of invasion of the primary lesion, and extranodal extension (ENE) in the setting of involved lymph nodes. Additionally, it clarifies the anatomical boundaries of the oral cavity for the purposes of stage assignment. This chapter highlights the key issues related to initial evaluation of patients affected by oral cavity carcinoma, and describes the hallmark changes introduced in the revised staging scheme for such malignancies.

Keywords: oral cavity, staging, prognosis, depth of invasion, extranodal extension

5.1 Introduction

Accurate and reproducible staging information is a critical component of high-quality care for patients diagnosed with malignant neoplasms. In addition to providing information on prognosis and guidelines for management for individual patients, the stage assignment provides consistency in describing disease burden across care settings, and allows comparison of patient outcomes between centers and across time periods. Moreover, cataloguing of data on a well-defined and established set of rules permits evolution in understanding the disease process over time. The first American Joint Committee on Cancer (AJCC) cancer staging manual was published in 1977 to accomplish these goals. Since then, the manual has been updated at regular intervals to incorporate new data and better reflect the contemporary population and the prevalent understanding of malignant diseases.

The AJCC staging system for malignancies of the oral cavity utilizes the Tumor, Node, Metastasis (TNM) staging system, which was first described by Denoix in 1952,[1] and relies on anatomic extent of involvement with malignant disease. While this remains an accurate predictor of disease behavior, there has been recognition that other biologic factors may have a substantial role as well. The eighth edition of the AJCC Cancer Staging Manual, effective January 1, 2018, incorporates phenotypic variables that represent adverse biology and clinical behavior, such as ENE in involved lymph nodes and depth of invasion (DOI) at the primary site, in cancers of the oral cavity. While incorporating these important variables, the staging system aims to balance accuracy, ease of use, and universal applicability in settings with variable availability of resources. This chapter highlights the key changes in the eighth edition of the AJCC Cancer Staging Manual for malignancies of the oral cavity and the rationale in support of these changes.

5.2 Overview of Changes in the Eighth Edition of the AJCC Staging Manual

AJCC Cancer Staging System is revamped at regular intervals. Frequency of revisions must strike a balance between reflecting current data and staying relevant to current clinical practices, and the burdens experienced by physicians, patients, cancer registries, and the health care systems on account of introduction of new staging parameters. Presently, the staging systems are updated once every 7 or 8 years.

The eighth edition significantly updates the staging information for cancers of the oral cavity by incorporating depth of primary tumor invasion. Previously, extrinsic tongue muscular involvement served as the surrogate marker for DOI, and was the standard that contributed to assignment of more advanced T classification. However, pathologists and clinicians struggled with how best to capture this feature, resulting in inconsistent data collection. The more reproducible standard of DOI has been incorporated based on a growing body of data supporting its importance.[2–4] ENE has been added to the N classification to reflect the negative impact of this finding on prognosis and recurrence.[2–4] Another important change is reflected in the definition of the staging boundaries of the oral cavity. These changes will be discussed in detail in the following sections.

5.3 Anatomic Considerations for Cancers of the Oral Cavity

A clear definition of anatomical confines is a prerequisite for accurately choosing the correct staging system and stage assignment when evaluating patients with a newly diagnosed malignancy. Malignant tumors are staged according to the site of their origin. In circumstances where the tumor extends to adjacent sites, the clinician must determine the epicenter of the neoplasm based on clinical examination, imaging studies, and sometimes molecular markers, in order to use the appropriate staging scheme. For example, squamous cell carcinoma (SCC) centered on the inner mucosa of the lower lip that has minor extension onto the cutaneous surface of the lip should be classified using the staging system for oral cavity, and not cutaneous SCC. Conversely, a lesion that is at the vermilion border and predominantly on the dry mucosa of the lower lip should be staged using the cutaneous staging system (Chapter 14 of the eighth edition of the AJCC Cancer Staging Manual).

Importantly, the definition of the anterior staging boundary of the oral cavity has been revised with the eighth edition of the AJCC staging manual. Previously, the vermilion border defined the line of demarcation between oral cavity and cutaneous structures. Under the old schema, tumors of the dry portion of the vermilion lip would have been classified as lip

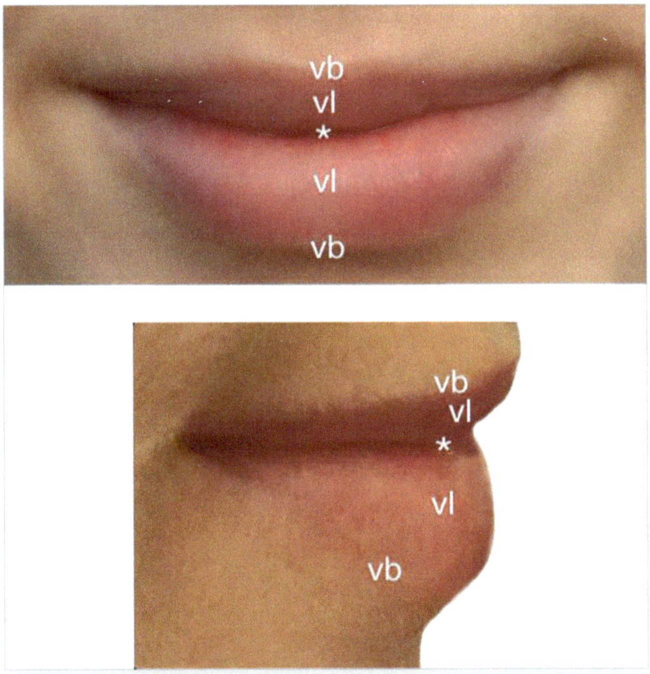

Fig. 5.1 Diagram of boundaries of the lip, as defined in the AJCC Staging Manual, eighth edition. The staging and anatomic boundaries of the oral cavity are now distinct. The vermilion border remains the anatomic boundary of the oral cavity. However, for staging purposes, the contact point of the lips, which separates the wet from the dry vermilion lip, is now defined as the staging boundary of the oral cavity. Malignancies arising anterior to this junction are staged according to the cutaneous malignancy chapter, and those arising posterior to this junction are staged according to the oral cavity chapter. (vb, vermilion border [anatomic boundary of oral cavity]; vl, vermilion lip; *, contact point of lips [*staging* boundary of oral cavity]).

tumors. However, the anterior boundary of the oral cavity has now been clarified as the location where the lips contact one another[2] (▶ Fig. 5.1). Any malignancy arising anterior to this wet–dry junction, even if it is located on the vermilion lip (red lip), should be classified as a cutaneous malignancy. Likewise, any malignancy arising from the wet lip, posterior to the wet–dry junction, should be classified as an oral cavity malignancy. This reclassification recognizes that tumors originating anterior to the contact point of the lips, even if they arise from the dry vermilion lip, share a common etiology with, and behave in a similar fashion to, cutaneous malignancies.

The posterior boundary of the oral cavity is located at its interface with the oropharynx. Superiorly, this is defined by the junction of the hard palate and the soft palate. Laterally, this is defined as the anterior faucial pillar. Inferiorly, the circumvallate papillae separate the oral tongue from the base of tongue (oropharyngeal tongue). This distinction now holds greater meaning, as oropharyngeal tumors may have a distinct etiology and biologic behavior with the rise of human papillomavirus (HPV) associated SCC in this region.

The most common location of regional nodal metastases from the oral cavity is to level I, II, and III cervical lymph node basins. Lungs are the most likely site of distant metastases, although bone, liver, and other soft-tissue sites may also be involved.

5.4 Evaluation

Workup of patients with known or suspected oral cavity malignancies should include a detailed history, physical examination, biopsy of primary or metastatic lesions, cross-sectional imaging studies, and an examination under anesthesia, as indicated.

Since the oral cavity can harbor a host of benign, premalignant, and malignant entities, clinicians should consider a wide differential when evaluating a patient with an oral lesion. While a full discussion on benign diseases of the oral cavity is beyond the scope of this book, details pertaining to premalignant lesions of the oral cavity are provided in Chapters 3 and 4.

5.4.1 History and Physical Examination

Clinicians should elucidate the duration of the lesion, its rate of growth, history of similar lesions in the past, associated lymphadenopathy, and symptoms associated with the presentation to hone the differential diagnosis. Patients may report symptoms such as ulceration, pain, foul breath, bleeding, dental loss, difficulty with chewing or swallowing, or symptoms suggestive of sensory, motor, and cranial nerve deficits. Concurrent oral health issues relevant to the workup of an oral cavity lesion include erosive lichen planus, history of recurrent aphthous stomatitis, Fanconi's anemia, history of radiation, and a history of any prior head and neck malignancies.

Clinicians should consider the patient's social history and role of the known risk factors for oral cavity malignancies, including smoking or chewing tobacco, alcohol use, betel nut chewing, and history of erosive lichen planus.[5,6] When applicable, the use of tobacco and alcohol should be quantified by pack-years and numbers of drinking days per week with number of drinks per day, respectively. A quit date, if present, should also be recorded.

Medical comorbidities should also be discussed, both in order to treat the patient as a whole and also to determine potential impact of baseline health on surgical risk, treatment options, and the survivorship experience. Medical conditions and their contribution to frailty is recognized as important risk factor for head and neck surgical patients.[7,8] Frailty can be estimated by a number of measures. The Modified Frailty Index is a measure of frailty that assesses 11 clinical variables and is represented as a score signifying degree of frailty. Another measure, the Johns Hopkins Frailty Index measures frailty as the presence of any one of a number of frailty-defining diagnoses,[7] grouped into 10 clusters, including malnutrition, dementia, severe vision impairment, decubitus ulcer, incontinence of urine, loss of weight, fecal incontinence, social support needs, difficulty in walking, and fall risk. While several other methods of measuring frailty have been tested, and validated, irrespective of the preferred tool, clinicians should consider frailty as an indicator of decline in physiologic reserve, which should be included as a key variable when formulating individualized treatment plans. Similarly, the presence of depression, anxiety, and other behavioral health issues or antidepressant use should be noted. The role of counseling and prophylactic use of antidepressants in reducing the incidence of major depression and their favorable impact on quality of life, especially in patients who require radiation therapy as part of their treatment, should be discussed and initiated when appropriate.[9,10]

A focused, yet detailed, head and neck examination should be performed. The primary tumor should be inspected carefully, paying attention to the boundaries of the tumor with respect to anatomical subsites. The dimensions of the tumor should be measured in centimeters and clearly recorded. When possible, clinical images may be added to the patient's medical record to facilitate objective record keeping of disease extent and collaboration with multiple specialties caring for the patient. The revised staging system makes it important to determine the tumor's DOI in millimeters. It is important to distinguish DOI from "tumor thickness," since DOI signifies the depth of tumor invasion into deep tissue and not the exophytic or heaped component of the tumor above the basement membrane. This distinction is discussed further below. It is readily acknowledged that exact determination of DOI may be clinically challenging, and may be further impacted by patient variables such as pain or trismus. However, clinicians should use their best clinical judgment in making a determination if the DOI for a particular oral malignant lesion is "thin" (≤ 5 mm), "intermediate" (> 5 mm but ≤ 10 mm), or "thick" (> 10 mm). In cases of clinical uncertainty, the staging rules and convention call for assigning the lower category when assessing DOI.

The examination of the neck should include inspection and careful palpation. Any suspicious or enlarged lymph nodes should be evaluated for number, size, location, consistency, fixation to surrounding tissues, and overlying skin changes. A comprehensive cranial nerve examination, including, but not limited to, the lingual nerve, the inferior alveolar nerve, and the hypoglossal nerve, should be performed. Involvement of cranial nerves carries important staging, and therefore prognostic information, as neck node involvement of these structures increases the clinical N category to 3b.

Flexible fiberoptic nasopharyngolaryngoscopy may be utilized to evaluate the airway, to evaluate the base of the tongue, and to examine for the presence of possible synchronous, second primary malignancies.

5.4.2 Imaging Studies

Imaging studies should be utilized in select patients to evaluate the primary tumor, the status of the cervical lymph nodes, and, when appropriate, to evaluate for the presence of distant metastases.

It is important to note that imaging is not indicated for superficial, localized T1–T2 oral lesions, with no clinical lymphadenopathy. For lesions involving the alveolar ridge, which are not mobile over the bone, a dental panoramic radiograph, dental plain films, or computed tomography (CT) of the mandible may further clarify concerns over bone involvement. Contrast-enhanced CT scan or magnetic resonance imaging (MRI) may assist the evaluation of the primary lesion by providing additional information on tumor depth, and its relationship to adjoining structures, including the mandible, maxilla, skull base, major vascular structures, neural foramina, and, in the case of MRI, cranial nerves. Reliable assessment of the primary lesion may be hobbled in some cases due to its small size or superficial nature, and proximity to dental restorations, which may distort image quality.

Imaging of the neck may be indicated when there is clinical suspicion for regional lymph node involvement, need for assessment of regional anatomy for surgical planning, and when clinical examination fails to provide information that may inform management choices. Ultrasonography can be particularly useful in characterizing cervical lymph nodes. When available in the office, clinician-performed ultrasound can provide critical and complementary information about regional nodal status and facilitate guided aspiration of target lesions when indicated. In the presence of pathologic nodes, cross-sectional imaging such as contrast-enhanced CT scan or MRI may help determine the size and number of nodes and help determine extent of surgery. While ENE may be suggested by imaging studies, radiological findings alone are not sufficient to satisfy the high bar set for clinical determination of ENE for staging purposes, and requires corroborating findings on clinical examination as described earlier in this chapter.

It is important to note that no imaging modality is sensitive enough to rule out the presence of occult cervical metastasis,[11] though CT scan may be more sensitive than MRI.[12] Therefore, when the risk of occult cervical metastasis is greater than 15 to 20%,[13] elective neck dissection is generally indicated.[14–16] Management of the neck nodes in oral malignancies is discussed further in Chapter 32 .

To evaluate for distant metastases, cross-sectional imaging of the chest is warranted in patients with three or more clinically positive lymph nodes, low jugular lymph nodes, bilateral lymph nodes, lymph nodes sized ≥ 6 cm, locoregional recurrence, and second primary tumors.[17,18] Localized (T1–T2, N0) oral cavity malignancies generally do not warrant cross-sectional imaging of the chest.[19]

In some instances, imaging studies may reveal the presence of a single pulmonary nodule.[20] The presence of an incidentally discovered pulmonary nodule during workup warrants further evaluation and characterization with appropriately chosen radiographic modalities and a directed biopsy when indicated. Differential diagnoses including benign and malignant entities must be considered, before determining if the finding of the pulmonary nodule would in fact influence the management of the oral cavity malignancy. In a single-institution retrospective study of 148 consecutive patients with newly diagnosed head and neck cancer (not limited to the oral cavity), 73 (49.3%) of the patients had an abnormal chest scan on initial workup. Of these patients, 45 (61.7%) ultimately were identified to have intrathoracic lesions that were benign, 22 (30.1%) malignant, and 6 (8.2%) indeterminate.[21] Of nodules that were ultimately proved malignant, only three were initially characterized as benign. Multidisciplinary care teams must consider the appearance and number of such lesions, findings from previous imaging studies, risk factors for primary or metastatic pulmonary neoplasm, goals of care, and other patient factors when deciding on management for patients who present with pulmonary lesions discovered during the workup of an oral cavity malignancy.

Studies have compared the diagnostic accuracy of chest CT scan to positron emission tomography with CT (PET-CT) in evaluating for distant pulmonary metastases. Brouwer et al, based on several retrospective series, suggested that PET-CT may have a higher sensitivity for pulmonary metastases.[22,23] This was studied prospectively in a multi-institutional study of 145 consecutive patients who underwent both chest CT scan and PET-CT.[24] Distant metastases were identified in 19 patients

(21%). Notably, the combination of chest CT scan with PET-CT was more accurate than either modality alone in the detection of distant metastases (positive predictive value, 86%; negative predictive value, 84%). Clinicians should consider patient care priorities and institutional protocols when choosing the appropriate imaging modality to assess for distant metastases.

5.4.3 Laboratory Evaluation

No specific laboratory evaluations are required for the workup of the oral cavity cancer patient. Elevated liver function tests secondary to liver metastases are a late finding and are not recommended for routine metastatic workup.[17] Preoperative thyroid function tests, complete blood count, basic metabolic panel, nutritional lab values, and coagulation studies may be considered but are not required for staging.

5.4.4 Preoperative Evaluation

For patients undergoing surgery, preoperative evaluation should be obtained. Depending on the patient's comorbidities and cardiac status, consultations with the patient's primary care physician, the anesthesiology team, and other collaborative specialists should be obtained as indicated. A full discussion on preoperative workup is beyond the scope of this chapter, and the reader is encouraged to read the latest guidelines for preoperative evaluation of patients undergoing noncardiac surgery.

5.5 Staging

The oral cavity staging system may be used for evaluation and staging of oral malignancies including SCC and its variants, and minor salivary gland malignancies.[2] As discussed earlier, the current staging paradigm utilizes the primary tumor, regional lymph nodes, and distant metastasis (TNM) categorization. These categories will be discussed in turn.

Notably, the staging schemas detailed below are only applicable to oral SCC and minor salivary gland malignancies. A comprehensive list of tumors that are staged according to this chapter is found in the AJCC staging manual, eighth edition,[2] and is not reproduced here. However, the following malignancies are not staged with these schemas: nonepithelial tumors of lymphoid tissue (i.e., lymphoma), nonepithelial tumors of soft tissue (including sarcomas), nonepithelial tumors of bone and cartilage, mucosal melanoma, and cutaneous SCC of the vermilion lip. A full discussion of these malignancies is beyond the scope of this chapter, but may be found elsewhere in this book (Section VII: Management of Nonsquamous Cell Cancers of the Oral Cavity).

5.5.1 Categorization of the Primary Tumor (T Category)

The categorization of the primary tumor in the eighth edition of the AJCC Cancer Staging Manual is primarily based on the size of primary tumor and DOI.[2] Additionally, anatomic extent of primary tumor is used to signify moderately advanced local disease (T4a) or very advanced local disease (T4b). The schema for T categorization is described below and summarized in ▸ Table 5.1.

Table 5.1 T categorization for oral cavity cancer[2,47]

T category	Criteria
Tx	Primary tumor cannot be assessed
Tis	Carcinoma in situ
T1	Tumor ≤ 2 cm, DOI ≤ 5 mm
T2	Tumor ≤ 2 cm, DOI > 5 mm or tumor > 2 cm but ≤ 4 cm, and DOI ≤ 10 mm
T3	Tumor > 2 cm and ≤ 4 cm with DOI > 10 mm or tumor > 4 cm with DOI ≤ 10 mm
T4	Moderately advanced or very advanced local disease
T4a	Moderately advanced local disease Tumor > 4 cm with DOI > 10 mm Tumor invades adjacent structures only (e.g., through cortical bone of the mandible or maxilla, or involves the maxillary sinus or skin of the face) Note: superficial erosion of bone/tooth socket (alone) by a gingival primary is not sufficient to classify a tumor as T4
T4b	Very advanced local disease Tumor invades masticator space, pterygoid plates, or skull base and/or encases the internal carotid artery

Abbreviation: DOI, depth of invasion (distinct from tumor thickness).

The descriptions of T4a and T4b categories have changed little from the Seventh Edition of the AJCC Cancer Staging Manual. One exception is that the "deep/extrinsic tongue muscle involvement" criterion that previously signified moderately advanced primary tumors (T4a), but proved to be an inconsistent and difficult-to-use metric, has been removed from the current staging scheme.

These key changes in assignment of T categories are detailed below.

Description and Rationale for Use of DOI in Staging Schema

The definition of T categories in staging of oral cavity malignancies had not been revised since early iterations of the system in 1970s. Kreppel et al showed that the current staging system is a poor predictor,[25] and updates were needed to incorporate emerging evidence regarding role of depth of tumor invasion.

Data suggest that DOI is an independent negative prognosticator for oral tongue cancers.[15,26–29] To clarify the issue, Ebrahimi et al retrospectively analyzed 3,149 surgically treated oral cavity patients from 11 institutions.[30] DOI was independently associated with disease-specific survival, even when controlling for pT category, pN category, decade of treatment, adjuvant radiation therapy, and other variables. A refined T categorization scheme was then developed, compared to the T categorization in the Seventh Edition of the AJCC Cancer Staging System, and to other proposed staging systems.[29,31] These data analyses were utilized in designing the new T categorization, as an amalgamation of the previous T categorization (primarily based on size) and DOI, and emphasize that both the horizontal and vertical dimensions of the tumor augur prognosis.

It is important to note that the terms "depth of invasion" and "tumor thickness" are not synonymous. DOI refers to the distance a tumor has invaded as measured from the basement

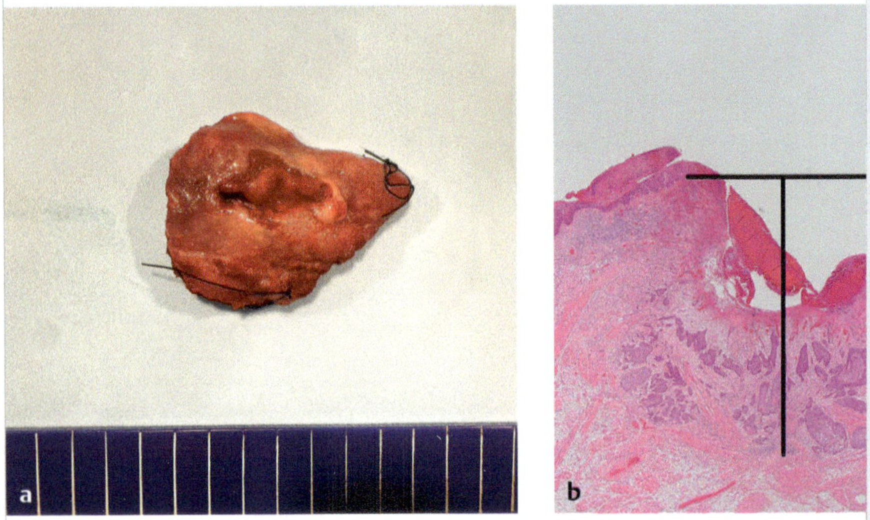

Fig. 5.2 Image of depth of invasion as compared to tumor thickness, for oral cavity malignancies. **(a)** Gross picture of surgical resection specimen of an ulcerated oral tongue squamous cell carcinoma. **(b)** Photomicrograph of surgically excised oral squamous cell carcinoma (hematoxylin and eosin stain, 4x). The transverse line indicates the basement membrane and the vertically oriented line identifies the plumb line (perpendicular to the horizon marked by the basement membrane) and extends to the invasive front of the malignancy in the deep soft tissue, thus measuring the depth of invasion. Depth of invasion does not include the exophytic component of the malignancy, or components above the horizon marked by the adjacent basement membrane. (These images are provided courtesy of Dr. John Gentry, MD and Dr. Shane Kohl, MD, Department of Pathology, Nebraska Methodist Hospital, Omaha, Nebraska.)

membrane to the deepest point tangent to the basement membrane (▶ Fig. 5.2). For example, an exophytic tumor may have a significantly larger tumor thickness than DOI, while an ulcerated tumor may actually have a larger DOI than its measured thickness. DOI more accurately predicts nodal involvement and prognosis than tumor thickness, although both are predictive, likely since it better reflects proximity of the tumor to the lymphatics and vasculature below.[26]

DOI should be clinically estimated at the time of initial examination. This clinical estimation should be noted into the record and utilized for clinical T classification. As previously discussed, when the determination of DOI is clinically challenging, clinicians should use their best judgment and determine if the DOI for a particular oral malignant lesion is "thin" (likely ≤ 5 mm), "intermediate" (> 5 mm but ≤ 10 mm), or "thick" (> 10 mm; ▶ Table 5.1).

Bone Involvement and T Categorization

As noted in ▶ Table 5.1, the presence of invasion of tumor through cortical bone automatically qualifies as a T4 tumor. The use of bone invasion as an independent prognosticator in oral SCCs is controversial, with some studies showing no effect, with others suggesting a significant impact on prognosis.[32–38] However, the disparity may result from differences in methodology; studies that specifically analyzed medullary (i.e., beyond cortical) invasion showed worse prognosis with bone invasion.[30,39,40] For this reason, the invasion must be through cortical bone (i.e., into the spongiosa/medullary cavity) rather than just into cortical bone in order to qualify for an increase in T categorization. This qualification, updated in the seventh edition of the AJCC Cancer Staging manual, has been retained in the eighth edition.

Other Locally Invasive Factors

Besides invasion through the cortical bone, other locally invasive factors may play an important role in prognosis, and therefore, in staging. Extension of invasive disease into specific adjacent soft tissue, skin, and neurovascular structures indicates a more advanced T category and worse prognosis. Therefore, it is important for the clinician to precisely evaluate for and document such findings, if present. For example, for patients affected by malignancies of the lip, invasions of the floor of the mouth, the inferior alveolar nerve, or the skin of the face indicate T4a disease. In such cases, assessment of sensation in the inferior alveolar/mental nerve distribution is significant. For other oral cavity cancers, involvement of the inferior alveolar nerve, though not specifically included as a criterion for T4a classification, should raise suspicion for invasion through the cortical bone of the mandible.

Very advanced local disease (▶ Table 5.1) is defined by involvement of the masticator space, the pterygoid plates, the skull base, and/or the internal carotid artery. These factors not only are poor prognostic signs, but also make meaningful surgical resection difficult, if not impossible. Presence of trismus should alert the clinician to the possibility of involvement of the pterygoid plates. However, trismus is not a specific sign, and may be pain related for some patients, suggesting involvement of the muscles of mastication rather than the actual pterygoid plates. Regardless, caution should be exercised in administering anesthesia to patients with trismus, as this can complicate endotracheal intubation, and require surgical airway management.

5.5.2 Categorization of the Cervical Lymph Nodes (N Category)

Involvement of the lymph nodes is one of the most important prognostic signs in oral cavity cancer. The nodal categorization of tumors has been updated in several ways for the eighth edition of the AJCC Cancer Staging Manual. First, the pathologic and clinical N categorizations are now distinct; second, ENE, formerly termed extracapsular extension, is now incorporated into the N categorization schema. ENE has been shown to portend a worse prognosis, independent of other variables,[41–43] and this is now reflected in the categorization scheme (▶ Table 5.2 and ▶ Table 5.3).[2,3] Incorporation of ENE into the new N categorization was validated using oral cavity patients in

Table 5.2 Clinical nodal categorization for oral cavity cancer (cN)[2]

N category	Criteria
Nx	Regional lymph nodes cannot be assessed
N0	No regional lymph node metastasis
N1	Metastasis in a single ipsilateral lymph node, ≤ 3 cm and ENE (–)
N2	Metastasis in a single ipsilateral lymph node > 3 cm but ≤ 6 cm in greatest dimension and ENE (–); *or* metastases in multiple ipsilateral lymph nodes, ≤ 6 cm in greatest dimension and ENE (–); *or* in bilateral or contralateral lymph nodes, ≤ 6 cm in greatest dimension, and ENE (–)
N2a	Metastasis in a single ipsilateral lymph node > 3 cm but ≤ 6 cm in greatest dimension and ENE (–)
N2b	Metastases in multiple ipsilateral lymph nodes, ≤ 6 cm in greatest dimension and ENE (–)
N2c	Metastases in bilateral or contralateral lymph nodes, ≤ 6 cm in greatest dimension and ENE (–)
N3	Metastasis in a lymph node larger than 6 cm in greatest dimension and ENE (–); *or* metastasis in any lymph node(s) with clinically overt ENE (+)
N3a	Metastasis in a lymph node > 6 cm in greatest dimension and ENE (–)
N3b	Metastasis in any lymph node(s) with clinically overt ENE (+)

Abbreviation: ENE, extra nodal extension

the National Cancer Database (NCDB) from 2010 to 2011 and tested against a dataset of patients from two institutions,[3] suggesting improved hazard discrimination and prognostication when ENE was incorporated into the N categorization scheme.

Therefore, all patients with oral cancer and associated lymphadenopathy must be evaluated for the presence or absence of ENE. Clinical assessment of ENE is primarily performed by physical examination.[3] The presence of a fixed node, involvement of a nearby nerve, or infiltration into neighboring muscle, soft tissue, or skin suggests ENE and automatically categorizes the mass as cN3b (▶ Table 5.2). Imaging studies may supplement clinical findings; for example, metastatic lymph nodes may be seen to invade adjacent skin, muscle, or vascular structures (▶ Fig. 5.3). However, importantly, imaging evidence alone is not sufficient to call clinical ENE without the associated clinical findings discussed earlier.[44,45]

The revised oral cavity cancer staging schema creates a novel system of pathologic lymph node categorization, which is distinct from the clinical categorization (▶ Table 5.3). In patients who undergo lymphadenectomy as part of their management, the pathologic information supersedes clinical information in assigning N categorization (▶ Table 5.3). For example, the presence of clinical ENE is classified as cN3b, while the presence of pathologic ENE may be classified as pN2a or pN3b, depending on the nodal size (▶ Table 5.3). The remainder of the N categorization is largely unchanged from the seventh edition of the AJCC Cancer Staging System and involves a combination of variables including node number (single or multiple positive lymph nodes), size (≤ 3 cm, or > 3 cm but ≤ 6 cm, or > 6 cm), and location (ipsilateral, contralateral, or bilateral).

To be classified as pathologic ENE, strict requirements must be met. The eighth edition of the AJCC Cancer Staging Manual

Table 5.3 Pathologic nodal categorization for oral cavity cancer (pN)[2,47]

N category	Criteria
Nx	Regional lymph nodes cannot be assessed
N0	No regional lymph node metastasis
N1	Metastasis in a single ipsilateral lymph node, ≤ 3 cm in greatest dimension and ENE (–)
N2	Metastasis in a single ipsilateral lymph node, ≤ 3 cm in greatest dimension and ENE (+); *or* > 3 cm but ≤ 6 cm in greatest dimension and ENE (–); *or* metastases in multiple ipsilateral lymph node(s), ≤ 6 cm in greatest dimension and ENE (–); *or* in bilateral or contralateral lymph nodes, ≤ 6 cm in greatest dimension, ENE (–)
N2a	Metastasis in single ipsilateral node ≤ 3 cm in greatest dimension and ENE (+); *or* a single ipsilateral node > 3 cm but ≤ 6 cm in greatest dimension and ENE (–)
N2b	Metastasis in multiple ipsilateral nodes, ≤ 6 cm in greatest dimension and ENE (–)
N2c	Metastasis in bilateral or contralateral lymph node (s), ≤ 6 cm in greatest dimension and ENE (–)
N3	Metastasis in a lymph node > 6 cm in greatest dimension and ENE (–); *or* metastasis in a single ipsilateral node > 3 cm in greatest dimension and ENE (+); *or* multiple ipsilateral, contralateral, or bilateral nodes, any with ENE (+) *or* a single contralateral node of any size and ENE (+)
N3a	Metastasis in a lymph node > 6 cm in greatest dimension and ENE (–)
N3b	Metastasis in a single ipsilateral node > 3 cm in greatest dimension and ENE (+); *or* multiple ipsilateral, contralateral, or bilateral nodes, any with ENE (+) *or* a single contralateral node of any size and ENE (+)

Abbreviation: ENE, extra nodal extension.

defines ENE as extension of metastatic carcinoma through the fibrous capsule into the surrounding connective tissue.[2] The presence or absence of a stromal reaction is not taken into consideration. Additionally, the extent of ENE should be noted as ≤ 2 mm or greater than 2 mm. However, any pathological ENE mandates the ENE + notation and thus affects the ultimate N category.

5.5.3 Categorization of Distant Metastases (M Category)

The presence of any distant metastases classifies a tumor as M1. Common locations for metastatic disease from the oral cavity include the lung (66%), bone (22%), and liver (10%).[17,46] The staging manual notes that metastases to level VII (superior mediastinal) lymph nodes, superior to the innominate artery, are not classified as distant metastases.

5.5.4 Other Prognostic Variables

Beside the conventional TNM parameters utilized in staging, and therefore prognosis, the collection of other variables, listed

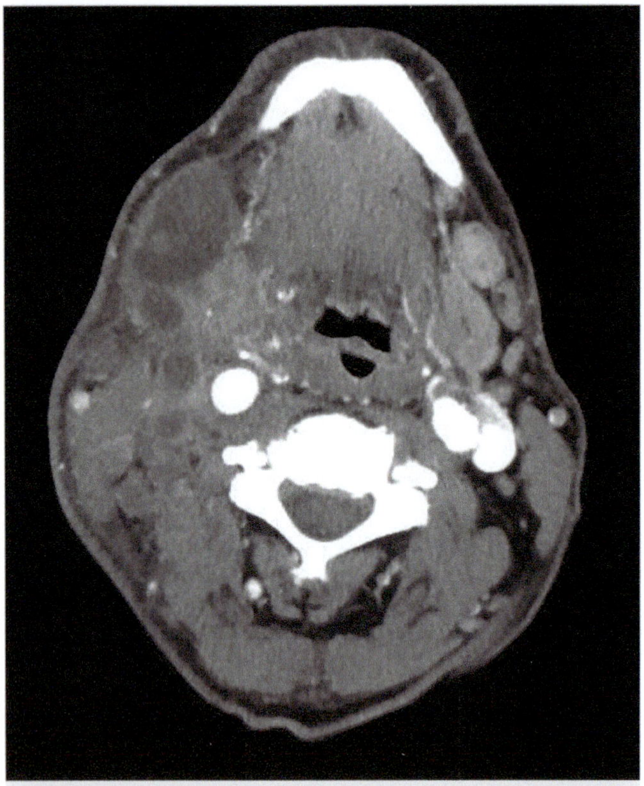

Fig. 5.3 Contrast-enhanced CT imaging (axial view) showing multiple enlarged cervical lymph nodes with peripheral enhancement and central necrosis and indistinct borders with likely ENE (extranodal extension). However, clinical designation of ENE cannot be determined by imaging findings alone, and requires congruent examination findings that demonstrate node fixation, or infiltration of neighboring skin, soft tissues, and/or neurovascular structures.

below, is recommended. These are variables that may influence prognosis and may be incorporated into future staging systems. The eighth edition of the AJCC Cancer Staging Manual recommends collecting information on comorbidities, performance status, tobacco abuse (in pack-years), alcohol abuse (quantified), nutrition status (weight loss of > 10% over 3 months), and depression.[10]

5.6 Conclusion

Patients affected by oral cavity carcinoma should undergo a comprehensive evaluation by health care teams experienced in management of head and neck malignancies. Management strategies may be determined not only by the nature and stage of disease but also by the baseline nutrition, frailty, and morbidity profile of the patient.

The eighth edition of the AJCC Cancer Staging System introduces major changes in the T and N category designations (▸ Table 5.4). It recognizes DOI of the primary lesion and ENE in case of involved lymph nodes as important indicators of T and N class, respectively. The new system allows distinct clinical and pathologic N classification schema. The new staging system is intended to provide improved hazard consistency, discrimination, and predictive ability for prognostication for patients

Table 5.4 AJCC (eighth edition) prognostic stage groups for oral cavity cancers[2,47]

T category	N category	M category	Stage group
Tis	N0	M0	0
T1	N0	M0	I
T2	N0	M0	II
T3	N0	M0	III
T0, T1, T2, T3	N1	M0	III
T4a	N0, N1	M0	IVA
T0, T1, T2, T3, T4a	N2	M0	IVA
Any T	N3	M0	IVB
T4b	Any N	M0	IVB
Any T	Any N	M1	IVC

Abbreviation: AJCC, American Joint Committee on Cancer.

undergoing management of oral cavity carcinoma. Additional variables such as tobacco and alcohol use, frailty status, nutritional parameters, evidence of depression, and others that have clinical implications should be recorded for possible inclusion in future revisions of the staging system.[47]

Key Points

- The eighth edition of the AJCC Cancer Staging System introduces major changes in the anatomical definition and staging of oral cavity cancers to enhance prognostication and better characterize the disease.
- Cancers originating at the contact surface between upper and lower lips, and those of the wet lip are classified as oral cavity cancers. However, cancers of the dry vermilion lip should be evaluated and staged based on skin cancer guidelines.
- In addition to size and tumor extent, T classification for oral cavity cancer utilizes DOI to assign T category and prognosis.
- DOI is distinct from tumor thickness (see text for details).
- Invasion of extrinsic tongue muscle is no longer used as a criterion for assigning T category.
- ENE is a key determinant of prognosis and contributes to determination of both cN and pN categories.
- Distinct clinical and pathologic N category schemas have been created.
- Determination of cENE (+) status is based on clinically unequivocal evidence of node fixation, invasion of skin, soft tissue, or neurovascular structures. Imaging studies by themselves are not sufficient in calling ENE, but may supplement clinical findings.
- Any evidence of ENE on pathologic examination should be recorded and its extent noted. All pENE increases the pN category.

References

[1] Denoix PF. Nomenclature classification des cancer. Bull Inst Natl Hyg. 1952; 7:743–748

[2] Ridge JA, Lydiatt WM, Patel SG, Ghossein RA, Shah JP. Lip and oral cavity. In: Amin MB, Edge SB, Greene FL, et al., eds. AJCC Cancer Staging Manual. 8th ed. New York, NY: Springer; 2017

[3] Lydiatt WM, Patel SG, O'Sullivan B, et al. Head and neck cancers—major changes in the American Joint Committee on Cancer Eighth Edition Cancer Staging Manual. CA Cancer J Clin. 2017; 67:122–137

[4] Huang SH, O'Sullivan B. Overview of the 8th Edition TNM Classification for Head and Neck Cancer. Curr Treat Options Oncol. 2017; 18(7):40

[5] Winn DM, Lee YC, Hashibe M, Boffetta P, INHANCE consortium. The INHANCE consortium: toward a better understanding of the causes and mechanisms of head and neck cancer. Oral Dis. 2015; 21(6):685–693

[6] Warnakulasuriya S, Kovacevic T, Madden P, et al. Factors predicting malignant transformation in oral potentially malignant disorders among patients accrued over a 10-year period in South East England. J Oral Pathol Med. 2011; 40(9):677–683

[7] Nieman CL, Pitman KT, Tufaro AP, Eisele DW, Frick KD, Gourin CG. The effect of frailty on short-term outcomes after head and neck cancer surgery. Laryngoscope. 2018; 128(1):102–110

[8] Wachal B, Johnson M, Burchell A, et al. Association of modified frailty index score with perioperative risk for patients undergoing total laryngectomy. JAMA Otolaryngol Head Neck Surg. 2017; 143(8):818–823

[9] Lydiatt WM, Denman D, McNeilly DP, Puumula SE, Burke WJA. A randomized, placebo-controlled trial of citalopram for the prevention of major depression during treatment for head and neck cancer. Arch Otolaryngol Head Neck Surg. 2008; 134(5):528–535

[10] Lydiatt WM, Bessette D, Schmid KK, Sayles H, Burke WJ. Prevention of depression with escitalopram in patients undergoing treatment for head and neck cancer: randomized, double-blind, placebo-controlled clinical trial. JAMA Otolaryngol Head Neck Surg. 2013; 139(7):678–686

[11] van den Brekel MW, van der Waal I, Meijer CJ, Freeman JL, Castelijns JA, Snow GB. The incidence of micrometastases in neck dissection specimens obtained from elective neck dissections. Laryngoscope. 1996; 106(8):987–991

[12] Curtin HD, Ishwaran H, Mancuso AA, Dalley RW, Caudry DJ, McNeil BJ. Comparison of CT and MR imaging in staging of neck metastases. Radiology. 1998; 207(1):123–130

[13] Weiss MH, Harrison LB, Isaacs RS. Use of decision analysis in planning a management strategy for the stage N0 neck. Arch Otolaryngol Head Neck Surg. 1994; 120(7):699–702

[14] D'Cruz AK, Vaish R, Kapre N, et al. Head and Neck Disease Management Group. Elective versus therapeutic neck dissection in node-negative oral cancer. N Engl J Med. 2015; 373(6):521–529

[15] Pentenero M, Gandolfo S, Carrozzo M. Importance of tumor thickness and depth of invasion in nodal involvement and prognosis of oral squamous cell carcinoma: a review of the literature. Head Neck. 2005; 27(12):1080–1091

[16] Lin MJ, Guiney A, Iseli CE, Buchanan M, Iseli TA. Prophylactic neck dissection in early oral tongue squamous cell carcinoma 2.1 to 4.0 mm depth. Otolaryngol Head Neck Surg. 2011; 144(4):542–548

[17] de Bree R, Deurloo EE, Snow GB, Leemans CR. Screening for distant metastases in patients with head and neck cancer. Laryngoscope. 2000; 110(3, Pt 1): 397–401

[18] Leemans CR, Tiwari R, Nauta JJ, van der Waal I, Snow GB. Regional lymph node involvement and its significance in the development of distant metastases in head and neck carcinoma. Cancer. 1993; 71(2):452–456

[19] Bisase B, Kerawala C, Lee J. The role of computed tomography of the chest in the staging of early squamous cell carcinoma of the tongue. Br J Oral Maxillofac Surg. 2008; 46(5):367–369

[20] Sercarz J, Ellison D, Holmes EC, Calcaterra TC. Isolated pulmonary nodules in head and neck cancer patients. Ann Otol Rhinol Laryngol. 1989; 98(2):113–118

[21] Zammit-Maempel I, Kurien R, Paleri V. Outcomes of synchronous pulmonary nodules detected on computed tomography in head and neck cancer patients: 12-year retrospective review of a consecutive cohort. J Laryngol Otol. 2016; 130(6):575–580

[22] Brouwer J, de Bree R, Hoekstra OS, et al. Screening for distant metastases in patients with head and neck cancer: is chest computed tomography sufficient? Laryngoscope. 2005; 115(10):1813–1817

[23] Brouwer J, Senft A, de Bree R, et al. Screening for distant metastases in patients with head and neck cancer: is there a role for (18)FDG-PET? Oral Oncol. 2006; 42(3):275–280

[24] Senft A, de Bree R, Hoekstra OS, et al. Screening for distant metastases in head and neck cancer patients by chest CT or whole body FDG-PET: a prospective multicenter trial. Radiother Oncol. 2008; 87(2):221–229

[25] Kreppel M, Drebber U, Rothamel D, et al. Prognostic impact of different TNM-based stage groupings for oral squamous cell carcinoma. Head Neck. 2011; 33 (10):1467–1475

[26] Tan WJ, Chia CS, Tan HK, Soo K-C, Iyer NG. Prognostic significance of invasion depth in oral tongue squamous cell carcinoma. ORL J Otorhinolaryngol Relat Spec. 2012; 74(5):264–270

[27] Ling W, Mijiti A, Moming A. Survival pattern and prognostic factors of patients with squamous cell carcinoma of the tongue: a retrospective analysis of 210 cases. J Oral Maxillofac Surg. 2013; 71(4):775–785

[28] Moore C, Kuhns JG, Greenberg RA. Thickness as prognostic aid in upper aerodigestive tract cancer. Arch Surg. 1986; 121(12):1410–1414

[29] Yuen APW, Lam KY, Wei WI, et al. A comparison of the prognostic significance of tumor diameter, length, width, thickness, area, volume, and clinicopathological features of oral tongue carcinoma. Am J Surg. 2000; 180 (2):139–143

[30] Ebrahimi A, Gil Z, Amit M, et al. International Consortium for Outcome Research (ICOR) in Head and Neck Cancer. Primary tumor staging for oral cancer and a proposed modification incorporating depth of invasion: an international multicenter retrospective study. JAMA Otolaryngol Head Neck Surg. 2014; 140(12):1138–1148

[31] Howaldt HP, Kainz M, Euler B, Vorast H. Proposal for modification of the TNM staging classification for cancer of the oral cavity. DOSAK. J Craniomaxillofac Surg. 1999; 27(5):275–288

[32] Soo KC, Spiro RH, King W, Harvey W, Strong EW. Squamous carcinoma of the gums. Am J Surg. 1988; 156(4):281–285

[33] Overholt SM, Eicher SA, Wolf P, Weber RS. Prognostic factors affecting outcome in lower gingival carcinoma. Laryngoscope. 1996; 106(11):1335–1339

[34] Ash CS, Nason RW, Abdoh AA, Cohen MA. Prognostic implications of mandibular invasion in oral cancer. Head Neck. 2000; 22(8):794–798

[35] O'Brien CJ, Adams JR, McNeil EB, et al. Influence of bone invasion and extent of mandibular resection on local control of cancers of the oral cavity and oropharynx. Int J Oral Maxillofac Surg. 2003; 32(5):492–497

[36] Muñoz Guerra MF, Naval Gías L, Campo FR, Pérez JS. Marginal and segmental mandibulectomy in patients with oral cancer: a statistical analysis of 106 cases. J Oral Maxillofac Surg. 2003; 61(11):1289–1296

[37] Patel RS, Dirven R, Clark JR, Swinson BD, Gao K, O'Brien CJ. The prognostic impact of extent of bone invasion and extent of bone resection in oral carcinoma. Laryngoscope. 2008; 118(5):780–785

[38] Mücke T, Hölzle F, Wagenpfeil S, Wolff K-D, Kesting M. The role of tumor invasion into the mandible of oral squamous cell carcinoma. J Cancer Res Clin Oncol. 2011; 137(1):165–171

[39] Fives C, Nae A, Roche P, et al. Impact of mandibular invasion on prognosis in oral squamous cell carcinoma four centimeters or less in size. Laryngoscope. 2017; 127(4):849–854

[40] Fried D, Mullins B, Weissler M, et al. Prognostic significance of bone invasion for oral cavity squamous cell carcinoma considered T1/T2 by American joint committee on cancer size criteria. Head Neck. 2014; 36(6):776–781

[41] Wreesmann VB, Katabi N, Palmer FL, et al. Influence of extracapsular nodal spread extent on prognosis of oral squamous cell carcinoma. Head Neck. 2016; 38 Suppl 1:E1192–E1199

[42] Myers J, Greenberg J, Mo V, Roberts D. Extracapsular spread: a significant predictor of treatment failure in patients with squamous cell carcinoma of the tongue. Cancer. 2001; 92 12:3030–3036

[43] de Juan J, García J, López M, et al. Inclusion of extracapsular spread in the pTNM classification system: a proposal for patients with head and neck carcinoma. JAMA Otolaryngol Head Neck Surg. 2013; 139(5):483–488

[44] Chai RL, Rath TJ, Johnson JT, et al. Accuracy of computed tomography in the prediction of extracapsular spread of lymph node metastases in squamous cell carcinoma of the head and neck. JAMA Otolaryngol Head Neck Surg. 2013; 139(11):1187–1194

[45] Prabhu RS, Magliocca KR, Hanasoge S, et al. Accuracy of computed tomography for predicting pathologic nodal extracapsular extension in patients with head-and-neck cancer undergoing initial surgical resection. Int J Radiat Oncol Biol Phys. 2014; 88(1):122–129

[46] Ferlito A, Shaha AR, Silver CE, Rinaldo A, Mondin V. Incidence and sites of distant metastases from head and neck cancer. ORL. 2001; 63(4):202–207

[47] Lydiatt WM, Head and Neck Section of the American Joint Committee on Cancer. Personal Communication. April 14, 2018

6 Photographic Documentation of the Oral Cavity

James H. Clark

Summary

Since the genesis of photography in the early 19th century, the application of this technology was swiftly recognized and embraced by the medical community. This chapter will address the role of photography in the management of oral pathology and address pitfalls and potential limitations faced when documenting the oral cavity utilizing a photographic approach.

Keywords: documentation, photographic, oral cavity

6.1 Introduction

Since the mid-1940s, photography has been described, predominantly dental and dermatologic, for documentation of lesions within the oral cavity.[1,2,3] Photography provides clinicians with a tool that can aid in medical consultation, documentation, and education.[2] The clinical use of photographs may reduce the need for verbose and potentially time-consuming description of the oral cavity. A picture can also help reduce inter- and intraobserver variation in descriptions.

The oral cavity, however, poses a multitude of challenges for photographers, including restricted space, limited light, and variability of both depth and planes. Attempts have been made to address these technical challenges by using light-field digital (LFD) cameras (also known as plenoptic cameras). Unlike the standard digital modality, LFD cameras capture data in regard to color, intensity, and the direction of light vector entering the camera. Using these data, offline software can then reconstruct a two-dimensional picture with the ability for the viewer to focus on different areas of interest within the picture after the image has been captured.[4] The need, however, for specialized equipment, associated expense, and comparative low resolution have limited the use of this technology for oral photodocumentation. Therefore, the focus of this chapter will be the usage of conventional digital photography and how to optimize image quality of the oral cavity.

6.2 Camera and Equipment

When taking pictures of the oral cavity, there are two features that are essential for it to be useful: first, sufficient resolution to record both soft- and hard-tissue details and, second, true color representation.[5]

The amount of detail seen on a picture is dependent on resolution, which is measured in pixels. A pixel refers to the smallest unit point within a digital picture that can be displayed and represented on a digital display. The pixels come together to make up the image. As such, the greater the number of pixels, the greater the amount of detail and the higher the resolution of the resulting picture. One megapixel (MP) corresponds to 1,216 × 912 pixels. There has been extensive discussion in the dermatology literature regarding the ideal photographic resolution required, with suggested values ranging from 0.4 to 1.3 MP.[6] This range falls well within the capacity of most new cameras currently available on the market, which typically have picture resolution starting at 3 MP.[6]

Picture resolution is, however, not the only factor determining the quality of an image; the capacity of lens and camera are also of equal importance. Poor lens quality or incorrect camera shutter speed, despite high-resolution capacity, will result in decreased quality as color and tissue texture can be lost.

Given these considerations, the choice of camera should therefore be determined by the need of the clinician, practicality of use, and cost, while also considering basic camera features such as adequate lens quality, shutter speed, and optimizing resolution. When making this investment, it is also important to remember that the images produced not only will serve as baseline for follow-up but are also part of the permanent medical-legal record, and therefore needs to be documented with precision.[5]

6.2.1 Digital Single-Lens Reflex Camera

Camera

Digital Single-Lens Reflex (DSLR) camera systems are considered the gold standard in dental photography.[7] A DSLR system is made up by the camera, lens, and flash system (see ▶ Fig. 6.1). There are two types of DSLR cameras available, with variable costs: semiprofessional and professional. The latter has additional features, the cost of which may not be justified for clinical use.[5] DSLR cameras tend to be modular, which allows the user to exchange the lens or flash system depending on the photographic needs.

Lens

Telephoto zoom lenses (TZL) are the most commonly used lenses for DSLR as they provide the user with an adjustable focal point. This allows the photographer to zoom in and provides closer framing of the object of interested without the shooter physically having to adjust where they are taking the photograph from.

Prime lens (PL) is a type of lens that has a fixed focal length. As a result, a user has to adjust the location from which he or she plans to take the picture (or use a prime lens with a different focal length) to ensure the object of interest is in focus and well framed. Traditionally, PL have been associated with increased picture quality and faster aperture.[8] The drawback, however, is the need to carry multiple lenses with different focal length, which is both cumbersome and expensive.

Macro Lenses (ML) are a fixed focal length lens designed to take pictures very up close and provides the photographer with images that are life size. The characteristics of ML are ideal for oral cavity photography, making ML popular among dentists. Review of the dental literature reveals a preference for an ML with a 100- or 105-mm focal length, which allows approximately 4- to 4.5-inch standoff.[7] An otolaryngologist—head and neck surgeon who uses a camera in both the clinic and the operating room, situations that require images to be taken from

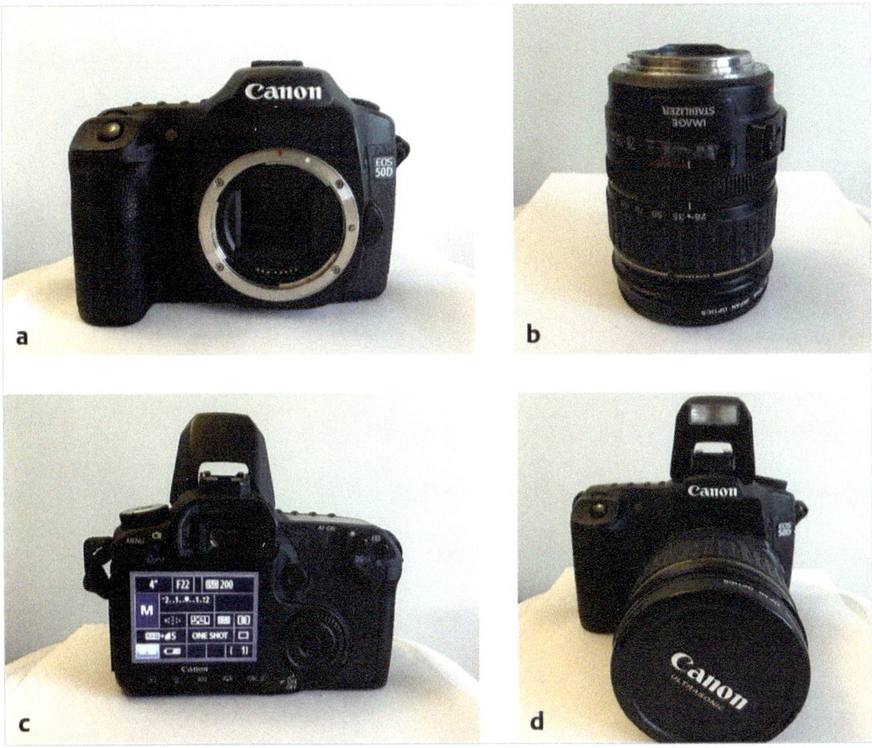

Fig. 6.1 **(a)** Digital single-lens reflex (DSLR) camera body. **(b)** A telephoto zoom lens is a type of lens with a variable focal length that can be used in combination with a DSLR camera body. Due to the modular design of DSLR camera body, the uses can alternate the type of lens used depending on his or her needs. **(c)** The DSLR camera body allows the photographer to use either the view finder or digital screen when taking pictures. **(d)** Many DSLR cameras (as shown above) have a built-in flash, but there are also a number of flash attachments available. (These images are provided courtesy of Alaa Ayyoub.)

different distances, would therefore need multiple fixed focal length lenses.

Flash/Lighting

Axial lighting (AL) is the most commonly used lighting by amateur photographers as most DSLR cameras have built-in flash units (▶ Fig. 6.1d). The built-in nature of this feature makes its use convenient and negates the need to carry additional equipment. AL, however, tends to create harsh shadows, uneven lighting, and possible asymmetric illumination. The built-in flash systems furthermore have a small range and most DSLR cameras do not permit flash intensity adjustment.[9]

Ring flash (RF) is a circular flash that mounts on the lens, and provides 360 degrees of illumination around the lens. The benefit of this is that it minimizes shadowing, which is particularly important when using fixed focal lenses such as PL and ML.[7,10] RF provides good light for when taking a picture within a cavity such as the oral cavity.[9] The use of RF increases the cost of the equipment as this is not a standard accessory for a DSLR to be equipped with and requires the user to carry additional equipment.

6.2.2 Point-and-Shoot Camera

The cost, bulk, and complicatedness of DSLR day-to-day use have seen many opting for a point-and-shoot camera (compact camera). Such devices are designed to fit in a pocket, easy to use, and are relatively inexpensive. Point-and-shoot cameras do produce a picture of inferior quality compared to a DSLR; however, the average image is acceptable for either clinical or publishing purposes.[6] When using a point-and-shoot camera, it is important to remember that some of these devices rely on parallax. Parallax refers to a view in the optical view finder that is not identical to that which is being recorded by the digital sensor. Clearly a mismatch in what is visualized in the optical view finder to what is being recorded by the digital sensor can have a significant impact when photographing images in the near field such as within the oral cavity.[5] This issue is largely overcome by using the digital view finder when taking the picture. Within the point-and-shoot camera market, there has also been an increase in the availability of crossover devices that incorporate features and functionality of DSLR cameras but are priced similar to point-and-shoot cameras.

6.2.3 Smartphone Cameras

With technological advancement and ubiquitous presence, smartphone cameras are increasingly being used in daily clinical practice. A number of studies have evaluated the clinical value of photographs taken on smartphones. These studies have consistently demonstrated that the quality of these images is sufficient to facilitate clinical diagnosis and patient care.[11–13] Milam et al conducted an anonymous questionnaire among 153 board-certified dermatologists in the United States. The results showed that 61.8% reported daily use of photography in clinical practice, of which 46% admitted to using a smartphone camera.[14] Haron et al published on the possible use of images taken by a mobile device to be used to detect oral cancer early in low-resource settings, reporting an overall sensitivity of 71% and specificity of 100%. Although this study had a number of design limitations including small sample size ($n = 16$), it does suggest that mobile phone cameras are sufficient for medical photography. There are, however, no available studies to date that compare conventional cameras and smartphone cameras for the purposes of medical documentation.

6.3 Photographic Documentation Method

***Standardization*:** When taking clinical photographs for documentation, the purpose is to demonstrate change (or stability) within the oral cavity. It is therefore important that all other aspects remain as stable as possible in terms of viewpoint, positioning, lighting, color, magnification, perspective, contrast, and background.[15] It is therefore our belief that the following principles should be embraced when taking a picture of the oral cavity.

***Views*:** Within other areas of otolaryngology subspecialization such as facial plastics, the clinical use of photographic documentation is routinely utilized and photographic standards have been established.[16] There is no current standard set of views for oral photography. We therefore suggest that a series of views should be taken when photographing the oral cavity as this will provide a comprehensive view of the patient's oral anatomy for photographic reconstruction of a three-dimensional space, while also providing a baseline from which future imaging can be compared (▶ Fig. 6.2). The clinician should ideally use the widest view setting. If using a smartphone, the device should be held vertically to avoid postacquisition editing that is common when pictures are taken in the horizontal or landscape format. Unless the clinician is an experienced photographer, it is recommended to leave the autofocus function on and utilize the automatic focus illuminator. The focus illuminator should be centered within the middle of the desired picture. To get a large area of interest, multiple pictures of separate segments might be required to maintain appropriate focus (see ▶ Fig. 6.3).

***Magnification*:** The importance of standardization of magnification in anatomical photography has resulted in the development of standardized scales such as the "Westminster scale." The latter has been widely adopted by medical photographers for commonly photographed anatomy.[17] The use of such scales

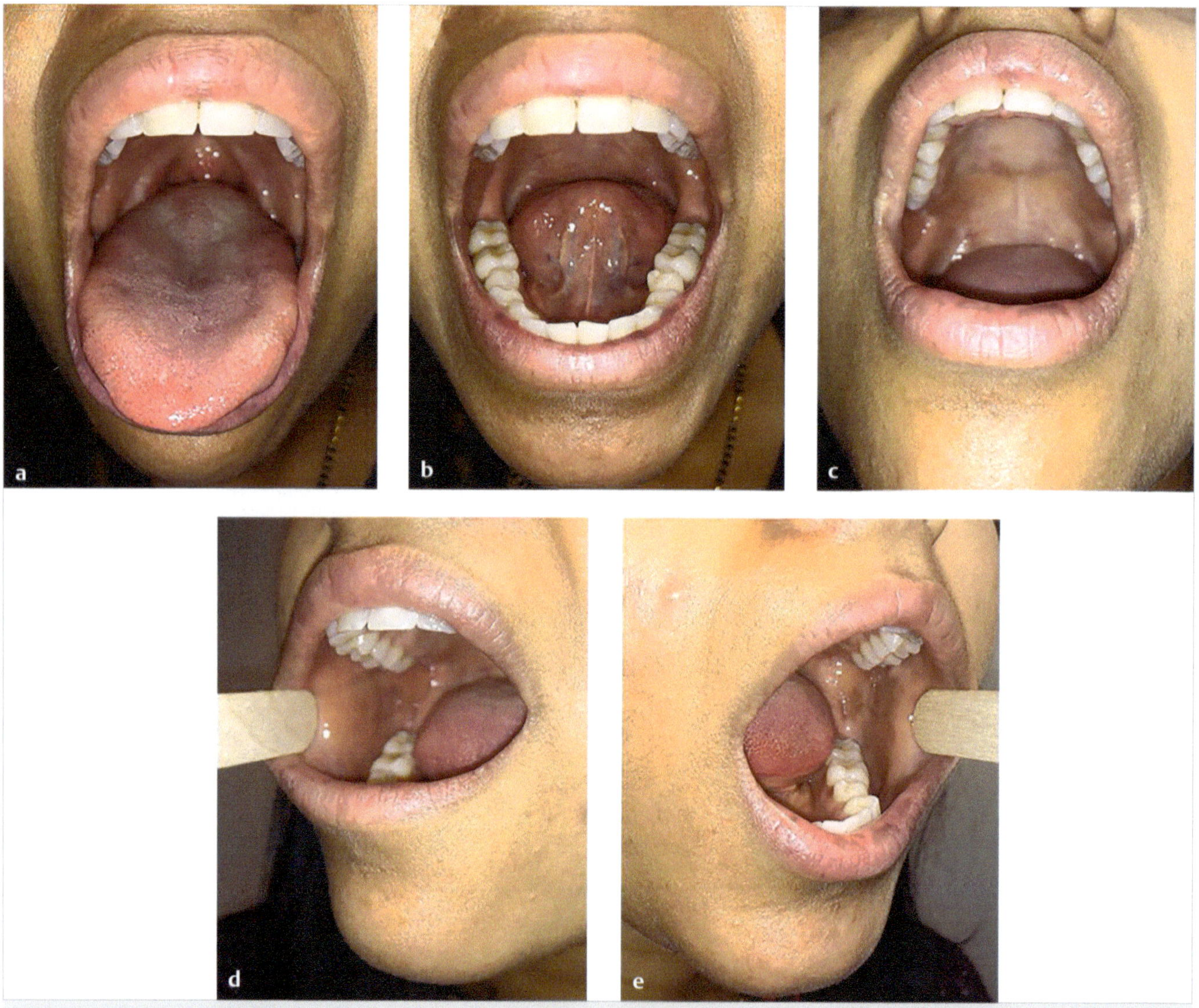

Fig. 6.2 When photographing the oral cavity, it is important to take multiple views to ensure that the images give the viewer a complete understanding of the patient's oral anatomy. We recommend the following five views: **(a)** frontal, **(b)** sublingual, **(c)** palate, **(d)** right buccal surface, and **(e)** left buccal surface.

allows for accurate comparison between images taken at different time points or by different photographers.[15,17] To our knowledge, no such standardization scale has been developed for intraoral photography and the importance of it can be seen in ▶ Fig. 6.4. Based upon our own practice and review of published manuscripts, we recommend that the camera be positioned between 6 and 8 inches away from the oral cavity and that no optical zoom be used.[18] Once the image is taken, the clinician can zoom in on the image and edit the photograph as desired.[18] If a clinician does utilize the zoom feature, it is recommended to note the amount of magnification within the documentation to ensure that similar settings are used at follow-up.

***Lighting*:** A significant challenge when photographing the oral cavity is the limited amount of light. To overcome this lack of light, the flash function should be utilized. Other outside sources of light such as headlamp should be avoided as these can lead to overexposure and potentially distort color. The light sensor that is located on the camera measures the light in the examination room rather than the oral cavity; therefore, it is recommended to manually turn the flash on rather than rely on the automatic flash function (▶ Fig. 6.5). The distance between the camera and the patient is important when using the flash. If the camera is too close, the flash can be reflected and wash out both anatomical and pathological features. Earlier we

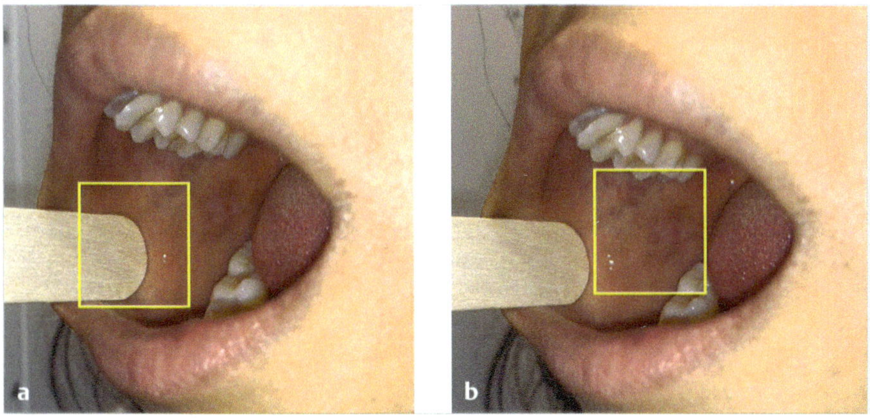

Fig. 6.3 **(a)** Within this image, the anterior aspect of the buccal surface is in focus, but the posterior aspect is blurred. **(b)** Within this image, the focal point has shifted posteriorly. As a result, the middle and posterior aspects of the buccal surface are better visualized in this image but with a loss of focus anteriorly.

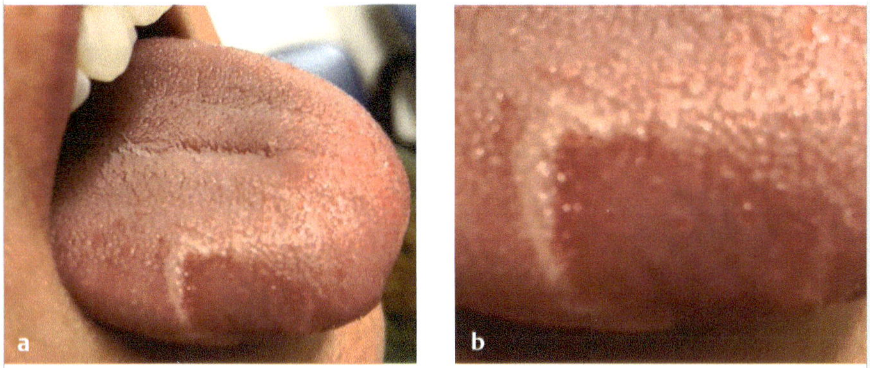

Fig. 6.4 **(a)** This image was taken without magnification and provides a clear image of a tongue ulcer in relation to the rest of the tongue. If the photographer is particularly concerned about a certain area, this area can then be enlarged from this original picture. **(b)** This image is taken with significant magnification and provides detailed view of the ulcer. Without image **(a)**, it would be impossible, however, to know the tongue location of the lesion. Furthermore, if these two pictures were taken during separate visits, it would be challenging to perform side-to-side clinical comparison as we can judge size.

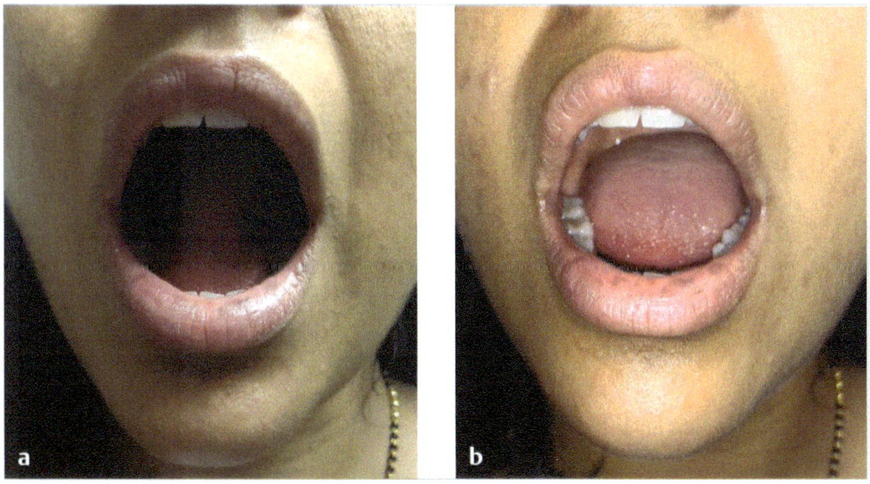

Fig. 6.5 Pictures taken in a well-lighted room. **(a)** The flash did not turn on automatically; as a result, little to none of the oral cavity is seen. **(b)** The flash was manually activated; as a result, the oral cavity is illuminated and visible.

identified some of the limitations of flash (shadowing) and touched very briefly on alternative flash system setups. The finer details of lighting and available flash technology are extensive and beyond the scope of this chapter, but it is readily available online for the interested reader.[19-21]

Depth of field: The variable depth within the oral cavity provides further challenge to the photographer. For example, images of the oral cavity will often have areas in focus and some areas out of focus. There is no simple solution to this and this is best overcome by taking multiple pictures from different views to allow the clinician to get a more complete understanding by combining the information from the different images.

6.4 Image Storage

Many electronic medical records allow pictures to be stored within the patient chart and can be easily accessed. The most common formatting used to save such files is as Joint Photographic Expert Group (JPEG) or Tagged Image File Format (TIFF). Kaliyadan et al identify TIFF as the default industrial standard for a cross-platform image format that can be opened by virtually all graphic applications. The disadvantage of TIFF files compared to JPEG, however, is that these larger files require more storage and potentially protracted uploading time.[6]

Many clinicians see the value of photographic imaging as a tool for teaching and further medical advancement. As a result, many clinicians choose to keep their own collection of medical images. In such a collection, the importance of meticulous cataloging is hard to overstate, where pictures should be clearly dated, filed by pathology process, and preferably have a system by which the clinician can identify the patient so that they are able to collect future disease progression and outcome data. Before creating such as database, it is important to review and ensure that such collections meet all medical and legal requirements.

6.5 Medical Legal Considerations

A study by Cheung et al investigated the patient perception of medical photographs being taken during an emergency room visit and found that 84% ($n = 100$) would give consent to having their image used for medical education.[22] Harting et al note that the law is, however, less clear on what is required to gain informed consent for pictures. Medical photography is generally classified as an editorial use unless the picture is not for "treatment purposes," in which case written consent is required.[2] It is, however, likely good practice and in the physicians' self-interests to gain written consent for all pictures taken particularly if the image is taken while the patient is asleep. The correct handling and storage of pictures is also important as many of the images could be considered a medical record and as such would fall within the realms of the Health Insurance Portability and Accountability Act (HIPPAA).

6.6 Conclusion

Photographic documentation can provide significant benefit in clinical practice, as it allows an easy and accurate way to document the oral examination. The images can also be used to assist in both patient and medical education. Here, we have described a number of easy methods to ensure optimum quality of captured images.

Key Points

- Photography of the oral cavity is a clinically useful tool that reduces the need for verbose and time-consuming description of the oral cavity. A picture can also help reduce inter- and intraobserver variation in interpretation and enable more precise follow-up for patients.
- The oral cavity presents a number of challenges for photography, but these can be overcome following some simple steps.
- The correct handling and storage of pictures is vital as many of the images can be considered a medical record and as such fall within the realms of the HIPAA.

References

[1] Clarke G. The Photograph. Oxford: Oxford University Press; 1997

[2] Harting MT, DeWees JM, Vela KM, Khirallah RT. Medical photography: current technology, evolving issues and legal perspectives. Int J Clin Pract. 2015; 69(4):401–409

[3] Payne WF. Photography of the oral cavity. J Biol Photogr Assoc. 1947; 15(3): 120–130

[4] Taheri A, Feldman SR. Can light-field photography ease focusing on the scalp and oral cavity? Skin Res Technol. 2013; 19(3):288–290

[5] Ahmad I. Digital dental photography. Part 1: an overview. Br Dent J. 2009; 206(8):403–407

[6] Kaliyadan F, Manoj J, Venkitakrishnan S, Dharmaratnam AD. Basic digital photography in dermatology. Indian J Dermatol Venereol Leprol. 2008; 74(5): 532–536

[7] Galloway SS, Easley J. Incorporating oral photography and endoscopy into the equine dental examination. Vet Clin North Am Equine Pract. 2013; 29(2): 345–366, vi

[8] Digital Photography School. Prime Lenses: An Introduction. Available at: https://digital-photography-school.com/prime-lenses-an-introduction/. Published April 3, 2007. Accessed October 27, 2018

[9] Barut C, Ertilav H. Guidelines for standard photography in gross and clinical anatomy. Anat Sci Educ. 2011; 4(6):348–356

[10] Ahmad I. Digital dental photography. Part 5: lighting. Br Dent J. 2009; 207(1): 13–18

[11] Eze N, Lo S, Bray D, Toma AG. The use of camera mobile phone to assess emergency ENT radiological investigations. Clin Otolaryngol. 2005; 30(3):230–233; discussion 233

[12] Boyce Z, Gilmore S, Xu C, Soyer HP. The remote assessment of melanocytic skin lesions: a viable alternative to face-to-face consultation. Dermatology. 2011; 223(3):244–250

[13] Boissin C, Fleming J, Wallis L, Hasselberg M, Laflamme L. Can we trust the use of smartphone cameras in clinical practice? Laypeople assessment of their image quality. Telemed J E Health. 2015; 21(11):887–892

[14] Milam EC, Leger MC. Use of medical photography among dermatologists: a nationwide online survey study. J Eur Acad Dermatol Venereol JEADV. 2018; 32(10):1804–1809

[15] Nayler JR. Clinical photography: a guide for the clinician. J Postgrad Med. 2003; 49(3):256–262

[16] Archibald DJ, Carlson ML, Friedman O. Pitfalls of nonstandardized photography. Facial Plast Surg Clin North Am. 2010; 18(2):253–266

[17] MIUK. Westminster Reproduction Ratios. November 2014. http://www.migroup.co.uk/westminster-reproduction-ratios/. Accessed July 29, 2018

[18] Joshipura DS, Joshipura S. A novel technique of digital photography for oral lesions. J Am Acad Dermatol. 2015; 73(1):e19–e20

[19] CreativeLive. The Ultimate Guide to Photography. Available at: https://www.creativelive.com/photography-guides. Accessed November 2, 2018

[20] Photography Life. Photography Tips for Beginners. Available at: https://photographylife.com/photography-tips-for-beginners. Accessed November 2, 2018

[21] ExpertPhotography. Photography for Beginners: A Complete Guide (Updated 2018). Available at: https://expertphotography.com/a-beginners-guide-to-photography/. Published November 6, 2011. Accessed November 2, 2018

[22] Cheung A, Al-Ausi M, Hathorn I, Hyam J, Jaye P. Patients' attitudes toward medical photography in the emergency department. Emerg Med J. 2005; 22 (8):609

7 Imaging of Oral Cavity Cancers

Majid Khan, Saudur Rahman, and Nafi Aygun

Summary
Radiologic imaging plays an important role in the assessment of oral cavity cancers. CT and MRI are complementary in evaluation of cancers in the subsites of the oral cavity and their routes of spread. Important features to assess on CT and MRI include but are not limited to the depth of invasion, extension across the midline, invasion of the neurovascular bundle, perineural spread, osseous invasion, and nodal metastasis.

Keywords: oral cavity cancer, squamous cell cancer, imaging of oral cavity cancer, staging of oral cavity cancer

7.1 Introduction

The oral cavity is the most ventral portion of the aerodigestive tract and has a complex anatomy with multiple anatomic subdivisions. The separation between the oral cavity and the oropharynx is very important. The squamous epithelium of the oral cavity derives from ectoderm, which tends to give rise to more differentiated and less aggressive lesions. In contrast, the squamous epithelium of the oropharynx derives from endoderm, which tends to give rise to poorly differentiated and aggressive carcinomas.[1]

The oral cavity is separated from the oropharynx by a ring of structures consisting of the circumvallate papillae, the hard and soft palate junction, and the anterior tonsillar pillars on both sides.[1] Please refer to the section on "Diagnosis and Evaluation" for a detailed description of the oral cavity anatomy and its subdivisions. The most common sites of involvement are the lower lip, lateral and ventral surface of the oral tongue, and the floor of the mouth.[1,2]

7.2 Epidemiology

Cancer of the oral cavity accounts for nearly 30% of all head and neck malignancies, and approximately 300,000 new cases of oral cavity cancers are diagnosed in the world every year.[3] The vast majority (almost 90%) of oral cavity malignancies are squamous cell carcinomas (SCCs), and the rest are comprised of minor salivary gland neoplasms, melanoma, lymphoma, and rare varieties of squamous cell and odontogenic tumors.[2,4]

Oral cavity cancer occurs most frequently in individuals older than 50 years of age, affecting men more frequently than women with a ratio of 2:1 to 3:1. In the United States, there is a higher incidence of oral cancer in the African American population. The main risk factors for the development of oral cavity cancer are tobacco and alcohol use.[2,5,6]

In the developed world, the overall incidence of oral cavity cancer has been declining since the 1970s due to the decrease in prevalence of tobacco use.[7,8] However, the prevalence of tobacco use is rising in the rest of the world, and the future burden of oral cavity cancer is expected to significantly increase in the lower-income countries, with an expected 80% increase in oral cavity cancers.[9]

Tobacco use is the most important risk factor for oral cavity cancer, and approximately 65% of oral cavity cancers are attributed to smoking tobacco. Tobacco use, including both smoking and chewing, confers a threefold to fivefold increased risk of oral cavity cancer, which is independent of alcohol use. However, the synergistic effect of alcohol and tobacco on increasing the risk of oral cavity cancer is well established, and results in almost threefold greater risk than the product of the individual effects of tobacco and alcohol.[6]

Additional risk factors include chewing betel quid leaves and areca nuts, which contribute to the high incidence of oral cavity cancers in Central and Southeast Asia. Prolonged ultraviolet (UV) exposure in regions with hot climates increases the risk of lip cancer.[10] Increased incidence of lip cancer has also been shown in renal transplant recipients on immunosuppressive therapy.[11]

Human papillomavirus (HPV) is now established as a major risk factor for oropharyngeal cancer in the developed world, but its role in oral cavity cancer is very limited. Multiple studies have shown that HPV does not often play a role in the pathogenesis of oral cavity cancer. In the United States, high-risk HPV type 16 deoxyribonucleic acid (DNA) has been detected in only 3 to 10% of oral cavity cancers, whereas it has been detected in nearly 60 to 80% of oropharyngeal cancers.[12,13] The difference in HPV prevalence in the oral cavity cancers and oropharyngeal cancers has implications for prevention, diagnosis, workup, treatment, and follow-up.[14]

Fanconi's anemia is a rare disorder that confers a 500- to 700-fold increased risk of developing head and neck SCC, most of which occur in the oral cavity. In patients who present with head and neck cancer that are younger and without typical risk factors of tobacco and alcohol use, Fanconi's anemia should be considered. Fanconi's anemia has an incidence of approximately 1:360,000 births, but the carrier frequency is believed to be as high as 1:100 in certain populations, such as Ashkenazi Jews, Spanish gypsies, and black South Africans. It is inherited in an autosomal recessive fashion, and it is the most common form of inherited aplastic anemia.[15]

7.3 Clinical Presentation

Oral cavity cancer is typically painless and asymptomatic at an early stage. As a result, patients with readily visible lip cancers present at an early stage. However, patients with intraoral cancers usually present when they are symptomatic and at a more advanced stage. Most common presenting symptoms are painful oral lesion, painful or bleeding ulcer, and loose teeth or ill-fitting dentures. Patients may also present with trismus (caused by pterygoid involvement), hypoesthesia (caused by perineural involvement), or otalgia (referred pain from cranial nerves [CNs] IX and X).[2,16,17]

On examination, tumors may appear as white, red, or speckled mucosal lesions, and advanced lesions classically have an ulcerated center with indurated or indistinct borders.[2] The most common locations for intraoral lesions are the lateral and ventral aspects of the oral tongue, and the floor of the mouth.[18]

A substantial percentage of patients have cervical lymphadenopathy at the time of initial presentation. Careful physical and radiologic evaluation of the cervical lymph node chains is important as the presence or absence of lymphadenopathy is the most important prognostic indicator in this disease.[17,19]

7.4 Diagnosis and Evaluation

Radiologic imaging plays an important role in evaluation and staging of oral cavity cancer. CT, MRI, and PET/CT are important in assessment of tumor size and depth of invasion (DOI), bone invasion, lymphadenopathy, presence of nodal extracapsular extension, perineural spread, second synchronous lesions, and distant metastases. In the section, we will present an overview of imaging modalities and patterns of spread for oral cavity cancers.

7.4.1 Computed Tomography

Contrast-enhanced CT is the most commonly utilized imaging modality for initial assessment of oral cavity cancer. CT is readily available and can be acquired very quickly, which limits motion artifact, and can be easily reformatted into coronal and sagittal planes. CT provides exquisite evaluation of cortical bone involvement. The disadvantages of CT include exposure to ionizing radiation and potential adverse reactions related to iodinated contrast agents, as well as streak artifact from dental amalgam and the mandible (▶ Fig. 7.1a). However, scanning in multiple planes can overcome the limitations related to streak artifacts.[2]

On CT, SCCs appear as homogeneous or heterogeneous soft-tissue attenuation lesions that demonstrate variable contrast enhancement. Early or more prominent enhancement of the tumor margins may be present, which is presumably related to higher vascularity at the periphery of the tumor. Necrotic areas demonstrate central hypodensity with peripheral enhancement. The peripheral enhancement can sometimes have similar attenuation as surrounding soft tissues, which can limit evaluation of the exact boundaries of the lesion.[2] On a technical note, it is important to perform the scan during optimum contrast enhancement of tissues. With the very fast modern scanners, it is possible to scan too early before the peak enhancement of the tumor occurs. In this regard, the timing of scanning with respect to contrast material injection is different in tumor assessment from other neck CT applications such as CT angiogram.

7.4.2 Magnetic Resonance Imaging

MR imaging offers better soft-tissue contrast and can complement CT in accurately delineating tumor extent and thickness. On conventional non-fat saturated T1-weighted images, SCC has intermediate signal intensity and generally demonstrates iso- to hypointensity compared to muscles of the floor of the mouth and tongue. Even though tumors have similar intensity to muscle on T1-weighted images, this sequence can still be very helpful to determine tumor margins as its boundaries may still be evident through disrupted internal structure of normal soft tissues. On T2-weighted images, SCC is typically heterogeneously hyperintense to normal muscle, making it more conspicuous, although it may be difficult to distinguish tumor from adjacent surrounding edema and inflammation resulting in overestimation of tumor size. On STIR (short tau inversion recovery) images, tumors have similar appearance as on T2-weighted images and may be more conspicuous, but STIR images are more prone to artifact and usually have lower spatial resolution. It should be noted that normal mucosal surfaces may have high signal intensity on STIR images.[2]

On gadolinium-enhanced T1-weighted images without fat saturation, SCC demonstrates variable enhancement and conspicuity (▶ Fig. 7.1c). Fat-saturated images can be helpful in distinguishing tumors from normal surrounding intrinsically hyperintense structures. However, some normal structures, such as salivary glands, also demonstrate increased conspicuity

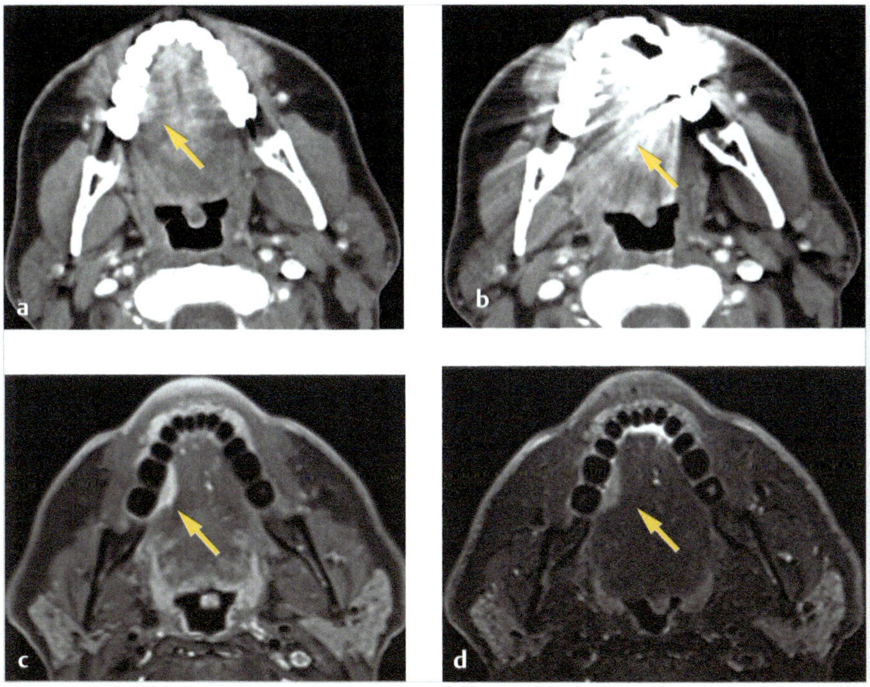

Fig. 7.1 Oral cavity cancer on CT versus MRI. **(a)** Axial contrast-enhanced CT shows enhancing right lateral oral tongue squamous cell carcinoma (SCC; *yellow arrow*), which is slightly obscured due to streak artifact from dental amalgam. **(b)** Axial contrast-enhanced CT image (inferior to a) shows near-complete obscuration of the mass due to the extensive streak artifact. **(c)** Axial contrast-enhanced T1 fat-saturated (FS) MRI sequence from the same patient at the same level as **(a)** shows improved visualization of the SCC. **(d)** Axial contrast-enhanced T1 FS MRI sequence at the same level as **(b)** shows much better visualization of the SCC compared to the CT.

on fat-saturated images, and should not be mistaken for pathology. Fat-saturated images require longer acquisition time, which may result in increased motion artifact. Susceptibility artifacts near bone or air limit evaluation of skull base foramina on the fat-saturated images.

MRI is superior to CT for assessment of perineural spread of disease, and medullary bone involvement (see below). MRI also has the advantage of reduced artifact from dental amalgam. However, MRI is more affected by motion artifact.[2]

7.4.3 Fluorodeoxyglucose PET/CT

Fluorodeoxyglucose (FDG) PET/CT has the potential to increase sensitivity for nodal disease, but studies have shown that it is generally not substantially superior to standard contrast-enhanced CT or MR imaging in detecting occult nodal metastases.[16,20–22] FDG-PET/CT is often utilized to detect an occult primary head and neck malignancy in the setting of a positive cervical lymph node. Finally, FDG-PET/CT is also useful in detecting second primary lesions and distant metastases. However, the positive predictive value for distant metastases is low, and often results in unnecessary additional imaging and biopsies. Therefore, FDG-PET/CT should be used for detection of distant metastases in the setting of advanced local disease with higher risk of distant metastases.[23,24]

7.4.4 Nodal Metastasis

The imaging assessment of cervical lymphadenopathy must include a determination of size, morphologic features, and margination of the node. The cardinal features of pathologic lymphadenopathy on imaging are large node size and presence of central necrosis. The usual size criterion as a maximal longitudinal diameter is 15 mm or greater for jugulodigastric nodes, and 10 mm or greater for other nodes. The usual size criterion as a minimal axial diameter is 11 mm for jugulodigastric nodes and 10 mm for other nodes. Clustering of three or more nonenlarged lymph nodes in the same lymphatic drainage area is considered suspicious for pathologic lymphadenopathy. A rounded appearance with loss of the normal reniform shape of a lymph node is also suspicious for nodal metastasis.[1,2,17]

Extracapsular spread (ECS) is an important finding as it results in an approximately 50% reduction in survival.[16,25] Imaging features of extracapsular spread on CT includes presence of an irregular, spiculated, blurred lymph node border; loss of fat plane around the node; irregular capsular enhancement; central nodal necrosis; and/or tumoral infiltration into soft tissue and vascular structures (▶ Fig. 7.2, ▶ Fig. 7.3, ▶ Fig. 7.4). On MR imaging, the ranked predictive criteria for extracapsular spread include high signal intensity in tissues surrounding a node on T2 STIR images, a poorly defined nodal border, irregular rimlike enhancement, and large nodal size.[1,26]

7.4.5 Perineural Spread

Perineural spread makes local and regional control of the disease particularly difficult by allowing tumor extension beyond the expected treatment margins. It is important for the radiologist to be alert to the possibility of perineural

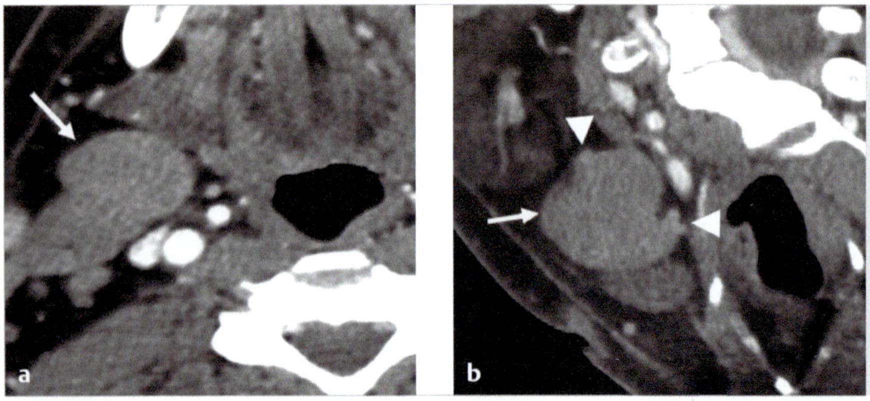

Fig. 7.2 Nodal metastasis with extracapsular extension (ECE). **(a)** Axial and **(b)** oblique coronal contrast-enhanced CT images show slight irregularity of the right level II nodal capsule (*arrows*) with a nodular soft tissue medial to the capsule (*arrowheads*) compatible with ECE. Pathology showed ECE measuring 12 mm.

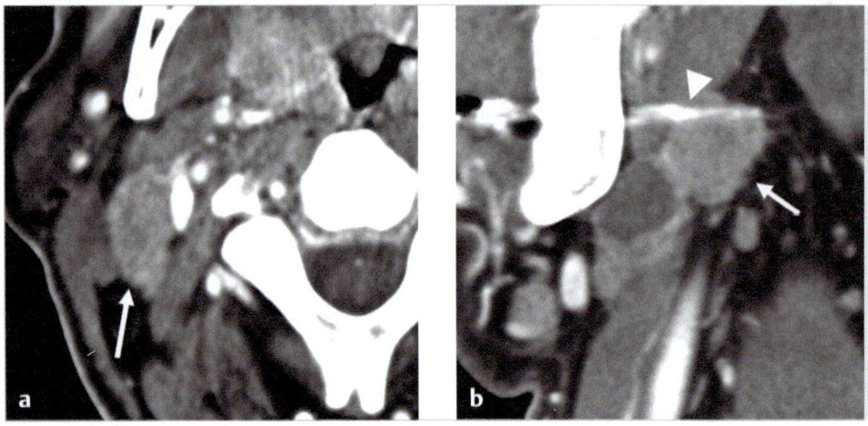

Fig. 7.3 Nodal metastasis with extracapsular extension (ECE). **(a)** Axial and **(b)** oblique coronal CT images show irregular nodal capsule contour with nodularity (*arrows*). The *arrowhead* in **(b)** points to artifact from dental amalgam. Pathology revealed ECE.

spread as it is often clinically silent. Perineural invasion is considered a characteristic of aggressive SCCs, and it is more common in subsites such as the floor of the mouth and hard palate, where the neurovascular bundles are particularly accessible.[1]

On CT, findings associated with perineural spread include foraminal enlargement and soft-tissue attenuation replacing fat attenuation within the foramina. MRI is superior to CT for direct assessment of perineural spread. Findings that are suspicious for perineural spread on MRI include enlargement, irregularity, and abnormal enhancement of the major cranial nerves and their branches. Replacement of high-intensity fat adjacent to the major skull base foramina and other fat-containing spaces such as the pterygopalatine fossa (PPF) by intermediate signal intensity tissue on unenhanced T1-weighted images are also suspicious findings. Indirect signs of nerve invasion such as muscle denervation may be seen as well. In the acute phase, a denervated muscle may appear swollen and hyperintense on T2-weighted images with increased enhancement. In the chronic phase, muscle denervation results in muscle atrophy and fatty replacement.[2]

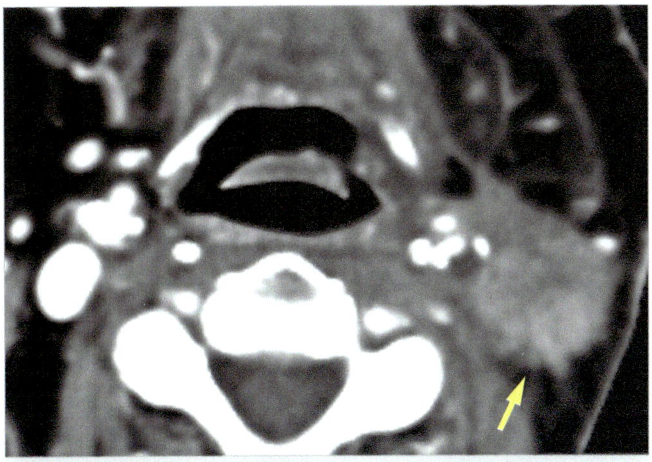

Fig. 7.4 Nodal metastasis with extracapsular extension (ECE). Axial contrast-enhanced CT shows left level II enlarged lymph node with irregular capsule with prominent spiculation (*yellow arrow*) and surrounding infiltration. Pathology revealed positive ECE.

7.4.6 Mandibular Invasion

Osseous invasion of oral cavity cancers upstages the disease to at least stage T4a, and presence or absence as well as the degree of osseous invasion alters treatment strategy. Tumors of the floor of the mouth, ventral surface of the tongue, gingiva, and retromolar trigone (RMT) may show early involvement of the mandible. Mechanism of invasion and routes of entry into the mandible have been studied, and the current understanding is that the tumor invades the mandible by direct extension through the periosteum rather than through lymphatic spread.[27] In the dentate mandible, tumors of the floor of the mouth and ventral surface of the tongue enter the mandible most commonly at the point of abutment rather than through the occlusal surface, neural foramina, or the periodontal membrane. The point of tumor abutment is commonly at the junction of the attached and reflected mucosa, and therefore, small cortical defects at the attachment of the mucosa to the bone are likely the weak points through which the tumor gains entry into the mandible.[28]

In the edentulous mandible, cortical irregularities in the occlusal surface of the mandible may serve as entry points for oral cancers into the mandible. Tumors of the gingiva and the RMT may also preferentially enter the mandible through the occlusal surface, which is commonly the point of abutment of these tumors with the mandible.[28–30]

Tumors invading the mandible can be managed with either a marginal or a segmental resection. If there is invasion of only the periosteum without gross cortical invasion, the tumor can be managed with a marginal mandibulectomy maintaining the integrity of the mandible. In general, tumors with gross cortical erosion or invasion of the medullary cavity require a segmental resection, which involves resection of the entire involved segment of the mandible necessitating a more complex reconstruction, requiring vascularized bone and soft tissue, often a fibular free flap.[17]

CT and MRI are complementary for evaluation of mandibular involvement. CT is superior to MRI for evaluation of subtle cortical erosion with high specificity and positive predictive value (90%), but limited sensitivity (50%; ▸ Fig. 7.5).[31] A pitfall in the evaluation of cortical erosion can occur in the body of the mandible when the plane of imaging is not along the long axis of the mandibular body (▸ Fig. 7.6).

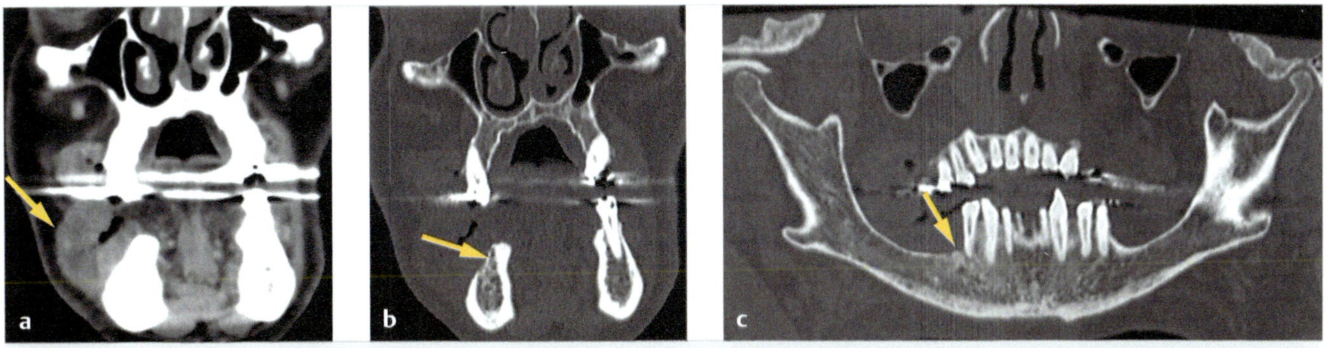

Fig. 7.5 Oral cavity squamous cell carcinoma (SCC) invading the mandible. **(a)** Coronal contrast-enhanced (CE) CT soft-tissue window shows right gingival SCC (*yellow arrow*). **(b)** Coronal CE CT bone window shows cortical erosion of the lingual cortex of the right mandibular body (*yellow arrow*). **(c)** Panoramic reformat created of the CE CT bone window shows improved visualization of the subtle cortical erosion of the right mandibular body (*yellow arrow*). Note the asymmetry compared to the normal contralateral side.

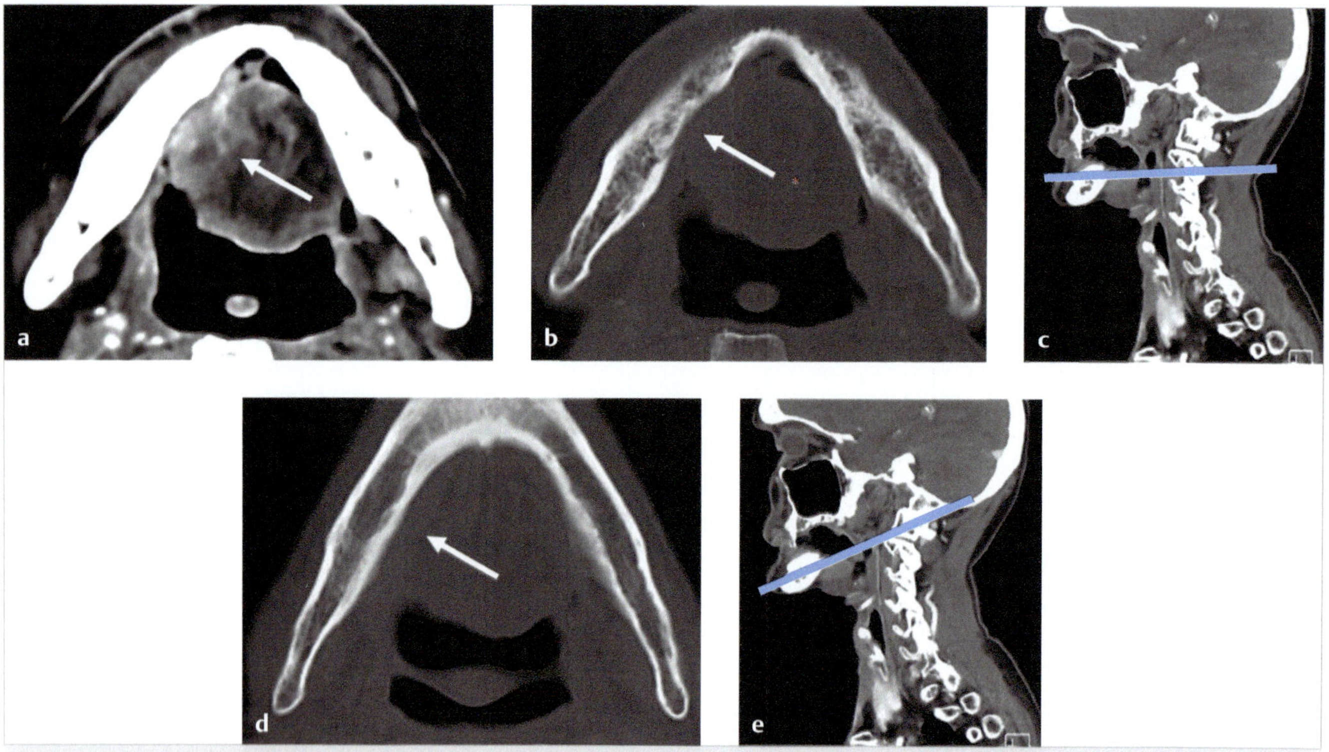

Fig. 7.6 Importance of evaluating the mandible in the right plane. **(a)** Axial contrast-enhanced CT shows the right floor of the mouth squamous cell carcinoma (*white arrow*) abutting the right mandibular body. **(b)** Axial CT bone window in the horizontal plane (**c**; *blue line*) shows possible cortical defect (*white arrow*) in the lingual cortex of the right mandibular body suggesting osseous invasion. **(d)** Axial CT bone window reformatted along the plane of the mandibular body (**e**; *blue line*) shows an intact cortex (*white arrow*) with no evidence of mandibular invasion. *, Images need to be looked at on both soft tissue and bone windows, because if bone is evaluated on soft tissue windows, then subtle osseous involvement can be missed.

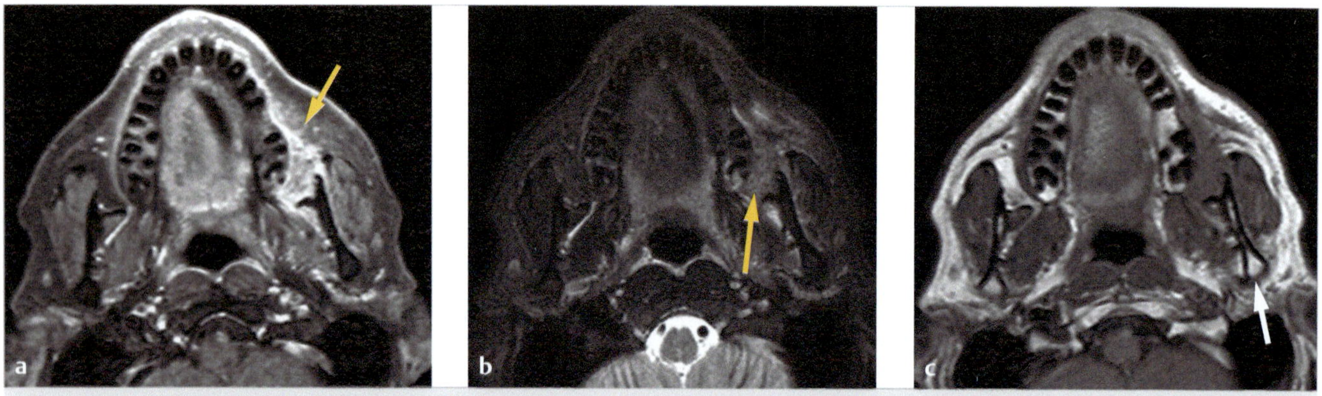

Fig. 7.7 High-sensitivity of mandibular invasion on MRI. Axial contrast-enhanced (CE) T1 fat-saturated (FS) MRI **(a)** and axial T2 short tau inversion recovery (STIR) MRI **(b)** show left gingival/retromolar trigone squamous cell carcinoma, which closely approximates the mandible cortex. However, the CE T1 FS, T2 STIR, and precontrast non-FS T1 MRI **(c)** show normal marrow signal within the adjacent mandible (*white arrow*). Partial resection of the mandible revealed no pathologic evidence of mandibular invasion. *Yellow arrows*, fat saturated post-contrast T1-weighted image makes it easier to assess enhancing tissue and the trajectory it is taking.

MR imaging is superior to CT for evaluation of the medullary cavity with high sensitivity (▸ Fig. 7.7), but low specificity.[32] Signs of marrow invasion on MR include T1 hypointensity replacing normal fatty marrow, loss of low-signal-intensity cortex, and contrast enhancement within the bone or along the inferior alveolar nerve. However, MR imaging suffers from low specificity in the setting of odontogenic disease, which can cause false-positive marrow replacement and even enhancement.[17,33]

7.5 Staging

Staging of oral cavity SCC and minor salivary gland carcinomas is based on the tumor, node, and metastasis (TNM) staging system, which has been revised in the eighth edition of the American Joint Committee on Cancer (AJCC) Cancer Staging Manual (▸ Table 7.1) with significant changes compared to the seventh edition.[34] Recent data have shown that DOI is a better prognostic indicator than tumor thickness for oral cavity cancers.[35]

Table 7.1 AJCC eighth edition: Lip and Oral Cavity Staging[34]

Primary tumor (T)	
TX	Primary tumor cannot be assessed
Tis	Carcinoma in situ
T1	Tumor ≤ 2 cm, ≤ 5 mm depth of invasion (DOI)
T2	Tumor ≤ 2 cm, DOI > 5 mm and ≤ 10 mm *or* tumor > 2 cm but ≤ 4 cm, and ≤ 10 mm DOI
T3	Tumor > 4 cm *or* any tumor > 10 mm DOI
T4a	Moderately advanced local disease
	(Lip) Tumor invades through the cortical bone, inferior alveolar nerve, floor of the mouth, or skin of face, i.e., chin or nose
	(Oral cavity) Tumor invades adjacent structures only (e.g., through cortical bone of the mandible or maxilla, or involves the maxillary sinus or skin of the face)
T4b	Very advanced local disease
	Tumor invades masticator space, pterygoid plates, or skull base and/or encases internal carotid artery
	Note: Superficial erosion alone of bone/tooth socket by gingival primary is not sufficient to classify a tumor as T4
Regional lymph nodes (N)	
NX	Regional lymph nodes cannot be assessed
N0	No regional lymph node metastasis
N1	Metastasis in a single ipsilateral lymph node, ≤ 3 cm in greatest dimension and ENE negative
N2	Metastasis in a single ipsilateral lymph node, ≤ 3 cm in greatest dimension and ENE positive; *or* greater than 3 cm but not greater than 6 cm in greatest dimension and ENE negative; or metastases in multiple ipsilateral lymph nodes, none more than 6 cm in greatest dimension and ENE negative; *or* metastasis in bilateral or contralateral lymph nodes, none more than 6 cm in greatest dimension and ENE negative
N2a	Metastasis in a single ipsilateral or contralateral lymph node 3 cm or less in greatest dimension and ENE positive; or metastasis in a single ipsilateral lymph node more than 3 cm but not more than 6 cm in greatest dimension and ENE negative
N2b	Metastasis in multiple ipsilateral lymph nodes, none more than 6 cm in greatest dimension and ENE negative
N2c	Metastasis in bilateral or contralateral lymph nodes, none more than 6 cm in greatest dimension and ENE negative
N3	Metastasis in a lymph node more than 6 cm in greatest dimension and ENE negative; or metastasis in a single ipsilateral lymph node more than 3 cm in greatest dimension and ENE positive; *or* metastasis in multiple ipsilateral, contralateral, or bilateral lymph nodes, with any ENE positive
N3a	Metastasis in a lymph node more than 6 cm in greatest dimension and ENE negative
N3b	Metastasis in a single ipsilateral node more than 3 cm in greatest dimension and ENE positive; *or* metastasis in multiple ipsilateral, contralateral, or bilateral lymph nodes, with any ENE positive
Distant metastasis (M)	
M0	No distant metastasis
M1	Distant metastasis

Abbreviation: ENE, extranodal extension.
Note: DOI is depth of invasion and not tumor thickness.

Pathologically, DOI is measured from the level of the basement membrane of the closest adjacent normal mucosa, and a "plumb line" is dropped from this plane to the deepest point of tumor invasion. DOI will now affect the T stage, which will increase by one level for every 5 mm increase in DOI. DOI supersedes not only tumor thickness, but also extrinsic tongue muscle involvement, which is no longer part of the criterion for T4 designation.

Patterns of invasion determine T4a or T4b stage of the lesion. Osseous invasion is the primary consideration for upstaging to T4a disease, or "moderately advanced" disease. T4b disease, or "very advanced" disease, refers to tumor invasion of the masticator space, pterygoid plates, or skull base; or tumor encasement of the internal carotid artery.

The criteria for nodal staging for oral cavity cancers are identical to the criteria for many other sites in the head and neck such as the pharynx and larynx. A significant change has been made to the N category of the staging system for head and neck cancers in the AJCC eight edition with inclusion of extranodal extension (ENE) as a prognostic variable for lymph node metastases. There is long-standing evidence that ENE profoundly affects prognosis for oral cavity cancers.[36] Current imaging modalities lack sensitivity and specificity in their abilities to detect early or minor ENE, and imaging evidence alone may be supportive but is not sufficient.[37] Therefore, only unambiguous ENE will be assigned a status of ENE positive, as determined by physical examination (invasion of skin, infiltration of musculature/dense tethering to adjacent structures, or dysfunction of a cranial nerve, the brachial plexus, the sympathetic trunk, or the phrenic nerve) and supported by radiological evidence.[34]

7.6 Anatomic and Imaging Considerations of Oral Cavity Cancers

The oral cavity is the most ventral portion of the aerodigestive tract and has a complex anatomy with multiple anatomic subdivisions. The separation between the oral cavity and the oropharynx is very important. The squamous epithelium of the oral cavity derives from the ectoderm, whereas the squamous epithelium of the oropharynx derives from the endoderm.[1] The oral cavity is separated from the oropharynx by a ring of structures consisting of the circumvallate papillae, the hard and soft palate junction, and the anterior tonsillar pillars on both sides.[1]

The oral cavity is bounded anteriorly by the lips, laterally by the cheeks, superiorly by the superior alveolar ridge and hard palate, and inferiorly by the inferior alveolar ridge and the mylohyoid muscle.[38] The oral cavity is anatomically subdivided into (1) the lips, (2) the floor of the mouth, (3) the oral tongue, (4) the RMT, (5) the upper and lower gingivae, (6) the buccal mucosa, and (7) the hard palate. Within the oral cavity, the most common sites of neoplastic involvement are the lower lip, lateral and ventral surface of the oral tongue, and the floor of the mouth.[1] Anatomic and imaging considerations for each subsite are discussed below.

7.6.1 The Lip

Anatomy

The lips are the anterior boundary of the oral cavity and are covered by keratinizing squamous epithelium on the outer surface, whereas the inner surface is covered by nonkeratinizing stratified squamous epithelium.[17] The lips are composed of the orbicularis oris muscle, which is primarily composed of muscle fibers from multiple facial muscles that insert into the lips. The motor innervation is derived from the facial nerve (CN VII), and the lymphatic drainage is to the submental and submandibular lymph nodes (levels IA and IB).[17,39]

Imaging Considerations

Although the lip is the most common site of involvement with cancer in the oral cavity (accounting for approximately 40% of cases),[1,17] it is rarely imaged because most cases present as small superficial lesions that are detected and well evaluated clinically with direct visualization. Cancers of the lip most commonly involve the lower lip, representing approximately 88 to 95% of cases, followed by the upper lip (2–7%), and the commissure (1%).[18] Lip cancers tend to arise from the vermilion border and spread superficially and laterally along the skin, or deep to the orbicularis oris muscle.[1,38]

Imaging is usually obtained for larger lesions with uncertain margins.[1,38] It is often difficult to differentiate early-stage lesion from the normal orbicularis oris muscle.[1] The most important features to assess on imaging include osseous extension and nodal metastasis. Osseous extension usually involves the buccal surfaces of the maxillary or mandibular alveolar ridges,[1,38] and osseous infiltration may allow for perineural spread along the alveolar nerves.[1]

7.6.2 Floor of the Mouth

Anatomy

The floor of the mouth is a crescent or **U**-shaped area of the oral cavity that is bordered by the lingual aspect of the lower gingiva anteriorly, the alveolar ridge of the mandible laterally, the insertion of the anterior tonsillar pillar into the tongue posteriorly, and the free inferior aspect of the tongue medially.[1] The inferior border and the main supporting structure of the floor of the mouth is the mylohyoid muscle with additional support from the anterior bellies of the digastric muscles and geniohyoid muscles (▶ Fig. 7.8c).[1,39] The mylohyoid muscle originates along the mylohyoid ridge of the inner surface of the mandible and inserts into the body of the hyoid posteriorly, and the midline fibrous raphe anteriorly,[1,17,39] which runs from the hyoid bone to the mandibular symphysis.[39] This forms the **U**-shaped sling, which is best demonstrated on coronal CT or MR imaging. The mylohyoid muscle separates the sublingual space from the submandibular space and it is innervated by the mylohyoid nerve, which is a branch of the inferior alveolar nerve (CN V3).[17]

The floor of the mouth is divided anteriorly in half by the lingual frenulum. The sublingual and submandibular glands drain into the floor of the mouth via the major sublingual (Bartholin's) ducts and the submandibular (Wharton's) ducts, respectively.[1] Within the sublingual space, the hyoglossus–styloglossus–palatoglossus muscle complex separates the

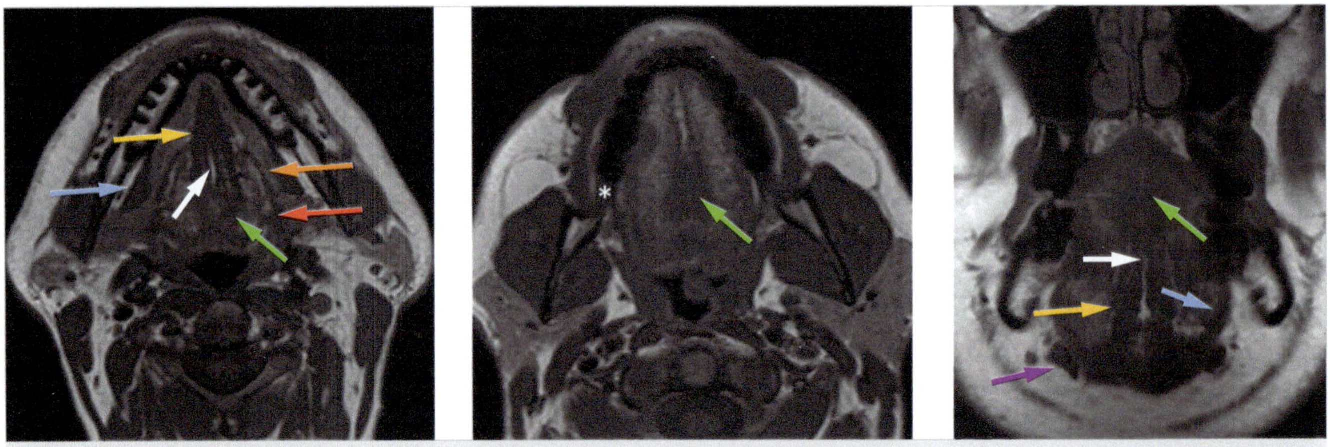

Fig. 7.8 Oral cavity anatomy. Axial noncontrast T1 and coronal T1 MRI images show genioglossus muscle (*yellow arrow*), mylohyoid muscle (*blue arrow*), lingual septum (*white arrow*), intrinsic tongue muscles (*green arrow*), RMT (*asterisk*), hyoglossus muscle (*orange arrow*), palatoglossus muscle (*red arrow*), and anterior belly of digastric muscle (*purple arrow*).

lingual artery, which courses medially, from the main lingual vein, the hypoglossal and lingual nerves, and Wharton's duct, which course laterally.[2]

Imaging Considerations

The floor of the mouth is a common site of oral cavity cancer. Primary malignancies in the floor of the mouth arise along the mucosal surface, sublingual space, and undersurface of the anterior two-thirds of the tongue. Carcinomas most often arise within 2 cm of the anterior midline[17] and tend to spread horizontally or superficially as the floor of mouth musculature forms a relative barrier to tumor spread.[2]

Superficial mucosal lesions are difficult to assess on imaging. However, imaging evaluation is important as clinical assessment of tumor depth and extent is difficult. Imaging evaluation should include tumor size and DOI. It is important to determine the extent of submucosal invasion, especially whether the tumor crosses the midline or not. There is a communication between the sublingual spaces anteriorly beneath the frenulum, which provides a route for contralateral spread of disease.[2] Involvement of the tumor across the midline, and involvement of the contralateral neurovascular bundle, precludes hemiglossectomy as a surgical option, and either a total glossectomy or nonsurgical treatment option is to be considered.[2,17,38] On CT, invasion of the neurovascular bundle can be suggested when there is loss of an intervening fat plane between the tumor and the enhancing lingual artery (▶ Fig. 7.9).

Due to their location, cancers in the floor of the mouth can obstruct the ostia of the submandibular ducts resulting in ductal dilatation or obstructive inflammatory changes of the submandibular gland. In fact, these changes can serve as signs of an occult floor of the mouth malignancy. The obstructive inflammatory changes should not be mistaken as tumor invasion of the submandibular gland, and MR imaging can be used to clarify in equivocal cases. In contradistinction, the sublingual glands are more prone to direct invasion by tumor rather than distal duct obstruction, likely due to their close proximity to the malignancies.[2]

Floor of the mouth cancers can extend anteriorly or laterally to invade the mandible. It is important to assess for signs of mandibular invasion, including subtle cortical erosions, which are better appreciated on CT. Mandibular involvement upstages the cancer to T4, and the extent of osseous invasion (cortical vs. marrow invasion) affects surgical management. MR imaging is useful to assess for marrow invasion.[31,32,40]

Tumors can extend posteriorly to involve the posterior oral tongue or the base of the tongue, the submandibular gland, or can directly extend inferiorly through the floor of the mouth or mylohyoid muscle, which are important factors for staging and surgical planning. Involvement of the extrinsic tongue muscles can also occur, although this finding no longer upstages the tumor to T4.[34] However, invasion of the skin of the face, the masticator and pterygoid spaces, and the skull base increase the T stage of the tumor to T4.

Lymphatic drainage of the floor of the mouth is predominantly through level I and II nodes.[2,17] Level IB and II nodes are frequently involved, with less frequent involvement of level IA. It is not uncommon for bilateral cervical nodal metastasis to be present. Increasing tumor thickness and presence of vascular invasion have been shown to increase the risk of nodal metastasis.[41–45]

7.6.3 Oral Tongue

Anatomy

The oral tongue represents the anterior two-thirds of the tongue, which is separated from the base of tongue by the circumvallate papillae. The base of the tongue is part of the oropharynx. The tongue is composed of intrinsic and extrinsic muscle fibers. The intrinsic muscles of the tongue include four interdigitating muscles: the superior and inferior longitudinal, transverse, and oblique muscles. The extrinsic tongue muscles originate from bony or soft-tissue attachments outside the tongue and their distal fibers interdigitate with the intrinsic tongue muscles. The four extrinsic muscles are the genioglossus, styloglossus, hyoglossus, and palatoglossus muscles, which originate from the genial tubercle of the inner mandible, anterior styloid process, cornua of the hyoid bone, and soft palate, respectively (▶ Fig. 7.10).[17]

The intrinsic and extrinsic tongue muscles are innervated by the hypoglossal nerve (CN XII), which courses through the sublingual space in between the mylohyoid muscle and the hyoglossus–styloglossus–palatoglossus muscle complex.[2,17] The palatoglossus muscle is also supplied by the vagus nerve (CN X) and the pharyngeal plexus. The sensory innervation of the anterior two-thirds of the tongue is by the lingual nerve, a branch of the trigeminal nerve (CN V), and gustatory fibers

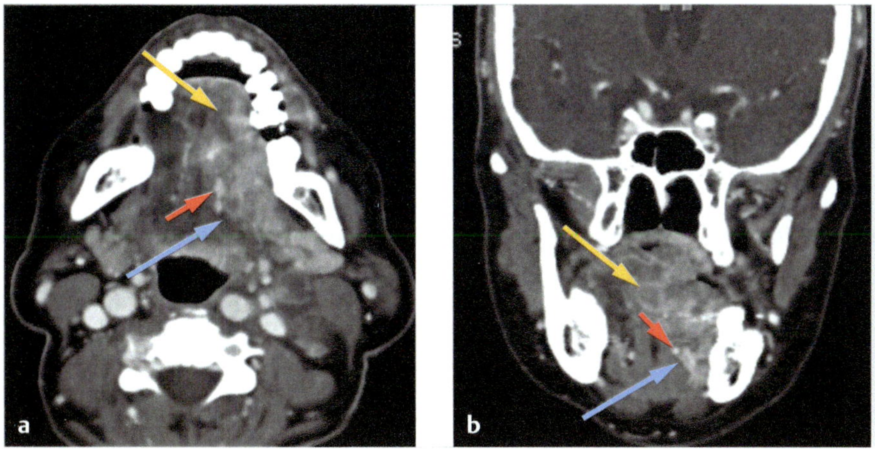

Fig. 7.9 Axial **(a)** and coronal **(b)** contrast-enhanced CT images show left tongue squamous cell carcinoma (*yellow arrows*) extending into the floor of the mouth. The mass is abutting the left lingual artery (*red arrows*) with loss of an intervening fat plane (*blue arrows*) suggesting invasion of the neurovascular bundle.

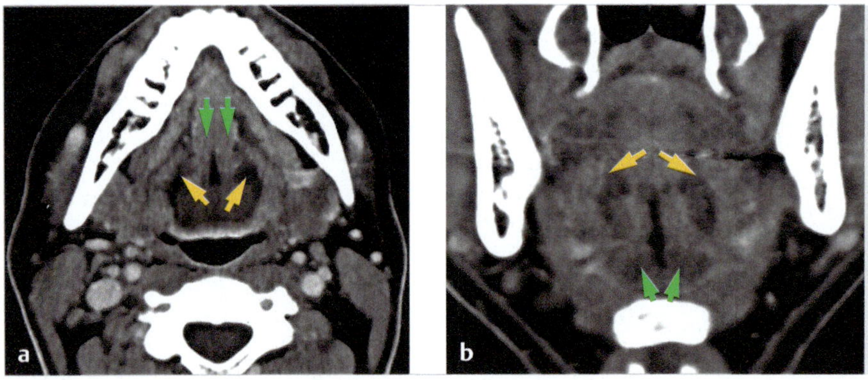

Fig. 7.10 Extrinsic muscles of the tongue. Axial **(a)** and coronal **(b)** contrast-enhanced CT images show normal genioglossus (*green arrows*) and hyoglossus muscles (*yellow arrows*).

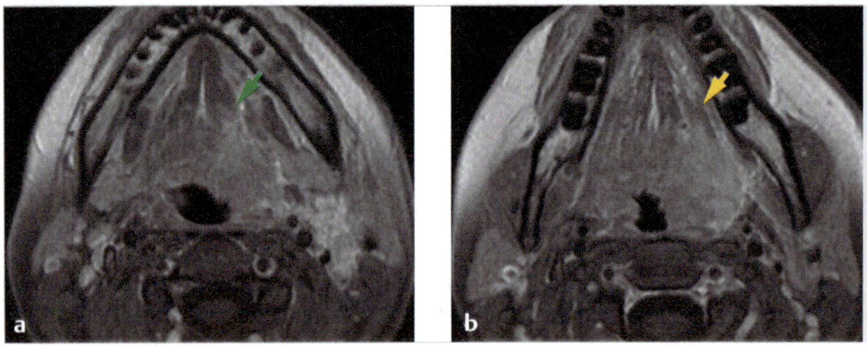

Fig. 7.11 Tongue squamous cell carcinoma (SCC) involving extrinsic tongue muscles. **(a)** Axial contrast-enhanced (CE) T1 fat-saturated (FS) MRI shows left tongue SCC with involvement of the left genioglossus muscle (*green arrow*). **(b)** Axial CE T1 FS MRI superior to **(a)** shows involvement of the left hyoglossus muscle (*yellow arrow*).

from the chorda tympani nerve, a branch of the facial nerve (CN VII).[17]

The primary lymphatic drainage is by the superficial mucosa and deep collecting system, both of which drain into anterior submandibular nodes (level IB). The superficial lymphatics drain into level IB and IIA nodes, whereas the deeper lymphatics of the oral tongue have drainage pathways to both sides of the tongue.[17]

Imaging Considerations

Nearly all oral tongue carcinomas occur along the lateral or ventral (undersurface) aspects of the tongue,[2,17] most frequently in the middle and posterior thirds of the oral tongue,[2] with approximately 75% of cases occurring on the posterolateral aspect of the oral tongue (▶ Fig. 7.1).[18] Diagnosis of superficial mucosal lesions is difficult on imaging. However, imaging evaluation of tongue cancer is important for assessment of submucosal extent and spread of tumor. Recent data have shown that DOI is a better prognostic indicator that tumor thickness for oral cavity cancers.[35] Pathologically, DOI is measured from the level of the basement membrane of the closest adjacent normal mucosa, and a "plumb line" is dropped from this plane to the deepest point of tumor invasion. While the tumor thickness can be measured with high accuracy by both CT and MRI, DOI is difficult to assess on imaging. Tumor thickness overestimates DOI in exophytic tumors, whereas it underestimates DOI in ulcerative tumors.

Imaging evaluation should include assessment for involvement of the extrinsic tongue muscles, although this finding no longer upstages the disease to T4.[34] Loss of fat planes between the extrinsic tongue muscles is often the only positive imaging finding (▶ Fig. 7.11). However, care must be taken not to suggest tumor involvement when tongue asymmetry is a result of fatty atrophy from denervation, which is a potential pitfall.[38] Tumors can spread along the extrinsic muscles to their sites of attachment, such as the mandible, hyoid bone, or styloid process (▶ Fig. 7.12).[2]

Evaluation of the midline lingual septum is very important as tumor extension across midline often precludes a hemiglossectomy as a surgical option and leads to either a total/subtotal glossectomy or nonsurgical treatment option.[2,17] Advanced tongue malignancies have defined routes of infiltration. Anterior third tumors tend to invade the floor of the mouth. Middle third tumors invade the tongue musculature and subsequently the floor of the mouth. If the tumor transgresses through the floor of the mouth, it can invade the mandible, skin of the face, and masticator and pterygoid spaces, all of which upstage the disease to T4 stage.[38] Posterior third tumors invade the anterior tonsillar pillar, tongue base, and glossotonsillar sulcus. Assessment of the tongue base is critical, as significant involvement of the tongue base may necessitate a total laryngectomy to prevent aspiration.[17,38]

Nodal metastasis is common with up to 35% of patients positive for nodal metastasis on presentation. Up to 30% of clinically N0 patients have occult metastasis.[46] The National Comprehensive Cancer Network (NCCN) guidelines recommend elective treatment of the clinically N0 neck if tumor depth is greater than 4 mm.[47] Although lymphatic drainage of the oral tongue primarily includes level IB and IIA nodes, studies have shown that up to 15% of lateral oral tongue cancers have a tendency toward "skip lesions," or nodal metastasis to level III or IV without involvement of levels I or II. Bilateral nodal involvement in oral tongue cancers is also frequent.[46,48]

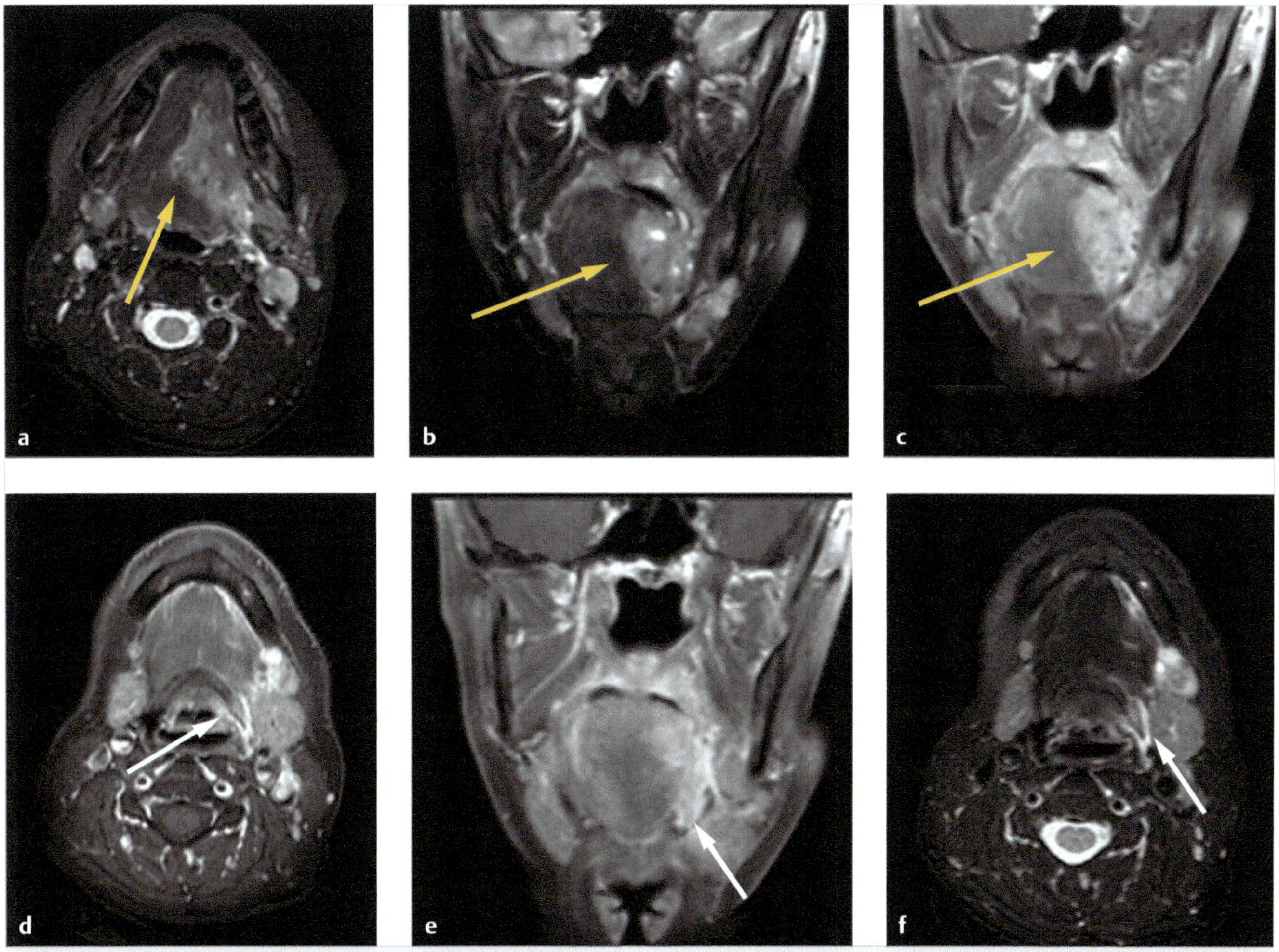

Fig. 7.12 Oral tongue squamous cell carcinoma (SCC) invading the hyoid bone. Axial and coronal T2 short tau inversion recovery (STIR; **a,b**) and coronal contrast-enhanced (CE) T1 fat-saturated (FS) MR images show large left oral tongue SCC (*yellow arrows*; **c**). Axial and coronal CE T1 FS MRI **(d–f)** and axial T2 STIR MR images show invasion of the left hyoid bone (*white arrows*).

7.6.4 The Retromolar Trigone

Anatomy

The RMT is a small triangle-shaped area of mucosa posterior to the last mandibular molar tooth overlying the anterior surface of the lower ascending ramus of the mandible (▶ Fig. 7.8).[1] It is continuous with the buccal mucosa laterally and the anterior tonsillar pillar medially. The superior extent is the maxillary tuberosity, and the anterior margin is the posterior aspect of the second mandibular molar tooth.[18]

The pterygomandibular raphe is a thick fibrous band that lies just beneath the mucosa of the RMT and provides attachment for the buccinator and superior pharyngeal constrictor muscles. This band connects the posterior mylohyoid line of the mandible to the hamulus of the medial pterygoid plate.[17] The pterygomandibular raphe is absent or incomplete in a substantial percentage of the adult population.[2]

Imaging Considerations

Cancers in the RMT may be primary or may be involved by direct extension from other subsites. Tumors in this location are relatively uncommon, accounting for approximately 5 to 12% of oral cavity cancers.[2] Cancers in the RMT usually present at an advanced stage and frequently involve the adjacent soft-tissue structures such as the anterior tonsillar pillar, soft palate, and lower gums. These tumors have a high propensity for early osseous invasion with reported rates of 12 to 53%.[49–51]

The RMT is an important site clinically as it serves as a crossroad for tumor spread in multiple directions to and from the oral cavity, oropharynx, buccal space, floor of the mouth, and masticator space. The tumor may spread posteriorly to the mandibular ramus, the masticator space, the superior constrictor muscles, and the mandibular branch of the trigeminal nerve. The tumor may also spread anteriorly along the alveolar ridge, and inferiorly along the mandible and the inferior alveolar nerve. If present, the tumor may also spread along the pterygomandibular raphe to the masticator space superolaterally involving the medial pterygoid muscle, which is often clinically evidenced by trismus, and the pterygoid process or the maxillary alveolus (▶ Fig. 7.13).[1,17] Involvement of the masticator space may allow perineural spread of the tumor along the lingual nerve, invasion of the skull base, and intracranial extension.[2]

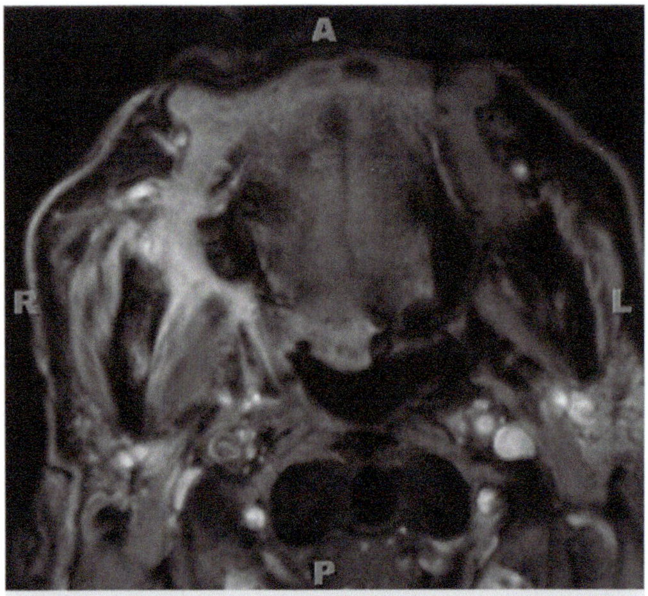

Fig. 7.13 Oral cavity cancer invading the pterygomandibular raphe. Axial contrast-enhanced fat-saturated T1 MRI shows involvement of the right masticator space from spread of the right oral cavity squamous cell carcinoma (not shown) via the pterygomandibular raphe.

7.6.5 The Upper and Lower Gingivae

Anatomy

The gingiva or "gums" represent the mucosal covering of the lingual (medial/inner) and buccal (lateral/outer) surfaces of the alveolar mandible and the maxilla. The junction between the gingival and the buccal mucosa lining the cheek is called the gingivobuccal sulcus.[17]

Imaging Considerations

Gingival or alveolar ridge cancers account for less than 10% of oral cavity cancers,[17] and the lower alveolar ridge is more frequently involved than the upper alveolar ridge.[2] Tumors of the lower alveolar ridge tend to spread medially to the floor of the mouth and laterally to the buccal and masticator spaces. In the upper alveolar ridge, tumors tend to spread medially to the palate, maxillary sinus, and nasal cavity.[38] Due to their close proximity to the underlying bone, osseous invasion of the mandible or maxilla is common. Mandibular involvement may allow perineural spread of the tumor along the inferior alveolar nerve.[2,18,38]

It can be difficult to distinguish a lateral gingival tumor from a buccal mucosal lesion on imaging. For CT, a "puffed cheek" technique separates the opposing mucosal surfaces and can be helpful in identifying the site of origin.[17,52] Due to long acquisition times, this technique is not feasible for MRI, and an alternative method is to pad the oral cavity at the site of the lesion with gauze.[38] These maneuvers are rarely necessary, however, as the superficial extent of tumor is readily assessable by the clinical examination. Inclusion of the clinical tumor subsite in the imaging order may assist the interpretation of the radiologist.

7.6.6 The Buccal Mucosa

Anatomy

The buccal mucosa covers the cheeks and lips and it is continuous with the buccal aspect of the gingiva of the maxillary and mandibular alveolar ridge, as well as the RMT.

Imaging Considerations

Carcinomas of the buccal mucosa tend to occur on the lateral walls, most frequently occurring adjacent to the third mandibular molar.[18] Verrucous carcinoma is a rare and nonaggressive form of SCC that mainly affects the buccal mucosa.[2,18] These tumors have a tendency for superficial spread and have a relatively good prognosis. However, invasive carcinomas can occur as well with submucosal extension.[2]

A relative lack of anatomic barriers allows buccal mucosa cancers to invade various structures within the buccal space including the buccinator muscle, Stensen's duct, and even the parotid gland if it extends posteriorly. Tumors may also extend to the RMT, the pterygomandibular raphe, and the underlying bone.[1,2,17,38] Buccal cancers can also extend submucosally to eventually involve the skin of the face.[17]

Lymphatic drainage of the buccal mucosa is primarily through level IB and IIA nodes. Anterior tumors metastasize to the submandibular level IB nodes, and posterior tumors metastasize to the high jugulodigastric or level IIA nodes.[1,18]

7.6.7 Hard Palate

Anatomy

The palate forms the roof of the mouth and is divided into the hard palate and the soft palate. The hard palate forms the superior margin of the oral cavity, and the inferior margin of the nasal cavity. It is a thin horizontal bone that spans the arch formed by the alveolar ridges and the upper teeth. The anterior two-thirds of the hard palate is formed by the palatine processes of the maxillae, and the posterior third of the hard palate is formed by the horizontal plates of the palatine bones. Posteriorly, the hard palate is contiguous with the soft palate, which is a subsite of the oropharynx.[17,52]

The mucosa covering the hard palate is thick and tightly bound to the periosteum of the underlying bones. Laterally, there is a submucosa that contains the neurovascular bundles that run in the roof of the mouth. The highest concentration of minor salivary glands in the oral cavity is found in the hard palate.[52]

The sensory innervation is from the greater palatine nerves and the nasopalatine branches of the maxillary nerve (CN V2). The paired greater palatine nerve runs through the greater palatine foramina, which are located medial to the posterior third molars within the lateral aspects of the bony palate. The incisive canal houses the nasopalatine nerves, which is found within the anterior hard palate, just posterior to the incisor teeth.[17,52]

Imaging Considerations

SCC of the hard palate is rare, accounting for approximately 0.5 to 6% of oral cavity cancers,[2] but still accounts for the most

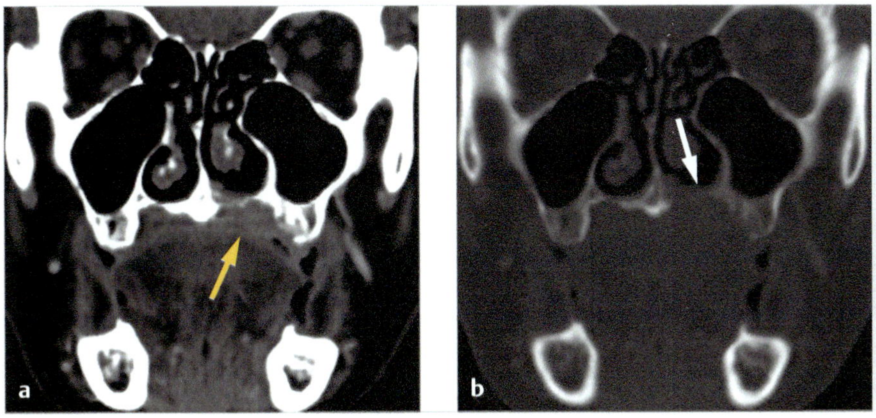

Fig. 7.14 Hard palate squamous cell carcinoma T4. **(a)** Coronal contrast-enhanced (CE) CT soft-tissue window shows soft-tissue mass (*yellow arrow*) arising from the left hard palate. **(b)** Coronal CE CT bone window shows cortical erosion of the left hard palate/maxilla (*white arrow*).

common malignancy of the hard palate. The hard palate is also a relatively frequent site of minor salivary gland tumors, including adenoid cystic, mucoepidermoid, and adenocarcinomas, which are a close second to SCC involvement in this region.[18] Oral cavity minor salivary gland tumors are most often found at the junction of the hard and soft palates.[17]

Due to their close proximity to the underlying bone, a major concern for hard palate cancers is osseous invasion (▶ Fig. 7.14), with possible extension into the maxillary sinus and nasal cavity. Tumors are difficult to identify on axial images due to the transverse orientation of the hard palate. Coronal and sagittal views are important for assessment of these lesions and any erosion of the underlying bone.[2,17]

Another major concern for hard palate cancers is perineural spread along the greater and lesser palatine nerves to the PPF, which provides a route for spread along the maxillary nerve to the gasserian ganglion and intracranial compartment. On CT, it is important to assess for widening of the greater palatine foramen, PPF, and foramen rotundum, which can be a sign of perineural spread. MR imaging is useful for direct evaluation of perineural spread of tumor.[1,2,17,38]

7.7 Conclusion

Radiologic imaging plays an important role in the assessment of oral cavity cancers. CT and MRI are complementary in evaluation of cancers in the subsites of the oral cavity and their routes of spread. Important features to assess on CT and MRI include, but are not limited to, the DOI, extension across the midline, invasion of the neurovascular bundle, perineural spread, osseous invasion, and nodal metastasis.

Key Points

- Radiologic imaging plays an important role in evaluation and staging of oral cavity cancer. CT, MRI, and PET/CT are important in assessment of tumor size, bone invasion, lymphadenopathy, presence of nodal extracapsular extension, perineural spread, second synchronous lesion, and distant metastases, and often complement each other especially in assessment of complex cases.
- CT provides good evaluation of oral tongue and exquisite evaluation of cortical bone involvement but may be limited in certain cases due to streak artifact from dental amalgam making tumor visualization hard. MR imaging offers better soft-tissue contrast and can complement CT in accurately delineating tumor extent and thickness.
- ECS is an important finding as it results in an approximately 50% reduction in survival. Both CT and MRI sensitivity and specificity are around 50 to 60% for ECS from meta-analysis studies and should be carefully looked at and reported.
- MRI is superior to CT for direct assessment of perineural spread although foraminal enlargement and soft-tissue attenuation replacing fat attenuation within the foramina on CT are important clues.
- Retromolar trigone and PPFs provide route for spread along the nerves and have connections between different neck spaces and also can lead to intracranial extension and should be very carefully evaluated on imaging once tumor involves/ extends to these spaces.

References

[1] Trotta BM, Pease CS, Rasamny JJ, Raghavan P, Mukherjee S. Oral cavity and oropharyngeal squamous cell cancer: key imaging findings for staging and treatment planning. Radiographics. 2011; 31(2):339–354

[2] Forghani R, Smoker WRK, Curtin HD. Pathology of the oral region. In: Som PM, Curtin HD, eds. Head and Neck Imaging. 5th ed. St. Louis, MO: Mosby; 2011:1643–1748

[3] Ferlay J, Soerjomataram I, Dikshit R, et al. Cancer incidence and mortality worldwide: sources, methods and major patterns in GLOBOCAN 2012. Int J Cancer. 2015; 136(5):E359–E386

[4] Cooper JS, Porter K, Mallin K, et al. National Cancer Database report on cancer of the head and neck: 10-year update. Head Neck. 2009; 31(6):748–758

[5] Lubin JH, Purdue M, Kelsey K, et al. Total exposure and exposure rate effects for alcohol and smoking and risk of head and neck cancer: a pooled analysis of case-control studies. Am J Epidemiol. 2009; 170(8):937–947

[6] Hashibe M, Brennan P, Benhamou S, et al. Alcohol drinking in never users of tobacco, cigarette smoking in never drinkers, and the risk of head and neck cancer: pooled analysis in the International Head and Neck Cancer Epidemiology Consortium. J Natl Cancer Inst. 2007; 99(10):777–789

[7] Thun M, Peto R, Boreham J, Lopez AD. Stages of the cigarette epidemic on entering its second century. Tob Control. 2012; 21(2):96–101

[8] Sturgis EM, Cinciripini PM. Trends in head and neck cancer incidence in relation to smoking prevalence: an emerging epidemic of human papillomavirus-associated cancers? Cancer. 2007; 110(7):1429–1435

[9] McCormack VA, Boffetta P. Today's lifestyles, tomorrow's cancers: trends in lifestyle risk factors for cancer in low- and middle-income countries. Ann Oncol. 2011; 22(11):2349–2357

[10] Kademani D. Oral cancer. Mayo Clin Proc. 2007; 82(7):878–887

[11] van Leeuwen MT, Grulich AE, McDonald SP, et al. Immunosuppression and other risk factors for lip cancer after kidney transplantation. Cancer Epidemiol Biomarkers Prev. 2009; 18(2):561–569

[12] Liang XH, Lewis J, Foote R, Smith D, Kademani D. Prevalence and significance of human papillomavirus in oral tongue cancer: the Mayo Clinic experience. J Oral Maxillofac Surg. 2008; 66(9):1875–1880

[13] Ha PK, Pai SI, Westra WH, et al. Real-time quantitative PCR demonstrates low prevalence of human papillomavirus type 16 in premalignant and malignant lesions of the oral cavity. Clin Cancer Res. 2002; 8(5):1203–1209

[14] Hashibe M, Sturgis EM. Epidemiology of oral-cavity and oropharyngeal carcinomas: controlling a tobacco epidemic while a human papillomavirus epidemic emerges. Otolaryngol Clin North Am. 2013; 46(4):507–520

[15] Lin J, Kutler DI. Why otolaryngologists need to be aware of Fanconi anemia. Otolaryngol Clin North Am. 2013; 46(4):567–577

[16] Zafereo ME. Evaluation and staging of squamous cell carcinoma of the oral cavity and oropharynx: limitations despite technological breakthroughs. Otolaryngol Clin North Am. 2013; 46(4):599–613

[17] Aiken AH. Pitfalls in the staging of cancer of oral cavity cancer. Neuroimaging Clin N Am. 2013; 23(1):27–45

[18] Wein RO, Weber RS. Malignant neoplasms of the oral cavity. In: Cummings C, ed. Otolaryngology head and Neck Surgery. 6th ed. Philadelphia, PA: Elsevier/Saunders; 2015:1359–1387

[19] Shah JP, Medina JE, Shaha AR, Schantz SP, Marti JR. Cervical lymph node metastasis. Curr Probl Surg. 1993; 30(3):1–335

[20] Menda Y, Graham MM. Update on 18F-fluorodeoxyglucose/positron emission tomography and positron emission tomography/computed tomography imaging of squamous head and neck cancers. Semin Nucl Med. 2005; 35(4): 214–219

[21] Pohar S, Brown R, Newman N, Koniarczyk M, Hsu J, Feiglin D. What does PET imaging add to conventional staging of head and neck cancer patients? Int J Radiat Oncol Biol Phys. 2007; 68(2):383–387

[22] Stuckensen T, Kovács AF, Adams S, Baum RP. Staging of the neck in patients with oral cavity squamous cell carcinomas: a prospective comparison of PET, ultrasound, CT and MRI. J Craniomaxillofac Surg. 2000; 28(6):319–324

[23] Cashman EC, MacMahon PJ, Shelly MJ, Kavanagh EC. Role of positron emission tomography: computed tomography in head and neck cancer. Ann Otol Rhinol Laryngol. 2011; 120(9):593–602

[24] Kim SY, Roh JL, Yeo NK, et al. Combined 18F-fluorodeoxyglucose-positron emission tomography and computed tomography as a primary screening method for detecting second primary cancers and distant metastases in patients with head and neck cancer. Ann Oncol. 2007; 18(10):1698–1703

[25] Johnson JT, Myers EN, Bedetti CD, Barnes EL, Schramm VL, Jr, Thearle PB. Cervical lymph node metastases. Incidence and implications of extracapsular carcinoma. Arch Otolaryngol. 1985; 111(8):534–537

[26] Kimura Y, Sumi M, Sakihama N, Tanaka F, Takahashi H, Nakamura T. MR imaging criteria for the prediction of extranodal spread of metastatic cancer in the neck. AJNR Am J Neuroradiol. 2008; 29(7):1355–1359

[27] Marchetta FC, Sako K, Murphy JB. The periosteum of the mandible and intraoral carcinoma. Am J Surg. 1971; 122(6):711–713

[28] Brown JS, Lowe D, Kalavrezos N, D'Souza J, Magennis P, Woolgar J. Patterns of invasion and routes of tumor entry into the mandible by oral squamous cell carcinoma. Head Neck. 2002; 24(4):370–383

[29] Montero PH, Patel SG. Cancer of the oral cavity. Surg Oncol Clin N Am. 2015; 24(3):491–508

[30] McGregor AD, MacDonald DG. Patterns of spread of squamous cell carcinoma within the mandible. Head Neck. 1989; 11(5):457–461

[31] Lane AP, Buckmire RA, Mukherji SK, Pillsbury HC, III, Meredith SD. Use of computed tomography in the assessment of mandibular invasion in carcinoma of the retromolar trigone. Otolaryngol Head Neck Surg. 2000; 122(5): 673–677

[32] Bolzoni A, Cappiello J, Piazza C, et al. Diagnostic accuracy of magnetic resonance imaging in the assessment of mandibular involvement in oral-oropharyngeal squamous cell carcinoma: a prospective study. Arch Otolaryngol Head Neck Surg. 2004; 130(7):837–843

[33] Imaizumi A, Yoshino N, Yamada I, et al. A potential pitfall of MR imaging for assessing mandibular invasion of squamous cell carcinoma in the oral cavity. AJNR Am J Neuroradiol. 2006; 27(1):114–122

[34] Lydiatt WM, Patel SG, O'Sullivan B, et al. Head and neck cancers—major changes in the american joint committee on cancer eighth edition cancer staging manual. CA: A Cancer Journal for Clinicians. 2017; 67(2):122–137

[35] Shim SJ, Cha J, Koom WS, et al. Clinical outcomes for T1-2N0-1 oral tongue cancer patients underwent surgery with and without postoperative radiotherapy. Radiat Oncol. 2010; 5:43

[36] Wreesmann VB, Katabi N, Palmer FL, et al. Influence of extracapsular nodal spread extent on prognosis of oral squamous cell carcinoma. Head Neck. 2016; 38 Suppl 1:E1192–E1199

[37] Prabhu RS, Magliocca KR, Hanasoge S, et al. Accuracy of computed tomography for predicting pathologic nodal extracapsular extension in patients with head-and-neck cancer undergoing initial surgical resection. International Journal of Radiation Oncology Biology Physics. 2014; 88(1):122–129

[38] Landry D, Glastonbury CM. Squamous cell carcinoma of the upper aerodigestive tract: a review. Radiol Clin North Am. 2015; 53(1):81–97

[39] Meesa IR, Srinivasan A. Imaging of the oral cavity. Radiol Clin North Am. 2015; 53(1):99–114

[40] Li C, Men Y, Yang W, Pan J, Sun J, Li L. Computed tomography for the diagnosis of mandibular invasion caused by head and neck cancer: a systematic review comparing contrast-enhanced and plain computed tomography. J Oral Maxillofac Surg. 2014; 72(8):1601–1615

[41] Close LG, Brown PM, Vuitch MF, Reisch J, Schaefer SD. Microvascular invasion and survival in cancer of the oral cavity and oropharynx. Arch Otolaryngol Head Neck Surg. 1989; 115(11):1304–1309

[42] Mohit-Tabatabai MA, Sobel HJ, Rush BF, Mashberg A. Relation of thickness of floor of mouth stage I and II cancers to regional metastasis. Am J Surg. 1986; 152(4):351–353

[43] Spiro RH, Huvos AG, Wong GY, Spiro JD, Gnecco CA, Strong EW. Predictive value of tumor thickness in squamous carcinoma confined to the tongue and floor of the mouth. Am J Surg. 1986; 152(4):345–350

[44] Wallwork BD, Anderson SR, Coman WB. Squamous cell carcinoma of the floor of the mouth: tumour thickness and the rate of cervical metastasis. ANZ J Surg. 2007; 77(9):761–764

[45] Huang SH, Hwang D, Lockwood G, Goldstein DP, O'Sullivan B. Predictive value of tumor thickness for cervical lymph-node involvement in squamous cell carcinoma of the oral cavity: a meta-analysis of reported studies. Cancer. 2009; 115(7):1489–1497

[46] Woolgar JA. Histological distribution of cervical lymph node metastases from intraoral/oropharyngeal squamous cell carcinomas. Br J Oral Maxillofac Surg. 1999; 37(3):175–180

[47] National Comprehensive Cancer Network. head and neck cancers (version 2.2017). Available at: https://www.nccn.org/professionals/physician_gls/pdf/head-and-neck.pdf. Accessed January 26, 2018

[48] Byers RM, Weber RS, Andrews T, McGill D, Kare R, Wolf P. Frequency and therapeutic implications of "skip metastases" in the neck from squamous carcinoma of the oral tongue. Head Neck. 1997; 19(1):14–19

[49] Ayad T, Guertin L, Soulières D, Belair M, Temam S, Nguyen-Tân PF. Controversies in the management of retromolar trigone carcinoma. Head Neck. 2009; 31(3):398–405

[50] Byers RM, Anderson B, Schwarz EA, Fields RS, Meoz R. Treatment of squamous carcinoma of the retromolar trigone. Am J Clin Oncol. 1984; 7(6): 647–652

[51] Huang CJ, Chao KS, Tsai J, et al. Cancer of retromolar trigone: long-term radiation therapy outcome. Head Neck. 2001; 23(9):758–763

[52] Smoker WRK, Som PM. Anatomy and imaging of the oral cavity and pharynx. In: Som PM, Curtin HD, eds. Head and neck imaging. 5th ed. St. Louis, MO: Mosby; 2011:1617–1642

8 Pathology and Cytopathology: Oral Malignant Mucosal Neoplasms

Lisa M. Rooper

Summary
This chapter discusses all aspects of the pathologic and cytopathologic evaluation of oral cavity squamous cell carcinoma and its precursor lesions, including diagnostic criteria for squamous dysplasia and squamous cell carcinoma, parameters used in histologic grading, common variants of squamous cell carcinoma, parameters used in pathologic tumor and lymph node staging, principles of margin evaluation, and other prognostically relevant elements of the pathology report.

Keywords: squamous cell carcinoma, oral cavity, pathology, histology, cytology, staging, margins

8.1 Introduction

More than 90% of malignancies that occur in the oral cavity are squamous cell carcinoma (SCC). While this statistic suggests a certain monotony to the pathologic examination of these lesions, it actually belies the rich variety of tumor morphology, grade, and variants included in this category as well as the challenging constellation of staging and prognostic variables that must be evaluated for each tumor. Correct and comprehensive pathological evaluation of these lesions forms the foundation for appropriate patient management and follow-up. This chapter provides an overview of the most relevant features and findings in the pathologic diagnosis and evaluation of oral cavity SCC and its precursors with an emphasis on new developments and priorities in the eighth edition of the AJCC Cancer Staging Manual[1] and the 2017 WHO Classification of Head and Neck Tumors.[2]

8.2 Precursor Lesions

Squamous dysplasia is well established as the main precursor of invasive SCC in the oral cavity. Pathologic diagnosis of dysplasia hinges upon assessment of both architectural and cytological atypia in squamous mucosa. As defined in the 2017 WHO Classification of Head and Neck Tumors, architectural changes that support a diagnosis of dysplasia include abnormalities in cellular stratification, loss of basal cell polarity, drop-shaped rete ridges, increased mitotic rate, the presence of superficial mitotic figures, single-cell keratinization, keratin pearl formation within rete ridges, and loss of epithelial cohesion.[3] Cytological changes that are seen in epithelial dysplasia include variation in nuclear size, variation in nuclear shape, variation in cell size, variation in cell shape, increased nuclear: cytoplasmic ratio, atypical mitotic figures, increased number and size of nucleoli, and nuclear hyperchromasia.[3] Unfortunately, there is no consistent threshold for determining how well developed or extensive these changes must be to differentiate dysplasia from hyperplastic and reactive processes.

The prognosis and management of squamous dysplasia is contingent upon the histologic grade that pathologists assign. Oral cavity dysplasia traditionally has been graded on a three-tiered system, with the atypia in mild dysplasia limited to the basal third of the epithelium, moderate dysplasia extending into the middle third of the epithelium, and severe dysplasia reaching the upper third of the epithelium (▶ Fig. 8.1).[3] Nevertheless, there is some flexibility in grading such that markedly increased cytological or architectural atypia, regardless of the epithelial stratum involved, supports an increased grade. The term carcinoma in situ can be used for full-thickness epithelial atypia but is essentially considered synonymous with severe dysplasia. Although a two-tiered system of just low-grade or high-grade dysplasia is now recommended for use in the larynx,[4] such a system has not yet been validated in the oral cavity. Given these flexible criteria, there is unsurprisingly poor interobserver agreement in the diagnosis and grading of squamous dysplasia.[5–8] Consequently, the prognostic implications of squamous dysplasia can vary widely between studies, with an overall rate of malignant transformation estimated at 12% in a large meta-analysis.[9] The likelihood of developing SCC is closely tied to histologic grade of dysplasia, being approximately 6% for mild dysplasia, 18% for moderate dysplasia, and 39% for severe dysplasia.[6] Nevertheless, pathologists must remember that SCC can arise even in the setting of mild or moderate dysplasia, in a pattern known as "drop" invasion.

A rarer precursor lesion to SCC that does not fit neatly into the category of squamous dysplasia is proliferative verrucous leukoplakia (PVL). PVL is a progressive, multifocal condition that can be very difficult to diagnose pathologically because of its variable and sometimes subtle histologic findings. At its earliest

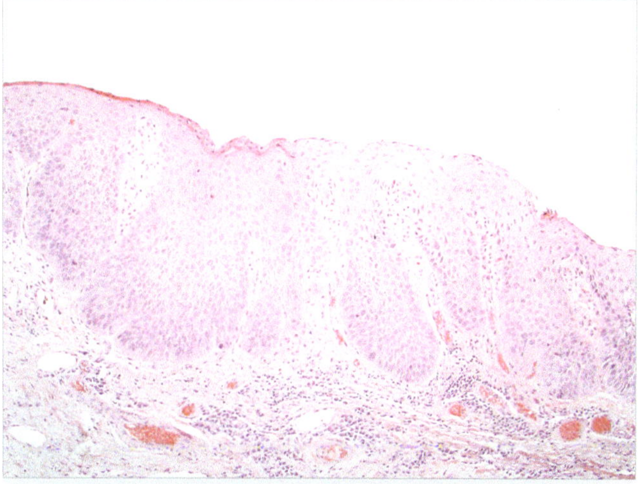

Fig. 8.1 The surface epithelium shows drop-shaped rete ridges, increased mitotic figures, nuclear pleomorphism, and nuclear hyperchromasia that extends to the upper third of the epithelium, consistent with severe squamous dysplasia.

stage, biopsy sampling of PVL may demonstrate only hyperkeratosis and verrucous hyperplasia. These lesions are frequently accompanied by interface mucositis, and may be mistaken for lichen planus or another reactive process.[3] As PVL progresses, however, lesions tend to develop more overtly dysplastic changes. Nevertheless, architectural atypia may be more marked than cytological atypia throughout the course of the disease. Pathologists must put these histologic changes in context of a clinical picture of recurrent and multifocal disease to help suggest this diagnosis. In contrast to conventional dysplasia, PVL has an approximately 50% risk of malignant transformation and can be associated with the development of both verrucous and conventional SCC.[10,11]

Several benign and reactive changes can pose a pitfall for pathologists when evaluating for squamous dysplasia. Broadly speaking, reactive changes in squamous epithelium comprise many features that overlap with dysplastic changes, including nuclear enlargement, mild nuclear membrane irregularity, prominent nucleoli, and increased mitotic figures; however, the presence of prominent inflammation and associated ulceration or granulation tissue can provide an important reminder to consider a reactive process. A wide range of insults can induce these reactive changes in squamous epithelium, including local trauma, inflammatory diseases such as lichen planus, and even unsampled underlying tumor. Candida infections can be especially treacherous in mimicking dysplasia because they can demonstrate marked architectural distortion, most notably elongation of the rete ridges, to accompany these reactive cytological alterations. Additionally, normal structures can also be mistaken for dysplasia in the oral cavity, particularly if a pathologist is not cognizant of anatomic site. Squamous epithelium surrounding the taste buds in fungiform papillae can demonstrate basal stratification that mimics dysplasia; recognition of sensory and sustentacular cells and underlying nerve fibers is essential to avoid this pitfall. Likewise, if approaching a pharyngeal site that is lined by respiratory epithelium, immature squamous metaplasia can be suggestive of disordered maturation. Seeing transition to adjacent respiratory mucosa and intermixed goblet cells can be helpful for detecting this benign process.

8.3 Squamous Cell Carcinoma

The pathologic diagnosis of SCC in the oral cavity hinges primarily on two features: the identification of invasive growth and the demonstration of squamous differentiation.[2] Histologically, oral cavity SCC is characterized by nests, cords, islands, and sheets of tumor cells that invade through the basement membrane to involve the subepithelial tissues and beyond. Invasion can be subtle in small and superficial tumors, and pathologists must meticulously evaluate the epithelial–stromal interface for small nests of infiltrative cells. However, infiltrative growth is not uniformly seen; invasion can also come in the form of broad, pushing-downward extension into stroma. Tumor cells can show varying evidence of squamous differentiation, manifesting as cytoplasmic keratinization with keratin pearl formation and intracellular bridges. In the highest-grade tumors, histologic hallmarks of squamous differentiation can be entirely absent, with sheets, nests, and cords of undifferentiated malignant cells. Immunohistochemical markers of squamous differentiation such as p40, p63, and CK5/6 may be necessary to establish the diagnosis in these cases.[12] Nonetheless, pathologists must remember that these markers are not entirely specific for squamous differentiation, being frequently seen in salivary tumors among others.[13,14]

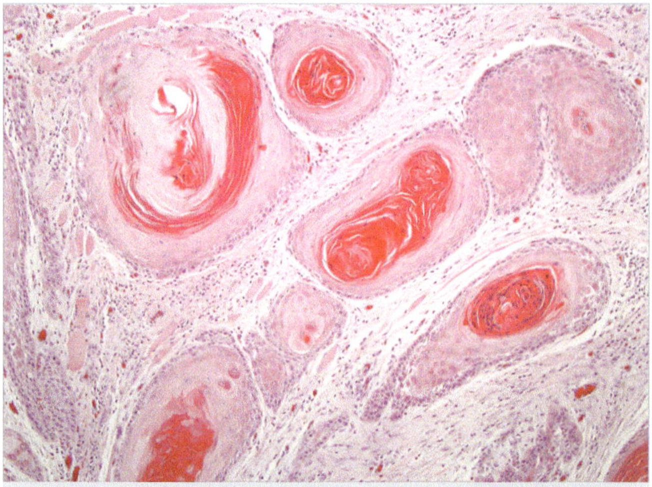

Fig. 8.2 Nests of squamous epithelium with exuberant keratin production and minimal cytologic atypia infiltrate through the skeletal muscle, diagnostic of well-differentiated squamous cell carcinoma.

Also analogous to squamous dysplasia, oral cavity SCC has traditionally been graded using a three-tiered system,[2] loosely based on the degree to which they resemble normal keratinizing squamous epithelium. In addition to the growth pattern and degree of keratinization, cytological atypia plays an important role in this classification. Well-differentiated SCC is characterized by obvious squamous differentiation, with large cells, prominent keratinization, and discernable intracellular bridges (▶ Fig. 8.2). These tumors frequently show minimal cytological atypia and some degree of maturation from basal-type peripheral cells to central keratinized cells, and can be difficult to distinguish from normal epithelium in small or tangentially embedded samples. Moderately differentiated SCC generally still show overt evidence of squamous differentiation, although keratin pearl formation and intracellular bridges might be focal compared to well-differentiated tumors. These tumors have more pronounced cytological atypia, including nuclear enlargement, nuclear pleomorphism, increased nuclear-to-cytoplasmic ratio, atypical mitotic figures, prominent nucleoli, and nuclear hyperchromasia; it is rarely difficult to discern that these tumors represent carcinoma (▶ Fig. 8.3). Finally, poorly differentiated SCC may have no overt histologic evidence of squamous differentiation, with nondescript to basaloid tumor cells that demonstrate minimal if any keratinization. These tumors also tend to have diffuse and well-developed cytological atypia (▶ Fig. 8.4). Although histologic grading does not always accurately reflect tumor prognosis,[15] it remains a key part of pathologic diagnosis.

Several benign processes can create findings that mimic well to moderately differentiated SCC. Necrotizing sialometaplasia poses a particular pitfall because it may present as an ulcerated lesion that also raises clinical suspicion for carcinoma. Histologically, this process is characterized by ischemic necrosis of minor salivary glands with resultant squamous metaplasia. Pathologists can distinguish necrotizing sialometaplasia from SCC due to its lobulated nature and contiguity with other

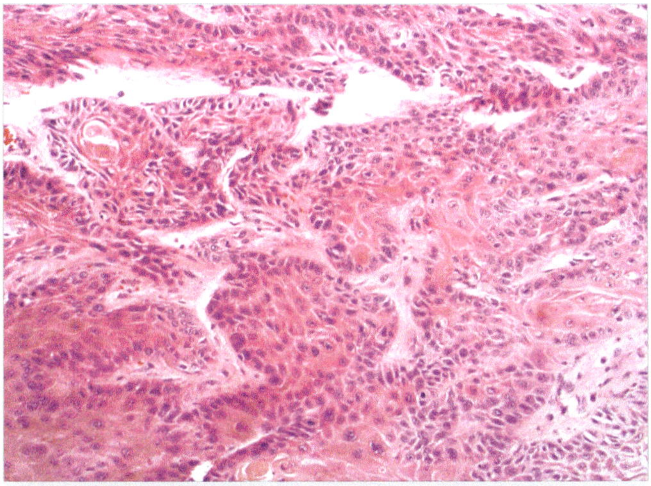

Fig. 8.3 Cords of markedly atypical cells with obvious squamous differentiation, including keratin pearls and intracellular bridges, are consistent with moderately differentiated squamous cell carcinoma.

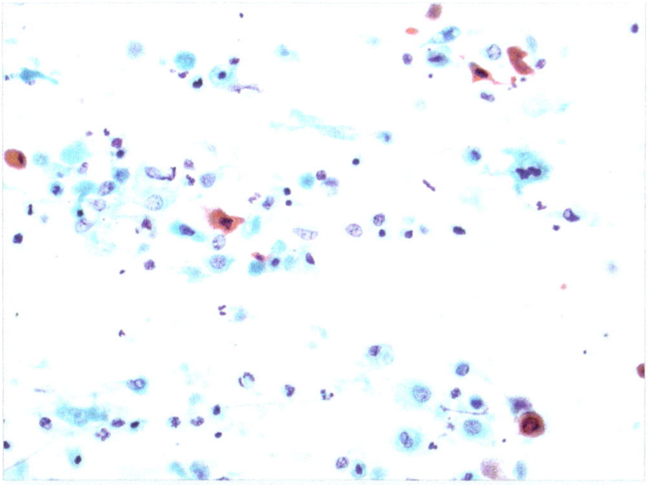

Fig. 8.5 Fine-needle aspiration specimens show sheets of malignant squamous cells with variable orangeophilia, nuclear hyperchromasia, nuclear enlargement, and nuclear membrane irregularities.

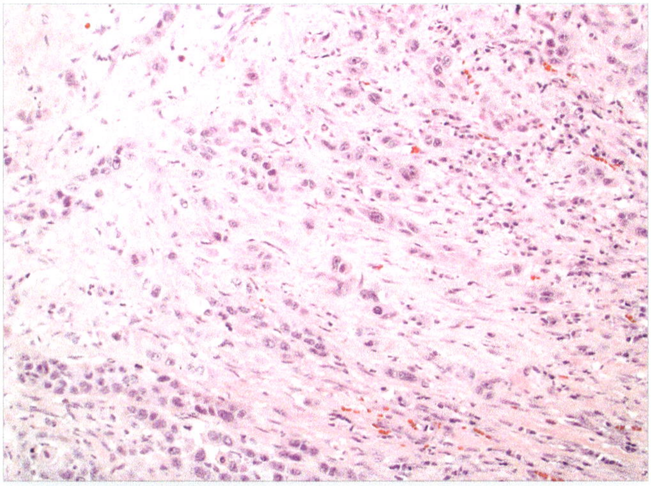

Fig. 8.4 Groups of malignant cells that entirely lack morphologic evidence of squamous differentiation can be seen in poorly differentiated squamous cell carcinoma.

salivary glands and ducts; however, marked reactive changes may pose a difficult differential diagnosis. Another important consideration is pseudoepitheliomatous hyperplasia, which can be induced by a wide range of reactive processes or tumors such as granular cell tumors or salivary gland neoplasms. In pseudoepitheliomatous hyperplasia, irregular tongues of squamous epithelium penetrate deeply into the subepithelium. These tongues of epithelium should lack the cytological atypia seen in SCC as well as significant abnormalities in cell cohesion and mitotic rate; however, abnormal keratinization is occasionally seen. Finally, normal structures can mimic SCC to the unwary observer. If specimen margins extend into the oropharynx, the reticulated epithelium of tonsillar tissue demonstrates an irregular stromal contour and numerous infiltrating lymphocytes that can be mistaken for invasive growth. Similarly, benign odontogenic remnants, including the juxtaoral organ of Chievitz in the retromolar area and rests of Serres in the gingival mucosa, can mimic invasive growth.

The histologic features of oral cavity SCC are mirrored in cytological sampling of these tumors. Cytopathological evaluation of oral cavity tumors occurs almost exclusively through fine-needle aspiration of cervical lymph node metastases; although epithelial brushings can be performed for primary diagnosis, this technique has inferior sensitivity compared to surgical biopsy.[16] As with histologic samples, fine-needle aspirates must be evaluated for squamous differentiation; however, without the benefit of tissue architecture, identification of cytological atypia takes precedence over invasive growth.[2] Squamous differentiation is generally easy to establish in common cytological preparations, with a characteristic robin egg blue color on Romanowsky-based stains and distinctive orangeophilic staining on Papanicolaou stains. Tumor cells can show varying degrees of cytological atypia, including nuclear hyperchromasia, nuclear enlargement, nuclear membrane irregularity, and atypical mitotic figures (▶ Fig. 8.5). Aspirates from lymph node metastases with cystic degeneration or treatment effect sometimes show only a mix of necrotic debris and rare parakeratinized cells, precluding a definitive diagnosis. Another important pitfall in cytological diagnosis of SCC is benign squamous-lined cysts such as branchial cleft cysts, which can raise misplaced concern for metastatic disease. However, these lesions should lack cytological atypia and have abundant foamy macrophages, indicative of their cystic nature.

8.4 Squamous Cell Carcinoma Variants

Several subtypes of SCC can rarely be seen in the oral cavity. In this site, the three variants that have equivalent or worse prognosis compared to conventional SCC are basaloid SCC, spindle cell (sarcomatoid) SCC, and adenosquamous carcinoma. Basaloid SCC is characterized by hyperchromatic cells with a high nuclear-to-cytoplasmic ratio, an adenoidal growth pattern, comedo-type necrosis, and prominent extracellular basement membrane-type material; it frequently raises diagnostic consideration of high-grade adenoid cystic carcinoma or neuroendocrine tumors.[17] It has overall similar prognosis to conventional SCC in the oral cavity but a higher rate of metastases.[18,19] Spindle cell (sarcomatoid) SCC frequently presents as a polypoid ulcerated lesion with overtly malignant spindled cells and variable morphologic and immunohistochemical evidence of squamous differentiation.[20] These tumors most commonly occur postradiation or as a second primary in the oral cavity and have a worse prognosis than conventional SCC.[21,22] Finally, adenosquamous carcinoma is characterized by biphasic architecture that encompasses a superficial squamous component and a deep glandular component.[23] These aggressive tumors also tend to have worse prognosis than conventional SCC.[24–26]

In contrast, verrucous carcinoma, papillary SCC, and carcinoma cuniculatum tend to have a better prognosis than conventional SCC in the oral cavity. Verrucous carcinoma is characterized by exophytic growth with prominent spires of parakeratin, minimal cytologic atypia, and a pushing pattern of invasion into underlying stroma.[27] Although verrucous carcinoma has the capacity for destructive local growth, it lacks true metastatic potential.[28,29] Papillary carcinoma also demonstrates exophytic growth, but its delicate fibrovascular cores are surrounded by overtly malignant squamous epithelium with notable cytological atypia.[30] Papillary carcinoma does have the potential for metastatic growth even in the absence of conventional invasion.[28,29,31] Finally, carcinoma cuniculatum is characterized by deeply invasive growth in a burrowing pattern with prominent tunnels of cytologically bland epithelium and prominent keratin production. Carcinoma cuniculatum has a tendency for local recurrence but only rarely metastasizes.[32]

8.5 Pathologic Staging and Prognostication

Pathologic tumor staging of oral cavity SCC has historically been based on tumor size and extent of involvement of adjacent structures, features that are well established to shape the prognosis in these lesions.[1] Along with these traditional elements, depth of invasion has been formally incorporated into the 8th edition of the AJCC oral cavity pathologic staging system.[1] The tumor thickness or depth of invasion have long been recognized as a vital prognostic feature in oral cavity SCC.[33,34] Although these two parameters are similar, there are slight differences in the techniques used for measurement. Depth of invasion is measured by drawing a "plumb line" from adjacent normal mucosa down to the deepest point of invasive growth.[1] In contrast, tumor thickness is measured from the mucosal surface of the tumor itself to the deepest point of invasive growth. Depth of invasion is currently regarded as the more accurate measurement because it does not underestimate the degree of tumor penetration in the cases with extensive ulceration. However, tumor thickness may be more accurate in tumors with predominantly exophytic growth.

Although not formally included in the AJCC staging system, many other factors carry prognostic significance in oral cavity SCC. Perineural and lymphovascular invasion are both well established to confer a negative prognosis in oral tumors.[35,36]

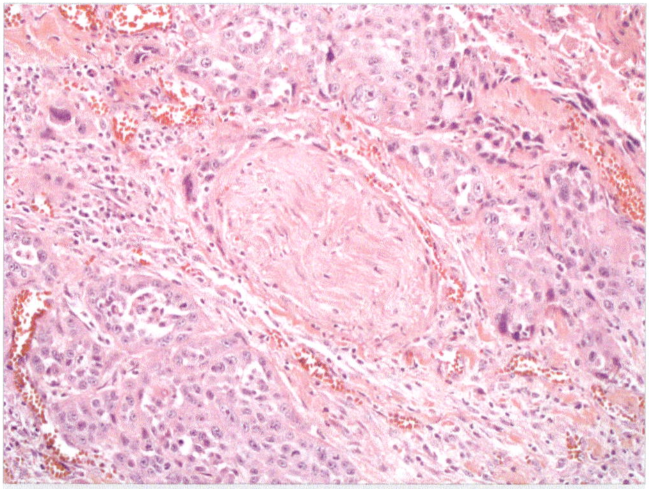

Fig. 8.6 A group of tumor cells is present within the perineurium of a small nerve fiber, supporting a diagnosis of perineural invasion.

Perineural invasion is associated with a higher rate of recurrent and metastatic disease in oral SCC,[37] with emerging evidence indicating that extratumoral perineural invasion has particularly adverse prognostic implications.[38] When diagnosing perineural invasion, it is essential that pathologists ignore tumor that is superficially abutting nerve bundles and consider only tumor directly involving the perineurium (▶ Fig. 8.6). Tumor that entirely surrounds the nerve seems to have a particularly bad prognosis.[39] Lymphovascular invasion is also associated with significantly decreased outcomes in oral SCC.[36] Pathologists should look for tumor plugs occupying lymphatic and venous spaces primarily at the edge of invasive tumors. These true foci of lymphovascular invasion must be distinguished histologically from tumor cells that were artifactually displaced into vascular spaces by a microtome and tumor nests surrounded by retraction artifact during processing. Because of their prognostic implications, both perineural and lymphovascular invasions are considered adverse risk features that merit additional therapy.[1]

Pattern of invasion is an emerging feature that has also been shown to have prognostic significance in oral cavity SCC, although it has not yet been formally incorporated into staging or treatment algorithms. Five separate histologic patterns of invasion have been described in oral cavity SCC, including[1] a pushing border,[2] finger-like growth,[3] large separate tumor islands of greater than 15 cells each,[4] small tumor islands of ≤ 15 tumor cells each, and[5] tumor satellites ≥ 1 mm away from the main tumor or each other.[15] When the worst pattern of invasion (WPOI) seen in each tumor is assessed, the presence of satellite nodules ≥ 1 mm away from the main tumor or each other, also known as WPOI-5, has been shown in multivariate analysis to have an adverse impact on prognosis.[15,40] However, this category includes islands of tumor involved in perineural or lymphovascular invasion and may reflect some prognostic overlap with those features.

8.6 Pathologic Assessment of Margins

In general, achievement of negative margins in oral cavity SCC is associated with lower rates of local recurrence and improved survival.[41–43] Pathologically, positive margins are defined by seeing tumor touching the inked or cauterized specimen edge of a resection specimen or identifying any tumor on a piece of tissue that is entirely designated as a margin. However, defining what constitutes an adequate margin in head and neck resections is still fraught with some uncertainty, with definitions that are highly dependent on anatomic site. In the oral cavity, margins of ≥ 5 mm are generally considered the minimal acceptable clearance and are associated with better outcomes than even negative but closer margins.[2] In some reports, margins of just 1 to 2 mm can be considered adequate if no further resection is possible; however, this circumstance is more common in the glottic larynx than oral cavity.[44] Severe squamous dysplasia at the resection margin is also correlated with a higher risk of local recurrence and second primary tumors.[45,46]

Recently, evidence has emerged that the techniques used to evaluate resections margins in low-stage SCC of the oral tongue can themselves influence patient outcomes. At the time of frozen section, margins from glossectomy specimens can be assessed in two ways. In the first method, the surgeon sends the entire resection specimen to pathology, and the pathologist grossly evaluates the entire specimen to select the areas where tumor most closely approaches margin for frozen section evaluation. This strategy allows precise quantitation of close margin intervals and accurate localization of positive margins. In the second method, the surgeon samples the mucosa of the tumor bed after resection, and the pathologist only performs frozen section on these tissue samples without gross evaluation of the resection specimen itself. This strategy is complicated by fragmentation of margins and difficulty orienting them with the main resection. Consequently, margins from the glossectomy specimen itself have been shown to be the only relevant prognostic factor in pT1–pT2, pN0 tumors; the tumor bed margins do not predict the risk of local recurrence.[47] Moreover, a multi-institutional study demonstrated a higher recurrence rate in the group of patients where only tumor bed margins were evaluated compared to patients where frozen sections were taken from the resection specimen itself.[48] If tumor bed margins are taken, it is recommended that they include only one tissue fragment that is large enough to account for the main specimen margins and are oriented by the surgeon with a designated true margin surface.[49] Regardless of method used at the time of frozen section, pathologists should report the final margins of the resection specimen.

8.7 Pathologic Evaluation of Lymph Node Metastases

Pathologic staging of lymph node metastases in the eighth edition of the AJCC Cancer Staging Manual is based on a combination of the number, size, and location of involved lymph nodes as well as the presence of extranodal extension (ENE).[1] The presence and extent of regional lymph node involvement is well established to be one of the most significant prognostic factors in oral cavity SCC, with positive lymph nodes associated with almost two times the risk of distant metastatic disease.[50] There is increasing evidence that surgical removal of at least 18 lymph nodes is associated with decreased rates of local-regional recurrence and improved survival.[51,52] Although no formal guidelines exist for the minimum extent of microscopic evaluation necessary in a lymph node dissection beyond that target, careful gross dissection with extensive tissue sampling is recommended to reflect the frequent presence of microscopic metastatic disease and even ENE in clinically negative necks.[53,54] On microscopic examination, it is generally straightforward to identify metastatic carcinoma without the need for routine ancillary staining in these tumors.

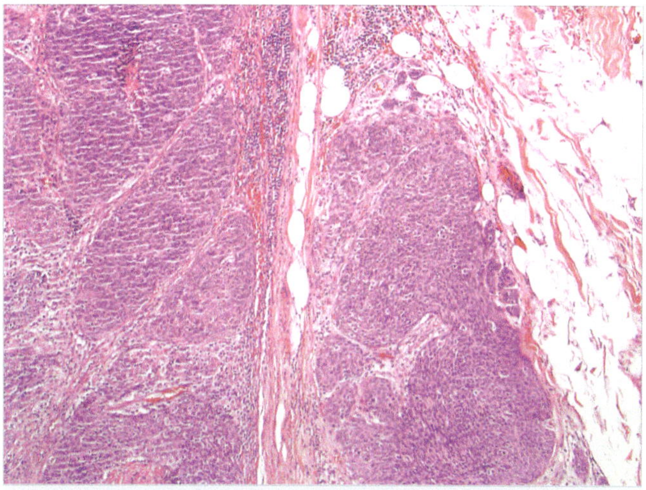

Fig. 8.7 A small plug of tumor extends beyond the fibrous lymph node capsule into the surrounding fibroadipose tissue, inducing a mild desmoplastic stromal response.

The inclusion of ENE in pathologic lymph node staging is a new addition to the eighth edition of the AJCC Cancer Staging Manual, with single unilateral nodes less than 3 cm with ENE classified as pN2a and all other nodes with ENE classified as pN3b.[1] Although there is some controversy about its value in the oropharynx, ENE is a well-validated prognostic factor in oral cavity SCC.[55] Indeed, the updated eighth edition of the AJCC classification including ENE has been shown to better predict prognosis in oral cavity SCC.[56] At the time of gross dissection, ENE can be suspected due to the presence of multiple matted lymph nodes or irregular tumor deposits in the fibroadipose tissue. Microscopically, ENE is defined by invasion of tumor cells beyond the lymph node capsule into surrounding fibroadipose tissue or adjacent structures; desmoplastic stromal response is frequently seen but is not required to diagnose ENE (▶ Fig. 8.7). However, assessing for ENE can be challenge due to irregular lymph node contours, capsular disruption, and variation in diagnostic criteria. Consequently, diagnosis of ENE has been shown to have poor interobserver agreement between pathologists.[57]

Although not yet required for staging oral cavity SCC, the eighth edition of the AJCC Cancer Staging Manual also recommends measurement of the distance ENE beyond the lymph node capsule.[1] This distance can be stratified into microscopic ENE (ENE_{mi}) for distances ≤ 2 mm and macroscopic ENE (ENE_{ma}) for distances greater than 2 mm, with a worse prognosis associated with a greater extent of ENE.[58,59] An alternate proposal to standardize assessment of ENE further subclassifies ENE levels, including (0) carcinoma limited to lymph node tissue, (1) carcinoma filling lymph node sinuses with thickened capsule, (2) carcinoma extending ≤ 1 mm beyond the lymph node capsule, (3) carcinoma extending greater than 1 mm beyond the lymph node capsule, and (4) carcinoma entirely obliterating nodal architecture.[60] These criteria, which were originally proposed for oropharyngeal SCC, modestly improved interobserver agreement in that site.[61] When applied to oral SCC, level 4 ENE with complete replacement of lymph nodes was shown to have a more adverse prognosis compared to more limited ENE.[59] However, this system has not been widely adopted in pathology practice.

Key Points

- The pathologic diagnosis of squamous dysplasia is based on a combination of architectural and cytological atypia and is graded by extent of epithelial involvement.
- The pathologic diagnosis of SCC requires both demonstration of invasive growth and squamous differentiation.
- Reactive processes and normal structures can mimic both squamous dysplasia and SCC.
- The basaloid, spindle cell, and adenosquamous variants are associated with similar or worse outcomes than conventional SCC in the oral cavity.
- The verrucous, papillary, and cuniculatum variants are associated with a better prognosis than conventional SCC in the oral cavity.
- Pathologic staging of oral cavity tumors is based on tumor size, depth of invasion, and extent of involvement of other structures.
- Perineural invasion, lymphovascular invasion, and pattern of invasion are also important prognostic factors in oral cavity SCC.
- Pathologic evaluation of margins in the oral cavity is best achieved by assessment of margins on the resection specimen rather than the tumor bed.
- Pathologic staging of lymph node metastases is based on size, laterality, and the presence of ENE.

References

[1] Ridge JA, Lydiatt WM, Patel SG, et al. Lip and oral cavity. In: Amin MB, ed. AJCC Cancer Staging Manual. 8th ed. Chicago, IL: American Joint Committee on Cancer, Springer; 2017:79–94

[2] Sloan P, Gale NKH, Lingen MW, et al. Malignant surface epithelial tumors. In: El-Naggar A, Chan JK, Grandis JR, Takata T, Slootweg PJ, eds. WHO Classification of Head and Neck Tumours. Lyon, France: International Agency for Research on Cancer; 2017:109–111

[3] Reibel J, Gale N, Hille J, et al. Oral potentially malignant disorders and oral epithelial dysplasia. In: El-Naggar A, Chan JK, Grandis JR, Takata T, Slootweg PJ, eds. WHO Classification of Head and Neck Tumours. Lyon, France: International Agency for Research on Cancer; 2017:112–115

[4] Gale N, Hille J, Jordan RC, Nadal A, Williams MD. Precursor lesions. In: El-Naggar A, Chan JK, Grandis JR, Takata T, Slootweg PJ, eds. WHO Classification of Head and Neck Tumours. Lyon, France: International Agency for Research on Cancer; 2017:91–93

[5] Fleskens SA, Bergshoeff VE, Voogd AC, et al. Interobserver variability of laryngeal mucosal premalignant lesions: a histopathological evaluation. Mod Pathol. 2011; 24(7):892–898

[6] Speight PM, Abram TJ, Floriano PN, James R, Vick J, Thornhill MH, et al. Interobserver agreement in dysplasia grading: toward an enhanced gold standard for clinical pathology trials. Oral Surg Oral Med Oral Pathol Oral Radiol. 2015; 120(4):474–82.e2

[7] Sperandio M, Brown AL, Lock C, et al. Predictive value of dysplasia grading and DNA ploidy in malignant transformation of oral potentially malignant disorders. Cancer Prev Res (Phila). 2013; 6(8):822–831

[8] Warnakulasuriya S, Reibel J, Bouquot J, Dabelsteen E. Oral epithelial dysplasia classification systems: predictive value, utility, weaknesses and scope for improvement. J Oral Pathol Med. 2008; 37(3):127–133

[9] Mehanna HM, Rattay T, Smith J, McConkey CC. Treatment and follow-up of oral dysplasia: a systematic review and meta-analysis. Head Neck. 2009; 31 (12):1600–1609

[10] Bagan JV, Jiménez-Soriano Y, Diaz-Fernandez JM, et al. Malignant transformation of proliferative verrucous leukoplakia to oral squamous cell carcinoma: a series of 55 cases. Oral Oncol. 2011; 47(8):732–735

[11] Upadhyaya JD, Fitzpatrick SG, Islam MN, Bhattacharyya I, Cohen DM. A retrospective 20-year analysis of proliferative verrucous leukoplakia and Its progression to malignancy and association with high-risk human papillomavirus. Head Neck Pathol. 2018; 12(4):500–510

[12] Bishop JA, Teruya-Feldstein J, Westra WH, Pelosi G, Travis WD, Rekhtman N. p40 (ΔNp63) is superior to p63 for the diagnosis of pulmonary squamous cell carcinoma. Mod Pathol. 2012; 25(3):405–415

[13] Owosho AA, Aguilar CE, Seethala RR. Comparison of p63 and p40 (ΔNp63) as basal, squamoid, and myoepithelial markers in salivary gland tumors. Appl Immunohistochem Mol Morphol. 2016; 24(7):501–508

[14] Rooper L, Sharma R, Bishop JA. Polymorphous low grade adenocarcinoma has a consistent p63+/p40–immunophenotype that helps distinguish it from adenoid cystic carcinoma and cellular pleomorphic adenoma. Head Neck Pathol. 2015; 9(1):79–84

[15] Brandwein-Gensler M, Teixeira MS, Lewis CM, et al. Oral squamous cell carcinoma: histologic risk assessment, but not margin status, is strongly predictive of local disease-free and overall survival. Am J Surg Pathol. 2005; 29(2):167–178

[16] Reddy CR, Kameswari VR, Prahlad D, Ramulu C, Reddy PG. Correlative study of exfoliative cytology and histopathology of oral carcinomas. J Oral Surg. 1975; 33(6):435–438

[17] Lewis JS, Gillison ML, Westra WH, Zidar N. Basaloid squamous cell carcinoma. In: El-Naggar A, Chan JK, Grandis JR, Takata T, Slootweg PJ, eds. WHO Classification of Head and Neck Tumours. Lyon, France: International Agency for Research on Cancer; 2017:85–86

[18] Fritsch VA, Gerry DR, Lentsch EJ. Basaloid squamous cell carcinoma of the oral cavity: an analysis of 92 cases. Laryngoscope. 2014; 124(7):1573–1578

[19] Xie S, Bredell M, Yang H, Shen S, Yang H. Basaloid squamous cell carcinoma of the maxillary gingiva: a case report and review of the literature. Oncol Lett. 2014; 8(3):1287–1290

[20] Bishop JA, Cardesa A, Helliwell TR, Hille J, Nadal A. Spindle cell squamous cell carcinoma. In: El-Naggar A, Chan JK, Grandis JR, Takata T, Slootweg PJ, eds. WHO Classification of Head and Neck Tumours. Lyon, France: International Agency for Research on Cancer; 2017:87–88

[21] Bice TC, Tran V, Merkley MA, et al. Disease-specific survival with spindle cell carcinoma of the head and neck. Otolaryngol Head Neck Surg. 2015; 153(6): 973–980

[22] Gerry D, Fritsch VA, Lentsch EJ. Spindle cell carcinoma of the upper aerodigestive tract: an analysis of 341 cases with comparison to conventional squamous cell carcinoma. Ann Otol Rhinol Laryngol. 2014; 123(8):576–583

[23] Prasad ML, Cardesa A, Helliwell TR, Hille J, Nadal A. Adenosquamous carcinoma. In: El-Naggar A, Chan JK, Grandis JR, Takata T, Slootweg PJ, eds. WHO Classification of Head and Neck Tumours. Lyon, France: International Agency for Research on Cancer; 2017:89

[24] Kass JI, Lee SC, Abberbock S, Seethala RR, Duvvuri U. Adenosquamous carcinoma of the head and neck: Molecular analysis using CRTC-MAML FISH and survival comparison with paired conventional squamous cell carcinoma. Laryngoscope. 2015; 125(11):E371–E376

[25] Masand RP, El-Mofty SK, Ma XJ, Luo Y, Flanagan JJ, Lewis JS, Jr. Adenosquamous carcinoma of the head and neck: relationship to human papillomavirus and review of the literature. Head Neck Pathol. 2011; 5(2):108–116

[26] Mehrad M, Trinkaus K, Lewis JS, Jr. Adenosquamous carcinoma of the head and neck: a case-control study with conventional squamous cell carcinoma. Head Neck Pathol. 2016; 10(4):486–493

[27] Zidar N, Cardesa A, Gillison ML, Helliwell TR, Hille J, Nadal A. Verrucous squamous cell carcinoma. In: El-Naggar A, Chan JK, Grandis JR, Takata T, Slootweg PJ, eds. WHO Classification of Head and Neck Tumours. Lyon, France: International Agency for Research on Cancer; 2017:84–85

[28] Mallick S, Breta M, Gupta SD, Dinda AK, Mohanty BK, Singh MK. Angiogenesis, proliferative activity and DNA ploidy in oral verrucous carcinoma: a comparative study including verrucous hyperplasia and squamous cell carcinoma. Pathol Oncol Res. 2015; 21(4):1249–1257

[29] Odar K, Gale N, Zidar N. Desmosomal proteins and microRNAs-markers for hybrid tumors (verrucous carcinoma with foci of squamous cell carcinoma). Ann Diagn Pathol. 2012; 16(2):157–158

[30] El-Mofty SK, Cardesa A, Helliwell TR, Hille J, Nadal A. Papillary squamous cell carcinoma. In: El-Naggar A, Chan JK, Grandis JR, Takata T, Slootweg PJ, eds. WHO Classification of Head and Neck Tumours. Lyon, France: International Agency for Research on Cancer; 2017:87
[31] Ding Y, Ma L, Shi L, Feng J, Liu W, Zhou Z. Papillary squamous cell carcinoma of the oral mucosa: a clinicopathologic and immunohistochemical study of 12 cases and literature review. Ann Diagn Pathol. 2013; 17(1):18–21
[32] Sun Y, Kuyama K, Burkhardt A, Yamamoto H. Clinicopathological evaluation of carcinoma cuniculatum: a variant of oral squamous cell carcinoma. J Oral Pathol Med. 2012; 41(4):303–308
[33] Ebrahimi A, Gil Z, Amit M, et al. International Consortium for Outcome Research (ICOR) in Head and Neck Cancer. Primary tumor staging for oral cancer and a proposed modification incorporating depth of invasion: an international multicenter retrospective study. JAMA Otolaryngol Head Neck Surg. 2014; 140(12):1138–1148
[34] Pentenero M, Navone R, Motta F, et al. Clinical features of microinvasive stage I oral carcinoma. Oral Dis. 2011; 17(3):298–303
[35] Woolgar JA. Histopathological prognosticators in oral and oropharyngeal squamous cell carcinoma. Oral Oncol. 2006; 42(3):229–239
[36] Jardim JF, Francisco AL, Gondak R, Damascena A, Kowalski LP. Prognostic impact of perineural invasion and lymphovascular invasion in advanced stage oral squamous cell carcinoma. Int J Oral Maxillofac Surg. 2015; 44(1):23–28
[37] Sinha N, Rigby MH, McNeil ML, et al. The histologic risk model is a useful and inexpensive tool to assess risk of recurrence and death in stage I or II squamous cell carcinoma of tongue and floor of mouth. Mod Pathol. 2018; 31(5): 772–779
[38] Miller ME, Palla B, Chen Q, et al. A novel classification system for perineural invasion in noncutaneous head and neck squamous cell carcinoma: histologic subcategories and patient outcomes. Am J Otolaryngol. 2012; 33(2):212–215
[39] Laske RD, Scholz I, Ikenberg K, et al. Perineural invasion in squamous cell carcinoma of the oral cavity: histology, tumor stage, and outcome. Laryngoscope Investig Otolaryngol. 2016; 1(1):13–18
[40] Brandwein-Gensler M, Smith RV, Wang B, et al. Validation of the histologic risk model in a new cohort of patients with head and neck squamous cell carcinoma. Am J Surg Pathol. 2010; 34(5):676–688
[41] Alicandri-Ciufelli M, Bonali M, Piccinini A, et al. Surgical margins in head and neck squamous cell carcinoma: what is "close"? Eur Arch Otorhinolaryngol. 2013; 270(10):2603–2609
[42] Hinni ML, Ferlito A, Brandwein-Gensler MS, et al. Surgical margins in head and neck cancer: a contemporary review. Head Neck. 2013; 35(9):1362–1370
[43] Liao CT, Chang JT, Wang HM, et al. Analysis of risk factors of predictive local tumor control in oral cavity cancer. Ann Surg Oncol. 2008; 15(3):915–922
[44] Weijers M, Snow GB, Bezemer DP, van dr Wal JE, van der Waal I. The status of the deep surgical margins in tongue and floor of mouth squamous cell carcinoma and risk of local recurrence; an analysis of 68 patients. Int J Oral Maxillofac Surg. 2004; 33(2):146–149
[45] Li Y, Bai S, Carroll W, et al. Validation of the risk model: high-risk classification and tumor pattern of invasion predict outcome for patients with low-stage oral cavity squamous cell carcinoma. Head Neck Pathol. 2013; 7(3): 211–223
[46] Weijers M, Snow GB, Bezemer PD, van der Wal JE, van der Waal I. The clinical relevance of epithelial dysplasia in the surgical margins of tongue and floor of mouth squamous cell carcinoma: an analysis of 37 patients. J Oral Pathol Med. 2002; 31(1):11–15
[47] Chang AM, Kim SW, Duvvuri U, et al. Early squamous cell carcinoma of the oral tongue: comparing margins obtained from the glossectomy specimen to margins from the tumor bed. Oral Oncol. 2013; 49(11):1077–1082
[48] Maxwell JH, Thompson LD, Brandwein-Gensler MS, et al. Early oral tongue squamous cell carcinoma: sampling of margins from tumor bed and worse local control. JAMA Otolaryngol Head Neck Surg. 2015; 141(12):1104–1110
[49] Prabhu AV, Sturgis CD, Lai C, et al. Improving margin revision: characterization of tumor bed margins in early oral tongue cancer. Oral Oncol. 2017; 75: 184–188
[50] Leemans CR, Tiwari R, Nauta JJ, van der Waal I, Snow GB. Regional lymph node involvement and its significance in the development of distant metastases in head and neck carcinoma. Cancer. 1993; 71(2):452–456
[51] Divi V, Harris J, Harari PM, et al. Establishing quality indicators for neck dissection: correlating the number of lymph nodes with oncologic outcomes (NRG Oncology RTOG 9501 and RTOG 0234). Cancer. 2016; 122(22):3464–3471
[52] Ebrahimi A, Clark JR, Amit M, et al. Minimum nodal yield in oral squamous cell carcinoma: defining the standard of care in a multicenter international pooled validation study. Ann Surg Oncol. 2014; 21(9):3049–3055
[53] Coatesworth AP, MacLennan K. Squamous cell carcinoma of the upper aerodigestive tract: the prevalence of microscopic extracapsular spread and soft tissue deposits in the clinically N0 neck. Head Neck. 2002; 24(3):258–261
[54] Suton P, Salaric I, Granic M, Mueller D, Luksic I. Prognostic significance of extracapsular spread of lymph node metastasis from oral squamous cell carcinoma in the clinically negative neck. Int J Oral Maxillofac Surg. 2017; 46(6): 669–675
[55] Johnson JT, Barnes EL, Myers EN, Schramm VL, Jr, Borochovitz D, Sigler BA. The extracapsular spread of tumors in cervical node metastasis. Arch Otolaryngol. 1981; 107(12):725–729
[56] Garcia J, Lopez M, Lopez L, et al. Validation of the pathological classification of lymph node metastasis for head and neck tumors according to the 8th edition of the TNM Classification of Malignant Tumors. Oral Oncol. 2017; 70:29–33
[57] van den Brekel MW, Lodder WL, Stel HV, Bloemena E, Leemans CR, van der Waal I. Observer variation in the histopathologic assessment of extranodal tumor spread in lymph node metastases in the neck. Head Neck. 2012; 34(6): 840–845
[58] Dünne AA, Müller HH, Eisele DW, Kessel K, Moll R, Werner JA. Meta-analysis of the prognostic significance of perinodal spread in head and neck squamous cell carcinomas (HNSCC) patients. Eur J Cancer. 2006; 42(12):1863–1868
[59] Prabhu RS, Hanasoge S, Magliocca KR, et al. Extent of pathologic extracapsular extension and outcomes in patients with nonoropharyngeal head and neck cancer treated with initial surgical resection. Cancer. 2014; 120(10): 1499–1506
[60] Lewis JS, Jr, Carpenter DH, Thorstad WL, Zhang Q, Haughey BH. Extracapsular extension is a poor predictor of disease recurrence in surgically treated oropharyngeal squamous cell carcinoma. Mod Pathol. 2011; 24(11):1413–1420
[61] Lewis JS, Jr, Tarabishy Y, Luo J, et al. Inter- and intra-observer variability in the classification of extracapsular extension in p16 positive oropharyngeal squamous cell carcinoma nodal metastases. Oral Oncol. 2015; 51(11): 985–990

9 Pathology: Oral Cavity Salivary Gland Malignancies

Elizabeth M. Kurian and Justin A. Bishop

Summary
Accurate diagnosis of minor salivary gland malignancies of the oral cavity determines prognosis and guides treatment. This chapter outlines the pertinent epidemiology, clinical presentation, and diagnostic histology. Pertinent associated molecular alterations are included, if applicable, with inclusion of the most common treatment considerations.

Keywords: mucoepidermoid carcinoma (MEC), adenoid cystic carcinoma (ACC), adenocarcinoma not otherwise specified, polymorphous adenocarcinoma (PAC), epithelial-myoepithelial carcinoma (EMC)

9.1 General Introduction

In the head and neck region, there are up to 750 minor salivary glands.[1] Minor salivary gland tumors represent a small subset (15–20%) of all salivary gland tumors, which in turn comprise only 3 to 5% of cumulative head and neck tumors.[2,3] The most common site of minor salivary gland tumors is the oral cavity. Unlike in major salivary glands, tumors of the minor salivary glands are predominantly malignant. The palate is the most common site of tumor involvement.[2,4–6] Based on geographic variability, the second most common site of involvement varies from tongue,[3,5] followed by either buccal mucosa or labial mucosa.[5–8]

Minor salivary gland malignancies affect all ages, with reported ranges of 6 to 96 years of age.[9] The mean age is 46 to 49 years.[3,5,9] The male-to-female ratio is 1.4:1 in Libyan and Indian study populations, with reported female predominance in the U.S. and Pakistan population studies.[5] The most common clinical presentation is a mass or swelling (72%), sometimes painful (13%) or less often as an ulcer (3%).[4] There are no known environmental associated risk factors (i.e., smoking, etc.), although genetic variants in deoxyribonucleic acid (DNA) double-strand break repair genes and germline *BRCA* mutations are associated with increased risk for salivary gland malignancies.[10]

The prevalence of histologic minor salivary gland carcinoma subtypes varies based on geography. Western countries (Australia,[8] United States, United Kingdom, Denmark) demonstrate a greater incidence of adenoid cystic carcinoma (ACC), followed by mucoepidermoid carcinoma (MEC). In contrast, this prevalence is reversed in some studies from India, Japan, United Kingdom, Australia, and the United States.[5,10] Overall, the most common malignant minor salivary gland tumors are MEC and ACC, followed by polymorphous adenocarcinoma (PAC) and adenocarcinoma not otherwise specified (NOS).[5,11]

In general, the primary treatment modality is complete surgical resection.[11] Chemotherapy is used only for palliative care.[1] Adjuvant or postoperative radiation therapy may be considered in cases with a positive surgical margin,[8,11,12] nodal metastases, high-grade carcinoma,[8,11,12] perineural invasion,[8,12] or in advanced malignancies with bone invasion.[9,12] In these cases, radiation may be effective for postoperative local control or as primary therapy for unresectable malignancies.[1,8] The rare minor salivary gland malignancies occurring in the pediatric population have a better overall survival and disease-free survival compared to adults.[11] Further details regarding the specific management of each subtype of oral cavity salivary gland malignancy can be found in Chapter 37. Overall, most studies show that clinical staging is the most important prognostic factor.[4]

9.2 Mucoepidermoid Carcinoma

9.2.1 Introduction

MEC is one of the most common intraoral minor salivary gland malignancies.[10] Histologically, it is composed of three cell types (mucinous, intermediate, and epidermoid cells) and classified into low-, intermediate-, and high-grade MEC.[10]

9.2.2 Epidemiology

The male-to-female ratio is 1:1.4; with an age range from 18 to 67 years (mean age of 60 years).[10] According to the WHO Classification of Head and Neck tumors, it is one of the most common salivary gland malignancies in young adults and children, and may be secondary to radiation exposure or prior treatment with chemotherapy (latency of 8 years).[10]

9.2.3 Clinical Presentation

While presentation is dependent on site, size, and grade,[10] it often presents as an asymptomatic dome or swelling. The most common site is the palate, followed by lower lip or alveolar mucosa.[7,10] A potential pitfall is when MEC may clinically mimic an intraoral mucocele.[10]

9.2.4 Diagnosis and Evaluation

MEC is characterized by three components, which include mucinous cells, intermediate-type cells, and epidermoid cells in variable proportions (▶ Fig. 9.1). The grading of these tumors accounts for solid versus cystic growth patterns, anaplasia, mitotic activity, necrosis, and invasiveness (i.e., perineural, lymphovascular, bone involvement, and/or metastasis).

Low-grade MECs are composed predominantly of a cystic component with a predominance of mucin, macrophages, and bland epithelioid cells. These lesions are usually well circumscribed.

Intermediate-grade MECs may show a mixture of solid and cystic components, without overt high-grade nuclear atypia, but are less well circumscribed. High-grade MECs are predominantly solid but must show at least focal intracellular mucin positivity to make the diagnosis.[10] According to the WHO classification, high-grade MECs should have at least one of the following: nuclear anaplasia, necrosis, increased mitotic rate, and perineural, lymphovascular, or bony invasion. The presence of keratinization is an unusual feature and may suggest squamous

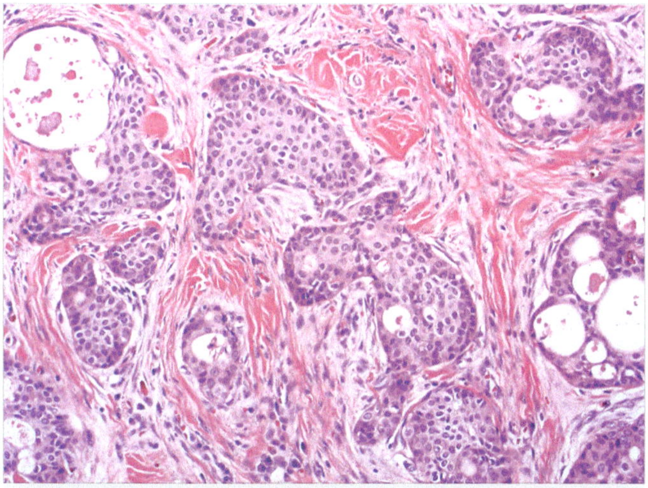

Fig. 9.1 Mucoepidermoid carcinoma consists of a mixture of epidermoid, mucinous, and intermediate cells growing as nests and microcysts.

carcinoma/non-MEC tumor (e.g., necrotizing sialometaplasia, pleomorphic adenoma with squamous metaplasia, sclerosing polycystic adenosis,[10] or epithelial-myoepithelial carcinoma [EMC] with squamous differentiation).

Ancillary studies such as a mucicarmine or periodic acid–Schiff (PAS) with diastase can highlight the mucin within the cytoplasm of the malignant cells. A p40 or p63 immunohistochemistry may be helpful to highlight epithelioid/intermediate cell components, or Ki-67 for better assessment of high mitotic activity within a poorly differentiated MEC. If there is extensive squamous differentiation, the differential diagnosis may also include squamous cell carcinoma of the oral mucosa. In high-grade MEC, at least focal mucin is required and keratinization would not be present.

Some variants of MEC include unicystic, sclerosing, ciliated, Warthin-like, oncocytic, clear cell, spindle cell, goblet cell aggressive, psammomatous, and sebaceous type.[13] These rare variants have no prognostic implications.[14] While these subtypes are rare in minor salivary glands, a brief review of the more histologically challenging variants are described for accurate recognition.

- Sclerosing mucoepidermoid carcinoma (SMEC) is characterized histologically by dense, central hyalinizing sclerosis that lacks an inflammatory response and may obscure classic histomorphologic features of mucin, intermediate cells, or the epidermoid component. The periphery of the tumor may show a mixed infiltrate of plasma cells, eosinophils, or lymphocytes. This is a rare variant with reports predominating in major salivary glands, and very few reports in minor salivary glands.[13]
- Ciliated MEC is defined by "macrocystic spaces punctuated by tubulopapillary proliferations of squamoid cells and ciliated columnar cells."[15] While the ciliated component may suggest benignity, the proliferation of squamous cells can be noted and ancillary molecular testing may assist with a definitive diagnosis.
- The oncocytic variant (OMEC) is characterized by the presence of polyhedral cells with granular eosinophilic cytoplasm that may be arranged in a cystic, organoid, or alveolar pattern with interspersed mucous cells. Few and/or variable squamoid cells and intermediate cells may be present. Only rare cases have been reported in minor salivary glands, all low grade ($n = 4$).[14] Immunohistochemistry for p63 or p40 is helpful in distinguishing OMEC from oncocytoma or oncocytic carcinoma, with diffuse staining typically seen in the former, and only patchy, peripheral staining in the latter.[14]

9.2.5 Molecular Testing

The gene fusions involving the *MAML2* gene (*CTRC1-MAML2* or CRTC3-MAML2) are found in the majority of MECs, of all grades (~75–80%).[15] This may be helpful in placing malignant cases into a definitive classification, when the histomorphologic diagnosis is elusive (i.e., poorly differentiated or variant MECs, etc.). Gene fusions involving *MAML2* are no longer thought to be a contributor to prognosis; therefore, routine *MAML2* testing for MEC is not required.[15]

9.2.6 Treatment Considerations and Approaches

Complete surgical excision is the primary treatment modality.

9.2.7 Key Points

- MEC is one of the most common intraoral salivary gland carcinomas.
- It is characterized histologically by variable proportion of epidermoid, mucinous, and intermediate-type cells, with associated gene fusions involving *MAML2*.
- Low-grade MECs are well circumscribed, have increased cystic component, and have a good prognosis (10-year survival of 90%).[10]
- High-grade MECs are poorly circumscribed, have a greater solid component, at least focal mucinous component, and more aggressive clinical course (10-year survival of 25%).

9.3 Adenoid Cystic Carcinoma

9.3.1 Introduction

Arising within the secretory glands, ACC is characterized histologically by two cell types (epithelial and myoepithelial cells). ACC has an aggressive clinical course with slow growth, neurotropism (less frequently lymphatic invasion), and propensity for metastatic disease.

9.3.2 Epidemiology

The male-to-female ratio is 1:1.5[10] with an age range of 20 to 78 years, most frequently occurring in older adults (age 60–79).[5,16] Local recurrence may occur, regardless of surgical margin status.[4] Distant metastasis is not uncommon, and ACC has an affinity for metastases to the lungs.[16] Late metastases may present as an isolated lesion and/or may present long after the primary diagnosis.[16] Complete resection is often challenging, and negative surgical margins are of prognostic benefit. Histologically, pathologic N-stage, perineural invasion, and ACC clinical stage are closely associated with the prognostic development of distant metastasis.[4,16]

9.3.3 Clinical Presentation

Frequent intraoral sites of ACC involvement include palate, floor of the mouth, alveolar, and buccal mucosa.[7]

9.3.4 Diagnosis and Evaluation

ACCs can be divided into three morphologic categories: (1) well-differentiated with tubular and cribriform mixed patterns and no solid components, (2) pure cribriform pattern (▶ Fig. 9.2), and (3) solid pattern predominating.[4] The pathologic review necessitates the assessment for key features such as perineural invasion and/or lymphovascular invasion.

In small biopsy evaluation, the presence of uniform glandular cells with a myxoid stroma lends to a morphologic differential diagnosis of PAC (formerly PLGA) versus ACC. In this setting, differential staining of p63 and p40 may be contributory to the diagnosis. ACC shows concordant staining with p40 and p63 (either both positive or both negative), whereas PAC is consistently p63 + /p40 (–).[17,18]

9.3.5 Molecular Testing

ACCs frequently have a reciprocal t(6;9) translocation, which results in impaired oncogene *MYB* fusion with transcription factor gene *NFIB* resulting in protein overexpression.[17] A small subset of ACCs harbor the alternate fusion *MYBL1-NFIB*.[19,20] All together, approximately 60 to 70% of ACCs harbor rearrangements of either *MYB* or *MYBL1*, and demonstrating one of these alterations is an effective strategy for distinguishing ACC from its mimickers.

9.3.6 Treatment Considerations and Approaches

The treatment for ACC is primarily complete surgical resection. On presentation, occasional patients may have nodal metastasis. Neck level IIa, II, or both are the most commonly involved locations.[4] For patients with close or positive surgical margins, nodal metastases, perineural, and/or lymphovascular invasion, postoperative radiation therapy may be given.[4]

9.3.7 Key Points

- ACC is composed of epithelial and myoepithelial cells, is highly neurotropic, and affects a wide age range.
- ACC has an aggressive clinical course with 80 to 90% of patients dying due to the disease in 10 to 15 years.[1]
- Tubular and cribriform ACCs have a better prognosis[21] and tend to spread by vascular rather than lymphatic system.[21]

9.4 Adenocarcinoma Not Otherwise Specified

9.4.1 Introduction

This category is exclusionary of known epithelial salivary gland carcinomas and is used to define gland-forming carcinomas of the salivary gland.

9.4.2 Epidemiology

The incidence of adenocarcinoma is approximately 10 to 15% of all salivary gland carcinomas. While most arise in major salivary glands, up to 40% occur within the minor salivary glands within the oral cavity[10]

9.4.3 Diagnosis and Evaluation

The histology of adenocarcinoma, NOS is quite variable, and may include proliferations of ducts in nests, cords, or solid sheets with or without cyst formations (▶ Fig. 9.3). The malignant cells may show a variety of types (i.e., clear, mucinous, oncocytic-appearing, plasmacytoid, columnar, or cuboidal). The

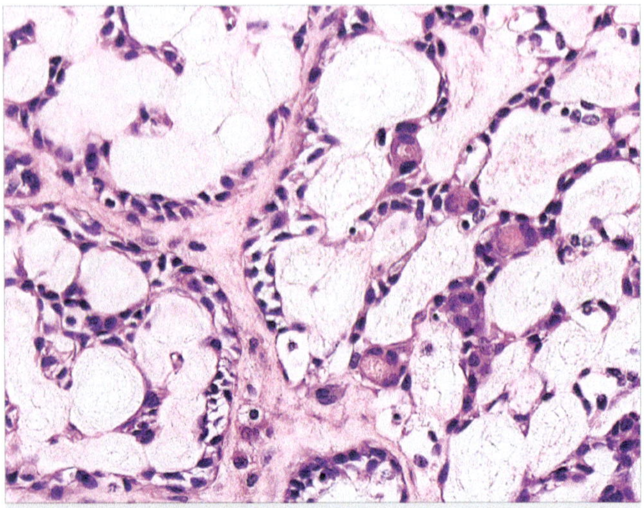

Fig. 9.2 Adenoid cystic carcinoma classically grows as cribriform structures with globules of abundant mucinous material.

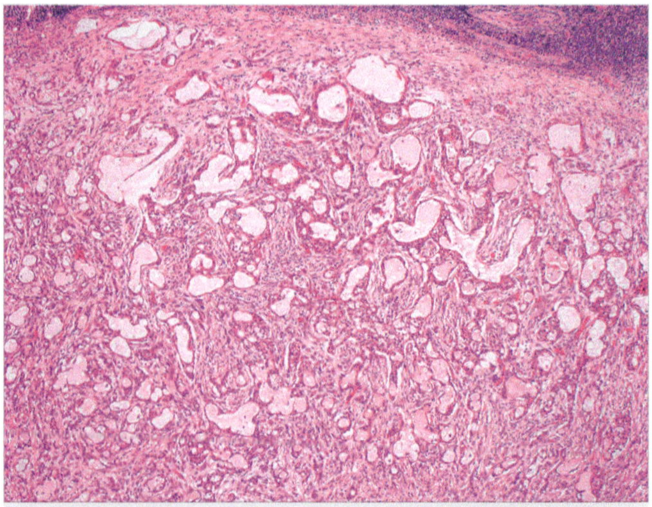

Fig. 9.3 Adenocarcinoma, not otherwise specified, is an infiltrative gland-forming neoplasm that cannot be better classified as another salivary gland tumor type.

grading of the carcinoma is based upon cellular atypia with a three-tier low-, intermediate or high-grade designation. As this is a diagnosis based on exclusion of known salivary carcinomas or metastases, immunohistochemical or special stains may be necessary. In the setting of a high-grade carcinoma, exclusion of salivary duct carcinoma (AR +, GCDFP +) and MEC (mucicarmine +, p40 +) or metastasis should be considered. In a low- to intermediate-grade carcinoma, differential considerations may include acinic cell carcinoma (DOG1 +, PAS/PAS-D +, mammaglobin–), PAC (p63 +, p40–),[18] and epithelial-myoepithelial lesions (myoepithelial component positive for SMA +, p40 +).

The WHO Classification of Head and Neck Tumors also indicated two aggressive subtypes, to include mucinous adenocarcinoma with variable cystic formation (formerly cystadenocarcinoma) and intestinal type (CK20 + and CDX2 +). Of note, the authors indicate uncertainty if this is a true variant versus a separate entity.[10]

9.4.4 Treatment Considerations and Approaches

The prognosis is dependent on size, site, and grade. The low- to intermediate-grade adenocarcinoma NOS has a better prognosis in contrast to the aggressive course of high-grade adenocarcinoma NOS,[21] as noted by 15-year respective survival rates of 54, 31, and 3%.[10] The cure rate is high after complete excision with infrequent recurrences and rare regional metastasis.[16]

9.4.5 Key Points

- Adenocarcinoma NOS is a diagnosis of exclusion, must rule out metastases and well-characterized/known salivary carcinomas.
- Grading is based on atypia (low, intermediate, high), and high-grade carcinomas carry a poor prognosis.

9.5 Polymorphous Adenocarcinoma

9.5.1 Introduction

Previously termed polymorphous low-grade adenocarcinoma (PLGA), the reports of a few aggressive and/or high-grade PACs required a name modification of the tumor. While generally a low-grade process, few cases may have necrosis, squamous differentiation, or high-grade cytologic atypia signaling high-grade transformation of the PAC.

9.5.2 Epidemiology

There is a high prevalence in women, with most of the patients aged 50 to 70 years or older.[7,10] Most studies do not report PAC as a recognized entity prior to 1984[6,8] for undetermined reasons. Prevalence may vary based on ethnic/environmental factors. One African population-based study reported that PAC composed 26% of malignant salivary gland tumors and was the most common malignancy.[6] Per the WHO Head and Neck Classification, PAC is "the second most common oral malignant salivary gland tumor, accounting for 26% of all carcinomas at this site."[10] In most other studies, PACs follow MEC and ACC, and in some cases adenocarcinoma NOS. For example, it was the third most common malignancy in an Indian study (3.3%, $n = 30$),[6] Australian study (20%, $n = 30$),[8] British study (23%, $n = 21$),[21] and Grecian study (9%, $n = 22$),[12] while it was fourth in a study from Pakistan (2.8%, $n = 70$).

9.5.3 Clinical Presentation

This usually presents as a painless mass, predominantly at the junction of the hard and soft palate. Other sites affected by PAC include the buccal mucosa, retromolar region, lip, and base of the tongue.[10]

9.5.4 Diagnosis and Evaluation

PACs are unencapsulated, poorly circumscribed neoplasms. Perineural invasion is common. The cytomorphology is bland but can vary in histologic patterns, and therefore may be confused for pleomorphic adenoma or adenocarcinoma.[19] Histologic patterns may include solid, papillary-cystic, cribriform, microcystic, lobular, or trabecular formation with variable mucinous or hyalinized stroma (▶ Fig. 9.4a). Some authors regard PACs with prominent cribriform, papillary, and glomeruloid patterns as a distinct entity known as "cribriform adenocarcinoma of the tongue and minor salivary glands," but under the current WHO classification these tumors are still included with the PAC group (▶ Fig. 9.4b).[10,22]

9.5.5 Molecular Testing

Most PACs harbor alterations of *PRKD1*, *PRKD2*, or *PRKD3*. Interestingly, PACs with conventional morphology usually harbor an E710D hotspot mutation in PRKD1, while most of cases morphologically classified as the cribriform adenocarcinoma of the tongue and minor salivary glands variant harbor rearrangements of *PRKD1*, *PRKD2*, or *PRKD3*.[23,24]

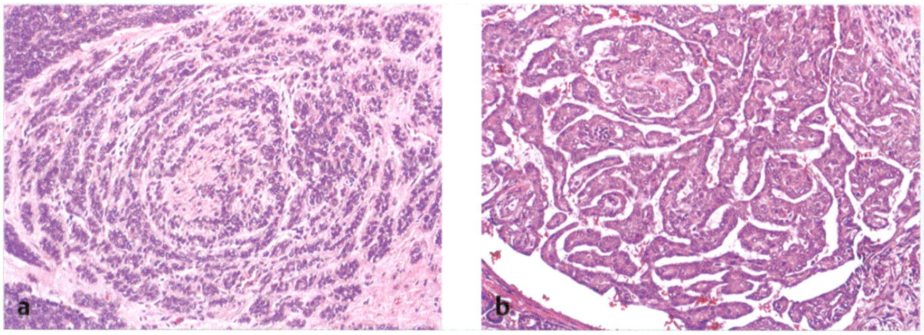

Fig. 9.4 **(a)** Polymorphous adenocarcinoma classically demonstrates a "targetoid" pattern of perineural invasion. **(b)** Cases of polymorphous adenocarcinoma with a prominent papillary pattern are sometimes referred to as "cribriform adenocarcinoma of the tongue and minor salivary glands."

9.5.6 Treatment Considerations and Approaches

Complete surgical excision is the primary treatment. The prognosis and survival rates are good, and generally local or distant recurrence is uncommon. The cribriform adenocarcinoma subtype has been reported to have a higher rate of cervical lymph node metastases; however, the survival of this subtype is still excellent.[25] In the rare cases of high-grade PAC transformation, the prognosis is poor.

9.5.7 Key Points

- PACs are more frequent in adults and generally low grade with good prognosis.
- The cytomorphology is bland with heterogeneous histologic patterns that can mimic other salivary lesions (e.g., pleomorphic adenoma or ACC, etc.).
- High-grade transformation is rare and is associated with poor prognosis.

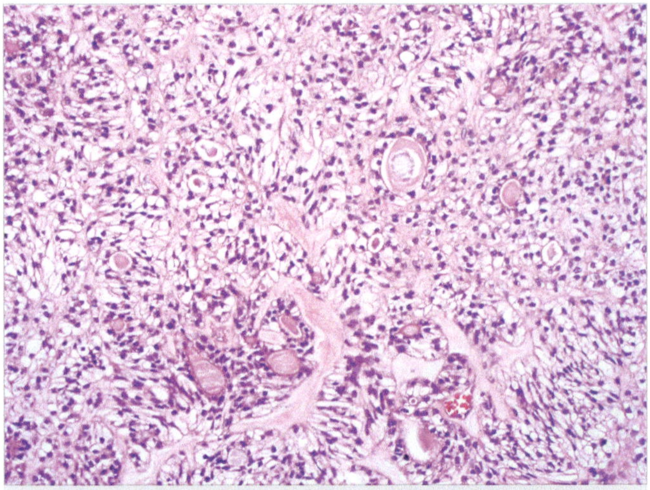

Fig. 9.5 Epithelial-myoepithelial carcinoma is a biphasic tumor, with a predominance of clear myoepithelial cells that surround eosinophilic ducts.

9.6 Epithelial-Myoepithelial Carcinoma

9.6.1 Introduction

EMC was first described by Donath et al in 1972.[26] This carcinoma is generally low grade arising from precursor epithelial and myoepithelial cells, which lend to a variegation of histomorphologic patterns. This subtype is rare (1%) among salivary malignancies with a prevalence for the parotid gland, but may also arise less frequently in the submandibular gland and minor salivary glands (e.g., base of the tongue, soft palate, etc.).[27]

9.6.2 Epidemiology

The mean age is 60 years, but it can also occur in children; it has a female predominance.

9.6.3 Clinical Presentation

EMC can present as an ill-defined submucosal mass and may have ulceration, but symptoms are dependent on the specific location of the tumor (e.g., dysphasia or speech difficulty if located on the tongue).[28]

9.6.4 Diagnosis and Evaluation

This neoplasm has no true capsule, but demonstrates expansile, pushing borders. Like ACC, the histology of EMC also includes two cells types; however, the proportion and variation of the appearance of the myoepithelial and epithelial cells makes this entity challenging. The myoepithelial cells are usually the outer layer of cells and contain abundant, clear cytoplasm, while the inner layer cells may resemble intercalated ducts (▶ Fig. 9.5).

Poor prognostic factors include large size, rapid tumor growth, and margin status (due to local recurrence).[28] Local recurrence is estimated to be about 30%, and distant metastases are rare.[27]

9.6.5 Treatment

Complete surgical resection is the main treatment. Overall survival is good, with one study indicating a 60-month survival of 91.3% ($n = 246$ patients inclusive of major and minor salivary glands).[27]

9.6.6 Key Points

- EMC is characterized by two cell components (epithelial and myoepithelial cells) in variable proportions and amenable to variable histologic appearances.
- The prognosis is good but dependent upon accurate pathologic assessment of tumor size, metastasis, and surgical margin status.

Chapter Overall Key Points

- Malignant minor salivary gland tumors are a small component of oral carcinomas, with MECs and ACCs being the most common.
- The most common location of minor salivary gland malignancies is the palate.
- Predominant treatment is compete surgical resection, and neck dissection if clinical metastases are present, with optional postsurgical radiation therapy.

References

[1] Stenman G, Persson F, Andersson MK. Diagnostic and therapeutic implications of new molecular biomarkers in salivary gland cancers. Oral Oncol. 2014; 50(8):683–690

[2] Vaidya AD, Pantvaidya GH, Metgudmath R, Kane SV, D'Cruz AK. Minor salivary gland tumors of the oral cavity: a case series with review of literature. J Cancer Res Ther. 2012; 8 Suppl 1:S111–S115

[3] Pandey M, Thomas S, Mathew A, Nair MK. Malignant tumours of the minor salivary glands: a survival analysis of 17 years from a tertiary referral cancer centre. J Postgrad Med. 2003; 49(1):25–28

[4] Lee SY, Shin HA, Rho KJ, Chung HJ, Kim SH, Choi EC. Characteristics, management of the neck, and oncological outcomes of malignant minor salivary gland tumours in the oral and sinonasal regions. Br J Oral Maxillofac Surg. 2013; 51(7):e142–e147

[5] Rahman B, Mamoon N, Jamal S, et al. Malignant tumors of the minor salivary glands in northern Pakistan: a clinicopathological study. Hematol Oncol Stem Cell Ther. 2008; 1(2):90–93

[6] Ramesh M, Krishnan R, Paul G. Intraoral minor salivary gland tumours: a retrospective study from a dental and maxillofacial surgery centre in salem, Tamil Nadu. J Maxillofac Oral Surg. 2014; 13(2):104–108

[7] Venkata V, Irulandy P. The frequency and distribution pattern of minor salivary gland tumors in a government dental teaching hospital, Chennai, India. Oral Surg Oral Med Oral Pathol Oral Radiol Endod. 2011; 111(1):e32–e39

[8] Hyam DM, Veness MJ, Morgan GJ. Minor salivary gland carcinoma involving the oral cavity or oropharynx. Aust Dent J. 2004; 49(1):16–19

[9] Lopes MA, Santos GC, Kowalski LP. Multivariate survival analysis of 128 cases of oral cavity minor salivary gland carcinomas. Head Neck. 1998; 20(8):699–706

[10] El-Naggar AK, Chan JKC, Grandis JR, Takata T, Slootweg PJ. WHO Classification of Head and Neck Tumours. 4th ed. 2017; Lyon: International Agency for Research on Cancer

[11] Galer C, Santillan AA, Chelius D, et al. Minor salivary gland malignancies in the pediatric population. Head Neck. 2012; 34(11):1648–1651

[12] Papadogeorgakis N, Parara E, Petsinis V, Pappa E, Nikolaidis A, Alexandridis K. A retrospective review of malignant minor salivary gland tumors and a proposed protocol for future care. Craniomaxillofac Trauma Reconstr. 2011; 4(1):1–10

[13] Lohiya PG, Chaudhary MS, Patil S, Agrawal SA. Sclerosing mucoepidermoid carcinoma of minor salivary gland. Contemp Clin Dent. 2014; 5(4):564–568

[14] Kumar R, Natarajan S, Sneha KS, Chitra NS, Boaz K, Manaktala N. Oncocytes in mucoepidermoid carcinoma of the palate: diagnostic challenges. Case Rep Dent. 2017; 2017:5741821

[15] Bishop JA, Cowan ML, Shum CH, Westra WH. MAML2 rearrangements in variant forms of mucoepidermoid carcinoma: ancillary diagnostic testing for the ciliated and warthin-like variants. Am J Surg Pathol. 2018; 42(1):130–136

[16] Kruse AL, Grätz KW, Obwegeser JA, Lübbers HT. Malignant minor salivary gland tumors: a retrospective study of 27 cases. Oral Maxillofac Surg. 2010; 14(4):203–209

[17] Argyris PP, Wetzel SL, Greipp P, et al. Clinical utility of myb rearrangement detection and p63/p40 immunophenotyping in the diagnosis of adenoid cystic carcinoma of minor salivary glands: a pilot study. Oral Surg Oral Med Oral Pathol Oral Radiol. 2016; 121(3):282–289

[18] Owosho AA, Aguilar CE, Seethala RR. Comparison of p63 and p40 (ΔNp63) as basal, squamoid, and myoepithelial markers in salivary gland tumors. Appl Immunohistochem Mol Morphol. 2016; 24(7):501–508

[19] Mitani Y, Liu B, Rao PH, et al. Novel MYBL1 gene rearrangements with recurrent MYBL1-NFIB fusions in salivary adenoid cystic carcinomas lacking t(6;9) translocations. Clin Cancer Res. 2016; 22(3):725–733

[20] Brayer KJ, Frerich CA, Kang H, Ness SA. Recurrent fusions in MYB and MYBL1 define a common, transcription factor-driven oncogenic pathway in salivary gland adenoid cystic carcinoma. Cancer Discov. 2016; 6(2):176–187

[21] Strick MJ, Kelly C, Soames JV, McLean NR. Malignant tumours of the minor salivary glands: a 20 year review. Br J Plast Surg. 2004; 57(7):624–631

[22] Skálová A, Gnepp DR, Lewis JS, Jr, et al. Newly described entities in salivary gland pathology. Am J Surg Pathol. 2017; 41(8):e33–e47

[23] Piscuoglio S, Fusco N, Ng CK, et al. Lack of PRKD2 and PRKD3 kinase domain somatic mutations in PRKD1 wild-type classic polymorphous low-grade adenocarcinomas of the salivary gland. Histopathology. 2016; 68(7):1055–1062

[24] Weinreb I, Zhang L, Tirunagari LM, et al. Novel PRKD gene rearrangements and variant fusions in cribriform adenocarcinoma of salivary gland origin. Genes Chromosomes Cancer. 2014; 53(10):845–856

[25] Michal M, Kacerovska D, Kazakov DV. Cribriform adenocarcinoma of the tongue and minor salivary glands: a review. Head Neck Pathol. 2013; 7 Suppl 1:S3–S11

[26] Donath K, Seifert G, Schmitz R. Diagnosis and ultrastructure of the tubular carcinoma of salivary gland ducts. Epithelial-myoepithelial carcinoma of the intercalated ducts. Virchows Arch A Pathol Pathol Anat. 1972; 356(1):16–31

[27] Vázquez A, Patel TD, D'Aguillo CM, et al. Epithelial-myoepithelial carcinoma of the salivary glands: an analysis of 246 cases. Otolaryngol Head Neck Surg. 2015; 153(4):569–574

[28] Dimitrijevic MV, Tomanovic NR, Jesic SD, Arsovic NA, Mircic AL, Krstic AM. Epithelial-myoepithelial carcinoma: review of clinicopathological and immunohistochemical features. Arch Iran Med. 2015; 18(4):218–222

Section IV

Pretreatment Considerations

IV

10 Pretreatment Dental Evaluation

Yee Seul Chun

Summary
A multidisciplinary approach to care is recommended for head and neck cancer patients in order to improve overall treatment outcomes. Dental providers should be included in this team and a complete oral/dental examination and any necessary dental treatment, such as extractions and restoration of restorable teeth, should be performed prior to radiation or chemotherapy. This process is critical in order to prevent serious oral problems that could result in delays or cessation of cancer treatments. Providers should educate patients on common oral side effects including mucositis, infections, xerostomia, taste changes, soft-tissue and/or bone necrosis, and exacerbation of dental and periodontal diseases. In addition, thorough home care instructions and fluoride supplementation should be incorporated into management due to increased caries risk and lifelong risk of osteoradionecrosis associated with radiation therapy to the head and neck region.

Keywords: dental, caries, osteoradionecrosis, extractions, periodontal disease, fluoride therapy

10.1 Introduction

The most common modalities used to treat head and neck cancer are comprised of surgery, radiation therapy, and chemotherapy. These aggressive cancer treatments not only act upon tumor cells, but also produce noxious effects to normal cells, including the oral mucosa and salivary glands. The short- and long-term effects of this toxicity on the oral cavity and dentition have been well documented.[1,2] Early evaluation and treatment by a trained dental team can diminish or prevent some of these oral complications, such as mucositis, oral infection, and osteoradionecrosis (ORN). It is therefore important that patients undergo a thorough dental evaluation prior to the initiation of head and neck cancer treatment.

10.2 Nonodontogenic Considerations

As the treatment of the cancer patient is multifaceted, communication between different providers to organize and coordinate care is critical in order to improve outcomes. A focus on the concept of a multidisciplinary team has therefore become increasingly prominent over the years. For head and neck cancer patients, this team often consists of head and neck cancer surgeons, reconstructive/plastic surgeons, radiation oncologists, medical oncologists, pathologists, speech and language therapists, dietitians, social workers, and dentists. Accordingly, it is important for the dental professional to take a multidisciplinary approach and communicate with other providers as there are numerous nonodontogenic factors to consider when constructing an initial dental treatment plan for head and neck cancer patients.

10.3 Diagnosis/Patient Prognosis

The patient's medical history, diagnosis, prognosis, and treatment plan should be obtained from the multidisciplinary team. If the patient prognosis is extremely poor or medical status extremely compromised, dental treatment may sometimes be deferred and the team may opt to address future dental sequelae as they arise.

10.4 Radiation Therapy Factors

A significant challenge to the dentist is the determination of what preexisting oral conditions or teeth require treatment in order to limit the risk of ORN following radiation therapy. ORN of the jaw is one of the most severe chronic side effects of radiation treatment to the head and neck region. First described by Regaud in Paris in 1922, ORN is defined as nonhealing exposed bone in a previously irradiated area present for over 3 months.[3] Other features include pain, halitosis, dysgeusia, food impaction in the area of exposed sequestra, pain, fractures, and fistulas.[4] It can occur in both dentate and edentulous patients, either spontaneously or following trauma, with most cases of ORN occurring after tooth extractions.[5]

As proper dental management is of utmost importance for the prevention of ORN, the dentist should receive from the radiation oncologist the general radiation plan prior to the initiation of treatment. Type of radiation, total cumulative dose, and intended field of direct radiotherapy should be considered when determining a dental treatment plan. All parts of the jaws are not necessarily included in the field of radiation and if the radiation dose to the area of the mandible or maxilla is less than 50 to 60 Gy, the risk of osteonecrosis has usually been considered lower (see Chapter 41 Radiotherapy Related Side Effects in the Treatment of Oral Cavity Malignancies).[6]

Conventional (two- and three-dimensional conformal radiotherapy) techniques can result in significant side effects and decreased quality of life. Over the last few decades, improvements have been made in radiotherapy for the treatment of cancer including intensity-modulated radiotherapy (IMRT), which manipulates photon and proton beams of radiation to conform to the shape of a tumor and reduce doses to normal tissues. Other advancements like volumetric intensity-modulated arc therapy and image-guided radiotherapy have also helped improve IMRT further.[7] There has been a reduction in the rates of ORN with these newer advances, which may be attributed to more conformal dose distributions that spare parts of the mandible that would have received a high dose with more conventional techniques. Salivary gland sparing with these advancements may also decrease the risk for development of dental caries.[8]

Finally, the scheduled time of commencement of radiotherapy and amount of time available for the dental assessment are important to take into consideration as this may influence prioritizing certain treatments if there are time constraints. In some cases, due to severity of the tumor and disease, dental treatment may be deferred so that radiation can proceed without delay. In such cases, the initial dental evaluation should be scheduled soon after cancer diagnosis in order to allow for sufficient time to complete any necessary dental treatment.

10.5 Patient-Related Factors

10.5.1 Patient Demographics

Certain demographic factors should be considered as they can *influence health care* outcomes. The socioeconomic status/finances of a patient should be considered as this may lead to difficulties with health care access. Of note, head and neck cancer patients to receive high doses of irradiation will have a lifelong risk of ORN should they require dental extractions in the future. If the patient lacks dental insurance or cannot afford regular and preventative dental care that is required, consideration may need to be given as to whether any teeth should remain in the proposed high-dose field of radiation. The age of a patient should also be considered, as younger patients must maintain disease-free dentition longer in order to avoid future complications.

10.5.2 Patient Compliance and Dexterity

Patients with a dental phobia, compromised manual dexterity, or a demonstrated lack of motivation to perform oral hygiene measures may require a more aggressive preradiation dental treatment plan. The provider may lean toward extracting all teeth in areas to receive high doses of radiation in these instances.

10.5.3 Patient Wishes for Dental Extraction

All clinicians should view the treatment planning process as a shared process and an educational experience for the patient. Treatment advantages, disadvantages, risks, and alternatives should all be reviewed. Alongside the actual indication and diagnosis of the teeth, the relevant wishes of the patient regarding tooth extraction should be considered when fabricating a treatment plan.

10.6 Oral Assessment before Treatment

Following a standard history, including medical diagnoses, a social and dental history, and current and recent complaints, a thorough oral and dental examination should be conducted. The purpose of the dental examination is to determine definitive diagnoses and prognoses for individual teeth in order to identify those that require aggressive or invasive dental treatment prior to chemotherapy and/or radiation treatment. Infection control should be instituted prior to cancer treatment in order to improve patient outcomes, as a healthy oral cavity has been shown to improve general comfort and result in fewer interruptions during treatment.[2]

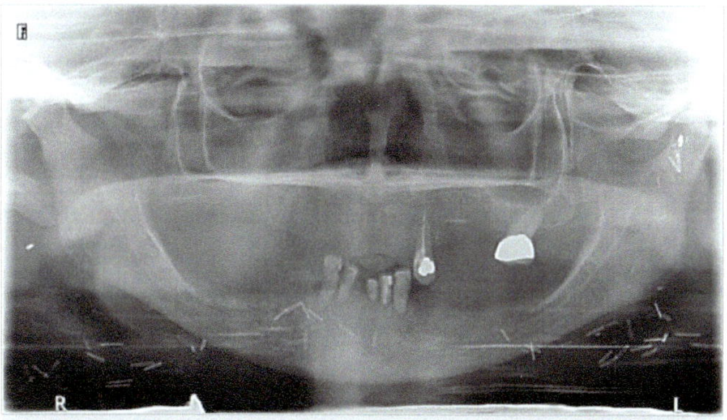

Fig. 10.1 Postsurgical panoramic radiograph of patient demonstrating need for full-mouth dental extractions prior to chemoradiation due to the presence of periodontal disease.

10.7 Radiographs

In addition to a clinical examination, a through dental evaluation should incorporate radiographic images. Select dental radiographs are a valuable diagnostic tool to aid in the assessment of areas for potential infection that may not be visually obvious. A panoramic radiograph and/or a full series of dental radiographs should be taken for dentate patients to assess for any bony pathology, screen for caries (tooth decay), and aid in the detection of periodontal disease (▶ Fig. 10.1). A panoramic radiograph should also be taken for edentulous patients in order to screen for any bony pathology, submucosal or intrabony root fragments, and impacted teeth.

10.8 Extraoral Examination

The dental evaluation begins with the overall appraisal of the patient and examination of the extraoral and perioral tissues. The patient's general physical status, appearance, gait, and mobility can be observed during movement in the office. Other components include the inspection of the head, face, eyes, and neck, noting any significant asymmetries or changes to the skin. A brief cranial nerve examination may also be conducted to screen for any neurologic deficits. Regional lymph node areas should also be palpated for enlargement, consistency, mobility, or tenderness. The lymph node examination should include the preauricular, postauricular, suboccipital, submandibular, submental, cervical, and supraclavicular lymph nodes. Cancer metastasis to lymph nodes may result in fixed, nontender, and firm enlarged nodes. In addition, the thyroid gland should be visually examined and palpated for enlargement. A temporomandibular joint (TMJ) examination may also evaluate for the presence of pain, clicking, popping, crepitus, deviations, and range of motion. Accordingly, a detailed TMJ examination including palpation of the muscles of mastication may be indicated.

10.9 Intraoral Examination

The intraoral examination involves a systematic assessment of the lips, labial and buccal mucosa, tongue, floor of the mouth, salivary glands, hard palate, soft palate, oropharynx, gingiva, and, of course, the dentition. All mucosal or facial tissues that seem to be abnormal should be palpated and changes in color or texture of the mucosa should be thoroughly investigated.

10.10 Odontogenic Considerations

10.10.1 Soft Tissue

Healthy gingiva is pink and stippled in appearance. The soft tissues should be examined for any localized or generalized edema, erythema, ulceration, or bleeding or be verified as within normal limits. Any soft-tissue abnormalities or swelling should be diagnosed and treated.

10.10.2 Caries, Fractures

Teeth with large caries or fractures should be considered for extraction prior to radiation, especially if they are in the proposed field of radiation. Smaller carious lesions should be treated with restorations prior to cancer treatment if time allows, although teeth with minor caries may not realistically require restorations before cancer treatment begins. If a patient has generalized tooth decay throughout the mouth and high caries risk, the dental provider may choose to be more aggressive in their overall treatment plan.

10.10.3 Root Canals

All previously endodontically treated teeth with periapical radiolucencies should be assessed for clinical signs and symptoms of current infection. A tooth may not heal as expected after initial treatment for a variety of reasons including complicated canal anatomy, fracture, and recontamination from delayed restoration of the tooth or recurrent decay. If the tooth is deemed restorable and time permits, endodontic retreatment of failed or nonhealing root canals may be performed. Poorly done or failing root canals with a guarded or worse long-term prognoses may be removed if they are in the direct field of radiotherapy.

10.10.4 Attrition

When protective enamel is lost due to attrition, teeth may develop hypersensitivity. In severely affected teeth, the progression of enamel and dentin destruction can produce frank or near pulpal involvement. For teeth with heavy attrition, the risk versus benefit of extraction should be considered.

10.10.5 Periodontal Disease

A complete periodontal examination and charting should be completed. Teeth may be considered for extraction if they have deep probing depths, furcation involvement, bony defects, or mobility as this indicates a poor long-term prognosis. Teeth with moderate to severe periodontal disease should be extracted if they are within the radiation field.

10.10.6 Impactions

Any impacted teeth (typically third molars) in the proposed field of radiation with associated pathology or communication with the oral cavity should be extracted prior to radiation. Partially impacted/erupted angled third molars can result in pericoronitis or induce caries on the distal aspect of the adjacent second molars. Full bony impacted teeth can often be left in place as there is no communication with the oral cavity.

10.10.7 Unopposed Teeth

Teeth that are unopposed or that will become unopposed after extraction of other teeth should similarly be evaluated for extraction due to potential for super-eruption and future loss of the tooth.

10.10.8 Tooth Position

The position of the tooth in the maxillary versus mandibular arch should be considered in the risk assessment and treatment decision. For example, ORN is hardly ever seen in the maxilla. Differences in anatomic structure and blood supply between the maxilla and mandible may explain this pattern.[9] A more aggressive treatment approach to odontogenic pathology in the field of radiation and in the mandible may be warranted during the preirradiation evaluation.

10.10.9 Prosthetics/Dentures

The fit of any existing prosthetic appliances should carefully be examined. Any sources of oral trauma and irritation such as ill-fitting dentures and other appliances should be identified and eliminated as these may be further aggravated from radiation or chemotherapy-induced mucositis. Furthermore, insult to the mucosa and underlying bone from ill-fitting prostheses can increase the susceptibility for ORN.[10]

It is important to remember that an aggressive approach to extractions may not always be desirable, as teeth play a significant role in masticatory efficiency and quality of life. Certain teeth may also be essential for successful retention of a prosthesis to replace a surgical defect as well.

10.11 Dental Treatment Prior to Cancer Treatment

There is evidence that patients on immunosuppressive chemotherapy, in conjunction with their radiation, can develop serious infectious complications from tooth infections, largely due to a decrease in neutrophils.[11] Furthermore, as the majority of cases of ORN occur in patients who were dentate in the mandible at tumor onset, proper preradiation dental management is key for its prevention.[5,12] Thus, elimination of oral disease and implementation of preventative measures designed to maintain maximum oral health should be completed before radiation and/or chemotherapy begins.

Patients should receive a comprehensive oral evaluation several weeks prior to chemoradiation in order to complete any necessary treatments. Pretreatment prophylaxis or scaling and restoration of carious lesions is advised. In order to allow for adequate healing, invasive dental procedures such as extractions should be ideally performed at least 14 days prior to radiation therapy and 10 days before myelosuppressive chemotherapy. However, the optimal schedule should be discussed with the radiation oncologist and/or medical oncologist, taking tumor progression and other treatment factors into consideration. In conjunction with extractions, adequate alveoloplasty, elimination of any sharp bony projections, and tori should be completed should the patient require dentures. Primary closure should be achieved if possible.[1,2] If possible, any teeth outside of the potential field of radiation that are symptomatic or have a poor prognosis should be extracted prior to radiation as well.

10.12 Patient Education

Patients should be advised about the potential effects of cancer treatment on their oral and dental structures with particular reference to mucositis, xerostomia, increased caries risk, and risk of ORN from postradiation extractions. Due to damage of the salivary glands during radiation, and the ensuing xerostomia that follows, head and neck cancer patients are at higher risk compared to average population for the development of caries (▶ Fig. 10.2). To combat the increase in caries susceptibility, and reduce the possibility of posttreatment extractions, patients must be provided with prevention advice, which should include a lifelong commitment to meticulous oral hygiene and frequent self-application of fluoride. Additionally, regular appointments (3-month recall visits) with a dentist and/or a dental hygienist whose role it is to reinforce the importance of prevention should be instituted.

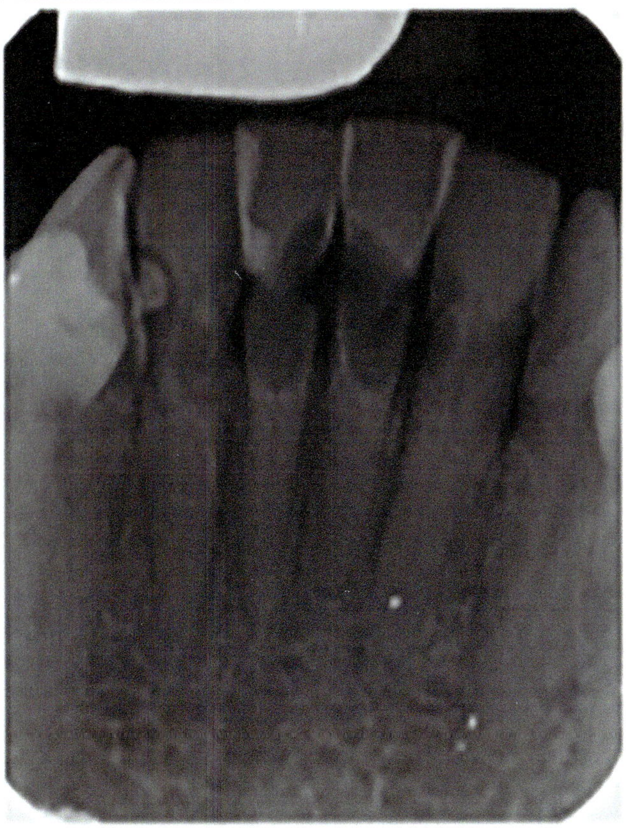

Fig. 10.2 Presence of postradiation cervical caries on mandibular anterior teeth.

During treatment with chemotherapy or head and neck radiation, advise patients to do the following:

- Brush teeth, gums, and tongue gently with a soft-bristle toothbrush and high fluoride/prescription toothpaste twice daily:
  - Review the modified bass technique.
  - If brushing causes discomfort, soften the bristles in warm water.
  - Use a fluoride toothpaste with a mild taste. Mint flavoring may irritate the mouth.
  - Floss teeth daily. If gums are sore or bleeding, avoid these areas especially if platelet count is low.
- Use fluoride gel/trays.
- Keep the mouth moisturized:
  - Drink a lot of water.
  - Suck ice chips.
  - Chew sugar-free gum or suck on sugar-free hard candies to stimulate the flow of saliva.
  - Add moisture to the air at night with a room humidifier.
  - Try saliva substitutes/moisturizing sprays/gels.
  - Consider prescription systemic sialogogues.
- Mucositis relief:
  - Ice chips.
  - Palifermin, sucralfate.
  - Application of topical anesthetics to prevent discomfort prior to eating.
  - Wear dentures only for meals.
  - Rinse your mouth with warm water with salt and/or baking soda (a teaspoon of each dissolved in 8 oz of warm water).
- Exercise the jaw muscles three times a day to prevent and combat jaw stiffness/trismus from radiation:
  - Open and close the mouth as far as possible; repeat 20 times.
- Stick to the recall schedule recommended by the dentist.
- Avoid:
  - Hot, spicy, acidic, sharp, or crunchy foods, which can all irritate your mouth.
  - Food high in sugar content, such as candy or soda, which increase caries incidence.
  - Excessive caffeine intake.
  - Tobacco (smoking cessation advice if applicable) and alcohol (including mouthwashes containing alcohol).

10.13 Supplemental Fluoride

The formation of a cavity is initiated by bacteria in plaque when they metabolize carbohydrates and produce an acid byproduct, demineralizing the tooth enamel. Demineralization involves the loss of calcium, phosphate, and carbonate from enamel. Fluoride has been shown to produce an anticaries effect by affecting homeostatic pathways and metabolic activity of cariogenic bacteria, reducing the acidification of plaque that results in demineralization. Furthermore, fluoride, along with calcium and phosphate, can remineralize weakened enamel and establish a crystal structure that is even more resistant to acidic dissolution than before.[13,14] Thus, fluoride reduces the incidence of dental caries and can reverse the progression of existing lesions.

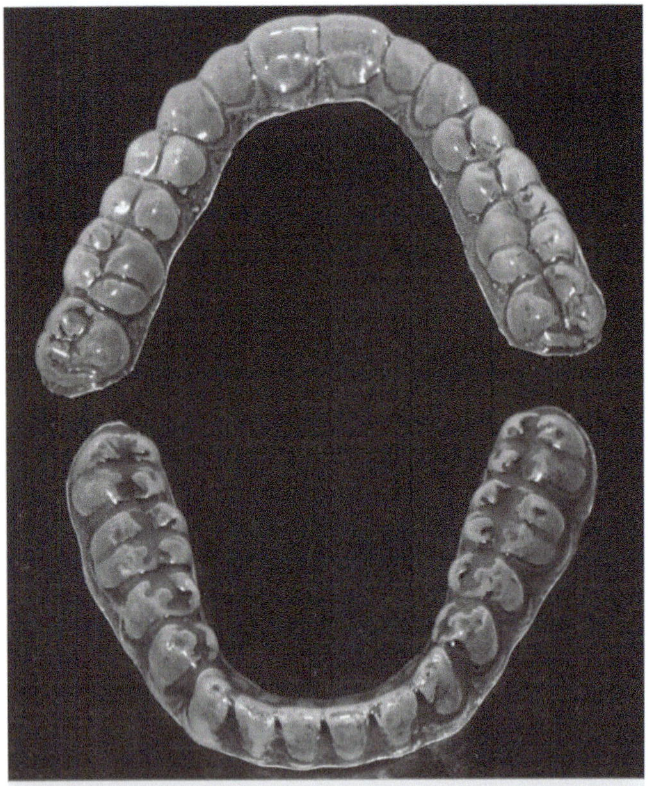

Fig. 10.3 Custom fluoride trays to aid in the prevention of caries.

Patients with radiation-induced salivary gland dysfunction should perform lifelong daily fluoride applications as a safe and effective means for reducing the incidence of caries. Daily topical 0.4% stannous fluoride (1,000 ppm of fluoride) or 1.1% sodium fluoride (5,000 ppm of fluoride) will typically be prescribed by the dental professional. Topical fluorides are available in multiple forms including toothpastes, varnishes, gels, foams, and mouth rinses.

Toothpaste is the most commonly used form of self-applied fluoride. For most people, brushing twice daily for about 2 minutes with a fluoridated toothpaste is recommended. For prescribed toothpaste, patients should use a thin ribbon of paste on the toothbrush, brush, and then spit out any excess, avoiding rinsing in order to prevent diluting the fluoride and reducing its preventative effects.

Additionally, the construction of custom, flexible topical fluoride trays for daily home application of fluoride is often advised (▶ Fig. 10.3). Trays should cover all tooth structures without irritating the gingival or mucosal tissues. A thin ribbon of fluoride gel should be placed in each tray and worn in place for at least 10 minutes. Trays should then be removed and excess gel expectorated. Refraining from eating or drinking for 30 minutes and rinsing with water afterward is suggested.

Professionally applied fluorides, which are more concentrated than the self-applied fluorides, may be applied regularly at recall visits. High-concentration fluoride varnish is painted onto the teeth and intended to hold a high concentration of fluoride in close contact with the teeth for several hours.[13]

Key Points

- Nonrestorable teeth should be removed and periodontal health maximized prior to chemoradiation therapy.
- Patients should be counseled about the short- and long-term dental complications of head and neck cancer treatments.
- Prevention is a critical management strategy of ORN.
- Patients should initiate a preventative dental care regimen with fluoride supplementation.

References

[1] National Cancer Institute. Oral Complications of Chemotherapy and Head/Neck Radiation. Available at: https://www.cancer.gov/about-cancer/treatment/side-effects/mouth-throat/oral-complications-hp-pdq. Accessed February 1, 2018

[2] National Institutes of Health consensus development conference statement: oral complications of cancer therapies: diagnosis, prevention, and treatment. J Am Dent Assoc. 1989; 119(1):179–183

[3] Regaud C. Sur la sensibilite du tissue osseux normal vis-avis des reyons X gamma et sur la mecanisme de l'osteoradionecrose. CR Soc Biol (Paris). 1922; 87:929–932

[4] Epstein JB, Wong FL, Stevenson-Moore P. Osteoradionecrosis: clinical experience and a proposal for classification. J Oral Maxillofac Surg. 1987; 45(2): 104–110

[5] Koga DH, Salvajoli JV, Alves FA. Dental extractions and radiotherapy in head and neck oncology: review of the literature. Oral Dis. 2008; 14(1):40–44

[6] Nabil S, Samman N. Incidence and prevention of osteoradionecrosis after dental extraction in irradiated patients: a systematic review. Int J Oral Maxillofac Surg. 2011; 40(3):229–243

[7] Bhide SA, Nutting CM. Advances in radiotherapy for head and neck cancer. Oral Oncol. 2010; 46(6):439–441

[8] Ben-David MA, Diamante M, Radawski JD, et al. Lack of osteoradionecrosis of the mandible after intensity-modulated radiotherapy for head and neck cancer: likely contributions of both dental care and improved dose distributions. Int J Radiat Oncol Biol Phys. 2007; 68(2):396–402

[9] Beumer J, Harrison R, Sanders B, Kurrasch M. Osteoradionecrosis: predisposing factors and outcomes of therapy. Head Neck Surg. 1984; 6(4):819–827

[10] Raguse J-D, Hossamo J, Tinhofer I, et al. Patient and treatment-related risk factors for osteoradionecrosis of the jaw in patients with head and neck cancer. Oral Surg Oral Med Oral Pathol Oral Radiol. 2016; 121(3):215–21.e1

[11] Hong CHL, Napeñas JJ, Hodgson BD, et al. Dental Disease Section, Oral Care Study Group, Multi-, national Association of Supportive Care in Cancer (MASCC)/International Society of Oral Oncology (ISOO). A systematic review of dental disease in patients undergoing cancer therapy. Support Care Cancer. 2010; 18(8):1007–1021

[12] Thorn JJ, Hansen HS, Specht L, Bastholt L. Osteoradionecrosis of the jaws: clinical characteristics and relation to the field of irradiation. J Oral Maxillofac Surg. 2000; 58(10):1088–1093, discussion 1093–1095

[13] Recommendations for using fluoride to prevent and control dental caries in the United States. Centers for Disease Control and Prevention. MMWR Recomm Rep. 2001; 50(Rr-14):1–42

[14] Marquis RE. Antimicrobial actions of fluoride for oral bacteria. Can J Microbiol. 1995; 41(11):955–964

11 Pretreatment Speech-language Pathology Evaluation

Kimberly Webster and Rina Abrams

Summary
It is highly recommended that patients meet with a speech-language pathologist (SLP) prior to treatment for oral cancer. Whether undergoing surgery, chemoradiation, or combined modality treatments, patients and families benefit from information on expected functional outcomes for speech and swallowing. Deficits can range widely, including articulation disorders, resonance imbalance, trismus, and oral and pharyngeal phase dysphagia. Clinical and instrumental swallowing examinations may be indicated. Baseline measurements of oral aperture are typical as well as measures of intelligibility and documentation of any speech or resonance difficulty. During the pretreatment evaluation, patients establish a relationship with an SLP, determine possible posttreatment deficits, and agree on a possible plan of posttreatment care. Additionally, nonsurgical patients benefit from learning prophylactic exercises to prevent radiation-related trismus and dysphagia. The effects on speech and swallowing depend largely on the location of tumor and treatment involved. Cancers can occur on lips, tongue, mandible, maxilla, alveolus, floor of mouth, retromolar trigone, or multiple sites in the oral cavity. Pretreatment evaluation can determine if there is any effect on speech or swallowing from the tumor itself and help patients and families understand how this anatomy and physiology will be affected with surgical excision of involved sites, reconstruction, and/or radiation treatment to these areas. Therapy can involve exercises, strategies, compensatory maneuvers, postures, oral prosthetics, dietary changes, and specialized feeding tools. Most importantly, patients can feel secure before they begin treatment that the goal is to re-establish functional speech and swallowing to the greatest possible extent.

Keywords: pretreatment evaluation, pretreatment counseling, dysphagia, dysarthria, trismus, oral motor examination, clinical swallow evaluation, fiberoptic endoscopic evaluation of swallowing, modified barium swallow study

11.1 Introduction

In the Unites States, there are approximately 3,800 patients diagnosed with oral cancer annually.[1] Patients with oral cancers have a significant risk of dysphagia and speech problems.[2,3] These deficits can be the result of tumor burden, surgery, and/or adjuvant radiation and chemotherapy. Speech-language pathology (SLP) intervention can be beneficial both pre- and postoperatively, as well as during the course of adjuvant treatments.[4–6]

The purpose of SLP involvement includes pretreatment counseling and evaluation and posttreatment intervention as indicated. Posttreatment considerations will be discussed in Chapter 44.

Pretreatment counseling has been a standardized part of head and neck cancer teams for many years. Although historically SLP pretreatment involvement began for total laryngectomy,[7] the value of pretreatment counseling is well documented for patients with oral cavity cancers as well.[4,5] Meeting with patients prior to cancer treatment allows the SLP to obtain baseline data on speech and swallowing, ease patients' and families' anxiety about what to expect, set appropriate and realistic posttreatment goals, introduce exercises or interventions, and establish rapport with the patient and family.[2,4,5,8,9]

More recently, involvement of a speech pathologist at the pretreatment stage has become standard for head and neck cancer patients undergoing radiation ± chemotherapy.[8,10] Introduction to prophylactic swallowing and oral exercises and pretreatment swallowing evaluations are the standard of care in most head and neck cancer centers and increasingly now in smaller, community hospitals providing chemoradiation therapy (CRT) for patients with head and neck cancer.[11] Prehabilitation is now common in cancer treatment and improves functional outcomes and compliance.[11,12]

Unfortunately, pretreatment evaluations by SLPs are not always standard protocol for patients with oral cancer. While patients undergoing total or subtotal glossectomy **(Video 11.1)** are referred more often for a pretreatment evaluation, those expected to have partial glossectomyies, floor of mouth resections, and palatal or mandibular resections do not often see an SLP until after surgery.[13] We believe the value of SLP involvement at the pretreatment stage can improve outcomes for the majority of patients undergoing surgical or nonsurgical treatment for oral cancer. Similar to patients undergoing CRT for oropharyngeal cancer or those requiring total laryngectomy, patients with oral cancer often have questions regarding posttreatment expected functional outcomes on speech and swallowing. Pretreatment evaluations can establish baseline function, help patients understand possible effects of surgery or CRT on speech and swallowing, and introduce exercises or interventions that may optimize speech and swallowing during and after treatment.[4,5,8,9] SLPs are often an important connection to other team members such as dieticians, dentists, prosthodontists, social workers, nurses, physical therapists, and certainly the physicians involved in definitive and adjuvant treatments. Additionally, multidisciplinary teams have been shown to be beneficial for patients with all types of head and neck cancer.[14,15] There has been an increase in the number of multidisciplinary teams where patients can see all their practitioners in one setting, rather than having individual evaluations. This has been shown to improve patient compliance and understanding of the SLP's role in their treatment.[14,15]

11.2 Incidence and Clinical Characteristics

There are few studies assessing the exact incidence of dysphagia and dysarthria in the oral cancer population; however, Colangelo and colleagues suggest that self-reported dysphagia and dysarthria are present in at least 34% of oral cancer patients prior to treatment.[13] Most studies combine head and neck cancers without differentiating between oral, oropharyngeal, and other cancers.[14,16,17] Further, since treatments are now often combined modalities, it is similarly hard to specify functional problems related to surgery versus chemoradiation. Additionally, many patients with speech or swallowing problems after oral cancer treatment may go unrecognized or untreated. Regardless, patients with oral cancer treated with surgery, nonsurgical treatment, or combined modalities can have deficits with any of the following: dysarthria or articulation problems, oral and/or pharyngeal dysphagia, resonance disorders, and trismus.[18]

11.3 Clinical Presentation and Anatomic Considerations

Clinical characteristics vary depending on tumor location and tumor size. As suspected, larger tumors result in greater deficits in speech and/or swallowing.[19] Dysarthria occurs when speech intelligibility is impacted, whereby speech is more difficult to understand, or unintelligible. Patients who have oral tongue tumors tend to experience the greatest speech disturbance of all the oral cancers.[20] This is because the tongue is our primary articulator. Anticipated speech and swallow deficits postoperatively are discussed with the patient during the initial preoperative visit. Patients are educated on likelihood of surgery having an impact on their articulation. The main point of preoperative education is for patients to understand that initial speech quality and articulation postoperatively will change and improve as edema decreases and lingual strength, tone, and range of movement increase.[4,21,22] This is usually gradual over weeks and months, and patients should understand preoperatively that realistic optimism is an ideal goal. Within the oral cavity, there are a variety of tumor locations, each with different potential impact of the tumor and its treatment on speech and swallowing, as briefly outlined below. Specific posttreatment considerations will be discussed further in Chapter 44.

Resection of cancers of the lip(s) will impact articulation of bilabial consonants (/p,b,w,m/), labiodental consonants (/f,v/), and fricatives that rely on lip rounding (/sh/).[23,24] The oral preparatory or oral phases of swallowing may be affected, resulting in incomplete lip closure and labial leakage.[21]

Resection of cancers of the alveolus or mandible may affect mastication. Unless severe, it is generally easy to compensate for partial alveolar or mandibular resections with little to no impact on speech and temporary impact on oral preparatory or oral phase of swallowing.[24,25]

Maxillary tumor resection can impact oral resonance and result in reduced oral pressure for chewing and swallowing.[26] These deficits are often temporary until an obturator can be made by a maxillofacial prosthodontist or a surgical flap is placed by a maxillofacial plastic surgeon.[24,27] Typically, patients with maxillary and mandibular tumors do not have preoperative dysarthria, with the exception of "muffled or mumbled speech," as the result of pain when speaking. In this instance, there is sometimes guarding or trying to move articulators minimally and keep mouth in a closed posture when speaking. The resulting impact on intelligibility is usually mild.[27]

Floor of mouth cancers and their treatment can affect swallowing since many of the laryngeal elevation muscles originate there.[28] Laryngeal elevation is an important component of airway protection.[25] Anterior and superior movement of the hyolaryngeal musculature allows for epiglottic inversion and airway protection before and during swallowing.[29] This may be seen as problems with thin liquid swallowing in the immediate postoperative period.[21]

Cancers of the retromolar trigone or areas requiring composite resection with or without adjuvant nonsurgical treatments may result in oral preparatory or oral phase problems.[24] As most of these cancers are unilateral, temporary postures and maneuvers are often helpful.[30]

Predicting impact on speech and swallowing for patients requiring partial glossectomy is directly related to the amount and location of tumor and resulting resection.[13] Tumors confined to the anterior tongue will result in speech deficits for lingual-alveolar consonants /t,d,n,l,s,z/ and "ʃ, dʒ, tʃ."[24,27] Oral preparatory and oral phases may be affected for swallowing. Unilateral deficits up to and including hemiglossectomy will have noticeable effects on consonant production requiring elevation of the lateral portion of the tongue (/s,z,sh,ch,j/).[24-27] Resulting dysarthria is often characterized by a lateral lisp. Similarly, loss of the bolus during the oral preparatory phase is common as is difficulty forming and transferring the bolus and oral residue after the swallow.[21] Large oral tongue tumors may result in significant lingual edema with limited tongue mobility and therefore reduced articulatory precision of lingual, linguadental, lingua-alveolar, and velar phonemes, including /t, d, n, l, s, z, k.g/.[24]

Total glossectomy results in much greater deficits for speech, with not only most consonants affected (other than bilabials), but impact on vowel production.[31] Despite the potentially large impact on specific sounds, speech can be quite intelligible for a patient undergoing total glossectomy.[32] This should be addressed in the preoperative session as many patients assume they "will never be able to speak." Patients are also educated on the use of augmentative and alternative communication options, which are beneficial in the immediate postoperative period and possibly long term. Similarly, patients can resume complete oral nutrition after total glossectomy with the right combination of reconstruction, speech/swallow therapy, prosthodontic intervention, and use of compensatory utensils and strategies.[29-33]

Patients who will be undergoing free-flap reconstruction are advised on the anticipated large "bulky" flap[34] and significant postoperative speech disturbances.[22,31] Regardless of the location of oral tumors, many patients with oral cancer require free-flap reconstruction[35] and therefore at least temporary speech deficits are anticipated.

If a tracheostomy is anticipated in conjunction with the surgery, the patient is educated on the anatomy and changes to physiology with the presence of a tracheostomy tube or cannula. We discuss the anticipated duration of the tracheostomy, downsizing, use of a speaking valve, and potentially the decannulation process. The amount of education, as with everything else during these sessions, varies depending on the patient and their family's comprehension, level of education, literacy, and emotional state as well as the exact anticipated surgery.

Trismus is tonic contraction of the muscles of mastication, mainly the pyterygoids.[36,37] It can be the result of tumor burden, surgery, and/or radiation. Intraoral opening is evaluated preoperatively by obtaining an interincisor or oral aperture measurement as discussed below. Trismus is not typically treated preoperatively, but rather only evaluated. Patients are educated on the potential development of trismus and types of treatments that could be expected postoperatively or throughout a course of radiation therapy (RT). As interincisor measurements vary widely, it is important to obtain a baseline measurement in the pretreatment evaluation.

11.4 Diagnosis and Evaluation

Pretreatment evaluations should include a history intake, evaluation of speech and swallowing, and discussion of posttreatment expected outcomes and rehabilitation or plan of care. As with any patient, performing a thorough chart review and obtaining a thorough patient history from the patient and family are important parts of the evaluation. When completing a chart review, it is important to note any comorbidities that may have caused a prior history of dysarthria, dysphagia, dysphonia, trismus, and/or resonance disorders. These comorbidities are potentially numerous, but we are typically searching for any past neurological diagnoses (i.e., history of cerebrovascular accident, traumatic brain injury, Parkinson's disease, etc.), prior history of radiation to the head and/or neck, pulmonary disorders that can impact respiratory function (i.e., chronic obstructive pulmonary disease, lung resections, etc.), any gastrointestinal problems such as reflux, and any history of oral, dental or mandibular dysfunction such as TMJ (temporomandibular joint) disease. There are a variety of interview questions to ask when obtaining a thorough case history, with a focus on prior and current deficits. We typically try to involve both the patient and caregivers/family members in this initial case history.[24]

Oral motor examinations are completed as part of the initial evaluation and a brief assessment of the following cranial nerves (CN): V, VII, IX, X, XI, and XII.[24,38] The concept behind assessing these particular nerves is to identify any deficits that may impact the patient's speech, oral, and/or swallow function. During the oral motor examination, we also measure intraoral opening to get a baseline measurement and rule out trismus. Intraoral measurements are obtained most accurately by utilizing a range of motion scale placed between the patient's gums or dentition (see ▸ Fig. 11.1). This measurement can also be obtained with a tape measure or ruler, but may be less accurate. There are limited normative data for interincisor aperture;[39,40] however, it is generally accepted to be greater than 35 or 40 mm within normal limits and greater than 30 mm within functional limits.

Typically, speech is not noticeably impaired preoperatively. If there are multiple noticeable errors and intelligibility deficits, a standardized articulation evaluation can be performed[27] to establish baseline intelligibility of phonemes, words, sentences, and/or connected speech. Standardized assessments (i.e., Frenchay Dysarthria Assessment[41] and Goldman-Fristoe Test of Articulation[42]) include objective scores that can be used for comparison purposes posttreatment. Alternatively, conducting a more informal measure of intelligibility and speech errors in conversational speech or a reading sample may be adequate. Overall, it is important to evaluate and document any pretreatment speech errors and try to determine if these are related to tumor presence or perhaps preexisting lifelong articulation errors. It is also worthwhile to document any language differences, dialectical or accent influences on someone's speech prior to treatment for oral cancer.

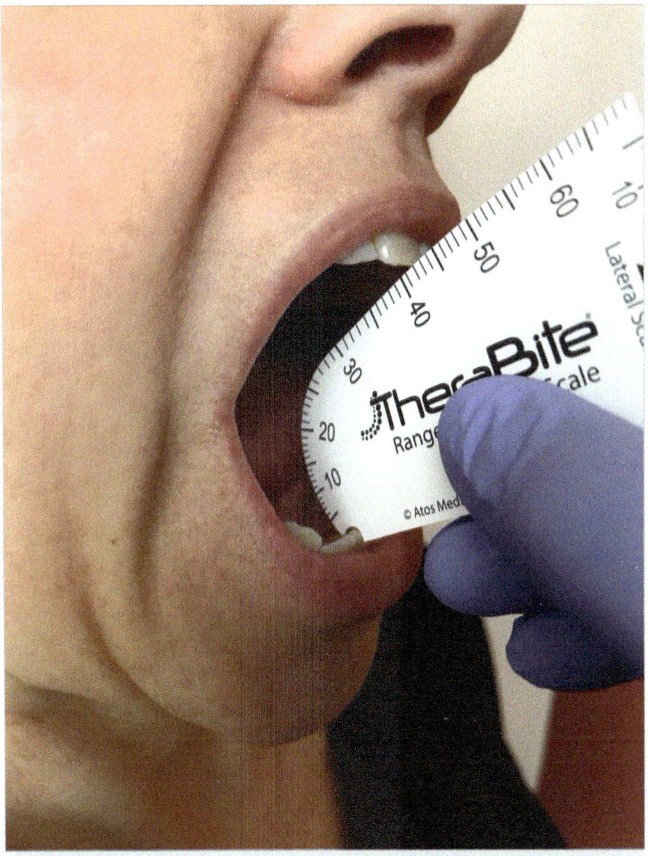

Fig. 11.1 Obtaining a jaw opening measurement using a TheraBite Jaw Range of Motion Scale.

Other baseline measurements during the oral motor examination can be obtained using the Iowa Oral Performance Instrument (IOPI).[43] It can be used to obtain baseline lip and tongue strength measurements in kilopascals (kPa). These measurements are obtained placing a bulb on the dorsal oral tongue, and cuing the patient to press their tongue against the hard palate (for tongue measurements) or placed in the midline and lateral aspects of the upper and lower lips. There are plentiful normative data for tongue pressures but only one study for lip pressures to date.[44–46] Regardless, this baseline measurement can be useful for comparison postoperatively.

A clinical swallow evaluation, or bedside swallow evaluation, is a subjective measure of a patient's swallowing function. Standard evaluations include incorporating ice chips, thin liquids with variation in volume (single sips, consecutive sips, cup vs. straw sips), thickened liquids as indicated, purees, soft solids, and/or regular solids. During a clinical swallow evaluation, the speech pathologist is assessing the oral and pharyngeal swallow.[47]

During the oral phase, we are easily able to assess labial seal, presence or absence of oral holding, and oral clearance. We are unable to fully assess lingual mobility, bolus propulsion, or ability to perform an oral hold with bolus trials during a clinical exam.[47]

During the pharyngeal phase of the swallow, we are clinically assessing for overt or covert signs and symptoms of penetration or aspiration, laryngeal elevation to palpation, and presence or absence of pharyngeal residue. These are all assessed subjectively while observing the patient eat and drink the abovementioned consistencies. We use this evaluation as more of a screening since silent aspiration is impossible to detect clinically and overall accuracy of detecting aspiration is less than 40%.[47,48] Aspiration cannot be discriminated from penetration during a clinical swallow evaluation. Overt signs and symptoms of penetration or aspiration include coughing, throat clearing, and wet vocal quality. More covert signs or indirect indicators of aspiration and dysphagia in general include watery eyes, sneezing, and variation in vital signs (i.e., drop in oxygen saturation).[47] Signs and symptoms of pharyngeal residue include the patient reporting sensation of presence of food or liquid remaining in their pharynx after swallowing (typically reported as "in the throat") and palpating or visualizing multiple swallows per single bolus. If there is a concern about any of these items mentioned earlier, instrumental evaluation is indicated.

In addition to a standard clinical swallow evaluation, if a patient has a tracheostomy tube, a blue dye clinical swallow evaluation can be performed. This is the same assessment as the clinical swallow, with the addition of food coloring to bolus trials. Typical food coloring is blue or green to allow for distinguishing discoloration of mucus from bolus trials. The concept behind a blue dye clinical swallow evaluation is to identify aspiration from tracheal secretions. If blue (or green) dye is expectorated or suctioned from the tracheostomy tube after oral feeding trials, it indicates definitive aspiration. The limitation of this assessment is that there is a high incidence of false negatives.[49] It is therefore a good clinical tool to use during a clinical swallow evaluation in addition to utilizing standard clinical skills.

If there is concern for aspiration or need to further view oral deficits, the SLP should subsequently proceed to instrumental examination (fiberoptic endoscopic evaluation of swallowing [FEES] or modified barium swallow study [MBS]). It is also pertinent to complete an instrumental examination in the event that the patient has a prior history of dysphagia, neurologic deficits, and/or prior radiation to the head or neck.[50] An instrumental examination such as a FEES[51,52] or the gold standard MBS[53] can give more objective information on baseline swallow function.[24] If there are oral deficits, MBS is more beneficial for assessing the oral phase.[26] If there are suspected pharyngeal deficits, both the FEES and MBS are useful assessments.[26]

Typically, a FEES is performed in a clinic room. The patient is seated upright. The nares may be sprayed with a topical anesthetic to reduce discomfort. The fiberoptic endoscope is passed through the nares by the SLP. It is helpful to visualize this examination on a video monitor while conducting it and to record it for review and archiving. Soft palate function and closure should be evaluated during both speaking and swallowing. The fiberoptic endoscope can then be advanced into the pharynx and is usually held steady at a level above the base of the tongue. Vocal fold motion and closure should be assessed during a speech task. PO trials are then presented to the patient. As with the clinical swallow evaluation, typically, several consistencies are evaluated. Using colored foods (i.e., milk, pudding, etc.) or placing a drop of green or blue food dye in the food and liquid can help with visualization and discrimination of the bolus from secretions. During a FEES examination, the SLP should assess base of tongue retraction, pharyngeal constriction, epiglottic tilt, airway protection, and clearance of the bolus as able. While visualization during the actual swallow is not possible, observing the pharynx and larynx before and after the swallow can give objective information on amount and symmetry of constriction, residue, and entry of bolus material into the laryngeal vestibule.[51–54]

MBS is preferred over a FEES in the event that the patient has significant oral deficits or the larynx is not adequately visualized with a FEES. Visualization during a FEES may be difficult secondary to the patient's anatomy or due to copious secretions.[51]

An MBS can be performed to objectively evaluate the oral, pharyngeal, and esophageal phases of swallowing. This examination involves coordination of a radiology appointment with a speech pathology appointment. The patient is seated in a chair or may be standing upright. He or she is presented with PO consistencies similar to the clinical swallow and FEES examinations, which are mixed with barium in order to be radiopaque. The SLP and radiologist evaluate as the bolus passes from the oral phase to the pharyngeal phase and into the esophagus. Ideally, the radiologist will complete at least one pass to the level of the stomach to observe movement of the bolus through the esophagus and into the stomach. The patient is evaluated in lateral projection, which is easiest to detect penetration or aspiration, and in the anteroposterior or frontal view, to evaluate symmetry of pharyngeal constriction, gross assessment of vocal fold closure, and symmetry. The amount and degree of residue in the valleculae and pyriform sinuses are assessed in lateral and frontal planes. The MBS, sometimes called a videofluoroscopic swallow study (VFSS), is considered the gold standard examination because one can observe swallowing as it naturally occurs from the bolus entering the oral cavity, being masticated, transferred posteriorly, entering into the pharyngeal phase, passing over the base of tongue as the epiglottis closes and larynx moves anteriorly and superiorly to protect the airway. Finally, one can visualize cricopharyngeal relaxation and assess for the ability of the bolus to pass to the esophageal phase.[54]

If the patient has had prior RT or chemoradiation (CRT), it is especially important to obtain the history regarding when RT/CRT occurred, to what areas (i.e., face, neck, pharynx, larynx, bilateral vs. unilateral, etc.), if they had a feeding tube during treatment, and if they were previously seen by SLP. It is also important to inquire whether these patients have lasting sequelae including dysphagia, xerostomia, dysgeusia, lymphedema, trismus, and fibrosis. With patients who have undergone prior RT/CRT to the head and neck, instrumental evaluation is indicated due to risks of silent aspiration post RT/CRT.[55–57] The remainder of the counseling session is similar to that for other patients who have not been previously treated with RT/CRT. Prior oral surgical resections should also be considered as there may be a degree of baseline altered anatomy and speech and/or swallowing dysfunction.

CN deficits should be taken into account if there was resection involving sacrifice of CNs. For oral cancer, we are particularly concerned with CN XII (hypoglossal) and occasionally CN VII (facial). When there are unilateral deficits, optimal placement of foods and liquids on the unaffected side can be extremely helpful. Certainly, if there is any history of CVA, Parkinson's disease, or other neurological history, this may impact speech and swallowing.[58,59]

The patient should always be asked if there is a prior history of dysphagia and details of this history should be obtained. All of these considerations would be indications to perform instrumental swallowing evaluations preoperatively, rather than just a clinical swallowing and oral motor evaluation.

11.5 Treatment Considerations and Approaches

In our institution, oral cancer patients are usually evaluated close to their surgery date and do not need to return for follow-up until after surgery unless they have extensive additional questions or concerns. Therapy is not necessarily indicated, given that speech and swallow functions are likely to change postoperatively.

However, postoperative treatment planning and goals are discussed in the preoperative evaluation. The anticipated need for swallowing, speech, and/or trismus therapy is reviewed with the patient. This has shown to be beneficial in improving postoperative patient compliance and understanding of their postoperative needs.[2,4,5,8,9] We have found that patients often ask if they will be able to speak or swallow, how "normal" their speech and swallowing will be, if people will understand them, and if they will be able to resume life and work functions. While the exact outcomes are often difficult to predict, patients are often reassured that with time and therapy, the goal is to establish the best possible speech and swallowing given the amount and nature of resection, reconstruction, and affected structures.[31] Meeting with other patients and/or seeing and hearing speech samples may also be helpful.

11.6 Surgical Options and Approaches

With lingual resections, there is often consideration of whether or not to utilize a free flap for reconstruction of the defect. The primary benefit of a flap in the case of oral tongue resections is both cosmetic and functional. It allows for improved ease of swallowing and can improve vocal resonance as well as potentially improved speech production.[19] This remains controversial regarding benefits of speech production, as some outcomes show increased scarring and reduced native tongue mobility when a flap is present.[20] One acute downside to flap reconstruction is the initial bulk of the flap, which significantly impacts speech and swallow function in the short term.[34] As the flap shrinks, this improves.[34] These are all topics that are discussed during a preoperative evaluation.

There are two options for reconstructing the maxilla in the event of maxillary resection, including a free flap or obturator.[60] There are benefits to both of these, as discussed in Section V, Chapters 26 and 30, and Section VIII, Chapter 39. Both are generally effective in reducing or eliminating nasal regurgitation when swallowing and nasal air emission when speaking.[60]

11.7 Conclusion

Preoperative SLP evaluations have been shown to be beneficial for many reasons, as discussed earlier. SLPs play a crucial role in the pre- and postoperative care of these oral cancer patients; therefore, establishing a relationship early on is essential and should be an integral component of the multidisciplinary intervention process.

Key Points

- Preoperative evaluations with SLP are recommended for the following:
  - To improve postoperative compliance.
  - To improve outcomes.
  - To improve patient understanding and reassure them that the goal is best possible functional outcomes.
  - To give subjective and objective baseline information on speech and swallowing.
  - To help patients to set realistic, appropriate goals for postoperative function.

References

[1] Weatherspoon DJ, Chattopadhyay A, Boroumand S, Garcia I. Oral cavity and oropharyngeal cancer incidence trends and disparities in the United States: 2000–2010. Cancer Epidemiol. 2015; 39(4):497–504

[2] Kalavrezos N, Cotrufo S, Govender R, et al. Factors affecting swallow outcome following treatment for advanced oral and oropharyngeal malignancies. Head Neck. 2014; 36(1):47–54

[3] Pauloski BR, Rademaker AW, Logemann JA, et al. Pretreatment swallowing function in patients with head and neck cancer. Head Neck. 2000; 22(5):474–482

[4] Lieberman A. Counseling issues: addressing behavioral and emotional considerations in the treatment of communication disorders. Am J Speech Lang Pathol. 2018; 27(1):13–23

[5] Dzioba A, Aalto D, Papadopoulos-Nydam G, et al. Head and Neck Research Network. Functional and quality of life outcomes after partial glossectomy: a multi-institutional longitudinal study of the head and neck research network. J Otolaryngol Head Neck Surg. 2017; 46(1):56

[6] Starmer H, Gourin C, Lua LL, Burkhead L. Pretreatment swallowing assessment in head and neck cancer patients. Laryngoscope. 2011; 121(6):1208–1211

[7] Shenson JA, Craig JN, Rohde SL. Effect of preoperative counseling on hospital length of stay and readmissions after total laryngectomy. Otolaryngol Head Neck Surg. 2017; 156(2):289–298

[8] Carroll WR, Locher JL, Canon CL, Bohannon IA, McColloch NL, Magnuson JS. Pretreatment swallowing exercises improve swallow function after chemoradiation. Laryngoscope. 2008; 118(1):39–43

[9] Landera MS, Odlum J, Lundy DS. Swallowing evaluation of the patient with head and neck cancer. Perspectives. 2013; 22(2):53–60

[10] Carnaby-Mann G, Crary MA, Schmalfuss I, Amdur R. "Pharyngocise": randomized controlled trial of preventative exercises to maintain muscle structure and swallowing function during head-and-neck chemoradiotherapy. Int J Radiat Oncol Biol Phys. 2012; 83(1):210–219

[11] Hansen K, Chenoweth M, Thompson H, Strouss A. Role of the speech-language pathologist (SLP) in the head and neck cancer team. In: Maghami E, Ho AS, eds. Multidisciplinary Care of the Head and Neck Cancer Patient. New York, NY: Springer; 2018:31–42

[12] Silver JK. Cancer prehabilitation and its role in improving health outcomes and reducing health care costs. Semin Oncol Nurs. 2015; 31(1):13–30

[13] Colangelo LA, Logemann JA, Rademaker AW. Tumor size and pretreatment speech and swallowing in patients with resectable tumors. Otolaryngol Head Neck Surg. 2000; 122(5):653–661

[14] Westin T, Stalfors J. Tumour boards/multidisciplinary head and neck cancer meetings: are they of value to patients, treating staff or a political additional drain on healthcare resources? Curr Opin Otolaryngol Head Neck Surg. 2008; 16(2):103–107

[15] Starmer H, Sanguineti G, Marur S, Gourin CG. Multidisciplinary head and neck cancer clinic and adherence with speech pathology. Laryngoscope. 2011; 121(10):2131–2135

[16] Rettig EM, D'Souza G. Epidemiology of head and neck cancer. Surg Oncol Clin N Am. 2015; 24(3):379–396

[17] Jakobsen KK, Grønhøj C, Jensen DH, et al. Increasing incidence and survival of head and neck cancers in Denmark: a nation-wide study from 1980 to 2014. Acta Oncol. 2018; 57(9):1143–1151
[18] Lazarus C, Logemann JA, Pauloski BR, et al. Effects of radiotherapy with or without chemotherapy on tongue strength and swallowing in patients with oral cancer. Head Neck. 2007; 29(7):632–637
[19] Joo YH, Hwang SH, Park JO, Cho KJ, Kim MS. Functional outcome after partial glossectomy with reconstruction using radial forearm free flap. Auris Nasus Larynx. 2013; 40(3):303–307
[20] Chuanjun C, Zhiyuan Z, Shaopu G, Xinquan J, Zhihong Z. Speech after partial glossectomy: a comparison between reconstruction and nonreconstruction patients. J Oral Maxillofac Surg. 2002; 60(4):404–407
[21] Namaki S, Tanaka T, Hara Y, Ohki H, Shinohara M, Yonhehara Y. Videofluorographic evaluation of dysphagia before and after modification of the flap and scar in patients with oral cancer. J Plast Surg Hand Surg. 2011; 45(3):136–142
[22] Matthews TW, Lampe HB. Treatment options in oral cancer. In: Doyle PC, Keith RL, eds. Contemporary considerations in the treatment and rehabilitation of head and Neck Cancer: Voice, speech, and swallowing. Austin, TX: Pro-Ed; 2005:153–170
[23] Borggreven PA, Verdonck-de Leeuw I, Langendijk JA, et al. Speech outcome after surgical treatment for oral and oropharyngeal cancer: a longitudinal assessment of patients reconstructed by a microvascular flap. Head Neck. 2005; 27(9):785–793
[24] Lazarus CL, Ward EC, Yiu EM. Speech and swallowing following oral, oropharyngeal, and nasopharyngeal cancers. In: Ward EC, van As-Brooks CJ, eds. Head and Neck Cancer: Treatment, Rehabilitation, and outcomes. San Diego, CA: Plural Publishing; 2014:103–122
[25] Tei K, Maekawa K, Kitada H, Ohiro Y, Yamazaki Y, Totsuka Y. Recovery from postsurgical swallowing dysfunction in patients with oral cancer. J Oral Maxillofac Surg. 2007; 65(6):1077–1083
[26] Logemann JA. Swallowing disorders after treatment for oral and oropharyngeal cancer. In: Logemann JA, ed. Evaluation and Treatment of Swallowing Disorders. Austin, TX: Pro-ed; 1942:251–277
[27] Leeper HA, Gratton DG, Lapointe HJ, Armstrong JEA. Maxillofacial rehabilitation for oral cancer: surgical, prosthodontic, and communication aspects of management. In: Doyle PC, Keith RL, eds. Contemporary considerations in the treatment and rehabilitation of head and Neck Cancer: Voice, speech, and swallowing. Austin, TX: Pro-Ed; 2005:261–314
[28] Koyama Y, Ota Y, Sakaizumi K, et al. Swallowing appliance: intraoral reshaping prosthesis for dysphagia secondary to oral floor cancer: a pilot study. Am J Phys Med Rehabil. 2014; 93(11):1008–1013
[29] Pearson WG, Jr, Hindson DF, Langmore SE, Zumwalt AC. Evaluating swallowing muscles essential for hyolaryngeal elevation by using muscle functional magnetic resonance imaging. Int J Radiat Oncol Biol Phys. 2013; 85(3):735–740
[30] Pauloski BR. Rehabilitation of dysphagia following head and neck cancer. Phys Med Rehabil Clin N Am. 2008; 19(4):889–928, x
[31] Keski-Säntti H, Bäck L, Lassus P, et al. Total or subtotal glossectomy with laryngeal preservation: a national study of 29 patients. Eur Arch Otorhinolaryngol. 2018; 275(1):191–197
[32] Lin DT, Yarlagadda BB, Sethi RK, et al. Long-term functional outcomes of total glossectomy with or without total laryngectomy. JAMA Otolaryngol Head Neck Surg. 2015; 141(9):797–803
[33] Logemann JA. Medical treatment for swallowing disorders. In: Logemann JA, ed. Evaluation and Treatment of Swallowing Disorders. Austin, TX: Pro-ed; 1942:345–354
[34] Kimura M, Takada K, Ishibashi K, et al. Quantitative analysis of chronological changes in the volume of flaps used for reconstruction of oral cavity defects. J Oral Sci. 2017; 59(4):499–503
[35] Vila PM, Rich JT, Desai SC. Defining Quality in Head and Neck Reconstruction. Otolaryngol Head Neck Surg. 2017; 157(4):545–547
[36] Buglione M, Cavagnini R, Di Rosario F, et al. Oral toxicity management in head and neck cancer patients treated with chemotherapy and radiation: Xerostomia and trismus (Part 2). Literature review and consensus statement. Crit Rev Oncol Hematol. 2016; 102:47–54
[37] Saunders NA, Coman WB, Guminski AD. Cancer of the head and neck. In: Ward EC, van As-Brooks CJ, eds. Head and Neck Cancer: Treatment, Rehabilitation, and Outcomes. San Diego, CA: Plural Publishing; 2014:1–26
[38] American Speech Language Hearing Association. https://www.asha.org/PRPSpecificTopic.aspx?folderid=8589942550&section=Assessment. Accessed February 25, 2018
[39] Gallagher C, Gallagher V, Whelton H, Cronin M. The normal range of mouth opening in an Irish population. J Oral Rehabil. 2004; 31(2):110–116
[40] Khare N, Patil SB, Kale SM, Sumeet J, Sonali I, Sumeet B. Normal mouth opening in an adult Indian population. J Maxillofac Oral Surg. 2012; 11(3):309–313
[41] Enderby P. Frenchay dysarthria assessment. Br J Disord Commun. 1980; 15 (3):165–173
[42] Goldman R, Fristoe M. Goldman-Fristoe test of articulation. Circle Pines, MN: American Guidance Service; 1986
[43] Northwest IOPI. Iowa Oral Performance Instrument: User's Manual. Carnation, WA: IOPI Northwest; 2005
[44] Adams V, Mathisen B, Baines S, Lazarus C, Callister R. A systematic review and meta-analysis of measurements of tongue and hand strength and endurance using the Iowa Oral Performance Instrument (IOPI). Dysphagia. 2013; 28 (3):350–369
[45] Solomon NP, Clark HM, Makashay MJ, Newman LA. Assessment of orofacial strength in patients with dysarthria. J Med Speech-Lang Pathol. 2008; 16(4): 251–258
[46] Vanderwegen J, Guns C, Van Nuffelen G, Elen R, De Bodt M. The influence of age, sex, bulb position, visual feedback, and the order of testing on maximum anterior and posterior tongue strength and endurance in healthy belgian adults. Dysphagia. 2013; 28(2):159–166
[47] Logemann JA. Evaluation of swallowing disorders. In: Logemann JA, ed. Evaluation and Treatment of Swallowing Disorders. Austin, TX: Pro-ed; 1942:135–185
[48] Aviv JE, Martin JH, Sacco RL, et al. Supraglottic and pharyngeal sensory abnormalities in stroke patients with dysphagia. Ann Otol Rhinol Laryngol. 1996; 105(2):92–97
[49] Fiorelli A, Ferraro F, Nagar F, et al. A new modified evans blue dye test as screening test for aspiration in tracheostomized patients. J Cardiothorac Vasc Anesth. 2017; 31(2):441–445
[50] Lazarus CL. Management of swallowing disorders in individuals with head and neck cancer. In: Doyle PC, Keith RL, eds. Contemporary considerations in the treatment and rehabilitation of head and Neck Cancer: Voice, Speech, and swallowing. Austin, TX: Pro-Ed; 2005:315–352
[51] Langmore SE, Schatz K, Olsen N. Fiberoptic endoscopic examination of swallowing safety: a new procedure. Dysphagia. 1988; 2(4):216–219
[52] Langmore SE. History of fiberoptic endoscopic evaluation of swallowing for evaluation and management of pharyngeal dysphagia: changes over the years. Dysphagia. 2017; 32(1):27–38
[53] Leder SB, Acton LM, Lisitano HL, Murray JT. Fiberoptic endoscopic evaluation of swallowing (FEES) with and without blue-dyed food. Dysphagia. 2005; 20 (2):157–162
[54] Logemann JA. A manual for Videofluoroscopic Evaluation of swallowing. Austin, TX: Pro-Ed; 1993:79–82
[55] Webster KT, Tippett D, Simpson M, et al. Speech-language pathology care and short- and long-term outcomes of oropharyngeal cancer treatment in the elderly. Laryngoscope. 2018; 128(6):1403–1411
[56] Starmer HM, Tippett D, Webster K, et al. Swallowing outcomes in patients with oropharyngeal cancer undergoing organ-preservation treatment. Head Neck. 2014; 36(10):1392–1397
[57] Starmer HM, Gourin CG. Is speech language pathologist evaluation necessary in the nonoperative treatment of head and neck cancer? Laryngoscope. 2013; 123(7):1571–1572
[58] Rugiu MG. Role of videofluoroscopy in evaluation of neurologic dysphagia. Acta Otorhinolaryngol Ital. 2007; 27(6):306–316
[59] Andrenelli E, Galli FL, Gesuita R, et al. Swallowing impairments in amyotrophic lateral sclerosis and myotonic dystrophy type 1: looking for the portrait of dysphagic patient in neuromuscular diseases. NeuroRehabilitation. 2018; 42(1):93–102
[60] Hagio M, Ishizaki K, Ryu M, Nomura T, Takano N, Sakurai K. Maxillofacial prosthetic treatment factors affecting oral health-related quality of life after surgery for patients with oral cancer. J Prosthet Dent. 2018; 119(4): 663–670

12 Nutrition for Oral Cancer Patients

Susan Hill and Steven S. Chang

Summary

Optimal nutrition is essential for all patients with head and neck cancer (HNC). More specifically, patients with oral cavity cancer (OCC) are at very high risk of suboptimal nutrition. Factors such as the site of the cancer and the types of treatment used can significantly affect a patient's nutritional status and put them at high risk for malnutrition. When the patient is malnourished, that increases susceptibility to a whole host of other issues that can affect tolerance to treatment and long-term survivability. Early nutrition intervention and continued involvement of the registered dietitian (RD) with this patient population across the continuum of care is recommended by the National Comprehensive Cancer Network (NCCN). The RD has the education and training to support the patient nutritionally throughout the treatment process and beyond to survivorship.

Keywords: malnutrition, nutritional status, muscle, high protein, high calorie, ERAS

12.1 Introduction

The relationship between cancer and malnutrition has long been known. Malnutrition can occur at all stages of the disease. Thirty to 90% of patients with head and neck cancers (HNCs) are affected by malnutrition.[1] Optimal nutrition is essential for everyone, and especially for the patient with oral cavity cancer (OCC). From the day of diagnosis, throughout the various treatments, and well into survivorship, poor nutrition is frequently a significant issue. Having treatment for OCC impacts the patient's ability to eat and drink. This can lead to impaired wound healing, increased length of hospital stay, poor quality of life (QoL), and interruptions to treatment.[2] Side effects of treatments also include swallowing difficulties, dry mouth, nausea, and a reduced appetite—rendering eating and drinking a significant challenge for a majority of these patients. The purpose of this chapter is to identify and address nutrition concerns in patients with OCC from diagnosis to survivorship.

12.2 NCCN Guidelines: Principles of Nutrition: Management and Supportive Care

The National Comprehensive Cancer Network (NCCN) Guidelines for Head and Neck Cancers recommend that the multidisciplinary evaluation of patients with HNC include a registered dietitian (RD) **before** *and* **after** treatment to assess the need for nutrition interventions (e.g., enteral support via feeding tubes).[3] Historically, and unfortunately still common today, the first time a patient with HNC would encounter an RD along the spectrum of care would be after a large weight loss had occurred or the patient had suffered significant side effects from cancer treatment and required hospital admission.[2] A proactive approach to nutrition in any patient with cancer is preferable to the commonly seen reactive approach, but especially the patient with OCC.

12.3 Diagnosis and Evaluation

12.3.1 Pretreatment Nutrition Evaluation

Part of a proactive approach to nutrition for patients with HNC is a pretreatment nutrition evaluation and intervention. The vast majority of this patient population will develop side effects from treatment that will affect his or her ability to maintain optimal nutrition status. They may begin with no identified issues, but pretreatment represents a good time to address not only any current nutrition issues, but also the potential nutrition issues expected to arise during treatment that can have serious implications.

The *screening* of *all* patients with HNC for malnutrition, especially those with OCC, early in the diagnosis process will help identify those patients at a higher nutritional risk. This screening allows for identification of patients who would benefit from a more extensive nutrition *assessment*. A nutrition screening is a brief evaluation to identify potential patients at high risk for malnutrition. A nutrition assessment is a more complex process meant to explore further their nutrition status.[4] Nutrition assessment is a detailed evaluation and interpretation of multiple factors, including height, weight, physical assessment, laboratory values, social issues, etc. This assessment seeks to identify those patients at risk of developing nutrition-related medical complications.

Although screening for malnutrition is not routinely done in the outpatient setting, it should be done for any patient with suspected HNC. There are numerous screening tools available and careful attention needs to be given to tools that have been validated for use with oncology patients. An ideal screening tool is one that can be administered quickly, can be interpreted by a variety of health care providers, and is useful across a range of cancer diagnoses.[5] The Academy of Nutrition and Dietetics' Evidence Analysis Library has reviewed and graded the most common nutrition screening tools available. Four tools were found to be appropriate for the oncology patient population: the Patient-Generated Subjective Global Assessment (PG-SGA),[6,7] the Malnutrition Screening Tool (MST),[8] Malnutrition Screening Tool for Cancer Patients (MSTC),[9] and the Malnutrition Universal Screening Tool (MUST).[10]

Of the four listed, the MST[8] has been favored as an easy to administer and interpret tool for early identification of potential malnutrition. This is a two-item, validated screening tool that includes weight loss and any recent change in appetite as its parameters. It is scored to determine their risk and can be used for both inpatient and outpatient across all age groups. A patient with a MST score of 2 or more is determined to be "at risk" and requires further nutrition assessment and intervention. Additionally, for any patient scoring 2 or more on the MST, an oral liquid nutrition supplement is recommended to help achieve a greater oral intake.

A comprehensive nutrition assessment is the next step in a complete pretreatment evaluation. The Evidence Analysis Library Oncology Working Group of the Academy of Nutrition and Dietetics states that "an adult oncology nutrition assessment should characterize and document the presence of (or expected potential for) altered nutrition status and nutrition impact symptoms (NIs) that may result in a measurable adverse effect on body composition, function, QOL or clinical outcome, and may also include indicators of malnutrition."[11] The key components of a nutrition assessment are grouped into five categories: food-/nutrition-related history; anthropometric measures; labs, medical tests, and procedures; nutrition-focused physical findings; and client medical/health/social history.

12.3.2 Food/Nutrition-Related History

This category includes not only the patient's diet history, but also the patient's medication history and any modifications they have made to their diet in order to consume adequate calories and protein. Are they able to eat whatever they want? Do they restrict any particular food or groups of food for any reason (e.g., meats or tough-to-chew foods, any foods containing sugar, only able to swallow liquids)? Are they eating the same amount of food they normally do or are they eating less? Is it taking them longer to eat? How many meals per day do they normally consume? Has this changed recently? Do they regularly drink alcohol? If so, what type of alcohol and how much? Are there any prescribed or over-the-counter medications that can affect their appetite either positively or negatively (e.g., appetite stimulants, narcotics, steroids)? Are they using any stool softeners/laxatives? If so, are these medications working? Do they need to modify the texture of any of the foods they are eating in order to make it easier to eat? Are they using only liquid oral nutritional supplements because they cannot tolerate solid foods of any type? If so, what type and how many per day?

These questions represent the majority of the nutrition assessment for this patient population. Considering where OCC is located and how the proposed treatment can alter these basic and life-sustaining activities, the functions of eating and drinking are at direct risk.

12.3.3 Anthropometric Measurements

This category includes the patient's height (actually measure this when able; do not rely on patient report), current weight, usual weight, and any weight changes over time (document weight lost over what time period). Any weight loss in this patient population has potential significance. Regardless of the patient's calculated body mass index (BMI) at assessment, unintentional weight loss has been associated with negative postoperative outcomes and functional decline.[12] When patients are unsure of any weight loss, ask if they have noticed their clothes fitting any differently (e.g., had to take in a notch or two on their belt buckle?). Other measurements can be taken such as triceps skin fold or mid-arm muscle circumference measured over time, though this is not commonly used in general practice.

12.3.4 Labs, Medical Tests, and Procedures

Although historically serum proteins such as albumin and prealbumin have been widely used by physicians, generally no laboratory data are a reliable predictor of nutritional status. The current consensus is that laboratory markers are not reliable by themselves; however, these could be used as a complement to a thorough physical examination.[13] Lab values pertaining to the patient's comorbidities, such as glycated hemoglobin for those with diabetes, still need attention as lack of proper glucose control can affect outcomes as well. One procedure/test that can be of value in nutrition assessment is the videofluoroscopic swallow study. Does the patient require education on diet modification regarding fluid viscosity or texture to avoid aspiration? Ensuring the safe consumption of nutrition is just as important as the nutrition itself, and the speech-language pathologist (SLP) is an important member of the multidisciplinary team (see Chapters 11 and 44).

12.3.5 Nutrition-Focused Physical Findings

A nutrition-focused physical examination will uncover any potential muscle wasting and other signs of malnutrition. For example, signs of temporal wasting or prominent clavicles can alert you to potential malnutrition. NIS, a variety of symptoms that can compromise oral intake, can be discovered during this part of the assessment as well.[14] Examples of NIS include nausea, vomiting, diarrhea, constipation, altered taste, depression, anxiety, and pain. Patients with HNC are likely to also experience dysphagia, mouth sores, xerostomia, dental problems, and difficulty chewing, which are also associated with reduced dietary intake.[14] Other issues to be aware of in this group of patients is trismus, tongue range of motion, fit of dentures if they have them, and tolerance to various food temperatures, acidity, and textures.

12.3.6 History: Medical/Health/Social

Understanding how the proposed treatment regimen will affect the patient nutritionally is a vital part of the nutrition assessment. Often a pretreatment nutrition assessment will not uncover any nutrition issues/deficiencies; however, the majority of these patients will likely develop nutrition issues as part of the proposed treatment. Educating the patient early in treatment is important to help avoid major nutrition issues in the future. Remember, a proactive approach is better than a reactive approach to the nutritional management of the patient with HNC.

A patient's social history is important to obtain in the HNC population. Knowing what support the patient has available to them and their living circumstances can help prevent potential complications. It can be a substantial challenge for patients to get to treatments or deal with dressing changes following a surgery if they live alone and lack friends or family who can help them. From a nutrition perspective, this is also a challenge, as many times the patient may not be motivated to prepare the foods necessary to maintain their nutritional status and will need to rely on their social supports to prepare foods. This is especially true if the patient is required to modify the texture of the foods they need to consume safely (e.g., pureed or ground foods). Nutritional supplements and tube feeding formulas can be a financial burden for the HNC patient. Most insurance companies do not cover the cost of the formulas if taken orally and some will only cover the cost of supplies like the 60-mL syringes used to administer the feeding.

Obtaining accurate alcohol intake history is vital. Malnutrition is significantly greater among alcohol users.[2] When patients are asked to stop drinking alcohol, a significant source of calories in their diet can be taken away. Micronutrients are also affected by chronic alcohol use, and a B-complex vitamin (especially thiamine) may be recommended.[15] The involvement of a behavioral health specialist can further motivate and support abstinence from alcohol.

Once all this information has been gathered, a nutrition plan is made for the patient. Regardless of the proposed treatment, nutrition plays an important role for patients with OCC. Preparing the patient for the upcoming treatment includes not only nutrition advice, but also education regarding what to expect from treatment that can affect the patient's nutritional status. A forewarned patient is forearmed.

12.4 Management

Nutritional goals for HNC:[11]

- Weight maintenance during and after treatment.
- Weight maintenance posttreatment until the patient is able to consume solid food safely.
- Successful, break-free completion of treatment.
- Minimal, if any, weight loss in overweight or obese patients until the patient is fully recovered from treatment and able to eat without difficulties.
- Weight maintenance during transitional feedings from enteral nutrition support to oral diet.

Goals are a good thing to have when treating this patient population. Of the five goals listed, four refer to weight maintenance or minimal weight loss for these patients. Weight loss in patients with HNC is not just loss of body fat but also potential muscle loss (somatic protein stores). It is important to make the patient aware of the potential loss of lean body mass so that they realize the importance of maintaining an adequate nutritional status from the start of the cancer journey, regardless of start weight or history of obesity. Now is not the time to consider weight loss a desired goal.

12.4.1 Pretreatment Nutrition Plan

Keeping in mind all the information that was gathered as part of the pretreatment nutrition assessment and the nutritional goals for these patients, a nutrition care plan is developed and shared with the patient. Spending the time necessary to review and explain the nutrition care plan to the patient is important for adherence and ultimately better outcomes. Use the teach-back method to assess for understanding of the main points of the care plan. Make sure written materials provided to the patient are clear and easy to read/understand and at the appropriate literacy level for the patient (e.g., within patient-facing medical information a fifth grade reading level is considered appropriate). Individualizing the nutrition care plan is important; however, there are some standard nutrition recommendations for all patients with HNC.

A high-calorie, high-protein diet is recommended as these patients are at a high risk of significant weight loss as a result of treatment. Additionally, patients with HNC have high protein needs for wound and tissue healing throughout treatment. A factor of 1.2 to 2.0 g of protein per kilogram of body weight per day has been suggested as a guide for protein goals in physically stressed patient populations, which is certainly true of this patient population.[12] As eating and drinking can become challenging for patients with OCC, patients need to make every bite and every sip count. Encourage the patient to begin these higher calorie/higher protein foods as soon as possible, preferably prior to treatment. Weight loss is a known complication for patients with OCC and the sooner it is addressed the better. Advise patients to eat when they feel hungry, not waiting until mealtime to eat. Other patients may not feel hungry and need to be reminded every couple of hours to eat. Most people have their best appetite in the morning, because they have not eaten all night; thus, encouragement to take in as many calories in the morning is prudent. Do not wait until later to choose high-calorie and high-protein foods. Box 12.1 lists some ideas to share with patients that can help them increase calorie and protein content in the food they are already eating.

Box 12.1 Ways to add calories and protein to foods

- Rather than serving broth, puree vegetable soup or bean soup as part of the liquid.
- Serve gravies or sauces made with pureed beans or blended soft/silken tofu over potatoes.
- Add butter or sour cream to mashed potatoes.
- Add powdered milk to liquid full fat milk. Ratio of 1 cup liquid milk to 1/3 cup powdered milk. Use this fortified milk wherever milk is required.
- Make ice cubes from milk or fruit nectar. Use these high-calorie ice cubes in smoothies or to keep drinks cold. As they melt, they will add calories and not water down the beverage.
- Choose creamy soups rather than broth-based soups.
- Have puddings and custards rather than gelatin desserts.
- Add sauces, gravies, or extra vegetable oil/butter to meals.
- Drink apricot or peach fruit nectars. They are less acidic than others.
- Drink fruit shakes or fruit smoothies made with yogurt or ice cream.
- Use a liquid nutritional supplement instead of milk to make a nutritious, high-calorie milkshake.
- Add sour cream, half and half, heavy cream, or whole milk to foods like mashed potatoes, sauces, gravies, cereals, soups, and casseroles. Consider adding mayonnaise to eggs, chicken, tuna, pasta, or potatoes to make a smooth, moist salad.
- Add avocado to dishes or smoothies.
- Add nut butters such as peanut butter to shakes and smoothies.

Use of a liquid nutrition supplement is also advised to begin as soon as possible. Which supplement is the best? The one the patient will drink that has the most calories and protein in the smallest liquid volume. Supplement companies will market various products to patients with cancer, but in the end the best supplement is the one the patient will consume on a consistent basis. Ideally, the "plus" version of supplements is recommended, as it typically contains the highest calories and/or protein in a smaller volume.

Educating the patient and caregivers on soft-texture foods early in the treatment process will also greatly benefit the patient with OCC. Oftentimes, patients with OCC will present with difficulty eating solid foods. Hard, chewy, dry, and tough foods are a great challenge and many times patients will have already eliminated these foods from their diet prior to the first visit with a specialist. Meat and other protein sources can be challenging for patients with OCC, so counseling them on alternative food choices and preparation techniques can help bring those vital sources of protein back into their daily diet. ▶ Table 12.1 provides examples of various foods to include and avoid when soft-texture foods are required by the patient. A discussion on the pureed diet, a more restrictive diet, will come later in this chapter.

To summarize, the general nutrition information that all patients with OCC should receive includes information about high-calorie/high-protein diet, recommendations to start a liquid nutrition supplement, and education regarding various soft-texture foods. The remainder of the nutrition care plan will depend on the cancer treatment modality that is recommended. Single modality versus bi-/tri-modality treatment requires further education and nutrition intervention.

Table 12.1 Recommendations for diet alterations

Food groups	Recommendations	Avoid
Beverages	2% or whole milk, juices, shakes, smoothies, eggnog, hot chocolate, soy milk, *fortified milk*,[a] liquid nutritional supplements.	Carbonated beverages, alcoholic beverages. Avoid filling up on low-calorie items like flavored waters.
Breads and bread products	Moisten bread products with gravies and margarine. Soft pancakes with margarine and syrup. Crackers well moistened in soup.	Toast and rough-textured breads, crusty breads, bagels, crackers, bread sticks.
Cereals	Cooked cereals made with *fortified milk*.[a] Cold cereals, well moistened with milk with little texture such as corn flakes and rice krispies	Very coarse cooked cereals that may contain flax seed or other seeds or nuts, Wholegrain dry or coarse cereals with nuts, seeds, dry fruit, and/or coconut
Dessert	Pudding, custard, soft fruit, or custard pies with bottom crust only. Soft moist cakes, ice cream, gelatin, soufflés, milk shakes. Soft, moist cookies that have been "dunked" in liquid. Yogurt.	Dry, coarse cakes and cookies. Anything with nuts, seeds, coconut, pineapple, or dried fruits.
Fats	Smooth sauces such as a white sauce or a cheese sauce. Butter, margarine, gravy, sour cream, mayonnaise, cream cheese, whipped topping, whipped cream.	Avoid any gravies or sauces with chunky additives (like large pieces of sausage in sausage gravy).
Fruits	Soft, canned or cooked fruits without seeds or skin. Fresh soft/ripe banana, applesauce, pureed fruit sauces.	Whole fruits with skin and seeds, dried fruits, fresh or canned pineapple.
Meats and meat substitutes. *Meat pieces should not exceed ¼ inch cube side and should be tender*	Moistened ground and cooked meats, poultry or fish (preferably meat with fat). Moist ground or tender meat should be served with gravy or a sauce. Casseroles with extra sauce. Moist macaroni and cheese, well-cooked pasta with meat sauce, tuna noodle casserole, moist meatloaf, meatballs. Tuna or egg salad without large chunks, celery, or onion. Cottage cheese, smooth quiche without large chunks. Poached, scrambled, or soft-cooked eggs. Well-cooked, moistened, slightly mashed beans and legumes. Melted cheese and cheese sauces. Cottage cheese.	Dry meats, tough meats (such as bacon, sausage, hot dogs). Dry casseroles or casseroles made with large chunks, peanut butter, pizza, nuts and seeds.
Potatoes and starches	Mashed potatoes with gravy. Well-cooked noodles in a sauce.	Baked potato with skin, cooked grains like rice and barley. Potato chips, French fried potatoes.
Soups	Soups with easy-to-chew or easy-to-swallow meats or vegetables (pieces should be < 0.5 inch).	Soups with large chunks of meats and vegetables.
Vegetables	All soft, well-cooked vegetables. Vegetables should be easily mashed with a fork.	Cooked corn and peas. Broccoli, cabbage, brussels sprouts, asparagus, or other fibrous, nontender, or rubbery cooked vegetables.
Miscellaneous	Jams and preserves without seeds, jelly. Sauces, salsas, etc., that may have small tender chunks. Soft, smooth chocolate bars that are easily chewed.	Seeds, nuts, coconut, sticky foods. Chewy candies such as caramel or licorice.

[a]For fortified milk, use ratio of 1 cup liquid milk to 1/3 cup powdered milk.

12.4.2 Nutrition Considerations with the Patient Treated with Surgical Resection

Preparing patients for surgery nutritionally is paramount. Enhanced Recovery after Surgery (ERAS) protocols have highlighted the importance of presurgical nutrition, in addition to re-examining the need for preoperative fasting and holding postoperative feeding for extended periods of time following surgery.[12] ERAS protocols not only address malnourished patients, but also improve outcomes for well-nourished patients. A meta-analysis of 38 trials reported reduced length of stay for those following ERAS protocols and a reduction in the risk of complications at 30 days after surgery by 30%.[16,17] It was recently reported in the Joint Consensus Statement on Nutrition Screening and Therapy within a Surgical Enhanced Recovery Pathway from the American Society for Enhanced Recovery and Perioperative Quality Initiative that for every $1 spent on nutrition therapy in hospitalized patients a savings of $52 in hospital costs was realized.[12] ERAS protocols encompass more than nutrition recommendations, but for the purpose of this chapter, only the nutrition components will be discussed.

Initially, ERAS protocols were developed for patients receiving treatment for colorectal malignancies, and many recommendations for other surgical sites have been based on that evidence. A 2017 Consensus Review and Recommendations article in JAMA Oto-HNS suggested ERAS protocols for Major Head and Neck Cancer Surgery with Free Flap Reconstruction.[12] Of the five nutritional care recommendations made, three had strong recommendations with moderate to high evidence for their use.

- All patients should have a preoperative comprehensive nutritional assessment and preoperative nutrition intervention is recommended for those identified as malnourished (strong recommendation with high evidence).
- Preoperative fasting should be minimized. For those patients able to safely consume oral liquids and solids, clear fluids should be permitted for up to 2 hours and solids for up to 6 hours prior to anesthesia (strong recommendation with high evidence for fluids, strong recommendation with low evidence for solids).
- Oral diet is the first choice for all patients as long as no evidence of aspiration is present. For those unable to tolerate an oral diet, a tube feeding should begin within 24 hours postoperative (strong recommendation with moderate evidence).[18]

The take-home message here is to feed the patient before and after surgery.[19] Withholding nutrition pre and postsurgically has been shown to exacerbate the surgical stress response, aggravate insulin resistance, exaggerate protein losses, and impair gastrointestinal function.[12] Although the recommendations are conditional and evidence low in the consensus statement, the use of a complex carbohydrate-rich beverage the night before and about 2 hours prior to surgery was given a strong recommendation by the American Society for Enhanced Recovery and Perioperative Quality Initiative.[12] Drinking a 50-g complex carbohydrate solution (maltodextrin based) about 2 to 3 hours prior to surgery helps decrease patient anxiety, thirst, hunger, and headaches.[12] Some studies also suggest drinking 100 g of this complex carbohydrate beverage the night prior to surgery.[12] For those who fear the possibility of aspiration under anesthesia, clear fluids taken up to 2 hours presurgery do not appear to increase gastric volumes, but could actually stimulate gastric emptying.[20] Further the demonstrated benefits of a preoperative complex carbohydrate drink has been shown to reduce the catabolic response to surgery, improve insulin resistance, and prevent postoperative hyperglycemia.[21] It should be noted that not all carbohydrate beverages are created equally. The complex carbohydrate beverage used in the studies was a 12.5% solution of maltodextrin.[22,23] Fruit juice and sports rehydration beverages are not good substitutes. Other presurgery beverages containing certain amino acids and omega-3 fatty acids have also been recommended, but concerns have been raised due to the heavy involvement of industry in sponsored studies, so there are insufficient data to provide a recommendation on their use.[22]

The decision to use a postoperative feeding tube should be based on the individual patient circumstance. For those patients with OCC whose surgery has altered their ability to safely swallow adequate nutrition or has included placement of a reconstructive flap, a Dobhoff tube is a reasonable option (vs. a gastrostomy/percutaneous endoscopic gastrostomy [PEG] tube), as the need for an alternate feeding route may be short and temporary.[16] A Dobhoff tube is a type of nasogastric feeding tube that is inserted into the stomach by way of the nasal passage and provides a safe route for not only nutrition, but also hydration and medication postsurgically to allow for better healing in the oral cavity. The feeding tube should remain in place until the patient has been evaluated by an SLP for the safety and efficiency of the patient's swallow. Should the patient develop long-term swallowing issues that either result in aspiration or a high risk for aspiration, then a gastrostomy/PEG tube should be considered.

Depending on the extent of the surgery to the oral cavity, some patients may be able to begin an oral diet following the procedure. A pureed or mechanically altered diet should be ordered for the patient. According to the National Dysphagia Diet guidelines, a pureed diet should consist of foods that are homogenous, very cohesive, puddinglike, requiring very little chewing or no chewing ability.[24] The mechanically altered foods should be cohesive, moist, semisolid foods, requiring some chewing.[24] The decision between the two diets is based on the patient's ability to control the food within the oral cavity. The patient may also require a thickened fluid as well, and once again an SLP should be involved at this point to help the multidisciplinary team make the appropriate diet choice.

Early postoperative feeding, within 24 hours of the procedure, whether via feeding tube or oral diet, has been shown to decrease postoperative complications, length of stay, and costs.[25] It is also recommended that a high-protein diet/formula be used during this time.[12] Protein turnover increases during the postoperative period. This elevated protein turnover is triggered by surgical stress, thus requiring a higher-than-normal intake of good-quality sources of protein.[26] It has also been suggested that concentrating on protein intake versus overall calorie intake is preferred postoperatively.[12] Most OCC patients who resume an oral diet postoperatively will most likely require some sort of high-protein oral liquid supplement to achieve these high-protein goals as many of the traditional forms of protein (meats and nuts) can be a challenge to chew and swallow immediately postsurgery.

12.4.3 Nutrition Considerations with the Patient Treated with Radiation with or without Chemotherapy

Radiation with or without chemotherapy is a common adjuvant treatment for OCC and can be a primary treatment for select patients. Educating the patient on what to expect during the course of treatment is very important from a nutrition standpoint. Radiation has a cumulative effect that can begin with mild irritation in the oral cavity and escalate to swelling, pain, and mouth sores requiring a feeding tube to be considered. For the first few weeks, the side effects are minor and the patient and caregiver may have a false sense of security regarding nutrition risks. As patients progress through the treatment, the side effects intensify and the patient's ability to even drink fluids can be impaired. These side effects can be made worse by the addition of chemotherapy. Ideally, the patient should not have any breaks in treatment; therefore, poor nutritional intake, uncontrolled pain, and dehydration should be avoided with appropriate nutrition assessment and planning.

A high-calorie, high-protein diet with high-calorie, high-protein oral liquid supplement should be started even before radiation, with or without chemotherapy, begins.[11] Patient education regarding the expected side effects of mucositis, xerostomia, pain with chewing, altered taste, and weight loss should be given early and the patient advised to begin with diet recommendations, even if they have not lost weight or are not experiencing any issues with eating. Patients will inevitably have problems, so being proactive is necessary. Explaining this to the patient can require a fine balance between sharing the honest information regarding what to expect and instilling fear in the patient. Putting this information in relatable terms can help improve compliance with the various recommendations (e.g., "this early diet intervention can help decrease potential muscle loss"). Use empowering language when discussing this with the patient (i.e., "This is what you can do to help yourself before treatment begins.").

A weekly visit with the RD and SLP is recommended while the patient is receiving radiation therapy for most HNC, and especially for OCC.[27,28] The combined side effects of dry mouth, altered taste, excess mucous, and pain due to mucositis make eating a chore and not a joy. It is at this point that the patient may benefit from restructuring cognitions about food, such that food is thought to be like medicine throughout treatment. It can taste bad and lack pleasure, but it is good for you. QoL can be compromised as eating becomes more problematic. Oral pain with eating may lead to selection of foods that do not aggravate the oral tissues, often at the expense of adequate nutrition. Nutritional deficiencies can be minimized by modifying the texture and consistency of the diet and by adding more frequent meals and snacks to increase calories and protein. In addition, a reminder to avoid extreme temperatures in food, and acidic and spicy foods, as well avoiding alcohol and tobacco use should be reinforced. Good oral hygiene is encouraged and rinsing with a solution of baking soda, salt, and water a couple of times a day can help with this.[29] Keeping a bottle of water with them at all times is also advised not only for hydration purposes, but also to help with the dry mouth that most develop. Weekly reinforcement and encouragement is necessary for many patients as they and their caregivers struggle with eating and drinking.

Proactive versus reactive feeding tube placement for a patient with OCC undergoing radiation therapy with or without chemotherapy is a subject where much debate has occurred and continues to occur. Certainly, if the patient has impaired swallowing prior to initiation of treatment, then a case could be made for a prophylactic feeding tube placement as the side effects of the treatment can continue to deteriorate the safety of oral intake.[30] Weekly monitoring of weight and the involvement of the RD at those weekly appointments can help delay or avoid a feeding tube.[27] The RD can investigate why the patient is not eating and drinking. Is there something the RD or SLP can suggest to help improve the patient's oral intake? It can be helpful to establish a threshold for weight loss with the patient at the start of treatment and review this throughout treatment. General clinical practice puts that threshold at about 10% loss of their body weight from baseline. Should a feeding tube be necessary, consider a short-term Dobhoff tube versus a gastrostomy/PEG tube.[27] Continue to encourage oral intake, even with the feeding tube, as long as oral intake is safe. Encourage patients to continue swallowing exercises. The goal is to keep the muscles used in swallowing strong and in continual use.

12.4.4 Posttreatment Nutrition Plan

Once the primary and adjuvant (if needed) treatment is complete, the role for nutrition interventions does not stop, but continues with the various short- and long-term side effects of treatment. This is especially true in patients who received radiation with or without chemotherapy. Dry mouth, taste changes, and pain with eating and swallowing take time to resolve and, for some patients, they may never regain 100% function. Regaining the weight lost during treatment is also a challenge for many of these patients. General clinical practice suggests that a reasonable goal for the first year following treatment is to maintain the current weight instead of pushing weight gain. Remind the patient that recovery takes time.[31] Those who lost a significant amount of weight (> 10%) during treatment tend to be the patients who struggle with weight following treatment. Encourage physical exercise and strength training to help regain muscle and endurance. A referral to physical therapy may be of assistance with these recommendations. Fatigue remains an issue for a period of time following the completion of treatment and this can affect nutrition, as patients do not have the energy to prepare or eat meals because of fatigue. Continue to encourage use of oral liquid nutrition supplements as part of their oral diet. If the patient required feeding via a tube, continue to work with them to wean off the tube and include softer and even pureed high-calorie, high-protein foods early in the day to maximize oral intake before use of the feeding tube. Resolution of dysgeusia (altered taste or loss of taste) following radiation treatment to the oral cavity takes months to years. Different taste sensations recover at different times.[32] It is helpful to advise the patient that the taste alterations can continue for months following treatment completion.[33] Taste alterations have been reported as an important symptom and an independent predictor of QoL for patients with HNC.[34] Encourage the patient to continue with good oral hygiene, use of the baking soda, salt, and water rinse, and to keep trying various flavors (sweet, salt, bitter, sour/tart). Hot and spicy foods are not recommended immediately posttreatment, but some patients may report that those tastes return the quickest.

QoL needs to be taken into consideration from the very beginning of the treatment process. Survival is usually the primary focus of the patient and caregiver on initial diagnosis—in their minds, cure is the goal, no matter the costs. As health care providers, we need to be aware of the whole picture through survivorship and help that patient and caregiver through these stages and changes. With OCC on the rise in younger individuals and the prognosis of those patients improving, the long-term effects of treatment on QoL are gaining more attention, as well as survivorship treatment planning.[35] Some of the key issues that affect QoL nutritionally include issues with eating, excessive secretions, dry mouth, low weight, disfigurement, and presence of a feeding tube.[36] During treatment, some of these issues are not as important to the patient as the goal of completing treatment in pursuit of cure. Then a new normal emerges and nutrition issues that were not as pressing suddenly take center stage. Functional problems associated with eating can remain for years following treatment, leading to compromised nutrition and QoL.[37] Depending on the extent of surgery and/or reconstruction the patient experienced, their ability to eat "normally" may have been altered and they may need to eat not only a modified texture/consistency diet, but also may also take twice as long to eat. Further, they may need to clear debris from their mouth manually if they do not have good tongue motion. Eating alone or at home in the kitchen with the immediate family may be acceptable, but what about going out to eat or gathering over holiday meals with family and friends? The patient may socially isolate themselves because of their difficulty eating, and that can lead to other behavioral issues that can further affect QoL. Eating is a very social activity and when the patient feels embarrassed or awkward, those around them may feel embarrassed and awkward as well. It takes a team of not only the RD, but also the SLP and the behavioral health specialist to help the patient and caregiver with these challenges. Discussing these concerns and then working with the patient to develop solutions to these issues goes a long way to improving the patient's QoL and helping the patient accept and embrace their new normal.

As mentioned earlier, the average age of the HNC patient population is getting younger and long-term survivorship issues need to be addressed. Physical exercise, preventative screening, attention to diet, and other chronic health conditions need to be part of the follow-up care these patients receive in addition to addressing some of the long-term side effects that may be present or later develop. Good dental care as well as continued abstinence from tobacco and alcohol are strongly encouraged.

12.5 Conclusion

It is important to identify and address nutrition concerns in patients with OCC from diagnosis to survivorship. It takes a multidisciplinary team to appropriately and effectively treat these patients, and the RD is a key member of this team. Life-sustaining activities such as eating and swallowing are greatly impacted by the various treatments for OCCs. Starting prior to active treatment, nutritional assessment and interventions play a pivotal role for positive patient outcomes throughout treatment, recovery, and survivorship.[28,37]

Key Points

- The majority of patients with OCC are at very high risk of suboptimal nutrition from diagnosis throughout the treatment process and into survivorship.
- Early nutrition intervention and continued involvement of the RD with this patient population across the continuum of care is recommended by the NCCN.
- Regardless of the patient's calculated BMI at diagnosis, malnutrition can be present if significant, unintentional weight loss has been experienced by the patient. This is associated with negative postoperative outcomes, functional decline, and poor tolerance to chemotherapy/radiation therapy.
- QoL needs to be taken into consideration from the very beginning of the treatment process. Initially, the patient may not be as concerned about QoL, but functional problems associated with eating can remain for years following treatment and these can affect nutritional status and QoL.
- It takes a multidisciplinary team to appropriately and effectively treat these patients, and the RD is a key member of this team.

References

[1] Magnano M, Mola P, Machetta G, et al. The nutritional assessment of head and neck cancer patients. European Archives of Oto-Rhino-Laryngology. 2015; 272(12):3793–3799

[2] Righini CA, Timi N, Junet P, Bertolo A, Reyt E, Atallah I. Assessment of nutritional status at the time of diagnosis in patients treated for head and neck cancer. Eur Ann Otorhinolaryngol Head Neck Dis. 2013; 130(1):8–14

[3] Forastiere A, Goepfert H, Goffinet D, et al. National Comprehensive Cancer Network. NCCN practice guidelines for head and neck cancer. Oncology (Williston Park). 1998; 12 7A:39–147

[4] Hensrud DD. Nutrition screening and assessment. Med Clin North Am. 1999; 83(6):1525–1546

[5] Biggs K. Malnutrition screening programs in adult cancer patients: clinical practice is hungry for evidence. Curr Oncol. 2012; 19(5):e305–e307

[6] Ferguson M. Patient-generated subjective global assessment. Oncology (Williston Park). 2003; 17(2) Suppl 2:13–14, discussion 14–16

[7] Bauer J, Capra S, Ferguson M. Use of the scored Patient-Generated Subjective Global Assessment (PG-SGA) as a nutrition assessment tool in patients with cancer. Eur J Clin Nutr. 2002; 56(8):779–785

[8] Ferguson ML, Bauer J, Gallagher B, Capra S, Christie DR, Mason BR. Validation of a malnutrition screening tool for patients receiving radiotherapy. Australas Radiol. 1999; 43(3):325–327

[9] Bauer J, Capra S. Comparison of a malnutrition screening tool with subjective global assessment in hospitalised patients with cancer: sensitivity and specificity. Asia Pac J Clin Nutr. 2003; 12(3):257–260

[10] Godfrey K. Implementation of the Malnutrition Universal Screening Tool. Nurs Times. 2004; 100(18):61–61

[11] Leser MLN, Begerson S, Trujillo E. Oncology Nutrition for Clinical Practice. New York, NY: Oncology Nutrition Dietetic Practice Group of the Academy of Nutrition and Dietetics; 2013

[12] Wischmeyer PE, Carli F, Evans DC, et al. Perioperative Quality Initiative (POQI) 2 Workgroup. American Society for Enhanced Recovery and Perioperative Quality Initiative Joint Consensus Statement on Nutrition Screening and Therapy within a Surgical Enhanced Recovery Pathway. Anesth Analg. 2018; 126(6):1883–1895

[13] Bharadwaj S, Ginoya S, Tandon P, et al. Malnutrition: laboratory markers vs nutritional assessment. Gastroenterol Rep (Oxf). 2016; 4(4):272–280
[14] Kubrak C, Olson K, Jha N, et al. Nutrition impact symptoms: key determinants of reduced dietary intake, weight loss, and reduced functional capacity of patients with head and neck cancer before treatment. Head Neck. 2010; 32 (3):290–300
[15] Day E, Bentham PW, Callaghan R, Kuruvilla T, George S. Thiamine for prevention and treatment of Wernicke-Korsakoff Syndrome in people who abuse alcohol. Cochrane Database Syst Rev. 2013(7):CD004033
[16] Coyle MJ, Main B, Hughes C, et al. Enhanced Recovery after Surgery (ERAS) for head and neck oncology patients. Clinical Otolaryngology. 2016; 41(2): 118–126
[17] Nicholson A, Lowe MC, Parker J, Lewis SR, Alderson P, Smith AF. Systematic review and meta-analysis of enhanced recovery programmes in surgical patients. Br J Surg. 2014; 101(3):172–188
[18] Dort JC, Farwell DG, Findlay M, et al. Optimal perioperative care in major head and neck cancer surgery with free flap reconstruction: a consensus review and recommendations from the Enhanced Recovery after Surgery Society. JAMA Otolaryngol Head Neck Surg. 2017; 143(3):292–303
[19] Carli F, Gillis C, Scheede-Bergdahl C. Promoting a culture of prehabilitation for the surgical cancer patient. Acta Oncol. 2017; 56(2):128–133
[20] McClave SA, Kozar R, Martindale RG, et al. Summary points and consensus recommendations from the North American Surgical Nutrition Summit. JPEN J Parenter Enteral Nutr. 2013; 37(5) Suppl:99S–105S
[21] Bilku DK, Dennison AR, Hall TC, Metcalfe MS, Garcea G. Role of preoperative carbohydrate loading: a systematic review. Ann R Coll Surg Engl. 2014; 96(1): 15–22
[22] Kratzing C. Pre-operative nutrition and carbohydrate loading. Proc Nutr Soc. 2011; 70(3):311–315
[23] Pogatschnik C, Steiger E. Review of preoperative carbohydrate loading. Nutr Clin Pract. 2015; 30(5):660–664
[24] McCullough G, Pelletier C, Steele C. National dysphagia diet: what to swallow? ASHA Leader. 2003; 8(20):16–27
[25] Ljungqvist O, Scott M, Fearon KC. Enhanced recovery after surgery: a review. JAMA Surg. 2017; 152(3):292–298
[26] Gillis C, Carli F. Promoting perioperative metabolic and nutritional care. Anesthesiology. 2015; 123(6):1455–1472
[27] Siddiqui F, Movsas B. Management of radiation toxicity in head and neck cancers. Semin Radiat Oncol. 2017; 27(4):340–349
[28] Isenring E, Capra S, Bauer J. Patient satisfaction is rated higher by radiation oncology outpatients receiving nutrition intervention compared with usual care. J Hum Nutr Diet. 2004; 17(2):145–152
[29] Shih A, Miaskowski C, Dodd MJ, Stotts NA, MacPhail L. A research review of the current treatments for radiation-induced oral mucositis in patients with head and neck cancer. Oncol Nurs Forum. 2002; 29(7):1063–1080
[30] Barnhart MK, Ward EC, Cartmill B, et al. Pretreatment factors associated with functional oral intake and feeding tube use at 1 and 6 months post-radiotherapy (+/– chemotherapy) for head and neck cancer. European Archives of Oto-Rhino-Laryngology. 2017; 274(1):507–516
[31] Isenring EA, Capra S, Bauer JD. Nutrition intervention is beneficial in oncology outpatients receiving radiotherapy to the gastrointestinal or head and neck area. Br J Cancer. 2004; 91(3):447–452
[32] Negi P, Kingsley P-A, Thomas M, Sachdeva J, Srivastava H, Kalra B. Pattern of gustatory impairment and its recovery after head and neck irradiation. Iran J Otorhinolaryngol. 2017; 29(95):319–327
[33] Rogers SN, Barber B. Using PROMs to guide patients and practitioners through the head and neck cancer journey. Patient Relat Outcome Meas. 2017; 8:133–142
[34] Alvarez-Camacho M, Gonella S, Ghosh S, et al. The impact of taste and smell alterations on quality of life in head and neck cancer patients. Qual Life Res. 2016; 25(6):1495–1504
[35] Ringash J. Survivorship and quality of life in head and neck cancer. J Clin Oncol. 2015; 33(29):3322–3327
[36] Rogers SN, Semple C, Babb M, Humphris G. Quality of life considerations in head and neck cancer: United Kingdom National Multidisciplinary Guidelines. J Laryngol Otol. 2016; 130 S2:S49–S52
[37] Crowder SL, Douglas KG, Yanina Pepino M, Sarma KP, Arthur AE. Nutrition impact symptoms and associated outcomes in post-chemoradiotherapy head and neck cancer survivors: a systematic review. J Cancer Surviv. 2018; 12(4): 479–494

Section V

Evaluation and Surgical Management of Subsite-specific Oral Squamous Cell Cancers

13 Squamous Cell Cancer of the Lip

John W. Werning

Summary
Our increased understanding of lip cancer has undergone an incremental evolution that permits head and neck cancer specialists to improve the treatment outcomes for our patients. Recognition that the biological behavior of lip cancer differs based on its origin from the wet or dry vermilion is essential to accordingly modify treatment and optimize outcomes. Multispecialty evaluation is essential so that every patient is afforded the most appropriate management for that patient's clinical situation, which may include alternatives to standard surgical management such as Mohs micrographic surgery, brachytherapy, and sentinel lymph node biopsy.

Keywords: actinic cheilitis, mucosal lip, dry vermilion

13.1 Introduction

The upper and lower lips, which are the central aesthetic feature of the lower third of the face, also serve important functions in facial expression, sucking, kissing, speech articulation, proprioception, hot–cold temperature differentiation, oral secretion management, and the establishment of a labial seal during the oral preparatory phase of swallowing. Alterations in their appearance or function can adversely impact self-esteem, societal acceptance, and quality of life. We are generally unaware of the aesthetic and functional importance of the lips until they are altered, but when they are altered, the impact can be life-changing.

As the point of transition between the skin of the face and the oral cavity, the lips are exposed to environmental agents that cause both skin cancer and oral cancer. Over the past decade, refinements in our understanding of the natural history and biological behavior of lip cancer have helped characterize the differences in diagnosis, management, and outcomes between cancers of the extraoral, or dry vermilion lip, and of the intraoral wet mucosal lip. This review compares and contrasts the treatment for and prognosis of cancers that arise from the mucosal lip and the dry vermilion.

13.2 Anatomy of the Lips

The external surface anatomy of the lips is comprised of the cutaneous lip and the dry vermilion. The boundaries of the upper cutaneous lip extend superiorly to the nostril sill and alar base, and laterally to the melolabial, or nasolabial sulcus. The upper lip is comprised of three aesthetic subunits: two lateral subunits, which extend from each philtral ridge to the melolabial sulcus, and the centrally located philtrum. The vermilion border, or mucocutaneous ridge, of the upper lip has a midline **V**-shaped indentation that terminates on either side at the philtral ridges known as Cupid's bow. In contrast, the lower cutaneous lip has one aesthetic unit that extends inferiorly to the labiomental crease. The cutaneous portion of the upper and lower lips terminates at the white roll, where the curvature of the vermilion creates a clearly delineated border.

In cross-section, the lip is a three-layered structure comprising the skin, orbicularis oris muscle, and lining intraoral mucosa. The vermilion region, or the true lip, has a rich vascular plexus that underlies a thin epithelial architecture that gives the vermilion its unique aesthetic appearance. The vermilion zone of the lip is covered by orthokeratinized stratified squamous epithelium that is firmly attached to the underlying orbicularis oris muscle, whereas the intraoral labial mucosa is nonkeratinized. The transition between the intraoral lining mucosa and the wet vermilion is termed the wet line.

The oral cavity, as defined by the American Joint Committee on Cancer (AJCC), "extends from the portion of the lip that contacts the opposed lip (wet mucosa) to the junction of the hard and soft palate above, to the line of circumvallate papillae below, and to the anterior tonsillar pillars bilaterally."[1] The **mucosal lip** is defined as the area that "begins at the junction of the wet and dry mucosa of the lip (the anterior border of the lip that comes into contact with the opposed lip) and extends posteriorly into the oral cavity to the attached gingiva of the alveolar ridge."[1] Previous editions of the AJCC Cancer Staging Manual included the **dry vermilion**, or that portion of the lip located external to the mucosal lip, in the chapter pertaining to the lip and oral cavity. However, cancers arising from the dry vermilion and the vermilion border are now designated as extraoral and are staged as cutaneous cancers.[2]

13.3 Incidence and Epidemiology

The estimated worldwide incidence of lip cancer in 2012 was 0.3 cases per 100,000 people annually—0.4/100,000 in males and 0.2/100,000 in females.[3,4] Papua New Guinea and Australia had the highest incidence rates of 8.9/100,000 and 2.6/100,000, respectively. In contrast, Eastern and Southeast Asia and sub-Saharan Africa had the lowest incidence rates. The incidence of lip cancer in the United states, based on data compiled by the Globocan Project, is between 0.4 and 0.9/100,000.[3] The estimated worldwide incidence of lip cancer is lower than oral cavity cancers (2.7/100,000) and oropharyngeal cancers (1.4/100,000).[3]

In the United States, squamous cell carcinoma (SCC) of the lip comprises approximately 20 to 25% of all cancers of the lip and oral cavity. Greater than 98% of the diagnosed lip cancers occur in the Caucasian population, and more than 60% of these are diagnosed in individuals older than 60 years of age.[5] Males comprise more than 80% of the individuals diagnosed. In a review of lip cancers entered into the Surveillance, Epidemiology, and End Results (SEER) database from 1973 through 2012, 90% of lip cancers arose from the lower lip, whereas cancers of the upper lip and labial commissure comprised 9 and 1%, respectively.[5] Other investigations, however, have documented that lower lip cancer comprises at least 95% of all diagnosed lip cancers.[6–8] Analysis of the SEER database also showed that 88.4% (1261/1426) of upper lip SCCs and 88.4% (12311/13928) of lower lip SCCs arose from the dry vermilion, or external portion of the lip.[5]

Numerous epidemiologic studies have documented the role of chronic sun exposure, or ultraviolet radiation, as the primary etiologic agent in SCC of the dry vermilion. Fishermen, farmers, foresters, and concrete workers who work outside have markedly higher incidence rates of lip cancer.[8–10] The relationship between cumulative sun exposure and lip cancer is also believed to explain the high incidence of lower lip cancer, since a greater surface area of the dry vermilion of the lower lip is exposed to sunlight relative to the upper lip vermilion.

In contrast, the etiology of mucosal lip SCC is believed to be caused by tobacco and alcohol use, similar to oral mucosal squamous carcinoma. However, epidemiologic evidence in support of this association is limited because the incidence rates of mucosal lip cancer and oral mucosal cancers in tobacco users have not been analyzed separately. Moreover, the association between chronic alcohol use and lip cancer has not been rigorously evaluated, so the causative role of alcohol use has been extrapolated from epidemiologic investigations of oral cancer patients and is largely presumptive.

Solid organ transplant recipients on immunosuppressive agents such as cyclosporine A and azathioprine have a risk of developing lip cancer that is 20 times greater than the general population.[11] Moreover, the risk of lip cancer has been shown to increase as the dose and duration of azathioprine therapy is increased.[12] Individuals who are immunosuppressed for other reasons, including human immunodeficiency virus infection, are also at increased risk.[13] Higher rates of lip cancer have also been associated with the use of antihypertensive agents, including hydrochlorothiazide and nifedipine, presumably because they are photosensitizers.[14]

13.4 Actinic Cheilitis

The precursor to lip cancer involving the dry vermilion, in approximately 95% of patients, is actinic cheilitis.[15] Ultraviolet radiation is the primary causative agent, and is more common in fair-skinned (Fitzpatrick I–III) individuals. Clinically, actinic cheilitis has a varied appearance, but is frequently characterized by areas of desiccation with a scaly appearance and rough surface texture, atrophic changes, and an increase in the prominence of vertical folds, or fissuring. Color variegation is frequently present with patchy areas of leukoplakia, erythroplakia, or erythroleukoplakia. The typically sharp delineation of the vermilion border may become obscured or retracted (▶ Fig. 13.1).[16] Ulcerations are frequently associated with more advanced disease.

Biopsy of the most concerning area should be performed whenever clinical examination is consistent with actinic cheilitis. Histopathologic evaluation can demonstrate a spectrum of pathology ranging from hyperkeratosis to dysplasia to invasive SCC. In the cases where carcinoma in situ or invasion is identified, biopsies of other less concerning areas along the surface of the lip may help clarify the indicated treatment (e.g., wedge resection with vermilionectomy). The exclusion of invasive cancer at the time of biopsy is of paramount importance since many of the treatment modalities that are used for actinic cheilitis ablate the epithelial surface in lieu of formal excision. However, choosing the most appropriate area for biopsy may be challenging because areas with a homogeneous appearance have been shown to demonstrate heterogeneous histologic changes.[17]

The rationale for the treatment of actinic cheilitis with dysplasia should be in part based on the risk of malignant transformation. Treatment is clearly indicated whenever the risk of evolution to malignancy is high, but excision or ablation may be optional if the risk of malignant progression is low, and may be based on patient factors, such as cosmetic concerns or patient discomfort.

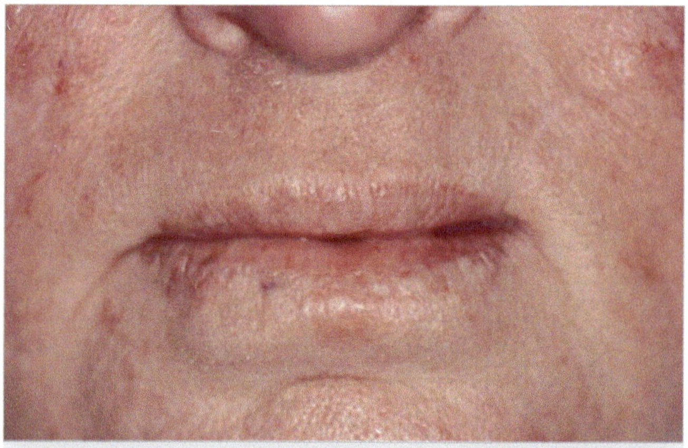

Fig. 13.1 Actinic cheilitis. The lips demonstrate atrophic changes with increased prominence of vertical folds, patchy color variegation, and obscuration of the vermilion border.

Several treatment modalities have been employed to treat actinic cheilitis, and the preferred modality is frequently based on that clinician's clinical experience and expertise. Vermilionectomy, or the lip shave, remains the standard by which the efficacy of other techniques must be compared since vermilionectomy is the only excisional procedure. Numerous other techniques have been used with varying success rates, including cryosurgery, 5-fluorouracil, imiquimod, photodynamic therapy, trichloroacetic acid chemical peel, electrodessication, carbon dioxide laser ablation, diclofenac, and dermabrasion.[18]

13.5 Natural History and Clinical Presentation

Clinicians should obtain a thorough history that reviews any symptoms that could be suggestive of invasive cancer, including dysesthesia or analgesia (e.g., the numb chin syndrome), a possible manifestation of perineural involvement. The medical history should be reviewed for conditions or medications that cause immunosuppression, as well as the use of photosensitizing antihypertensive medications. Documentation of the extent of sun exposure and the amount of tobacco and alcohol use is essential to identify possible etiologies.

Lip cancer is usually detected in its early stages due to its conspicuous anatomic location. Cancers arising from the dry vermilion that arise from areas involved by actinic cheilitis tend to be slow growing. Surface changes that are thought to be due to actinic cheilitis may in fact be involved by early invasive cancer that remains undiagnosed until vermilionectomy is performed. Subtle actinic-appearing changes, if untreated, may slowly progress to a raised irregular exophytic lesion, an indurated subcutaneous/submucosal lesion, or an ulcerated lesion. Each of these clinical manifestations is highly suggestive of invasive cancer.

Mucosal SCC arising from the wet mucosa frequently begins as an area of leukoplakia or erythroplakia. The involved mucosa may have a patchy appearance with areas of normal-appearing mucosa. Ulceration or submucosal induration increases the concern for invasive cancer. All of these clinical presentations mandate biopsy of the most concerning area. Biopsy of a necrotic central ulceration may result in a false-negative biopsy result, so biopsy of viable tissue surrounding the central ulceration is preferred.

Clinical evaluation requires careful inspection of the surface anatomy of the lip to characterize any changes of the dry and wet vermilion. Examination for mottling, color and textural changes, fissuring, ulcerations, induration, and obscuration of the vermilion border and normal lip anatomy should be performed. Incisional or punch biopsy is preferred over shave biopsy, which could lead to the incorrect diagnosis of a noninvasive in situ lesion.

Physical examination of the lip and neck is sufficient for smaller lesions, whereas axial imaging should be considered for lesions measuring more than 2 cm in diameter. Computed tomography (CT) with contrast provides valuable information about the extent of soft-tissue involvement, mandibular or maxillary invasion, maxillary sinus involvement, and the presence of cervical and intraparotid lymphadenopathy. Information pertaining to retrograde perineural involvement of the trigeminal nerve and mandibular marrow invasion is ideally assessed with magnetic resonance imaging. Cone beam CT may be used to provide complimentary information about cortical bone destruction that is not appreciated on standard CT scan imaging.

13.6 Staging Lip Cancer

Squamous carcinomas arising from the mucosal lip are staged with the staging system for the lip and oral cavity.[1] In contrast, squamous carcinomas originating from the vermilion border or the external dry vermilion of the upper and lower lips are now staged according to the staging system for cutaneous SCC of the head and neck.[2] These changes in staging reflect the disparate etiology and biological behavior of oral mucosal cancers and cutaneous cancers. Consequently, the definitions of the primary tumor (T) in the most recent edition of the AJCC Cancer Staging Manual differ for the mucosal lip and the dry vermilion.[1,2] Here is a comparison of the T stage criteria for each site:

- T1 mucosal lip is ≤ 2 cm maximum diameter (MD), ≤ 5 mm depth of invasion (DOI), measured from the level of the basement membrane of the adjacent intact squamous mucosa, *whereas* T1 external lip is < 2 cm.
- T2 mucosal lip is ≤ 2 cm, DOI > 5 mm, and ≤ 10 mm **or** > 2 cm but ≤ 4 cm and ≤ 10 mm DOI, *whereas* T2 external lip is ≥ 2 cm but < 4 cm.
- T3 mucosal lip is > 4 cm **or** any tumor with DOI > 10 mm, *whereas* T3 external lip is ≥ 4 cm **or** minor bone erosion, perineural invasion (PNI), or deep invasion (> 6 mm or beyond the subcutaneous fat).

Adoption of the updated AJCC TNM (tumor size, node involvement, and metastasis status) staging criteria published in the eighth edition may assign a particular cancerous lesion to a different stage group based on its site of origin in the mucosal or the cutaneous vermilion of the lip. For example, a 1.5-cm lesion with 6-mm DOI that is clinically N0M0 would be assigned to prognostic stage group II as a mucosal lip lesion versus stage I as a vermilion border lesion. In contrast, a 2.5-cm lesion with 8-mm DOI that is cN0M0 would be designated as a stage II mucosal lip cancer versus a stage III external lip cancer. While the updated staging criteria reflect our current understanding of lip cancer, they will also result in stage migration that limits our ability to extrapolate treatment outcomes from the existing peer-reviewed literature to the updated stage groups.

The presence of extranodal extension (ENE) is a criterion that is now used to designate N stage for lip cancers of the mucosal lip and dry vermilion. If there is clinically overt ENE based on physical examination and/or radiographic imaging, the N stage is designated as N3b. The criteria for pathological ENE, however, differ between oral mucosal cancers and cutaneous SCCs of the head and neck. Cancers arising from the mucosal lip receive pathological ENE (+) status *only* if there is macroscopic ENE, which is defined as "either extranodal extension apparent to the naked eye at the time of dissection or extension > 2 mm beyond the lymph node capsule microscopically."[1] In contrast, cutaneous SCCs of the head and neck region, including the dry vermilion, are designated as ENE (+) if there is "extension through the lymph node capsule into the connective tissue."[2]

13.7 Predictors of Regional Metastasis

In general, the likelihood of metastatic cervical lymphadenopathy is related to primary tumor size. Most retrospective case series document metastasis rates of less than 15% in lesions measuring 4 cm or less. Zitsch et al documented cervical metastasis in 7% of patients 2 cm or less in diameter versus 16% in larger cancers.[19] In a retrospective review of 617 patients, lymph node metastasis occurred in 7.9% of T1–T2 lesions and in 27.9% of patients with T3–T4 lesions.[20] Another series of 299 patients found lymph node involvement in 5.6% of T1–T2 lesions and 17.6% for T3 cancers.[21] In a more recent retrospective investigation, however, the rate of cervical metastasis was 9% in 23 lip cancers measuring 2 to 3 cm in diameter versus 43.7% in 16 lip cancers greater than 3 cm but ≤ 4 cm in diameter.[22]

Numerous investigators have documented an increased incidence of nodal metastasis when tumor thickness (TT) exceeds 4 to 5 mm.[23–25] There are, however, limited data in the peer-reviewed literature pertaining to DOI and the risk of regional metastasis for mucosal lip cancers. Hence, using DOI as a criterion for designating T stage in mucosal lip cancers is largely based on the extrapolation of data obtained from other oral mucosal sites and requires further investigation. Cutaneous lesions with greater than 6 mm DOI or PNI of large caliber nerves (> 0.1 mm) have a greater than 15% risk of regional metastasis.[26,27] In a study of cutaneous SCC in 615 patients by Brantsch and colleagues, there was a direct correlation between TT and the nodal metastatic rate (NMR): TT = 2.0, NMR = 0%; TT = 2.1 to 6 mm, NMR = 4%; TT > 6 mm, NMR = 16%.[26]

The association between the site of the lip cancer and the likelihood of cervical metastasis has also been evaluated. A large retrospective review of 1,036 lip cancers found that 31% of cancers involving the commissure metastasized to the cervical lymph nodes, which was significantly greater than cancers arising from the upper or lower lip.[7] A subsequent retrospective series, however, did not confirm any relationship between primary tumor location and regional metastasis.[28]

Other independent risk factors for metastasis include poor differentiation, PNI, lymphovascular invasion, and desmoplasia.[19,26,29,30] A low histopathological grade at the invasive tumor front is associated with a low rate of metastasis.[31] A histologic risk assessment grading system that estimates the risk of regional lymph node metastasis for lip cancer has been evaluated.[31] The *histologic risk assessment* model scores three morphological parameters: worst pattern of invasion (WPOI), ranging from a pushing border (type 1) to "tumor satellites ≥ 1 mm away from main tumor or next closest satellite" (type 5); lymphocytic infiltrate ranging from a "dense complete host response" (type 1) to "little or no host response" (type 3); and PNI, with no invasion, tumor wrapping around nerves less than 1 mm in diameter, or large nerves ≥ 1 mm in diameter.[32] The relationship between the risk assessment score and regional lymph node metastasis is highly significant.[31] Nodal metastasis to the parotid gland has also been associated with the presence of lymphovascular invasion in cutaneous SCCs.[33]

13.8 Surgical Management

Prior to surgical treatment of lip cancer, the patient should be extensively counseled regarding the planned surgical procedure and the possibility of intraoperative modifications that may be necessitated to achieve clear margins (CMs), as well as the possible reconstructive techniques that may need to be employed. Since the extent of lip resection can dramatically impact the reconstructive plan and the patient's ultimate appearance and quality of life, the patient must have a clear understanding of the potential impact on oral competence and social acceptance. Individuals who wear removable dentures must be counseled that postoperative microstomia may prevent their use.

Careful preoperative assessment with inspection and palpation permits the surgeon to appreciate the three-dimensional nature of the cancer, the planned resection, and the resultant soft-tissue defect. Lip cancer resection should be performed en bloc with the intent to achieve negative, or clear, margins during the initial resection.

For cancers of the mucosal lip, "a clear margin is defined as the distance from the invasive tumor front that is 5 mm or more from the resected margin."[1] In contrast, the margins that should be achieved for squamous carcinomas arising from the dry vermilion are based on the available evidence for high-risk cutaneous SCC lesions. Cutaneous squamous carcinoma arising within the high-risk "mask area" of the face have a higher rate of local recurrence (LR) when standard surgical excision with narrow excision margins are obtained. Hence, a "clear" margin (CM) is achieved using the following criteria that are based on the MD of the lesion: MD < 1 cm and CM ≥ 4 mm; MD ≥ 1 but ≤ 1.9 cm and CM ≥ 6 mm; and MD ≥ 2 cm and CM ≥ 9 mm.[2] Mohs micrographic surgery (MMS) may also be performed and is a recommended surgical option for high-risk areas such as the lip since complete margin assessment is possible with maximal tissue conservation.

Locally advanced lip cancers, however, frequently have both cutaneous and mucosal involvement, and have an inherently higher risk of LR and regional metastasis. Wider tumor-free margins are essential to maximize local control and to minimize the need for adjuvant radiotherapy with or without chemotherapy. Multiple variables impact the surgeon's ability to achieve widely CMs in these circumstances, including adjacent soft-tissue involvement of the cheek, chin, and nasal soft tissues, extensive intraoral mucosal involvement, mandibular or maxillary involvement, and retrograde PNI. Since external beam radiation and brachytherapy (BT; brachy means "short distance" in Greek) alone are viable management options that may provide comparable rates of local control, it is paramount for the cancer surgeon to preoperatively consider the implications of incomplete surgical resection of a lip cancer that will require adjuvant treatment.

While a 5-mm microscopically tumor-free margin is generally accepted as a CM for oral mucosal cancers, the ideal tumor-free margin that is required to achieve local control following standard surgical excision is less well defined for lip cancers. The size of the margin can dramatically impact the extent of lip resection that is resected, and larger lip resections can markedly alter the reconstructive approach (▶ Fig. 13.2, ▶ Fig. 13.3, ▶ Fig. 13.4, ▶ Fig. 13.5, ▶ Fig. 13.6). The 2018 National Comprehensive Cancer Network (NCCN) guidelines for head and neck cancers state that the achievement of clear resection margins requires the excision of surrounding normal-appearing mucosa, "often 1.5–2 cm of visible and palpable normal mucosa."[34] This recommendation raises an important question: Is resection of lip cancer with 1.5-cm mucosal margins, resulting in defects measuring at least 3 cm greater than the grossly appreciated

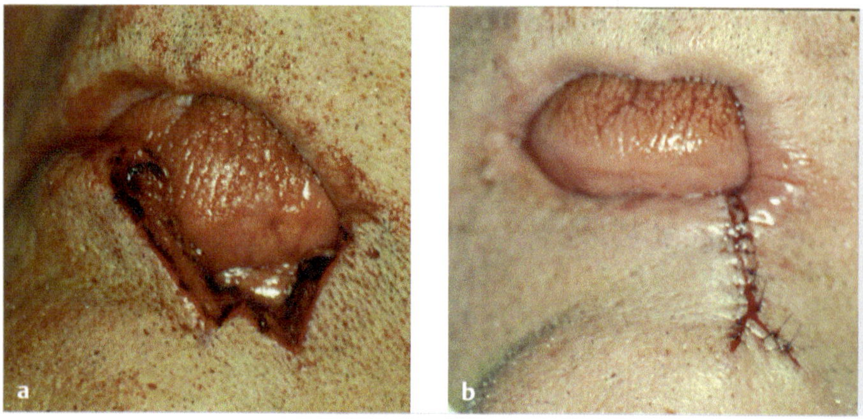

Fig. 13.2 (a, b) Wedge excision with inverse M-plasty to facilitate closure.

extent of the primary tumor, appropriate? The answer to this question remains unresolved. The excision of lip cancers with 10-mm mucosal margins that are immersed in 10% buffered formalin shrink by 41 to 47.5%: 20% shrinkage occurs immediately following resection and 14% additional shrinkage occurs within 24 hours of formalin fixation.[35] In a retrospective study from Germany that evaluated the outcomes of 105 patients who underwent lip cancer resection (71.4% were lesions ≤ 2 cm,

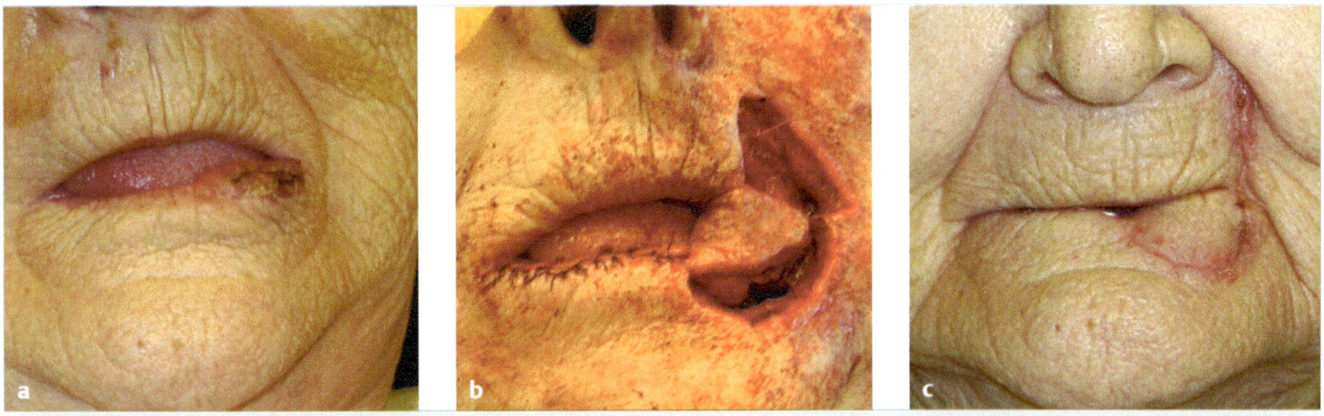

Fig. 13.3 (a–c) Invasive lower lip cancer that extends to the labial commissure with adjacent actinic cheilitis. Resection of the lip cancer and vermilionectomy of the entire lower lip was performed. Reconstruction was achieved with a circumoral Estlander flap and a labial mucosal advancement flap to reconstruct the vermilion.

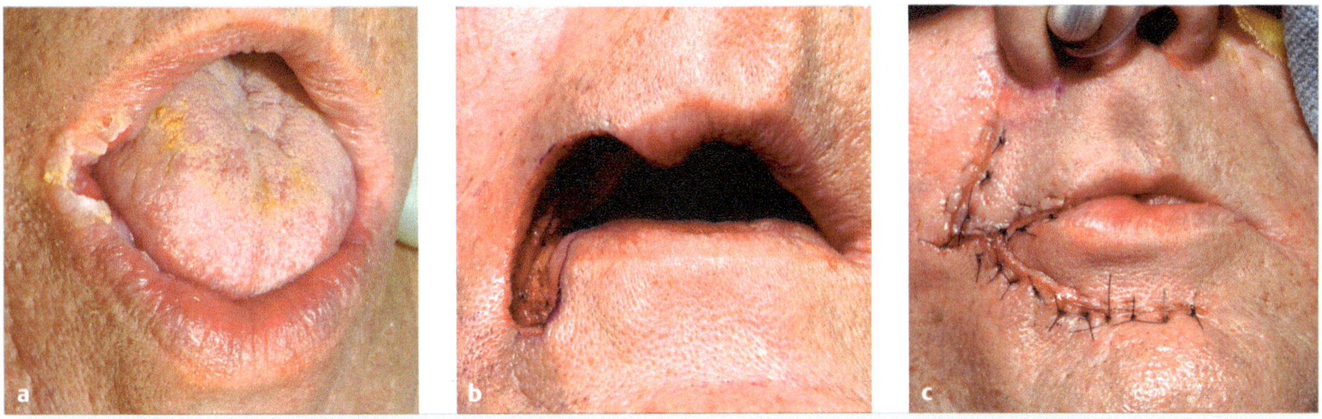

Fig. 13.4 (a–c) Invasive cancer of the labial commissure. Resection resulted in a complex defect that involved the medial cheek and cutaneous lower lip. A modified circumoral advancement-rotation flap was designed, incorporating the melolabial fold and the mental crease into the design.

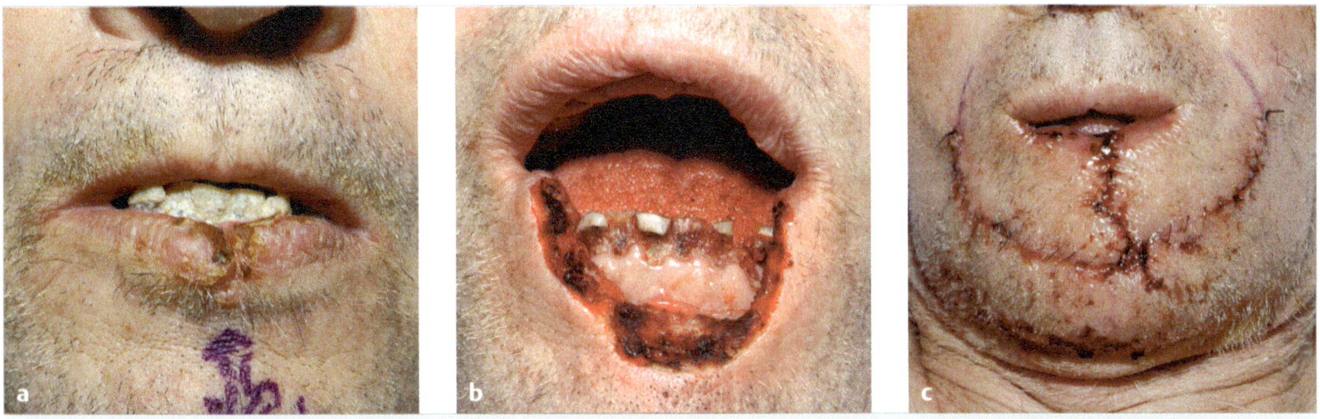

Fig. 13.5 (a–c) Infiltrating lower lip cancer that required resection of 75% of the vermilion lip and much of the cutaneous lip. A Karapandzic flap was utilized to reconstruct the defect with resultant microstomia.

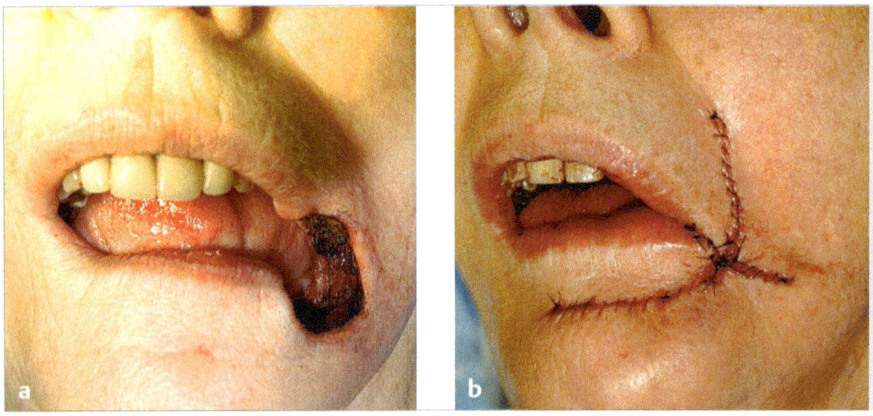

Fig. 13.6 (a, b) Resection of labial commissure cancer with a complex defect of the lips and lower cheek. Reconstruction was achieved with a modified circumoral advancement-rotation flap.

24.8% were lesions > 2 cm but ≤ 4 cm), a "histological resection margin" (not a microscopically tumor-free margin) of 7.5 mm resulted in a 20% LR rate and poorer recurrence-free survival.[36] In contrast, investigators from the Netherlands achieved a 97% 2-year local control rate for SCC of the lower lip ≤ 2 cm in diameter when a 3-mm margin of "clinically uninvolved tissue" was resected in concert with intraoperative frozen section (IFS) analysis.[37] Investigations of cutaneous SCCs that are resected using IFS to confirm negative margins have, however, demonstrated positive margins in 10 to 20% of cases on final pathological assessment.[38,39]

Sentinel lymph node biopsy or elective neck dissection (END) of lymph node levels I to III is indicated when the risk of occult nodal metastasis (ONM) exceeds 15 to 20%.[40] Sentinel lymph node biopsy has a false-negative rate of approximately 5%.[40] In a literature review of 378 elective supraomohyoid neck dissections, the pooled estimate of occult metastasis was 17%.[41]

Therapeutic neck dissection and parotidectomy, if indicated, should be performed when there is evidence for pathologic lymphadenopathy on axial imaging. Approximately 25% of patients who have lip cancer involving the middle third of the lower lip and are clinically node positive have bilateral cervical metastatic disease.[19] Superficial parotidectomy and/or dissection of the external jugular nodes may be necessary if axial imaging suggests nodal metastatic involvement. Adverse pathologic features that may be indications for postoperative adjuvant therapy include close or positive margins, PNI, lymphovascular invasion, ENE, multiple lymph node metastases, transcortical bone invasion, and WPOI. PNI involving nerves ≥ 0.1 mm in caliber have worse outcomes in squamous cancers of the dry vermilion or vermilion border.[27,42]

Positive margins should be re-resected whenever feasible. Adjuvant radiotherapy is indicated for positive margins, PNI, and multiple node lymph metastases, and platinum-based chemotherapy may also be indicated for positive margins or ENE.

13.9 Radiation Therapy

External beam radiation therapy (EBRT) and BT are both efficacious treatment modalities for lip cancer and may be preferred if radiotherapy can provide similar oncologic outcomes with preservation of lip cosmesis and function, if the patient is a poor surgical candidate, or the patient does not want surgical resection. Treatment of cT1–T2N0 lesions with EBRT are directed solely to the primary site with a total dose of 66 to 70 Gy in fractions of approximately 2 Gy/d, 5 days a week as a continuous course. Treatment of T3–T4 lesions with EBRT is performed with parallel-opposed fields that treat the lip lesion and the level I and II cervical nodes.

BT for lip cancer entails the interstitial placement of plastic tubes or rigid needles in a geometric arrangement to achieve uniform dose distribution under anesthesia followed by placement of ^{192}Ir typically using an automated remote after-loading technique that minimizes radiation exposure to the clinician. Patients treated with BT should expect the development of acute mucositis with confluent ulcerations and bleeding. BT may be delivered at a low-dose rate (LDR) of 0.4 to 1 Gy/h, or at a high-dose rate (HDR) of more than 12 Gy/h. In general, LDR-BT has been supplanted by HDR-BT, since HDR-BT provides comparable rates of local control with lower complication rates.[43,44] Late complications such as soft-tissue or bone necrosis are experienced in approximately 15% of patients treated with LDR.[43] BT may also be used as a boost following EBRT in selected cases.

13.10 Outcomes of Therapy

There are no prospective clinical trials that have evaluated the efficacy of different treatment modalities for lip cancer. Standard surgical excision of lip cancer is associated with excellent local control rates. At the University of Missouri, 424 patients with lip cancer who underwent surgical excision with negative margins had a determinate survival rate of 94%.[7] Similarly, de Visscher et al documented a 3% rate of LR following excision of T1–T2 lesions with IFS analysis.[37] Comparable outcomes have been documented by other retrospective studies.[45]

Since positive margins are present on final pathological analysis in at least 10% of excised cutaneous SCCs, which are negative during frozen section examination, MMS is preferred for high-risk areas such as the lip.[2,38,39] A meta-analysis of studies reviewing outcomes for cutaneous SCCs treated with MMS found a 3.1% LR rate: increased LR occurred with poorly differentiated cancers and lesions greater than 2 cm in diameter.[46]

Treatment of lip cancer with EBRT using orthovoltage photons or electrons is an established treatment modality with excellent control rates. Investigators from Sydney, Australia, evaluated the outcomes of 93 patients with cT1–T2N0 lip cancer treated with EBRT: the rate of LR was 5%, and 5-year recurrence-free survival was 90%.[47] LR developed in 4% of 83 T1 lip cancers treated with EBRT in another series from the Netherlands.[48] Favorable treatment outcomes following EBRT have been confirmed by other retrospective studies.[49–51]

LDR and HDR BT both provide excellent rates of local control. In a retrospective series from France, 237 patients with lower lip cancer were treated with ^{192}Ir LDR-BT with the following T stages: T1, 67%; T2, 25%; and T3–T4, 8%.[52] The 5-year rates of local control and disease-specific survival (DSS) were 95 and 91%, respectively. Similar outcomes have been realized with HDR-BT. An outcome analysis of 102 patients treated with HDR-BT documented a 94.6% local control rate and a 93.2% DSS rate. Local control rates, by T stage, were as follows: T1, 100%; T2, 93.9%; and T4, 80%.[43,44] Skin involvement was the only pathologic variable associated with recurrence on multivariate analysis.

END improves survival in patients with occult nodal metastatic disease. In a systematic review that evaluated outcomes following END (five studies) and without END (eight studies), mean DSS was 96.2 and 87.8%, respectively.[41] The challenge for clinicians, of course, is to select those patients who are at risk of ONM for END to minimize the number of unnecessary neck dissections.

Most of these findings are based on the treatment outcomes for lower lip cancers ≤ 4 cm in diameter, and the outcomes for cancers of the upper lip and commissure are based on very limited retrospective data. While some investigations have documented worse outcomes for upper lip cancers, a recent study could not substantiate these findings.[28] Cancers that involve the commissure are typically larger lesions that extend to the commissure, and isolated commissure involvement is uncommon. Critical evaluation of oncologic outcomes in retrospective series for more advanced lip cancer is generally limited by the confounding impact of unmeasured adverse prognostic features such as ONM and perineural/lymphovascular invasion as well as the variability in treatment approach between studies, all of which pose limitations for pooled analyses.

13.11 Risk Factors for Local Recurrence and Worse Survival

Based on the differences in biological behavior between cancer arising from the mucosal lip and cutaneous SCC arising from the dry vermilion, the prognostic factors for oral cancerous lesions and cutaneous SCCs of the head and neck region are discussed.

There is a strong association between maximal tumor size and outcomes following treatment for oral cancer and cutaneous SCC. Five-year determinate survival for lip cancers less than 1 cm in diameter demonstrated 94% survival versus 62% survival for cancers greater than 4 cm ($p < 0.01$) in the University of Missouri series.[7] Cutaneous SCCs greater than 2 cm in size have higher rates of nodal metastasis and worse DSS.[26,42,53,54] Moreover, the risk of death is increased by more than 400% when cutaneous SCCs are ≥ 4 cm in size.[55]

DOI is a risk factor for increased LR and poorer DSS for cancers of the wet or dry vermilion. The correlation between DOI and the risk of regional metastasis in oral cancer has been extensively studied. Moreover, numerous investigations have confirmed that higher rates of LR, nodal metastasis, and death are associated with increased TT and DOI in cutaneous SCC, including high-risk sites such as the lip.[26,53,54] A systematic review of 36 studies of cutaneous SCC that included lip cancers confirmed that TT greater than 2 mm was associated with an increased risk of LR and metastasis, and invasion beyond subcutaneous fat increased the risk of disease-specific death.[54]

Poorer outcomes are associated with PNI in lip cancers of mucosal and cutaneous origin. Cutaneous SCCs with PNI involving nerves less than 0.1 mm in caliber (small dermal nerve fibers) have not been associated with worse outcomes, whereas the presence of tumor cells within the nerve sheath of nerves ≥ 0.1 mm is associated with nodal metastasis and death.[42,56] Although the relative prognostic impact of small-caliber PNI and large-caliber PNI remains undefined for cancers of the mucosal lip and oral cavity, the adverse prognostic import of large-caliber PNI is likely.

WPOI is predictive of increased local-regional recurrence and DSS in oral cancers. The rate of local-regional recurrence is higher than 40% when WPOI-5 is present.[32] Poorly differentiated cutaneous SCCs have markedly increased rates of LR, nodal metastasis, and worse DSS.[27,42,53,54,57] Desmoplasia, which is characterized by the production of dense connective tissue with low cellularity, disorganized vasculature, and an infiltrative growth pattern, is associated with worse outcomes in cutaneous SCC.[26,58,59] MMS resulted in markedly lower rates of LR when compared to standard surgical excision (80 vs. 9%) in one retrospective series of 73 cutaneous SCCs with desmoplasia.[59]

Lymphovascular invasion in cutaneous SCCs of the head and neck region is associated with cervical lymph node metastasis and intraparotid lymph nodal metastasis.[33,60,61]

Other risk factors that are associated with poorer outcomes for both oral and cutaneous SCCs include ENE, transcortical bone invasion, positive margins, and immunosuppression.

Most retrospective investigations have demonstrated worse survival in patients diagnosed with cancer of the upper lip or commissure. In a review of 1,036 lip cancers treated between 1940 and 1987 that included 39 cases of upper lip cancer and 7 cancers limited to the commissure, cancers of the upper lip and labial commissure demonstrated worse DSS.[7] More recently, investigators from the Netherlands retrospectively evaluated 1,105 SCCs of the lip that were treated between 2004 and 2014, including 126 upper lip cancers.[28] There were no differences in 5-year overall survival, and 10-year relative survival (the ratio of observed to expected survival) was 94 and 90% for upper and lower lip cancers, respectively, which was not statistically significant.

Key Points

- The lip represents the convergence of the mucosa and skin, and therefore cutaneous and mucosal cancers may impact the anatomic subsite.
- The staging, treatment and prognosis of lip cancer is impacted by its origin from the inner mucosal lip or external dry vermilion.
- Sun exposure, tobacco and alcohol, and immunosuppression are independent risk factors.
- Surgery is the mainstay of treatment.

References

[1] Ridge JA, Lydiatt WM, Patel SG, et al. Lip and oral cavity. In: Amin MB, ed. AJCC Cancer Staging Manual. 8th ed. Chicago, IL: Springer International Publishing; 2017:79–94
[2] Califano JA, Lydiatt WM, Nehal KS, et al. Cutaneous squamous cell carcinoma of the head and neck. In: Amin MB, ed. AJCC Cancer Staging Manual. 8th ed. Chicago, IL: Springer International Publishing; 2017:171–181
[3] Shield KD, Ferlay J, Jemal A, et al. The global incidence of lip, oral cavity, and pharyngeal cancers by subsite in 2012. CA Cancer J Clin. 2017; 67 (1):51–64
[4] Ferlay J, Soerjomataram I, Dikshit R, et al. Cancer incidence and mortality worldwide: sources, methods and major patterns in GLOBOCAN 2012. Int J Cancer. 2015; 136(5):E359–E386
[5] Han AY, Kuan EC, Mallen-St Clair J, Alonso JE, Arshi A, St John MA. Epidemiology of squamous cell carcinoma of the lip in the United States: a population-based cohort analysis. JAMA Otolaryngol Head Neck Surg. 2016; 142(12): 1216–1223
[6] de Visscher JG, Schaapveld M, Otter R, Visser O, van der Waal I. Epidemiology of cancer of the lip in the Netherlands. Oral Oncol. 1998; 34(5):421–426
[7] Zitsch RP, III, Park CW, Renner GJ, Rea JL. Outcome analysis for lip carcinoma. Otolaryngol Head Neck Surg. 1995; 113(5):589–596
[8] Spitzer WO, Hill GB, Chambers LW, Helliwell BE, Murphy HB. The occupation of fishing as a risk factor in cancer of the lip. N Engl J Med. 1975; 293(9):419–424
[9] Acquavella J, Olsen G, Cole P, et al. Cancer among farmers: a meta-analysis. Ann Epidemiol. 1998; 8(1):64–74
[10] Pukkala E, Söderholm AL, Lindqvist C. Cancers of the lip and oropharynx in different social and occupational groups in Finland. Eur J Cancer B Oral Oncol. 1994; 30B(3):209–215
[11] Engels EA, Pfeiffer RM, Fraumeni JF, Jr, et al. Spectrum of cancer risk among US solid organ transplant recipients. JAMA. 2011; 306(17):1891–1901
[12] Na R, Laaksonen MA, Grulich AE, et al. High azathioprine dose and lip cancer risk in liver, heart, and lung transplant recipients: a population-based cohort study. J Am Acad Dermatol. 2016; 74(6):1144–1152 e1146
[13] Grulich AE, Vajdic CM. The epidemiology of cancers in human immunodeficiency virus infection and after organ transplantation. Semin Oncol. 2015; 42 (2):247–257
[14] Friedman GD, Asgari MM, Warton EM, Chan J, Habel LA. Antihypertensive drugs and lip cancer in non-Hispanic whites. Arch Intern Med. 2012; 172 (16):1246–1251
[15] Câmara PR, Dutra SN, Takahama Júnior A, Fontes K, Azevedo RS. A comparative study using WHO and binary oral epithelial dysplasia grading systems in actinic cheilitis. Oral Dis. 2016; 22(6):523–529
[16] Spyridonos P, Gaitanis G, Bassukas ID, Tzaphlidou M. Evaluation of vermillion border descriptors and relevance vector machines discrimination model for making probabilistic predictions of solar cheilosis on digital lip photographs. Comput Biol Med. 2015; 63:11–18
[17] Menta Simonsen Nico M, Rivitti EA, Lourenço SV. Actinic cheilitis: histologic study of the entire vermilion and comparison with previous biopsy. J Cutan Pathol. 2007; 34(4):309–314
[18] Shah AY, Doherty SD, Rosen T. Actinic cheilitis: a treatment review. Int J Dermatol. 2010; 49(11):1225–1234
[19] Zitsch RP, III, Lee BW, Smith RB. Cervical lymph node metastases and squamous cell carcinoma of the lip. Head Neck. 1999; 21(5):447–453
[20] Vartanian JG, Carvalho AL, de Araújo Filho MJ, Junior MH, Magrin J, Kowalski LP. Predictive factors and distribution of lymph node metastasis in lip cancer patients and their implications on the treatment of the neck. Oral Oncol. 2004; 40(2):223–227
[21] Cowen D, Essomba M, Richaud P, Renaud-Salis JL, Pigneux J. Treatment of cervical lymph nodes in lip cancers. Bull Cancer Radiother. 1990; 77(2):111–117
[22] Vanderlei JP, Pereira-Filho FJ, da Cruz FA, et al. Management of neck metastases in T2N0 lip squamous cell carcinoma. Am J Otolaryngol. 2013; 34(2):103–106
[23] Onercl M, Yilmaz T, Gedikoğlu G. Tumor thickness as a predictor of cervical lymph node metastasis in squamous cell carcinoma of the lower lip. Otolaryngol Head Neck Surg. 2000; 122(1):139–142
[24] de Visscher JG, van den Elsaker K, Grond AJ, van der Wal JE, van der Waal I. Surgical treatment of squamous cell carcinoma of the lower lip: evaluation of long-term results and prognostic factors: a retrospective analysis of 184 patients. J Oral Maxillofac Surg. 1998; 56(7):814–820, discussion 820–821
[25] Najim M, Cross S, Gebski V, Palme CE, Morgan GJ, Veness MJ. Early-stage squamous cell carcinoma of the lip: the Australian experience and the benefits of radiotherapy in improving outcome in high-risk patients after resection. Head Neck. 2013; 35(10):1426–1430
[26] Brantsch KD, Meisner C, Schönfisch B, et al. Analysis of risk factors determining prognosis of cutaneous squamous-cell carcinoma: a prospective study. Lancet Oncol. 2008; 9(8):713–720
[27] Karia PS, Han J, Schmults CD. Cutaneous squamous cell carcinoma: estimated incidence of disease, nodal metastasis, and deaths from disease in the United States, 2012. J Am Acad Dermatol. 2013; 68(6):957–966
[28] Pietersma NS, de Bock GH, de Visscher JG, Roodenburg JL, van Dijk BA. No evidence for a survival difference between upper and lower lip squamous cell carcinoma. Int J Oral Maxillofac Surg. 2015; 44(5):549–554
[29] Cherpelis BS, Marcusen C, Lang PG. Prognostic factors for metastasis in squamous cell carcinoma of the skin. Dermatol Surg. 2002; 28(3):268–273
[30] Jackson JE, Dickie GJ, Wiltshire KL, et al. Radiotherapy for perineural invasion in cutaneous head and neck carcinomas: toward a risk-adapted treatment approach. Head Neck. 2009; 31(5):604–610
[31] Santos HB, Silva AL, Cavalcante LH, Alves PM, Godoy GP, Nonaka CF. Histopathological grading systems and their relationship with clinical parameters in lower lip squamous cell carcinoma. Int J Oral Maxillofac Surg. 2014; 43(5): 539–545
[32] Brandwein-Gensler M, Teixeira MS, Lewis CM, et al. Oral squamous cell carcinoma: histologic risk assessment, but not margin status, is strongly predictive of local disease-free and overall survival. Am J Surg Pathol. 2005; 29(2): 167–178
[33] Durham AB, Lowe L, Malloy KM, et al. Sentinel lymph node biopsy for cutaneous squamous cell carcinoma on the head and neck. JAMA Otolaryngol Head Neck Surg. 2016; 142(12):1171–1176
[34] Pfister DG, Spencer S, Adelstein D, et al. NCCN Guidelines Head and Neck Cancers. Version 2.2018. Washington, PA: NCCN; 2018
[35] Egemen O, Bingöl D, Orman Ç, Sayilgan AT, Özkaya Ö, Akan M. Quantification of the surgical margin shrinkage in lip cancer: determining the relation between the surgical and histopathologic margins. J Craniofac Surg. 2014; 25 (6):2152–2155
[36] Schüller M, Gosau M, Müller S, et al. Long-term outcome and subjective quality of life after surgical treatment of lower lip cancer. Clin Oral Investig. 2015; 19(5):1093–1099
[37] de Visscher JG, Gooris PJ, Vermey A, Roodenburg JL. Surgical margins for resection of squamous cell carcinoma of the lower lip. Int J Oral Maxillofac Surg. 2002; 31(2):154–157
[38] Chambers KJ, Kraft S, Emerick K. Evaluation of frozen section margins in high-risk cutaneous squamous cell carcinomas of the head and neck. Laryngoscope. 2015; 125(3):636–639
[39] Castley AJ, Theile DR, Lambie D. The use of frozen section in the excision of cutaneous malignancy: a Queensland experience. Ann Plast Surg. 2013; 71 (4):386–389
[40] Sollamo EMJ, Ilmonen SK, Virolainen MS, Suominen SH. Sentinel lymph node biopsy in cN0 squamous cell carcinoma of the lip: a retrospective study. Head Neck. 2016; 38 Suppl 1:E1375–E1380
[41] Bhandari K, Wang DC, Li SC, et al. Primary cN0 lip squamous cell carcinoma and elective neck dissection: systematic review and meta-analysis. Head Neck. 2015; 37(9):1392–1400
[42] Schmults CD, Karia PS, Carter JB, Han J, Qureshi AA. Factors predictive of recurrence and death from cutaneous squamous cell carcinoma: a 10-year, single-institution cohort study. JAMA Dermatol. 2013; 149(5):541–547
[43] Guinot JL, Arribas L, Tortajada MI, et al. From low-dose-rate to high-dose-rate brachytherapy in lip carcinoma: Equivalent results but fewer complications. Brachytherapy. 2013; 12(6):528–534
[44] Guinot JL, Arribas L, Vendrell JB, et al. Prognostic factors in squamous cell lip carcinoma treated with high-dose-rate brachytherapy. Head Neck. 2014; 36 (12):1737–1742
[45] Biasoli ER, Valente VB, Mantovan B, et al. Lip cancer: a clinicopathological study and treatment outcomes in a 25-year experience. J Oral Maxillofac Surg. 2016; 74(7):1360–1367
[46] Rowe DE, Carroll RJ, Day CL, Jr. Prognostic factors for local recurrence, metastasis, and survival rates in squamous cell carcinoma of the skin, ear, and lip. Implications for treatment modality selection. J Am Acad Dermatol. 1992; 26 (6):976–990
[47] Thanh Pham T, Cross S, Gebski V, Veness MJ. Squamous cell carcinoma of the lip in Australian patients: definitive radiotherapy is an efficacious option to surgery in select patients. Dermatol Surg. 2015; 41(2):219–225

[48] de Visscher JG, Botke G, Schakenraad JA, van der Waal I. A comparison of results after radiotherapy and surgery for stage I squamous cell carcinoma of the lower lip. Head Neck. 1999; 21(6):526–530

[49] Gooris PJ, Maat B, Vermey A, Roukema JA, Roodenburg JL. Radiotherapy for cancer of the lip. A long-term evaluation of 85 treated cases. Oral Surg Oral Med Oral Pathol Oral Radiol Endod. 1998; 86(3):325–330

[50] Cerezo L, Liu FF, Tsang R, Payne D. Squamous cell carcinoma of the lip: analysis of the Princess Margaret Hospital experience. Radiother Oncol. 1993; 28 (2):142–147

[51] Hollen TR, Morris CG, Kirwan JM, Amdur RJ, Werning J, Vaysberg M, Mendenhall W. Squamous cell carcinoma of the lip: a retrospective analysis of the University of Florida experience. Int J Radiat Oncol Biol Phys. 2013; 87:S612

[52] Beauvois S, Hoffstetter S, Peiffert D, et al. Brachytherapy for lower lip epidermoid cancer: tumoral and treatment factors influencing recurrences and complications. Radiother Oncol. 1994; 33(3):195–203

[53] Jambusaria-Pahlajani A, Kanetsky PA, Karia PS, et al. Evaluation of AJCC tumor staging for cutaneous squamous cell carcinoma and a proposed alternative tumor staging system. JAMA Dermatol. 2013; 149(4):402–410

[54] Thompson AK, Kelley BF, Prokop LJ, Murad H, Baum CL. Risk factors for cutaneous squamous cell carcinoma recurrence, metastasis, and disease-specific death s: a systematic review and meta-analysis. JAMA Dermatol. 2016; 152 (4):419–428

[55] Clayman GL, Lee JJ, Holsinger FC, et al. Mortality risk from squamous cell skin cancer. J Clin Oncol. 2005; 23(4):759–765

[56] Karia PS, Morgan FC, Ruiz ES, Schmults CD. Clinical and incidental perineural invasion of cutaneous squamous cell carcinoma: a systematic review and pooled analysis of outcomes data. JAMA Dermatol. 2017; 153 (8):781–788

[57] Brougham ND, Dennett ER, Cameron R, Tan ST. The incidence of metastasis from cutaneous squamous cell carcinoma and the impact of its risk factors. J Surg Oncol. 2012; 106(7):811–815

[58] Breuninger H, Schaumburg-Lever G, Holzschuh J, Horny HP. Desmoplastic squamous cell carcinoma of skin and vermilion surface: a highly malignant subtype of skin cancer. Cancer. 1997; 79(5):915–919

[59] Salmon PJ, Hussain W, Geisse JK, Grekin RC, Mortimer NJ. Sclerosing squamous cell carcinoma of the skin, an underemphasized locally aggressive variant: a 20-year experience. Dermatol Surg. 2011; 37(5): 664–670

[60] Moore BA, Weber RS, Prieto V, et al. Lymph node metastases from cutaneous squamous cell carcinoma of the head and neck. Laryngoscope. 2005; 115(9): 1561–1567

[61] Gore SM, Shaw D, Martin RC, et al. Prospective study of sentinel node biopsy for high-risk cutaneous squamous cell carcinoma of the head and neck. Head Neck. 2016; 38 Suppl 1:E884–E889

14 Reconstruction of the Lip

Carl M. Truesdale, Andrew W. Joseph, and Shaun C. Desai

Summary
The human lip has many important functions and dynamic, complex anatomic relationships. The ideal reconstruction requires a strong understanding of the techniques available to the surgeon. The proper selection of technique demands a nuanced review of the literature as well as meticulous planning and execution. It is important to optimize both the function and appearance of lips in oral reconstruction.

Keywords: lip reconstruction, lip cancer, lip flap

14.1 Introduction

The lip is a major defining feature of the human face. It is a complex, dynamic soft-tissue structure that represents a major facial aesthetic subunit. The lip has many functions, including speech production, tactile sensation, facial expression, communication, and maintenance of an oral seal. Facial surgeons are often tasked with reconstructing various defects in this region. A thorough understanding of lip anatomy is important to enable the best reconstructive outcome. This chapter is a review of the reconstructive options available for surgeons who repair defects of the lip.

14.2 Background

As with many modern surgical reconstruction techniques, lip reconstruction has a rich and far-reaching history. Early reports of lip repairs are included in an ancient book *Sushruta Samhita*-written by Sushruta sometime between 600 and 1,000 BC.[1,2] Advances in lip reconstruction were relatively stagnant until the 16th century, when Italian surgeon Gaspare Tagliacozzi developed reconstructive techniques using pedicled arm flaps to the nose and lip.[3] Later, in the 18th and 19th centuries, cross-lip techniques were pioneered by Johann Gustaaf Hjertzeel, Sabattini, Abbe, and Estander.[4,5] In the 19th century, German Victor von Bruns introduced the vermilionectomy for lip malignancy in early H- and T-plasty and superiorly based flaps for lower lip reconstruction. It was also during this time period that Dieffenbach may have first introduced vermillion reconstruction using a pedicled cheek mucosa.[6] More recently, Walton and Bunkis[7] and Sakai et al[8] were the first to publish microsurgical reconstructive techniques of the upper and lower lips. These pioneers established the basis for our modern techniques.

14.3 Anatomic Considerations/ Relevant Anatomy

The face can be divided into vertical thirds from menton to trichion. The lip is positioned in the bottom third of the face, situated between the menton and the subnasale. The lip is bounded by the nose superiorly, labiomental crease inferiorly, and melolabial crease bilaterally. The lip is one of the seven aesthetic units of the face. The surgical anatomy can further be divided into the white lip and red lip. In contrast to lip mucosa, which is pink, the vermillion represents the darker colored fleshy folds and exists as a dry transition zone between the skin and mucous membrane. The upper vermillion is usually thinner than lower vermillion in both men and women.[9] The upper lip is also on average 15 to 17% larger than the lower lip.[9,10]

14.3.1 The Upper White Lip

The upper lip can be further broken down into the philtral dimple, philtrum columns or ridges, melolabial/nasolabial folds, Cupid's bow, and vermilion border (see ▸ Fig. 14.1). The Cupid's bow is located at the midline upper lip and is classically **V**-shaped. The philtral columns or ridges represent the vertical raised tissue extending from the apices of the Cupid's bow to the nose. The philtral dimple is the depression between the columns. The upper lip can similarly be divided into the philtrum centrally and two lateral upper lip components to the right and left of the philtrum.[11]

14.3.2 The Vermillion

The vermillion is distinct in that it is devoid of minor salivary glands or eccrine glands, which are normally found throughout the oral cavity and its epithelium is thinner than that of oral mucosa. The rich vascular bed and a thin layer of keratinized stratified squamous epithelium of the vermillion are also responsible for its more red/rosy color.[12] The wet line (also known as the red line) represents the distinct transition between the intraoral labial mucosa and the transition zone of the vermillion. The tubercle or procheilon is the area of the upper lip that is prominent centrally.

14.3.3 Lip Function

The lips play a vital role in many aspects of our daily lives. They are important for tactile sensation, oral communication, and facial expression. The lips have a critical role in forming bilabial and labiodental sounds. Bilabial sounds "b," "m," "w," and "p" are formed from the action of both lips. Labiodental sounds "f," "v," and "c" are formed from the interaction of the lips and teeth.[13] The lips also shape the mouth, creating a visual cue that aids communication for deaf or hearing-impaired patients in particular. One of the other vital functions of the lips is to prevent leakage of fluid or air. Without this type of oral competence, the patient will lack the ability to form the natural food/ liquid barrier primarily at the lower and lateral lip regions, thus resulting in drooling. Lip adduction and food bolus containment is also necessary to initiate the oral phase of swallowing. A strong understanding of the lip functions and components, including nervous, muscular, arterial, mucosa, skin, and vascular components, must be mastered in order to optimize reconstruction.

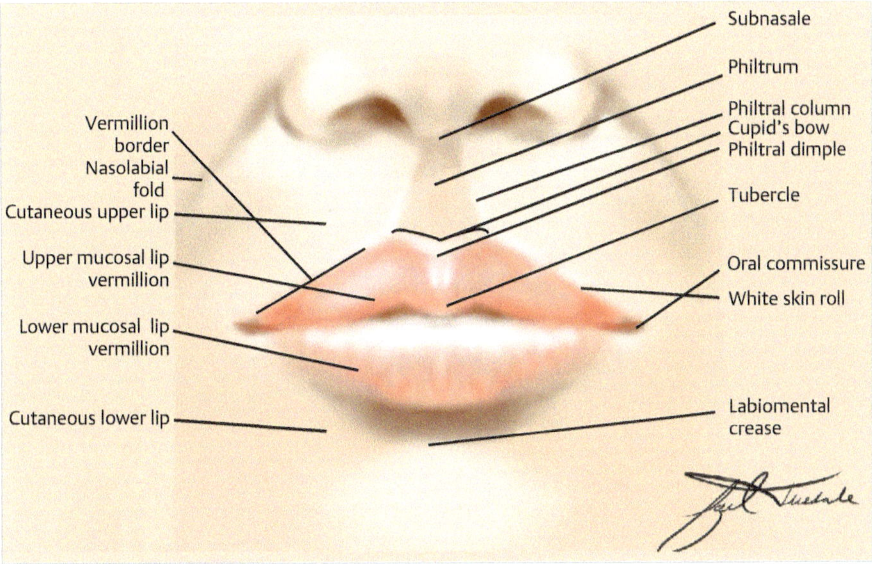

Fig. 14.1 Diagram of normal lip anatomy.

14.3.4 Nervous Components

The lips contain a high density of nervous system structures. In fact, when studying the homunculus or pictorially mapped representation of brain sensation, the lips are proportioned larger than almost any body part. This is due to the many brain cells dedicated to lip sensation and movement. The motor innervation of the lip is provided by the facial nerves, which generally enter the facial muscles on the deep surface.[14]

The sensory afferents are provided by the maxillary and mandibular divisions of the trigeminal nerve. The mental branch of the mandibular division provides sensation to the lower lip, which is important when judging food temperature and texture. Disruption of the nervous afferents and efferent may result in dyskinetic motion or inadvertent lip injury due to lack of sensation (e.g., biting, burns).

14.3.5 Muscular Components

The lip has several muscular components. The main muscle of the lip is the orbicularis oris, which provides the major sphincter control of the mouth. The varied muscle fiber orientation allows for dynamic expression and shaping of complex movements. The risorius, depressor anguli oris, depressor labii inferior, mentalis, buccinator, zygomaticus major, zygomaticus minor, nasalis, and depressor septi all attach to the orbicularis oris. Muscles of facial expression also insert adjacent to the oral commissure, forming a complex of muscle and connective tissue known as the modiolus.

As with any muscle group in the body, knowing the origin, insertion points, and muscle orientation allows one to predict the muscle's action and vector forces. The deep perioral musculature provides oral cavity sphincter function, in contrast to the fine control allowed by the superficial muscles. Orbicularis oris muscle fibers decussate at the midline and insert into the dermis 5 mm from the midline, thus creating the philtral columns.[15] The philtral groove has no dermal attachment and therefore appears concave.[15]

14.3.6 Arterial and Venous Supply

The arterial supply to the lips is primarily based off the facial artery system, a branch of the external carotid artery. The facial artery divides to form the inferior labial artery and superior labial artery. The proximal facial artery crosses the mandible to reach the face deep to the risorius/zygomaticus major and superficial to the buccinator muscle. The superior labial artery gives off the angular artery, which continues its course superiorly. This artery has several points of anastomosis to the contralateral side and buccal artery branches. The artery has a variable course either between the orbicularis muscle or between the muscle and mucosa.[16] Classically, it is found between 1 and 2 cm from the oral commissure.[17] The artery has been found to travel through the orbicularis oris muscle in half of patients and been found higher in the central parts of the upper lip.[12]

The inferior labial artery branches from the facial artery near the oral commissure. It runs deep to the depressor angularis oris and to the orbicularis oris. This artery also forms an anastomosis with the contralateral side. The inferior labial artery may not always be present. Dissection studies have demonstrated variability in the presence of this artery from 10 to 64%.[16,18]

There are additional vascular contributions to the lip from the maxillary artery. Both the buccal artery and the inferior alveolar artery are terminal branches of the maxillary artery and supply the lip region. The mental branch of the inferior alveolar artery finds its path to the lower lip after it courses along the mental foramen with the mental nerve. The buccal artery courses from the infraorbital region to the superficial face, paralleling the facial artery across the lateral oral region.

The veins draining the lip travel with the arterial supply and in the upper lip may be included in the "danger triangle," which may drain to the cavernous sinus via the ophthalmic veins from facial veins.[19] This is the reason that infections in the upper lip region have the theoretical ability to cause intracranial infections.

14.3.7 Lymphatic Drainage

The lymphatic patterns of the lips must also be understood given the oncologic implications of many lip defects that result from malignancy. The lymphatic drainage from the latter upper lip drains to the submandibular nodes, periparotid nodes, and possibly to the submental nodes.[20] The upper and middle lip may drain to the submandibular, periparotid, and submental nodes. The lower lip drains bilaterally to the submental nodes in the center and submandibular and perifacial nodes laterally.[20]

14.4 Reconstructive Procedures by Defect and Anatomical Site

14.4.1 Partial-Thickness Red Lip Defect (Vermillion Reconstruction)

Superficial lesions of the vermillion may be treated with vermilionectomy without sacrifice of deeper muscular layers. These defects present a unique clinical challenge for surgeons. The human eye is attracted to contrast in both color and shape; the vermillion has both of these attributes. Irregularities in the vermillion border are amplified as the human eye is drawn to the lips in conversation. Meticulous reapproximation of the oral/red lip interface minimizes what might otherwise be conspicuous repairs.

Primary Closure

Defects across the vermillion border and into the cutaneous (white) lip may be closed primarily. Again, it is important to closely and accurately reapproximate the vermillion border. A common technique to allow for the identification of the vermillion edge is the placement of hatch marks with a scalpel blade sharply, although the authors prefer marking with methylene blue or a skin marking pen. Vertical mattress sutures are often utilized at the vermillion border to optimize outcome.

Pedicled Mucosal Grafts

Mucosa from the tongue may be pedicled to the lip mucosa and later divided, producing good results. Numerous authors have described the use of dorsal tongue sutured to the vermilionectomy defect. The dorsal aspect of the tongue is used to prevent subsequent tongue tethering and nerve injury. The flap is then divided 3 to 4 weeks after inset. The tongue mucosa subsequently becomes smooth and closely resembles the normal red lip. The resultant lip flap is prone to drying and generally improves with time.[21] Free mucosal grafts from various donor sources have also been successfully accomplished for large defects of the upper and lower vermillion.[22]

Mucosal Advancement Flaps

Mucosal advancement flaps have been used for more than 150 years for reconstruction of lip defects. Mucosal defects may be closed after vermilionectomy by advancing the vestibular or buccal mucosa to the cutaneous lip.[6,23] The mucosa may be undermined and freed in a submucosal plane with releasing incisions in the oral cavity to gain length. This reconstructive technique can produce very good cosmetic results, but tissue thinning and internal lip rotation are occasional sequelae. Volume deficiency may be addressed with fat or filler injections, but lip rotation is best addressed by anticipating and preventing it at the time of the primary operation. This reconstruction can also impart an unnatural wet appearance to portions of the vermillion, as well as result in a deeper red appearance. It is important to preoperatively counsel patients regarding these expected changes.

Vermillion Mucosal V–Y Advancement Flap

This technique can be used to advance small to medium-sized areas of mucosa to close vermillion defects. With this technique, a wedge-shaped portion of the mucosa is designed to be equal or slightly larger in width to the size of the defect, and then tapers to the apex of the V within the oral vestibular mucosa. The mucosal flap is generally elevated along with the orbicularis oris muscle underlying the flap in order to preserve vascularity. Although this technique transfers well-vascularized tissue, it has the risk of producing a trap door deformity, an area of raised or bulging tissue that can result from lymphatic or venous obstruction, scar hypertrophy, or excessive fatty or redundant tissue.

Cross-Lip Mucosal Flap

It has been proposed that disproportion between the upper and lower lip contributes significantly to the lip deformity following reconstruction.[24] By borrowing tissue from the larger and more redundant lower lip, this size disparity can be minimized. This is the main principle behind the cross-lip mucosal flap, which is a technique that can be used to repair large upper vermillion defects. The flap is raised from the contralateral lower lip mucosa onto the buccal mucosa beyond the commissure and pedicled at the midline. Following this, the vermillion flap is then sutured to the upper lip defect. The pedicle is divided in 7 to 10 days and trimmed. The upper and lower lips are then closed.[25]

Facial Artery Musculomucosal Flap

The upper or lower lip vermillion may be reconstructed with this robust composite flap in a bilateral or unilateral manner. Intraoral mucosa is harvested from the lateral cheek as a composite flap along with the axial blood supply from the facial artery, lateral to the buccinator.[26] The flap is designed after using a doppler to identify the course of the facial artery, with its course marked along the mucosa with a pen. After the trajectory of the facial artery is marked, the borders of the flap are designed such that the flap is centered over the artery. This flap may be inferior or superiorly based depending on orientation and vascular supply. We often find it useful to make mucosal incisions with a colorado-tipped monopolar cautery. Following mucosal incision and muscular division, the distal (or proximal facial artery in superiorly based flaps) is identified and ligated. The flap is raised with the mucosa, submucosa and small amount of buccinator muscle. Satisfactory lip volume is achieved with this technique. Careful attention should be paid not to injure Stensen's duct and to restrict the anterior aspect of the flap to 1 cm posterior to the commissure to ensure no external cosmetic deformity (▶ Fig. 14.2).

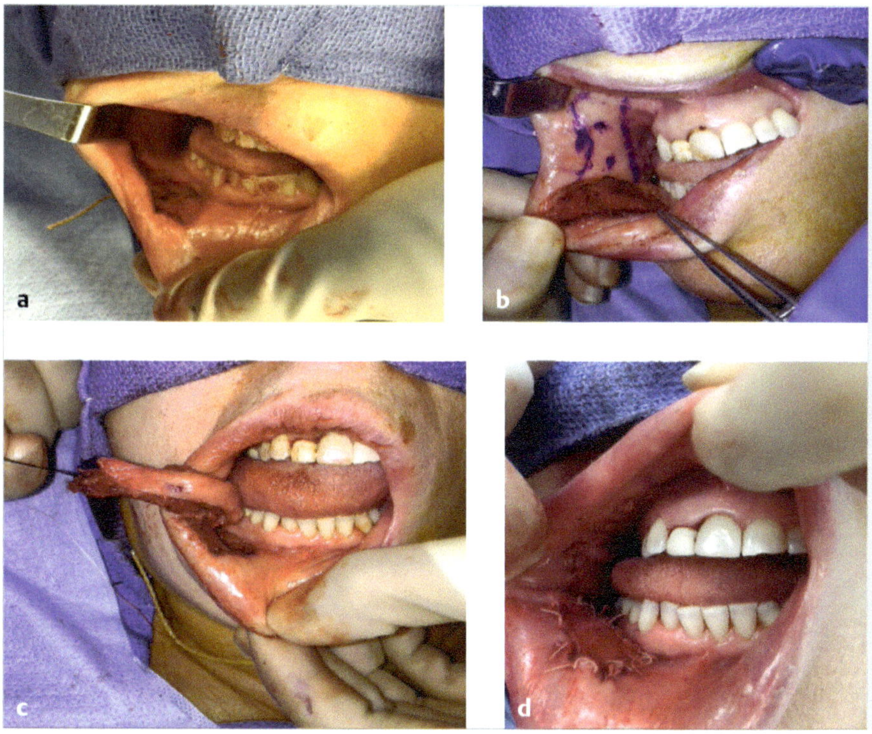

Fig. 14.2 **(a)** Vestibular mucosal lip defect after tumor resection. **(b)** Facial artery musculomucosal flap (FAMM) marked out with dots representing facial artery Doppler signal. Note the anterior border of the flap is marked 1 cm posterior to the oral commissure and the posterior border of the flap is anterior to Stensen's duct. **(c)** FAMM flap dissected out and pedicled off of facial artery. **(d)** FAMM flap insetted into place by rotating 180 degrees into lip defect.

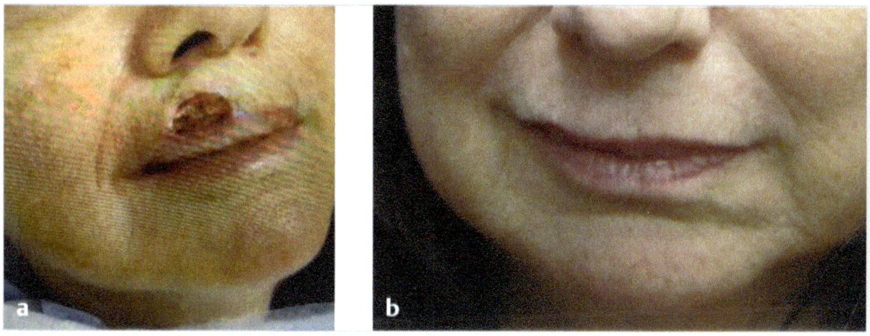

Fig. 14.3 **(a)** Preoperative photograph of partial-thickness white and red lip defect after Mohs procedure. **(b)** Patient reconstructed with full-thickness skin graft with dermabrasion (6 weeks afterward) for white lip and vermillion advancement flap for red lip. Unfortunately, the patient developed slight asymmetry and lack of volume to the red lip from the vermillion advancement flap.

14.4.2 Partial-Thickness Cutaneous Reconstruction

Lip soft-tissue defects that do not involve the deeper muscular layers may be closed with little lip function implications. A focus on cosmetic outcome is the primary emphasis when reconstructing these defects. Again, the principles of respecting aesthetic subunits must be followed. All of the following closures involve dissection of skin and subcutaneous tissues overlying the muscles of facial expression/orbicularis oris.

Primary Closure

Cutaneous lip lesions may be primarily closed with tissue advancement. The defect may be made fusiform in nature and then closed without standing cutaneous cones. The closure must be oriented parallel to relaxed skin tension lines.[27] These lines usually are perpendicular to the underlying muscle direction. In young patients, the surgeon may study pictures of the patient's older relatives to best determine the direction of closure.[27] This closure technique has the disadvantage of flattening the Cupid's bow or distortion of the vermillion border. Some authors suggest up to 50% of the cutaneous upper lip may be closed primarily.[17] To avoid extension into the chin for a lengthy closure, an M-plasty may be designed.

Skin Grafts and Secondary Intention

These reconstructive techniques have limited role in the reconstruction of partial-thickness defects given their poor aesthetic outcomes compared with local flaps. Full- and split-thickness skin grafts require that the skin undergo imbibition, which requires immobility, which is difficult to achieve in the dynamic region of the lip. Poor color and texture match is usually seen with these flaps in the lip region. Although variable in outcome, full-thickness skin grafts have been used to reconstruct the central philtral subunit defect with a satisfactory outcome.[28] A bolster, oftentimes made of xeroform, is recommended to help protect the skin graft as it achieves neovascularization in the first 5 to 7 days (▶ Fig. 14.3).

Secondary intention is rarely advocated in the region of the lips given skin contraction and distortion produced, which is unwanted in the lip area.[29] It has been suggested that small defects that do not involve the vermillion and are at an acceptable distance from the vermillion line may heal well by secondary intention such as the nasolabial or labiomental creases.[30]

Local Flap Reconstruction

Simple Advancement Flaps

Skin from the lateral upper lip, lower lip, and the medial cheek may be advanced into the medial lip region. The dissection is carried down to the fascia overlying the muscles of facial expression. Often a standing cutaneous cone may need to be excised for closure. The commissure may be pulled medially with this advancement, which over time becomes less noticeable.[17,29]

H-Plasty Flap

Cutaneous defects of the upper and lower lip may be closed centrally through the use of H-plasty. This modified advancement flap allows dissection of cutaneous/subcutaneous tissue above the muscular layers to the defect in a flanking manner that meets in the middle. Four lateral Burow's triangles may be removed to facilitate flap advancement by taking advantage of laxity of the medial cheek tissue. In the upper lip, incisions for advancement may be extended to the nasolabial crease and vermillion border. There may be a resultant blunting of the philtral columns. In the lower lip, an H-plasty may be used above the labiomental crease in a curvilinear incision.

O–T Flap

This is a modification of the H-plasty flap. This technique is used to advance flanking tissue into the circular defect. A standing cutaneous cone may be freed from the defect to allow for midline closure. Like the H-plasty, two Burow's triangles may be resected at the ends of horizontal incisions extended from the defect. This technique may be used effectively for smaller defects at the aesthetic boundaries such as the vermillion.[31]

V–Y Island Flap

Lateral upper and lower lip defects may be addressed with a subcutaneous pedicled V–Y island flap. Surgeons must pay particular attention to the vermillion and commissure to avoid vector displacement. Design of the flap may utilize the natural nasolabial fold with advancement occurring along this natural border. As will most local flaps, substantial subcutaneous undermining is necessary to prevent puckering and allow for tension-free closure.

Melolabial Flaps

Large lateral upper and lower lip cutaneous defects may be reconstructed by use of various types of melolabial flaps. Melolabial flaps take advantage of adjacent cheek laxity, which provides a valuable area for tissue recruitment. The melolabial flap is most commonly designed as a subcutaneous pedicled island advancement flap or a transposition flap, although interpolated flaps are also utilized in select cases. Melolabial transposition flaps may be superiorly or inferiorly based as the medial cheek skin in this area has a robust vascular supply from the adjacent angular artery.[29,32] It is important to recognize that there may be blunting of the melolabial crease with use of this flap, although this may be mitigated by incorporating a lateral incision to form a new crease.

Design of a melolabial island flap begins by cutting a template to the exact size of the skin defect. In some cases, it may be necessary to enlarge the size of the defect in order to allow the flap to be advanced along the vermillion border and provide for a more natural appearance with resultant scars better hidden at the anatomical subunit border. Defects that abut the alar base may require the defect to be extended adjacent to the alar groove. Next, the template is used to mark the proposed flap along the medial cheek just lateral to the melolabial fold. The subcutaneous pedicled island flap utilizes the relatively mobile medial cheek fat in order to form the subcutaneous pedicle, while medial cheek skin abutting the melolabial fold and remaining upper lip skin are utilized as the skin flap. The skin immediately adjacent to the defect is carefully undermined a short distance in the subcutaneous plane in order to separate it from the underlying orbicularis oris. The skin is next incised along the periphery of the skin flap, while taking care to maintain an adequate subcutaneous pedicle to the central third of the flap. The flap is then advanced into position, fixated to the skin surrounding the defect. The secondary defect is generally closed along the melolabial crease in a V–Y fashion.

Note Flap

For small, lateral cutaneous lip defects, the note flap is a good reconstructive option. With this flap, a circular defect is reconstructed by extending an incision tangentially from the defect. This ultimately takes on an appearance similar to that of a musical eighth note. To design the flap, a line is measured tangential from the defect along relaxed tension-free lines for a length of 1.5x the diameter of the defect. Next, a second incision is made from the end of the first tangential cut and angled at 50 to 60 degrees, ultimately creating a triangular shaped flap. The flap is then raised in a subcutaneous plane with the tip de-epithelialized and sutured into the defect.[33] There may or may not be a standing cutaneous cone that may need to be excised from the defect.[17]

Conversion to Full Thickness

In some cases, partial-thickness defects may be converted to full-thickness defects in order to improve the ultimate appearance. The decision to convert a partial-thickness defect into a full-thickness one is often based on the observed involvement of the vermillion border. Following conversion to a full-thickness wedge defect, the wound may often be closed in a primary fashion.

14.4.3 Full-Thickness Defect Reconstruction

Full-thickness defects of the lips may be categorized based on the total defect size, location (upper lip vs. lower lip), and whether the defect involves or abuts the oral commissure. Each of these characteristics helps determine optimal treatment strategy. Closure of all full-thickness defects will involve four primary tissue layers, including mucosa, a muscular orbicularis oris layer, a subcutaneous layer, and the skin layer. The importance of a meticulous closure cannot be overemphasized. The authors often find it helpful to use a fine-tipped marking pen or methylene blue to mark the vermillion border prior to distortion from infiltration of local anesthetic or prior to soft-tissue manipulation. Closure should meticulously reapproximate each tissue layer as indiscriminate closure can often lead to unsatisfying results for the patient and surgeon alike. Given the potential intraoral contamination of the deep wound in full-thickness defects, attention is given to oral hygiene postoperatively. Often mouth rinses with chlorhexidine gluconate may be encouraged after meals in the first postoperative week. Also, to minimize stress placed on the reconstruction, a soft or liquid diet may be advised. Early in wound healing as the layered tissues obtain their initial strength during early remodeling, it is important to minimize stress on the wound with talking or large oral movements in this phase. Steri-strips may be used to help reinforce the wound closure with skin adhesive.

Lip Replantation

Some authors have successfully replanted lips in the context of traumatic avulsion. A multi-institutional review of the topic demonstrated that the technique is feasible, but it may not have the optimal functional and/or cosmetic result.[34,35] This technique involves the reanastomosis of the avulsed lip's vascular supply to its corresponding labial artery and vein if possible. In most cases, the vein may not be identified and venous anastomoses cannot take place, which results in venous congestion of the avulsed segment, which oftentimes requires adjuvant leech therapy, anticoagulation, and antispasmodics.[34] Drawbacks of this technique ranged from hypertrophic scar, long operative time (average 5.6 hours), increased blood loss, longer hospital stay, an acute setting requirement for cold ischemia time, a necessity for institutional microsurgical expertise, and cost.[34]

Wedge Resections

Full-thickness defects that comprise one-third of the lip or less (although some authors have described up to one half of the lip width) and do not involve the oral commissure may often be closed by converting the defect into a **V**-shaped (wedge) defect. The lower lip has very good cosmetic outcomes given the increased soft tissue when this technique is employed. The wedge excision may be completed in V, W, or T design. All three layers of the lip are reapproximated with attention given again to the reapproximation of the orbicularis oris and vermillion border. The lower lip often tolerates larger reconstructions using this technique, as do older patients. When planning the incisions for the defect, the surgeon should ensure that the final orientation of the scar is parallel to the relaxed skin tension lines or "smoker's lines." When planning the incisions, defects situated near the midline should have relatively symmetric limbs of the **V**-shaped defect (and perhaps oriented along the philtral columns). On the lower central lip, the authors prefer a "W" incision to help minimize the dog-ear, and the ability to hide cutaneous extension in the labiomental crease. Conversely, those situated more laterally may be modified in order to allow the final scar to be more rotated and parallel to the radially oriented relaxed skin tension lines around the orbicularis oris. When possible, it is ideal to limit extension of the incision into the chin subunit as this will allow for a more aesthetically pleasing result. It is occasionally necessary with midline upper lip defects to supplement closures with perialar crescentic and nasolabial crease extensions to allow for closure (T closure).

Lip-Switch Procedures

Lip-switch (cross-lip) procedures are most useful for full-thickness defects that involve greater than one-third of the lip, but less than two-thirds of the lip. The Abbe flap and the Estlander flap are the most commonly utilized cross-lip flaps and both are based on the superior and inferior labial arteries.

The Abbe flap has been employed for greater than 150 years to reconstruct both upper and lower lip defects. The Abbe flap is an interpolated flap that involves transfer of a triangular portion of a donor lip tissue to a defect situated in the corresponding portion of the opposite lip. The Abbe flap may be used equally well for reconstruction of superior or inferior lip defects. Flap design is begun by assessment of the width of the lip defect and making note of the affected aesthetic subunits. Reconstruction of upper lip defects are often more challenging, and may require transfer of flaps of equal width when an entire anatomic subunit is affected. For example, reconstruction of defects of the philtrum should be reconstructed by transferring an equal-width central lower lip flap. After precise measurement and assessment of the defect, a triangularly shaped interpolated tissue flap is outlined on the opposite lip. As noted earlier, it is important to consider that final scars should be positioned parallel to the radially oriented relaxed skin tension lines. In most cases, the Abbe flap may be based on either a medial or a lateral vascular pedicle, and the decision is often based on ease of transfer and anticipated degree of postoperative obstruction of the mouth. Next, a full-thickness incision is made through the boundary of the **V**-shaped donor flap, with the exception of the anticipated entry point for the vascular pedicle. The superior and inferior labial arteries consistently course along the vermillion border within the submucosal layer in the majority of cases (77–87%), but in some patients it may course through the superficial orbicularis oris muscle.[36] Therefore, in order to preserve the vascular pedicle, the dissection should proceed no deeper than the orbicularis oris muscular layer at the level of the vermillion border on the pedicled portion of the flap. After completing the incisions, the flap is transferred to the opposite lip and suture fixated into position. Similar to other interpolated flaps, the Abbe flap is generally left pedicled for 3 to 4 weeks, after which the pedicle may be divided during a second procedure and the inset of the flap completed.

The Estlander flap is similar to the Abbe flap, but it is usually a one-stage cross-lip flap that is employed for full-thickness defects that abut the oral commissure. With the Estlander flap, a triangular-shaped donor flap is based medially off of the contralateral labial artery, and the flap is advanced around the commissure into the defect (▶ Fig. 14.4). Some have described preservation of the ipsilateral labial artery, which might be advantageous in the cases where the contralateral labial artery is of uncertain integrity, perhaps from previous surgery.[37] By

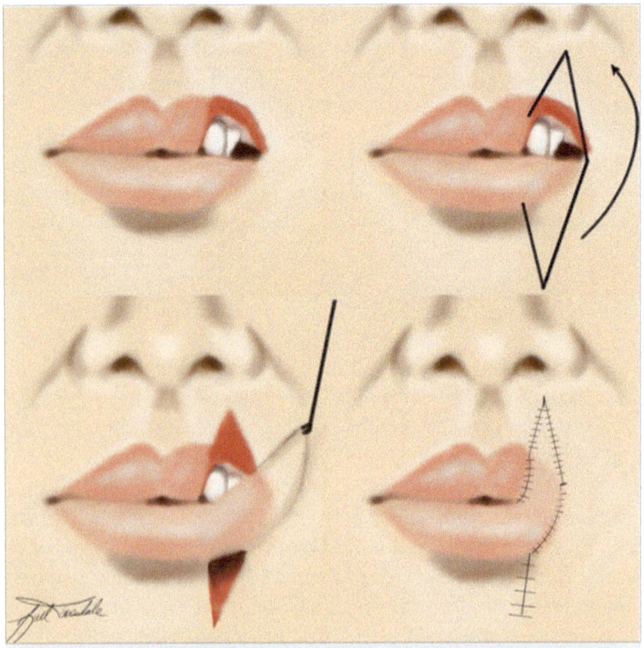

Fig. 14.4 Diagram for the markings of an Estlander flap for an upper lip/oral commissure defect.

nature of the transfer of the Estlander flap across the oral commissure, this structure becomes blunted. It is for this reason that a commissure plasty procedure is many times required following the traditional Estlander flap. In order to avoid disruption of the commissure, some surgeons have excluded transfer across the commissure and instead perform this as a two-stage interpolated flap, much like a laterally situated Abbe flap (many have termed this an Abbe–Estlander flap). In the case of the Estlander flap, the donor flap is usually designed to reconstruct at least half of the defect width. Although the original descriptions of the Abbe flap involved a radially oriented scar, some have modified the incisions in order to situate donor scars within the melolabial crease when possible.[38]

There are many important limitations to cross-lip flaps. Although the cross-lip flaps involve transfer of muscle tissue, there is at the very least temporary denervation, which may result in oral incompetence and anesthesia within the transferred areas. It has been shown that patients often obtain a degree of recovery of motor function in transferred tissue, although the extent of this may not be clear in every case.[11,39] Therefore, some patients will have resultant adynamic segments of their lip following these flaps, which can have functional and aesthetic consequences. Furthermore, hypesthesia is a temporary inconvenience for all patients and may be a permanent sequelae for some. Another notable drawback to these flaps is significant tendency for the development of a trapdoor deformity, which may be related to circumferential scar tissue formation and/or disruption of lymphatic outflow.

Defects Greater than Two-Thirds of the Lip

Stairstep Flap

Full-thickness lower lip defects up to two-thirds of the lip length may be reconstructed using an advancement of inferiorly based tissue. With the stairstep incision (also called the staircase procedure), the tissue is advanced with a series of stairstep incisions (horizontal and vertical) oriented along an oblique 45-degree angle beginning in the inferior lateral lip travelling in the superomedial direction.[40–42] The horizontal incisions of each stairstep are half the length of vertical incisions. The rectangles produced from the incisions are removed. The inferiorly based tissue is then slid superiorly. The flap is used for either midline or lateral defects. Extension into the mentum may be avoided by extending the stairstep beyond the labiomental crease. The stairsteps allow for increased advancement length and geometric breaking of the scar. At the inferior/lateral aspect of both incisions, a Burow triangle is excised.

Rotation-Advancement Flaps (Gillies' Fan Flap)

Gillies and Millard first described this flap as a modification of von Bruns, which uses an inferiorly based nasolabial flap.[23] The flap is similar to the Estlander flap, but more nasolabial tissue is rotated into the defect. This flap may be used to reconstruct lateral lip defects or total/subtotal lib defects with bilateral flaps.[43]

This technique involves the advancement of skin and muscle to create a neocommissure. Skin and lip tissue is rotated and advanced medially with releasing incisions as needed for skin closure. An incision is carried along full thickness medial to the defect and extended laterally around the commissure to the melolabial fold. The vermillion is then reapproximated along with all layers of the defect. The main disadvantage to this flap is the denervation of orbicularis oris to a variable degree and microstomia.[23,32]

Karapandzic Flap

The Karapandzic flap allows the closure of large full-thickness defects of the white and red lip.[44] The flap has been used successfully for the upper (half upper lip length defect) and lower lips (two-thirds lip defect and more). Central lower lip defects are the best candidates for reconstruction with this technique. The bilateral flaps may be advanced centrally similarly to the H-plasty with circumoral incisions that extend along the nasolabial crease. Separate flap incisions are made through the skin and mucosa only to allow preservation of the muscle and neurovascular structures. Blunt dissection is then performed through the subcutaneous tissue and division of neurovascular structures is avoided. One of the advantages of this flap is that it allows for the preservation of the sensory and motor nerves to the lip. The main disadvantage of the flap is the amount of microstomia that results from the reconstruction. Furthermore, the oral commissures will be blunted with this technique.

Bernard–Von Burow Flap

Large full-thickness defects may also be reconstructed using a technique described by Bernard and Von Burow.[23] With this technique, cheek tissue is advanced medially elevated in a full-thickness manner with excision of planned triangles (Burow's triangles) for closure.[45] This technique may be utilized for closure of upper or lower lip defects. A modification of the original technique was devised by Webster in order to make Burow's triangles more crescentic and allow for them to more naturally lie within the melolabial and labiomental creases (▶ Fig. 14.5).

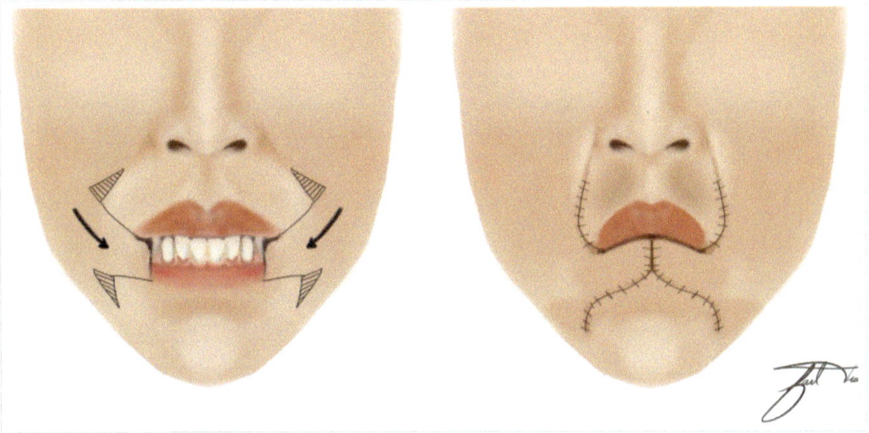

Fig. 14.5 The Webster modification of the Bernard–Von Burow flap for larger full-thickness lower lip defects.

Temporoparietal Flap

This flap has been used to reconstruct large full-thickness defects of both the upper and lower lips.[46] The flap may be transferred as either pedicled interpolated flap or free flap. The temporoparietal fascia and the overlying scalp are transferred as hair-bearing skin. In males, this may be advantageous to recreate the mustache and camouflage reconstruction. The flap has a good cosmetic, speech, and mastication outcomes. Gillies first used this flap for lip and eye brown defects.[46] The arterial supply is the superficial temporal artery. A full-thickness skin graft may be used for the underside of the flap/neomucosal layer. If the flap is pedicled, the division may be completed at least 3 weeks after inset. In its free-flap form, this interposition graft required saphenous vein grafting. Sensory input into this graft is accomplished via the auriculotemporal nerve scaffolding.[47]

14.4.4 Free Flaps

Upper and Lower Lip Reconstruction

Forearm Free Flap

Microvascular free-flap reconstruction is used for large full-thickness defects of the lip. The radial artery and cephalic vein are harvested with free tissue and anastomosed to various vascular bundles in the head and neck.[8] The radial artery free flap is most often used to reconstruct lower lip defects. These may include the palmaris longus tendon, which can be used for suspension to the orbicularis oris muscle.[48] The reconstruction has the theoretical potential for allowing sensation and preservation of oral competence. Sensation to the free tissue is provided by the microneural anastomosis of a cutaneous nerve of the forearm to the mental nerve. This technique has the advantage of providing pliable skin and soft-tissue coverage to the mandible in a single staged procedure. The disadvantages include cost, flap failure, need for microsurgical expertise, hospital stay, skin color, and texture mismatch. One adjunct that can significantly improve aesthetic outcome is medical tattoos, which can help achieve the color and shape of natural vermillion.[49]

Other Lower Lip Free Flaps

The scapular free flap, lateral arm free flap, and anterolateral thigh free flap have all been used for soft-tissue free tissue transfer to the lower lip.[50–52] Nonetheless, these flaps all result in largely adynamic segments of soft tissue. Due to this drawback, some have described the use of the gracilis muscle tissue for lip reconstruction. The process is multistaged and includes harvesting the flap with the pedicle delayed. The lip is prepared with neomucosa and tendinous substrate for sphincter attachment. Finally, the tissue is transferred, tendinous tissue attached to neomodiolus, and motor nerve anastomosed to the marginal mandibular branch of the facial nerve for motor function.[53] Nonetheless, the radial forearm free flap remains the workhorse at many institutions.

14.4.5 Commissuroplasty

Alterations of the commissure are common following reconstructive surgeries, facial trauma, and burn injuries. A simple repair described by Converse and Wood-Smith involves a horizontal full-thickness cut into the commissure with skin triangle excision, and subsequent mucosal advancement through various local flaps such as rhombic rearrangement or simple advancement.[12,54] It must be noted that the technique does suffer a disadvantage of potentially causing oral incompetence as the muscular layers and modiolus are altered.

Vermillion-cutaneous scars or misalignments may be reoriented with Z-plasty. Dermabrasion also has the ability to smooth raised scars in the lip area in the postoperative period. Lip expanders/implants may be used to bulk the postoperative lip deficit with good cosmetic outcome. Nonetheless, despite a number of described techniques to address the oral commissure, reconstructions of this area remain challenging.

14.5 Surgical Sequelae

Reconstructive lip procedures can lead to a variety of sequelae including flap failure, infection, fistula formation, nerve injury/lip weakness, perioral incompetence, articulation difficulty, and poor cosmetic appearance of scars. The most devastating of these sequelae is full flap loss. Fortunately, due to the robust perfusion to the face, it is rare for well-planned flaps to have a complete failure, although partial loss and epidermolysis may infrequently occur in patients who are active smokers or those with previous history of radiation to the operative bed. Oftentimes in these situations of partial flap necrosis, local wound care is sufficient to ultimately allow for a satisfactory outcome.

From a practical standpoint, a familiarity with scar management techniques is imperative for the reconstructive lip surgeon. It is not uncommon for scars within the melolabial area to require formal scar revision, and it is therefore useful to counsel patients prior to the initial operation that lip reconstruction is often a staged process. In addition to formal scar revision, dermabrasion is also commonly employed. Scars that heal with a fibrous band or nodularity can often be improved with vigilant massage multiple times a day, as well as injection of steroid in appropriate patients.

Key Points

- Lip reconstruction should be individualized and is largely based on unique patient and clinical characteristics such as defect size and location, defect thickness, timing of repair, prognosis, aesthetic and functional goals, available areas for tissue recruitment, and medical comorbidities.
- The bulk of reconstructive lip procedures involve local flaps, although the full gamut of the reconstructive ladder may be required.
- Facial aesthetic units are respected when designing reconstructive treatment plans. Meticulous attention to reconstruction of the white roll, vermillion border, philtral columns, Cupid's bow, and individual tissue layers will allow for optimal functional and aesthetic outcomes.

References

[1] Johnston-Saint P. An outline of the history of medicine in India. Indian Med Rec. 1929; 49:289–299

[2] Hauben DJ. Sushruta Samhita (Sushruta'a Collection) (800–600 B.C.). Pioneers of plastic surgery. Acta Chir Plast. 1984; 26(2):65–68

[3] Keil G. The history of plastic surgery (author's transl). Laryngol Rhinol Otol (Stuttg). 1978; 57(7):581–591

[4] Al-Benna S, Steinstraesser L, Steinau H-U. The cross-lip flap from 1756 to 1898. Reply to "The Sabattini-Abbé flap: a historical note.". Plast Reconstr Surg. 2009; 124(2):666–667, author reply 667–668

[5] Estlander J. Eine Methode Aus Er Einen Ippe Substanzverluste Der Anderen Zu Ersetzein. Arch Klin Chir. 1872; 14:622

[6] Roldán JC, Teschke M, Feinendegen DL. The vermilionectomy and the subsequent lower lip reconstruction were introduced by Victor von Bruns and not by von Langenbeck or von Esmarch as reported previously. Plast Reconstr Surg Glob Open. 2016; 4(5):e699

[7] Walton RL, Bunkis J. A free occipital hair-bearing flap for reconstruction of the upper lip. Br J Plast Surg. 1983; 36(2):168–170

[8] Sakai S, Soeda S, Endo T, Ishii M, Uchiumi E. A compound radial artery forearm flap for the reconstruction of lip and chin defect. Br J Plast Surg. 1989; 42(3):337–338

[9] Farkas LG, Katic MJ, Hreczko TA, Deutsch C, Munro IR. Anthropometric proportions in the upper lip-lower lip-chin area of the lower face in young white adults. Am J Orthod. 1984; 86(1):52–60

[10] Anic-Milosevic S, Mestrovic S, Prlić A, Slaj M. Proportions in the upper lip-lower lip-chin area of the lower face as determined by photogrammetric method. J Craniomaxillofac Surg. 2010; 38(2):90–95

[11] Burget GC, Menick FJ. Aesthetic restoration of one-half the upper lip. Plast Reconstr Surg. 1986; 78(5):583–593

[12] Neligan PC. Strategies in lip reconstruction. Clin Plast Surg. 2009; 36(3):477–485

[13] Ladefoged P, Maddieson I. The Sounds of the World's Languages. Oxford: Blackwell; 1996:102

[14] Coppit GL, Lin DT, Burkey BB. Current concepts in lip reconstruction. Curr Opin Otolaryngol Head Neck Surg. 2004; 12(4):281–287

[15] Briedis J, Jackson IT. The anatomy of the philtrum: observations made on dissections in the normal lip. Br J Plast Surg. 1981; 34(2):128–132

[16] Pinar YA, Bilge O, Govsa F. Anatomic study of the blood supply of perioral region. Clin Anat. 2005; 18(5):330–339

[17] Renner GJ. Reconstruction of the lip. In: Baker SR, ed. Local Flaps in Facial Reconstruction. Philadelphia, PA: Mosby Elsevier; 2007:475–524

[18] Mağden O, Edizer M, Atabey A, Tayfur V, Ergür I. Cadaveric study of the arterial anatomy of the upper lip. Plast Reconstr Surg. 2004; 114(2):355–359

[19] Pannu AK, Saroch A, Sharma N. Danger triangle of face and septic cavernous sinus thrombosis. J Emerg Med. 2017; 53(1):137–138

[20] Larson DL, Coers CR, III, Rodin AE, Parcansky GM, Corujo MR, Lewis SR. Lymphatics of the upper and lower lip. A clinical and experimental study. Am J Surg. 1967; 114(4):525–529

[21] McGregor IA. The tongue flap in lip surgery. Br J Plast Surg. 1966; 19(3):253–263

[22] Müller-Richter UDA, Weyandt GH, Woeckel A, Kübler AC. Vermilion reconstruction with genital mucosa. Plast Reconstr Surg Glob Open. 2016; 4(5):e701

[23] Hauben DJ. Victor von Bruns (1812–1883) and his contributions to plastic and reconstructive surgery. Plast Reconstr Surg. 1985; 75(1):120–127

[24] Brown JB, McDowell F. Secondary repair of cleft lips and their nasal deformities. Ann Surg. 1941; 114(1):101–117

[25] Wagner JD, Newman MH. Bipedicled axial cross-lip flap for correction of major vermilion deficiency after cleft lip repair. Cleft Palate Craniofac J. 1994; 31(2):148–151

[26] Pribaz J, Stephens W, Crespo L, Gifford G. A new intraoral flap: facial artery musculomucosal (FAMM) flap. Plast Reconstr Surg. 1992; 90(3):421–429

[27] Lemperle G, Holmes RE, Cohen SR, Lemperle SM. A classification of facial wrinkles. Plast Reconstr Surg. 2001; 108(6):1735–1750, discussion 1751–1752

[28] Tromovitch TA, Stegman SJ, Glogau RG, eds. Defects of the lips. In: Flaps and Grafts in Dermatologic Surgery. Chicago, IL: Yearbook Medical Publ; 1989:169–181

[29] Renner GJ, Zitsch RP, III. Reconstruction of the lip. Otolaryngol Clin North Am. 1990; 23(5):975–990

[30] Zitelli JA. Secondary intention healing: an alternative to surgical repair. Clin Dermatol. 1984; 2(3):92–106

[31] Larrabee YC, Moyer JS. Reconstruction of Mohs defects of the lips and chin. Facial Plast Surg Clin North Am. 2017; 25(3):427–442

[32] Pepper J-P, Baker SR. Local flaps: cheek and lip reconstruction. JAMA Facial Plast Surg. 2013; 15(5):374–382

[33] Walike JW, Larrabee WF, Jr. The "note flap.". Arch Otolaryngol. 1985; 111(7):430–433

[34] Walton RL, Beahm EK, Brown RE, et al. Microsurgical replantation of the lip: a multi-institutional experience. Plast Reconstr Surg. 1998; 102(2):358–368

[35] James NJ. Survival of large replanted segment of upper lip and nose. Case report. Plast Reconstr Surg. 1976; 58(5):623–625

[36] Ahmadi SK, Rahpeyma A, Rezvani HN. Vermilion lower lip cross flap: an anatomic study on 22 fresh cadavers. Ann Maxillofac Surg. 2012; 2(2):107–110

[37] Genc S, Ugur SS, Arslan IB, Tuhanioglu B, Demir A, Selcuk A. Lower lip reconstruction with Abbe-Estlander flap modification: preserving the same side vascular pedicle. Eur Arch Otorhinolaryngol. 2012; 269(12):2593–2594

[38] Templer J, Renner G, Davis WE, Thomas JR. "How I do it": plastic surgery. Practical suggestions on facial plastic surgery. A modification of the Abbe-Estlander flap for defects of the lower lip. Laryngoscope. 1981; 91(1):153–156

[39] Rea JL, Davis WE, Rittenhouse LK. Reinnervation of an Abbe-Estlander and a Gillies fan flap of the lower lip: electromyographic comparison. Arch Otolaryngol. 1978; 104(5):294–295

[40] Blomgren I, Blomqvist G, Lauritzen C, Lilja J, Peterson LE, Holmström H. The step technique for the reconstruction of lower lip defects after cancer resection. A follow-up study of 165 cases. Scand J Plast Reconstr Surg Hand Surg. 1988; 22(1):103–111

[41] Johanson B, Aspelund E, Breine U, Holmström H. Surgical treatment of non-traumatic lower lip lesions with special reference to the step technique. A follow-up on 149 patients. Scand J Plast Reconstr Surg. 1974; 8(3):232–240

[42] Kuttenberger JJ, Hardt N. Results of a modified staircase technique for reconstruction of the lower lip. J Craniomaxillofac Surg. 1997; 25(5):239–244

[43] Ducic Y, Athre R, Cochran CS. The split orbicularis myomucosal flap for lower lip reconstruction. Arch Facial Plast Surg. 2005; 7(5):347–352

[44] Karapandzic M. Reconstruction of lip defects by local arterial flaps. Br J Plast Surg. 1974; 27(1):93–97

[45] Mazzola RF, Lupo G. Evolving concepts in lip reconstruction. Clin Plast Surg. 1984; 11(4):583–617

[46] Kim JC, Hadlock T, Varvares MA, Cheney ML. Hair-bearing temporoparietal fascial flap reconstruction of upper lip and scalp defects. Arch Facial Plast Surg. 2001; 3(3):170–177

[47] David SK, Cheney ML. An anatomic study of the temporoparietal fascial flap. Arch Otolaryngol Head Neck Surg. 1995; 121(10):1153–1156

[48] Sadove RC, Luce EA, McGrath PC. Reconstruction of the lower lip and chin with the composite radial forearm-palmaris longus free flap. Plast Reconstr Surg. 1991; 88(2):209–214

[49] Furuta S, Hataya Y, Watanabe T, Yuzuriha S. Vermilionplasty using medical tattooing after radial forearm flap reconstruction of the lower lip. Br J Plast Surg. 1994; 47(6):422–424

[50] Granick MS, Newton ED, Hanna DC. Scapular free flap for repair of massive lower facial composite defects. Head Neck Surg. 1986; 8(6):436–441

[51] Reinert S. The free revascularized lateral upper arm flap in maxillofacial reconstruction following ablative tumour surgery. J Craniomaxillofac Surg. 2000; 28(2):69–73

[52] Upton J, Albin RE, Mulliken JB, Murray JE. The use of scapular and parascapular flaps for cheek reconstruction. Plast Reconstr Surg. 1992; 90(6): 959–971

[53] Lengelé BG, Testelin S, Bayet B, Devauchelle B. Total lower lip functional reconstruction with a prefabricated gracilis muscle free flap. Int J Oral Maxillofac Surg. 2004; 33(4):396–401

[54] Converse JM, Wood-Smith D. Techniques for repair of defects of the lips and cheeks. In: Converse JM, ed. Reconstructive Plastic Surgery. Philadelphia, PA: W.B. Saunders Company; 1977:1544–1594

15 Squamous Cell Cancer of the Oral Tongue

Zain Rizvi and Maie A. St. John

Summary
Oral tongue cancer is the most common subsite in the oral cavity. While smoking and alcohol use are contribute factors, nonsmoking, non-drinking and young patients are increasingly affected by this disease. Surgery with adjuvant treatment remain a mainstay for treatment. A better understanding of this disease as well as innovations in approaches continue to evolve treatment of oral tongue cancer.

Keywords: oral tongue cancer, glossectomy, neck dissection

15.1 Epidemiology, Etiology, and Genomics

Oral tongue cancer is the most common intraoral cancer in most countries worldwide, with squamous cell carcinoma continuing to be the most common type of tongue cancer.[1] The average age of diagnosis is 64 years with most patients frequently diagnosed with early-stage lesions (T1 or T2).[1] Epidemiologic studies suggest that black males have a higher incidence of oral tongue cancer and alongside low-income patients, are more often diagnosed with advanced disease.[2]

Historically, alcohol and tobacco use has been associated with the development of oral cancer, with the risk of cancer related to the amount of tobacco or alcohol consumed. Synergistic effects exist between tobacco and alcohol such that combined use boosts the risk of developing cancer when compared to controls.[3] In smokers, the incidence of cancer in the head and neck is higher in males when compared to females. Use of smokeless tobacco and betel nut has also been implicated as etiologic factors in the development of oral tongue cancer, with smokeless tobacco imparting a fourfold increased risk of oral cavity cancer.[3] Even after diagnosis and treatment of oral cavity cancer, smoking cessation imparts further risk reduction of developing a second primary lesion. Moore demonstrated that the second primary rate after treatment of an oral cavity cancer went from 6% in former smokers to 40% in continuing smokers.[4] Yet, despite smoking cessation and improved public health awareness, epidemiologic data suggest increased incidence of oral tongue cancer in population subgroups, particularly in young patients.[5,6]

Though smoking and alcohol use remain significant risk factors for oral tongue cancer, epidemiologic studies reveal an increase in the number of nonsmoking nondrinking (NSND) patients diagnosed with oral tongue squamous cell carcinoma.[7] Oral trauma and inflammation have been proposed as risk factors for this subset of patients.[8] Indeed, the lateral aspect of the oral tongue is the most common site of oral tongue cancer and is twice as common in nonsmokers.[9] This suggests that dental trauma, bruxism, caries, or inflammation at the lateral tongue border leading to chronic inflammation may lead to malignant transformation. Furthermore, studies have shown a relationship between ill-fitting dentures and defective teeth and the development of oral cancer.[8] Taken together, this does support a role for chronic inflammation and the development of cancer in nonsmoking patients.

Base of tongue cancers associated with human papillomavirus (HPV) have been well described, yet studies by different groups have failed to demonstrate the same causative factors for oral tongue cancers. Prior studies have shown that HPV deoxyribonucleic acid (DNA) is present in a greater proportion of oral cavity specimens with squamous cell carcinoma than in matched noncarcinoma controls, suggesting that this may be an independent factor for the development of carcinoma.[10] HPV and its surrogate marker p16, have been identified in oral tongue squamous cell carcinoma in varying frequencies, from 11 to 55%.[11] However, when defined as transcriptionally active HPV, the rate significantly decreases, suggesting that HPV may not be as significant in the etiology of these tumors as compared to oropharyngeal cancers.[12,13] Other studies suggest that in contrast to base of tongue cancers, different HPV subtypes (such as HPV beta-5) may be involved in oral tongue cancer, though the exact etiologic role remains to be determined.[9] Some preliminary studies have suggested that HPV status in oral tongue cancer may be associated with an overall worse prognosis though this remains an area of active investigation.[7,11] Furthermore, unlike the base of tongue and oropharyngeal subsites, HPV status in oral tongue cancer has yet to alter treatment strategies, specifically with regard to de-escalation or conservation therapy.

There has been increasing interest in studying the subset of young NSND patients developing oral tongue cancer, possible etiologic factors, and clinical implications.[11] HPV detection remains low in the young NSND cohort as is the case for all oral tongue cancers, and when present it is predictive of an overall worse prognosis.[11] This implies multiple transformative events leading to aggressive tumor biology. Other studies suggest this population has recurrence and survival similar to smokers, suggesting a unifying biology albeit through alternative molecular mechanisms. Genomically, the mutational landscape of tumors isolated from young NSND tongue cancer patients is similar to that of tumors isolated from older, smoking patients.[14] Mutation of *p53* is relatively rare in nonsmokers when compared to smokers, as is the overall rate of loss of heterozygosity and allelic alterations, though it is common in young NSND patients.[15]

Jeon et al have shown that young tongue cancer patients (< 40 years old) demonstrate a higher rate of distant metastasis and worse prognosis.[16] Other studies have shown that some young female patients with a high degree of immune checkpoint regulator PDL-1 expression had a decreased risk of recurrence and improved survival.[17] This expanding group of patients represents a unique subtype requiring further studies to better understand the epidemiologic risk factors and the molecular mechanisms to develop targeted therapy.

Whole-exome sequencing and banked databases such as the Cancer Genome Atlas (TCGA) database have expanded our genomic understanding of oral tongue cancer. Oral tongue cancer predominantly represents HPV-negative disease and often carries *p53* loss and *CDKN2A* inactivation. While these tumors are quite heterogeneous, *NOTCH1* was noted to be a frequently mutated gene as well as copy number changes in *NOTCH2/NOTCH3*.[14,18] Numerous signaling pathway alterations are also encountered, including those involved with growth and cell cycle regulation, oxidative stress, and differentiation.[14] Clinically distinct behavior has been noted in tumors with and without alterations in the epidermal growth factor receptor (EGFR) pathway. Src family kinases are also altered in relation to EGFR signaling and represent a therapeutic target in oral tongue cancer.[18] Translational studies have also implicated dysregulation of immune checkpoints in head and neck cancer. PD-1 blockade increases T-cell proliferation and IFN-y production in tumors, and when combined with a toll-like receptor agonist enhanced granulocyte-macrophage vaccine (TEGVAX) causes regression of HPV-negative head and neck cancer growth in vivo.[19] Though preliminary, these studies have the potential to provide the basis for molecularly tailored therapy for head and neck cancer patients.

15.2 Clinical Presentation

Cancer of the oral tongue most commonly presents as pain followed by an ulcer or swelling on the tongue. Early, small lesions may go undetected until a critical size is reached that prompts symptoms and medical visits. As tumor size evolves and adjacent structures become involved, other complaints such as bleeding, tongue immobility, dysarthria, and dysphagia may develop. Regional disease may present as a neck mass. Certain clinical clues such as complaints of ear pain, dysphagia, voice changes, and trismus may suggest involvement of other subsites, such as the oropharynx.

An examination of the oral tongue should include evaluation of sensation and mobility. Any deficits should prompt concern for perineural invasion of the lingual and hypoglossal nerves. The fixed tongue should also trigger investigation into mandibular, floor of the mouth, or retromolar trigone involvement, significantly altering both staging and treatment. Furthermore, trismus may be a harbinger of pterygoid or masseter involvement and should be investigated carefully.[20]

Premalignant lesions such as leukoplakia, erythroplakia, submucous fibrosis, lichen planus, and others may be noted by the patient or other practitioners during routine examinations. These have various underlying etiologies such as ill-fitting dentures, smoking, as well as inherited conditions such as xeroderma pigmentosa, and should be treated as premalignant lesions until proven otherwise. Rate of conversion to malignancy is variable and may be compounded by exposures, heritable disorders, and comorbidities.[21] Typically, erythroplakia has a higher transformation rate to malignancy (reported from 15 to 50%) when compared to leukoplakia, the most common lesion of this class.[21,22] A full discussion precludes the scope of this chapter; however, these lesions remain a critical biologic entity to recognize. Various treatment strategies have been employed and include surgical excision as well as topical and systemic agents. Complete surgical excision is often superior to biopsy so as to avoid the possibility of "geographic miss." Should a lesion prove to contain high-grade dysplasia or microinvasive carcinoma, excision remains the gold standard. Adjuncts such as laser treatment of wide fields have also been performed invariably with success.[21] Recurrence rates have also been noted to occur between 10 and 30% following appropriate treatments and emphasize ongoing multidisciplinary surveillance, including the patient self-surveillance.[23] Photodynamic therapy, cryotherapy, retinoic acid, COX-2 (cyclooxygenase-2) inhibitors, and even metformin have been trialed with varying success in treatment and suppression of premalignant lesions and may be considered as treatment adjuncts.

In patients with previously treated head and neck cancer, diagnosis of recurrent or new lesions of the oral tongue may prove difficult. Clinically, during surveillance, worsening or new symptoms similar to their original presentation should tip the clinician to a through physical examination for new lesions. Pain is often the most sensitive indicator of recurrence and patients should be queried as to whether they are taking pain medications as this may mask new-onset pain. Some symptoms may be difficult to separate from treatment sequelae—such as numbness from prior surgery, or mucositis and pain from radiation. Patients previously treated for oral tongue cancer can most commonly fail locoregionally and these sites should be examined closely.[24]

15.3 Diagnosis and Evaluation

Initial diagnosis for oral tongue cancers centers on tissue biopsy, which can often be performed with local anesthesia in the clinic. Histologic characteristics such as degree of keratinization, nuclear polymorphism, and perineural and perivascular invasion combined with tumor biomarkers such as p53, Ki-67, cyclin-D1, WGFR, STAT3, VEGF, and HOXB7 aid in diagnosis and treatment.[25]

While classic squamous cell carcinoma can be readily identified on histopathology, certain controversies exist. In patients with prior surgical or radiation treatment of an oral tongue lesion, there may be extensive atypia, metaplasia, and inflammation, resulting in difficulty in diagnosing persistent, recurrent, or new disease. Another diagnostic conundrum may be microinvasive disease. Should adequate biopsies be performed, microinvasive disease may alter management in terms of extent of resection and need for treatment of the neck, as depth of invasion has been correlated with regional disease.[26] Necrotizing sialometaplasia can be mistaken for squamous cell carcinoma and requires close consultation with head and neck pathologists to differentiate this benign condition from malignancy.[27]

For surgical planning, tumor mapping may be performed by either in-office examination or operative endoscopy. For small, accessible lesions, office examination may be sufficient to plan for surgical resection, with careful attention being paid to the floor of the mouth, base of the tongue, retromolar trigone, oropharynx, and mandibular periosteum. Palpation should be performed to identify deeply invasive lesions or those that cross the midline as resection may not only impart substantial functional deficits but also require increasingly advanced reconstructive efforts.

For tumors located posteriorly or for patients who do not tolerate a full bimanual office examination, operative endoscopy may be necessary. Historically, panendoscopy was performed to evaluate for synchronous lesions. While this has been demonstrated to be safe,[28,29] recent reviews have found a relatively low rate of synchronous primary lesions in patients with early-stage oral tongue cancers.[30] With an increased proportion of NSND patients, the role of panendoscopy and synchronous primary rate may be evolving. In practice, endoscopy can be combined at the time of surgical intervention.

Evaluation of the neck should also be completed during diagnostic workup. In-office examination of the neck may reveal palpable adenopathy, particularly in levels 1, 2, and 3, which represent the first echelon of lymphatic drainage from the oral tongue and thus are the most frequently involved regional metastatic site.[31] Imaging is a useful adjunct for staging and surgical planning for both primary and regional sites. CT and MRI have distinct advantages and may be complementary. While CT scan offers excellent bony definition, MRI offers improved resolution of soft tissue and may be used to help assess for perineural invasion, changes in bone marrow signal suggestive of invasion, and intracranial involvement.[32] Ultimately, individual patient disease factors may dictate which imaging modality is best suited to answer a given clinical question. Both CT and MRI may also be used to evaluate the neck for regional metastasis, although ultrasound has been demonstrated to have improved accuracy in assessment of lymph nodes with greater detail of architecture.[33] Furthermore, image-guided biopsy of abnormal lymph nodes may be easily performed at the time of ultrasound examination.[33]

PET/CT can be used for metastatic staging of oral tongue cancer patients; however, studies specifically evaluating the utility of PET/CT in early oral tongue cancer are limited. Studies examining both early- and late-stage head and neck cancer patients did show downstream alterations in treatment in a significant proportion of both patient groups, though this study included subsites with much higher risk of metastatic disease.[34] While routine PET/CT may be of limited utility for early-stage primary disease, the utility of PET/CT in far advanced, recurrent, or persistent disease may be extremely helpful.[35] Current National Comprehensive Cancer Network (NCCN) guidelines recommend PET scan for patients with stage III/IV disease, as prior studies demonstrate clear upstaging and alteration of this group of patients.[35] PET/CT should also be considered in patients undergoing primary nonsurgical treatment or in patients who are to receive adjuvant therapy to have an index marker of uptake before and after treatment.[34]

15.4 Anatomic Considerations

When planning surgical resection of oral tongue squamous cell carcinoma, consideration must be given toward functional anatomy. Patients should be counseled with regard to functional deficits, which may be predicted during initial examination and tumor localization. Lesions that cross the midline may require total glossectomy to achieve oncologic margins and remove nonviable remnant tongue. Suspected hypoglossal nerve involvement preoperatively should allow the oncologic surgeon to expect invasive disease, perineural invasion, and need for resection extending toward the tongue base.[36]

Functionally, the oral tongue is a neuromuscular organ important for articulation, deglutition, and taste, all of which can be impacted during and after treatment.[37] Consequently, functional loss and impairment of the tongue due to surgical resection and reconstruction, or secondary to chemotherapy or radiation, can be attributed to loss of bulk, shape, mobility, and sensation.[38] Typically the oral tongue predominantly plays a role in speech articulation, while the base of the tongue has a larger role in swallowing and bolus propulsion though both roles may be affected during treatment.[38] The neurovascular anatomy of the tongue can be seen in ▶ Fig. 15.1.

15.5 Functional Considerations: Swallowing

The tongue is critical for initiation of the swallow process. During deglutition, the oral tongue is chiefly involved in the preparatory and oral stage of swallow.[39] In the preparatory stage, the tongue is involved in lateral rolling to coordinate bolus formation and mastication. Once the bolus is prepared, the oral stage of swallow begins. Again, the neuromuscular function of the tongue lifts and squeezes the bolus against the palate, and coordinated movement allows for wavelike propulsion of the bolus from the oral cavity toward the oropharynx.[39] Treatment of malignancy through surgery, radiation, or chemotherapy will affect coordination of these events, thus altering the swallow function.[40]

15.6 Functional Considerations: Speech

The tongue also plays a critical role in speech articulation. Specifically, the coordinated movement of the tongue helps shape the oral cavity chamber during phonation during both vowel and consonant formation.[41] In the context or partial glossectomy, only time to follow-up was correlated with speech articulation regardless of age, T stage, or need for radiation, suggesting continued improvement with time and recovery.[42] Another study suggested

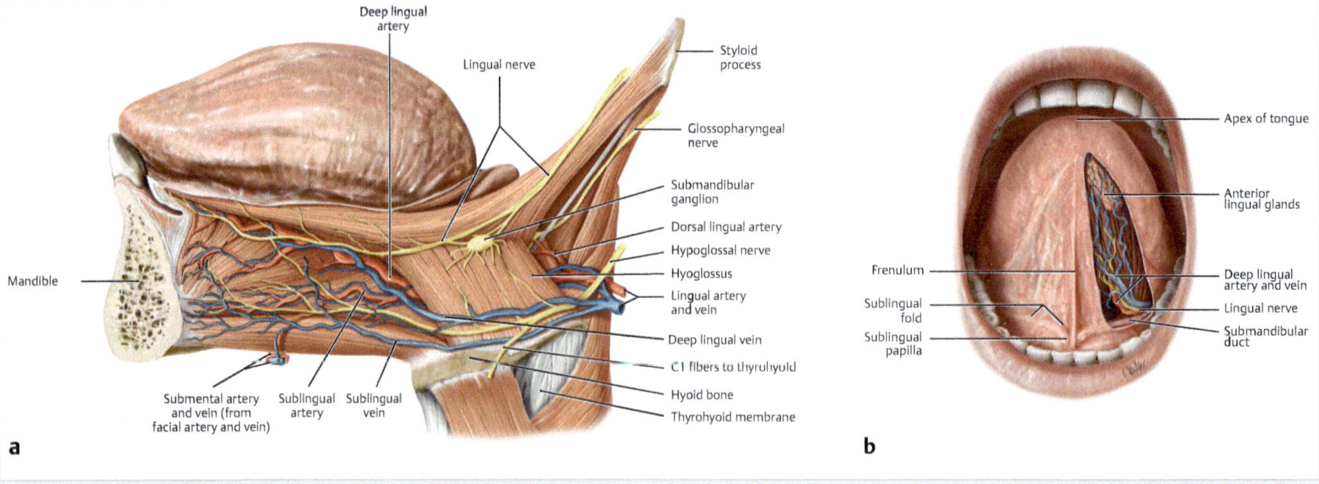

Fig. 15.1 Neurovascular anatomy of the tongue. **(a)** Left lateral view. **(b)** View of the inferior surface of the tongue. (Source: Baker EW. Head and Neck Anatomy for Dental Medicine. 1st Edition. New York: Thieme Medical Publishers; 2010. Based on: Schuenke M, Schulte E, Schumacher U. Illustrations by Voll M and Wesker K.)

the amount of radiation delivered to the base of the tongue and velum did impact velopharyngeal function and thus nasality and the dynamic resonating sound chamber of the oral cavity.[43]

When treating oral tongue squamous cell carcinoma, attention must also be focused on the neck in regard to lymphatic drainage patterns. A study by Shah demonstrated that neck levels I, II, and III are the first echelon of lymphatic drainage of the oral tongue, with only a 9% occult metastasis rate in level IV.[31] Level V was rarely found to have pathologic disease during elective or therapeutic neck dissections in primary oral cavity cancers.[31] Furthermore, risk of nodal disease is correlated to depth of invasion of the primary tumor, with studies supporting an increase in nodal disease in tumors greater than 2 to 4 mm.[26,44] Lesions that cross the midline have a propensity for bilateral lymphatic spread and warrant evaluation and potential treatment of the contralateral neck.[31]

15.7 Surgical Considerations and Approaches

Traditionally, resection of early-stage oral tongue cancer can be done transorally. Large tumors with posterior extension or those involving adjacent anatomic subsites may require a more advanced approach and should be identified during initial workup. Larger tumors can be approached by means of mandibulotomy or lower cheek flap with lip split as well as a visor flap with degloving.[44] These may be combined with mandibulectomy should a composite resection be required. A visor approach allows for access to the anterior oral tongue and may allow for resection of deeply invasive tumors while avoiding a lip-splitting incision though numbness occurs due to division of the mental nerve. A lower cheek flap provides excellent exposure to the anterior and lateral oral cavity including the deep musculature, floor of the mouth, cheek, and mandible, allowing for composite resection.[44] Finally, a lip-splitting incision with or without paramedian manidbulotomy may be needed to resect large tumors with posterior extension toward the base of the tongue and the oropharynx.[45] Complications of mandibulotomy include hardware exposure (most common), malocclusion, nonunion, osteonecrosis, and temporomandibular joint dysfunction.[46,47] During any of these approaches, a marginal mandibulectomy may also be deployed to preserve continuity of the mandible. A pull-through combines a transoral–transcervical approach by resecting the specimen transcervically in combination with neck dissection. This allows resection of deeply invasive tumors that do not involve the bony cortex of the mandible by resecting the oral tongue, floor of the mouth, periosteum, as well as deep tongue musculature en bloc.[48]

The goal of surgery for the primary lesion is to achieve negative surgical margins though clinical and pathologic definitions may vary. A 5-mm margin is widely accepted as a clear margin on final pathology.[49] However, histopathologic studies examining local recurrence-free survival (LRFS) and close-margin status propose a cutoff of 2.2 mm as this was the variable most closely related to LRFS.[49] One promising area of surgical innovation is the identification and management of intraoperative margins. Real-time, intraoperative optical imaging has the potential to improve surgery success in achieving negative margins, thereby decreasing the need for additional surgeries.[50] While a comprehensive review of all imaging modalities is beyond the scope of this chapter, this exciting area of innovation warrants a brief review.

Several innovative optical imaging techniques to include Raman spectroscopy, confocal microscopy, and fluorescence imaging have been developed for intraoperative tumor margin guidance. Ideally, these innovations improve localization at both the gross and microscopic levels. Most recently, dynamic optical contrast imaging (DOCI) has been developed at UCLA (University of California-Los Angeles) as a novel modality for intraoperative tumor margin delineation.[51] DOCI can rapidly distinguish head and neck squamous cell carcinoma from normal tissue, yielding wide-field visual contrast consistent with histology. DOCI can now be used as an intraoperative instrument for directed frozen section analysis, and ultimately for real-time intraoperative tumor margin demarcation. Significant advances have been achieved in real-time optical imaging strategies and hold great promise in achieving the highest percentage of negative surgical margins. The extended surgical approaches are demonstrated in ▶ Fig. 15.2 and ▶ Fig. 15.3.

15.8 Role of Neck Dissection

For the N0 neck, some debate exists regarding empiric treatment. Studies have compared a wait-and-wait approach and upfront elective neck dissection (END) for early (T1 and T2) primary cancers. Close follow-up with interval ultrasound has been shown to be equivalent to upfront neck dissection in terms of survival, though a strict follow-up regimen was absolutely required.[52] Randomized control trials comparing END to observation with salvage for neck recurrence following no treatment have had mixed results, though recent studies have demonstrated improved survival with END.[53] Some bias may exist as some of these studies also had a higher proportion of END patients undergo adjuvant radiation. However, this may also represent a distinct advantage of END: it is not only therapeutic but also diagnostic by allowing for accurate staging. Should concerning findings such as extracapsular extension be present, adjuvant radiation or chemoradiation may be considered.[54]

Other studies have attempted to evaluate if tumor thickness may be prognostic. One such study suggests comprehensive therapy for tumors with greater than 4 mm of thickness as rates of nodal disease and survival rates change significantly beyond this depth of invasion[55] Sentinel lymph node biopsy has also been compared to END with promising results. It has been demonstrated to be safe, and, in limited trials, at least equal to END.[56] The summary of these discordant studies is that a proportion of patients with N0 disease likely have unfavorable biology and benefit from therapeutic intervention by means of surgery or radiation. Current standard of care recommends treatment of the neck for patients with N0 disease at the time of tumor treatment. However, future studies of ultrasound follow-up, sentinel node biopsy, and biomarkers will help delineate which patients would benefit most from neck dissection and those who can be observed while still ensuring the best possible outcomes.

For the clinically positive neck, current guidelines dictate neck treatment.[31,54] Typically, a modified radical neck dissection can be performed, though some studies suggest that END of the primary echelon of lymphatics (levels I, II, and III) may be oncologically sound.[54] However, data also suggest that lateral oral tongue lesions, even in N0 necks, had a 15.8% rate of skip metastases, whereby patients had lesions in level III or IV without disease in level I or II.[57] As such, these authors recommend

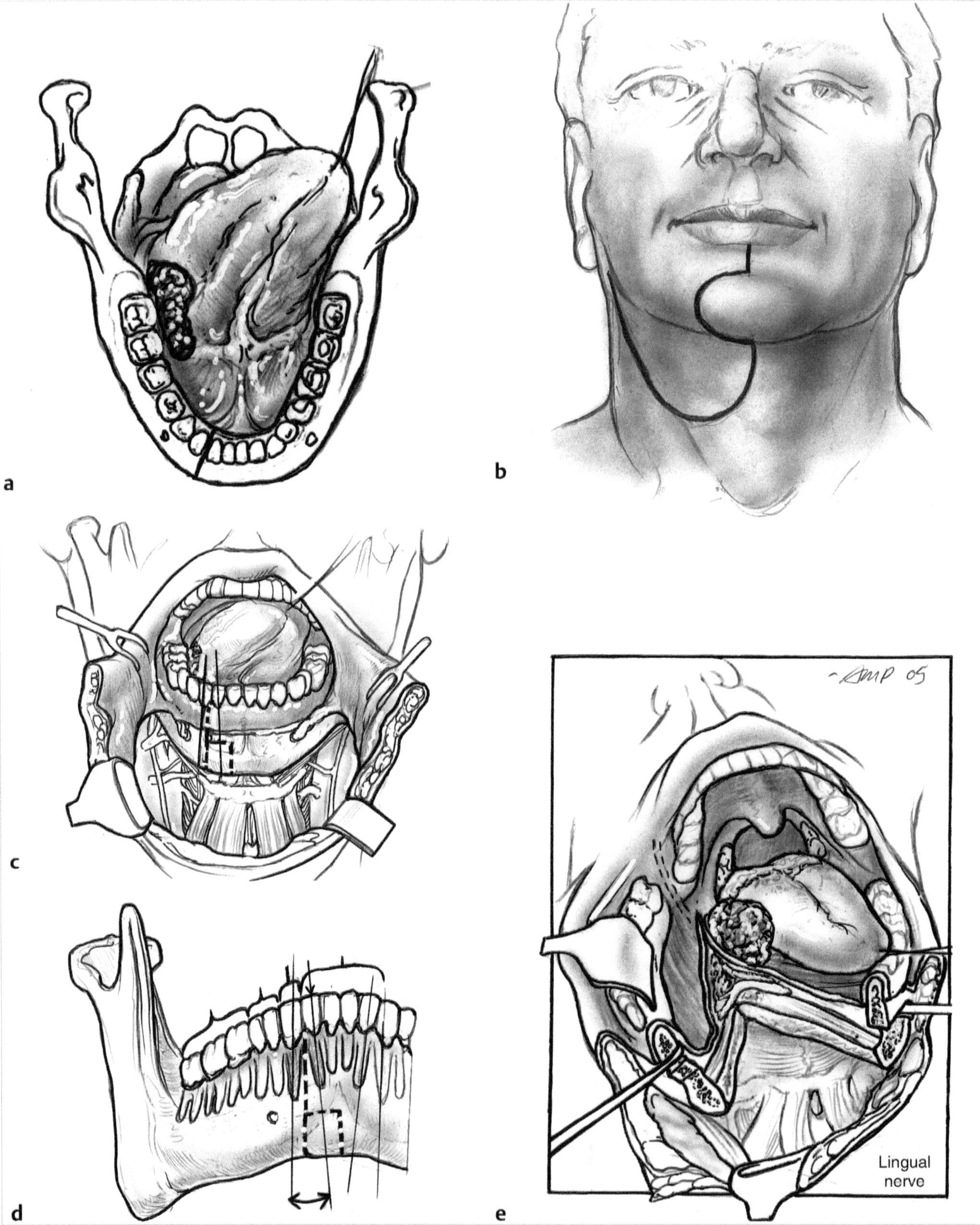

Fig. 15.2 Extended surgical approaches—lip split and mandibulotomy. **(a)** Tumor involving the lateral tongue and floor of mouth (FOM) is depicted. **(b)** A lip split with or without mandibulotomy may be considered. An apron incision can be connected to a lip-splitting incision. Depicted here is a planned incision around the chin, however a "zig-zag" pattern through the chin can be used instead to camouflage the scar and aid in abnormal contracture. **(c)** The mucosal incision is extended into the labial vestibular sulcus, the mandibular periosteum is elevated, and a cheek flap is raised to the region of the planned osteotomy. The paramedian osteotomy is placed anterior to the mental foramen between the lateral incisor and the canine. The straight and stair-step osteotomies are depicted. **(d)** The angle of divergence between the mandibular lateral incisor and canine is greater than between the incisors. However, a tooth-sparing osteotomy should be considered only when adequate alveolar crestal bone exists to house both tooth roots following the osteotomy. **(e)** The mandible is lateralized and the soft tissues of the FOM are divided, preserving the lingual nerve whenever possible. Excellent access is gained by this approach to facilitate circumferential tumor resection and reconstruction. (Source: Treatment. In: Werning J, ed. Oral Cancer, Diagnosis, Management and Rehabilitaion.1st Edition. Thieme; 2007.)

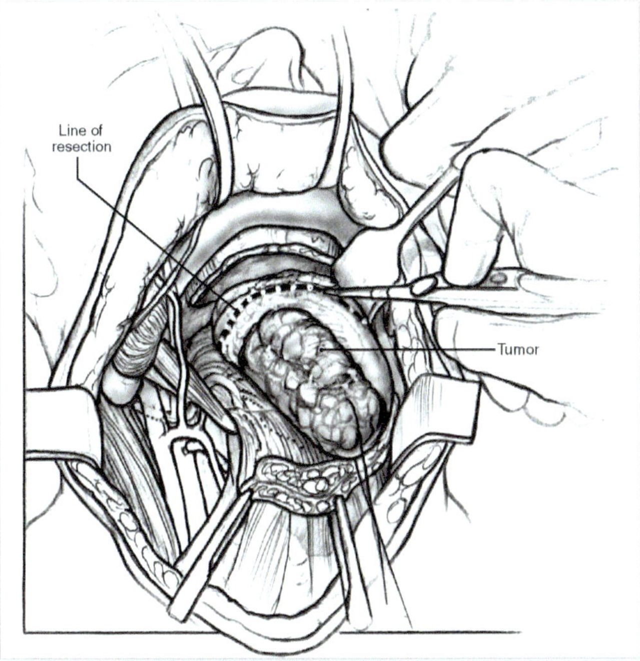

Fig. 15.3 Extended surgical approaches—visor or manibular Lingual Release Approach. After raising a subplatysmal apron flap, a mucosal incision is made in the floor of mouth along the mandibular sulcus. The suprahyoid musculature is divided at the site of attachment of the mandible. The external and internal incision are connected, leaving a cuff of mucosa intraorally for later reconstruction. The tongue and any attached floor of mouth tissue may be pulled into the cervical region for access to the entire tumor and facilitate reconstruction (Source: Treatment. In: Werning J, ed. Oral Cancer, Diagnosis, Management and Rehabilitaion. 1st Edition. Thieme; 2007.)

modified radical neck dissection for oral tongue cancer, as a survival benefit was noted over supraomohyoid neck dissection.[57] Studies of sentinel lymph node biopsy also show an increased rate of positive sentinel nodes outside the field of planned limited neck dissection, supporting a role for comprehensive neck dissection.[56] For lesions that involve or cross the midline, bilateral neck dissection is indicated given the high incidence of bilateral lymphatic spread.[54]

15.9 Surgical Sequelae

Short- and long-term effects on swallowing and articulation following treatment and reconstruction for oral tongue cancer are to be expected. Though there is some heterogeneity in studies examining function after surgery and reconstruction, initial staging and tumor size are related to overall quality of life after treatment.[58] Some perioperative functional deficits may be predicted on patient and disease factors. Prior radiation, volume of base of tongue resection, and hypoglossal nerve sacrifice are predictive of aspiration and need for gastrostomy tube following resection and free-flap reconstruction of oral cavity and oropharyngeal tumors.[59] Taste disorders also occur following treatment and are correlated to the extent of resection.[60]

Typically for partial glossectomy patients, primary closure may be employed though some advocate placement of a skin graft for floor of mouth involvement to prevent tethering of the tongue remnant to the floor of the mouth or the alveolar ridge.[61] For hemiglossectomy or larger defects, local or free-flap reconstruction is advocated.[61] However, in some studies that have examined functional deficits following surgery with and without reconstruction, mixed findings preclude consensus on optimal reconstruction with regard to function.[38] Some studies have demonstrated improved tongue mobility, articulation, and speech intelligibility for hemiglossectomy patients whose defect reconstructed with a free flap when compared to healing by secondary intention, while partial glossectomy defects demonstrated improved speech function when closed primarily.[38,62] With deglutition and hemiglossectomy or larger defects, a general consensus suggests that free-flap reconstruction provides tissue volume to assist with bolus preparation and propulsion, though specific ability to tolerate oral intake may vary.[38]

Key Points

- While smoking and alcohol use continue to be significant etiologic factors for tongue cancer, a new increasing cohort of NSND patients with newly diagnosed tongue cancer must be recognized.
- Genomic analysis has revealed mutations in p53, NOTCH1, and EGFR pathway alterations, which may be exploited for targeted therapy. The role of HPV in oral tongue cancer is not clearly defined though early studies do not suggest a strong link between oral tongue cancer and HPV.
- Surgical margins are related to LRFS. Technologies are rapidly evolving to help develop real-time intraoperative margin control.
- Studies suggest improvement in survival with END for early oral tongue cancers though sentinel lymph node biopsy or ultrasound surveillance may be used in the future for patients with low-risk tumor biology.
- Surgical sequelae are directly related to the articulation and deglutition function of the tongue. This may be predicted preoperatively based on tumor size, location, patient symptoms, and type of reconstruction used.

References

[1] Moore SR, Johnson NW, Pierce AM, Wilson DF. The epidemiology of tongue cancer: a review of global incidence. Oral Dis. 2000; 6(2):75–84
[2] Gerson SJ. Oral cancer. Crit Rev Oral Biol Med. 1990; 1(3):153–166
[3] Sankaranarayanan R, et al. Oral cancer: prevention, early detection, and treatment. In: Gelband H, Jha P, Sankaranarayanan R, Horton S, eds. Cancer: Disease Control Priorities. 3rd ed. Vol. 3. Washington, DC: The International Bank for Reconstruction and Development/The World Bank; 2015:85–100
[4] Moore C. Cigarette smoking and cancer of the mouth, pharynx, and larynx. A continuing study. JAMA. 1971; 218(4):553–558
[5] Patel SC, Carpenter WR, Tyree S, et al. Increasing incidence of oral tongue squamous cell carcinoma in young white women, age 18 to 44 years. J Clin Oncol. 2011; 29(11):1488–1494
[6] Ng JH, Iyer NG, Tan MH, Edgren G. Changing epidemiology of oral squamous cell carcinoma of the tongue: a global study. Head Neck. 2017; 39(2):297–304
[7] Tota JE, Anderson WF, Coffey C, et al. Rising incidence of oral tongue cancer among white men and women in the United States, 1973–2012. Oral Oncol. 2017; 67:146–152
[8] Singhvi HR, Malik A, Chaturvedi P. The role of chronic mucosal trauma in oral cancer: a review of literature. Indian J Med Paediatr Oncol. 2017; 38(1):44–50
[9] Perry BJ, Zammit AP, Lewandowski AW, et al. Sites of origin of oral cavity cancer in nonsmokers vs smokers: possible evidence of dental trauma carcinogenesis and its importance compared with human papillomavirus. JAMA Otolaryngol Head Neck Surg. 2015; 141(1):5–11

[10] Hobbs CG, Sterne JA, Bailey M, Heyderman RS, Birchall MA, Thomas SJ. Human papillomavirus and head and neck cancer: a systematic review and meta-analysis. Clin Otolaryngol. 2006; 31(4):259–266
[11] Dediol E, Sabol I, Virag M, Grce M, Muller D, Manojlović S. HPV prevalence and p16INKa overexpression in non-smoking non-drinking oral cavity cancer patients. Oral Dis. 2016; 22(6):517–522
[12] Liang XH, Lewis J, Foote R, Smith D, Kademani D. Prevalence and significance of human papillomavirus in oral tongue cancer: the Mayo Clinic experience. J Oral Maxillofac Surg. 2008; 66(9):1875–1880
[13] Poling JS, Ma XJ, Bui S, et al. Human papillomavirus (HPV) status of non-tobacco related squamous cell carcinomas of the lateral tongue. Oral Oncol. 2014; 50(4):306–310
[14] Pickering CR, Zhang J, Neskey DM, et al. Squamous cell carcinoma of the oral tongue in young non-smokers is genomically similar to tumors in older smokers. Clin Cancer Res. 2014; 20(14):3842–3848
[15] Koch WM, Lango M, Sewell D, Zahurak M, Sidransky D. Head and neck cancer in nonsmokers: a distinct clinical and molecular entity. Laryngoscope. 1999; 109(10):1544–1551
[16] Jeon JH, Kim MG, Park JY, et al. Analysis of the outcome of young age tongue squamous cell carcinoma. Maxillofac Plast Reconstr Surg. 2017; 39(1):41
[17] Hanna GJ, et al. Tumor PD-L1 expression is associated with improved survival and lower recurrence risk in young women with oral cavity squamous cell carcinoma. Int J Oral Maxillofac Surg. 2018; 47(5):568–577
[18] Su SC, Lin CW, Liu YF, et al. Exome sequencing of oral squamous cell carcinoma reveals molecular subgroups and novel therapeutic opportunities. Theranostics. 2017; 7(5):1088–1099
[19] Fu J, Malm IJ, Kadayakkara DK, Levitsky H, Pardoll D, Kim YJ. Preclinical evidence that PD1 blockade cooperates with cancer vaccine TEGVAX to elicit regression of established tumors. Cancer Res. 2014; 74(15):4042–4052
[20] Teguh DN, Levendag PC, Voet P, et al. Trismus in patients with oropharyngeal cancer: relationship with dose in structures of mastication apparatus. Head Neck. 2008; 30(5):622–630
[21] van der Waal I, Scully C. Oral cancer: comprehending the condition, causes, controversies, control and consequences. 4. Potentially malignant disorders of the oral and oropharyngeal mucosa. Dent Update. 2011; 38(2):138–140
[22] Reichart PA, Philipsen HP. Oral erythroplakia: a review. Oral Oncol. 2005; 41 (6):551–561
[23] Ribeiro AS, Salles PR, da Silva TA, Mesquita RA. A review of the nonsurgical treatment of oral leukoplakia. Int J Dent. 2010; 2010:186018
[24] da Silva SD, Hier M, Mlynarek A, Kowalski LP, Alaoui-Jamali MA. Recurrent oral cancer: current and emerging therapeutic approaches. Front Pharmacol. 2012; 3:149
[25] Rivera C, Venegas B. Histological and molecular aspects of oral squamous cell carcinoma [review]. Oncol Lett. 2014; 8(1):7–11
[26] Peng KA, Chu AC, Lai C, et al. Is there a role for neck dissection in T1 oral tongue squamous cell carcinoma? The UCLA experience. Am J Otolaryngol. 2014; 35(6):741–746
[27] Joshi SA, Halli R, Koranne V, Singh S. Necrotizing sialometaplasia: a diagnostic dilemma! J Oral Maxillofac Pathol. 2014; 18(3):420–422
[28] Clayburgh DR, Brickman D. Is esophagoscopy necessary during panendoscopy? Laryngoscope. 2017; 127(1):2–3
[29] Shahangian A, Damrose EJ. Bronchoscopy in panendoscopy: review and assessment. J Laryngol Otol. 2015; 129(12):1220–1223
[30] Koo K, Harris R, Wiesenfeld D, Iseli TA. A role for panendoscopy? Second primary tumour in early stage squamous cell carcinoma of the oral tongue. J Laryngol Otol. 2015; 129 Suppl 1:S27–S31
[31] Shah JP. Patterns of cervical lymph node metastasis from squamous carcinomas of the upper aerodigestive tract. Am J Surg. 1990; 160(4):405–409
[32] Dammann F, Bootz F, Cohnen M, Hassfeld S, Tatagiba M, Kösling S. Diagnostic imaging modalities in head and neck disease. Dtsch Arztebl Int. 2014; 111 (23–24):417–423
[33] Ahuja AT, Ying M, Ho SY, et al. Ultrasound of malignant cervical lymph nodes. Cancer Imaging. 2008; 8:48–56
[34] Ha PK, Hdeib A, Goldenberg D, et al. The role of positron emission tomography and computed tomography fusion in the management of early-stage and advanced-stage primary head and neck squamous cell carcinoma. Arch Otolaryngol Head Neck Surg. 2006; 132(1):12–16
[35] Fleming AJ, Jr, Smith SP, Jr, Paul CM, et al. Impact of [18F]-2-fluorodeoxyglucose-positron emission tomography/computed tomography on previously untreated head and neck cancer patients. Laryngoscope. 2007; 117(7):1173–1179
[36] Calabrese L, Giugliano G, Bruschini R, et al. Compartmental surgery in tongue tumours: description of a new surgical technique. Acta Otorhinolaryngol Ital. 2009; 29(5):259–264
[37] Barringer DA, Hutcheson KA, Sturgis EM, Kies MS, Lewin JS. Effect of induction chemotherapy on speech and swallowing function in patients with oral tongue cancer. Head Neck. 2009; 31(5):611–617
[38] Ji YB, Cho YH, Song CM, et al. Long-term functional outcomes after resection of tongue cancer: determining the optimal reconstruction method. Eur Arch Otorhinolaryngol. 2017; 274(10):3751–3756
[39] Palmer JB, Rudin NJ, Lara G, Crompton AW. Coordination of mastication and swallowing. Dysphagia. 1992; 7(4):187–200
[40] Ha J, Sung IY, Son JH, Stone M, Ord R, Cho YC. Analysis of speech and tongue motion in normal and post-glossectomy speaker using cine MRI. J Appl Oral Sci. 2016; 24(5):472–480
[41] Van Lierde K, Galiwango G, Hodges A, Bettens K, Luyten A, Vermeersch H. Impact of tongue reduction on overall speech intelligibility, articulation and oromyofunctional behavior in 4 children with Beckwith-Wiedemann syndrome. Folia Phoniatr Logop. 2012; 64(2):55–63
[42] Lee DY, Ryu YJ, Hah JH, Kwon TK, Sung MW, Kim KH. Long-term subjective tongue function after partial glossectomy. J Oral Rehabil. 2014; 41(10):754–758
[43] Jacobi I, Navran A, van der Molen L, Heemsbergen WD, Hilgers FJ, van den Brekel MW. Radiation dose to the tongue and velopharynx predicts acoustic-articulatory changes after chemo-IMRT treatment for advanced head and neck cancer. Eur Arch Otorhinolaryngol. 2016; 273(2):487–494
[44] Shah JP, Gil Z. Current concepts in management of oral cancer: surgery. Oral Oncol. 2009; 45(4–5):394–401
[45] Yu GY, Zhang L, Guo CB, Huang MX, Mao C, Peng X. Pre-mental foramen mandibulotomy for resecting tumors of tongue base and parapharyngeal space. Chin Med J (Engl). 2005; 118(21):1803–1807
[46] Dziegielewski PT, Mlynarek AM, Dimitry J, Harris JR, Seikaly H. The mandibulotomy: friend or foe? Safety outcomes and literature review. Laryngoscope. 2009; 119(12):2369–2375
[47] Rao LP, Shukla M, Sharma V, Pandey M. Mandibular conservation in oral cancer. Surg Oncol. 2012; 21(2):109–118
[48] Scheunemann H. Pull-through surgery in mouth floor: tongue neoplasms. Acta Stomatol Belg. 1975; 72(2):229–230
[49] Zanoni DK, Migliacci JC, Xu B, et al. A proposal to redefine close surgical margins in squamous cell carcinoma of the oral tongue. JAMA Otolaryngol Head Neck Surg. 2017; 143(6):555–560
[50] Frangioni JV. New technologies for human cancer imaging. J Clin Oncol. 2008; 26(24):4012–4021
[51] Tajudeen BA, Taylor ZD, Garritano J, et al. Dynamic optical contrast imaging as a novel modality for rapidly distinguishing head and neck squamous cell carcinoma from surrounding normal tissue. Cancer. 2017; 123(5):879–886
[52] Yuen AP, Ho CM, Chow TL, et al. Prospective randomized study of selective neck dissection versus observation for N0 neck of early tongue carcinoma. Head Neck. 2009; 31(6):765–772
[53] D'Cruz AK, Vaish R, Kapre N, et al. Head and Neck Disease Management Group. Elective versus therapeutic neck dissection in node-negative oral cancer. N Engl J Med. 2015; 373(6):521–529
[54] Forastiere A, Goepfert H, Goffinet D, et al. National Comprehensive Cancer Network. NCCN practice guidelines for head and neck cancer. Oncology (Williston Park). 1998; 12 7A:39–147
[55] O'Brien CJ, Lauer CS, Fredricks S, et al. Tumor thickness influences prognosis of T1 and T2 oral cavity cancer: but what thickness? Head Neck. 2003; 25(11):937–945
[56] Fan SF, Zeng ZY, Peng HW, Guo ZM, Wang SL, Zhang Q. Sentinel lymph node biopsy versus elective neck dissection in patients with cT1-2N0 oral tongue squamous cell carcinoma. Oral Surg Oral Med Oral Pathol Oral Radiol. 2014; 117(2):186–190
[57] Huang SF, Kang CJ, Lin CY, et al. Neck treatment of patients with early stage oral tongue cancer: comparison between observation, supraomohyoid dissection, and extended dissection. Cancer. 2008; 112(5):1066–1075
[58] Agarwal SK, Munjal M, Koul R, Agarwal R. Prospective evaluation of the quality of life of oral tongue cancer patients before and after the treatment. Ann Palliat Med. 2014; 3(4):238–243
[59] Smith JE, Suh JD, Erman A, Nabili V, Chhetri DK, Blackwell KE. Risk factors predicting aspiration after free flap reconstruction of oral cavity and oropharyngeal defects. Arch Otolaryngol Head Neck Surg. 2008; 134(11):1205–1208
[60] Tomita S, Terao Y, Hatano T, Nishimura R. Subtotal glossectomy preserving half the tongue base prevents taste disorder in patients with tongue cancer. Int J Oral Maxillofac Surg. 2014; 43(9):1042–1046
[61] Hurvitz KA, Kobayashi M, Evans GR. Current options in head and neck reconstruction. Plast Reconstr Surg. 2006; 118(5):122e–133e
[62] Villaret AB, Cappiello J, Piazza C, Pedruzzi B, Nicolai P. Quality of life in patients treated for cancer of the oral cavity requiring reconstruction: a prospective study. Acta Otorhinolaryngol Ital. 2008; 28(3):120–125

16 Reconstruction of the Oral Tongue

Peter S. Vosler

Summary
Reconstruction of the oral tongue is essential for restoration of speech and swallowing function following resection of both benign and malignant tumors. This chapter outlines the pertinent anatomy, principles of reconstruction, and the reconstructive options based on the location and size of the ablative defect. Locoregional and free-flap reconstruction options and functional outcomes of each flap are discussed.

Keywords: tongue reconstruction, locoregional flaps, free flaps, oral tongue resection, articulation, swallow function

16.1 Introduction

Reconstruction of the oral tongue is critical for maintenance of quality of life as the oral tongue is essential for articulation, mastication, and swallowing. Extirpation of benign and, more often, malignant tumors is the indication for reconstruction in the majority of cases. The type of reconstruction depends on the type and extent of the tumor, involvement of other subsites of the oral cavity and oropharynx, and patient factors including comorbid conditions, body habitus, and prior radiation therapy. Overall, the goal of reconstruction is to close the oral defect and restore volume to the oral tongue to assist with articulation and swallowing.

16.2 Diagnosis and Evaluation

Consideration of several factors is essential to determine the type of reconstruction necessary for an individual patient. Tumor location is an important consideration for tongue reconstruction, as removal of tumors of the tip of the oral tongue tends to produce more difficulties with articulation than tumors involving the lateral tongue. Size of the tumor and involvement of other oral cavity or oropharyngeal subsites will influence the decision of the type and extent of reconstruction. Finally, prior radiation therapy of the oral cavity and neck will limit the use of local and regional flaps, thus limiting the reconstructive options.

Physical examination of the oral cavity should consist of determining the location of the tumor, involvement of adjacent subsites such as the floor of the mouth, mandibular alveolus, retromolar trigone, and base of tongue, and estimation of the depth of the tumor. The ipsilateral buccal mucosa is evaluated for the presence of tumor and scars for consideration of regional flap reconstruction. The presence or absence of teeth is also important for reconstructive planning. The laxity of cervical skin, the presence of scars from prior surgeries or injuries, and radiation fibrosis should be assessed to determine the feasibility of local and regional flap reconstruction. For anticipated defects greater than 50% of the oral tongue, or if multiple subsites are involved, free-flap reconstruction is preferred. Allen's test of the patient's nondominant hand, palpation of the lateral thigh skin, evaluation of the skin and subcutaneous tissue overlying the abdomen, and palpation of the skin and muscle overlying the latissimus dorsi muscle are performed to determine the best potential free-flap donor site.

Diagnostic imagining is imperative for comprehensive determination of tumor involvement and tumor thickness. MRI provides the best soft-tissue resolution; however, CT scan can provide adequate resolution for tumor extirpation and reconstruction, and it is the preferred modality to asses for bone invasion.

16.3 Anatomic Considerations

16.3.1 Oral Tongue Musculature

The oral tongue consists of intrinsic and extrinsic muscles covered by a mucosal membrane. The subsites of the oral tongue include the tip and the body of the tongue. The body of the tongue is divided into dorsal and ventral components in the axial plane, and into lateral halves in the sagittal plane separated by the median sulcus. The posterior aspect of the oral tongue is the terminal sulcus, indicated by the circumvallate papillae.

There are four intrinsic muscles of the tongue: superior longitudinal, inferior longitudinal, transverse, and vertical muscles. They have no bony insertion and act to alter the shape of the tongue. The extrinsic muscles include the genioglossus, hyoglossus, styloglossus, and palatoglossus. These muscles originate outside the tongue and insert within it to change tongue position. Deep to the extrinsic muscles is the mylohyoid muscle, which provides a diaphragm for the oral cavity contents. While it is not a muscle of the tongue, involvement of the mylohyoid and removal for safe oncologic margin affects the reconstructive design due to the potential for ptosis of the oral cavity contents postoperatively.

16.3.2 Vasculature

The main blood supply is from bilateral lingual arteries arising from the external carotid artery. The lingual arteries travel deep to the styloglossus muscle traveling superomedially and then altering course traveling anteroinferiorly. The main branches of the lingual artery are the dorsal lingual artery, the deep lingual, and the sublingual arteries. The dorsal lingual artery supplies the base of the tongue, while the latter two supply the oral tongue. Knowledge of the vascular anatomy of the tongue is important for both the ablative surgeon and the reconstructive surgeon. Adequate hemostatic control of the dorsal lingual artery is imperative to prevent potential catastrophic hemorrhage postoperatively.

16.3.3 Nerves

The major motor innervation to the tongue is the hypoglossal nerve. The only exception is the palatoglossus, which is innervated by the vagus nerve. The sensory innervation of the tongue via the lingual nerve is a more important consideration for the reconstructive surgeon if there is a plan for tongue sensory reinnervation. This will be discussed in more depth in section 16.4.5.

16.4 Surgical Considerations and Approaches

16.4.1 Reconstructive Options

The type of tongue reconstruction depends on the location and the size of the defect. Often, small benign and malignant lesions can be left to heal by secondary intention. Small defects in the ventral tongue and floor of mouth should not be allowed to heal by secondary intention, as there is the potential risk of scarring and tethering of the tongue. Skin grafts are an option and are well reported in the literature.[1] Skin grafts require bolsters to ensure graft viability on the dynamic tongue musculature, and with their use airway compromise must be avoided.

Defects that leave a large surface area of the tongue exposed but not large enough to produce a significant reduction of tongue volume greater than approximately one-third of the tongue[2] can be partially or completely closed primarily with absorbable sutures. Mobilization of local tongue mucosa and musculature with a local flap is also an option to aid in closure. However, too much tissue rearrangement results in impaired function with no correction for the loss of tongue volume.

There are many regional pedicled flaps and free flaps that are available for defects spanning one-third to one-half of the oral tongue. The regional pedicled flaps include the submental artery island flap, facial artery myomucosal flap, supraclavicular artery island flap, temporalis muscle flap, and the pectoralis major myocutaneous flap. Free flaps such as the radial forearm free flap (RFFF), the anterolateral thigh (ALT), and the gracilis myocutaneous free flap can also be used for both smaller defects of one-third to one-half of the oral tongue.

For defects greater than or equal to half of the tongue, larger volume flaps such as the ALT, latissimus dorsi, thoracodorsal artery perforator, upper lateral arm, or rectus abdominis free flaps are necessary to fill dead space. Pectoralis major myocutaneous pedicled flaps can also be used, but are generally reserved for salvage cases. Please refer to ▶ Table 16.1 for a list of tissue options for oral tongue reconstruction based on defect size and location.

16.4.2 Principles of Reconstruction

There are several principles important to consider when reconstructing the oral tongue. These are comprehensively described by Chepeha et al, and are summarized in the following text.[3]

Table 16.1 Regional and free-flap options for tongue reconstruction

Defect size	Reconstruction	Flap type	Comments
< 33%	Primary closure		Optimal choice for limited defects to decrease operative time
	Local flap	L	Judicious use to prevent reducing tongue function for overcorrection
	FAMM	LR	Ideal for restoring mucosal lining of tongue. Not an option for dentate patients due to pedicle compromise
	FAMM	LR	See above
	SPIF	LR	Good regional option with little donor site morbidity. Potential concern for oncologic control
	SCAIF	LR	Good pedicle length. Potential for peripheral skin paddle necrosis
	Temporalis	LR	Temporal donor site defect, need for zygoma osteotomy for inset
33–50%	Pectoralis major	LR	Donor site defect–functional and cosmetic implications. Generally reserved as a salvage option or patients with significant comorbidities
	RFFF	FF	Good for midsize defect with thin fasciocutaneous flap. Can harvest with fat to increase volume. Donor site morbidity due to skin graft and healing issues
	ALT	FF	Limited donor site morbidity. May have too much subcutaneous tissue for appropriate reconstruction based on patient body habitus
	Rectus abdominis	FF	Potential postoperative ileus and hernia
	TDAP	FF	Perforator difficult to identify; may have to convert to latissimus dorsi free flap, which increases volume significantly
	Pectoralis major	LR	See above
	ALT	FF	Usually a good option for subtotal and total glossectomies given adequate volume available
	Latissimus dorsi	FF	Limited donor site morbidity. Good tissue volume
	TDAP	FF	See above
> 50%	Upper lateral arm	FF	Decent volume available. Potential donor site morbidity if radial nerve injured
	Rectus abdominis	FF	See above
	Gracilis	FF	Potential for motor innervation. There is limited use of this flap in the literature
	Gastrocnemius	FF	Potential for motor innervation. There is limited use of this flap in the literature

Abbreviations: ALT, anterolateral thigh free flap; FAMM, facial artery myomucosal flap; FF, free flap; LR, locoregional flap; RFFF, radial forearm free flap; SCAIF, supraclavicular artery island flap; SPIF, submental artery perforator island flap; TDAP, thoracodorsal artery perforator flap.

- Eliminate the dead space caused by the ablation. Overcorrect for the eventual volume loss due to scar and atrophy over time, as well as the further decrease in volume if adjuvant radiation therapy is planned. Expect an approximately 20% reduction in size with no radiation therapy, and approximately 40% reduction with radiation therapy.[4] The reconstruction and the native tongue should be in contact with all the mucosal surfaces of the mouth when the mouth is closed. This is important for swallowing and better secretion control, and it aids in removal of residual food following eating.
  - Ensure proper bulk with tongue base resections to ensure neotongue contact with the pharyngeal walls and soft palate.[5]
- Ensure premaxillary contact. It is particularly important for the native tongue (if it was not sacrificed due to tumor involvement) to be in contact with the premaxilla for articulation. Reconstruction of the floor of the mouth and adequate volume of the flap are essential to ensure the native tongue will reach the premaxilla.
- Optimize the function of the remaining native tongue. The purpose of the tongue is to clear food and secretions from the mouth, and articulation. Ensure the tongue is not tethered to the floor of the mouth or mandible by using thin tissue to reconstruct the floor of the mouth. Evidence demonstrates that protrusion of the tongue greater than 0.8 cm improves the range of solids consumed and comfort eating in public, and tongue elevation greater than 1.5 cm improves the range of liquids consumed.[3]
- Tongue size, mandibular height, and presence or absence of dentition are all considerations when determining volume requirements of the reconstruction.
- Ensure optimal sensation of the reconstructed tongue. This is somewhat controversial and is discussed in section 16.4.5. However, the underlying rationale is increased sensation leads to better functional outcome.
- Laryngeal suspension in total or subtotal glossectomy is important to help reduce the risk of aspiration.[6]

16.4.3 Flap Design

Hemiglossectomy Defect Designs

Flap design should incorporate all of the aforementioned principles based on the extent of resected tongue. Restoration of tongue bulk and mobility of the tongue is paramount to successful reconstruction of a hemiglossectomy defect. The introduction of the biolobed, sensate radial forearm flap by Urken and Biller with the addition of vascularized subcutaneous fat if necessary based on the size of the defect provides adequate bulk, and it has a floor of mouth component that prevents tethering of the tongue.[7] The concern with this design is partial necrosis of the flap from disruption of the microvasculature of the distal flap on the lobe not adjacent to the pedicle.

A rectangle template for hemiglossectomy defects incorporates the principles of the biolobed flap into a simple design without any concern for partial flap necrosis from devascularization.[3] The principle of this design is to place the thicker tissue and fat pad overlying the brachioradialis to reconstruct the bulk of the tongue, and to place the thinner tissue overlying the flexor carpi radialis and palmaris longus tendons along the floor of mouth reconstruction. The shortcoming of this design is that the nondominant hand is not always oriented properly for reconstruction. This results in increased donor site morbidity when the dominant forearm is harvested.

A more simplistic but equally effective design is a simple oval that accounts for the loss of bulk in hemiglossectomy defects. This design simply measures the anteroposterior and dorsoventral defects in the minimally protruded tongue. A shortcoming of this design is that it results in tongue tethering if there is a significant floor of mouth component of the defect.

The ALT free flap is also a viable option for reconstruction of hemiglossectomy defects in the appropriate patient population. Reconstruction using an individualized "ABC" flap design, where "A" represents the tip, "B" is the body of the tongue and floor of mouth reconstruction, and "C" the tongue base, results in improved swallowing function compared to a common oval design ALT flap.[8]

Subtotal or Total Glossectomy Defects

Defects that involve greater than half of the oral tongue and those that extend to the base of the tongue require increased tissue volume for adequate reconstruction. The flaps traditionally used for this extent of reconstruction are outlined in ▶ Table 16.1. The most common flaps used for subtotal or total glossectomy in the literature include the ALT and recuts abdominis free flaps.[6,9–11]

A "money pouch–like" design of a rectus abdominis myocutaneous free flap describes outlining a skin paddle 20% larger than the tongue defect and an additional de-epithelialized section of the flap folded under the flap along with muscle bulk to increase the overall volume. This flap is inset from the base of the tongue to the anterior mouth, which forms a "money pouch–like" shape. This design allows for the neotongue to be in contact with the hard palate when the mouth is closed.[9]

For thin patients without substantial adipose tissue, a two-island rectus abdominis myocutaneous flap has been described. This design involves harvesting a skin paddle to reconstruct the neotongue with the harvest of a de-epithelialized second paddle to fold under the cutaneous portion to increase volume.[11] This design is not specific to the rectus abdominis flap as it can be used with the ALT and latissimus dorsi flaps as well.

Regardless of the flap choice, the most important consideration with flap design is to produce a protuberant tongue. Evaluation of 30 patients who underwent subtotal or total glossectomy and reconstruction with ALT or rectus abdominis free flaps revealed that patients with a semiprotuberant or protuberant tongue had improved speech intelligibility, improved swallowing function, and less weight loss than patients with depressed tongues. It was concluded that flaps should be designed 30% larger than the defect and the larynx should be resuspended to prevent flap prolapse and reduce the risk of aspiration.[6]

16.4.4 Functional Evidence for Flap Choice

The choice of flap is multifactorial based on location and size of the defect. An added level of sophistication should incorporate functional determinants. Comparison of RFFF reconstruction versus primary closure of defects from pT3 lesions averaging

41.6 versus 39.1% of the oral tongue resected, respectively, revealed improved quality-of-life scores involving swallowing, speech, and social eating in the free-flap reconstruction group.[12] Similarly, swallowing function was found to be nearly normal in patients who had RFFF reconstruction as measured by videofluoroscopy. Swallowing was noticeably impaired with primary closure only.[13] Data from these papers suggest reconstruction improves functional outcome compared to primary closure with defects larger than 33% of the tongue.

Evaluation of RFFFs compared to local tongue tissue rearrangement revealed no difference in intelligibility of 100 Chinese words. However, a majority of these patients had T1 or T2 lesions, and there was no assessment of swallowing function.[14] There was a difference in speech intelligibility between patients with T1 and T3 lesions regardless of reconstructive method, indicating that the volume of intrinsic tongue muscle resected is more closely related to function.

RFFF compared to the regional submental island perforator flap demonstrated similar speech and swallowing outcome between the two groups. The submental island perforator group did have decreased operative time and decreased hospital length of stay compared to the RFFF patients.[15] Concern has been raised regarding the oncologic safety of using the submental island perforator flap for reconstruction of oral cavity malignancies due to transfer of occult metastatic disease. However, a retrospective review of 50 patients that had submental flaps for oral cavity reconstruction demonstrated a 10% occult metastatic node rate in level 1 with no local recurrences.[16] This suggests that this flap is a viable option for reconstruction.

Functional comparison of other regional flaps to the RFFF demonstrates improved speech intelligibility with RFFF compared to the pectoralis major flap. There was no difference in swallowing function between the two groups.[17] Reconstruction using the less-bulky supraclavicular artery island flap produced similar functional results compared to RFFF reconstruction with fewer donor site complications in the supraclavicular artery island flap cohort.[18] This indicates the supraclavicular artery island flap is a good option for oral tongue reconstruction. Although not found in this study, it should be noted that peripheral and complete necrosis of the supraclavicular artery island flap has been reported.[19]

Direct comparison of RFFFs and ALT flaps for hemiglossectomy defects revealed no differences in tongue mobility, speech intelligibility, or swallowing function between the two flaps.[20,21] A meta-analysis examining 12 papers including 198 RFFFs and 168 ALT free flaps revealed no differences in speech, swallowing, or the appearance of the tongue between the two flaps. The only significant finding was decreased donor site morbidity for the ALT.[22,23] It should be noted that the majority of papers in the meta-analysis were published from groups in China and Taiwan, with only one paper from the United States. This is an important factor as body mass index and thigh bulk are variable in different patient populations that effect flap choice with the RFFF preferred for hemiglossectomy defects, while the increased bulk of the ALT is useful for subtotal and total glossectomies.

16.4.5 Flap Reinnervation

The act of speaking and deglutition involves the coordination of motor control and sensory input. It is reasonable to hypothesize that providing innervation to the flap with both motor nerve input to harvested muscle and sensory nerve input would improve functional outcomes. There is evidence that reinnervation of sensory nerves from the flap to the lingual nerve improves sensation.[24,25] Despite improved sensation of the flap, there is no definitive evidence that enhanced flap sensation improves function measured by speech and swallowing evaluation.[24,26] Sensation is also reported to return in flaps that have no reinnervation, suggesting that a limited amount of sensation may be all that is needed to improve function. Speech and swallowing function postreconstruction is likely predominately mediated by the amount of native tongue sacrificed and the final volume of the reconstruction rather than a return to baseline sensation.

There are a few studies examining the effect of motor reinnervation of free flaps to reconstruct the oral tongue using ALT with vastus lateralis, gracilis, and gastrocnemius flaps.[25,27,28] These studies all report good swallowing function in the majority of patients; however, there is no direct comparison to patients with nonmotor innervated flaps, and they all have small cohorts of 6, 10, and 6 patients. It is difficult to extrapolate meaningful conclusions with such small sample sizes and lack of a control group. More investigation is thus warranted.

16.5 Perioperative Management

Postoperative flap management has become relatively standardized over the past nearly four decades. Our protocol for free-flap reconstruction is for flap checks every hour for the first 24 hours, every 2 hours for the second 24 hours, and every 4 hours thereafter. Pedicled regional flaps require no monitoring, and have been shown to have decreased hospital stay compared to free-flap reconstruction.[15] However, all patients with oral tongue reconstruction require initial inpatient management to ensure a safe airway, proper nutritional intake, and satisfactory healing to avoid the development of fistula or infection.

16.6 Surgical Sequelae

The short-term surgical sequelae include potential aspiration depending on the extent of the tongue excised for tumor removal and local wound issues such as fistula and potential neck abscess. These are all closely monitored during the hospital stay. Patients with free-flap reconstruction typically are hospitalized for 5 to 10 days depending on the type of reconstruction and their ability to safely ingest an oral diet.

Subsequent posthospital care involves local wound care to free flap and local flap donor sites and continued work with speech-language pathology for speech and swallow rehabilitation. As discussed earlier, RFFF reconstruction tends to have more donor site complications than ALT reconstruction. This is predominately due to the split-thickness skin graft used to cover the forearm defect with dehiscence of the graft overlying the flexor carpi radialis tendon. The ALT donor site can develop dehiscence of the incision and seroma formation given the activity of the lower extremities and the size of the surgical incision required for harvest.

Key Points

- Reconstruction of the oral tongue following tumor extirpation is imperative for improved speech and swallowing function.
- The type of reconstruction is related to the size of the defect. The appropriate reconstructive option should consider functional outcome, patient comorbidities in relation to operative time, and potential donor site morbidity.
- The principles of oral tongue reconstruction, including restoration of sufficient volume for premaxilla, palatal, and pharyngeal contact of the reconstructed tissue, should be followed.
- Perform laryngeal suspension in patients who have had lingual release for tumor resection to help prevent postoperative aspiration.
- Reinnervation of flaps improves sensation; however, the functional implications are yet to be known.

References

[1] Schramm VL, Jr, Johnson JT, Myers EN. Skin grafts and flaps in oral cavity reconstruction. Arch Otolaryngol. 1983; 109(3):175–177

[2] Hartig GK. Free flaps in oral cavity reconstruction: when you need them and when you don't. Int J Radiat Oncol Biol Phys. 2007; 69(2) Suppl:S19–S21

[3] Chepeha DB, Teknos TN, Shargorodsky J, et al. Rectangle tongue template for reconstruction of the hemiglossectomy defect. Arch Otolaryngol Head Neck Surg. 2008; 134(9):993–998

[4] Tarsitano A, Battaglia S, Cipriani R, Marchetti C. Microvascular reconstruction of the tongue using a free anterolateral thigh flap: three-dimensional evaluation of volume loss after radiotherapy. J Craniomaxillofac Surg. 2016; 44(9): 1287–1291

[5] Urken ML, Moscoso JF, Lawson W, Biller HF. A systematic approach to functional reconstruction of the oral cavity following partial and total glossectomy. Arch Otolaryngol Head Neck Surg. 1994; 120(6):589–601

[6] Kimata Y, Sakuraba M, Hishinuma S, et al. Analysis of the relations between the shape of the reconstructed tongue and postoperative functions after subtotal or total glossectomy. Laryngoscope. 2003; 113(5):905–909

[7] Urken ML, Biller HF. A new bilobed design for the sensate radial forearm flap to preserve tongue mobility following significant glossectomy. Arch Otolaryngol Head Neck Surg. 1994; 120(1):26–31

[8] Wang L, Liu K, Shao Z, Shang Z-J. Individual design of the anterolateral thigh flap for functional reconstruction after hemiglossectomy: experience with 238 patients. Int J Oral Maxillofac Surg. 2016; 45(6):726–730

[9] Kiyokawa K, Tai Y, Inoue Y, Yanaga H, Mori K, Nakashima T. Functional reconstruction of swallowing and articulation after total glossectomy without laryngectomy: money pouch-like reconstruction method using rectus abdominis myocutaneous flap. Plast Reconstr Surg. 1999; 104(7):2015–2020

[10] Leymarie N, Karsenti G, Sarfati B, Rimareix F, Kolb F. Modification of flap design for total mobile tongue reconstruction using a sensitive antero-lateral thigh flap. J Plast Reconstr Aesthet Surg. 2012; 65(7):e169–e174

[11] Sakuraba M, Asano T, Miyamoto S, et al. A new flap design for tongue reconstruction after total or subtotal glossectomy in thin patients. J Plast Reconstr Aesthet Surg. 2009; 62(6):795–799

[12] Canis M, Weiss BG, Ihler F, Hummers-Pradier E, Matthias C, Wolff HA. Quality of life in patients after resection of pT3 lateral tongue carcinoma: microvascular reconstruction versus primary closure. Head Neck. 2016; 38(1):89–94

[13] Hsiao H-T, Leu Y-S, Chang S-H, Lee J-T. Swallowing function in patients who underwent hemiglossectomy: comparison of primary closure and free radial forearm flap reconstruction with videofluoroscopy. Ann Plast Surg. 2003; 50 (5):450–455

[14] Sun J, Weng Y, Li J, Wang G, Zhang Z. Analysis of determinants on speech function after glossectomy. J Oral Maxillofac Surg. 2007; 65(10):1944–1950

[15] Paydarfar JA, Patel UA. Submental island pedicled flap vs radial forearm free flap for oral reconstruction: comparison of outcomes. Arch Otolaryngol Head Neck Surg. 2011; 137(1):82–87

[16] Howard BE, Nagel TH, Donald CB, Hinni ML, Hayden RE. Oncologic safety of the submental flap for reconstruction in oral cavity malignancies. Otolaryngol Head Neck Surg. 2014; 150(4):558–562

[17] Su W-F, Hsia Y-J, Chang Y-C, Chen S-G, Sheng H. Functional comparison after reconstruction with a radial forearm free flap or a pectoralis major flap for cancer of the tongue. Otolaryngol Head Neck Surg. 2003; 128(3):412–418

[18] Zhang S, Chen W, Cao G, Dong Z. Pedicled supraclavicular artery island flap versus free radial forearm flap for tongue reconstruction following hemiglossectomy. J Craniofac Surg. 2015; 26(6):e527–e530

[19] Padiyar BV, Azeem Mohiyuddin SM, Sagayaraj A, Merchant S. Usefulness of supraclavicular flap in reconstruction following resection of oral cancer. World J Otorhinolaryngol Head Neck Surg. 2017; 4(2):148–152

[20] de Vicente JC, de Villalaín L, Torre A, Peña I. Microvascular free tissue transfer for tongue reconstruction after hemiglossectomy: a functional assessment of radial forearm versus anterolateral thigh flap. J Oral Maxillofac Surg. 2008; 66 (11):2270–2275

[21] Hsiao H-T, Leu Y-S, Liu C-J, Tung K-Y, Lin C-C. Radial forearm versus anterolateral thigh flap reconstruction after hemiglossectomy: functional assessment of swallowing and speech. J Reconstr Microsurg. 2008; 24(2):85–88

[22] Chen H, Zhou N, Huang X, Song S. Comparison of morbidity after reconstruction of tongue defects with an anterolateral thigh cutaneous flap compared with a radial forearm free-flap: a meta-analysis. Br J Oral Maxillofac Surg. 2016; 54(10):1095–1101

[23] Noel CW, Vosler PS, Hong M, et al. Motor and sensory morbidity associated with the anterolateral thigh perforator free flap. Laryngoscope. 2018; 128(5): 1057–1061

[24] Baas M, Duraku LS, Corten EML, Mureau MAM. A systematic review on the sensory reinnervation of free flaps for tongue reconstruction: does improved sensibility imply functional benefits? J Plast Reconstr Aesthet Surg. 2015; 68 (8):1025–1035

[25] Ozkan O, Ozkan O, Derin AT, et al. True functional reconstruction of total or subtotal glossectomy defects using a chimeric anterolateral thigh flap with both sensorial and motor innervation. Ann Plast Surg. 2015; 74(5):557–564

[26] Loewen IJ, Boliek CA, Harris J, Seikaly H, Rieger JM. Oral sensation and function: a comparison of patients with innervated radial forearm free flap reconstruction to healthy matched controls. Head Neck. 2010; 32(1):85–95

[27] Calabrese L, Saito A, Navach V, et al. Tongue reconstruction with the gracilis myocutaneous free flap. Microsurgery. 2011; 31(5):355–359

[28] Grinsell D, Yue BYT. The functional free innervated medial gastrocnemius flap. J Reconstr Microsurg. 2014; 30(7):451–456

17 Squamous Cell Cancer of the Floor of Mouth

Zenon Yeung, Eddy W.Y. Wong, and Jason Y.K. Chan

Summary

The floor of the mouth (FOM) is the second most common site of malignancy in the oral cavity; however, it receives limited focus in current literature. Cancer of the FOM represents a challenging area to approach and treat given its unique location and proximity to critical structures that are involved in speech and swallowing. Its lack of a physical barrier permits early invasion to lymphatics and adjacent neurovascular structures. Invasion of FOM cancer to the anterior arch of the mandible makes resection and subsequent reconstruction technically demanding. The limited surgical access, coupled with the small space increase the likelihood of positive margins, and the propensity for cervical metastases make this area challenging for surgeons.[1–3] Through this chapter, we hope to focus on an approach to ablative resections to the FOM that will provide sound oncologic outcomes and minimal morbidities.

Keywords: floor of the mouth cancer, oral cavity cancer, squamous cell carcinoma, approach to floor of the mouth, mandibulotomy, mandibulectomy, mandibular invasion

17.1 Epidemiology

The floor of the mouth (FOM) represents the second most common site of malignancies in the oral cavity after the oral tongue and the most common histology is squamous cell carcinoma (SCC). FOM SCC tends to affect older (~60 years old), Caucasian males[2,4]; however, it is not uncommon in younger persons. Traditional risk factors including smoking, chewing tobacco, spitting tobacco, and regular alcohol intake combine synergistically to increase the risk of FOM cancers. In an analysis of the Surveillance, Epidemiology, and End Results (SEER) database of 14,010 patients with FOM SCC, patients most commonly presented with early stage I or II disease (59.5%). The survival rate for patients with stages I, II, III, and IV are 90, 80, 65, and 30%, respectively.

17.2 Clinical Presentation

Patients with an FOM SCC commonly present with a mass or a painful ulcer with an irregular border (▸ Fig. 17.1, ▸ Fig. 17.2). There may be surrounding coexistent leukoplakia or erythroplakia. These lesions will continue to enlarge if neglected by patients, giving rise to more advanced symptoms including ankyloglossia with involvement of the tongue musculature, hypoglossal nerve, or mucoperiosteum of the mandible, paresthesias of the FOM and tongue with involvement of the lingual nerve, sialadenitis with involvement of the duct openings or sublingual gland, halitosis from a necrotic tumor, and referred pain to the ear. In addition, patients may initially present with a neck mass from regional lymph node metastases or even direct extension of tumors into the submental or submandibular region.

17.3 Diagnosis and Evaluation

Screening through a variety of methods including cytological brush, oral saliva, oral rinse evaluations of proteomics, gene microarray, methylation, and other assays have been described; however, there have been no robust clinical trials to validate that these tests are superior to a thorough clinical examination. For a definitive diagnosis, a tissue biopsy is still needed. This can be readily achieved under local anesthetic, followed by a punch biopsy of the edge of the tumor and normal tissue.

A thorough history and examination should be performed in all these patients, beginning with an inquiry about the presenting symptoms including pain, paresthesia, ear pain, dysphagia, odynophagia, voice change, dysarthria, trismus, bleeding, weight loss, lower lip/chin numbness, loose dentition, and preexisting dentures. This should be followed by specific questions about their past medical history and surgical history, allergies, social network and support, tobacco use, and alcohol consumption. These factors all influence the preoperative counseling and optimization of patients. It is our practice to routinely refer patients with ≥ 10% weight loss to a dietitian for optimization of nutrition prior to surgery. The choice of surgical reconstruction, particularly if a segmental mandibulectomy is required, is dependent on the patient's comorbidities, their willingness to undergo the surgery, and their social background and support. These factors also significantly influence the postoperative management of the patient in terms of rehabilitation and progression through to adjuvant therapies including radiotherapy and chemotherapy.

The physical examination should include a complete head and neck examination. A thorough examination, in particular, with bimanual palpation of the lesion should be attempted to ascertain the size. Laterally, fixation of the tumor through involvement of the periosteum may indicate underlying involvement of the mandible. The medial extent of the tumor edge should also be evaluated, focusing on the extent of involvement of the oral tongue. Loose dentition, particularly, adjacent to the tumor should be noted for potential invasion of the mandible. Trismus should also be noted as this will influence the choice of surgical access, which will be discussed later. The neck should then be systematically examined for the clinical determination of regional spread. This is then followed by an examination of the ear and nose. Flexible laryngoscopy should be routinely performed to evaluate for potential posterior extension of the tumor, synchronous primaries, and the status of the airway. Following this if reconstruction with a pedicled or free flap is being considered, the appropriate donor sites should be assessed, as discussed in Chapter 18.

Further evaluation involves imaging with computed tomography (CT) and magnetic resonance imaging (MRI), the two most common modalities utilized. CT is commonly used to delineate cortical bony involvement and lymph node metastases, whereas MRI is utilized to evaluate for soft-tissue invasion, perineural spread, and extension into medullary bone. CT has been shown to have a sensitivity ranging from 63 to 86% and a specificity ranging from 68 to 100% for detecting cortical bone

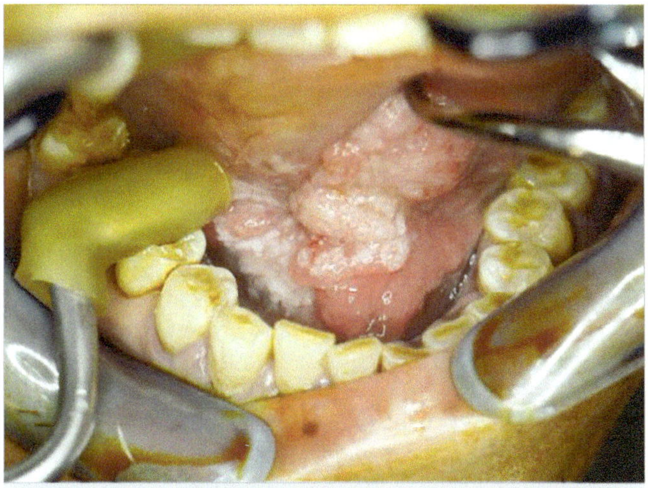

Fig. 17.1 Cancer of the right floor of the mouth extending across the frenulum and toward the ventral surface of tongue.

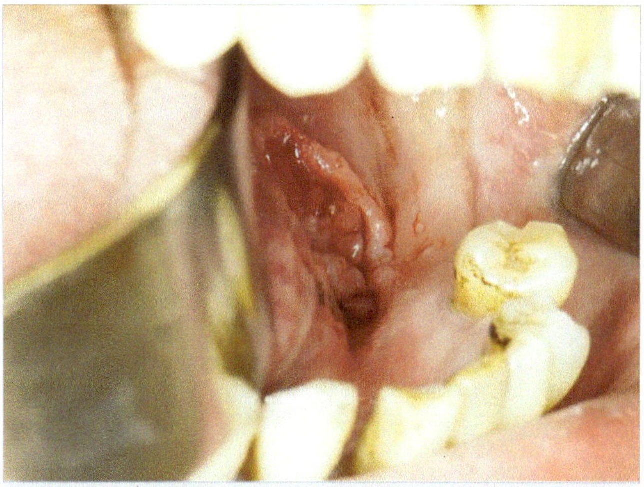

Fig. 17.2 Cancer of the left posterior floor of the mouth involving the left anterior tonsil pillar and the lateral border of tongue.

invasion.[5–7] Cone beam CT may offer an alternative with a smaller machine, less expensive cost, an upright patient position, and a lower radiation dose, and this may have a better sensitivity (range 91–94%) at the expense of specificity (range 59–97%) for the evaluation of cortical bone invasion.[5–7] The use of PET-CT in the staging of patients is not uniform but may find a particular role in patients with advanced disease, to evaluate for distant metastases as these patients would not be candidates for curative surgical treatment and alternative options should be considered.

17.4 Relevant Anatomy

The FOM is a horseshoe-shaped area inferior to the ventral surface of tongue that is covered by a thin mucous membrane made up of nonkeratinized stratified squamous epithelium. It is bounded anteriorly and laterally by the lingual surface of the mandible and its overlying mucoperiosteum, medially by the lateral surface of the tongue. The posterior extent of the FOM extends laterally to the base of the anterior tonsillar pillar. The FOM is connected to the ventral surface of the tongue by a midline mucosal fold called the frenulum. On each side of the frenulum (from superior to inferior) are the deep lingual vein, the sublingual ridge, and the sublingual caruncles. Medially at the sublingual caruncles, the submandibular duct openings (Wharton's duct) can be identified.

Inferiorly, the FOM is bounded by the muscular diaphragm consisting of the mylohyoid, geniohyoid, and the genioglossus muscles. Medial to the mylohyoid muscle are the sublingual gland, submandibular duct, hypoglossal nerve, and lingual nerve. The submandibular gland lies at the posterior free edge of the mylohyoid with the deep lobe situating deep to the mylohyoid muscle.

The FOM is innervated by the lingual nerve (CN V3). Lymphatic drainage of the anterior FOM is via the submental nodes that then drain bilaterally to the submandibular nodes and deep cervical nodes (Level I–III). Lymphatic drainage of the posterior FOM is toward ipsilateral submandibular nodes and then deep cervical nodes.

17.5 Surgical Considerations

Although the locoregional control of early FOM SCC is similar for surgery and primary irradiation, radiotherapy has a longer duration of treatment (typically daily for 6–7 weeks) and is associated with a significantly higher risk of complications including xerostomia, dysphagia, dysarthria, and osteoradionecrosis; therefore, FOM SCC like the rest of the oral cavity is best managed by primary surgery.

Again, intraoperatively it is useful, with the patient fully relaxed, to carefully examine the FOM SCC with good lighting and bimanual palpation, as this is sometimes difficult in the clinic to fully appreciate the extent of the lesion with the patient in pain. In general, superficial and small lesions that do not extend to the extrinsic tongue muscles can typically be resected transorally, whereas deeply infiltrating lesions with invasion to the underlying muscular diaphragm of the FOM require a visor flap with a pull-through approach or a mandibulotomy with lip split approach if trismus is significant. If there is mandibular invasion noted preoperatively or intraoperatively, a segmental mandibulectomy is needed.

For small lesions of the anterior FOM, most can be approached transorally. Whether or not to routinely excise the sublingual gland is controversial. Steinhart and Kleinsasser advocated that the sublingual gland should be routinely excised for oncological clearance because it is commonly infiltrated in cancer of the FOM.[8,9] However, Clark et al found that only 4.2% of patients who had no gross sublingual gland involvement had microscopic disease on histopathological examination. Routinely sacrificing the sublingual gland not only puts the lingual nerve, hypoglossal nerve, and submandibular duct at risk, but also increases the risk of fistula formation and neck wound complications to 25% compared to 14% of patients who did not undergo sublingual gland excision.[9,10]

With more extensive lesions, a combined transoral and transcervical approach utilizing a visor flap and pull-through technique is needed, the caveat being the absence of bony involvement. A lip-splitting procedure, followed by a paramedian mandibulotomy (▶ Fig. 17.3) in general is not required for

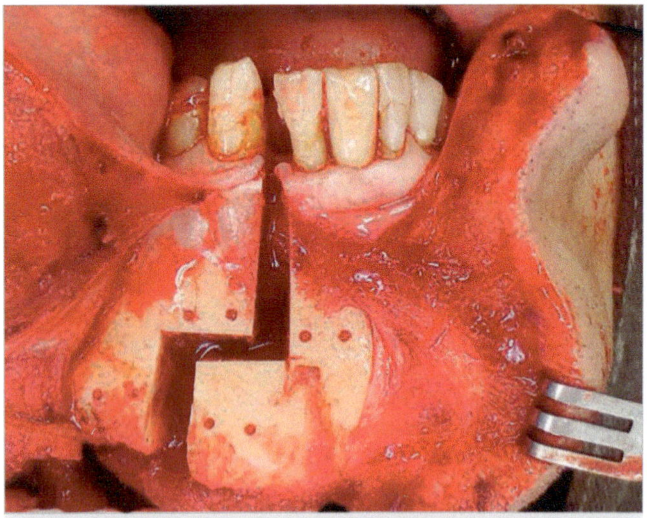

Fig. 17.3 Lip-splitting paramedian mandibulotomy.

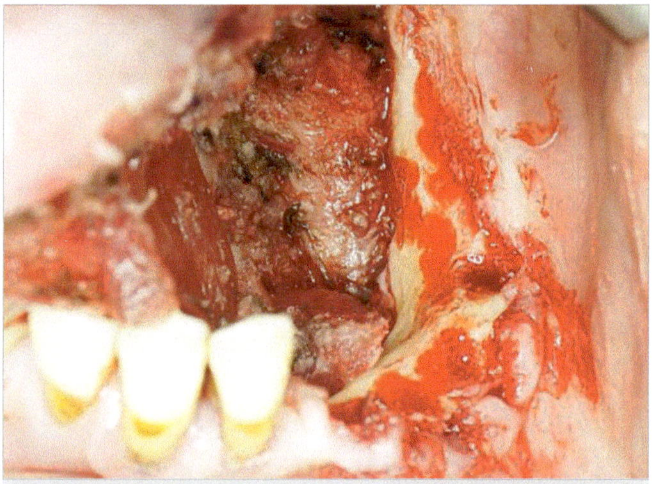

Fig. 17.5 The same patient as in ▶ Fig. 17.2, after resection of the left posterior floor of the mouth tumor and marginal mandibulectomy to achieve sufficient resection margin.

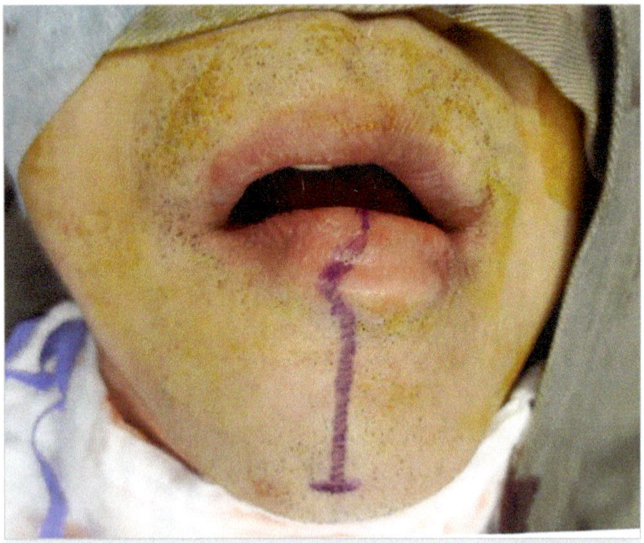

Fig. 17.4 Marking for a lower lip-splitting incision.

lesions that only involve the anterior FOM. But this technique can be useful for patients who have significant trismus, involvement of the posterior FOM, or significant involvement of the tongue base or retromolar trigone. This involves a lower lip-splitting incision (▶ Fig. 17.4) that can be straight or curvilinear, and extends inferiorly and laterally to join the transverse incision for a neck dissection. Marginal mandibulectomy may be performed to achieve sufficient resection margin if there is involvement of the periosteum or cortical erosion (▶ Fig. 17.5). In the absence of marrow or inferior alveolar canal invasion, marginal mandibulectomy is sufficient.[11,12] There are multiple routes of tumor entry into the mandible. Once the tumor breaches the soft tissue and periosteum of the mandible, in dentate patients, tumor cells migrate into the dental sockets and into the mandible. In edentulous patients, the alveolus typically undergoes atrophy, and tumor cells can quickly grow into the dental defect to invade into the inferior alveolar canal. Hence in edentulous patients with reduced mandibular bone height and more advanced marrow involvement, segmental mandibulectomy may be necessary.

When marginal mandibulectomy is performed, curvilinear incisions should be used to avoid the acute angles that may precipitate a mandibular fracture. Curvilinear incisions also facilitate subsequent dental fillings. Alternatively, a burr may be used to drill down the bone if only the periosteum of the lingual aspect of the mandible is involved. The majority of patients require an oblique marginal mandibulectomy including resection of the upper rim and medial cortex of the mandible due to the pattern of invasion by the tumor. Vertical or horizontal (rim) mandibulectomies are less commonly performed.[11] Marginal mandibulectomy is contraindicated in patients who have previously irradiated mandible as this carries a high risk of osteoradionecrosis. Segmental mandibulectomy followed by osseocutaneous free-flap reconstruction should be performed instead. If there is gross cortical bone and/or medullary bone involvement, or if an edentulous patient would be expected to have less than 1-cm bone height after a marginal mandibulectomy, then a segmental mandibulectomy should be performed.

When performing a paramedian mandibulotomy, in our practice the osteotomy is made via a step osteotomy between the lateral incisors and canine (▶ Fig. 17.3). Alternatively, the canine can be extracted and osteotomy performed through the socket if there is not adequate space between the teeth to perform the osteotomy without injuring the tooth roots. A step osteotomy gives better stability and alignment to the osteotomy site, preventing nonunion and malunion of the osteotomy site. To ensure accurate alignment and dental occlusion, miniplates and locking screws are prepared on the intact mandible before completing osteotomy. The osteotomy site is first marked with a marking pen, then sagittal saw. Two miniplates are bent according to the contour of the outer cortex of the mandible, screw holes are drilled, and locking screws applied. Miniplate and screw holes are then removed and the osteotomy completed. Dental wires can also be applied to improve fixation and therefore healing of mandibulotomy site. If miniplate and screws are

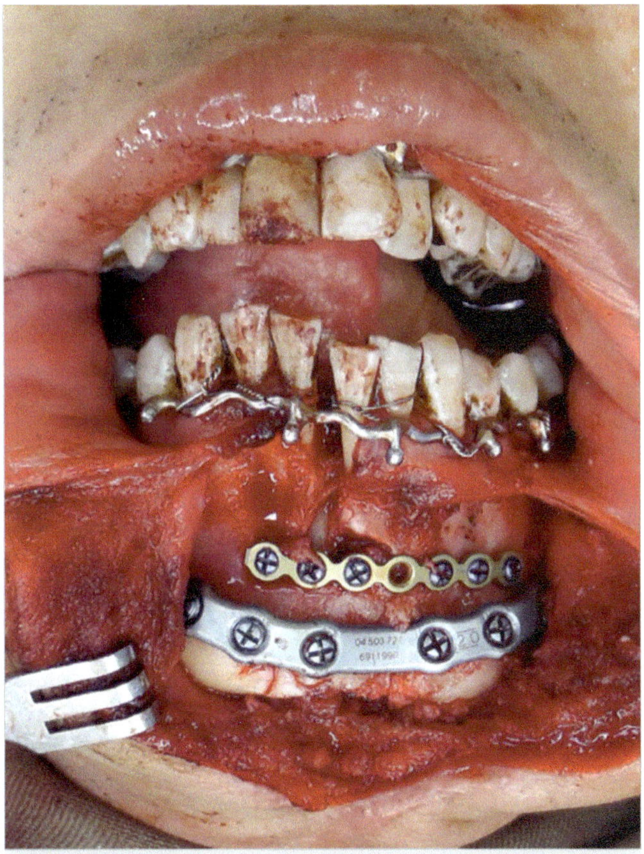

Fig. 17.6 This patient suffered from malunion of mandibulotomy site. Dental wire, miniplates, and screws were reapplied to ensure stability for bone union.

used, it is important to have watertight closure with or without flap coverage. Implant exposure or extrusion can lead to infection, nonunion, malunion (▶ Fig. 17.6), or osteomyelitis of the mandible. Previous irradiation also increases the risk of subsequent osteomyelitis and poor healing of mandibulotomy. In a patient with previous irradiation involving the mandible, a mandibulotomy should be avoided if possible to avoid higher risks of malunion, nonunion, and osteoradionecrosis; if a mandibulotomy must be performed in these patients, adequate soft-tissue coverage of the implant with well-vascularized tissue is crucial to minimize complications.

When performing surgical resections transorally, it is important that the lingual nerve is identified and protected during resection of the FOM lesion in order to preserve sensation and taste of the tongue. The lingual nerve is relatively superficial and has a close relationship with the submandibular duct. When the submandibular ducts need to be transected, this should be done obliquely if they are identified positively to ensure a sufficient circumference at the opening that can be sutured to the FOM mucosa using absorbable sutures. Transposition of submandibular duct should be performed particularly when the ipsilateral submandibular gland is not excised. It has been shown to reduce the incidence of postoperative pain or sialocele from 33 to 13% after excision of cancer of the FOM or lateral tongue.[9,13]

Given that cervical metastases occur in up to 53% of patients including occult nodal metastases in ≥ 20% of patient, a selective supraomohyoid neck dissection is indicated in all cases with clinically N0 disease. If the lesion involves or approaches the midline, then bilateral neck dissections should be performed given the rich lymphatic supply. For patients with node-positive disease, N2b or greater a modified radical neck dissection should be performed to address the neck.

17.6 Surgical Sequelae

The sequelae resulting from surgery for FOM SCC include both the consequences of the route of access to remove the FOM SCC and the consequences of the tumor removal itself. In terms of surgical access, a mandibulotomy provides excellent surgical access in patients who have trismus or extensive involvement posteriorly involving the tongue base and retromolar trigone. However, a mandibulotomy is not without risks that may include temporomandibular joint disruption or lingual nerve injury from forceful retraction and manipulation of the joint. Nonunion or malunion (▶ Fig. 17.6) of the mandibulotomy site occurs in up to 7% of patients, which can be caused by insufficient immobilization or infection of the osteotomy site. A visor approach to resection of the FOM gives a better cosmetic outcome; however, both mental nerves may be injured, resulting in temporary or permanent numbness of the lower lip and chin.

Following resection of the FOM, the main concern is potential scarring of the FOM with resultant tethering of the oral tongue and the subsequent effects on speech and swallowing. To mitigate this in smaller transoral oral resections, a skin graft can be used, as discussed in Chapter 18. The key to successful skin grafting of the FOM defect requires an adequately sized and piecrusted skin graft, adequate immobilization, and meticulous hemostasis. The skin graft is sewn to the FOM mucosa and a bolster dressing is tied over the skin graft to ensure immobilization and prevent hematoma formation underneath the skin graft.

Sialocele can occur following injury to the ipsilateral or contralateral sublingual gland or their ducts, resulting in leakage of saliva. The submandibular gland is excised during neck dissection; therefore, it rarely causes sialocele unless the contralateral submandibular duct is injured. Sialocele usually presents as a painless cystic swelling after surgery. Aspiration yields clear yellow fluid that has high amylase content. Small collections may resorb spontaneously. Larger collections may require repeated aspiration using aseptic technique. Anticholinergics are often ineffective and commonly cause side effects, for example, dry mouth, blurred vision, urinary retention, and constipation.

Key Points

- A bimanual palpation of the lesions both preoperatively and intraoperatively is important in deciding on the surgical management of these patients.
- Lesions involving the midline or close to the midline must undergo a bilateral neck dissection.
- A lip split with mandibulotomy for access should be avoided where possible to minimize the postoperative morbidity including malunion, nonunion, or osteoradionecrosis.
- A segmental mandibulectomy should be performed when there is extensive cortical bone or medullary bone involvement.

- For superficial and early-stage lesions of the FOM, particular care should be taken to prevent injury to the lingual nerve.

References

[1] Fives C, Nae A, Roche P, et al. Impact of mandibular invasion on prognosis in oral squamous cell carcinoma four centimeters or less in size. Laryngoscope. 2017; 127(4):849–854

[2] Hicks WL, Jr, Loree TR, Garcia RI, et al. Squamous cell carcinoma of the floor of mouth: a 20-year review. Head Neck. 1997; 19(5):400–405

[3] Luryi AL, Chen MM, Mehra S, Roman SA, Sosa JA, Judson BL. Positive surgical margins in early stage oral cavity cancer: an analysis of 20,602 cases. Otolaryngol Head Neck Surg. 2014; 151(6):984–990

[4] Saggi S, Badran KW, Han AY, Kuan EC, St John MA. Clinicopathologic characteristics and survival outcomes in floor of mouth squamous cell carcinoma: a population-based study. Otolaryngol Head Neck Surg. 2018; 159(1):51–58

[5] Czerwonka L, Bissada E, Goldstein DP, et al. High-resolution cone-beam computed tomography for assessment of bone invasion in oral cancer: comparison with conventional computed tomography. Head Neck. 2017; 39(10): 2016–2020

[6] Dreiseidler T, Alarabi N, Ritter L, et al. A comparison of multislice computerized tomography, cone-beam computerized tomography, and single photon emission computerized tomography for the assessment of bone invasion by oral malignancies. Oral Surg Oral Med Oral Pathol Oral Radiol Endod. 2011; 112(3):367–374

[7] Hakim SG, Wieker H, Trenkle T, et al. Imaging of mandible invasion by oral squamous cell carcinoma using computed tomography, cone-beam computed tomography and bone scintigraphy with SPECT. Clin Oral Investig. 2014; 18 (3):961–967

[8] Steinhart H, Kleinsasser O. Growth and spread of squamous cell carcinoma of the floor of the mouth. Eur Arch Otorhinolaryngol. 1993; 250 (6):358–361

[9] Patel K, Claiborne S, Mehrotra A, Nisi K, Kademani D. Early floor of mouth cancer. In: Bell RB, Andersen PE, Fernandes RP, eds. Oral, Head and Neck Oncology and Reconstructive Surgery. Amsterdam: Elsevier; 2018:420–427

[10] Clark JR, Franklin JH, Naranjo N, Odell MJ, Gullane PJ. Sublingual gland resection in squamous cell carcinoma of the floor of mouth: is it necessary? Laryngoscope. 2006; 116(3):382–386

[11] Genden EM, Rinaldo A, Jacobson A, et al. Management of mandibular invasion: when is a marginal mandibulectomy appropriate? Oral Oncol. 2005; 41 (8):776–782

[12] Genden EM, Ferlito A, Silver CE, et al. Contemporary management of cancer of the oral cavity. Eur Arch Otorhinolaryngol. 2010; 267(7):1001–1017

[13] Wong DW, Kamisetty A, Lowe D, Rogers SN. Frequency and outcomes of submandibular gland obstruction following resection of squamous cell carcinomas in the vicinity of the submandibular duct. Ann R Coll Surg Engl. 2014; 96 (8):602–605

18 Floor of Mouth Reconstruction

Tim J. Phillips and Michael G. Moore

Summary
The floor of the mouth is a pliable mucosally lined surface spanning from the lower aspect of the ventral tongue to the fixed gingiva of the lingual surface of the mandibular alveolar ridge. Reconstruction of this area is critical following tumor resection in order to optimize postoperative function. The redundancy of this region provides freedom of motion of the tongue relative to the adjacent, rigid mandible. Repair options range from simple primary closure to complex reconstruction with composite free tissue transfer with the ultimate goal being to provide a healed epithelial-lined surface to minimize tethering of the adjacent tongue and allow for more natural speech and swallowing rehabilitation.

Keywords: floor of mouth, articulation, sialodochoplasty, reconstruction, speech, radial forearm free flap, anterolateral thigh free flap, skin graft

18.1 Introduction

The floor of the mouth is a pliable mucosally lined surface that provides redundancy and freedom of movement of the oral tongue from the immobile mandibular arch. This flexibility allows the tongue to manipulate the food bolus during mastication and deglutition and also freely press against the gums, palate, lips, and teeth during speech to allow for clear articulation. It is fairly uncommon for defects resulting from oral cavity cancer resections to be limited just to the floor of the mouth. Many defects extend to involve the adjacent tongue and/or mandible and consequently have different reconstructive requirements. Reconstruction of such defects involving multiple sites will be covered in Chapter 31 entitled "Reconstruction of Multisite Defects." Here we focus specifically on defects limited to the floor of the mouth, with or without associated communication with a concomitant neck dissection wound.

18.2 Diagnosis and Evaluation

18.2.1 Defect Evaluation

For the purposes of planning, evaluation of the primary tumor is essential for determining the likely approach that will be needed for reconstruction. Examination of the tumor's proximity to the adjacent mandible and tongue is crucial, and bimanual palpation with one hand on the lesion and one in the submental/submandibular region will allow the surgeon to get a better sense of any endophytic component of the disease and the likelihood of needing a resection of the floor of mouth muscular sling to achieve adequate oncologic margins. Imaging with CT can assist in evaluating for bone erosion and to look for pathologic lymphadenopathy, but such images often provide little detail on the soft-tissue extent of the primary tumor, especially when significant dental artifact is present. When needed, MRI can be employed to provide additional soft-tissue detail on invasion into the floor of the mouth and tongue musculature and also can provide information on perineural invasion and mandibular involvement.

Intraoperatively, in determining the appropriate reconstruction following tumor removal of the floor of the mouth, the process starts with a careful analysis of the wound. Defects can range from simple mucosal loss with minimal associated muscle resection to larger composite defects with oral glossectomy and/or segmental mandibulectomy. For the purposes of this chapter, emphasis will be placed on defects limited to the floor of the mouth. In these instances, attention should be paid to look at the amount and location of mucosal surface area lost, the depth of the defect and extent of resection of the underlying floor of mouth musculature, and whether or not there is an associated defect of the adjacent mandible and/or the tongue musculature. Additional factors should include the status of the patient's dentition, whether or not they had undergone prior surgery or radiation therapy, and if the submandibular duct papilla is affected (in situations where the gland is preserved).

As mentioned earlier, one of the critical factors to assess in floor of mouth reconstruction is the integrity of the underlying muscular sling. The mylohyoid muscle and hyoglossus muscles not only serve to suspend the larynx and support tongue movement, but, in the context of a floor of mouth resection, also can serve as a barrier, separating the oral cavity from the underlying neck dissection wound. In defects where this muscular layer has been removed, particular emphasis must be placed on achieving a watertight closure of the floor of the mouth, resuspending the tongue and/or hyoid bone, and providing adequate bulk to obliterate the created submental dead space. In addition, the surgical approach to the resection also must be taken into account. For example, for individuals undergoing a lingual release to allow for their resection, the detached musculature of the anterior floor of the mouth may need to be resuspended to the mandible to minimize posterior tongue displacement and to optimize postoperative function.

18.2.2 Donor Site Evaluation

Of all of the potential reconstructive approaches for lesions limited to the floor of the mouth, only the radial forearm free flap (RFFF) requires special preoperative evaluation. In such instances, typically the nondominant arm is assessed utilizing the modified Allen's test.[1] Using this approach, both the radial and ulnar arteries are occluded with digital pressure and the hand is pumped multiple times to remove blood from the hand and fingers. The ulnar pressure is then released and the hand is assessed for refill of blood to the thumb and index finger over the next 15 seconds. Inadequate filling signifies an incomplete palmar arch circulation and is termed a "positive Allen test." In such individuals, an alternative donor site should be found. For equivocal or delayed filling, the palmar arch can be formally assessed with Doppler testing[2,3] or pulse oximetry[4] to further assess the safety of graft harvest.

When considering patients for an anterolateral thigh (ALT) flap, outside of inquiring about prior hip surgery or vascular surgery of the lower extremity, the other primary consideration is the patient's body habitus and fat distribution. For floor of mouth repair, it is ideal to have minimal subcutaneous fat to allow for a more supple flap and less restriction of motion of the adjacent tongue.

18.3 Anatomic Considerations/ Relevant Anatomy

Anatomically, the floor of the mouth extends from the lingual surface of the fixed gingiva of the mandible to the ventral surface of the tongue, with its posterior extent defined by the glossotonsillar fold (▶ Fig. 18.1).

Its inferior support is made up of a complex muscular sling including the mylohyoid muscle as well as additional contributions from the genioglossus, geniohyoid, and hyoglossus muscles. Lying deep to the mucosa and on top of the muscular floor are the sublingual glands, a network of veins, and the lingual nerves, as well as the paired submandibular ducts, which terminate near the midline at their respective papillae. Just beneath these structures course the terminal branches of the hypoglossal nerve providing motor function to the tongue musculature.

The mucosal surface of the floor of the mouth is redundant, creating a gravity-dependent sulcus that serves as a reservoir for food and liquid and also helps provide laxity and freedom to allow the tongue to move independently from the adjacent, more rigid mandible. Such tongue mobility is critical during mastication for food manipulation (▶ Fig. 18.2). It also allows for optimal bolus formation and transit to the oropharynx early during deglutition as the tongue moves toward the hard palate. With regard to speech, adequate tongue mobility is necessary to allow for articulation and clear pronunciation. More specifically, consonant sounds such as “K” and “T” can be particularly challenging in the absence of full tongue-tip mobility.

18.4 Surgical Considerations and Approaches

18.4.1 Management of the Sublingual and Submandibular Glands

The floor of the mouth, as previously discussed, contains the paired sublingual glands that empty either into the adjacent submandibular duct or through a network of smaller ducts directly to the surface above. In instances of floor of mouth resection, when possible, care should be made to minimize burying of sublingual salivary tissue in an attempt to avoid ranula formation. This may require removal of portions of the gland that have been unroofed.

Management of the submandibular ducts, when the associated gland has not been removed, requires reimplantation of the ducts by way of a sialodochoplasty. To accomplish this, the duct is ideally cannulated with a lacrimal probe to identify its tract. Once the mucosal resection is completed, the duct can be marsupialized with fine scissors or a scalpel. An initial absorbable anchoring suture is placed through the apex of the superficial aspect of the proximal portion of the duct to the adjacent mucosal edge, with additional sutures being placed to tack the other portions of the wall open to maximize patency. If needed, an angiocatheter can be placed for 1 to 2 weeks as a stent. ▶ Fig. 18.3 demonstrates a well-healed result of a bilateral submandibular duct sialodochoplasty following resection of an anterior floor of mouth carcinoma in situ.

18.4.2 Goals of Reconstruction and Development of a Reconstructive Algorithm

The primary goals of floor of mouth repair include the following:

- Create a watertight closure of the floor of the mouth.
- Replace missing mucosal areas with an epithelial-lined surface to allow for redundancy.
- Provide adequate bulk and support for the adjacent tongue musculature.

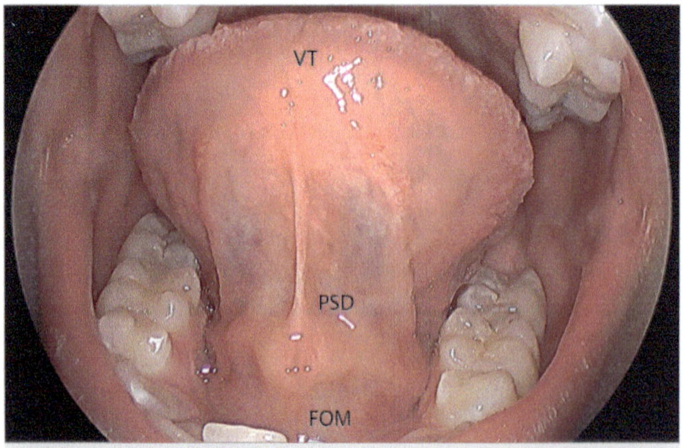

Fig. 18.1 This transoral photograph of the oral cavity demonstrates the relationship of the floor of mouth mucosa (FOM) with the mandible, ventral tongue (VT), and paired submandibular ducts (PSD).

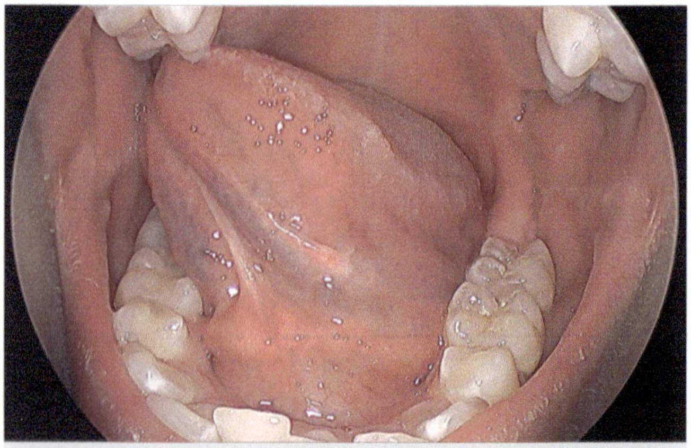

Fig. 18.2 This intramural photograph shows how the redundant floor of mouth mucosa allows for mobility of the oral tongue. This range of motion is critical for speech and articulation and assist with food manipulation during mastication.

To accomplish these goals, methods can range from simple to complex. Very limited surface defects with no communication with the neck can be closed primarily or left open to heal by secondary intention. For more significant resections, options include split-thickness skin grafts, local tissue rearrangement, regional rotational flaps, and free tissue transfer. For all graft inset and intraoral closure, absorbable sutures are typically employed using 3–0 vicryl sutures in either a simple or a horizontal mattress fashion. In situations where there is adequate cuff of mobile floor of mouth mucosa to allow for repair, the fixed gingiva on the lingual surface of the mandible can be resected to allow for circumdental sutures (dentulous patients) or repair to the fixed gingiva on the top of the alveolar ridge. This allows for more robust tissue to support the stitch and also prevents the suture line from being in the gravity-dependent sulcus of the floor of the mouth.

18.4.3 Reconstructive Techniques

Local Tissue Closure

In instances where there is limited mucosal loss and no communication with the adjacent neck dissection wound, the defect can be closed primarily or left to heal using secondary intention. In such circumstances, it is critical to ensure that there is adequate mobile mucosa still remaining in this portion of the floor of the mouth and also that the defect does not significantly extend onto the lateral tongue in order to minimize tethering and associated oral dysphagia and dysarthria. This is especially important in dentulous patients as the resulting tongue deviation on protrusion will often result in significant trauma to the adjacent mucosal surface.

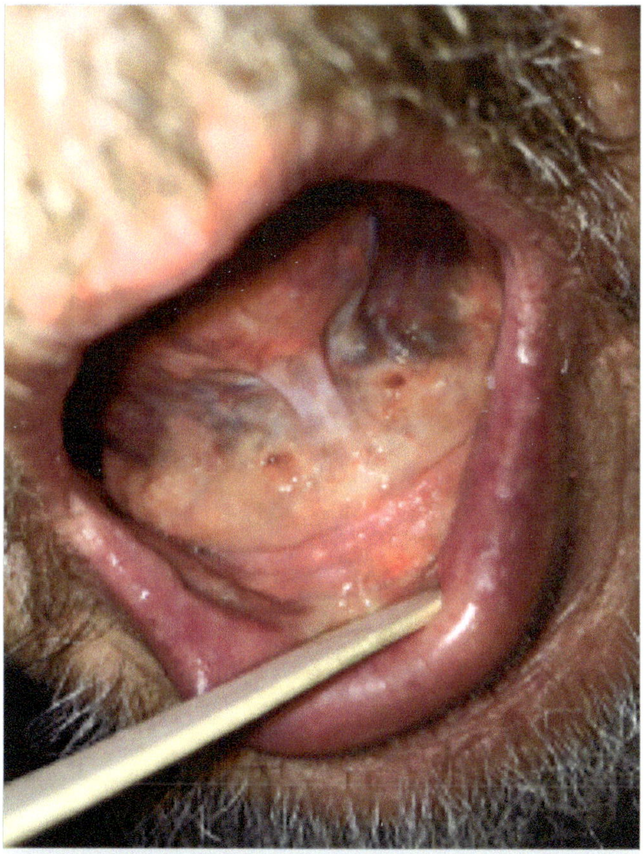

Fig. 18.3 This is a transoral view of a patient who underwent a resection of an anterior floor of mouth carcinoma in situ involving both of the submandibular duct papillae. The healed sites of the bilateral sialodochoplasties can be seen on this photo taken 6 months after surgery.

Skin Graft Closure

For larger mucosal defects that lack significant bone exposure or communication with the neck wound, a split-thickness skin graft can be employed. The purpose of the graft is to create an epithelial surface to minimize associated contracture and limitations in tongue mobility. In these instances, the graft is typically harvested as a split-thickness autograft from the thigh using a dermatome with the depth of harvest being between 0.015 and 0.0175 inches. The graft is then conservatively pie crusted to avoid fluid accumulating deep to the graft and interfering with the initial imbibition phase of healing. In all instances, it is critical to harvest a graft of adequate size to allow for significant redundancy. Once secured in place with absorbable sutures, a bolster should be secured to apply pressure to the graft, keeping it flush with the underlying muscular wound bed. The bolster can then be removed in the office on postoperative day 7. When needed, a sialodochoplasty can also be performed, placing the duct at the periphery of the graft or through a hole created within it. ▶ Fig. 18.4 shows a floor of mouth defect that was repaired with a split-thickness skin graft.

Regional Flap Closure

Locoregional flaps (LrFs) have regained popularity for closure of head and neck defects. There are multiple options for LrFs, each with their own benefits and disadvantages. LrFs are often touted

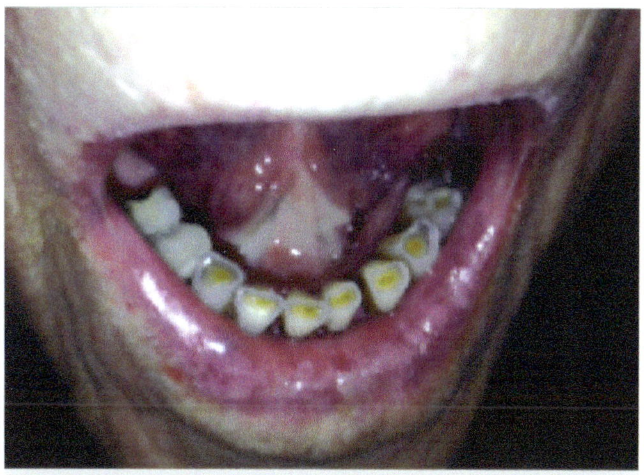

Fig. 18.4 This is a transoral photograph taken 6 months after a patient underwent resection of a small T1N0M0 squamous cell carcinoma of the anterior floor of the mouth with split-thickness skin graft repair. The maintenance of the laxity of the region with the graft allows for excellent tongue mobility.

as an equivalent replacement for a free flap. However, although LrFs offer the ability to close large defects with robust, vascularized tissue, without the need for microvascular expertise, they still suffer from a few shortcomings and lack the adaptability that is offered by free flaps. Specifically, they can be limited by the length and degree of rotation of their vascular pedicle and may be affected by defect size and location. The benefits of LrF over free flaps include quicker harvest, less operative time,[5–7] shorter hospital stay, and decreased health care costs.[8]

Submental Island Flap

The submental island flap is a commonly used regional flap for reconstruction of the oral cavity. Its vascular supply is the submental artery that branches off the facial artery. The skin can easily be rotated into the oral cavity to fill defects.[9] One of the main critiques of the submental island flap for reconstruction after oral cavity cancer is risk of leaving pathological nodal disease in level I of the neck. However, if level I is shown to be clinically negative for disease, the submental island flap can still be used and the harvest of the flap allows for an appropriate level Ia and Ib neck dissection without compromising the flap pedicle.[10] A retrospective study by Howard et al showed that patients undergoing a submental island flap after oral cancer resection did not have an increased risk of locoregional recurrence.[11]

The submental island flap can provide a large skin paddle of up to 11 × 11 cm[9] and the pedicle length is 5 cm, but it can be longer if the facial artery and vein are ligated distal to the takeoff of the submental vessels.[12] The boundaries of the skin that can be harvested include the lower border of the mandible to the hyoid and from angle to angle of the mandible. Although variations in harvest technique are described, the general steps are as follows:[9,11,12]

- The skin paddle is designed to fit the necessary defect.
- The skin incision through the inferior edge of flap is performed and subplatysmal flaps are elevated.
- The marginal mandibular nerve is found and preserved.
- The facial artery is found as it traces over the mandible and then the submental arteries are identified branching off the facial and are traced to the anterior belly of the digastric.
- The level I neck dissection can be completed, preserving the facial and submental vessels.
- The anterior flap incision can be made and the mandibular attachment of the anterior belly of the digastric can be divided to help protect the pedicle. The depth of the flap dissection is to the mylohyoid muscle with branches of the submental artery supplying the mylohyoid needing to be ligated.
- Once the flap is elevated, if necessary, any remaining nodal contents can be cleared carefully from the adjacent pedicle before being rotated into oral cavity for inset.
- The donor site can be closed primarily.

Facial Artery Musculomucosal Flap

The facial artery myomucosal (FAMM) flap is another well-described flap for reconstruction of the oral cavity.[13] Indications for its use would be to cover smaller defects on the side of the floor of the mouth ipsilateral to the flap, as the size of the flap is generally limited to a width of 3 cm. Contraindications for the flap would be large defects, spread of disease onto buccal mucosa, or compromise of facial artery due to nodal disease or surgical resection.[13,14]

The harvest of the FAMM flap is done entirely transorally. The limits of the flap are within 1 cm of the oral commissure and anterior to Stensen's duct. It can be raised as a superiorly[14] or inferiorly based flap[13] with the limits of the harvest being the inferior and superior gingival sulci. The key step is to identify the facial artery and this can be done at the anterior or posterior incision of the flap. The artery lies deep to the buccinator muscle and the flap is harvested in a plane deep to the artery. The artery must stay attached to the more superficial tissues to maintain vascularity and the venous drainage is based on submucosal venous plexus. Once the flap is harvested, it can be rotated into position. The pedicle can be ligated between from 13 and 21 days after inset; however, techniques have been described to tunnel the pedicle to avoid needed ligation.[15] Closure of the defect site can be done primarily if it is under 3 cm. If it is too large to close primarily, it can be left to granulate or closed using a buccal fat pad transposition flap.

Supraclavicular Island Flap

The supraclavicular island flap is a popular LrF being used with increased frequency by head and neck surgeons and has shown application in floor of mouth reconstruction.[5,16] It offers the benefit of a fast and relative easy harvest, can reconstruct large defects, has little hair, and is rarely affected by metastatic disease.[17] Contraindications for the flap would be if the defect cannot be reached by the pedicle, if the pedicle is absent, or if the pedicle is compromised during the neck dissection.[16,17]

The harvest of the flap begins with using a Doppler to identify the supraclavicular artery, which is a branch of the thyrocervical trunk. It can be located in the triangle created by the sternocleidomastoid muscle, clavicle, and external jugular vein. The artery can then be marked out heading laterally over the supraclavicular fossa eventually crossing the clavicle. The length of the skin that can be taken has been described to extend reliably up to 5 cm past the most distal portion of the pedicle Doppler signal.[6] However, the longer the flap, the greater the risk of necrosis. Using the triangle previously mapped out as a fulcrum point, a gauze or something similar can be used to estimate the length of flap needed to reach the defect site. Once the pedicle is designed, skin incisions are made. The distal portion of the flap can be raised supra- or subfascially to the fascia overlying the deltoid muscle. The flap is raised up in this plane up to the pedicle found medial to the inferolateral border of the trapezius muscle. The flap is then tunneled through the neck to the oral cavity. The superficial plane of dissection above the clavicle is in the supraplatysmal plane to avoid injury to the contributing vascularity.[16,17]

Platysma Flap

The platysma flap is a less frequently used regional flap, but it offers a reliable myocutaneous reconstruction option for oral cavity reconstruction.[7,18–20] It can be used even if a neck dissection is being performed on the ipsilateral side.[19] Its use is typically contraindicated in a previously radiated neck or if there is neck disease involving the overlying platysma. Debate remains whether the facial artery needs to remain intact to ensure flap survival, but ideally the submental artery and veins are left in continuity with the flap.[19,21]

Flap elevation begins with designing the skin paddle over the lateral neck. The paddle is then incised staying supraplatysmal. Supraplatysmal skin flaps are then raised to the mandible. Next the skin paddle is raised with the underlying platysma, raising a subplatysmal flap. The external jugular vein is ligated distally and left attached to the platysma to allow for retrograde venous drainage and ideally the submental branches of the facial artery and vein are left in continuity with the flap to allow for optimal vascularity. The flap can then be inset into the oral cavity defect. The donor site scar is similar to that of a standard neck dissection.[19,21]

Nasolabial Flap

The nasolabial flap is a well-known pedicled option for nasal and facial reconstruction; however, it has also been described for intraoral defects.[22] The benefits of the flap are that the incision lines are well hidden and do not interfere with the neck dissection, and it is within the same surgical field. The disadvantages of using the flap for floor of mouth defects are that it can only be used on smaller defects, it is not an option for dentulous patients, and that a second-stage pedicle takedown procedure is required.

The flap is raised in the same manner as one would for reconstructing facial defects. The flap is raised superficial to the facial musculature. The maximum dimensions are 3.5 × 9 cm.[22,23] Once the flap is raised, a tunnel is bluntly dissected into the oral cavity to avoid damage to the facial nerve and artery. The flap is then rotated into the defect site. The portion of the flap that is in the tunnel is de-epithelized in order to avoid buried epithelium.[23]

Free Tissue Closure

Free tissue transfer is the most complex reconstructive option for floor of mouth defects. Although there are no definite indications for free-flap reconstruction, common reasons include the following: large defects with minimal remaining mobile floor of mouth mucosa attached to the fixed gingiva, resection after radiation failure, or composite reconstruction resulting in a through-and-through defect into an associated neck dissection wound. Many options exist for free-flap reconstruction, each with their own advantages and disadvantages. Generally, when reconstructing the floor of the mouth a flap should be chosen that has a thin and pliable skin paddle, a decent length vascular pedicle, and the option of incorporating soft tissue into the flap to add bulk. The two most common soft-tissue flaps used to reconstruct the floor of the mouth are the radial forearm and anterolateral free flap.

Radial Forearm Free Flap

The RFFF is the most commonly described free flap for FOM reconstruction.[24–26] The pliable skin paddle allows the flap to be inset into most defects without being too bulky to inhibit eating, swallowing, and speech. The pedicle, based on the radial artery, associated venae comitantes, and the cephalic vein, is fairly long, which allows access to vessels on both sides of the neck if needed. Often with FOM resections, a dead space is created inferior to the free flap where the contents of the level I neck dissection were removed. In such instances, subcutaneous tissue in the proximal forearm can be incorporated into the RFFF to fill this space, described as the "beavertail" modification (▸ Fig. 18.5). This tissue can also be utilized to increase the bulk to the reconstruction in patients undergoing a partial glossectomy as a part of their resection.

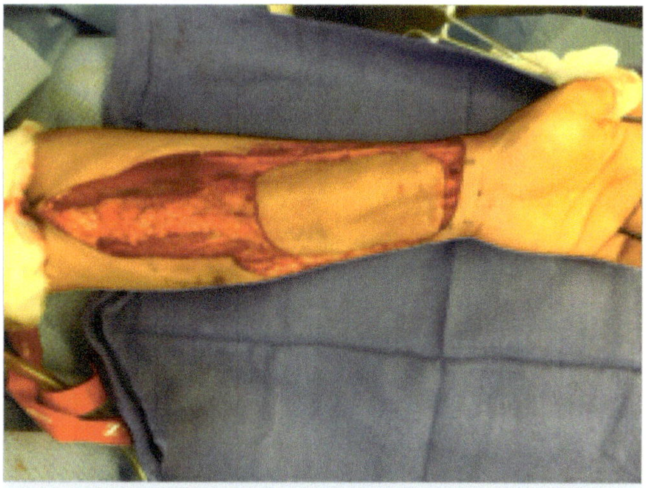

Fig. 18.5 When raising a radial forearm free flap, if additional bulk is needed, the subcutaneous fat can be harvested along with the proximal pedicle ("beavertail modification"). This can be used to obliterate any submental dead space resulting from the resection.

An additional adaption of flap design is the use of a bilobed skin paddle to allow for one apex to be inset into the floor of the mouth and the other relining the ventral tongue to allow for optimal mobility of the adjacent tongue[26] (▸ Fig. 18.6). The associated donor site is typically closed with a split- or full-thickness skin graft, with primary closure of the proximal incision.[27]

Anterolateral Thigh Free Flap

The ALT free flap is another commonly used flap in floor of mouth reconstruction. It offers the possibility of a large, modifiable skin paddle with soft-tissue bulk and a pedicle length of 8 cm.[28] The artery is the descending branch of the lateral circumflex femoral and the venous drainage is through paired venae comitantes.[29–31] A benefit of the ALT over RFFF is the availability of increased bulk and decreased donor site morbidity. However, in defects limited to the floor of the mouth, this increased bulk can sometimes be detrimental and may even limit tongue mobility and cause mass effect on the oral and oropharyngeal airway. An additional disadvantage is the potential for variability of the perforator vascular supply that can result in an increased challenge with harvest.[32] When using the ALT for floor of mouth reconstruction, the thigh skin should be examined prior to harvest to assess the thickness. In thin patients such as those in the East Asian population where it was initially described,[30] the skin can be appropriately thin. It should also be noted that the skin paddle is often thinner with less subcutaneous fat in the distal portion of the leg, while thicker more proximally. Therefore, the skin paddle could be designed to incorporate the distal skin, if perforating vessel anatomy allows.

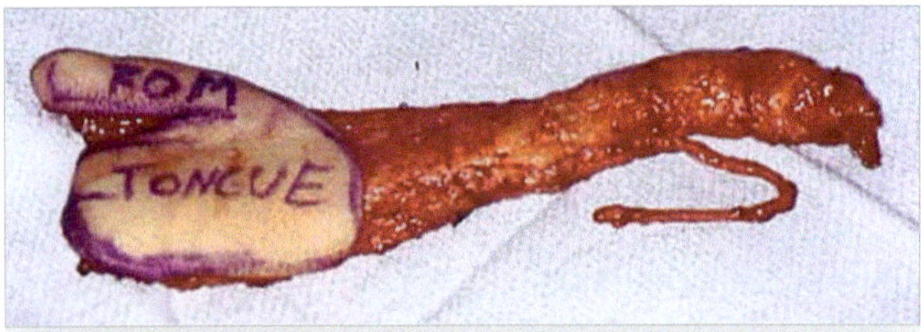

Fig. 18.6 This image depicts a radial forearm free flap with a bilobed skin paddle. Such a design can be used for defects involving the floor of the mouth as well as the adjacent ventral or lateral tongue to optimize mobility of the anterior tongue. (Reproduced with permission of Dr. Neal Futran.)

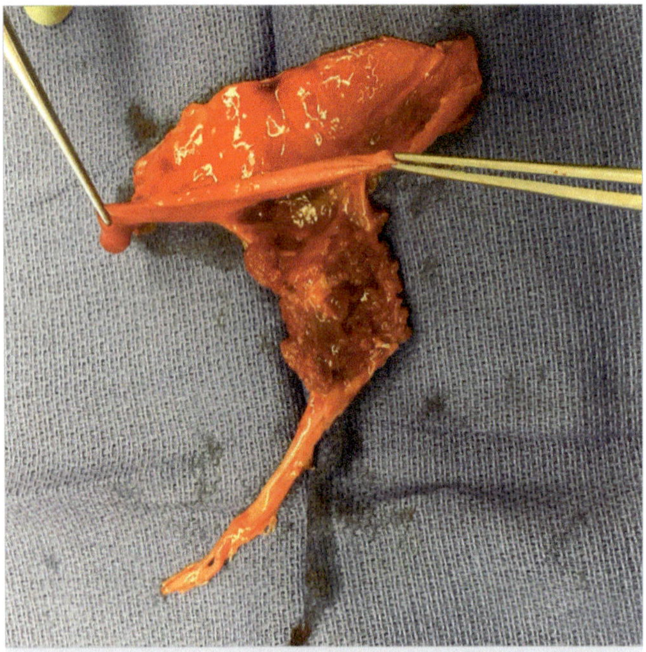

Fig. 18.7 The fascia lata myofascial flap is a modification of the anterolateral thigh free flap that can be used to reline the floor of the mouth and fill the submental dead space in instances where the thigh is too bulky to incorporate skin. Such reconstructions are more prone to contracture than skin-containing free flaps. (Reproduced with permission of Dr. Arnaud Bewley.)

If the skin paddle is deemed too thick, a fascia lata myofascial flap can be considered. Using the vastus lateralis as a free myofascial tissue flap has been described for FOM and tongue reconstruction.[33] It offers the benefits of the ALT without the bulkiness associated with the skin paddle (▶ Fig. 18.7). Downsides of the fascia-only flap have been shrinkage and contracture of the flap. Harvesting a larger flap and/or innervating the flap to prevent muscle atrophy may compensate for this.[33]

Ulnar Free Flap

Another free flap utilized for FOM reconstruction is the ulnar artery free flap. It offers many of the advantages of the RFFF with few disadvantages. It provides a large, pliable, and thin skin paddle. It is also often free of hair, unlike the RFFF. If needed, bone can also be harvested with it.[34] It results in a similar donor defect as the RFFF; however, there is a lower reported rate of tendon exposure compared to the RFFF. One disadvantage is that the ulnar nerve and artery are closely related, with the artery giving multiple branches to vascularize the nerve. This vascular pattern mandates a more delicate elevation of the flap, compared to the RFFF.[35]

Other Free Flap Options

Less commonly used flaps for isolated floor of mouth defects include the scapular and parascapular fasciocutaneous flaps. While these flaps can provide versatile options for a large variety of bony and soft-tissue defects, the thickness of skin on the back make them less ideal for this type of repair. Moreover, due to the location on the shoulder, the ability to perform a two-team approach to optimize efficiency is more limited.

18.5 Perioperative Management

Postoperative care following floor of mouth reconstruction should be tailored based on the extent of the oncologic resection and repair. For limited resections with primary closure or wounds left open to granulate without communication to the neck wound, patients can be allowed to start an oral diet immediately postoperatively. Often full liquids or a soft mechanical diet is ideal to start, advancing when appropriate. In such instances, chlorhexidine mouth rinse can be used three times daily and after food to provide topical antibacterial coverage.

In instances where a split-thickness skin graft is used, a xeroform bolster can be placed to keep the graft flush with the underlying wound bed. These patients should be maintained on a liquid diet or with a nasogastric tube for nutrition, with regular antibiotic mouth rinse. The bolster can then be removed in the office around 1 week postoperatively, at which time the diet can be slowly advanced.

For regional or free tissue transfer repair, patients should be covered with 24 hours of perioperative systemic antibiotic coverage for gram-positive, gram-negative, and anaerobic organisms.[36,37] Unless contraindicated for medical reasons, 24 hours of postoperative steroids should also be used to minimize associated edema and the risk for pedicle compression. To allow for initial healing of intraoral suture line, patients are typically restricted to nothing per os (NPO) for 5 to 7 days postoperatively, providing nutrition via a nasogastric tube. Following this initial period, if the suture line remains intact, they should be assessed by a speech and swallowing team regarding the safety for starting oral intake.

18.5.1 Speech and Swallowing Rehabilitation

Following removal of floor of mouth tumors and the subsequent reconstruction, optimal speech and swallowing function necessitates continued therapy to assist in recovering tongue strength and range of motion. In most instances, it is appropriate to work in conjunction with a certified speech-language pathologist. Prior to initiating therapy, as detailed earlier, it is important for there to be a detailed assessment of the integrity of the healing of the wound to ensure that such exercises will not result in wound separation or disruption of healing. This is of particular importance in patients undergoing split-thickness skin graft placement as the success of the graft depends on a stable vascularized wound bed with minimal shear forces placed across the area for the first week after placement. Similar measures are also taken after regional or free-flap reconstruction in order to minimize the risk of fistula formation. After this initial period of observation, the patient should start regular active exercises that are meant to optimize tongue protrusion and lateral movement.

18.6 Surgical Sequelae

18.6.1 Head and Neck Sequelae

Following reconstruction of the floor of the mouth, the largest impact tends to be speech and swallowing function, with particular detriment in certain types of fine articulation, as described earlier. Additional side effects can include obstruction of submandibular duct drainage (in patients where the glands are preserved) or drooling, related to the loss of the natural floor of mouth sulcus. An additional consideration is the challenge for dental rehabilitation in patients with missing or extracted teeth. Due to blunting of the floor of the mouth and the consequent relative loss of height of the mandibular alveolar ridge, maintenance of partial or complete lower dentures can be particularly challenging. In some instances, delayed debulking procedures may be needed to optimize the gingival contour.

18.6.2 Donor Site Sequelae

One of the biggest critiques of the RFFF is the donor site morbidity,[38] which generally requires a skin graft from the thigh for skin closure.[39] This causes additional donor site discomfort, the risk of tendon exposure, and, in some individuals, loss of strength and dexterity in the donor hand.[38] Several techniques have been described to avoid the donor site morbidity including skin graft harvesting from the planned donor site prior to flap elevation[40] and closure with adjacent tissue rearrangement.[41]

For ALT free flaps, the donor defect can typically be closed primarily. The most common morbidities include lateral thigh paresthesia (24%) and musculoskeletal dysfunction (4.8%) and seroma (2.4%) formation postoperatively.[42] Compartment syndrome is very rare. It has been found that suprafascial dissection and preservation of the lateral femoral cutaneous nerve branches decreases paresthesias and improves patient satisfaction.[42,43]

Key Points

- The floor of the mouth is a mucosally lined subsite that allows laxity and freedom of tongue movement from the adjacent mandible.
- Defect analysis should include an assessment of the amount and location of mucosa lost, whether or not the submandibular ducts are involved, the amount of floor of mouth musculature resected, and if there is a communication with the underlying neck wound.
- Goals of reconstruction include obtaining a watertight closure, maintaining redundancy of the floor of the mouth, and providing adequate bulk and support.
- Small and intermediate defects can be closed primarily or with skin grafting.
- Larger defects and those with communication with the neck require an LrF or a free flap for repair.
- A commonly used LrF for floor of mouth repair is the submental island flap.
- The RFFF provides excellent pliable skin for repair with minimal bulk.
- The ALT free flap can be used in instances where more soft-tissue volume is required.
- Following an initial period of healing, rehabilitation through the direction of a speech-language pathologist can optimize postoperative speech and swallowing function.

References

[1] Ejrup B, Fischer B, Wright IS. Clinical evaluation of blood flow to the hand. The false-positive Allen test. Circulation. 1966; 33(5):778–780

[2] Ciria-Lloréns G, Gómez-Cia T. Hand blood supply in radial forearm flap donor extremities: a qualitative analysis using doppler examination. J Hand Surg [Br]. 2001; 26(2):125–128

[3] Dost P, Rudofsky G. Doppler ultrasonography as a pre-operative aid to base the forearm flap on the radial or ulnar artery. Clin Otolaryngol Allied Sci. 1993; 18(5):355–358

[4] Barbeau GR, Arsenault F, Dugas L, Simard S, Larivière MM. Evaluation of the ulnopalmar arterial arches with pulse oximetry and plethysmography: comparison with the Allen's test in 1010 patients. Am Heart J. 2004; 147(3):489–493

[5] Welz C, Canis M, Schwenk-Zieger S, Spiegel JL, Weiss BG, Pilavakis Y. Oral cancer reconstruction using the supraclavicular artery island flap: comparison to free radial forearm flap. J Oral Maxillofac Surg. 2017; 75(10): 2261–2269

[6] Granzow JW, Suliman A, Roostaeian J, Perry A, Boyd JB. Supraclavicular artery island flap (SCAIF) vs free fasciocutaneous flaps for head and neck reconstruction. Otolaryngol Head Neck Surg. 2013; 148(6):941–948

[7] Wang KH, Hsu EK, Shemen LJ. Platysma myocutaneous flap for oral cavity reconstruction. Ear Nose Throat J. 2010; 89(6):276–279

[8] Forner D, Phillips T, Rigby M, Hart R, Taylor M, Trites J. Submental island flap reconstruction reduces cost in oral cancer reconstruction compared to radial forearm free flap reconstruction: a case series and cost analysis. J Otolaryngol Head Neck Surg. 2016; 45:11

[9] Eskander A, Strigenz D, Seim N, Ozer E. Submental artery island flap with simultaneous level I neck dissection. Head Neck. 2018; 40(4):842–845

[10] Thomas S, Varghese BT, Ganesh SA, et al. Oncological safety of submental artery island flap in oral reconstruction: analysis of 229 cases. Indian J Surg Oncol. 2016; 7(4):420–424

[11] Howard BE, Nagel TH, Donald CB, Hinni ML, Hayden RE. Oncologic safety of the submental flap for reconstruction in oral cavity malignancies. Otolaryngol Head Neck Surg. 2014; 150(4):558–562

[12] Sebastian P, Thomas S, Varghese BT, Iype EM, Balagopal PG, Mathew PC. The submental island flap for reconstruction of intraoral defects in oral cancer patients. Oral Oncol. 2008; 44(11):1014–1018

[13] Ayad T, Kolb F, De Monés E, Mamelle G, Temam S. Reconstruction of floor of mouth defects by the facial artery musculo-mucosal flap following cancer ablation. Head Neck. 2008; 30(4):437–445

[14] Berania I, Lavigne F, Rahal A, Ayad T. Superiorly based facial artery musculomucosal flap: a versatile pedicled flap. Head Neck. 2018; 40(2):402–405

[15] Duranceau M, Ayad T. The facial artery musculomucosal flap: modification of the harvesting technique for a single-stage procedure. Laryngoscope. 2011; 121(12):2586–2589

[16] Trautman J, et al. Supraclavicular flap repair in the free flap era. ANZ J Surg. 2018; 88(6):540–546

[17] Granzow JW, Suliman A, Roostaeian J, Perry A, Boyd JB. The supraclavicular artery island flap (SCAIF) for head and neck reconstruction: surgical technique and refinements. Otolaryngol Head Neck Surg. 2013; 148(6):933–940
[18] Künzel J, Iro H, Psychogios G, Zenk J, Koch M. Closure of defects after resection of tumors of the oral cavity and the pharynx: medium- to long-term oncologic and functional results with the myocutaneous platysma flap. Eur Arch Otorhinolaryngol. 2013; 270(9):2537–2545
[19] Manni JJ, Bruaset I. Reconstruction of the anterior oral cavity using the platysma myocutaneous island flap. Laryngoscope. 1986; 96(5):564–567
[20] Bande C, Joshi A, Gawande M, Tiwari M, Rode V. Utility of superiorly based platysma myocutaneous flap for reconstruction of intraoral surgical defects: our experience. Oral Maxillofac Surg. 2018; 22(1):45–51
[21] Eckardt AM. Platysma myocutaneous flap: its current role in reconstructive surgery of oral soft tissue defects. J Korean Assoc Oral Maxillofac Surg. 2013; 39(1):3–8
[22] Ducic Y, Burye M. Nasolabial flap reconstruction of oral cavity defects: a report of 18 cases. J Oral Maxillofac Surg. 2000; 58(10):1104–1108, discussion 1108–1109
[23] Mebeed AH, Hussein HA, Saber TKh. Critical appraisal of nasolabial flap for reconstruction of oral cavity defects in cancer patients. J Egypt Natl Canc Inst. 2009; 21(1):33–42
[24] Matthews RN, Hodge RA, Eyre J, Davies DM, Walsh-Waring GP. Radial forearm flap for floor of mouth reconstruction. Br J Surg. 1985; 72(7):561–564
[25] Henry A, McCaul JA. Osseocutaneous radial forearm flap with beavertail modification; a case report of a novel, single, reconstructive free flap for the tongue, floor of mouth and mandible. Int J Surg Case Rep. 2016; 28:270–273
[26] Ko AB, Lavertu P, Rezaee RP. Double bilobed radial forearm free flap for anterior tongue and floor-of-mouth reconstruction. Ear Nose Throat J. 2010; 89 (4):177–179
[27] Zuidam JM, Coert JH, Hofer SO. Closure of the donor site of the free radial forearm flap: a comparison of full-thickness graft and split-thickness skin graft. Ann Plast Surg. 2005; 55(6):612–616
[28] Kim JW, Kim DY, Ahn KM, Lee JH. Surgical implications of anatomical variation in anterolateral thigh flaps for the reconstruction of oral and maxillofacial soft tissue defects: focus on perforators and pedicles. J Korean Assoc Oral Maxillofac Surg. 2016; 42(5):265–270
[29] Boahene K, Richmon J, Sultan B, Fakhry C, Byrne P. A novel step in the anterolateral thigh free flap harvest. Otolaryngol Head Neck Surg. 2010; 142(6): 909–910
[30] Song YG, Chen GZ, Song YL. The free thigh flap: a new free flap concept based on the septocutaneous artery. Br J Plast Surg. 1984; 37(2):149–159
[31] Demirkan F, Chen HC, Wei FC, et al. The versatile anterolateral thigh flap: a musculocutaneous flap in disguise in head and neck reconstruction. Br J Plast Surg. 2000; 53(1):30–36
[32] Lee YC, Chen WC, Chou TM, Shieh SJ. Anatomical variability of the anterolateral thigh flap perforators: vascular anatomy and its clinical implications. Plast Reconstr Surg. 2015; 135(4):1097–1107
[33] Wang L, Liu K, Shao Z, Shang ZJ. Reconstruction of the tongue and mouth floor with the myofascial vastus lateralis free flap after cancer ablation. Int J Oral Maxillofac Surg. 2016; 45(8):951–954
[34] Lin CH, Liao CT, Lin CH, Tan BK, Lee CT. Ulnar forearm osteocutaneous flap harvesting using Kapandji procedure for pre-existing complicated fibular flap on mandible reconstruction-cadaveric and clinical study. Ann Plast Surg. 2015; 74 Suppl 2:S152–S157
[35] Wax MK, Rosenthal EL, Winslow CP, Bascom DA, Andersen PE. The ulnar fasciocutaneous free flap in head and neck reconstruction. Laryngoscope. 2002; 112(12):2155–2160
[36] Dort JC, Farwell DG, Findlay M, et al. Optimal perioperative care in major head and neck cancer surgery with free flap reconstruction: a consensus review and recommendations from the enhanced recovery after surgery society. JAMA Otolaryngol Head Neck Surg. 2017; 143(3):292–303
[37] Rodrigo JP, Alvarez JC, Gómez JR, Suárez C, Fernández JA, Martínez JA. Comparison of three prophylactic antibiotic regimens in clean-contaminated head and neck surgery. Head Neck. 1997; 19(3):188–193
[38] Orlik JR, Horwich P, Bartlett C, Trites J, Hart R, Taylor SM. Long-term functional donor site morbidity of the free radial forearm flap in head and neck cancer survivors. J Otolaryngol Head Neck Surg. 2014; 43:1
[39] Emerick KS, Deschler DG. Incidence of donor site skin graft loss requiring surgical intervention with the radial forearm free flap. Head Neck. 2007; 29(6): 573–576
[40] Riecke B, Assaf AT, Heiland M, et al. Local full-thickness skin graft of the donor arm: a novel technique for the reduction of donor site morbidity in radial forearm free flap. Int J Oral Maxillofac Surg. 2015; 44(8):937–941
[41] Jaquet Y, Enepekides DJ, Torgerson C, Higgins KM. Radial forearm free flap donor site morbidity: ulnar-based transposition flap vs split-thickness skin graft. Arch Otolaryngol Head Neck Surg. 2012; 138(1):38–43
[42] Collins J, Ayeni O, Thoma A. A systematic review of anterolateral thigh flap donor site morbidity. Can J Plast Surg. 2012; 20(1):17–23
[43] Chen YC, Scaglioni MF, Carrillo Jimenez LE, Yang JC, Huang EY, Lin TS. Suprafascial anterolateral thigh flap harvest: a better way to minimize donor-site morbidity in head and neck reconstruction. Plast Reconstr Surg. 2016; 138 (3):689–698

19 Squamous Cell Carcinoma of the Buccal Mucosa

Anthony P. Tufaro and Christine G. Gourin

Summary

Buccal cancers represent an aggressive oral cavity subsite with a propensity for early spread because of a lack of anatomic barriers, early nodal involvement, and difficulty achieving wide margins. Treatment is primarily surgical and often requires reconstruction and adjuvant therapy. Rehabilitation of swallowing and trismus is key in mitigating late dysphagia.

Keywords: buccal cancer, oral cancer, surgery, reconstruction

19.1 Epidemiology

Oral cancer comprises 3 to 4% of all cancers and 3 to 4% of all cancer deaths globally.[1] Carcinomas arising from the buccal mucosa are a subsite of oral cavity cancers that show marked geographic differences in incidence and presentation. Cancer of the buccal mucosa is relatively uncommon in North America and Western Europe, accounting for only 6% of all oral cavity cancers and 0.2% of all cancers in the United States in 2018.[1] However, the incidence of oral cancer is significantly higher in the Indian subcontinent and southern Asia, where oral cancer is the most common cancer, comprising more than 30% of all cancer cases, with the buccal mucosa the most common site for oral cavity cancer.[2–4] In India, buccal carcinoma is the most common cancer in men and the third most common cancer in women.

Squamous cell cancer comprises 95% of buccal cancers, with the remainder of buccal tumors arising from minor salivary glands.[5] There is a male predominance for this disease, with a male-to-female ratio of 3 to 4:1 in most large series.[4,6–11] While it has been suggested that the incidence in females is greater in North American compared to Asian populations, contemporary data demonstrate a male predominance in the West that is similar to that reported in Asian countries.[1,2,12–14] Buccal cancer most commonly presents in patients in the sixth or seventh decade of life; however, large series from India and Taiwan demonstrate a younger age at diagnosis, which likely reflects differences in tobacco product use, the primary etiologic agent.[3,6,11]

Tobacco use has been documented in more than 70% of patients, regardless of geographic origin, and the combined use of alcohol with tobacco has a well-known synergistic effect in the development of mucosal cancers in North America.[4,8,13] In Asia, hand-rolled tobacco products called bidis and betel quid, a combination of tobacco leaves and betel nut, are popular masticatory products that are associated with the development of buccal carcinoma.[6,7,14] In India, betel nut users have an incidence of buccal carcinoma about eight times greater than the general population, and immigrants from India to Western countries have a higher rate of buccal cancer than the host population.[2] Betel nut is a paste made primarily of the fruit of the areca palm, which is mixed with tobacco, powdered lime, and a number of other irritants and chewed.[15] It is said that the use of betel nut can induce a mild state of euphoria. Over 90% of Indian patients with buccal carcinoma have a history of betel nut use. Patients who use these products present with buccal mucosal carcinoma at a much younger age, usually younger than 50 years of age. These malignancies are most frequently located on the occlusal line or the lower gingivobuccal sulcus, which is the site where the betel nut bolus is placed. Reverse smoking, a popular habit in Asia, also induces keratosis in addition to the carcinogenic risks associated with smoking. As is often seen in the development and progression of malignancy, inflammation plays a very significant role. The agents that are mixed together with the tobacco cause a significant inflammatory response in the mucosa and submucosa, which then leads to a dense fibrosis and keratosis of the usually soft pliable tissues of the cheek. This can lead to the development of oral submucosal fibrosis as well as leukoplakia and other precancerous changes.[16]

Oral submucosal fibrosis has been associated with the development of buccal cancer. This condition is characterized by fibroelastic changes resulting in mucosal atrophy and the development of fibrotic bands that lead to scarring and trismus. Oral submucosal fibrosis is associated with tobacco and betel nut use, and appears to have a genetic predisposition, occurring more commonly in young Indian men.[17,18] Overall, the risk of malignant transformation in oral submucosal fibrosis is 8%, and oral submucosal fibrosis is associated with a 19-fold increase in the risk of oral cancer, with cancer arising in this setting more invasive and with a greater risk of metastases.[5]

Several precancerous oral lesions have been associated with the development of buccal squamous cell cancer.[5] Leukoplakia, which is often found on the buccal mucosa prior to a diagnosis of invasive squamous cell carcinoma, is a clinical term defined as a white patch or plaque that cannot be characterized clinically or pathologically as any other disease.[19] This lesion is usually associated with smoking and alcohol use. The prevalence of leukoplakia worldwide is between 2 and 3%. Dysplastic changes are seen in only 2 to 5% of patients. The overall rate of malignant transformation for leukoplakia is 3.5%; however, proliferative verrucous leukoplakia is reported to have a malignant transformation rate of 61% and is associated with multiple contiguous or noncontiguous areas of the oral cavity with verrucous features on biopsy.[5,19] Erythroplakia, which has the appearance of a velvety, bright red painless area or patch, is commonly associated with dysplasia and carcinoma in situ, with malignant transformation occurring in more than 50% of cases.[5]

Patients with oral lichen planus or oral lichenoid lesions involving the buccal mucosa have an increased risk for developing buccal cancer. Lichen planus and oral lichenoid lesions are common, immunologically mediated diseases of the oral mucosa, characterized by reticular white patches in atrophic mucosa that may have erosive or ulcerated areas and are associated with a malignant transformation rate of 1 to 3%, with an increased risk for the erosive subtype.[20,21] These lesions usually arise in middle-aged white females with histology characterized by lymphocytic infiltration, but there is no gender predisposition for malignant transformation, with males and females affected equally.[21] The risk of buccal cancer is increased in patients with lichenoid changes who use tobacco or alcohol. Verrucous carcinoma is a well-differentiated variant of buccal squamous cell carcinoma with a wartlike, verrucous appearance. These tumors may arise from preexisting oral lichenoid lesions and proliferative verrucous leukoplakia and may represent a continuum of these diseases, with a history of these precursor lesions in one-third of patients.[22]

19.2 Clinical Presentation

Patients with buccal carcinoma uncommonly present with pain or bleeding from the primary site in the early stages of the disease. The origins of the disease are often insidious unless there is concurrent infection or bleeding associated with a mucosal ulceration, and symptoms are generally not present until the tumor is at an advanced stage. The clinical presentation is often associated with a nonhealing mucosal ulceration, fullness or swelling of the cheek, trismus that can restrict the patient's normal daily functions of eating and speaking, or a mass in the submental or submandibular area, which is often indicative of nodal metastasis (▶ Fig. 19.1a). These clinical presenting signs indicate more advanced stage disease. Multiple areas of leukoplakia and other mucosal and submucosal changes may be associated with the inflammatory insult of topical irritants such as tobacco, alcohol, betel nut may be detected on routine dental evaluation and are usually asymptomatic. Risk factors for malignant transformation include presence of dysplasia, duration of the leukoplakia, and a size greater than 2 cm in a nonsmoker. Erythroplakia is associated with dysplasia and carcinoma in situ in more than 50% of cases.[5] Dysplasia is classified by degree from mild, moderate, severe, and finally carcinoma in situ, with many pathologists considering severe dysplasia and carcinoma in situ to be equivalent. Biopsies of these areas are indicated and are necessary to adequately plan the primary resection.

The incidence of early primary site disease varies widely, with the incidence of patients presenting with primary tumors ≤ 4 cm ranging from 18 to 91% in the literature.[3–5,8,10,12,15,23–26] However, the incidence of advanced primary site disease is higher in underdeveloped countries. In the largest series to date of 665 patients with buccal cancer treated at Tata Memorial Hospital in India, the primary tumor size was greater than 4 cm in 82% of cases.[8] Advanced tumor presentations are felt to be related to socioeconomic reasons with lack of access to care, as well as the relative lack of symptoms compared to other oral cancer sites in early stages of disease. Tumor thickness, rather than size, appears to be of greater importance for buccal cancer and increases the risk of early disease spread and local recurrence.[9,12,27] The buccal space has limited anatomic barriers to tumor spread, and thus even early-stage disease may involve the buccinator muscle in more than a third of cases and lead to trismus.[4] Careful examination, including bimanual palpation and imaging, is required to adequately assess the extent of local disease.

Trismus is an uncommon presenting symptom that usually indicates advanced primary site disease. Trismus may result from pain from the primary ulcerative lesion, infiltration of the underlying buccinator muscle, or indicate involvement of the pterygoid muscles due to the proximity of the buccal mucosa to the retromolar trigone and mandible. While early-stage disease may result in trismus from pain, the likelihood of trismus increases with primary tumor stage, and skin and bone involvement is present in 41 to 67% of patients presenting with large primary tumors.[25,26] It is very important to evaluate the overlying facial skin and the possible need for full-thickness resection (▶ Fig. 19.1b). The skin and subcutaneous tissue should be easily mobile over the mass. Erosion into the overlying skin with ulceration or fixation is a sign of very advanced disease. Dimpling of the skin, or "peau d'orange," is caused by cutaneous lymphatic edema causing swelling. The epidermis is fixed to the dermis, limiting the ability to swell and causing the classic dimpling effect. Failure to adequately evaluate the depth of invasion and proximity to the dermis will lead to early local recurrence in the skin and inability to clear disease. Facial paralysis is a sign of deep infiltration through the buccinator muscle, extending beyond the buccal space, and is associated with very advanced disease.

At the time of initial diagnosis, nearly 50% of patients will present with cervical metastasis.[8,26] The incidence of nodal involvement increases with increasing primary tumor stage, and is present in less than 10% of tumors ≤ 2 cm in size, and in approximately 50% in tumors greater than 4 cm.[4] The exception is verrucous carcinoma, which has a markedly lower incidence of cervical metastasis, reported at 2% in the largest series to date.[28] In general, patients who present with cervical metastasis, more posterior tumors of the buccal mucosa, ulcerated lesions, large tumors, and more poorly differentiated squamous cell carcinoma have a poorer prognosis even with multimodality therapy.[4,8,24]

19.3 Diagnosis and Evaluation

The evaluation of the patient with buccal cancer begins with a careful history and complete head and neck examination, followed by biopsy of the primary site. Particular attention should be paid to not only the extent of mucosal involvement, but also the depth of the tumor, in light of the propensity of buccal

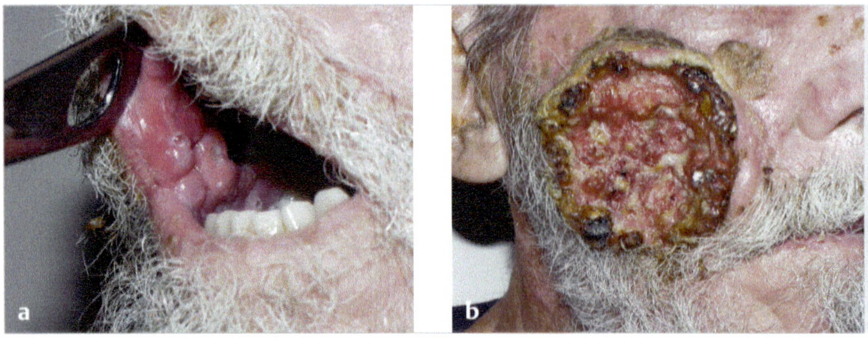

Fig. 19.1 (a) Buccal cancer. The proximity of the buccal mucosa to the lips, Stensen's duct, buccinator muscle, subcutaneous fat, and skin makes both extirpation and reconstruction challenging. **(b)** Advanced buccal cancer with direct extension into the overlying skin.

carcinoma to demonstrate deep infiltration because of a lack of barriers in the buccal space to tumor infiltration. The importance of depth of invasion rather than tumor diameter alone has recently been recognized as a prognostic variable in the eighth edition of the American Joint Committee on Cancer (AJCC) Tumor Staging Manual as a significant predictor of outcome in oral cancer with advanced depth an indicator of more aggressive disease[29] (Chapter 5). The buccal space is involved in 70% of buccal carcinoma on imaging.[30] Attention should also be paid to involvement of the skin as well as facial nerve function. Dimpling of the skin, or "peau d'orange," can be difficult to differentiate from direct tumor infiltration and should be taken into account when assessing the extent of the tumor. Tumors may approach or cross the midline of the face, with an increased risk of contralateral nodal involvement.[26]

The National Comprehensive Cancer Network (NCCN) guidelines for oral cavity cancer workup and staging recommend obtaining imaging studies using CT scan with contrast and/or MRI with contrast of primary site and neck as particularly important for staging and planning therapy.[31] CT provides better evaluation of osseous involvement but provides less soft-tissue detail than MRI and is more susceptible to dental artifact (▶ Fig. 19.2). Given the proximity of the buccal mucosa to the dentition, MRI is preferred when dental artifact is present.[32,33] Imaging is particularly important in evaluation of the extent of buccal carcinoma, which has a propensity for both superficial and deep spread of adjacent structures. Radiologic demonstration of tumor infiltration and spread has been reported in 59% of cases, with involvement of other subsites of the oral cavity in 73%, involvement of the buccal space in 70%, infiltration of the masticatory muscles in 58%, and skin involvement in 39% of cases.[30] Fluorodeoxyglucose positron emission tomography (FDG PET) is a functional, rather than an anatomic, imaging study and has inferior resolution to anatomic imaging in evaluating the primary site and neck. In patients with stage III to IV disease, up to 20% of patients may have distant metastases at presentation.[11] FDG PET may alter management through detection of distant disease but is not indicated for staging the clinically N0 neck.[31,33]

The status of regional lymph nodes has prognostic significance and has been reported in numerous studies to be the most significant predictor of survival and recurrence in buccal cancer.[11,14] A greater incidence of clinically positive nodes is reported in studies from non-Western countries than in Western countries, primarily because of a greater incidence of advanced T stage at presentation.[14] Shah[34] described the prevalence of nodal metastases as 34% in patients with clinically N0 disease and 76% in patients with clinical N+disease, with the majority of metastatic nodes located in levels I to III. The proximity of the buccal mucosa to facial nodes increases the likelihood of occult level I nodal disease, with level I most commonly involved in clinically N0 patients.[35] In clinically N0 patients, levels IV and V are involved less than 5% of the time. This observation is the basis for elective supraomohyoid neck dissection for this oral subsite in N0 patients, which removes neck levels I to III.

Extranodal extension (ENE) has long been recognized as an adverse pathologic feature in regional nodal metastases and was incorporated into nodal staging as a prognostic variable in the eighth edition of the AJCC[29] (Chapter 5). Pathologic ENE is defined as metastatic disease that breaches the capsule of the lymph node, with extension into the adjacent soft tissue. Clinically apparent ENE is defined as overt evidence of extension such as invasion of skin, infiltration of muscle, fixation to adjacent structures, or dysfunction of adjacent cranial nerves, the brachial plexus, or phrenic nerve. Radiologic findings of indistinct nodal margins or irregular nodal capsular enhancement may suggest ENE, but alone are not sufficient because of lack of specificity and sensitivity in detecting early ENE and overestimating ENE in cases of brisk stromal inflammation. Clear infiltration of adjacent fat or muscle is the strongest imaging features supporting ENE.[36]

Speech and swallowing evaluations are recommended by the NCCN guidelines for "at-risk" patients.[31] In patients with buccal cancer, trismus following treatment is a significant concern, as is dysphagia when radiation therapy is employed in treatment, and pretreatment evaluation as well as ongoing swallow therapy and support should be part of the multidisciplinary care of the buccal cancer patient. One group has reported that 53% of patients present with trismus at the time of diagnosis, which then increased to 87% postsurgery.[37]

19.4 Anatomic Considerations/ Relevant Anatomy

The buccal mucosa extends from the skin–vermillion junction of the lips extending posteriorly to the anterior tonsillar pillars and glossotonsillar folds. This represents an area of 50 to 60 cm² (▶ Fig. 19.3). The buccal mucosa extends to the upper

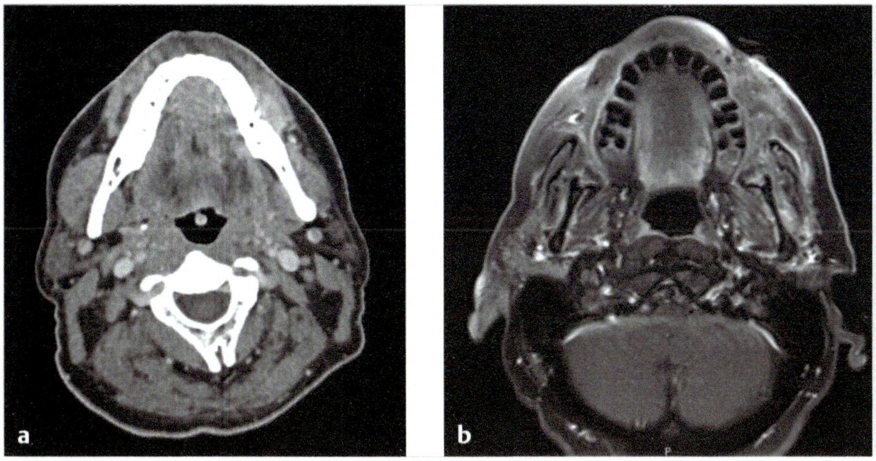

Fig. 19.2 (a) CT scan and **(b)** MRI scan of a left buccal cancer. CT provides less soft-tissue detail than MRI and is more susceptible to dental artifact.

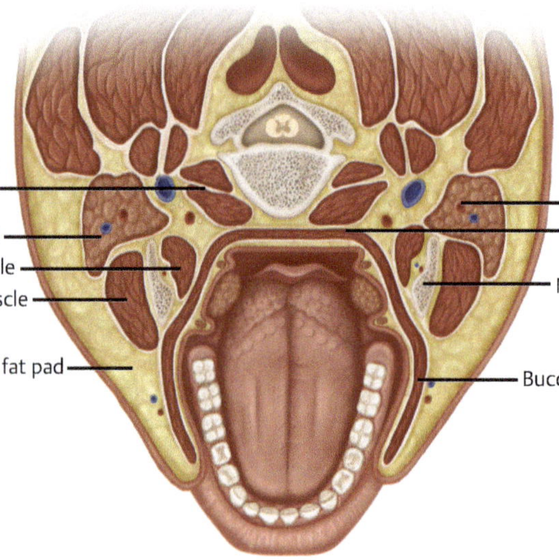

Fig. 19.3 Anatomy of the buccal space. The buccal mucosa is a thin layer lining the oral cavity, deep to which is the buccal fat pad, masticatory muscles, and in close proximity to the mandible and maxilla.

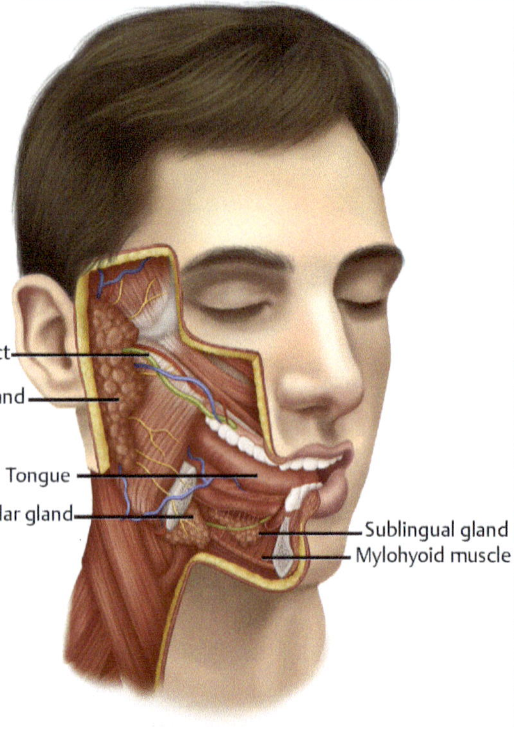

Fig. 19.4 The buccal mucosa is penetrated by Stensen's duct, which is the drainage system for the parotid gland. The duct runs on the lateral border of the masseter and turns medially through the buccinator to enter the oral cavity through the mucosa adjacent to the first and second maxillary molars.

and lower gingivobuccal sulci and connects with the maxillary and mandibular alveolar ridges. Due to the overlapping nature of the areas, it can be difficult at times to discern if the lesion originated on the alveolar process and extended onto the buccal mucosa or vice versa. In patients who are oral tobacco or betel nut users, the mucosal insult/carcinoma is most commonly found below the occlusal plane. The mucosa and submucosa overlie the buccinator and orbicularis oris muscles. There are scattered mucous glands throughout the mucosal field. The entire construct is penetrated by Stensen's duct, which is the drainage system for the parotid gland. The duct runs on the lateral border of the masseter and turns medially through the buccinator to enter the oral cavity through the mucosa adjacent to the first and second maxillary molars (▶ Fig. 19.4). The primary lymphatic drainage is via the perivascular submandibular nodes. There is also drainage through the submental, parotid, and deep jugular nodes.

The unique laminated nature of the buccal cavity, extending from buccal mucosa, submucosa, buccinator muscle, subcutaneous fat, and skin, makes both extirpation and reconstruction challenging. These delicate tissues must be able to "slide" over each other to enable normal or near-normal mouth opening, mastication, and phonation. Surgery and/or radiation therapy will negatively impact this delicate anatomic construct and often lead to irreversible trismus. Trismus is defined as an oral/interincisal opening of less than 35 mm. Patients with buccal cancer often present with trismus prior to the diagnosis of malignancy. This limitation of interincisal opening poses a significant functional problem for both the patient and the examining physician and can lead to underestimation of clinical disease, but should be considered a harbinger of very advanced disease.

The proximity of the buccal mucosa to adjacent oral cavity structures such as the maxilla, the retromolar trigone, and mandible, dentition, and lip increases the risk of mucosal spread to these sites. The thin layer of mucosal covering the maxilla and mandible overlays the periosteal covering of these structures, which may be involved and require incorporation in surgical planning.

19.5 Surgical Considerations and Approaches

Buccal cancer remains primarily a surgical disease, with surgery preferred for early and advanced-stage resectable disease.[31]

Unlike other head and neck sites, organ preservation is not part of the initial management of buccal cancer. Functional outcomes of surgery are very good, but usually require free tissue transfer to reconstruct all but the smallest defects because of the unique anatomy of the buccal mucosa. Radiation therapy alone has been used for early-stage disease or advanced unresectable disease, or those with significant comorbidities that preclude surgical care. There is a relative paucity of studies comparing radiation therapy to surgery with most series showing improved locoregional control with surgery.[32] Interstitial brachytherapy and external beam radiation therapy may be equally effective in the control of small primary tumors; however, the side effects of lifelong xerostomia, temporary or permanent dysgeusia, advanced dental caries, soft-tissue fibrosis, as well as the risk of jaw osteoradionecrosis suggest that most patients benefit from surgical excision. Advanced-stage disease requires multimodality therapy. While primary chemoradiation in a clinical trial setting has been reported to be effective in disease control,[38] current guidelines recommend surgical treatment followed by adjuvant therapy based on adverse histologic features.[31]

Buccal cancer is an aggressive disease, characterized by a higher rate of locoregional failure than other oral cancer subsites.[13,14] As a thin structure with a relative paucity of underlying soft tissue, buccal cancers can readily invade the adjacent buccinator muscle, buccal fat space, and other adjacent structures. Adequate resection is defined as sufficient clearance to achieve clear frozen and permanent surgical margins, which correlates with a resection margin of at least 5 mm between tumor and normal tissue in the resected specimen.[32] Resection margins less than 5 mm are considered close, and have been shown to correlate with increased recurrence and poorer survival.[39] Buccal cancer is itself a risk factor for a twofold increased risk of having a positive margin.[9] Local recurrence occurs in approximately 50% of patients with buccal cancer, even with clear resection margins.[10,24,27,40,41]

The unique elasticity of the buccal mucosa often affects the surgical planning of an adequate surgical margin, particularly with performance of a transoral resection. During maximal mouth opening, the elasticity of the buccal mucosa causes stretching of the adjacent mucosa, which can result in overestimation of the extent of the margin of tissue resected. It has been calculated that margins need to be 32% larger to account for this effect and avoid inadequate resection.[42] Similarly, after resection, formalin fixation can result in up to 30% shrinkage of the soft-tissue margin.[43] Thus, the extent of resection should incorporate a resection of 1.5 to 2 cm of surrounding normal mucosa to obtain an adequate resection margin, and may necessitate resection of skin, adjacent lip, or muscles of mastication.

Small T1 lesions can be resected and closed primarily with local tissue rearrangement or a small skin graft.[15,44] The use of local tissue, which initially may be tight, will replace the defect with "like" tissues. The laminated nature of the cheek will be reconstructed, and a more functional result attained. These tumors usually will not violate the buccinator muscle. The muscle fascia can be taken as the deep margin and the mucosa, submucosa, and submucosal fat can be mobilized into the defect, thus reconstructing the multiple layers of the cheek. All skin grafts tend to contract and can cause contractures, which will get worse with radiation therapy. Full-thickness skin grafts will contract less than split-thickness grafts, due to the presence of a thicker dermal layer. However, a full-thickness graft requires a very rich vascular bed, which may not be present in a patient with previous surgery or radiation therapy.

Once the decision to use a full- or split-thickness graft is made, the steps to ensure 100% take of the graft are the same. Loss of any or all of the graft will dictate that the wound will heal by secondary intention. This leads to contraction of the wound leading to pathological contracture, which is an ongoing problem without an easy solution. To ensure complete take of the buccal skin graft, a tie-over bolster should be used. The graft is secured at the mucosal margins with interrupted chromic or other absorbable sutures. It is desirable to augment the bolster with through-and-through buccal mattress sutures, usually done with chromic sutures. The sutures can be tied on the skin over a cotton dental roll or a piece of petrolatum gauze rolled into a sausage shape. This will avoid necrosis on the skin and the sutures will increase complete contact of the graft with the bed and insure excellent take of the graft. The bolster and the transbuccal sutures can be removed at 7 days. Initially the buccal surface will be deeply indented in the area of resection, but will fill in over time.

Larger tumors will require larger resections. The laminated nature of the cheek will need to be resected and an adequate reconstruction cannot be accomplished with local tissue. The option of a skin graft will remain if the cheek skin is intact. A composite resection of buccal mucosa, buccinator, and skin will require a complex reconstruction. A thin, pliable free tissue transfer will be needed. This technique may be needed even if the cheek skin is intact. The two surgical teams should work in concert to decrease operative time. Based on size, the defect may require a "folded" flap to give internal lining and skin coverage. Initially, this will produce a very bulky construct that will thin out over time. Following the patient's radiation therapy and perhaps a year after the initial surgery, the flap can be elevated, thinned, and re-inset. The flap will be insensate and will not animate and with the loss of the buccinator there will be a tendency for the patient to be unable to mobilize the food bolus onto the occlusal surface. The skin will eventually mucosalize in the oral cavity. The use of pedicled local and regional flaps for reconstruction of larger defects of the buccal tissues is for the most part of historical significance. For patients who cannot tolerate the prolonged surgical time associated with free tissue transfers, temporalis muscular flaps and pectoralis major myocutaneous flaps have been described and can be used in selected circumstances.

The problem of involvement of Stensen's duct, be it with tumor invasion or resection as part of the surgical margin, must be recognized at the initial operation and addressed. The duct should be cannulated and dissected free. A frozen section margin of the duct should be sent to pathology while preparing the repositioning of the structure. The duct can be freed up to the anterior border of the masseter and cannulated with a lacrimal probe or other instrument. It should be opened longitudinally for a few millimeters to give a "fish-mouth" effect, opening the drainage of the duct and avoiding a stricture. A stent, angiocatheter, or other soft pliable device should be placed and sutured into the cheek. If the duct cannot be repositioned, it should be ligated.

Reconstruction of larger defects and will result in cosmetic and functional disability, particularly if adjuvant radiation therapy is employed. All patients should be counseled prior to treatment that physical therapy and speech and swallowing therapy will be an ongoing process that will require their active participation in an effort to return the patient to a full and active life. Trismus is a common sequela of treatment requiring ongoing stretching and swallowing therapy.

In patients who are clinically N0, observation, elective neck dissection, sentinel node biopsy, or elective neck radiation have all been employed. In patients with early-stage cancers, the NCCN guidelines recommend either elective neck dissection at the time of surgical resection or observation for N0 patients.[31] However, several studies including a prospective randomized controlled trial that demonstrate that elective neck dissection, compared to observation with therapeutic neck dissection for nodal relapse, was associated with greater rates of overall survival (80 vs. 68%) and disease-free survival (70 vs. 46%).[31,45] The argument for observation in early-stage disease is that up to 70% of patients will be found to be truly node negative and could be spared surgery. However, locoregional recurrence rates are higher in patients who undergo observation compared to elective neck dissection, ranging from 25 to 100% versus 7 to 33%, with corresponding statistically significant differences in overall survival.[13,23,46] Knowledge of pathological nodal status allows patients with occult cervical metastasis to be upstaged and may influence treatment recommendations. Neck dissection for oral cancer is covered in more detail in Chapter 32.

Patients with advanced-stage buccal cancer have a higher incidence of occult nodal metastasis, and should undergo elective neck dissection at the time of primary site surgery. Patients with clinically N + disease should undergo therapeutic neck dissection encompassing at least levels I to IV. The incidence of nodal metastases in level V is reported at less than 5% and most patients will require postoperative radiation therapy.[34,35] An in-continuity neck dissection that sacrifices contiguous structures between the primary tumor and neck such as the parotid duct, the parotid gland, lower branches of the facial nerve, mandible, adjacent musculature, and cheek skin has been shown to be associated with a lower rate of locoregional recurrence and may be appropriate for larger tumors.[40] Patients with large tumors that approach or cross midline with ipsilateral neck disease are at increased risk of contralateral neck disease, which needs to be incorporated in treatment planning.[26]

19.6 Surgical Sequelae

Overall 5-year survival rates for buccal cancer range from 34 to 69%, with recurrence rates of approximately 50%.[10,11,13,14,24,27,40,41] Local recurrence rates are approximately 50% even with clear margins, underscoring the importance of other adverse features unique to this disease.[10,41] Isolated regional recurrence in the absence of local recurrence is uncommon, with up to 80% of recurrence local only.[11] While skin involvement is a sign of advanced disease by itself it has not been found to be a prognostic factor for recurrence.[3] Distant metastases develop in 7 to 20% after treatment.[11,23] The largest North American series to date reported 5-year overall survival rates of 78 to 90% for stage I, 66 to 83% for stage II, 52 to 69% for stage III, and 43 to 53% for stage IV disease, with worse survival observed in patients with nodal involvement, ENE, perineural invasion, and poor histologic grade.[3,4,6,13] The likelihood of surgical salvage decreases with stage, with up to 69% of early-stage tumors able to be salvaged, but fewer than 40% amenable to salvage when regional recurrence is present.[15] Successful surgical salvage is possible in less than 10% and adversely influenced by larger tumor stage, nodal disease, poorly differentiated histologic grade, and a disease-free interval of less than 6 months.[4,11,15]

Postoperative radiation therapy for early-stage disease is indicated when adverse prognostic features are found on surgical pathology, specifically involvement of more than one lymph node, close surgical margins, perineural invasion, or lymphovascular spread, and may improve outcomes in buccal carcinoma.[11] There has only been one randomized controlled trial of postoperative radiation therapy versus surgery alone, limited to patients with stage III or IV disease in whom the addition of postoperative radiation therapy improved disease-free survival from 38 to 68%.[47] In early-stage disease, institutional studies have not shown improvements in 5-year disease-specific survival with the addition of postoperative radiation therapy compared to surgery alone, but surgery with or without postoperative radiation therapy was superior to radiation therapy alone, perhaps reflecting patient selection.[11,14,48,49]

Patients with advanced-stage oral cancer are usually offered surgery with postoperative radiation therapy, with nodal status being the primary determinant of failure.[11,13,14,47] Postoperative radiation therapy is recommended for any patient with advanced primary or nodal stage disease, nodal involvement of levels IV or V, perineural invasion, or lymphovascular spread.[31] Radiation therapy is also recommended for positive margins when reresection is not feasible, or ENE, but for these two high-risk features, adjuvant chemoradiation is preferred. Because of the high recurrence rates associated with buccal cancer, postoperative radiation therapy is recommend for all but favorable early-stage disease. Adjuvant treatment for oral cancer is covered in more detail in Chapter 35 and 36.

19.7 Conclusion

Buccal cancers represent an aggressive oral cavity subsite with a propensity for early spread because of a lack of anatomic barriers, early nodal involvement, and difficulty achieving wide margins. Treatment is primarily surgical and often requires reconstruction and adjuvant therapy. Despite this, locoregional recurrence rates are high. The incorporation of depth of invasion and ENE into current staging paradigms will likely upstage many patients who present with this disease and may expand the indications for adjuvant therapy.

Key Points

- Buccal cancer is an aggressive oral cavity subsite.
- Nodal disease is present in 50% of patients at presentation.
- Treatment is primarily surgical.
- Small lesions can be reconstructed with skin grafts.
- A composite resection of buccal mucosa, buccinator, and skin will require a complex reconstruction.
- Postoperative radiation therapy is indicated for stage III or IV disease, or when perineural invasion is present.

- Postoperative chemoradiation is indicated for ENE or a positive surgical margin.
- Trismus can be a significant problem after treatment.
- Early, aggressive swallowing rehabilitation is advised to mitigate late dysphagia.

References

[1] Siegel RL, Miller KD, Jemal A. Cancer statistics, 2018. CA Cancer J Clin. 2018; 68(1):7–30

[2] Shield KD, Ferlay J, Jemal A, et al. The global incidence of lip, oral cavity, and pharyngeal cancers by subsite in 2012. CA Cancer J Clin. 2017; 67(1):51–64

[3] Bobdey S, Sathwara J, Jain A, Saoba S, Balasubramaniam G. Squamous cell carcinoma of buccal mucosa: an analysis of prognostic factors. South Asian J Cancer. 2018; 7(1):49–54

[4] Huang CH, Chu ST, Ger LP, Hou YY, Sun CP. Clinicopathologic evaluation of prognostic factors for squamous cell carcinoma of the buccal mucosa. J Chin Med Assoc. 2007; 70(4):164–170

[5] Ganesh D, Sreenivasan P, Öhman J, et al. Potentially malignant oral disorders and cancer transformation. Anticancer Res. 2018; 38(6):3223–3229

[6] Jan JC, Hsu WH, Liu SA, et al. Prognostic factors in patients with buccal squamous cell carcinoma: 10-year experience. J Oral Maxillofac Surg. 2011; 69(2): 396–404

[7] Pathak KA, Nason R, Talole S, et al. Cancer of the buccal mucosa: a tale of two continents. Int J Oral Maxillofac Surg. 2009; 38(2):146–150

[8] Nair S, Singh B, Pawar PV, et al. Squamous cell carcinoma of tongue and buccal mucosa: clinico-pathologically different entities. Eur Arch Otorhinolaryngol. 2016; 273(11):3921–3928

[9] Luryi AL, Chen MM, Mehra S, Roman SA, Sosa JA, Judson BL. Positive surgical margins in early stage oral cavity cancer: an analysis of 20,602 cases. Otolaryngol Head Neck Surg. 2014; 151(6):984–990

[10] Sieczka E, Datta R, Singh A, et al. Cancer of the buccal mucosa: are margins and T-stage accurate predictors of local control? Am J Otolaryngol. 2001; 22(6):395–399

[11] Lin CS, Jen YM, Cheng MF, et al. Squamous cell carcinoma of the buccal mucosa: an aggressive cancer requiring multimodality treatment. Head Neck. 2006; 28(2):150–157

[12] Urist MM, O'Brien CJ, Soong SJ, Visscher DW, Maddox WA. Squamous cell carcinoma of the buccal mucosa: analysis of prognostic factors. Am J Surg. 1987; 154(4):411–414

[13] Diaz EM, Jr, Holsinger FC, Zuniga ER, Roberts DB, Sorensen DM. Squamous cell carcinoma of the buccal mucosa: one institution's experience with 119 previously untreated patients. Head Neck. 2003; 25(4):267–273

[14] Bachar G, Goldstein DP, Barker E, et al. Squamous cell carcinoma of the buccal mucosa: outcomes of treatment in the modern era. Laryngoscope. 2012; 122 (7):1552–1557

[15] Iyer SG, Pradhan SA, Pai PS, Patil S. Surgical treatment outcomes of localized squamous carcinoma of buccal mucosa. Head Neck. 2004; 26(10):897–902

[16] Anand R, Dhingra C, Prasad S, Menon I. Betel nut chewing and its deleterious effects on oral cavity. J Cancer Res Ther. 2014; 10(3):499–505

[17] Ray JG, Ranganathan K, Chattopadhyay A. Malignant transformation of oral submucous fibrosis: overview of histopathological aspects. Oral Surg Oral Med Oral Pathol Oral Radiol. 2016; 122(2):200–209

[18] Kiran Kumar K, Saraswathi TR, Ranganathan K, Uma Devi M, Elizabeth J. Oral submucous fibrosis: a clinico-histopathological study in Chennai. Indian J Dent Res. 2007; 18(3):106–111

[19] Warnakulasuriya S, Johnson NW, van der Waal I. Nomenclature and classification of potentially malignant disorders of the oral mucosa. J Oral Pathol Med. 2007; 36(10):575–580

[20] Giuliani M, Troiano G, Cordaro M, et al. Rate of malignant transformation of oral lichen planus: a systematic review. Oral Dis. 2019; 25(3):693–709:epub ahead of print

[21] Aghbari SMH, Abushouk AI, Attia A, et al. Malignant transformation of oral lichen planus and oral lichenoid lesions: a meta-analysis of 20095 patient data. Oral Oncol. 2017; 68:92–102

[22] Thomson PJ, Goodson ML, Smith DR. Potentially malignant disorders revisited-The lichenoid lesion/proliferative verrucous leukoplakia conundrum. J Oral Pathol Med. 2018; 47(6):557–565

[23] Dillon JK, Villing A, Jones S, Futran N, Brockhoff H, Ward B. What is the role of elective neck dissection in the treatment of patients with buccal squamous cell carcinoma and clinically negative neck findings? J Oral Maxillofac Surg. 2017; 75(3):603–608

[24] Sagheb K, Blatt S, Kraft IS, et al. Outcome and cervical metastatic spread of squamous cell cancer of the buccal mucosa, a retrospective analysis of the past 25 years. J Oral Pathol Med. 2017; 46(6):460–464

[25] Ghoshal S, Mallick I, Panda N, Sharma SC. Carcinoma of the buccal mucosa: analysis of clinical presentation, outcome and prognostic factors. Oral Oncol. 2006; 42(5):533–539

[26] Mair M, Nair S, Thiagarajan SK, Agrawal J, Nair D, Chaturvedi P. Skin involvement and ipsilateral nodal metastasis as a predictor of contralateral nodal metastasis in buccal mucosa cancers. Indian J Cancer. 2016; 53(3):394–396

[27] Zaman SU, Aqil S, Sulaiman MA. Predictors of locoregional recurrence in early stage buccal cancer with pathologically clear surgical margins and negative neck. Acta Otorrinolaringol Esp. 2018; 69(4):226–230

[28] Alonso JE, Kuan EC, Arshi A, St John MA. A population-based analysis of verrucous carcinoma of the oral cavity. Laryngoscope. 2018; 128(2):393–397

[29] Lydiatt WM, Patel SG, O'Sullivan B, et al. Head and neck cancer: major changes in the American Joint Committee on Cancer Eighth Edition cancer staging manual. Ca Cancer J Clin. 2017; 67:122–137

[30] Xu SS, Li D, Zhou Y, Sheng B, Zeng C, Zhong SX. Pathways involved in the spread of buccal carcinoma on contrast-enhanced multislice CT. Dentomaxillofac Radiol. 2015; 44(2):20140111

[31] National Comprehensive Cancer Network. NCCN Guidelines for head and neck cancer care. Available at: http://www.nccn.org/professionals/physician_gls/pdf/head-and-neck.pdf. Accessed May 1, 2017

[32] Gill A, Vasan N, Givi B, Joshi A. AHNS Series: do you know your guidelines? Evidence-based management of oral cavity cancers. Head Neck. 2018; 40(2): 406–416

[33] Arya S, Rane P, Deshmukh A. Oral cavity squamous cell carcinoma: role of pretreatment imaging and its influence on management. Clin Radiol. 2014; 69(9):916–930

[34] Shah JP. Patterns of cervical lymph node metastases from squamous carcinomas of the upper aerodigestive tract. Am J Surg. 1990; 116:432–435

[35] Shah JP, Candela FC, Poddar AK. The patterns of cervical lymph node metastases from squamous carcinoma of the oral cavity. Cancer. 1990; 66(1):109–113

[36] Glastonbury CM, Mukherji SK, O'Sullivan B, Lydiatt WM. Setting the stage for 2018: how the changes in the American Joint Committee on Cancer/Union for International Cancer Control Cancer Staging Manual Eighth Edition impact radiologists. AJNR. 2017; 38:2231–2237

[37] Agarwal P, Shiva Kumar HR, Rai KK. Trismus in oral cancer patients undergoing surgery and radiotherapy. J Oral Biol Craniofac Res. 2016; 6 Suppl 1:S9–S13

[38] Foster CC, Melotek JM, Brisson RJ, et al. Definitive chemoradiation for locally-advanced oral cavity cancer: a 20-year experience. Oral Oncol. 2018; 80: 16–22

[39] Hinni ML, Ferlito A, Brandwein-Gensler MS, et al. Surgical margins in head and neck cancer: a contemporary review. Head Neck. 2013; 35(9):1362–1370

[40] Xie L, Zhang Y, Huang W, Chen J, Yu J, Zhou X. In-continuity neck dissection: long-term oncological outcomes in squamous cell carcinoma of the buccal mucosa. J Oral Maxillofac Surg. 2018; 76(5):1107–1116

[41] Lubek JE, Dyalram D, Perera EH, Liu X, Ord RA. A retrospective analysis of squamous carcinoma of the buccal mucosa: an aggressive subsite within the oral cavity. J Oral Maxillofac Surg. 2013; 71(6):1126–1131

[42] Tsai PT, Shieh YS, Wu CT, Lee SP, Chen YW. Buccal mucosa elasticity influences surgical margin determination in buccal carcinoma resection. J Oral Maxillofac Surg. 2016; 74(9):1900.e1–1900.e7

[43] Mohiyuddin SMA, Padiyar BV, Suresh TN, et al. Clinicopathological study of surgical margins in squamous cell carcinoma of buccal mucosa. World J Otorhinolaryngol Head Neck Surg. 2016; 2(1):17–21

[44] Montero PH, Patel SG. Cancer of the oral cavity. Surg Oncol Clin N Am. 2015; 24(3):491–508

[45] D'Cruz AK, Vaish R, Kapre N, et al. Head and Neck Disease Management Group. Elective versus therapeutic neck dissection in node-negative oral cancer. N Engl J Med. 2015; 373(6):521–529

[46] Huang SF, Chang JT, Liao CT, et al. The role of elective neck dissection in early stage buccal cancer. Laryngoscope. 2015; 125(1):128–133

[47] Mishra RC, Singh DN, Mishra TK. Post-operative radiotherapy in carcinoma of buccal mucosa, a prospective randomized trial. Eur J Surg Oncol. 1996; 22(5): 502–504

[48] Brown JS, Shaw RJ, Bekiroglu F, Rogers SN. Systematic review of the current evidence in the use of postoperative radiotherapy for oral squamous cell carcinoma. Br J Oral Maxillofac Surg. 2012; 50(6):481–489

[49] Dixit S, Vyas RK, Toparani RB, Baboo HA, Patel DD. Surgery versus surgery and postoperative radiotherapy in squamous cell carcinoma of the buccal mucosa: a comparative study. Ann Surg Oncol. 1998; 5(6):502–510

20 Buccal Reconstruction

David Chen, Kofi Boahene, David W. Eisele, and Carole Fakhry

Summary
Reconstruction of the buccal region following tumor resection poses a unique challenge with important aesthetic and functional considerations. The buccal region plays a major role in mouth opening, chewing, swallowing, speech, as well as facial movement. The optimal reconstructive technique is largely based on the size of the primary defect. Smaller defects may be closed primarily or with a local flap, while larger defects may require a regional or free flap to preserve function. Trismus is one of the most common sequelae following buccal tumor resection and reconstruction, especially in patients who have undergone or are planned to undergo radiation therapy. There are multiple nonoperative as well as operative treatments for trismus, with microvascular free tissue transfer playing an important role in creating long-lasting improvement in mouth opening.

Keywords: buccal defects, oral vestibular reconstruction

20.1 Introduction

Reconstruction of the buccal region following resection of an oral malignancy constitutes a challenging problem from both a functional and an aesthetic standpoint. Functionally, the buccal region plays a crucial role in oral phase swallowing, speech, mastication, and facial movement. Facial expression, along with the contour of the face and appearance of the oral commissure, can also introduce aesthetic complexities in reconstruction. Successful reconstruction of the buccal region is aimed at restoring a barrier that encloses the oral cavity while supporting the functional and aesthetic components listed above.

20.2 Anatomy

The buccal region is roughly defined anteriorly by the oral commissure, posteriorly by the ramus of the mandible, superiorly by the zygomatic process of the maxilla, inferiorly by the inferior border of the mandible, medially by the maxillary and mandibular alveolus, and laterally by the skin of the cheek. The key anatomic components are comprised of skin, oral mucosa, buccal fat pad (BFP), facial and buccal vessels, parotid duct, as well as the facial nerve and associated musculature. Each of these elements must be considered in characterizing a defect and planning for an appropriate reconstruction

The muscles of facial expression in the buccal region include the orbicularis oris, risorius, zygomaticus major and minor, buccinator, and depressor anguli oris. These muscles are all enveloped by the superficial muscular aponeurotic system (SMAS) and are innervated by the buccal branches of the facial nerve, with contributions from the zygomatic and marginal mandibular branches. The facial nerve branches travel just deep to the SMAS and innervate the muscles of facial expression, with the exception of the buccinator, from their deep surface.

The arterial supply of the buccal regions is derived from the buccal branch of the internal maxillary artery as well as the facial artery. Venous drainage is comprised of the pterygoid plexus and facial vein. Sensory innervation is supplied by branches of the maxillary and mandibular branches of the trigeminal nerve.

The parotid duct exits from the anterior aspect of the parotid gland and courses superficial to the masseter muscle. At the anterior border of the masseter, it turns medially and pierces the BFP, buccinator fascia, and buccinator muscle before exiting into the oral cavity via a papilla opposite the second maxillary molar.

20.3 Functional Considerations

The various components of the buccal region play a major role in the functions of mouth opening, chewing, swallowing, speech, as well as facial movement, all of which may be impacted by tumor resection. In simple terms, the buccal mucosa serves as a passive barrier that helps enclose the oral cavity and, in conjunction with the action of the lips, prevents leakage of saliva and other oral contents. The ability to seal the oral cavity is also necessary to generate a positive air pressure gradient for plosive speech and a negative pressure gradient for sucking. The muscles of facial expression, in addition to accomplishing their namesake, are involved in the transit of food during mastication and deglutition. Facial reanimation, as it pertains to the buccal region, is therefore an important consideration for reconstruction of buccal defects that involve the facial musculature and nerve branches. Specific techniques for facial reanimation, however, are beyond the scope of this chapter.

One of the most common functional consequences of surgical resection and reconstruction for buccal cancer is the development of trismus, defined as a mouth opening limited to 35 mm or less.[1] The reported incidence of trismus following treatment of oral cancer varies, but may be seen in as many as 86% of patients following radiation therapy or surgery.[2,3] Reduced mouth opening may result from scarring of the muscles of mastication and buccal soft tissue, and/or tissue loss following radiation therapy or surgery. In addition, native buccal mucosa has a high degree of inherent elasticity that is difficult to replicate through any form of tissue transfer. By itself, trismus may contribute to difficulty with oral intake, chewing, swallowing, speaking, as well as dental issues from poor oral hygiene.[3] Therefore, reducing the risk of trismus should be one of the primary considerations when choosing a reconstructive technique.

20.4 Options for Reconstruction

The choice for an optimal reconstructive plan is largely dictated by size and location of the primary defect. Squaquara et al classify the size of intraoral defects into small (≤ 4 cm diameter), medium (≤ 7 cm diameter), and large (> 7 cm diameter).[4] When measuring the size of the defect, the superior to inferior dimension will generally be the most important in determining mouth opening.[5] Small defects may be closed primarily or, for superficial defects, either left to heal by secondary intention or repaired with a split-thickness skin graft. However, with increasing defect diameter and soft-tissue involvement, the risk of trismus increases.[4] Numerous options for reconstruction using local and regional flaps have been reported in the literature. For large and complex defects, free tissue transfer remains the most versatile option for reconstruction, although it is not without its drawbacks.[6,7]

20.4.1 Local Flaps

A simple mucosal advancement flap may be sufficient to repair smaller buccal defects. The use of a posteriorly based buccinator musculomucosal flap has also been reported.[8] These flaps have the advantage of utilizing native buccal tissue, as well as potentially preserving sensation to the buccal surface. Excessive harvesting of buccal mucosa, however, may result in trismus as well as damage to the parotid duct.[5]

For slightly larger defects, the BFP can be harvested and used as a pedicled flap (▶ Fig. 20.1). The BFP is found in the masticator space in between the buccinator and masseter muscles, and has a relatively rich blood supply consisting of branches of the internal maxillary artery, transverse facial branch of the superficial temporal artery, and facial artery. Mucosalization of the BFP typically takes place over several weeks, and so an additional skin graft is usually not necessary. Buccal fat has the advantage of being easily harvested. However, it provides minimal bulk and can retract substantially, making it unsuitable for medium or large defects.[9,10]

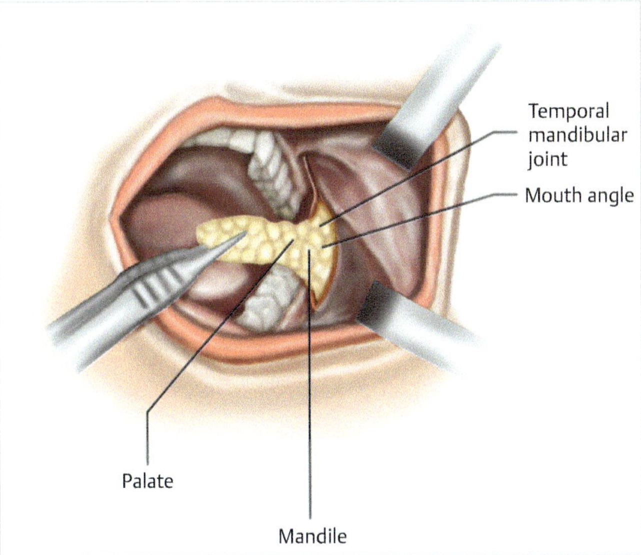

Fig. 20.1 Buccal fat pad flap.

The facial artery musculomucosal (FAMM) is robust pedicled flap with an axial blood supply based off of the facial artery (▶ Fig. 20.2). It is designed just anterior to the parotid duct and consists of mucosa, submucosa, part of the buccinator muscle, the facial artery, and a rich submucous venous plexus. The FAMM flap may be inferiorly (anterograde flow) or superiorly (retrograde flow) based, depending on the location of the defect.[11]

Various tongue flap designs, including the double-door and lateral tongue flap, have also been described for the closure of buccal defects (▶ Fig. 20.3). These flaps are generally versatile and reliable, but require a second-stage surgery, as the flap pedicle tethers the tongue and must be divided after the initial inset. During the postoperative period, trauma to the pedicle can occur from the teeth, as well as excessive movement of the tongue. Dysarthria is also a potential sequela, although this can usually be avoided if the mobility of the tongue tip is maintained.[12–14]

20.4.2 Regional Flaps

The platysma muscle can be used for buccal reconstruction as either a submental flap or island platysma flap (▶ Fig. 20.4). Both flaps can be harvested either as muscle alone or as a musculocutaneous flap, and are based off of the submental artery. The submental flap is designed across the midline in the submental area, and can be used to reconstruct full-thickness defects of the cheek. If skin is included, the patient should be counseled on the potential for development of intraoral hair. In contrast, the island platysma flap is designed over a hairless area at the distal aspect of the sternocleidomastoid muscle. It is generally thinner and more ideal for mucosal defects.[15,16]

A nasolabial island flap can be raised and tunneled intraorally to close buccal defects (▶ Fig. 20.5). This flap is based off of

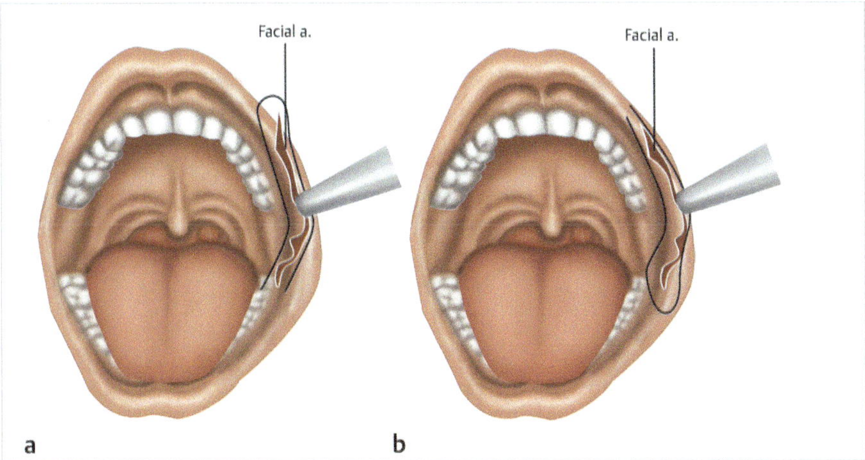

Fig. 20.2 Inferiorly based (**a**) and superiorly based (**b**) facial artery musculomucosal flaps.

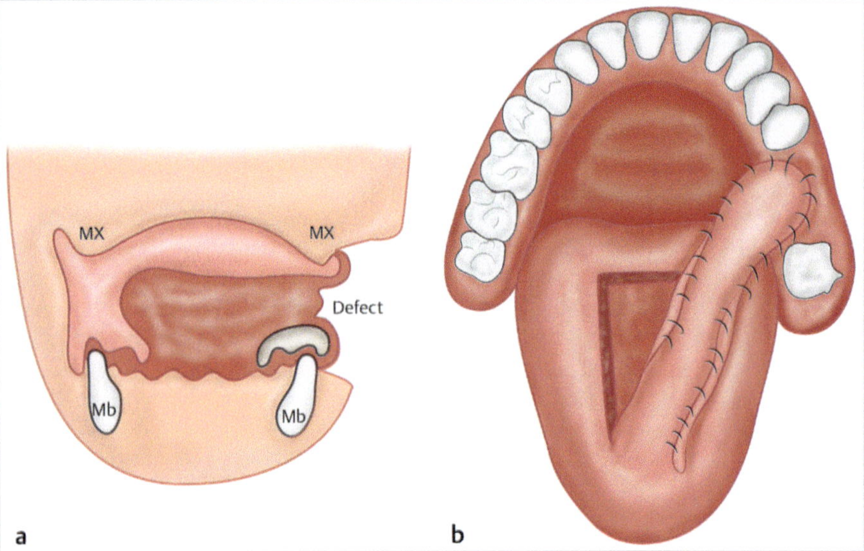

Fig. 20.3 Double-door (a) and lateral tongue (b) flaps.

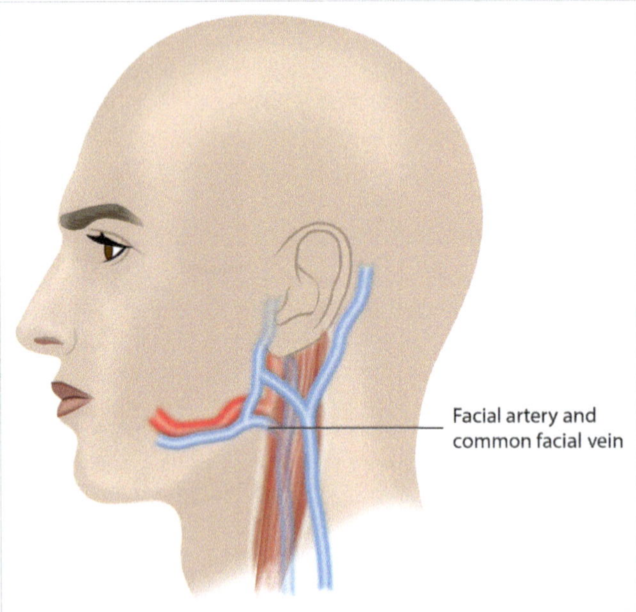

Fig. 20.4 Submental island or platysma island flap based off of the submental artery.

subcutaneous blood supply from the facial, transverse facial, and angular vessels. Facial artery ligation does not appear to affect the viability of the flap, as its arterial supply is derived from multiple vessels. A superiorly based flap is typically used for defects centered above the occlusal line, whereas an inferiorly based flap is used for defects centered below.[17]

The pectoralis major flap, trapezius flap, and supraclavicular flap may be used to reconstruct larger intraoral defects when free tissue transfer is either unfeasible or the patient is not a suitable candidate. These flaps may be harvested either as muscle only or as a myocutaneous flap. The trapezius can be harvested as one of a combination of three different flaps: the superior trapezius flap based off of paraspinous perforators, the lateral island trapezius flap based off of the transverse cervical artery, and the vertical trapezius flap based off of the dorsal scapular artery. The superior trapezius flap is unique in that its blood supply is unaffected by neck dissection. For intraoral reconstruction, it can reach the posterior part of the cheek. The lateral island trapezius flap is the least reliable of the three trapezius flaps. It may be used to reconstruct the lateral oral cavity although its primary use is for external defects of the lateral and anterior neck. The vertical trapezius flap is thin and pliable, with a large arc of rotation that makes it the most versatile of the three trapezius flaps (▶ Fig. 20.6).[4]

A supraclavicular fasciocutaneous island flap may be harvested based off of the transverse cervical artery, which arises from the thyrocervical trunk or, less commonly, directly from the subclavian artery (▶ Fig. 20.7). The venous drainage for this flap occurs through the superficial cervical veins, rather than the venae comitantes of the transverse cervical artery. Given the thin size of the pedicle, the supraclavicular flap may be tunneled into the buccal defect with minimal donor site morbidity and better cosmesis compared to the pectoralis major and trapezius flaps. However, the thyrocervical trunk must be preserved and remain undamaged by prior or concurrent neck dissection. Furthermore, limitations in pedicle length and variations in vascular anatomy may limit its reach to the buccal area.[18]

20.4.3 Free Flaps

For large intraoral defects, microvascular free tissue transfer is perhaps the most versatile reconstructive option.[19] Free flaps afford superior outcomes for postoperative mouth opening when compared to skin grafts and locoregional flaps, as well as increased volume to maintain facial contour.[20,21] In addition, the use of locoregional flaps may be complicated by the presence of nodal metastases near the donor site, as well as radiation therapy sequelae to the donor site prior to surgery, both of which are obviated with free tissue transfer.

The radial forearm free flap (RFFF) and anterolateral thigh free flap (ALTFF) are the most common free flaps used for

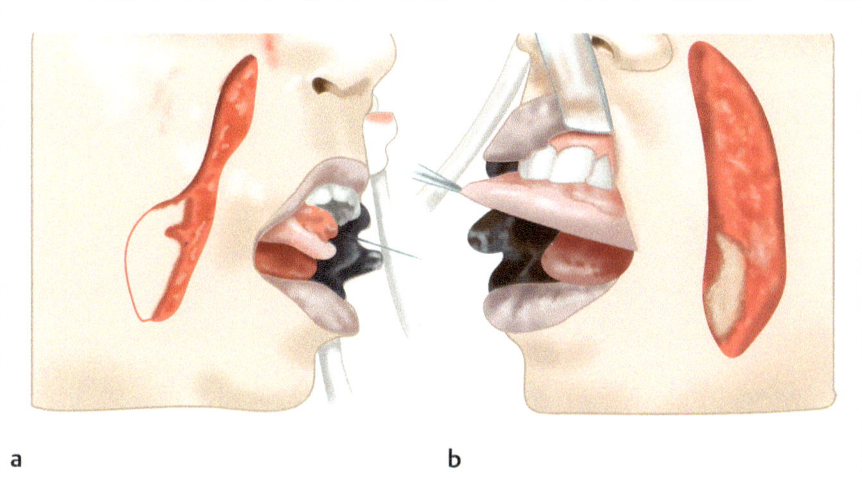

Fig. 20.5 (a, b) Intraoral nasolabial flap.

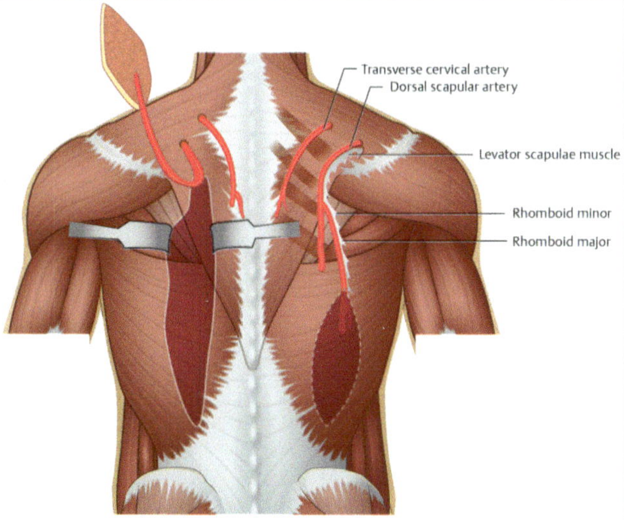

Fig. 20.6 Vertical trapezius flap based off of dorsal scapular artery.

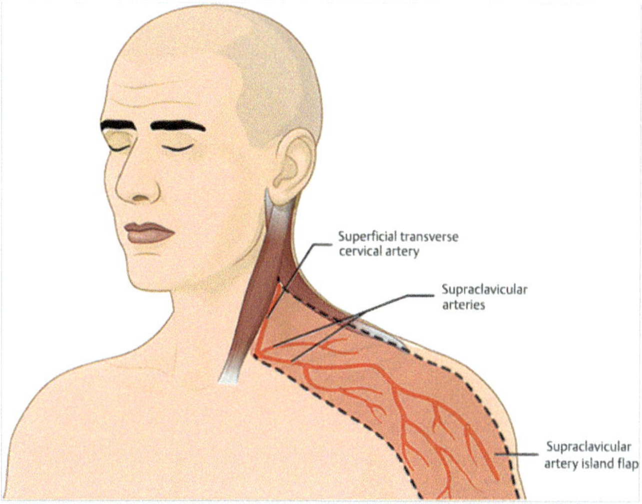

Fig. 20.7 Supraclavicular island flap.

buccal reconstruction (▶ Fig. 20.8). The advantages of the RFFF include its thinness and pliability, which make it an excellent replacement for buccal mucosa.[7] It has also been described as a folded flap for repair of full-thickness defects of the cheek.[22] For larger defects with greater volume deficit, an ALTFF may be more ideal.[23] The overall success rates for oral cavity reconstruction are similar for both flaps.[23,24]

The potential drawbacks of free flaps include the need for a microvascular-trained surgeon, increased operative time, and more extensive postoperative monitoring. In addition, patients with multiple comorbidities may not be suitable candidates to undergo microvascular free tissue transfer.

20.5 Additional Considerations

Scarring, contracture, and volume loss are all factors that must be considered when deciding on a plan for reconstruction of the buccal region. These factors are exacerbated in patients who undergo postoperative radiation therapy. The prevalence of trismus is estimated to be over 25% in patients who have undergone conventional radiation therapy and over 30% in patients who have undergone concurrent chemoradiation.[3] As such, for these patients the optimal reconstructive strategy is one that provides additional volume support as well as maximizes mouth opening. Trismus in the setting of radiation therapy can be caused by direct contracture of the buccal soft tissue as well as scarring of the muscles of mastication within the field of radiation. Nonoperative management of trismus includes physical therapy exercises, the use of a tongue depressor plate, mechanical stretching aids, pentoxifylline, or injection of steroids, fibrinolytic agents, or botulinum toxin. Surgical management usually entails a combination of scar release, masticatory muscle myotomy, coronoidectomy, and microvascular free tissue transfer. Free tissue transfer is especially important to create long-lasting improvement in mouth opening, as it introduces healthy, nonirradiated, and well-perfused tissue.[25,26] There is also some evidence to suggest that masticator myotomy and coronoidectomy at the time of tumor resection may improve postoperative mouth opening at least 3 years out.[27]

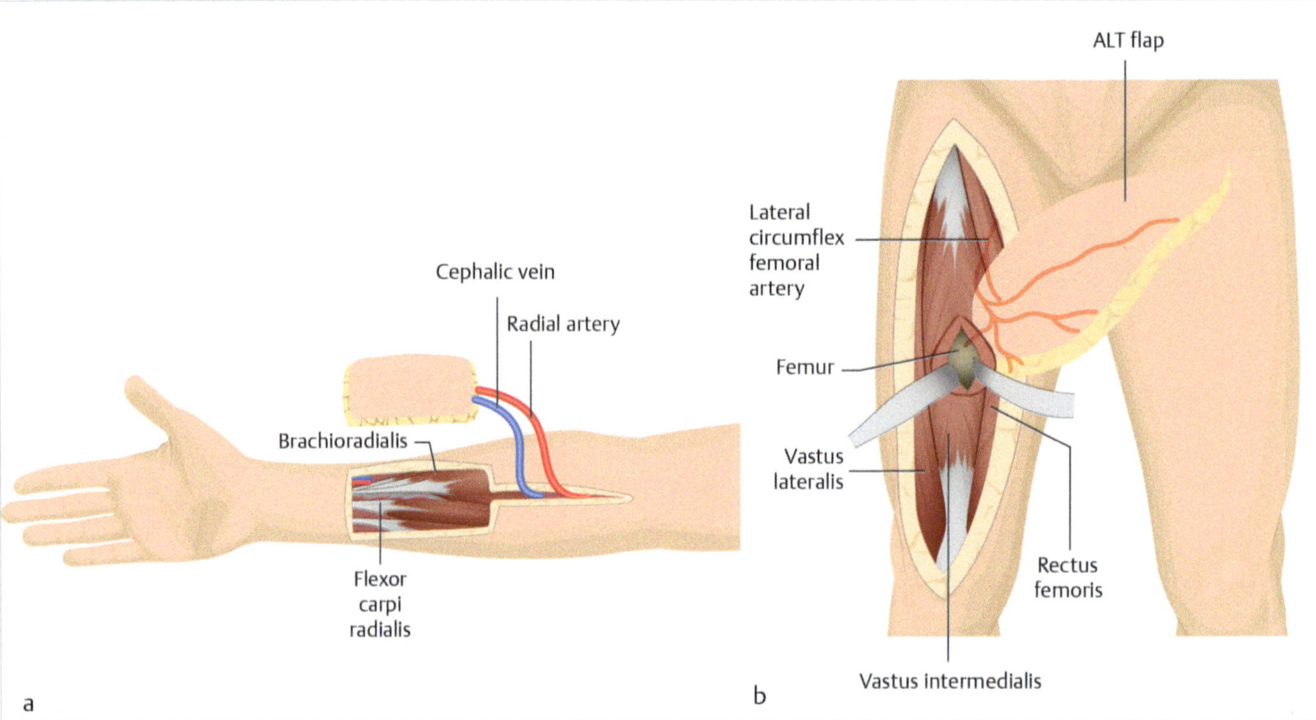

Fig. 20.8 Radial forearm free flap (**a**) and anterolateral thigh free flap (**b**).

Key Points

- Reconstruction of the buccal region following tumor resection poses a unique challenge with important aesthetic and functional considerations.
- Trismus is one of the most common sequelae following buccal tumor resection and reconstruction, especially in patients who have undergone or are planned to undergo radiation therapy.
- The optimal reconstructive technique is largely based on the size of the primary defect. Reconstructive options range from healing by secondary intention to microvascular free tissue transfer.

References

[1] Dijkstra PU, Huisman PM, Roodenburg JL. Criteria for trismus in head and neck oncology. Int J Oral Maxillofac Surg. 2006; 35(4):337–342

[2] Agarwal P, Shiva Kumar HR, Rai KK. Trismus in oral cancer patients undergoing surgery and radiotherapy. J Oral Biol Craniofac Res. 2016; 6 Suppl 1:S9–S13

[3] Bensadoun RJ, Riesenbeck D, Lockhart PB, Elting LS, Spijkervet FK, Brennan MT, Trismus Section, Oral Care Study Group, Multinational Association for Supportive Care in Cancer (MASCC)/International Society of Oral Oncology (ISOO). A systematic review of trismus induced by cancer therapies in head and neck cancer patients. Support Care Cancer. 2010; 18(8):1033–1038

[4] Squaquara R, Kim Evans KF, Spanio di Spilimbergo S, Mardini S. Intraoral reconstruction using local and regional flaps. Semin Plast Surg. 2010; 24(2): 198–211

[5] Ying B, Ye W, Zhu S, Zhu H, Hu J, Zhang Y. Buccal reconstruction with the mouth floor mucosal flap. J Craniofac Surg. 2012; 23(4):1143–1145

[6] Zhou T, Zhang L, Sun G, Hu Q. Ablation of buccal cancer and functionality buccal reconstruction using an individuation anterolateral thigh flap. J Craniofac Surg. 2018; 29(4):e396–e398–; Epub ahead of print

[7] Fang QG, Li ZN, Zhang X, Liu FY, Xu ZF, Sun CF. Clinical reliability of radial forearm free flap in repair of buccal defects. World J Surg Oncol. 2013; 11:26

[8] Licameli GR, Dolan R. Buccinator musculomucosal flap: applications in intraoral reconstruction. Arch Otolaryngol Head Neck Surg. 1998; 124(1):69–72

[9] Colella G, Tartaro G, Giudice A. The buccal fat pad in oral reconstruction. Br J Plast Surg. 2004; 57(4):326–329

[10] Hasibul K, Nakai F, Nakai Y, et al. Intra oral reconstruction with buccal fat pad: recent applications of autologous tissue transplantation as a local flap. JPRAS. 2016; 10:33–39

[11] Pribaz J, Stephens W, Crespo L, Gifford G. A new intraoral flap: facial artery musculomucosal (FAMM) flap. Plast Reconstr Surg. 1992; 90(3): 421–429

[12] von Domarus H. The double-door tongue flap for total cheek mucosa defects. Plast Reconstr Surg. 1988; 82(2):351–356

[13] Cunha-Gomes D, Joshi P, Bhathena H, Kavarana NM. The lateral tongue flap: a salvage option for reconstruction of buccal recurrences. Acta Chir Plast. 1999; 41(1):7–10

[14] Johnson PA, Banks P, Brown AE. Use of the posteriorly based lateral tongue flap in the repair of palatal fistulae. Int J Oral Maxillofac Surg. 1992; 21(1):6–9

[15] Martin D, Pascal JF, Baudet J, et al. The submental island flap: a new donor site. Anatomy and clinical applications as a free or pedicled flap. Plast Reconstr Surg. 1993; 92(5):867–873

[16] Szudek J, Taylor SM. Systematic review of the platysma myocutaneous flap for head and neck reconstruction. Arch Otolaryngol Head Neck Surg. 2007; 133(7):655–661

[17] Lazaridis N, Tilaveridis I, Karakasis D. Superiorly or inferiorly based "islanded" nasolabial flap for buccal mucosa defects reconstruction. J Oral Maxillofac Surg. 2008; 66(1):7–15

[18] Chen W, Zhang D, Yang Z, et al. Extended supraclavicular fasciocutaneous island flap based on the transverse cervical artery for head and neck reconstruction after cancer ablation. J Oral Maxillofac Surg. 2010; 68(10):2422–2430

[19] Song M, Chen F, Guo Z, et al. Application of various flaps to intraoral reconstruction of buccal defects after resection of buccal mucosa carcinoma. Chin J Cancer. 2009;28:663-667. J Oral Maxillofac Surg. 2010; 68: 2422–2430

[20] Chien CY, Hwang CF, Chuang HC, Jeng SF, Su CY. Comparison of radial forearm free flap, pedicled buccal fat pad flap and split-thickness skin graft in reconstruction of buccal mucosal defect. Oral Oncol. 2005; 41(7):694–697
[21] Fang QG, Safdar J, Shi S, et al. Comparison studies of different flaps for reconstruction of buccal defects. J Craniofac Surg. 2013; 24(5):e450–e451
[22] Liu F, Wang L, Pang S. Reconstruction of full-thickness buccal defects with folded radial forearm free flaps: a retrospective clinical study. Medicine (Baltimore). 2017; 96:e7344
[23] Kesting MR, Hölzle F, Wales C, et al. Microsurgical reconstruction of the oral cavity with free flaps from the anterolateral thigh and the radial forearm: a comparison of perioperative data from 161 cases. Ann Surg Oncol. 2011; 18 (7):1988–1994
[24] Liu WW, Li H, Guo ZM, et al. Reconstruction of soft-tissue defects of the head and neck: radial forearm flap or anterolateral thigh flap? Eur Arch Otorhinolaryngol. 2011; 268(12):1809–1812
[25] Chang YM, Deek NF, Wei FC. Trismus secondary release surgery and microsurgical free flap reconstruction after surgical treatment of head and neck cancer. Clin Plast Surg. 2016; 43(4):747–752
[26] Mardini S, Chang YM, Tsai CY, Coskunfirat OK, Wei FC. Release and free flap reconstruction for trismus that develops after previous intraoral reconstruction. Plast Reconstr Surg. 2006; 118(1):102–107
[27] Tsai CC, Wu SL, Lin SL, Ko SY, Chiang WF, Yang JW. Reducing trismus after surgery and radiotherapy in oral cancer patients: results of an alternative operation versus traditional operative. J Oral Maxillofac Surg. 2016; 74(5):1072–1083

21 Squamous Cell Cancer of the Alveolar Ridge

Theresa Guo and Karen T. Pitman

Summary
Squamous cell cancer of the alveolar ridge is primarily a surgically treated disease. These tumors are generally associated with smoking and use of alcohol, but can also be related to chewing carcinogens and chronic inflammation related to poor dental health. Tumors are often closely associated with dentition, and dental roots represent potential routes of bony invasion. Knowledge of dental anatomy and dental status of the patient impact surgical decision making. The primary surgical approach to upper alveolar ridge tumors is infrastructure maxillectomy, while lower alveolar ridge tumors are resected with marginal or segmental mandibulectomy.

Keywords: alveolar ridge, hard palate, infrastructure maxillectomy, marginal mandibulectomy, segmental mandibulectomy, oral cavity

21.1 Introduction

The alveolar ridge is defined as the bony ridge of the maxilla and mandible that harbors the tooth roots. It may also be described as the upper and lower gum, or gingiva. Along the maxilla, it is bounded anteriorly by the maxillary buccal vestibule and posteriorly by the hard palate to the pterygopalatine arch. The inferior alveolar ridge is bounded anteriorly by the mandibular buccal vestibule and posteriorly by the free mucosa of the floor of mouth; it extends along the ramus, ending at the retromolar trigone. The gingiva comprises the primary mucosa that lines the alveolar ridge. This is a nonkeratinized mucosa that forms the characteristic lining mucosa of a part of the oral cavity. Given that the mucosa in this region is in close proximity to the bone with minimal soft tissue, bony invasion can be common. As will be discussed in this chapter, in-depth knowledge of dental anatomy can aid decision-making when considering surgery in this region, help understand patterns of tumor spread, and help preserve dental and palate function. Disease in this region is commonly identified by oral dentists or oral surgeons, who also assist in comprehensive care of these patients including in reconstruction with obturators or dental implants.

21.2 Epidemiology

The oral cavity is the most common site of squamous cell carcinoma of the head and neck, particularly human papillomavirus (HPV) negative disease. Within the oral cavity, alveolar ridge cancers comprise about 7–12% of oral cavity cancers.[1,2]

Median age of diagnosis of alveolar ridge carcinoma is 66 years of age.[3] With regard to patient's gender, unlike other lesions of the oral cavity or oropharynx, there is a similar rate of presentation between men and women, with about 53–58% of patients being women.[3–5] Smoking and alcohol use are major risk factors for oral cavity cancer with higher risk associated heavy smoking and alcohol use. It is believed that inhaled carcinogens tend to mix into the saliva and come in contact with dependent regions of the oral cavity such as the floor of mouth or lateral tongue. In contrast, chewed carcinogens (chewing tobacco, betel nut) come in direct contact with the mucosa and may increase the risk of buccal or gingival cancers.[6] In addition, some risk factors that are specific to the alveolar ridge are a diet with low vegetable intake, poor oral hygiene, and periodontal disease which may contribute to chronic inflammation and cell turnover.[7]

With regard to oral hygiene, there is also some evidence that the oral microbiome may play a role in carcinogenesis in patients with oral cavity. A study in Taiwan found that patients with periodontitis have increased risk (1.79 adjusted hazard ratio) of developing oral cancer.[8] This may be a result of direct effects of bacterial toxins which impact cell growth, stimulate chronic inflammation, or affect the host microenvironment and immune system. *Porphyromonas gingivalis* is a known contributor to periodontal disease, resulting in microbial imbalance and chronic inflammation. In addition, *P. gingivalis* also inhibits apoptosis and has been shown to suppress the tumor suppressor p53.[9] Similar to other oral cavity cancers, tumors of the alveolar ridge are generally not associated with HPV.

Epidemiology of alveolar ridge cancer is similar to that of other oral cavity sites. The incidence in the past 30 years has overall decreased in the United States.[10] However, there is global variation in incidence. India has the highest incidence of oral cavity cancer, about 15–20%. Other risk factors, such as betel nut chewing, play an important role in the risk for oral cavity cancer in Asia, and as such, incidence of oral cavity cancer is actually rising in many Asian countries.[7] Betel nut chewing may be a more significant risk factor for oral cavity cancer than alcohol or tobacco use (adjusted odds ratio [OR] 6.9).[11]

21.3 Clinical Presentation

Clinical presentation of alveolar ridge lesions can vary significantly based on the location as well as patient factors (▶ Fig. 21.1). Early lesions are often asymptomatic and can be detected by routine oral examination.[1] As lesions progress, the patient may experience pain (about 30–40%) that can manifest as dental pain, burning pain, gingival pain, or ear pain.[12] Additional presenting complaints include bleeding (from ulceration), loose teeth, problems with denture fit, numbness of the teeth or lips, and trismus (secondary to pterygoid involvement).

Some patients may also present after transformation of premalignant lesions. Oral leukoplakia is a descriptive diagnosis, referring to a white "patch" or "plaque." Among these lesions, dysplasia or carcinoma occurs in up to 17–25% of lesions.[13,14] Some studies have suggested that leukoplakia lesions that arise in the floor of mouth, ventrolateral tongue or retromolar trigone, and soft palate have higher rates of transformation to malignancy, which were correlated with loss of heterozygosity in these subsites.[15]

Tumors of the alveolar ridge may present at any stage (T1–T4), with or without clinically evident nodal disease. One study reviewing 155 cases of lower alveolar ridge carcinoma showed

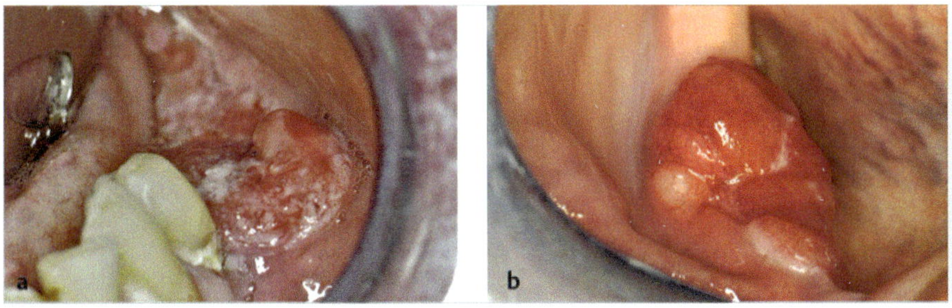

Fig. 21.1 Carcinoma of gingiva **(a)** surrounding dentition and **(b)** alveolar ridge in edentulous region.[12]

that most tumors were diagnosed as T2 lesions (45%).[3] Furthermore, most patients (82%) had clinically N0 neck at the time of presentation. In the upper alveolar ridge, the rates of clinically positive nodes are slightly higher—4% in T1 lesions, 10–15% in T2/3 lesions, and 25% in T4 lesions.[4]

21.4 Diagnosis and Evaluation

Evaluation should focus on assessment of factors that will determine definitive treatment. These factors include pathology, extent of tumor including involvement of adjacent structures, bony invasion, native bony stock, dental status, nodal disease burden, and distant metastasis. This assessment will help to determine the first steps in surgical treatment including marginal versus segmental mandibulectomy, extent of bony resection for maxillary lesions, need for neck dissection, and potential need for reconstruction. Clinical evaluation should assess tumor size, extension to other subsites (floor of mouth, lip, oral tongue, palate), nerve involvement (V2 or V3 numbness, tongue weakness), fixation to the bone (which may be suggestive of invasion), and dental status (will be discussed below).

Diagnosis is made from clinical biopsy of suspicious lesions. In the oral cavity, alveolar ridge lesions are generally accessible and amenable to biopsy in the clinic, unless significant trismus is present. Biopsies should be performed using punch technique rather than shave technique to allow for assessment of depth of invasion. Evaluation of bony or periosteal invasion may not be possible from in-office biopsy, but may be enough to secure a diagnosis of malignancy to guide further treatment.

Recently the American Joint Committee on Cancer (AJCC) 8th edition staging manual included changes to T staging for oral cavity tumors to include depth of invasion. These changes were made to reflect the correlation between depth of invasion and aggressive biologic tumor behavior.

Imaging: Computed tomography (CT) with contrast is the mainstay of imaging for cancers involving the alveolar ridge, and offers the best sensitivity and specificity for bony invasion compared to panorex or bone scan.[16] However, evaluation can still be challenging due to irregularities of the dental socket and artifact from dental amalgam;[17] therefore, clinical evaluation remains important.[18] If there is question of soft tissue invasion into the intrinsic tongue musculature, magnetic resonance imaging (MRI) can provide additional insight. Both of these modalities can also identify cervical lymph adenopathy. In addition, chest imaging should be performed for staging to rule out distant metastases or second primary, particularly in patients with a history of smoking.

Bony invasion: Evaluation of bony invasion is critical for surgical decision-making. In histologic studies, the routes of bony invasion are shown to come from direct extension from the primary tumor.[19] Notably, tumors of the alveolar ridge are more likely to have bony invasion compared to other oral cavity tumors, and this generally occurs at the occlusal ridge.[19,20] Two patterns of invasion have been observed: erosive and infiltrative. The erosive pattern shows a broad tumor front that pushes into the bone, with a well-defined border. The infiltrative pattern shows a more irregular tumor front with finger-like extensions into the bone. In a study of 68 patients, 60% of patients had erosive pattern of bony invasion. Patients with infiltrative pattern of bony invasion were more likely to have positive bony margins, and had a significantly worse 3-year overall survival.[21]

Routes of bony invasion can also be impacted by the existing bony stock. The most common site of bony invasion is along the occlusal ridge.[22] Entry into the bone occurs in this region as it lacks a thick cortical bony barrier. In dentulous patients, this may track along the dental sockets. In edentulous patients, the occlusal ridge is at a lower height and more easily accessed (▶ Fig. 21.2). In addition, invasion in the lingual and buccal cortical plates may also occur due to thinner bone stock. Nerve foramina represent another area where a defect in the cortical bone allows tumors to directly access medullary bone, and patients with nerve involvement are likely to have bony involvement, especially in edentulous patients.[23] In patients with history of irradiation, cortical bony invasion is more common, and tends to be less predictable, occurring in multiple foci (▶ Fig. 21.2).

Dental status and bone height also impact surgical decision-making. If there is involvement of the periosteum, at least a marginal mandibulectomy should be performed. However, only dentate patients with healthy bone stock should be considered for possible marginal mandibulectomy procedures. In these patients, average height of the mandible is higher in the parasymphyseal region (38 mm) compared to the molar region (26 mm). Therefore, invasion in the molar region requiring > 10 mm bony resection leaves insufficient height for a stable marginal mandibulectomy.[20] As will be discussed in surgical approaches, rim or sagittal marginal mandibulectomy approaches may be considered.

In the edentulous patient, the duration of edentulous status impacts the height and strength of the mandibular bone stock, as atrophy occurs over time. Segmental mandibulectomy is recommended if any bony resection is required. Due to inadequate bone stock, the risk of pathologic fracture is high. However, if the bony resection is lateral, the mandible may be left "swinging" without bone or plated reconstruction. In this case, soft tissue coverage is important to prevent tethering or trismus. Midline mandibulectomy however necessitates rigid

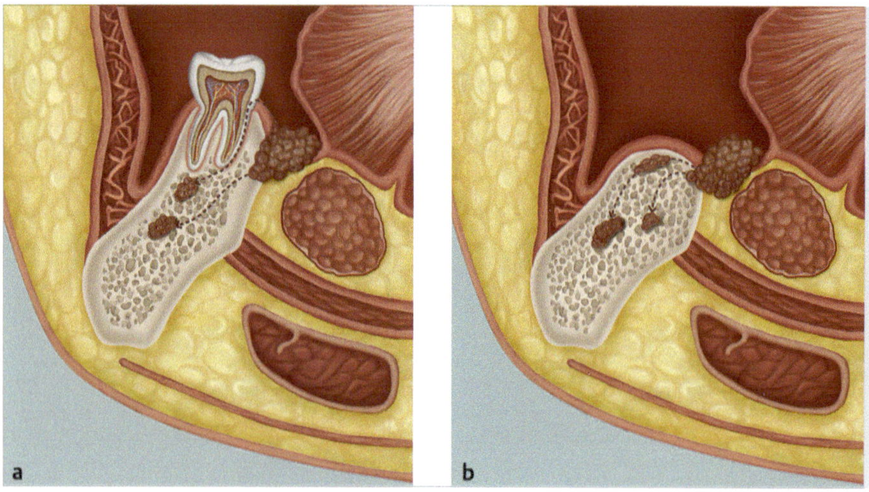

Fig. 21.2 (a, b) Routes of bony invasion in dentulous and edentulous patients.

reconstruction, to prevent significant retrognathia and subsequent airway compromise, as the tongue musculature and tongue base attach to the mandible anteriorly.

Lastly, history of radiation is an important factor to consider. As discussed previously, the patients with history of radiation tend to have less predictable and multifocal regions of bony tumor invasion. In addition, previously radiated bone has decreased vascular supply within the marrow and is at risk of poor wound healing and higher risk of pathologic fracture. Therefore, segmental mandibulectomy is recommended if any bony resection is required.

21.5 Anatomic Considerations/ Relevant Anatomy

An understanding of dental anatomy is helpful in documentation and treatment planning for alveolar ridge disease. Recall that numbering of teeth begins at the right third molar from #1 and is then numbered clockwise to #32. There are three molars on each side, in both the maxilla and mandible, although the third molar or wisdom tooth is not always erupted. Medial to the molars are the first and second premolars, followed by canine, lateral incisor, and central incisor. Each tooth has enamel which is the hardest surface layer, primarily composed of calcium phosphate. Underneath the enamel is dentin, which is more porous—thus symptoms of pain or sensitivity of teeth may be a sign of exposed dentin from enamel erosion. Within the dentin is the pulp containing vasculature and nerve fibers of the tooth root. The length of tooth roots is generally between 1.0 and 1.5 cm with canines having the longest roots. Knowledge of tooth roots can be helpful in planning osteotomy incisions or drilling bone for plating.

Additional landmarks in the maxilla that are of particular importance are the anterior and posterior ethmoidal arteries, skull base, and lacrimal fossa. The lacrimal fossa contains the lacrimal duct and opens in the medial orbit bounded by the anterior and posterior lacrimal crest. The nasolacrimal duct then travels along the anteriomedial wall of the maxillary sinus and empties in the inferior nasal meatus. The anterior ethmoidal foramen is located posterior to the lacrimal crest, while the posterior ethmoidal artery enters 36 mm from the lacrimal crest (and 12 mm from the anterior ethmoidal artery). The optic canal lies 6 mm behind the posterior ethmoidal artery. The frontoethmoidal suture line marks the superior boundary of any bony dissection to avoid injury to the cribiform plate. Recall that posterior to the maxilla is the pterygopalatine fossa, which contains the internal maxillary artery, pterygopalatine ganglion, and maxillary nerve (V2).

In the mandible, blood supply is primarily from the inferior alveolar artery (which takes off from internal maxillary artery), facial artery, and lingual artery. The innervation is supplied by the inferior alveolar nerve, which enters on the lingual surface of the mandibular ramus through the mandibular foramen and exits through the mental foramen at the second premolar. The lingual nerve runs medially within the floor of mouth in close proximity to the mandible and should be identified during intraoral dissection.

21.6 Surgical Consideration and Approaches

When performing surgery in the oral cavity, surgeons should seek to maintain the key functions of the oral cavity of swallowing, mastication, speech, and saliva production without compromising oncologic resection. Surgery remains the mainstay of disease control in oral cavity squamous cell carcinoma in both the primary and recurrent setting.

In addition, surgery offers patients the possibility of single modality treatment, if tumors are in early stage such as T1 or T2 and N0. However, notably in the alveolar ridge, due the mucosa's close proximity to bone, bony invasion may occur early, even in smaller tumors. Surgical resection allows for decrease of radiation dosing from a treatment dose (66–70 Gy) to an adjuvant dose (44–66 Gy), especially in the setting of negative margins and no adverse features.[24] Radiation treatment, especially in the oral cavity region, is not without risk, including severe xerostomia, mucositis, and high risk for osteoradionecrosis of the bone. Rates of osteoradionecrosis are higher following radiation of over 55–70 Gy, and in patients with alveolar ridge tumors or requiring mandibular surgery.[25,26] However, with the advent of intensity-modulated radiation therapy (IMRT), rates of osteoradionecrosis have decreased over time.[27]

Assessment of bony invasion is critical in evaluation of the extent of resection required. If no gross bony invasion is seen on imaging, evaluation of the periosteum should be performed intraoperatively. If there is no involvement of the periosteum, then a subperiosteal dissection can be performed, with the periosteum taken as a negative margin. However, if there is periosteal involvement, either marginal or segmental mandibulectomy with bony resection should be performed. In the past, it was believed that the lymphatics of oral lesions drained through the mandibular periosteum to reach the neck. As such, it was believed that a segmental mandibulectomy was necessary to remove all surrounding periosteum and truly clear disease. Then, Marchetta and McGregor determined that bony invasion was a result of direct extension into the bone.[22,23,28] Therefore, they instead advocated for marginal mandibulectomy in cases of tumors involving the periosteum, reserving segmental mandibulectomy for patients with gross bony invasion. Some surgeons have also advocated for marginal mandibulectomy for limited bone invasion[29] and have shown local control rates of 75–80%, which are slightly lower, but not significantly different from local control rates for segmental mandibulectomy (80–95%).[30,31]

With regard to airway management, a tracheostomy should be considered for every patient with mandibular reconstruction. If lesions are superficial and only require subperiosteal resection or marginal mandibulectomy, then airway is less likely to be compromised. However, in resections involving the anterior mandible, tongue base prolapse can cause significant airway obstruction. If bony reconstruction is not performed, patients may become tracheostomy dependent.[29] In patients with maxilla resection and reconstruction, generally the tissue sits superior and anterior, and therefore does not cause significant airway obstruction. History of prior radiation or lymph node resections requiring internal jugular vein sacrifice are also risk factors for postsurgical upper airway edema, which should be considered.

If tracheostomy is not performed, nasotracheal intubation provides improved access to the oral cavity and assessment of occlusion for mandibular resections. Care should be taken to secure the tube with silk suture or tape, and nasal ala should be padded to prevent alar necrosis. For maxillectomy resections, contralateral nasal or orotracheal intubation may allow for improved visualization. Tracheostomy may be performed at the beginning of a case to allow for freedom of surgical access during expiration of the tumor. Many patients can be decannulated in the immediate postoperative period (within 5–7 days).

Temporary placement of feeding tube is prudent, if the patient does not have prior gastrostomy tube. Depending on reconstructive needs, the patient may be recommended for limited oral diet to allow for surgical site healing and prevention of fistula. The exception may be in patients where primary mucosal closure is performed over periosteal or marginal mandibulectomy resections. In addition to allowing for surgical site healing, patients may have significant oral phase dysphagia due to surgical site swelling and tissue bulk that may limit oral nutrition. Poor nutrition status and low serum albumin level postoperatively can increase risk of wound infection after oral cavity surgery.[32]

Neck dissection, as previously discussed, should be performed in patients with clinically evident neck disease, and elective neck dissection should be considered in N0 patients as well. In general, elective neck dissection is recommended if risk of occult cervical metastasis is greater than 20%.[33] For patients with N0 disease, occult nodal disease is still significant, especially in patients with T3 and T4 lesions. In the lower alveolar ridge, occult disease is found in 14–17% of patients with T1/2 lesions and 44% of patients with T3/T4 lesions,[3] and positive nodes are found in levels I–III. Similarly, in the upper alveolar ridge, occult nodal disease resides primarily in levels I–II,[5,34] and the rates have been reported to be between 20 and 30%, with slightly lower rates (20%) in patients with T1 and T2 disease.[35,36] In patients with clinically positive neck disease, a complete neck dissection should be performed, as nodal disease may be present in levels I–V.[3,34]

For tumors of the maxilla and alveolar ridge, there has been some evidence that elective neck dissection improves overall disease-free survival, particularly for higher T stages.[36,37] Given the relatively higher rates of occult nodal disease and potential for survival benefit, if the neck is to be opened for exploration of neck vessels for free flap reconstruction, elective neck dissection should be performed regardless of T stage, including levels I–III.

Perioperative antibiotics should be given prior to surgery given the clean-contaminated nature of the surgical field which universally involves intraoral mucosa. Prior studies showed similar outcomes in patients treated with ampicillin/sulbactam and clindamycin.[38] More recent studies have shown higher rates of surgical wound infection in head and neck reconstruction that used clindamycin, due to incomplete gram negative coverage.[39,40] Given the recent data, patients should be treated with ampicillin/sulbactam or second-generation cephalosporin with metronidazole for penicillin allergic patients.

21.7 Maxilla—Upper Alveolar Ridge

Lesions of the upper alveolar ridge or hard palate may be addressed by an infrastructure or inferior maxillectomy approach, as long as tumors do not extend through the maxillary sinus or nasal cavity. Preoperative consultation with a prosthodontist can allow for an obturator to be fashioned prior to surgery. Prior to making incisions or osteotomies, the extent of the tumor and surgical margins should be marked. Local anesthesia with epinephrine should be applied prior to incisions in both the skin and mucosa after incisions are planned. For midface degloving approach, intranasal injections including the caudal septum and topical vasoconstriction will aid in dissection and visualization.

21.8 Infrastructure Maxillectomy

In the infrastructure maxillectomy, resection bony cuts define the main margins medially (along the hard palate), superiorly (along the floor of the maxillary sinus), and laterally, which may extend to the lateral extent of the maxilla (▶ Fig. 21.3). Prior to incisions, the extent of tumor and planned bony cuts should be visualized and marked. Intraoral dissection or midface degloving should allow adequate access without skin incisions unless resection extends superiorly toward the orbital floor. Mucosal incision is carried out along the anterior labial

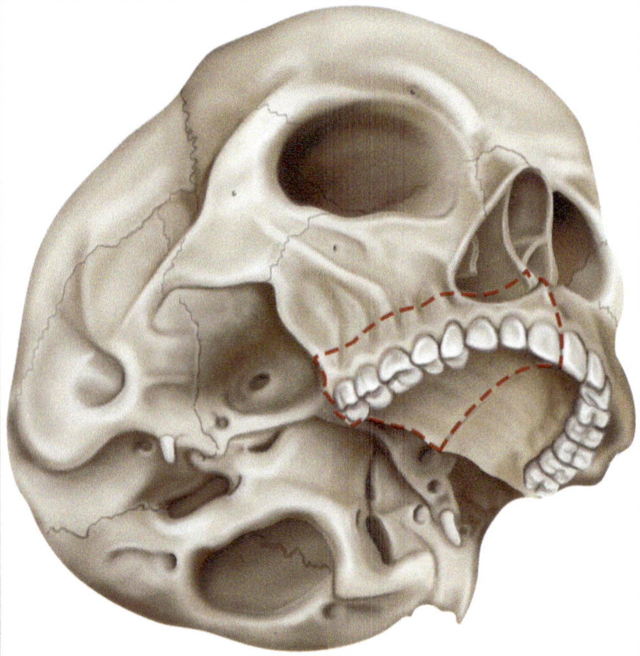

Fig. 21.3 Bony cuts for infrastructure maxillectomy resection.

sulcus to the bone. For a midface degloving, this can be carried across midline to extend bilaterally to canines on each side. The posterior portion of the incision on the side of the resection can be curved superiorly to allow for reduced tension during retraction. The soft tissue is then elevated off the maxillary bone and infraorbital nerve is identified. This should be preserved in an infrastructure resection. A full transfixion incision can be performed to release the soft tissue and allow for degloving access, if resection extends bilaterally. For unilateral access, the nasal cavity can be entered through the lateral nasal wall, with care to avoid injury to the inferior turbinate.

Next, hard palate incisions can be planned based on tumor location and extent. Mucosa is scored with cautery and then carried down to the bone. The mucosa is released with periosteal elevator to create a tract for planned osteotomies. If the patient is dentate, the tooth at the planned osteotomy should be extracted. Posteriorly, the mucosa of the soft palate can be released from the hard palate.

All soft tissue work should be completed before osteotomies are made. First a Caldwell-Luc anterior maxillary antrostomy is made inferior to the infraorbital nerve. This allows access to the maxilla and evaluation of tumor extent superiorly. Next, osteotomy is performed through the lateral maxillary wall up to the posterior maxillary wall, or may be curved if only a portion of the maxilla is to be removed. Then the medial osteotomy is performed, to connect with the nasal vestibule, with care not to injure the septum or inferior turbinate to avoid bleeding. Next a posterior osteotomy is performed to free the maxilla from the pterygoid plates. After this, the hard palate osteotomies are performed. If the resection extends across midline, the nasal septum will need to be released from the nasal floor. The specimen is then down fractured and released. Posterior soft tissue release may be performed with a heavy curved mayo scissors. Packing and pressure may be applied to help achieve hemostasis after the specimen is removed. Internal maxillary artery can get divided or sheared during specimen removal and this should be identified and ligated if resection extends to the pterygopalatine fossa.

The defect may be left to granulate with a plan for obturator placement. The primary functional consequence is oroantral fistula. Alternatively, local flaps (such as nasolabial, temporalis, palatal) may be used to fill the defect, or free flap reconstruction may be considered for larger resections such as radial forearm to obliterate the fistula, or fibular/osseocutaneous forearm to restore bony stock.

21.9 Lower Alveolar Ridge—Mandible

When evaluating tumors of the lower alveolar ridge, dental status, history of radiation, or bony stock of the mandible dictates the surgical extent and approach. Marginal mandibulectomy may be considered in patients with periosteal disease but no gross bony invasion. Generally, only dentulous, non-radiated patients have mandibular bony stock to be candidates for marginal mandibulectomy procedures without the risk of pathologic fracture. Furthermore, radiated and edentulous patients have higher risk of medullary bone invasion. If a segmental mandibulectomy is planned in a dentate patient, occlusion status should be assessed preoperatively with the goal of restoring occlusion when possible. Assisted three-dimensional CT reconstruction, custom plates, or custom bone saw guides for bony reconstruction may be helpful. In addition, prebending and drilling plates prior to planned osteotomies can assist in restoring preoperative occlusion and position of the mandible.

21.10 Marginal Mandibulectomy

Once a patient has been determined to be a candidate for a marginal mandibulectomy, the patient should be assessed for his or her mouth opening, as this will impact the ability to approach the resection through a strictly transoral approach. Depending on the location of the lesion, the bone may be shaved with a saw with a sagittal cut (▶ Fig. 21.4a) or along the rim where bony cuts should be made beyond the tooth roots if present (▶ Fig. 21.4b, c) ▶ Fig. 21.4). If lesions are primarily on the lingual surface of the mandible, these lesions may be addressed with a sagittal marginal bony cut for removal of the inner cortex. Sagittal mandibulectomy can be challenging with a high risk of fracture during the procedure if not carefully executed and weak points of the mandible are encountered. A curved osteotomy cut can help maximize remaining bone stock and help prevent fracture of remaining bone. Patients should be counseled of the possibility of fracture and need for plating. Tooth roots should be fully removed with any dentition. Bone grafting or placement of bone dust may help the bone achieve greater bony strength during the healing process.

21.11 Segmental Mandibulectomy

For laterally based tumors along the mandible, the lateral cheek approach provides excellent unilateral exposure while protecting important anatomic structures of the cheek soft tissue such

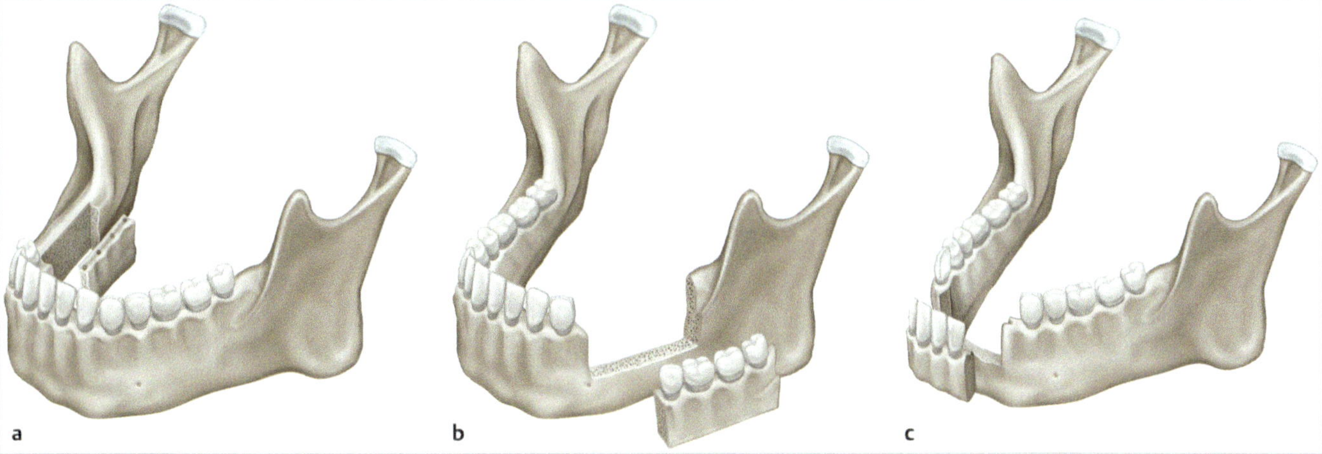

Fig. 21.4 (a–c) Marginal mandibulectomy approaches.

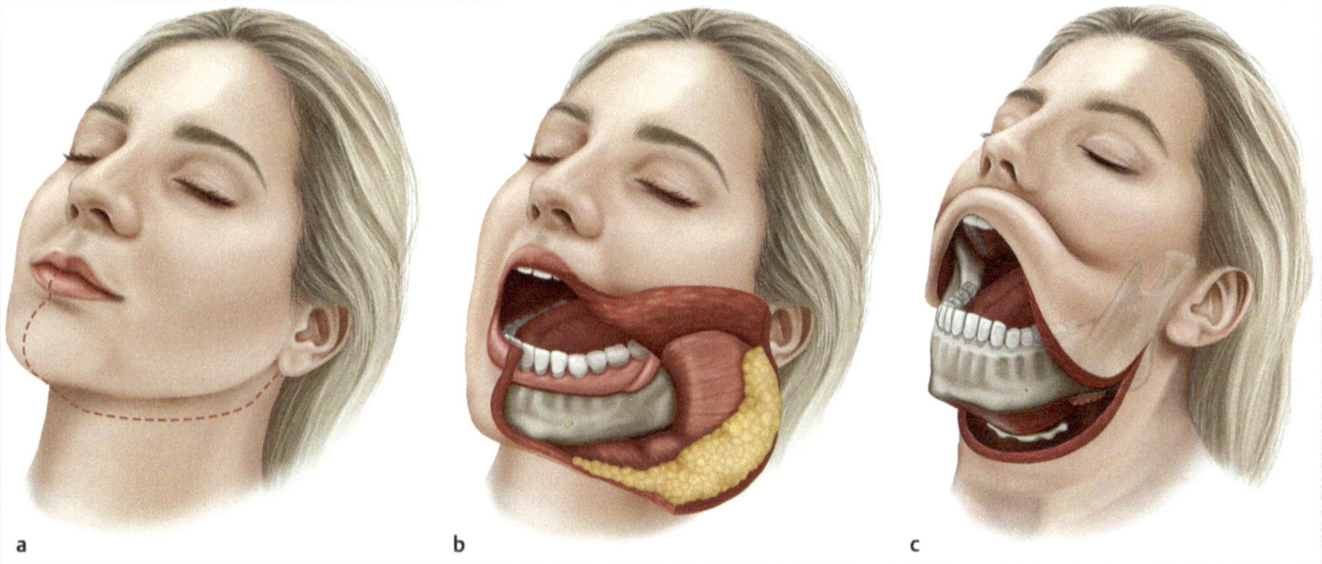

Fig. 21.5 (a–c) Lateral neck and visor approaches to the mandible.

as facial artery and marginal mandibular branch of the facial nerve (▶ Fig. 21.5a, b). This involves a vertical lip split with extension of the incision along the mentum to connect with a neck incision that will allow for exposure of levels I and II for neck dissection. Skin incision should run 2 fingerbreadths below the mandible to protect the marginal mandibular nerve. Marginal mandibular nerve should be identified to allow for adequate resection of level I lymph nodes while protecting the nerve.

Intraoral incision should be made (with adequate mucosa margin) along the labial sulcus. This incision should leave adequate gingival mucosa along the remaining mandible to allow for closure. The soft tissue is then raised along the periosteum to expose the bone. When possible, the mental nerve (not pictured) may be identified and kept intact if oncologically sound, although this may be more difficult in lateral mandibulectomy. The bone is then freed circumferentially to prepare for osteotomies. Along the lingual surface of the mandible it may be pertinent to identify lingual nerve within the floor of mouth to avoid injury. Bone cuts may be performed between tooth roots, but if dentition is poor or tooth roots are exposed extraction is recommended. If bony reconstruction is planned, plates should be bent and drilled to fit the native mandible before bony cuts are made, especially in the dentulous patient.

For tumors near the midline, a visor approach may be ideal (▶ Fig. 21.5c). This incision avoids a lip split and provides access to the anterior mandible. Incision may be planned at the level of the hyoid and two fingerbreadths below the mandible, to avoid injury to the marginal mandibular nerves. The dissection is carried out in a subplatysmal plane up to the mandible in the midline. Within this plane, the marginal mandibular nerve may be encountered. It universally travels superficial to the facial vessels which may be identified near the facial notch. These may require ligation to achieve additional mobility and care to preserve vessel integrity may facilitate free flap reconstruction, if needed. Note that skin laxity may play a role in the ability to retract the soft tissue superiorly. As the mandible and bone is encountered, again mental nerve should be identified and preserved when possible; adequate dissection and release of the nerve from the bone will allow additional mobility of the skin flap. Once the mandible periosteum is identified, soft tissue should be released in the subperiosteal plane to release the bone. At this point, the intraoral mucosa cuts within the vestibule as well as floor of mouth should be assessed to ensure adequate mucosal margins. These mucosal cuts can be carried to the subperiosteal plane and joined with the previously dissected plane from below. Connection of these planes beginning near the midline protects the mental nerves from injury. Once the bone has been released circumferentially, bony cuts may be planned.

A composite resection may also be performed through this approach in conjunction with a neck dissection. Similar surgical approaches may be taken and the specimen is removed en bloc with the neck dissection.

21.12 Surgical Sequelae

In the short-term postoperative period, patients may experience significant challenges with regard to breathing, swallowing, and speech. Generally, dysphagia is temporary, as resection of bony alveolar ridge tends to preserve the soft tissue, posterior pharynx, and cranial nerves (with the exception of V2 and V3). However, in the immediate postoperative period, patients will often remain nil per os (NPO) to allow for surgical site healing of any reconstruction. This is particularly important for mandibular resection and reconstruction, as saliva and food tend to rest inferiorly along suture lines and are at higher risk of infection or salivary leak. Maxillary reconstruction may cause dysphagia secondary to bulk, preventing swallow of oral bolus, but this generally improves. Some patients may require tracheostomy which is often temporary, particularly for patients who undergo midline mandibular resection and reconstruction (▶ Fig. 21.5). Tissue bulk will push the tongue base posteriorly, and most patients will have a relative retrognathia that exacerbates airway obstruction. As tissue swelling subsides, many patients can be decannulated during the first 1–2 weeks after surgery.

Other longer term sequelae include nonunion of reconstructed bone, malocclusion, temporal mandibular joint ankylosis, and trismus. These may be addressed in subsequent follow-up procedures. Lastly, patients may undergo postoperative radiation, which is recommended within 6 weeks after surgery. Radiation may contribute to trismus with stiffening of pterygoid muscles. Osteoradionecrosis is a risk factor in these patients, and may put them at risk of exposed hardware, recurrent infections or fistulas, or need for revision surgery. Patients should be monitored in follow-up for regions of non-healing which may be a sign of recurrent disease or osteoradionecrosis.

Key Points

- Alveolar ridge tumors occur within the oral cavity and are associated with chewing carcinogens (chewing tobacco and betel nut) in addition to smoking and alcohol use.
- Dental status, history of radiation, and mandibular bone stock impact surgical decision-making, and impact risk for bony invasion.
- Elective neck dissection, levels I–III, should be performed for patients with alveolar ridge cancers with T3/T4 disease and should be considered in patients with T2 disease. Complete neck dissection, levels I–V, should be performed in any patient with clinical positive neck disease.
- Bone should be resected if there is periosteal involvement.
- Edentulous patients and those who have undergone radiation likely require segmental mandibulectomy, if any mandibular bony resection is needed.
- All soft tissue work should be completed before bony osteotomies are made.
- Reconstruction is often required. For infrastructure maxillectomy defects, an obturator may be fashioned. For segmental mandibulectomy defects, midline resections require rigid reconstruction. Lateral mandibulectomy defects may be left swinging in the edentulous patient.

References

[1] Mashberg A, Merletti F, Boffetta P, et al. Appearance, site of occurrence, and physical and clinical characteristics of oral carcinoma in Torino, Italy. Cancer. 1989; 63(12):2522–2527

[2] Hirata RM, Jaques DA, Chambers RG, Tuttle JR, Mahoney WD. Carcinoma of the oral cavity: an analysis of 478 cases. Ann Surg. 1975; 182(2):98–103

[3] Eicher SA, Overholt SM, el-Naggar AK, Byers RM, Weber RS. Lower gingival carcinoma: clinical and pathologic determinants of regional metastases. Arch Otolaryngol Head Neck Surg. 1996; 122(6):634–638

[4] Lin HW, Bhattacharyya N. Survival impact of nodal disease in hard palate and maxillary alveolus cancer. Laryngoscope. 2009; 119(2):312–315

[5] Os AD, Karakullukcu B, Leemans CR, et al. Management of the clinically N0 neck in squamous cell carcinoma of the maxillary alveolus and hard palate. Head Neck. 2016; 38(12):1794–1798

[6] Natarajan E, Eisenberg E. Contemporary concepts in the diagnosis of oral cancer and precancer. Dent Clin North Am. 2011; 55(1):63–88

[7] Krishna Rao SV, Mejia G, Roberts-Thomson K, Logan R. Epidemiology of oral cancer in Asia in the past decade—an update (2000–2012). Asian Pac J Cancer Prev. 2013; 14(10):5567–5577

[8] Wen BW, Tsai CS, Lin CL, et al. Cancer risk among gingivitis and periodontitis patients: a nationwide cohort study. QJM. 2014; 107(4):283–290

[9] Ferguson BL, Barber S, Asher IH, Wood CR. Role of oral microbial infections in oral cancer. Dent Clin North Am. 2017; 61(2):425–434

[10] Chaturvedi AK, Anderson WF, Lortet-Tieulent J, et al. Worldwide trends in incidence rates for oral cavity and oropharyngeal cancers. J Clin Oncol. 2013; 31(36):4550–4559

[11] Ko YC, Huang YL, Lee CH, Chen MJ, Lin LM, Tsai CC. Betel quid chewing, cigarette smoking and alcohol consumption related to oral cancer in Taiwan. J Oral Pathol Med. 1995; 24(10):450–453

[12] Bagan J, Sarrion G, Jimenez Y. Oral cancer: clinical features. Oral Oncol. 2010; 46(6):414–417

[13] Waldron CA, Shafer WG. Leukoplakia revisited: a clinicopathologic study 3256 oral leukoplakias. Cancer. 1975; 36(4):1386–1392

[14] Bouquot JE, Gorlin RJ. Leukoplakia, lichen planus, and other oral keratoses in 23,616 white Americans over the age of 35 years. Oral Surg Oral Med Oral Pathol. 1986; 61(4):373–381

[15] Zhang L, Cheung KJ, Jr, Lam WL, et al. Increased genetic damage in oral leukoplakia from high risk sites: potential impact on staging and clinical management. Cancer. 2001; 91(11):2148–2155

[16] Close LG, Merkel M, Burns DK, Schaefer SD. Computed tomography in the assessment of mandibular invasion by intraoral carcinoma. Ann Otol Rhinol Laryngol. 1986; 95(4 Pt 1):383–388

[17] Shaha AR. Preoperative evaluation of the mandible in patients with carcinoma of the floor of mouth. Head Neck. 1991; 13(5):398–402

[18] Werning JW, Byers RM, Novas MA, Roberts D. Preoperative assessment for and outcomes of mandibular conservation surgery. Head Neck. 2001; 23(12): 1024–1030

[19] Tsue TT, McCulloch TM, Girod DA, Couper DJ, Weymuller EA, Jr, Glenn MG. Predictors of carcinomatous invasion of the mandible. Head Neck. 1994; 16 (2):116–126

[20] Brown JS, Griffith JF, Phelps PD, Browne RM. A comparison of different imaging modalities and direct inspection after periosteal stripping in predicting the invasion of the mandible by oral squamous cell carcinoma. Br J Oral Maxillofac Surg. 1994; 32(6):347–359

[21] Wong RJ, Keel SB, Glynn RJ, Varvares MA. Histological pattern of mandibular invasion by oral squamous cell carcinoma. Laryngoscope. 2000; 110(1):65–72

[22] McGregor AD, MacDonald DG. Routes of entry of squamous cell carcinoma to the mandible. Head Neck Surg. 1988; 10(5):294–301

[23] McGregor AD, MacDonald DG. Patterns of spread of squamous cell carcinoma within the mandible. Head Neck. 1989; 11(5):457–461

[24] Head and Neck Cancers. National Comprehensive Cancer Network Guidelines 2018; Version 2.2018:https://www.nccn.org/professionals/physician_gls/pdf/head-and-neck.pdf. Accessed June 20, 2018

[25] Bedwinek JM, Shukovsky LJ, Fletcher GH, Daley TE. Osteonecrosis in patients treated with definitive radiotherapy for squamous cell carcinomas of the oral cavity and naso- and oropharynx. Radiology. 1976; 119(3):665–667

[26] Lee IJ, Koom WS, Lee CG, et al. Risk factors and dose-effect relationship for mandibular osteoradionecrosis in oral and oropharyngeal cancer patients. Int J Radiat Oncol Biol Phys. 2009; 75(4):1084–1091

[27] Ben-David MA, Diamante M, Radawski JD, et al. Lack of osteoradionecrosis of the mandible after intensity-modulated radiotherapy for head and neck cancer: likely contributions of both dental care and improved dose distributions. Int J Radiat Oncol Biol Phys. 2007; 68(2):396–402

[28] Marchetta FC, Sako K, Murphy JB. The periosteum of the mandible and intraoral carcinoma. Am J Surg. 1971; 122(6):711–713

[29] Genden EM, Rinaldo A, Jacobson A, et al. Management of mandibular invasion: when is a marginal mandibulectomy appropriate? Oral Oncol. 2005; 41 (8):776–782

[30] O'Brien CJ, Adams JR, McNeil EB, et al. Influence of bone invasion and extent of mandibular resection on local control of cancers of the oral cavity and oropharynx. Int J Oral Maxillofac Surg. 2003; 32(5):492–497

[31] Dubner S, Heller KS. Local control of squamous cell carcinoma following marginal and segmental mandibulectomy. Head Neck. 1993; 15(1): 29–32

[32] Liu SA, Wong YK, Poon CK, Wang CC, Wang CP, Tung KC. Risk factors for wound infection after surgery in primary oral cavity cancer patients. Laryngoscope. 2007; 117(1):166–171

[33] Wein ROW. R.S. Malignant neoplasms of the oral cavity. In: Cummings, ed. Cummings Otolaryngology: Head and Neck Surgery. Philadelphia, PA: Elsevier Mosby; 2005:1591–1607

[34] Shah JP, Candela FC, Poddar AK. The patterns of cervical lymph node metastases from squamous carcinoma of the oral cavity. Cancer. 1990; 66(1): 109–113

[35] Simental AA, Jr, Johnson JT, Myers EN. Cervical metastasis from squamous cell carcinoma of the maxillary alveolus and hard palate. Laryngoscope. 2006; 116(9):1682–1684

[36] Givi B, Eskander A, Awad MI, et al. Impact of elective neck dissection on the outcome of oral squamous cell carcinomas arising in the maxillary alveolus and hard palate. Head Neck. 2016; 38 Suppl 1:E1688–E1694

[37] Poeschl PW, Seemann R, Czembirek C, et al. Impact of elective neck dissection on regional recurrence and survival in cN0 staged oral maxillary squamous cell carcinoma. Oral Oncol. 2012; 48(2):173–178

[38] Johnson JT, Kachman K, Wagner RL, Myers EN. Comparison of ampicillin/sulbactam versus clindamycin in the prevention of infection in patients undergoing head and neck surgery. Head Neck. 1997; 19(5):367–371

[39] Weber RS, Raad I, Frankenthaler R, et al. Ampicillin-sulbactam vs clindamycin in head and neck oncologic surgery: the need for gram-negative coverage. Arch Otolaryngol Head Neck Surg. 1992; 118(11):1159–1163

[40] Pool C, Kass J, Spivack J, et al. Increased surgical site infection rates following clindamycin use in head and neck free tissue transfer. Otolaryngol Head Neck Surg. 2016; 154(2):272–278

22 Reconstruction of Alveolar Ridge

Andrea L. Hanick, Michael G. Roskies, and Jamie A. Ku

Summary

Defects of the alveolar ridge can lead to significant loss of function and poor aesthetic outcomes for head and neck cancer patients. The ideal reconstruction of the alveolar ridge improves both the form and function of the head and neck cancer patient, specifically restoring articulation of speech, potential for dental implants, and adequate cosmesis. Restoration of the alveolar ridge may be achieved with free grafts, locoregional flaps, or may require microvascular techniques for free tissue transfer. In considering restorative options, the advancements in new dental and oral surgery techniques should be employed to provide optimal results to patients.

Keywords: alveolar ridge, reconstruction, oral cavity cancer, flaps, free flaps

22.1 Introduction

The approach to reconstruction of the alveolar ridge is multidisciplinary, involving head and neck reconstructive surgeons, oral surgeons, prosthodontists, and speech-language pathologists. As described by Chen and Zhang in 1992, the goal of reconstruction of the alveolar ridge is twofold: to restore contour and to restore continuity.[1] Adequate reconstruction requires bony structural support and viable soft tissue coverage of the substructure. The ideal reconstruction of the alveolar ridge improves both the form and function for the head and neck cancer patient, specifically by restoring articulation of speech, potential for dentition, and adequate cosmesis.[2]

The concepts pertaining to the reconstruction of the alveolar process overlap with those for segmental and marginal mandibular defects. As such, this chapter will focus principally on soft tissue reconstructive options, allogenic materials, and tissue-engineered constructs.

22.2 Anatomic Considerations/ Relevant Anatomy

The alveolar ridge presents unique reconstructive challenges due to its specific anatomic features (▶ Fig. 22.1). Defined by the thickened ridge of bone that contains dental alveoli (tooth sockets), the alveolar process is located at the superior surface of the mandible and the inferior surface of the maxilla. Important components of this bone include the periodontal ligament and the compact lamina dura to which it attaches.

The blood supply to the alveolar process and teeth originates from the internal maxillary artery, which gives rise to the inferior alveolar artery, supplying the mandibular alveolus, and the posterior and anterior branches of the superior alveolar artery, supplying the maxillary alveolus. The innervations of the superior and inferior alveoli and teeth are the maxillary and mandibular divisions of the trigeminal nerve, respectively. In the edentulous patient, the alveolar portion of the mandible gradually resorbs, putting the inferior alveolar nerve at increased risk of injury during any surgical intervention.

The alveolar process of the maxilla contains the opposing maxillary dentition. The bony projections are bordered by corresponding soft tissue sulci laterally, the gingivobuccal and gingivolabial sulci. Medially, the tongue articulates against the dentition and alveolar ridge, contributing to speech clarity. The alveolar ridges provide horizontal projection to the overlying lip soft tissue, creating normal facial contour. The tissue of the buccal and upper gingival mucosa is tightly bound to the alveolar ridges and this covering overlies bone of variable thickness and structural integrity.

Overall, any defect of the alveolar ridge can lead to significant loss of function and poor aesthetic outcomes for head and neck cancer patients. Loss of dentition or of occlusal surface area for restorative dental prosthetics may lead to weight loss and decreased quality of life.[3,4] Loss of support for facial soft tissue has ramifications for speech, articulation, and oral competence. Finally, the aesthetic value of both dentition and bony support for facial soft tissue leading to alterations in social smile, facial profile, and projection should not be overlooked.

22.3 Diagnosis and Evaluation

22.3.1 Patient Selection

In preparing for reconstruction of the alveolar ridge, it is crucial to consider the patient's specific presentation, including comorbidities, body mass index (BMI), mental status, desire for dentition, size and location of the tumor, previous surgery, prior radiation, and need for postoperative radiation therapy. The surgeon must evaluate the status of current dentition and the preoperative mandibular bone height.

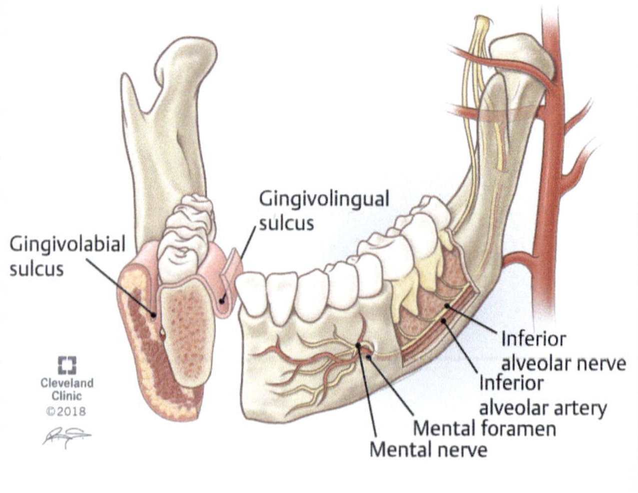

Fig. 22.1 Mandibular alveolar ridge anatomy. (Reproduced with permission, Cleveland Clinic Center for Medical Art & Photography ©2018. All Rights Reserved.)

22.3.2 Evaluation of Defect and Determining Reconstructive Options

As with any preoperative evaluation, the status of the tumor, including anatomic location, size, extent of invasion, and amount of bony involvement or destruction, must be carefully assessed. Specifically, when considering the alveolar ridge, reconstructive requirements will be radically different depending upon location and extent of disease. A small defect restricted to the ridge will be repaired much differently, utilizing local tissue rearrangement or free grafts, when compared to an extended defect that requires restoration of adjacent soft tissue structures, which might require a free tissue transfer for reconstruction.

As with all oral cavity defect reconstruction, areas of importance to reconstitute include the gingivolabial sulcus, gingivobuccal sulcus, and lateral tongue gutter or floor of mouth. These anatomic structures are challenging to recreate, and blunting, excess bulk, and/or scarring of these areas may lead to difficulties with speech and swallowing as well as improper fitting of dental restorative prosthetics. Often times, delayed secondary revision surgeries or vestibuloplasties are required.

22.4 Surgical Considerations and Approaches

22.4.1 Approaches to the Alveolar Ridge

Depending on the exposure necessary for both the oncologic excision of the tumor and the reconstruction of the defect, surgical approaches to the alveolar ridge include transoral, transcervical, and mandibular split, or a combination of the latter approaches. Reconstruction can include skin graft, local or regional flaps, or free tissue transfer. The location of facial, angular, and superficial temporal vessels may allow for more minimal access procedures when free flaps are employed.[5]

22.4.2 Ideal Characteristics for Reconstruction of the Alveolar Ridge

An ideal reconstruction of the alveolar ridge would provide thin and pliable soft tissue to allow optimal fit into the oral cavity without persisting excess bulk, conform to underlying bony structures, and be sufficiently durable to support the functions of the ridge, including mastication. Specific to the alveolar ridge, the ideal reconstruction allows for dental rehabilitation with implants or prosthodontics for both function and cosmesis. In the case of bony deficit, an osseous component to the reconstruction may be required to restore ridge height and provide a stable platform for soft tissue reconstruction. The ideal reconstruction creates minimal donor site morbidity and is able to be harvested distal to the site of resection, allowing for a two-team surgical approach. In the oral cavity, reconstruction of the alveolar ridge provides a barrier to infection by covering surgically exposed structures with viable soft tissue to prevent saliva and oral flora from extending into the neck. In addition, soft tissue coverage improves postoperative pain. The ideal reconstruction is able to integrate with surrounding soft tissue and mucosalize over time to mimic surrounding tissues. The complexity of this region creates surgical challenges and often no single ideal approach exists to meet all the above goals simultaneously. Thus, reconstructive planning depends on patient's wishes, patient-specific anatomy, and surgeon's preference within a multidisciplinary team.

22.5 Reconstructive Options

22.5.1 Secondary Intention, Primary Closure, and Buccal Advancement Flap

For very small, superficial defects, healing by secondary intention may be an option in some patients. However, coverage of the defect with soft tissue improves wound healing and decreases postoperative discomfort. Unfortunately, primary closure of gingival edges recruited from both the lingual and buccal sides of the defect is often not feasible after an oncologic extirpative surgery for alveolar ridge tumors. In select cases of a small, easily accessible, and soft tissue only defect of the alveolar ridge, a buccal advancement flap may be employed to free more local tissue for coverage. Branches of the maxillary artery (buccal artery, anterior, middle, and posterior superior alveolar arteries) richly supply the buccal mucosa, and leaving a broad base to the elevated mucopericondrial flap allows for a sufficient vascularity to the flap. Lengthening incisions can be made through the periosteum at the flap base when needed.[6] The primary drawback to this flap is blunting of the vestibule, which can require revision vestibuloplasty. However, in most cases, this improves with time as the buccal mucosa accommodates to the shape of the underlying bone.

22.5.2 Free Grafts: Full and Split Thickness Skin Grafts, Dermal Matrix Substitutes, and Bone Grafts

Skin Grafts

Full and split thickness skin grafts can be used to cover small defects of the alveolar ridge that are unable to be covered by local advancement of surrounding tissue. These options are possible over a well-vascularized wound bed, such as the periosteum or the bone marrow. Free skin grafts have minimal chance to grow over bare cortical bone surfaces, as the graft initially survives by diffusion of nutrients from fluids and blood in the wound bed into the graft until neo-vascularization and integration occurs. Convenient sites for full thickness skin graft harvest include the pre and postauricular skin (for small defects), supraclavicular skin, and the skin of abdomen or groin (for larger defects). Drawbacks of the use of skin grafts primarily include the potential for wound retraction and the relatively thin and delicate nature of the skin grafts that puts the graft's healing at risk on occlusive surfaces. Nonetheless, a temporary barrier serves as an advantage during healing, and some surgeons may opt for skin grafts, even while assuming they may eventually fail to incorporate.

Dermal Matrix Substitutes

Cadaveric-derived acellular, nonimmunogenic dermal substitutes, originally used for skin grafting, have gained popularity in bony defect coverage within the oral cavity.[7,8] Girod et al demonstrated that acellular dermal matrix (ADM) had advantages over split thickness skin graft (STSG) in limited oral cavity mucosal defects, including decreased surgical time and donor-site morbidity with improved quality of life.[9] The bipolar organization of ADM allows for epithelial cell migration along the basal lamina and fibroblast/angiogenic cell migration along the dermal matrix.[10] Studies examining their use in bone coverage along the alveolar ridge have demonstrated good incorporation, increased gingival thickness, and keratinization of tissue with an acceptable cosmetic result.[7,11–13] Certain skin substitutes provide temporary wound coverage, barrier protection, and may secrete cytokines and growth factors that promote epithelialization (e.g., Dermagraft ®), while others restore the epidermal barrier to become integrated within the wound (e.g., Alloderm ®).

It is important to note that, as with native skin grafts, skin substitute grafts will only be able to promote cell growth and heal wounds in a well-vascularized recipient site. For example, these products may be placed over periosteum, peritenon (fascial layer around tendon providing vascular supply to overlying skin graft), fascia, and muscle. However, cortical bone would need to be drilled down to expose marrow in order to support grafted material and allow for epithelialization.

Bone Block Grafting

Bone grafts, either autogenic or allogenic, are employed for the restoration of the alveolar ridge when severe resorption has occurred or a large marginal bone defect has been created. A variety of free bone grafts have been used to successfully add contour and bulk to the alveolar ridge. Deproteinized bovine bone graft material as well as deproteinized cadaveric human bone graft material have been used for alveolar ridge augmentation.[14] However, autogenic bone graft remains the gold standard, when available. Autogenic block bone grafts can be taken intraorally from the chin or mandibular ramus, or can be harvested distantly from the anterior iliac crest or rib. Autogenous bone can be harvested as block graft from the anterior iliac crest[1] and can be implanted en bloc or as particulate to restore alveolar ridge height and depth when deficient after oncologic resection. Free bone grafts may also be used as second stage reconstruction after fibular free flap mandibular reconstruction when the bony contour remains insufficient for dental restoration.

Jacotti et al described the use of allogenic block grafts wrapped in allogenic pericardial membrane for the atrophic mandible needing dental implantation.[15] After grafting, there was histologic evidence of healthy lamellar bone which was reliably used for dental rehabilitation. Krasny et al have similarly described the use of allogenic, frozen, radiation-sterilized block grafts for the restoration of atrophic alveolar ridge prior to dental rehabilitation with implants.[16]

Current research has focused on synthetic substitutes for allogenic bone graft material. Calcium phosphate ceramics (alone or in combination with calcium sulfate), calcium sulfate hemihydrate, and hydroxyapatite have been demonstrated to be viable options for reconstruction of the alveolar ridge in the case of bone loss after dental extractions and may be useful for smaller bony alveolar ridge defects.[17–19] It should be noted that for patients who have been radiated, or for whom radiation is planned, bone graft and synthetic graft material should be wrapped with vascularized tissue in the form of a free flap, for example, a free fascia lata flap wrapped around a block bone graft. Without a reliable blood supply, graft material will be unlikely to integrate in these patients.

22.5.3 Local Pedicled Flaps: Palatal Island Rotational, Buccal Fat Pad, and Facial Artery Musculomucosal (FAMM) Flaps

Palatal Island Rotational Flap

The palatal island rotational flap was introduced for cleft palate repair by Millard in 1962, and its indications for use were expanded by Gullane for reconstruction of other oral cavity defects in 1977.[20] This flap is pedicled off the paired greater palatine arteries, branches of the descending palatine artery. Notably, one artery is sufficient to supply a palatal mucoperichondrial flap that spans the midline of the palate. The flap is raised sharply from the bone of the hard palate, and incisions are designed based on the anatomy of the extirpative defect. The procedure has limited donor site morbidity, as the hard palate granulates in and heals secondarily.[21] This rotational flap is best used to reconstruct posterior maxillary alveolar ridge defects while anterior maxillary alveolar ridge defects are unable to be reached due to geometry of rotation and limited pedicle length.

Buccal Fat Pad Pedicled Flap

The buccal fat pad pedicled flap offers a vascularized source of soft tissue that is easily accessible through the oral cavity and can be mobilized to provide soft tissue coverage for alveolar ridge defects.[22] While initially utilized primarily for closure of oroantral fistulas, the buccal fat pad has been demonstrated to be useful in the closure of defects after oncologic resection of oral cancer, including those involving the alveolar ridge.[23,24] The buccal fat pad has several advantages over other sources of tissue adjacent to the alveolar ridge that make it an excellent reconstructive tool.[25] Anatomically, the buccal fat pad is lobulated and easily mobilized while maintaining excellent vascularity. This robust blood supply makes it advantageous when compared to free graft in cases of compromised wound bed vascularity or wound healing concerns, such as radiated fields or in diabetic patients. In addition, the buccal fat pad can supply enough tissue to cover approximately 10 cm^2 and does not seem to significantly atrophy with age, thus remaining a viable option in the elderly.[26] A limitation of this flap is that, although it easily reaches more posterior alveolar ridge defects of the maxilla and mandible, even with maximal mobilization of the vascular pedicle, it will not adequately reach more anterior defects.

Surgical technique begins with identification of Stenson's duct to ensure the duct is not harmed during the procedure. Next, a mucosal flap is elevated and the buccinator muscle is divided to identify the fat pad. Gentle delivery of the fat pad allows the fat pad to herniate through the muscles and rotate into position without injuring the vascular supply. This may be allowed to epithelialize or used in combination with other local flaps or graft materials for a superficial layer, such as a skin graft or even dermal matrix substitutes.[6]

Facial Artery Musculomucosal (FAMM) Flap

The facial artery musculomucosal (FAMM) flap is perhaps the best suited of the smaller rotational flaps to reconstruct soft tissue alveolar ridge deficits. The FAMM flap was initially designed as a combination of the concepts of the nasolabial and buccal mucosal flaps as described by Pribaz et al in 1992.[27] It is based off of the facial artery and can be designed on either antegrade or retrograde flow through the artery, making it geometrically versatile for oral cavity reconstruction. It provides a thin, pliable soft tissue covering for alveolar ridge reconstruction that has a robust vascular pedicle.[28] One limitation of this flap is that the width of the flap is usually limited to less than 2 cm due to the need to close the donor site primarily while leaving enough laxity to prevent scarring and trismus.[29]

Briefly, surgical technique begins with first identifying the course of the facial artery, typically using doppler ultrasound. The position of the posterior cut is limited by the need to remain anterior to Stenson's duct, and the anterior cut should be at least 1 cm posterior to the oral commissure. The width of the flap should be planned based on the size of the defect. However, it is limited to less than or equal to 2 cm to avoid tension during primary closure of the donor site. The facial artery is isolated by making an incision through mucosa, submucosa, and buccinator, usually at the most distal aspect of the flap. The vascular pedicle is then traced and the flap elevated to include buccinator, submucosa, and mucosa, taking care to keep the facial artery closely adhered to the elevated flap. The flap can then be rotated into place to use for the reconstruction of the alveolar ridge (▶ Fig. 22.2).[30] A modification of this flap includes the use of the angular artery branch of the facial artery as the vascular pedicle to create a superiorly based flap.[31]

22.5.4 Regional Pedicled Flaps: Traditional, Supraclavicular Artery Island, and Submental Artery Island Flaps

Traditional Soft Tissue Regional Flaps

Traditionally, soft tissue coverage of the maxilla and mandible could be accomplished by a variety of regional flaps, derived from but not limited to the deltopectoral, pectoralis major, and platysma systems. Benefits to regional flaps include avoidance of the need for microvascular techniques while being able to provide abundant vascularized soft tissue. In the context of alveolar ridge reconstruction, a major disadvantage of these flaps is overall bulkiness that may be ill-suited to the reconstruction of smaller defects. This section will focus on a select few regional pedicled flaps that are more ideal for the coverage of alveolar ridge defects.

Supraclavicular Artery Island Flap (SCAIF)

The supraclavicular artery island flap (SCAIF) can be harvested as a thin fasciocutaneous soft tissue flap for coverage of head and neck defects, including reconstruction of the oral cavity and alveolar ridge. This flap is an axial regional flap based off of the supraclavicular artery, a branch of the transverse cervical artery, and is drained by two venae comitantes. The flap is designed along the patient's shoulder with relative boundaries of the clavicle, trapezius, and deltoid muscle. The flap pedicle is predictably located in an anatomic triangle made up of the posterior border of the sternocleidomastoid, the external jugular vein, and the clavicle. Once the pedicle is identified, dissection proceeds distal to proximal in either a suprafascial or subfascial plane. Mobility and pliability are improved by pedicle skeletonization down to the origin at the transverse cervical artery as well as selective deepithelization.[32] Additionally, distal viability can be aided by harvest beyond the supraclavicular system to the anastomosis with the branches of the posterior circumflex humoral artery.[33] Benefits of this flap have been reported to be reliable pedicle anatomy, short harvest time, and minimal donor site morbidity with ability to primarily close harvest site.[34] Caution should be taken in patients who have had previous neck dissections including levels IV and V as well as in patients with significant postradiation changes.

Submental Artery Island Flap

Initially described in 1993 by Martin et al, the submental artery island flap is a useful regional flap for soft tissue coverage for moderate sized defects of the alveolar ridge.[35] The blood supply is derived from the submental branch of the facial artery, and it is drained through the facial vein system. The pedicle runs deep to the anterior belly of digastric muscle in 70% of the cases, while it runs superficial to the muscle in the remaining 30% of the cases. It courses superficial to the mylohyoid muscle in level Ia and gives off perforators that pierce the platysma muscle to supply the submental region. Pedicle length has been estimated to be 8 cm, an advantage for oral cavity reach. Surgical technique begins with flap design; the flap can span the entire

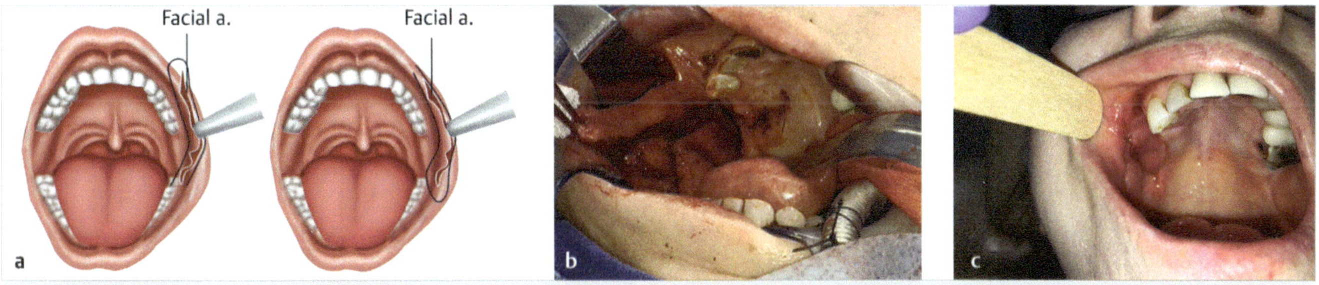

Fig. 22.2 Facial artery musculomucosal (FAMM) flap. **(a)** The illustration on the left demonstrates antegrade flap and right demonstrates retrograde flap. **(b)** Intraoperative flap elevation. **(c)** Postoperative result after 3 weeks.

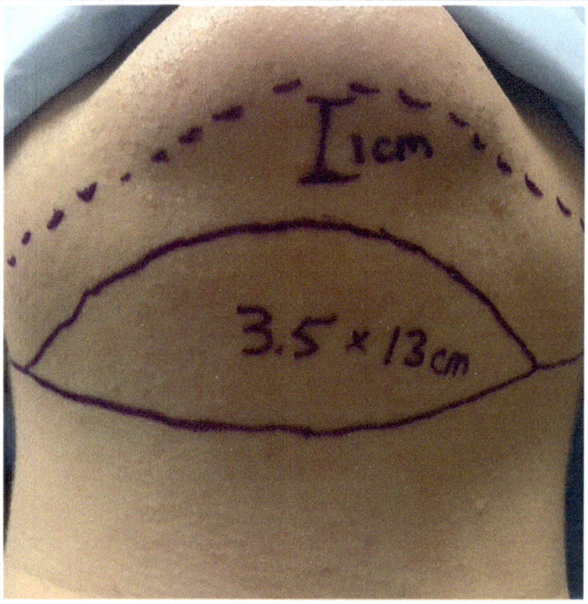

a

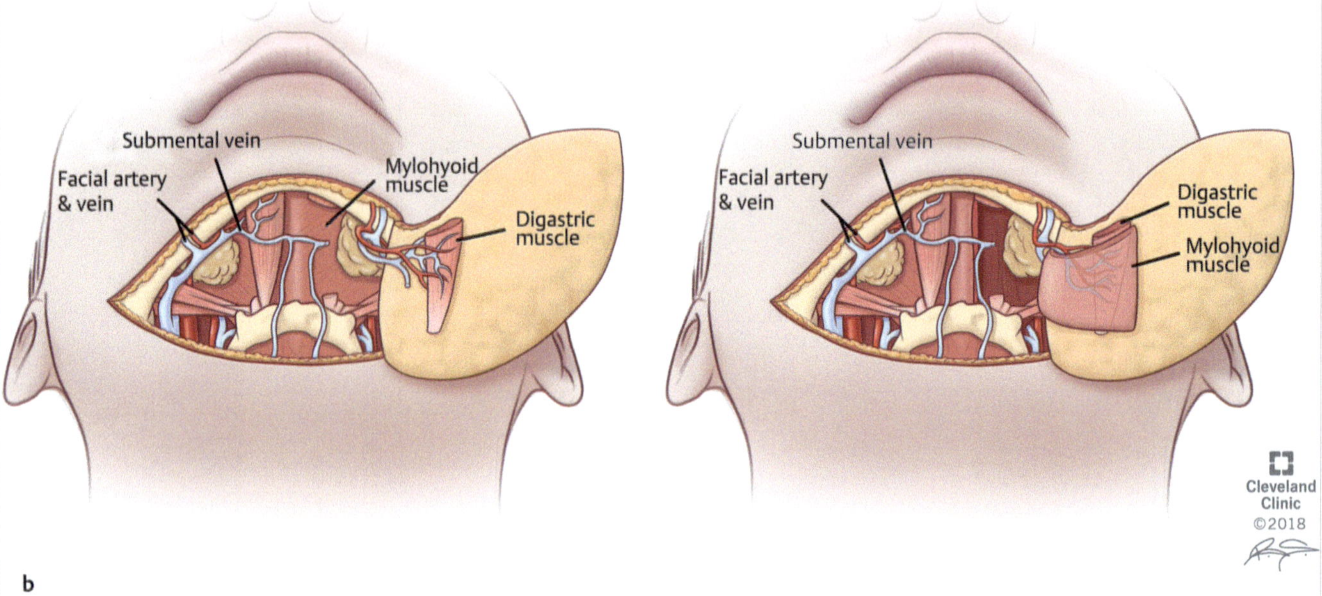

b

Fig. 22.3 Submental artery island flap. **(a)** Flap design demonstrating skin paddle spanning the submental region from angle of mandible to opposite angle. **(b)** The submental artery island flap may also be raised to incorporate a portion of mylohyoid to protect the pedicle. (Reproduced with permission, Cleveland Clinic Center for Medical Art & Photography ©2018. All Rights Reserved.)

anterior submandibular region from angle to angle (▶ Fig. 22.3). The maximum flap width can be estimated with a skin pinch test to ensure primary closure will be possible, and can be as large as 18 × 7 cm. The anterior incision is positioned 1–1.5 cm posterior to the mandible to minimize scar visibility. First, dissection proceeds to the level of the submandibular gland on the ipsilateral side of the planned pedicle, and the facial and submental vessels are identified and protected. Care is taken to preserve the marginal mandibular branches of the facial nerve during dissection by early identification. Subsequently, dissection proceeds to raise the flap in a subplatysmal plane beginning on the contralateral side; at the midline, dissection is carried down to the anterior belly of the digastric muscle, which is released from the mandible and the hyoid. Finally, dissection is taken to the level of the mylohyoid muscle where the pedicle can either be dissected from the muscle, or the mylohyoid muscle can be included in the flap by detaching it from the mandible, hyoid, and geniohyoid muscle. It has been argued that including the mylohyoid muscle protects the vascular pedicle and facilitates efficient, safe flap harvest.[36] To increase pedicle length, the facial artery and vein can be ligated distal to the take-off of the pedicle as needed. The wound is closed primarily.

Specific risks to this regional flap include injury to the marginal mandibular division of the facial nerve; however, several studies have reported a low rate of injury (0–17%). Most importantly, there has been debate in the literature as to whether, in the head and neck cancer patient, the dissection of the submental neck for flap harvest and inset poses too great a risk for recurrence or disease spread to recipient soft tissue bed, even in the absence of known nodal metastasis.[37,38]

22.5.5 Free Tissue Transfer

Free tissue transfer has become the standard for head and neck reconstruction and, in many cases, has replaced locoregional flaps for large- and even medium-sized defects requiring a robust source of vascularized tissue. Free flaps can be successful even in poor transplant beds that have been compromised by scar, radiation, repeat operation, and trauma, as they bring along the vascular supply from the donor site. Moreover, as improvements in microsurgical techniques and the implementation of two-team approaches for oncologic resection and flap harvest have shortened operative time, free flaps have become a feasible reconstructive option for some patients previously considered poor candidates, such as the elderly.[39]

In the oral cavity, and for the alveolar ridge in particular, soft tissue coverage of underlying maxillary or mandibular bone requires durable soft tissue coverage without excessive bulk, a balance that is at times difficult to achieve.

Soft Tissue Flaps: Anterolateral Thigh Free Flap, Radial Forearm Free Flap, and Ulnar Artery Perforator Free Flap

Anterolateral Thigh Free Flap

The anterolateral thigh (ALT) free flap has become an increasingly popular choice for large head and neck ablative defects, including defects of the alveolar ridge, when significant soft tissue bulk is needed. The ease of harvest using a two-team approach, the long pedicle length, the low donor site morbidity, and the reliable vascular supply from septocutaneous or musculocutaneous perforators of the lateral circumflex femoral artery makes this flap a popular option.[40,41] The ALT free flap has been described to have advantages over the more commonly performed radial forearm free flap, including less donor site morbidity, fewer postoperative healing complications in some series, and increased availability of tissue bulk.[42,43] Naturally, high body mass index and significant thickness of the thigh are reasons why smaller alveolar ridge defects may not be ideally reconstructed with an ALT flap. However, even with the intrinsically larger bulk of the thigh compared to the forearm, the ALT flap is versatile in that it can be harvested as a thin fasciocutaneous flap or can be secondarily debulked. Several studies have described further modifications of the flap to a thinned ALT (tALT) in which removal of subcutaneous fat to the level of the subdermal plexus is performed.[44]

A variation of the ALT free flap, the adipofascial or fascia lata free flap, has been shown to be uniquely useful for oral cavity and specifically alveolar ridge reconstruction.[45] The flap is harvested as a perforator based flap without muscular or cutaneous components, although a cutaneous paddle may be included to aid in intraoperative manipulation of the flap and for monitoring of the reconstruction, if preferred. This thin, pliable flap mucosalizes primarily in the oral cavity, which has advantage over skin containing flaps, which are more bulky, hair-bearing, less compliant, and nonsecretory.

Radial Forearm Free Flap

The radial forearm free flap is a fasciocutaneous flap that is versatile for use in alveolar ridge reconstruction; specifically in small- to medium-sized soft tissue defects where underlying bony support remains intact, this soft tissue free flap is optimal. First introduced by Yang et al in 1981, it is now one of the most commonly utilized free flap for head and neck reconstruction.[46] It offers a thin, pliable, and relatively hairless soft tissue covering for oral cavity. The flap is supplied by perforators from the radial artery.[47] Advantages of this flap include a long pedicle length with good caliber, a consistent anatomy, the potential of a two-team approach. One potential drawback of the radial forearm flap is the donor site morbidity including potential paresthesias and tendon exposure. In addition, this flap harvest site often cannot be closed primarily and typically requires the harvest of a skin graft, which creates a secondary donor site.[48]

Ulnar Artery Perforator Free Flap

The ulnar artery perforator (UAP) flap was first described by Lovie et al in 1984 and then further delineated by Yu et al.[49,50] It is supplied by perforators of the ulnar artery, which runs distally between tendons of the flexor digitorum superficialis (FDS) and the flexor carpi ulnaris (FCU) in close proximity to the ulnar nerve. The skin of the ulnar forearm is innervated by the medial antebrachial cutaneous nerve and can be included in a sensate flap.

Compared to the radial forearm free flap, it has many advantages including: less hair-bearing tissue, an inconspicuous scar, the possibility of primary closure, less tendon exposure, and improved graft take when a skin graft is used.[50] Additionally, some studies have shown that the radial artery is the dominant blood supply to the hand.[51] This flap offers ideal anatomy for use in alveolar ridge reconstruction, as it is thin and pliable. Relative disadvantages of this free flap include a comparatively shorter pedicle length than the radial artery based flap and somewhat thicker tissue compared to the radial forearm. However, there are patients in whom slightly thicker tissue may be considered an advantage.

The technique of flap harvest is demonstrated in **Video 22.1** and ▸ Fig. 22.4. Briefly, a straight line is drawn between the medial epicondyle of the humerus and the pisiform of the wrist (WE line). Perforators A, B, and C are marked slightly ulnar to this line at a distance of 7, 12, and 16 cm from the pisiform, respectively. The distal skin cut is made approximately 5 cm from the pisiform crease; this detail may benefit patients functionally, allowing them to continue to wear watches and jewelry below the level of any surgical scaring. Starting on the radial side, suprafascial dissection proceeds, past the FDS tendon, until the perforators are found. The ulnar neurovascular pedicle is then exposed by incising the fascia on its radial side and retracting the FDS. After the distal end is ligated and clipped, the pedicle is carefully dissected proximally off the

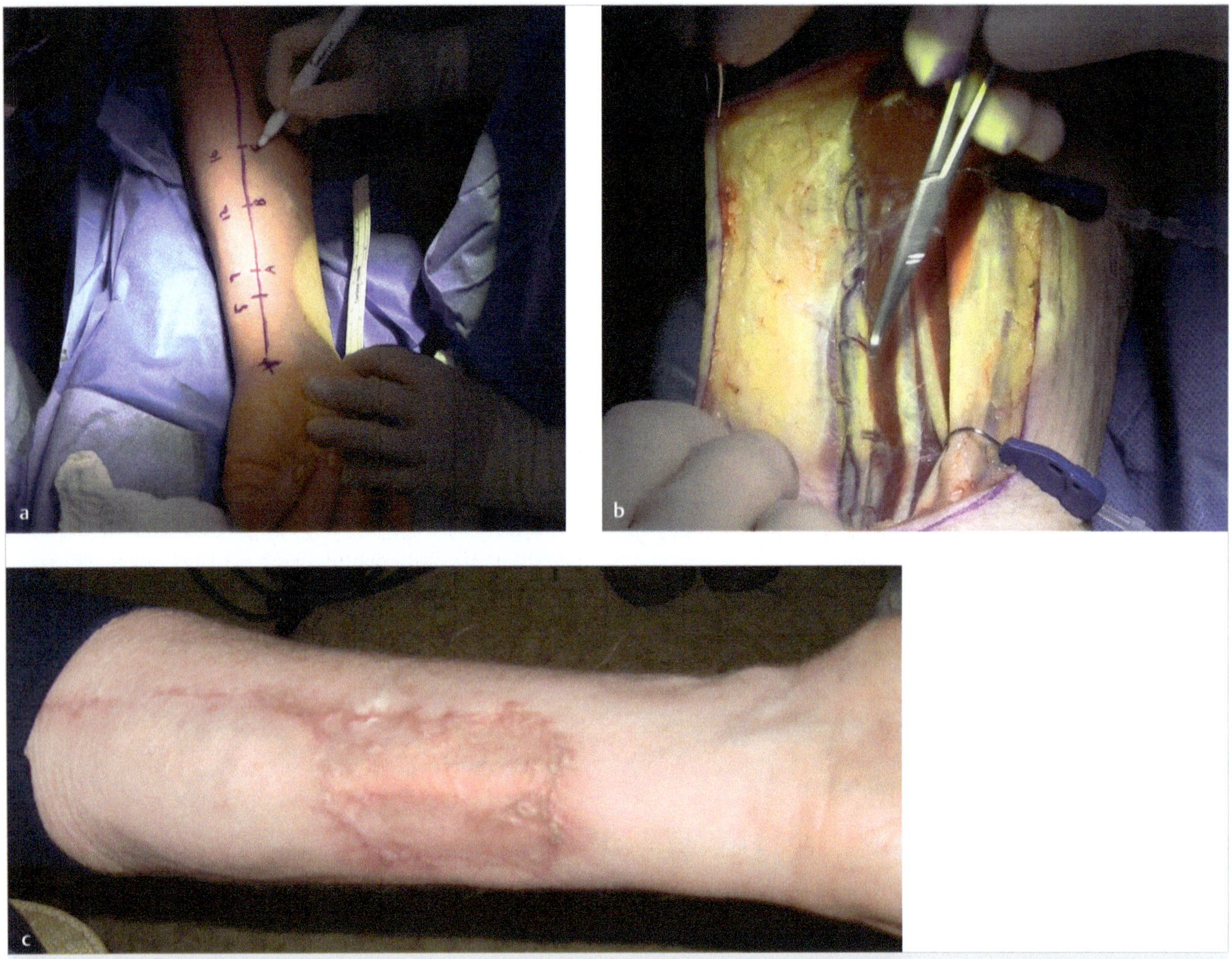

Fig. 22.4 Ulnar artery perforator flap. (a) Flap design with perforators marked along the wrist-elbow (WE) line between the medial epicondyle of the humerus and the pisiform of the wrist. (b) Perforator vessels identified intraoperatively. (c) Postoperative donor site with skin grafting.

ulnar nerve as it travels through the FDS and the flexor digitorum profundus muscles to the bifurcation with the common interosseous artery. The proximal skin cut is then made, paying particular attention to preserving the septum and perforators between the FCU and FDS.

Osseous Free Flaps: Osteocutaneous Radial Forearm and Fibula Free Flaps

While more detailed descriptions of osseous free flaps will be provided in the context of reconstruction for mandibulectomy defects, the following condensed descriptions reflect the most relevant details of alveolar ridge reconstruction.

Osteocutaneous Radial Forearm Free Flap

As a modification to the previously described radial forearm free flap, an osteocutaneous free flap can be raised off the radial vessels. This modification involves the identification and preservation of perforators to the radius traveling from the radial artery in a fascial septum. These perforators are preserved along with a small muscle cuff of flexor pollicis longus to improve periosteal perfusion. The available length of bone is limited to less than 10 cm, and less than 50% of the width of the radius should be taken to preserve stability and prevent postoperative fracture. Osteotomies should be angled or "boat-shaped." Many surgeons advocate plating the donor radius to decrease the risk of postoperative fracture.

Fibula Free Flap

Fibula free flaps are now frequently used for complex mandibular reconstruction in the head and neck cancer patient. The osseofasciocutaneous fibula free flap was initially described in 1975 by Taylor et al and then applied to mandibular reconstruction by Hidalgo in 1989.[52] This flap has many advantages in large-scale, comprehensive reconstruction including the potential for a two-team approach during surgery, the generous length of bone available to reconstruct bony facial deficits, and the option to simultaneously provide soft tissue for oral cavity reconstruction. In addition, one major advantage in relation to alveolar ridge reconstruction is the potential to provide viable bone for dental rehabilitation with dental implants.

Specific to the reconstruction of the alveolar ridge is the dental rehabilitation performed in conjunction with mandibular reconstruction with osseous free flaps. Dental implants may be placed into alveolar ridges that have previously been reconstructed with osseous free flaps.[53–55] It has also been proposed that the primary placement of dental implants into the bone during the initial reconstruction allows for osseointegration and eliminates the need for a secondary oral surgery for implant placement after primary healing.[56,57] The technique described includes placement of implants after the osseous free flap (iliac crest, scapula, or fibula) has been revascularized with microvascular anastomosis, followed by unroofing of the implants under local anesthetic after time has elapsed for healing, and finally loading with the dental prosthesis, approximately 4 months after implant placement. However, care must be taken to select patients with sufficient vascular supply and with limited risk for osteoradionecrosis. In addition, selection of patient candidates should take into account the need for potential post operative radiation therapy which may compromise osseointegration and make patients poor candidates for upfront dental implantation. Some patients may be at too great a risk for late onset vascular compromise to the grafted fibular bone with the addition of dental implants.

22.6 New Advances

In discussion of the wide variety of reconstructive options for the alveolar ridge, it is useful to consider literature generated in the context of nononcologic pathologies primarily treated by dentists and oral surgeons, such as alveolar clefts and bone loss related to tooth extraction, as similar principles and concepts may be relevant to the head and neck cancer patient.[58] Innovations in treating and ameliorating these benign pathologies can be applied to restore form and function, especially as tertiary therapies in the oncologically cured patient after extirpation of disease and primary healing has occurred.

22.6.1 Dental Rehabilitation

The range of dental prosthesis and technologies available to restore dentition is beyond the scope of this chapter and will be discussed further in Chapter 39. Briefly, dental rehabilitation requires the previously described establishment of soft tissue coverage to the occlusal surfaces of the maxilla and mandible. It will also require bony support structure for the same. The implantation of permanent dentition with dental implants, when feasible, over removable obturator or denture devices has become the gold standard.

It is important to be mindful that, for the majority of patients, dental rehabilitation first requires revision surgery to any primary reconstructive effort in order to prepare the site for potential prosthodontic treatment. For example, bulky flaps may need to be thinned or soft tissue may even need to be replaced with thinner alternatives such as skin graft in order to improve the definition of bony landmarks, deepen sulci, and reduce soft tissue laxity or redundancy for improved stability of prosthetics. The removal of redundant or bulky soft tissue may also be required to improve access to bone in which dental implants can be placed.

As mentioned previously, it is vital to evaluate the patient's candidacy for dental implants when considering reconstructive options. Patients who have been previously radiated, or who will require post operative radiation therapy, will have poorer outcomes related to osseointegration of dental implants and higher risk of implant failure due to bone vascularity and healing potential. In addition, for patients who have undergone fibular free flap reconstruction require sufficient union between the remnant native mandible bone and the transplanted fibula bone prior to consideration of loading any dental implant hardware. Additionally, it is important to consider that dental rehabilitation including dental implantation may not be covered by the patient's insurance and, thus, can be a prohibitively expensive undertaking.

22.6.2 Implants and Biomaterials, Tissue Engineering, and Three-Dimensional Printing

The dental literature is replete with ample techniques for alveolar ridge reconstruction including free gingival onlay grafts, autografting (i.e., palatal muscosal grafts, bone block grafts), dermal matrix substitution, and distraction osteogenesis.[59,60] More recent technology has afforded opportunities to use tissue engineering to improve outcomes for alveolar ridge augmentation.

Growth factors, including platelet rich plasma (PRP), bone morphogenic proteins, and enamel matrix proteins continue to be investigated, usually in combination with bone or soft tissue graft techniques, to establish their efficacy in wound healing and tissue restoration. PRP has shown promise, although with variable results, when used in combination with allogenic or xenogenic bone grafts to promote wound healing and improve bone regeneration.[61–64] More recently, platelet rich fibrin (PRF) has been suggested to have further advantages over PRP due to the lack of need to use an anticoagulant in the preparation, which was purported to hinder wound healing.[17,63]

Three-dimensional printing techniques have improved the ability to more closely mimic trabecular bony architecture with biocompatible synthetic materials that may be useful for mandibular and alveolar ridge reconstruction. For example, polyetheretherketone (PEEK) can be printed into three-dimensional implants that are then impregnated with biomaterials, such as bone marrow derived and adipose derived stem cells. These implants have been demonstrated to sufficiently integrate in a rabbit model with marginal mandibular defects.[65–67]

22.7 Perioperative Management

Postoperatively, patients in whom alveolar ridge reconstruction has been completed may have restrictions in immediate postoperative functioning. For example, often patients may be asked to avoid mastication, eat only a soft diet, or even eat nothing by mouth for some period to allow for healing and stabilization of the reconstruction. In this case, alternative nutritional methods such as nasogastric feeding may be required.

Mouth care and oral hygiene are also uniquely important to these patients. Chlorhexidine oral rinse has been demonstrated to decrease oral cavity bacteria in head and neck patients.[68,69] Thus, it is commonly used after oral cavity reconstruction. Alternatively, salt and soda or normal saline rinses are also prescribed to postoperative patients to soothe and assist with oral hygiene after oral cavity surgery. Gentle mechanical cleansing with soft swabs may be necessary to clean desquamating debris from skin bearing flaps.

In patients on whom free tissue transfer has been performed, often the monitoring of the free flap requires some length of postoperative hospital stay to allow for serial evaluations of the health of the transferred tissue. The oral cavity can be visualized easily for assessment of flap health, and frequently pencil Doppler is used to monitor blood flow through the flap.

Key Points

- The alveolar ridge is anatomically and functionally complex, making reconstruction both challenging and critical to patient's postoperative outcomes.
- A wide spectrum of reconstructive tools may need to be employed during each patient's reconstruction, which should be tailored to the patient's unique oncologic defect and postoperative goals.
- Local tissue rearrangement, locoregional flaps, free grafts, and free tissue transfer techniques have all been used successfully for alveolar ridge reconstruction.
- The successful reconstruction of the alveolar ridge allows for dental rehabilitation; however, dental rehabilitation will take various forms based on each patient's preference and individual factors.
- Often, dental rehabilitation will require revision surgeries and/or augmentation of the bony alveolar ridge.

References

[1] Chen Z, Zhang Y. Primary reconstruction of the mandibular alveolar ridge following resection. Int J Oral Maxillofac Surg. 1992; 21(5):253–255

[2] Donald PJ. Surgical rehabilitation following anterior resection for oral cavity carcinoma. Laryngoscope. 1981; 91(11):1941–1956

[3] Nakamura M, Ojima T, Nakade M, et al. Poor oral health and diet in relation to weight loss, stable underweight, and obesity in community-dwelling older adults: a cross-sectional study from the JAGES 2010 project. J Epidemiol. 2016; 26(6):322–329

[4] Emami E, de Souza RF, Kabawat M, Feine JS. The impact of edentulism on oral and general health. Int J Dent. 2013; 2013:498305

[5] Revenaugh PC, Fritz MA, Haffey TM, Seth R, Markey J, Knott PD. Minimizing morbidity in microvascular surgery: small-caliber anastomotic vessels and minimal access approaches. JAMA Facial Plast Surg. 2015; 17(1): 44–48

[6] Batra H, Jindal G, Kaur S. Evaluation of different treatment modalities for closure of oro-antral communications and formulation of a rational approach. J Maxillofac Oral Surg. 2010; 9(1):13–18

[7] Cummings LC, Kaldahl WB, Allen EP. Histologic evaluation of autogenous connective tissue and acellular dermal matrix grafts in humans. J Periodontol. 2005; 76(2):178–186

[8] Wainwright D, Madden M, Luterman A, et al. Clinical evaluation of an acellular allograft dermal matrix in full-thickness burns. J Burn Care Rehabil. 1996; 17(2):124–136

[9] Girod DA, Sykes K, Jorgensen J, Tawfik O, Tsue T. Acellular dermis compared to skin grafts in oral cavity reconstruction. Laryngoscope. 2009; 119(11): 2141–2149

[10] Livesey SA, Herndon DN, Hollyoak MA, Atkinson YH, Nag A. Transplanted acellular allograft dermal matrix: potential as a template for the reconstruction of viable dermis. Transplantation. 1995; 60(1):1–9

[11] Aichelmann-Reidy ME, Yukna RA, Evans GH, Nasr HF, Mayer ET. Clinical evaluation of acellular allograft dermis for the treatment of human gingival recession. J Periodontol. 2001; 72(8):998–1005

[12] Novaes AB, Jr, Grisi DC, Molina GO, Souza SL, Taba M, Jr, Grisi MF. Comparative 6-month clinical study of a subepithelial connective tissue graft and acellular dermal matrix graft for the treatment of gingival recession. J Periodontol. 2001; 72(11):1477–1484

[13] Fowler EB, Breault LG. Ridge augmentation with a folded acellular dermal matrix allograft: a case report. J Contemp Dent Pract. 2001; 2(3):31–40

[14] Hämmerle CH, Karring T. Guided bone regeneration at oral implant sites. Periodontol 2000. 1998; 17:151–175

[15] Jacotti M, Wang H-L, Fu J-H, Zamboni G, Bernardello F. Ridge augmentation with mineralized block allografts: clinical and histological evaluation of 8 cases treated with the 3-dimensional block technique. Implant Dent. 2012; 21(6):444–448

[16] Krasny M, Krasny K, Fiedor P, Zadurska M, Kamiński A. Long-term outcomes of the use of allogeneic, radiation-sterilised bone blocks in reconstruction of the atrophied alveolar ridge in the maxilla and mandible. Cell Tissue Bank. 2015; 16(4):631–638

[17] Yerke LM, Jamjoom A, Zahid TM, Cohen RE. The effect of platelet-rich fibrin, calcium sulfate hemihydrate, platelet-rich plasma and resorbable collagen on soft tissue closure of extraction sites. J Funct Biomater. 2017; 8(2):E17

[18] Fairbairn P, Leventis M, Mangham C, Horowitz R. Alveolar ridge preservation using a novel synthetic grafting material: a case with two-year follow-up. Case Rep Dent. 2018; 2018:6412806

[19] Horowitz RA, Mazor Z, Miller RJ, Krauser J, Prasad HS, Rohrer MD. Clinical evaluation alveolar ridge preservation with a beta-tricalcium phosphate socket graft. Compend Contin Educ Dent. 2009; 30(9):588–590, 592, 594 passim, quiz 604, 606

[20] Gullane PJ, Arena S. Palatal island flap for reconstruction of oral defects. Arch Otolaryngol. 1977; 103(10):598–599

[21] Genden EM, Lee BB, Urken ML. The palatal island flap for reconstruction of palatal and retromolar trigone defects revisited. Arch Otolaryngol Head Neck Surg. 2001; 127(7):837–841

[22] Egyedi P. Utilization of the buccal fat pad for closure of oro-antral and/or oro-nasal communications. J Maxillofac Surg. 1977; 5(4):241–244

[23] Manuel S, Kumar S, Nair PR. The versatility in the use of buccal fat pad in the closure of oro-antral fistulas. J Maxillofac Oral Surg. 2015; 14(2):374–377

[24] Rapidis AD, Alexandridis CA, Eleftheriadis E, Angelopoulos AP. The use of the buccal fat pad for reconstruction of oral defects: review of the literature and report of 15 cases. J Oral Maxillofac Surg. 2000; 58(2):158–163

[25] Kim M-K, Han W, Kim S-G. The use of the buccal fat pad flap for oral reconstruction. Maxillofac Plast Reconstr Surg. 2017; 39(1):5

[26] Arce K. Buccal fat pad in maxillary reconstruction. Atlas Oral Maxillofac Surg Clin North Am. 2007; 15(1):23–32

[27] Pribaz J, Stephens W, Crespo L, Gifford G. A new intraoral flap: facial artery musculomucosal (FAMM) flap. Plast Reconstr Surg. 1992; 90(3):421–429

[28] Ayad T, Xie L. Facial artery musculomucosal flap in head and neck reconstruction: a systematic review. Head Neck. 2015; 37(9):1375–1386

[29] Yu P. Chapter 2: Oral cavity reconstruction. In: Hanasono M, Robb G, Skoracki R, Yu P, eds. Reconstructive Plastic Surgery of the Head and Neck Current Techniques and Flap Atlas. New York, New York: Thieme; 2016

[30] Duranceau M, Ayad T. The facial artery musculomucosal flap: modification of the harvesting technique for a single-stage procedure. Laryngoscope. 2011; 121(12):2586–2589

[31] Berania I, Lavigne F, Rahal A, Ayad T. Superiorly based facial artery musculomucosal flap: a versatile pedicled flap. Head Neck. 2018; 40(2):402–405

[32] Granzow JW, Suliman A, Roostaeian J, Perry A, Boyd JB. The supraclavicular artery island flap (SCAIF) for head and neck reconstruction: surgical technique and refinements. Otolaryngol Head Neck Surg. 2013; 148(6):933–940

[33] Atallah S, Guth A, Chabolle F, Bach C-A. Supraclavicular artery island flap in head and neck reconstruction. Eur Ann Otorhinolaryngol Head Neck Dis. 2015; 132(5):291–294

[34] Chiu ES, Liu PH, Friedlander PL. Supraclavicular artery island flap for head and neck oncologic reconstruction: indications, complications, and outcomes. Plast Reconstr Surg. 2009; 124(1):115–123

[35] Martin D, Pascal JF, Baudet J, et al. The submental island flap: a new donor site. Anatomy and clinical applications as a free or pedicled flap. Plast Reconstr Surg. 1993; 92(5):867–873

[36] Patel UA, Bayles SW, Hayden RE. The submental flap: a modified technique for resident training. Laryngoscope. 2007; 117(1):186–189

[37] Amin AA, Sakkary MA, Khalil AA, Rifaat MA, Zayed SB. The submental flap for oral cavity reconstruction: extended indications and technical refinements. Head Neck Oncol. 2011; 3:51

[38] Sebastian P, Thomas S, Varghese BT, Iype EM, Balagopal PG, Mathew PC. The submental island flap for reconstruction of intraoral defects in oral cancer patients. Oral Oncol. 2008; 44(11):1014–1018

[39] Grammatica A, Piazza C, Paderno A, Taglietti V, Marengoni A, Nicolai P. Free flaps in head and neck reconstruction after oncologic surgery: expected outcomes in the elderly. Otolaryngol Head Neck Surg. 2015; 152(5):796–802

[40] Song YG, Chen GZ, Song YL. The free thigh flap: a new free flap concept based on the septocutaneous artery. Br J Plast Surg. 1984; 37(2):149–159

[41] Graboyes EM, Hornig JD. Evolution of the anterolateral thigh free flap. Curr Opin Otolaryngol Head Neck Surg. 2017; 25(5):416–421

[42] Kesting MR, Hölzle F, Wales C, et al. Microsurgical reconstruction of the oral cavity with free flaps from the anterolateral thigh and the radial forearm: a comparison of perioperative data from 161 cases. Ann Surg Oncol. 2011; 18 (7):1988–1994

[43] Collins J, Ayeni O, Thoma A. A systematic review of anterolateral thigh flap donor site morbidity. Can J Plast Surg. 2012; 20(1):17–23

[44] Loreti A, Di Lella G, Vetrano S, Tedaldi M, Dell'Osso A, Poladas G. Thinned anterolateral thigh cutaneous flap and radial fasciocutaneous forearm flap for reconstruction of oral defects: comparison of donor site morbidity. J Oral Maxillofac Surg. 2008; 66(6):1093–1098

[45] Revenaugh PC, Haffey TM, Seth R, Fritz MA. Anterolateral thigh adipofascial flap in mucosal reconstruction. JAMA Facial Plast Surg. 2014; 16(6):395–399

[46] Yang GF, Chen PJ, Gao YZ, et al. Forearm free skin flap transplantation: a report of 56 cases. 1981. Br J Plast Surg. 1997; 50(3):162–165

[47] Timmons MJ. The vascular basis of the radial forearm flap. Plast Reconstr Surg. 1986; 77(1):80–92

[48] Loeffelbein DJ, Al-Benna S, Steinsträßer L, et al. Reduction of donor site morbidity of free radial forearm flaps: what level of evidence is available? Eplasty. 2012; 12:e9

[49] Lovie MJ, Duncan GM, Glasson DW. The ulnar artery forearm free flap. Br J Plast Surg. 1984; 37(4):486–492

[50] Yu P, Chang EI, Selber JC, Hanasono MM. Perforator patterns of the ulnar artery perforator flap. Plast Reconstr Surg. 2012; 129(1):213–220

[51] Tonks AM, Lawrence J, Lovie MJ. Comparison of ulnar and radial arterial blood-flow at the wrist. J Hand Surg [Br]. 1995; 20(2):240–242

[52] Hidalgo DA. Fibula free flap: a new method of mandible reconstruction. Plast Reconstr Surg. 1989; 84(1):71–79

[53] Carbiner R, Jerjes W, Shakib K, Giannoudis PV, Hopper C. Analysis of the compatibility of dental implant systems in fibula free flap reconstruction. Head Neck Oncol. 2012; 4:37

[54] Chiapasco M, Biglioli F, Autelitano L, Romeo E, Brusati R. Clinical outcome of dental implants placed in fibula-free flaps used for the reconstruction of maxillo-mandibular defects following ablation for tumors or osteoradionecrosis. Clin Oral Implants Res. 2006; 17(2):220–228

[55] Kramer F-J, Dempf R, Bremer B. Efficacy of dental implants placed into fibula-free flaps for orofacial reconstruction. Clin Oral Implants Res. 2005; 16(1):80–88

[56] Urken ML, Buchbinder D, Weinberg H, Vickery C, Sheiner A, Biller HF. Primary placement of osseointegrated implants in microvascular mandibular reconstruction. Otolaryngol Head Neck Surg. 1989; 101(1):56–73

[57] Urken ML, Buchbinder D, Costantino PD, et al. Oromandibular reconstruction using microvascular composite flaps: report of 210 cases. Arch Otolaryngol Head Neck Surg. 1998; 124(1):46–55

[58] Horowitz R, Holtzclaw D, Rosen PS. A review on alveolar ridge preservation following tooth extraction. J Evid Based Dent Pract. 2012; 12(3) Suppl: 149–160

[59] Miller PD, Jr. Concept of periodontal plastic surgery. Pract Periodontics Aesthet Dent. 1993; 5(5):15–20, 22, quiz 22

[60] Miller PD, Jr, Allen EP. The development of periodontal plastic surgery. Periodontol 2000. 1996; 11:7–17

[61] Bezerra BT, Pinho JNA, Figueiredo FED, Brandão JRMCB, Ayres LCG, da Silva LCF. Autogenous bone graft versus bovine bone graft in association with platelet-rich plasma for the reconstruction of alveolar clefts: a pilot study. Cleft Palate Craniofac J. 2019; 56(1):134–140

[62] Del Corso M, Vervelle A, Simonpieri A, et al. Current knowledge and perspectives for the use of platelet-rich plasma (PRP) and platelet-rich fibrin (PRF) in oral and maxillofacial surgery part 1: periodontal and dentoalveolar surgery. Curr Pharm Biotechnol. 2012; 13(7):1207–1230

[63] Miron RJ, Fujioka-Kobayashi M, Bishara M, Zhang Y, Hernandez M, Choukroun J. Platelet-rich fibrin and soft tissue wound healing: a systematic review. Tissue Eng Part B Rev. 2017; 23(1):83–99

[64] Eskan MA, Greenwell H, Hill M, et al. Platelet-rich plasma-assisted guided bone regeneration for ridge augmentation: a randomized, controlled clinical trial. J Periodontol. 2014; 85(5):661–668

[65] Roskies MG, Fang D, Abdallah M-N, et al. Three-dimensionally printed polyetherketoneketone scaffolds with mesenchymal stem cells for the reconstruction of critical-sized mandibular defects. Laryngoscope. 2017; 127(11):E392–E398

[66] Roskies M, Jordan JO, Fang D, et al. Improving PEEK bioactivity for craniofacial reconstruction using a 3D printed scaffold embedded with mesenchymal stem cells. J Biomater Appl. 2016; 31(1):132–139

[67] Fang D, Roskies M, Abdallah M-N, et al. Three-dimensional printed scaffolds with multipotent mesenchymal stromal cells for rabbit mandibular reconstruction and engineering. Methods Mol Biol. 2017; 1553:273–291

[68] Bidra AS, Tarrand JJ, Roberts DB, Rolston KV, Chambers MS. Antimicrobial efficacy of oral topical agents on microorganisms associated with radiated head and neck cancer patients: an in vitro study. Quintessence Int. 2011; 42 (4):307–315

[69] Malhotra N, Rao SP, Acharya S, Vasudev B. Comparative in vitro evaluation of efficacy of mouthrinses against Streptococcus mutans, Lactobacilli and Candida albicans. Oral Health Prev Dent. 2011; 9(3):261–268

23 Squamous Cell Cancer of Retromolar Trigone

Vishal Gupta, Kimberly E. Wooten, Hassan Arshad, and Wesley L. Hicks Jr.

Summary

The retromolar trigone (RTM) is the mucosal space located between third molar of the mandible and maxillary tuberosity. Carcinomas of the RMT often remain asymptomatic for prolonged periods resulting in advanced clinical disease at presentation. Unfortunately, even early T stage disease (T1/T2) of the RMT can have a high local recurrence rate due to undetected extension to surrounding anatomic areas. Accurate diagnosis and staging require thorough clinical examination and appropriate imaging workup. Surgical therapy is the first line of management and can be technically challenging to resect and reconstruct.

Keywords: retromolar trigone (RMT), pterygomandibular raphe (PMR), submucosal fibrosis, buccal space, mandibulectomy, microvascular reconstruction

23.1 Introduction

The cancers of retromolar trigone (RMT) are prevalent in regions of the world where there is tobacco and/or betel nut use. Because of potential late presentation and under staging, they can have a poor clinical outcome.

23.2 Anatomic Considerations

The RMT is a triangular area of mucosa, overlying the mandibular ramus, immediately posterior to the 3rd molars (▸ Fig. 23.1).[1] The base of the triangle is posterior to the last mandibular molar and the apex is in continuity with the maxillary tuberosity behind the last upper molar. RMT is bounded laterally by the gingival buccal mucosa and medially by anterior tonsillar pillar (▸ Fig. 23.2). Pterygomandibular raphe (PMR), which is a central fibrous band extending from pterygoid hamulus superiorly to mylohyoid line inferiorly, lies under this triangular fold of mucosa (▸ Fig. 23.3).[1] PMR provides attachment to buccinators and superior constrictor muscles.

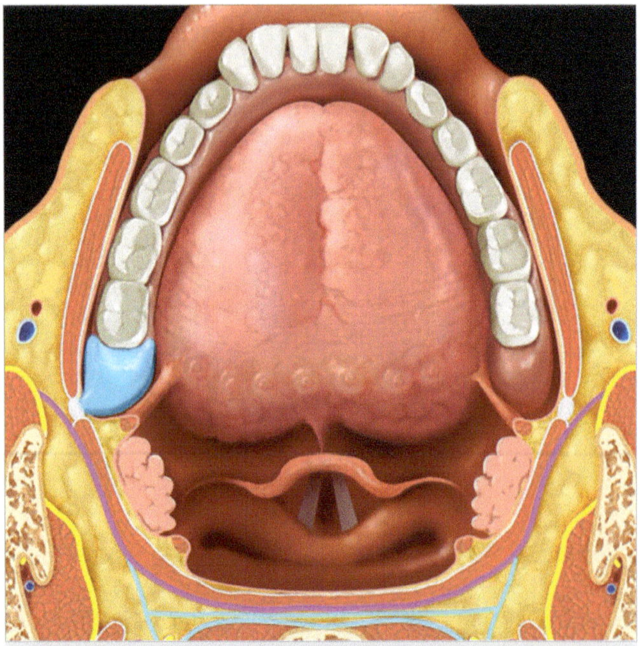

Fig. 23.1 Axial diagram of the mandible showing the retromolar trigone (RMT) area in crescent blue pattern.

23.3 Clinical Presentation

The cancers involving this subsite of oral cavity are notorious for indolent growth and late presentation. Cancers of this area may present as isolated ulcerative or endophytic lesions and may present with involvement of adjacent structures, that is, buccal mucosa or tonsillar fossa. Patients often present with advanced stage disease presenting with trismus as an initial presenting symptom (▸ Fig. 23.4).

Due to proximity to the maxilla, mandible, and pterygomandibular raphe (PMR), the cancer of RMT has propensity for local invasion of these sites. Although superficial extension is not difficult to diagnose, the extent of involvement can be difficult to accurately discern. One or more adjacent subsites are involved in 73 to 84% of cases reported.[3,4] The most common sites of

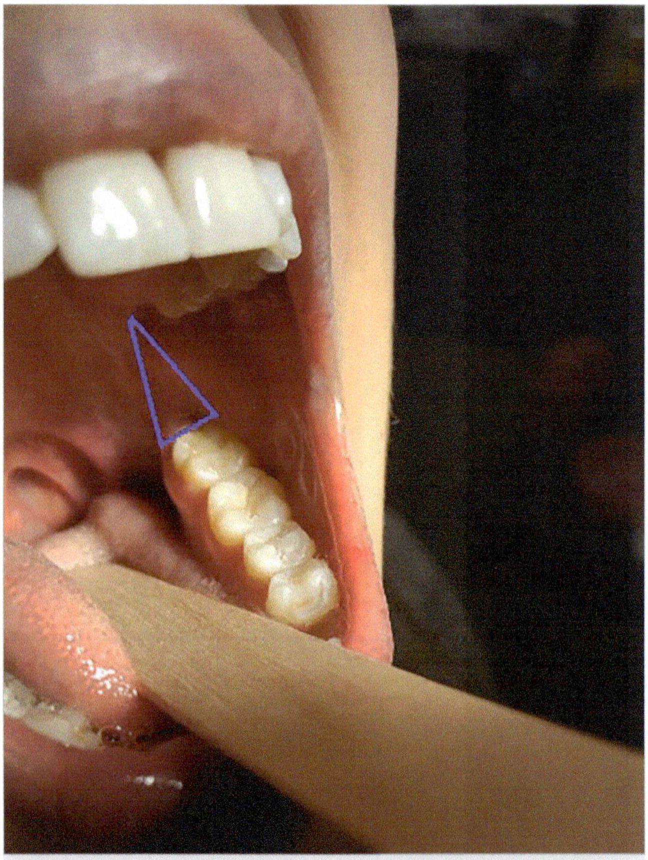

Fig. 23.2 Peroral view of retromolar trigone (RMT) area.

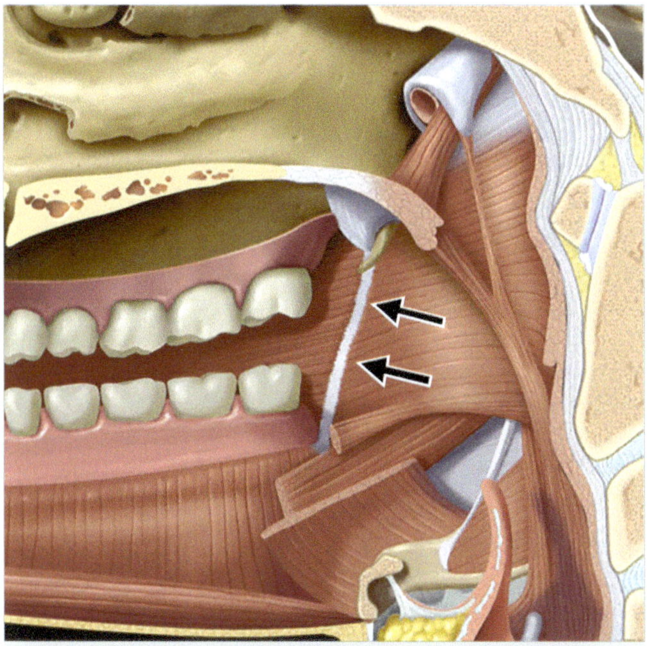

Fig. 23.3 Sagittal diagram showing the pterygomandibular raphe (PMR) extending from the hamulus of the medial pterygoid plate to the mandibular mylohyoid ridge.

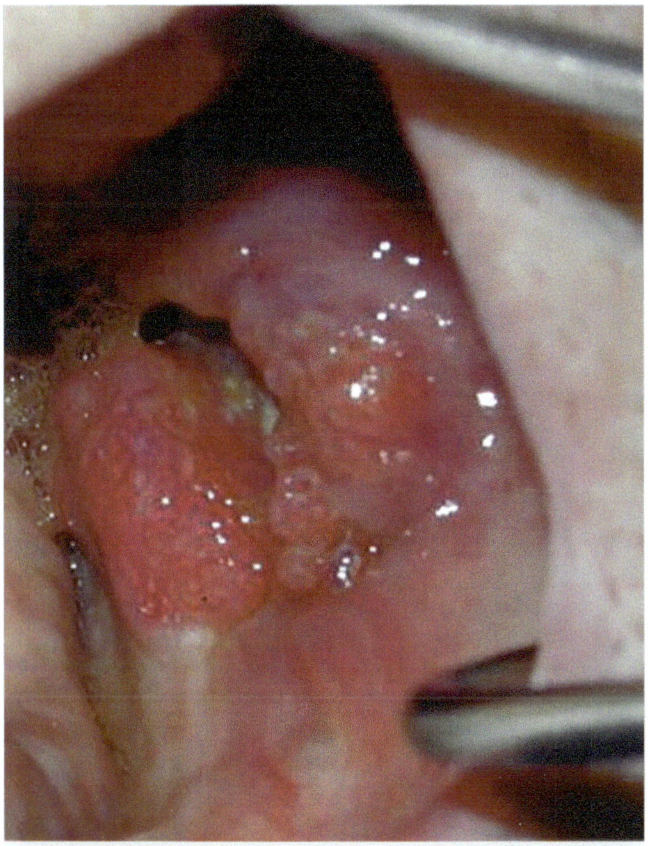

Fig. 23.4 Clinical appearance of cancer of retromolar trigone (RMT) at presentation.[2]

local involvement are reported to be the anterior tonsillar pillar (80%), the soft palate (59%), and the lower gum (37%).[5,6] The cancers of RMT are also known to have particular propensity toward bone involvement. The largest survey regarding bone invasion in RMT cancers was reported by Byers et al.[4] In a series of 110 patients with RMT involvement, they reported 14% incidence of histopathologic bone invasion. In another study examining all oral cancer sites, Gilbert et al[7] reported bone invasion in 3 out of 17 patients with RMT cancer. Brown et al[8] reported 75% incidence (9/12 cases) of bony involvement.

23.4 Epidemiology and Causes

Oral and pharyngeal cancers, together, constitute the sixth most common cancer in the world. There is wide geographical variation in the incidence of oral cancer, with the areas of South and Southeast Asia (India, Sri Lanka, Pakistan, and Taiwan), parts of Western (France) and Eastern Europe (Hungry, Slovenia, and Slovakia), parts of Latin America and the Caribbean (Puerto Rico, Brazil, and Uruguay), and Pacific regions (Papua New Guinea and Melanesia) characterized by higher incidence than the rest of the world. In countries like India, Sri Lanka, Pakistan, and Bangladesh, oral cancer is the most common cancer and constitutes 25% of all new cancers.[9] According to an estimate by American Cancer Society, there will be 51,540 new cases of oral cavity and pharyngeal cancer in United States in 2018. Approximately 10,030 will die of the disease in 2018.[10]

Etiology of oral cancer including RMT is multifactorial. Cigarette smoking remains the most important risk factor for oral cavity cancer including RMT. Concomitant alcohol use has synergistic effect, further increasing the risk of oral cavity cancer by 10- to 15-fold. Regular alcohol consumption is associated with the increased risk of oral cancer including retromolar subsite of oral cavity. In this dose dependent association, people consuming 4–5 drinks daily are at two to three times higher risk of oral cancer than nondrinkers.[11]

Betel nut chewing is one of key factors causing the increase in the incidence of retromolar cancers in Southeast Asia. International Agency for Research on Cancer classifies betel quid as oral carcinogen with evidence of dose–response relationship.[12] About 600 million people are exposed to the habit of betel nut chewing making it the fourth most-consumed drug after nicotine, ethanol, and caffeine.[13]

Parker et al reported higher incidence of oral and pharyngeal cancer in the area of the world with high prevalence of betel-quid chewing.[14] According to a study by Yeole et al in 2001, oral cancers among Parsi subgroup of population in Mumbai, India was significantly lower than non-Parsi population. Parsis are known to be nonsmoker and also avoid chewing betel quid due to religious reasons, although both of these addictions are very common in Mumbai, India. They reported that, in 1995, annual age-adjusted incidence rates (per 100,000) of cancers at several sites were lower among Parsi men than among the male population of Mumbai as a whole: tongue and mouth, 4.5 versus 11.9; pharynx, 2.6 versus 10.6; esophagus, 2.6 versus 8.7; stomach, 2.8 versus 6.6; larynx, 2.2 versus 7.2; and lung, 4.2 versus 12.6.[15]

Betel nut quid is known to induce fibroblast dysfunction and fibrosis causing a premalignant condition called submucosal fibrosis.[13] Oral submucosal fibrosis (OSF) is characterized by hypovascularity of mucosa leading to blanching, staining, and trismus. The fibroblast dysfunction and fibrosis are caused by the main constituents of betel nut quid, i.e., arecoline and copper. Paymaster[16] described slow growth of squamous cell carcinoma (SCC) in one-third of the patients with OSF. Malignant transformation rate of OSF has been reported to be in the range of 7–13%. On long-term follow-up, studies have reported a transformation rate of 7.6% over a period of 17 years.[17] Pindborg et al[18] and Murti et al[19] in two separate studies reported malignant transformation of OSF in oral cancer in 4.5% of their study populations.

Deficiencies in non-starchy vegetables, fruits, and foods containing carotenoids has been reported to be associated with oral cancer.[11] Role of various micronutrients is not very clear. It has been theorized that plant-based foods contain substances with antioxidant and anticarcinogenic properties. These nutrients could play an important role in amending the carcinogenic effects of tobacco smoke, alcohol consumption, and betel quid chewing.

23.5 Diagnosis

Most cancers arising in retromolar area are SCCs. The lesions could be ulcerative, exophytic, or infiltrative in nature. A thorough history and physical examination is crucial for initial diagnosis and staging. Cancers of RMT have a very complex spatial relationship with surrounding structures. They can spread in several directions through direct extension as well as can involve the mandibular bone or have a perineural extension via the inferior alveolar nerve. Although the presence of trismus may raise the suspicion of pterygoid muscle involvement, it may be due to the inflammation of pterygoid musculature. It is important to assess the space from where the pathology has originated, tumor size, and if there is trans-spatial extension or invasion of deep structures. History and physical examination should evaluate the factors such as lifestyle habits (including alcohol consumption, smoking, and use of drugs), comorbid conditions (including nutritional status, chronic obstructive lung disease, and liver function), and a detailed family history. All of these factors may affect the management of primary disease.

23.5.1 Clinical Examination

Detailed clinical examination performed in an upright position is a vital part of the management of retromolar cancers. This should not only involve inspection, but also palpation of the mucosa and underlying soft tissue. It is the practice of our institute to evaluate all new cancer patients with flexible fiberoptic laryngoscope and document the examination as videos. This allows for adequate assessment of various subsites of the head and neck that are not easily evaluated by direct visualization.

23.5.2 Imaging

It is often difficult to diagnose cortical bone and periosteal invasion based on clinical examination. Due to apposition of mucosal surfaces in oral cavity and oropharynx, early stage small lesions can be missed or its true depth may not be accurately delineated. It is extremely important for any imaging study to evaluate the local as well as regional/distal extent of the tumors for appropriate surgical or nonsurgical management.

Computed tomography (CT) and magnetic resonance imaging (MRI) scans are complementary in the evaluation of retromolar cancers. CT is considered to be a good first-line imaging test to assess the extent of RMT lesion. On contrast enhanced CT, the lesion appears as enhancing mass in the area of RMT. It is difficult to pick up small lesions due to opposition of mucosal surfaces. "Puffed-cheek" technique is reported to be helpful in the detection of small doubtful lesions. Erdogan et al[20] evaluated 11 patients in a prospective study to compare the effectiveness of conventional CT and puffed-cheek CT in detecting the presence and extent of oral malignant tumors. They reported that the puffed-cheek CTs provided additional information about the true size and extent of the tumor than the conventional CT. Puffed-cheek maneuver is easily taught and is easy to comply with. Initially, the patients were asked to hold breath while puffing their cheeks. But it was also possible to puff out the cheeks and continue breathing quietly further improving the compliance as well as quality of the study.

Bone windows of CT scan can be used to evaluate the erosion of cortical bone adjacent to the tumor. These windows may also be able to show findings suggestive of aggressive periosteal reaction, pathological fractures, and abnormal attenuation in bone marrow. Lane et al[21] reviewed the records of patients with biopsy proven retromolar cancer. They compared the preoperative CT findings with histopathologic findings during surgery. They reported that preoperative CT scan failed to detect bone invasion in 27% of the patients. In the study, the sensitivity of CT for bone involvement in RMT was reported to be 50%, with a negative predictive value of 61.1%. The positive predictive value was reported to be 91.1%. The inaccuracy of CT scan in detecting bone involvement is significant in treatment planning. Arya et al[22] investigated the accuracy of 16 section multidetector computed tomography (MDCT) in assessing mandibular invasion in RMT cancers. MDCT involves replacing the linear array of detector elements used on typical conventical and helical CT scanners with two-dimensional array of detector elements. This permits acquisition of multiple slices simultaneously and with increased speed. They reported sensitivity, specificity, and accuracy of 16 section MDCT for mandibular, cortical, and marrow invasion as 94, 90, and 91.8% and 83, 92, and 89%, respectively. The accuracy for detection of inferior alveolar canal invasion was reported to be 100%.

Crecco et al[23] evaluated the diagnostic accuracy of magnetic resonance images to find out both the T stage and establish the spatial relationship between the tumors and surrounding structures in RMT area. In this study, preoperative MRI staging data correlated with pathology in 19 of 22 patients with overall accuracy of 86%. MRI is able to provide exact T staging of tumors due to better soft tissue contrast. MRI images are also less affected by dental amalgam compared to CT and have high sensitivity for marrow infiltration and perineural spread.

Vidiri et al[24] retrospectively compared the diagnostic accuracy of MRI and MDCT. Thirty-six surgical patients with histologically proven SCC of oral cavity who performed both a preoperative MRI and MDCT were retrospectively analyzed.

Although, MRI showed higher sensitivity compared to MDCT, findings were not statistically significant. Wiener et al[25] retrospectively reviewed 52 patients with histologically proven primary SCC of oral cavity who underwent both 16-slice MDCT and MRI. Results of radiological assessment were correlated with the intraoperative and histopathological findings. They reported MRI to be better for T staging compared to MSCT due to underestimation of tumor size by MSCT.

Advantages of preoperative MDCT are ability to use multiplanar reformatting at a faster speed of scanning and better patient compliance. When used optimally, it also has high accuracy in detecting mandibular invasion. MRI images are less likely to be degraded by dental amalgam, have more accurate T staging, and have high sensitivity for marrow infiltration and perineural spread. Genden et al[26] recommended a panoramic radiograph and CT scan for all patients presenting with a tumor of RMT. In patients with trismus, extensive soft tissue involvement, and/or change of sensation including pain, MRI scanning was recommended.

23.6 Surgical Considerations and Approaches

23.6.1 Surgical Considerations

Malignancies of the RMT create a challenge for the surgeon. RMT cancers tend to spread to at least one adjacent site in more than 75% of cases,[3-5] very often to the anterior tonsillar pillar, the soft palate, and the lower gum.[6] Their anatomical location and close proximity to those structures also means that cancers of this region can easily spread in many directions, including:[27]

- Anterolaterally to the buccinator muscle and cheek.
- Posterolaterally to the buccal fat and masticator muscle.
- Posteromedially to the tongue.
- Posteriorly to the anterior tonsillar pillar/oropharynx.
- Superiorly via the PMR to the maxilla.
- Inferiorly to the mandible and inferior alveolar nerve.

Additionally, cancers of the RMT lie directly on the anterior ramus of the mandible, and develop early invasion of the bone.[3-5] CT and/or MRI imaging modalities are useful for identifying bony invasion and should always be employed during initial assessment. The decision to perform a marginal or segmental mandibulectomy should be carefully considered—bone involvement can be assessed intraoperatively by judiciously stripping the periosteum and evaluating the bone. The periosteum can be sent for frozen assessment. If the periosteum is not involved, a marginal mandibulectomy may be an appropriate resection.[28]

Segmental resections may cause severe functional deficits and associated cosmetic challenges, whereas marginal mandibular resections may increase the risk of fractures.[28,29] Mandibular conservation has been advocated because of the improved function and aesthetics. Pascoal et al[30] reported on mandibular conservation and found that there was no difference in survival rate when comparing segmental versus marginal mandibulectomy for carcinoma of the RMT, and that conserving the ascending ramus of the mandible did not increase recurrence rate. Several authors agree that mandibular preservation has control rates equal to that of segmental mandibulectomy and should be based on the extent of invasion.[29,31-33] However, it is recommended that segmental mandibulectomy be performed for gross invasion of the cortex or bone marrow or limited invasion in the setting of an atrophic mandibular bone.[29,34]

It is generally accepted that marginal mandibulectomy should avoided in the irradiated mandible, as the pattern of invasion is via direct extension along multiple points along the cortex instead of the occlusal surface; thus, extensive and diffuse invasion of the mandibular body is expected.[28,29] In these patients, segmental mandibulectomy is performed. Thus, consideration of pre- or postoperative adjuvant radiation is critical for appropriate surgical treatment.

As mentioned in previous sections, RMT cancer frequently spreads along the pterygomandibular raphae, and from here can continue upward and involve the pterygoid muscle, plate, or directly invade the maxillary sinus from its lateral wall. Infratemporal fossa clearance may be an important component for complete resection, particularly in advanced disease. Hao et al[35] demonstrated in their series that tumor of RMT involved the maxilla in 22% of patients, more commonly than the mandible, which was involved in 18% of patients.

Resection of RMT cancers may involve structures critical for maintenance of speech and swallowing. Hence, careful preoperative evaluation is essential to minimize deficits and to preserve function.

23.6.2 Surgical Approaches

The surgical treatments for carcinomas of the RMT have evolved over the past half century. Surgery became first line therapy when Barbosa[36] reported on the "retromolar operation" in 1959. Although this included a hemimandibulectomy with en bloc resection of the pterygoid and masseter muscles and ipsilateral neck dissection, the extensive operation was deemed superior to radiation at the time. Kowalski et al[3] applied this technique to 114 patients with carcinoma of the RMT over a span of 30 years. Forty percent of the patients were classified as early stage disease (T1–T2). Unfortunately, the rate of local recurrence was 27.2%, which prompted the authors to conclude that more extensive resection was appropriate in patients with advanced cancers, or when the tumor demonstrated histologic criteria suggestive of aggressiveness (PNI or vascular emboli). However, in more recent years, several authors have advocated less extensive resections, particularly for early stage disease,[35] but as far as the extent of surgery is concerned, there is no clear consensus. Some support segmental resections, while others promote mandibular conservation in these patients. Deo et al[37] advocate that in view of the propensity for mandibular invasion, all advanced RMT cancers should be treated with hemimandibulectomy, which can also facilitate adequate infratemporal fossa clearance.

The surgical approach to SCC of RMT is dependent upon the primary tumor's size, site, infiltrative depth, and proximity to the mandible or maxilla.[38] Preoperative clinical assessment is indicated to accurately define the extent of the tumor, and should include an examination under anesthesia. In addition, adequate clinical and radiographic evaluation is critical to determine bone invasion. At our institution, we recommend preoperative CT scan if there is concern regarding mandibular or maxillary invasion. An MRI may be useful if there is also high suspicion of other soft tissue or nerve invasion.

Early, small tumors of the RMT can often be approached transorally. A 1.5 to 2 cm superficial resection margin is generally adequate; however, for tumors that penetrate through the cheek skin, a larger margin is preferred (2–3 cm).

The access to RMT can be more challenging for larger tumors, but traditionally, a midline mandibulotomy is employed. However, this maneuver is associated with significant morbidity: lip splitting, which can lead to unsightly scarring; injury to the inferior alveolar nerve, and mandibular nonunion or malunion. Patients may require a nasogastric or percutaneous feeding tube (we use the latter at our institution), and a temporary tracheostomy to avoid airway compromise in the postoperative period. Upper and lower cheek flaps minimize some of this morbidity, and can provide appropriate access in some cases. Access to the maxilla can be achieved through a Weber-Ferguson incision.

Horta et al[34] composed a table to categorize the commonly used surgical approaches for cancer of the RMT (▶ Table 23.1); a pictoral diagram 1 is included below.

Table 23.1 Most commonly used surgical approaches for retromolar trigone cancer

Approach	Description
Per oral	• Reserved for smaller T1 or T2 lesions, which are easily accessible • Exposure is obtained via a side mouth gag or self-retaining retractor. If further exposure is needed, an Army-Navy retractor can be placed in the region of the oral commissure
Upper or lower cheek flap approach	• The cheek flap (labiotomy) approach may be upper or lower depending on the precise location of the tumor • It is particularly useful for posteriorly located tumors • All of the soft tissue of the cheek is raised from the mandible until it meets the tumor. The mental nerve can be preserved in small or anteriorly located tumors
Lower lip splitting and marginal mandibulotomy approach	• More suitable for posterior RMT tumors in patients who also present with trismus • A midline lower labiotomy is performed. The lower cheek flap is reflected until it meets the tumor
Paramidline mandibulotomy and marginal mandibulectomy	• Good exposure for RMT, floor of mouth, and soft palate • It can be performed anterior to the mental foramen preserving cheek skin sensation
Upper lip splitting	• Upper lip splitting can involve only an upper lip split or can extend to a full Weber-Ferguson incision. The upper cheek flap can then be elevated off the anterior surface of the maxilla to the maxillary tuberosity
Segmental mandibulectomy (paramidline to subcondyle)	• Indicated in patients with gross cortical invasion or evidence of bone marrow infiltration of the mandible

Source: Horta et al.[34]
Abbreviation: RMT, retromolar trigone.

23.7 Management of the Neck

The presence of pathologic nodes is a poor prognostic indicator in RMT cancers, as well as for other SCCs of the oral cavity. Histologically, positive lymph nodes are found in anywhere from 26 to 80% of patients with tumors of the RMT.[4,35,39] The best predictor for neck metastasis is the depth of invasion, which is indistinct from other subsites of the oral cavity.[34,38] Therefore, it should be used to guide treatment decisions. In a recently published report, a depth of invasion between 3 and 4 mm confers a 20% incidence of nodal metastasis in carcinomas of the RMT.[40] For tumor depth greater than 4 mm, elective dissection should be performed, and as this recent report suggests, it should also be considered for a depth of 3 mm at this anatomical site. When an ipsilateral selective neck dissection is performed for clinically N0 necks, patients are treated with at least a supraomohyoid neck dissection. Dissection of level 2b should be included if the lesion extends to the oropharynx.

The role of sentinel lymph node biopsy in early oral cancers for N0 necks is expanding, and could potentially be used as a reliable staging procedure for patients with early stage disease, as more recent studies have demonstrated no differences in recurrence or overall survival.[41–44] However, the current standard of care is an ipsilateral neck dissection. There are a few anecdotal accounts of contralateral spread in the literature; therefore, bilateral neck dissection is recommended only if the lesion crosses midline in the oral cavity or oropharynx.

Thus, in correlation with cancers of the oral cavity, nodal status is an important prognostic indicator for RMT cancers, and when indicated, an ipsilateral selective neck dissection should be included in any surgical resection for curative intent.[5]

23.8 Surgical Sequelae

Surgical defects of RMT tumors, because of their location and early extension, can be significant. In 2006, Goldie et al described which important structures could be involved in the resection and demonstrated not only the resultant deficits, but also the functional concerns after surgery.[45]

Multiple structures—including the lingual nerve, submandibular duct, and palatoglossus—are at particular risk. This could affect sensation, speech, swallowing, and tongue movements. The functional intraoral Glasgow scale (FIGS)[46] is a point system to assess pre- and postoperative ability to speak, chew, and swallow in patients who have had extensive oral and oropharyngeal cavity resection, and has been used to evaluate postoperative function in patients who were treated for cancer of RMT.

Not surprisingly, more advanced tumor stage was related to greater functional impairment, which remained during and after rehabilitation.[46] Long-term complications also included poor speech understandability and oropharyngeal swallow ability.

Extensive resection of soft palate can lead to velopharyngeal insufficiency (Genden), although obturator or free flap reconstruction can minimize or correct this functional deficit.

Short-term sequelae are frequently related to surgery and include hematoma, seroma, wound infection, wound breakdown, minor flap necrosis and dehiscence, salivary fistula, abscess, chyle leak, facial and/or shoulder weakness, and reduced range of motion (ROM) and pain. Additionally, tracheostomy tube placement may be indicated during the surgery, and a feeding tube may be necessary during the postoperative period, as the patient may have limited oral mobility and dysphagia.

Long-term complications, either related to surgery or a result of adjuvant treatment, can be both functionally and physically debilitating. Problems with trismus, chewing, and swallowing, including velopharyngeal insufficiency (VPI), may result from prolonged percutaneous gastrostomy (PEG) tube dependency. Obstacles with tongue movement and xerostomia may limit the patient's ability to speak. Poor cosmesis may be a long-term sequelae, especially after free flap or mandibular reconstruction. In the latter event, long-term issues such as hardware exposure or osteoradionecrosis may develop, and require more surgical treatment.

It is important that all of these patients have access to psychological assessment. Many have anxiety and depression related to the functional implications of surgery. Many are embarrassed when eating and drinking, and they are often dissatisfied with their conversational speech and appearance after surgery. The adjustment period to a new normal way of everyday interaction may be significant for many patients.

23.9 Adjuvant Treatment

Surgery remains the mainstay of treatment for carcinomas of the RMT. While some early studies suggested that T1 or T2 lesions can be treated with radiation with equal rates of locoregional control,[4] current research does not support primary radiotherapy as first line therapy in patients who can tolerate surgical resection. Outcomes are most favorable when surgery is combined with adjuvant radiotherapy (pre- or postoperative).[5,47] Primary radiotherapy has a higher incidence of locoregional failure than when radiotherapy is combined with surgery. For patients who are unsuitable or unable to tolerate primary surgical treatment, combined chemoradiotherapy is now the standard in that patient population, and it has improved outcome compared to radiotherapy alone.

Key Points

- Squamous cell cancers of RMT are notorious for their indolent course and late presentation.
- Even the early stage cancer can have a rapid microscopic extension to surrounding soft tissue and bones with high recurrence rate.
- The location of the RMT allows early spread of cancer in multiple directions to nearby structures.
- Surgical resection is based upon the extent of tumor, and may involve bony structures.
- Early evaluation with imaging to determine bony involvement is important for surgical planning.
- A selective neck dissection should be included in surgical resection for curative intent.
- Free flap reconstruction for advanced disease is mainstay for treatment, and improves functional and cosmetic outcomes.
- Functional and cosmetic long-term sequelae can be substantial.

References

[1] Trotta BM, Pease CS, Rasamny JJ, Raghavan P, Mukherjee S. Oral cavity and oropharyngeal squamous cell cancer: key imaging findings for staging and treatment planning. Radiographics. 2011; 31(2):339–354

[2] Binahmed A, Nason RW, Abdoh AA, Sándor GKB. Population-based study of treatment outcomes in squamous cell carcinoma of the retromolar trigone. Oral Surg Oral Med Oral Pathol Oral Radiol Endod. 2007; 104(5):662–665

[3] Kowalski LP, Hashimoto I, Magrin J. End results of 114 extended "commando" operations for retromolar trigone carcinoma. Am J Surg. 1993; 166(4):374–379

[4] Byers RM, Anderson B, Schwarz EA, Fields RS, Meoz R. Treatment of squamous carcinoma of the retromolar trigone. Am J Clin Oncol. 1984; 7(6):647–652

[5] Huang C-J, Chao KSC, Tsai J, et al. Cancer of retromolar trigone: long-term radiation therapy outcome. Head Neck. 2001; 23(9):758–763

[6] Ayad T, Gelinas M, Guertin L, et al. Retromolar trigone carcinoma treated by primary radiation therapy: an alternative to the primary surgical approach. Arch Otolaryngol Head Neck Surg. 2005; 131(7):576–582

[7] Gilbert S, Tzadik A, Leonard G. Mandibular involvement by oral squamous cell carcinoma. Laryngoscope. 1986; 96(1):96–101

[8] Brown JS, Griffith JF, Phelps PD, Browne RM. A comparison of different imaging modalities and direct inspection after periosteal stripping in predicting the invasion of the mandible by oral squamous cell carcinoma. Br J Oral Maxillofac Surg. 1994; 32(6):347–359

[9] Warnakulasuriya S. Global epidemiology of oral and oropharyngeal cancer. Oral Oncol. 2009; 45(4–5):309–316

[10] Siegel RL, Miller KD, Jemal A. Cancer statistics, 2018. CA Cancer J Clin. 2018; 68(1):7–30

[11] Petti S. Lifestyle risk factors for oral cancer. Oral Oncol. 2009; 45(4–5):340–350. Epub 2008 Jul 1031

[12] IARC Working Group on the Evaluation of Carcinogenic Risks to Humans. Betel-quid and areca-nut chewing and some areca-nut derived nitrosamines. IARC Monogr Eval Carcinog Risks Hum. 2004; 85:1–334

[13] Wollina U, Verma SB, Ali FM, Patil K. Oral submucous fibrosis: an update. Clin Cosmet Investig Dermatol. 2015; 8:193–204

[14] Cancer incidence in five continents. Volume VIII. IARC Sci Publ. 2002(155): 1–781

[15] Yeole BB, Kurkure A, Advani S, Lizzy S. An assessment of cancer incidence patterns in Parsi and non Parsi populations, Greater Mumbai. Asian Pac J Cancer Prev. 2001; 2(4):293–298

[16] Paymaster JC. Cancer of the buccal mucosa; a clinical study of 650 cases in Indian patients. Cancer. 1956; 9(3):431–435

[17] Tilakaratne WM, Klinikowski MF, Saku T, Peters TJ, Warnakulasuriya S. Oral submucous fibrosis: review on aetiology and pathogenesis. Oral Oncol. 2006; 42(6):561–568

[18] Pindborg JJ, Murti PR, Bhonsle RB, Gupta PC, Daftary DK, Mehta FS. Oral submucous fibrosis as a precancerous condition. Scand J Dent Res. 1984; 92(3): 224–229

[19] Murti PR, Bhonsle RB, Pindborg JJ, Daftary DK, Gupta PC, Mehta FS. Malignant transformation rate in oral submucous fibrosis over a 17-year period. Community Dent Oral Epidemiol. 1985; 13(6):340–341

[20] Erdogan N, Bulbul E, Songu M, et al. Puffed-cheek computed tomography: a dynamic maneuver for imaging oral cavity tumors. Ear Nose Throat J. 2012; 91(9):383–384, 386

[21] Lane AP, Buckmire RA, Mukherji SK, Pillsbury HC, III, Meredith SD. Use of computed tomography in the assessment of mandibular invasion in carcinoma of the retromolar trigone. Otolaryngol Head Neck Surg. 2000; 122(5): 673–677

[22] Arya S, Rane P, Sable N, Juvekar S, Bal M, Chaukar D. Retromolar trigone squamous cell cancers: a reappraisal of 16 section MDCT for assessing mandibular invasion. Clin Radiol. 2013; 68(12):e680–e688

[23] Crecco M, Vidiri A, Angelone ML, Palma O, Morello R. Retromolar trigone tumors: evaluation by magnetic resonance imaging and correlation with pathological data. Eur J Radiol. 1999; 32(3):182–188

[24] Vidiri A, Guerrisi A, Pellini R, et al. Multi-detector row computed tomography (MDCT) and magnetic resonance imaging (MRI) in the evaluation of the mandibular invasion by squamous cell carcinomas (SCC) of the oral cavity. Correlation with pathological data. J Exp Clin Cancer Res. 2010; 29(1):73–73

[25] Wiener E, Pautke C, Link TM, Neff A, Kolk A. Comparison of 16-slice MSCT and MRI in the assessment of squamous cell carcinoma of the oral cavity. Eur J Radiol. 2006; 58(1):113–118

[26] Genden EM, Ferlito A, Shaha AR, Rinaldo A. Management of cancer of the retromolar trigone. Oral Oncol. 2003; 39(7):633–637

[27] Purohit BS HR, Op de beeck K. Imaging in squamous cell carcinoma of the retromolar trigone. 2014

[28] Wax MK, Bascom DA, Myers LL. Marginal mandibulectomy vs segmental mandibulectomy: indications and controversies. Arch Otolaryngol Head Neck Surg. 2002; 128(5):600–603

[29] Rao LP, Shukla M, Sharma V, Pandey M. Mandibular conservation in oral cancer. Surg Oncol. 2012; 21(2):109–118

[30] Pascoal MBN, Chagas JF, Alonso N, et al. A mandibulectomia marginal no tratamento dos tumores de loja amigdalina e região retromolar. Rev Bras Otorrinolaringol. 2007; 73:180–184

[31] Dubner S, Heller KS. Local control of squamous cell carcinoma following marginal and segmental mandibulectomy. Head Neck. 1993; 15(1):29–32

[32] Ord RA, Sarmadi M, Papadimitrou J. A comparison of segmental and marginal bony resection for oral squamous cell carcinoma involving the mandible. J Oral Maxillofac Surg. 1997; 55(5):470–477, discussion 477–478

[33] Nishi H, Shinozaki T, Tomioka T, Maruo T, Hayashi R. Squamous cell carcinoma of the retromolar trigone: treatment outcomes. Auris Nasus Larynx. 2018; 45(2):337–342

[34] Horta R, Nascimento R, Silva A, Amarante J. The retromolar trigone: anatomy, cancer treatment modalities, reconstruction, and a classification system. J Craniofac Surg. 2016; 27(4):1070–1076

[35] Hao SP, Tsang NM, Chang KP, Chen CK, Huang SS. Treatment of squamous cell carcinoma of the retromolar trigone. Laryngoscope. 2006; 116(6):916–920

[36] Barbosa JF. Cancer of the retromolar area; a study of twenty-eight cases with the presentation of a new surgical technique for their treatment. AMA Arch Otolaryngol. 1959; 69(1):19–30

[37] Deo SV, Shukla NK, Kallianpur AA, Mohanti BK, Thulkar SP. Aggressive multimodality management of locally advanced retromolar trigone tumors. Head Neck. 2013; 35(9):1269–1273

[38] Shah JP, Gil Z. Current concepts in management of oral cancer—surgery. Oral Oncol. 2009; 45(4–5):394–401

[39] Antoniades K, Lazaridis N, Vahtsevanos K, Hadjipetrou L, Antoniades V, Karakasis D. Treatment of squamous cell carcinoma of the anterior faucial pillar-retromolar trigone. Oral Oncol. 2003; 39(7):680–686

[40] Brockhoff HC, II, Kim RY, Braun TM, Skouteris C, Helman JI, Ward BB. Correlating the depth of invasion at specific anatomic locations with the risk for regional metastatic disease to lymph nodes in the neck for oral squamous cell carcinoma. Head Neck. 2017; 39(5):974–979

[41] Wiseman SM, Loree TR, Hicks WL, Jr, Rigual NR. Sentinel lymph node biopsy in SCC of the head and neck: a major advance in staging the N0 neck. Ear Nose Throat J. 2002; 81(3):156–160, 163

[42] Monroe MM, Lai SY. Sentinel lymph node biopsy for oral cancer: supporting evidence and recent novel developments. Curr Oncol Rep. 2014; 16(5):385

[43] Pribaz J, Stephens W, Crespo L, Gifford G. A new intraoral flap: facial artery musculomucosal (FAMM) flap. Plast Reconstr Surg. 1992; 90(3): 421–429

[44] Cigna E, Rizzo MI, Greco A, et al. Retromolar trigone reconstructive surgery: prospective comparative analysis between free flaps. Ann Surg Oncol. 2015; 22(1):272–278

[45] Goldie SJ, Soutar DS, Shaw-Dunn J. The effect of surgical resection in the region of the retromolar trigone. J Plast Reconstr Aesthet Surg. 2006; 59(12): 1263–1268

[46] Goldie SJ, Jackson MS, Soutar DS, Shaw-Dunn J. The functional intraoral Glasgow scale (FIGS) in retromolar trigone cancer patients. J Plast Reconstr Aesthet Surg. 2006; 59(7):743–746

[47] Bayman NA, Sykes AJ, Bonington S, et al. Primary radiotherapy for carcinoma of the retromolar trigone: a useful alternative to surgery. Clin Oncol (R Coll Radiol). 2010; 22(2):119–124

24 Reconstruction of the Retromolar Trigone

Jennifer Christenson and Ryan J. Li

Summary
The goal of reconstruction of the retromolar trigone after cancer resection is to provide bone coverage, reducing contracture that risks trismus, and maintaining occlusion when applicable. Such efforts should be able to withstand adjuvant radiotherapy as well. The surgical reconstructive options are wide-ranging and can be tailored to individual patient considerations, include comorbid status, health of tissue at donor site, and prospect of future dental rehabilitation. Thoughtful reconstruction should be paired with expert rehabilitative services of speech and swallow specialists.

Keywords: reconstruction, oral cancer, free tissue transfer, trismus

24.1 Introduction

Squamous cell carcinoma of the retromolar trigone (RMT) is relatively uncommon, comprising approximately 6% of all cancers of the oral cavity.[1] Cancers of this subsite have a tendency to present in an advanced stage with a propensity for bony invasion.[2] This leads to lower rates of locoregional control and overall survival.[1,2] It is generally accepted that treatment for squamous cell carcinoma in this location is surgical, and adjuvant therapy is indicated in cases of advanced disease. If a functional reconstruction can be achieved via a simple approach, it should be attempted first.[3] Although local pedicled flaps can provide similar tissue, shorter operative times, and potentially lower morbidity, free tissue transfer is considered the gold standard in the reconstruction of RMT. For every patient, the goals of care, nature of the defect, and patient-specific risks must be evaluated.

24.2 Diagnosis and Evaluation

Collaboration among the involved surgeons in preoperative ablative and reconstructive planning is essential. RMT lesions are often easily visualized through oral examination. Flexible nasopharyngolaryngoscopy or mirror examination should be performed to evaluate for oropharyngeal tumor extension. The mucosa of the RMT lies directly on the anterior surface of the mandibular ramus, and bony invasion may occur quite early.[1] Patients should be assessed preoperatively with computed tomography (CT) to estimate the extent of invasion and anticipate whether a bony defect will be present after resection. Allen's testing of both hands should be performed. If a fibular osseous or osteocutaneous (OC) free tissue transfer is needed for a planned segmental mandibulectomy, lower extremity CT angiography or ultrasound duplex study is recommended to evaluate the quality of lower extremity vessels, and to identify potential poor collateral blood flow. Three-dimensional virtual surgical planning may also be utilized for bony reconstruction.

24.3 Anatomic Considerations/ Relevant Anatomy

The RMT describes the small area posterior to the 3rd mandibular molar. Gingival and buccal mucosa overlie a segment of the mandibular ramus bounded by the temporal crest, anterior border of the ramus, and posterior socket of the lower third molar.[4] Superiorly, temporalis muscle fibers attach to the coronoid process and medially, the medial pterygoid muscle inserts onto the medial angle and body of the ramus.[5] This subsite of the oral cavity is bounded by the buccal mucosa laterally, the mandibular alveolar ridge anteroinferiorly, the anterior tonsillar pillar medially, the mandibular ramus deep to the mucosa, and the maxillary alveolar ridge anterosuperiorly.

Because malignant lesions of this area typically require a 1 cm gross mucosal margin during ablation—which inevitably contracts to a smaller margin—the surgical defect can become quite large and functionally significant. If a segmental mandibulectomy is performed in the setting of cortical invasion, then an OC flap should be used—for which fibula, scapula, and potentially radial forearm OC flaps are options. In patients who are not surgical candidates for an OC free flap, allowing the mandible to swing often produces acceptable functional outcomes with soft tissue-only reconstruction. Elsewhere in this book, mandibular reconstruction is described in further detail. If a marginal mandibulectomy is performed, a soft tissue-only reconstruction is indicated.

The goals of RMT reconstruction include preservation of masticatory and optimal speech and swallow functions. Although bony surfaces like the hard palate can often heal well by secondary intention, exposed bone along the RMT should be covered by a soft tissue flap for several reasons. Healing by secondary intention along the RMT leads to unacceptable fibrosis and potentially debilitating trismus.[6] In this regard, free tissue transfer is an ideal method of reconstruction, choosing thin and pliable soft tissue of appropriate volume.[4] However, various other reconstructive options are available and may be more appropriate based on the patient's clinical state and stated goals. Various options along the reconstructive ladder, including advantages and disadvantages of each method, are described below. Comprehensive technical details of specific flaps are beyond the scope of this chapter.

24.4 Surgical Considerations and Approaches

24.4.1 Skin Grafts

Split or full thickness skin grafts may be considered for small defects of the RMT if a vascular bed is still present over mandibular cortex. Without a vascular bed, skin grafts serve only as a short-term biological dressing.[4] With low morbidity, an appropriately sized graft can be bolstered to the surgical bed, and may promote neovascularization and reepithelialization from the wound edges.[7] Advantages include an abundance of donor tissue, ease of harvest and inset, and the resultant short operative time. In certain patients who have submucosal fibrosis—for example, due to betel nut chewing—poor vascularity will reduce skin graft viability.[8] Disadvantages of skin grafts include donor site pain, lack of tissue bulk, and wound contracture across the entire surgical bed that will result in trismus. To avoid donor site complications, acellular dermal matrix grafts can be used in place of skin for similar results; however, a vascularized wound bed is often lacking after RMT cancer excisions.[9] As discussed next, skin grafting is rarely a first-line option for quick reconstruction, given the availability of various pedicled local and regional flaps.

24.4.2 Local and Regional Pedicled Flaps

Local and regional flaps are an excellent reconstructive option in patients who have multiple medical comorbidities that preclude longer periods of general anesthesia required for free tissue transfer. With the majority of oral cancer patients presenting in the sixth decade of life and upward, medical comorbidities, functional status, and vessel quality become major considerations. Pedicled flaps are reliable options requiring minimal specialized equipment, training, and postoperative vascular monitoring. Many local and regional pedicled flaps have been described in RMT reconstruction including the buccinator musculomucosal flap (BMF), facial artery musculomucosal flap (FAMM), palatal island flap, tongue propeller flap, submental island flap, superficial temporal artery island flap, melo- and nasolabial flaps, platysma island flap, supraclavicular artery island flap (SCAIF), and pectoralis musculocutaneous flap (PMMC). Several of these reconstructive options are described in further detail below.

Buccinator Musculomucosal Flap (BMF)

The posteriorly-based BMF provides well-vascularized tissue for reconstruction of small RMT defects.[10] This flap provides similar, sensate tissue that is easy to harvest in close proximity to the RMT defect, facilitating tension-free insetting for small defects. The flap is pedicled upon the buccal artery and vein, which enter the buccinator muscle at the posterior-inferior muscle edge on its lateral side, medial to the buccopharyngeal fascia. These are vascular tributaries of the internal maxillary system.[5,10,11] Preservation of the buccopharyngeal fascia protects the more lateral facial nerve branches, and prevents herniation of the buccal fat pad into the surgical wound. The superior limit of the flap lies 3 mm inferior to Stenson's duct and the anterior limit lies 1 cm posterior to the oral commissure. This flap can be harvested to a maximal height and length of approximately 4 × 7 cm. The donor site defect may be closed through primary closure or left to heal by secondary intention.

Facial Artery Musculomucosal Flap (FAMM)

The FAMM is a reliable and versatile flap first described by Pribaz et al in 1992, extrapolating from techniques used to harvest nasolabial and buccal flaps.[12] The flap is pedicled upon the facial artery running axially. A superiorly-based FAMM receives retrograde facial arterial flow, and begins within the ipsilateral gingivolabial sulcus adjacent to the nasal alar margin. An inferiorly-based FAMM begins adjacent to the RMT and receives anterograde facial arterial flow. Careful design requires a broad mucosal base during elevation, as the venous outflow of the FAMM is via submucosal tributaries. The maximal dimensions of this flap are approximately 3 × 8 cm, which can be rotated over a gentle axis to cover the RMT and adjacent defects. As with the BMF, the Stenson's duct is protected, in this case posterior to the flap margin. Flaps greater than 3 cm in width may have a higher risk of symptomatic cheek contracture, and thus should be avoided.[13] The rotation of the FAMM into the RMT does not require crossing a dentate area, an issue that poses challenge in other oral cavity sites. The donor site can be closed primarily with acceptable contracture with the above dimension limits.

Palatal Island Flap

The palatal island flap was first described by Gullane and Arena in 1977 for local oral cavity reconstruction after oncologic resection.[14] The flap is raised as an axial mucosal flap based on the ipsilateral greater palatine vessels. It can be rotated 180 degrees.[3] Further mobilization can be achieved by removing the hamulus of the medial pterygoid plate. Nearly the entire hard palate mucosa can be transferred for reconstruction, with healing of the donor site by secondary intention. An alternative local flap should be considered for patients with a prior radiation volume including the hard palate, or prior hard palate surgery. This flap can be utilized for RMT patients even with full dentition. Because this flap requires the borrowing of maxillary mucosa to reconstruct a mandibular defect, alternative flaps may have a lower risk of promoting trismus.

Deep Lingual Artery Axial Propeller Flap

Although there is concern that borrowing tissue from the intrinsic tongue poses an unacceptable risk to oral function,[3] the deep lingual artery axial propeller flap is feasible for RMT reconstruction.[15] This flap is based on the ipsilateral deep lingual vessels and includes a long musculomucosal paddle. Retrograde dissection of the pedicle is performed to its origin between the genioglossus and hyoglossus muscles. The flap can span the entire length of the tongue and is approximately 6 mm thick with a maximal height of 4 cm. After harvest the donor site can be closed primarily or allowed to close secondarily. Depending on the RMT defect, intervening mucosa between the recipient and donor site may require excision, or incorporation into the flap advancement. This flap provides excellent soft tissue and reach to the RMT; however, the risk of tongue contracture, dehiscence from tongue movement, and speech impairment may again be greater than alternatives.

Superficial Temporal Artery Island Flap

The superficial temporal artery island flap can be raised as a fasciocutaneous or temporoparietal fascial flap based on either the anterior or posterior terminal branches of the superficial temporal artery.[16] The branches of the artery are mapped using a handheld Doppler probe, with the flap centered over the desired pedicle. The pedicle is dissected proximally into the parotid gland, a safe dissection that passes posterior to uppermost facial nerve divisions. After blunt dissection between the masseteric and zygomatic muscles below the zygomatic arch, this pliable flap can be tunneled medially into the oral cavity. If fasciocutaneous in design, the bridging skin segment will require deepithelialization. Flaps as large as 8 × 16 cm can be harvested, and the incisional scar can be camouflaged well within hair-bearing skin. This flap has a reliable vascular supply, but its use may have been limited due to probable contracture and resulting trismus.

Supraclavicular Artery Island Flap (SCAIF)

The SCAIF is a robust, pedicled fasciocutaneous regional flap that has regained popularity in recent years.[7] This axial flap is supplied by the supraclavicular artery, a terminal confluence of transverse cervical arterial tributaries. The pedicle runs reliably within 1–2 cm of the posterior clavicular border, and can be followed with Doppler probe. The accompanying venous outflow runs in the same plane as the external jugular vein. The skin paddle can be designed as large as 12 × 35 cm, and is easily deepithelialized for tunneling to the RMT and surrounding defect. The SCAIF is elevated in a subfascial plane over the deltoid muscle from distal to proximal. The proximal pedicle can be precisely skeletonized for mobilization, or broadly protected. Complications include wound dehiscence with wider skin paddles, although defects as wide as 8 cm can be closed primarily. Surgical drains should be placed given the large potential space formed after harvest. Distal flap loss has been reported in 8–15% of cases.[17,18] The use of intraoperative Novadaq SPY fluorescence imaging can aid in predicting distal flap viability. While studies have reported distal flap viability up to 5 cm beyond the detectable pedicle Doppler signal, intraoperative perfusion imaging techniques such as SPY are likely more precise estimators. With ease of harvest, a long and wide skin paddle, and low donor site morbidity, this flap is an excellent alternative to free tissue transfer for RMT reconstruction. Patients with multiple comorbidities and poor vascular status may have a more expeditious reconstruction via this approach.[19]

Pectoralis Major Musculocutaneous Flap (PMMC)

The PMMC is a classic reconstructive workhorse in head and neck surgery. This flap has a robust and predictable vascular pedicle (pectoral branch of thoracoacromial trunk) that is directly visualized throughout harvest. While the PMMC may be too bulky for most soft tissue RMT defects, it can provide excellent bulk and cutaneous coverage for larger defects that require mandibular resection. In many edentulous or frail patients, bony reconstruction for posterior mandibular defects adds no functional or cosmetic value over soft tissue coverage. ▶ Fig. 24.1a–h illustrates a patient who underwent composite resection of an RMT mass with angle and ramus mandibulectomy. Preoperatively, he was fully reliant on a pureed and liquid consistency diet. During this procedure he underwent complete dental extraction. The defect was successfully reconstructed with a PMMC allowing the mandible to swing. The soft tissue reconstruction maintained his facial contours, and he enjoyed excellent oral excursion.

The reach and arc of rotation of the PMMC is maximized by extensive thinning of pectoralis muscle overlying the vascular pedicle, especially at the clavicular attachment. As with all pedicled flaps, skeletonization of the pedicle is only for optimal mobilization of the flap, as loss of this soft tissue envelope may increase the risk of pedicle kinking. Careful hemostasis involves tamponade (e.g., via oversew) of the transected humeral muscular head, and patients should be monitored postoperatively for donor site hematoma. Primary closure of skin defect (if one is present) is uniformly achieved by extensive suprafascial undermining of neighboring skin. Surgical drains are placed given the large potential space created.

24.4.3 Free Flaps

Free tissue transfer is the most versatile option for RMT reconstruction, with numerous modifications to thickness, contour, and tissue composition available. Despite these advantages, a successful microvascular program is resource intensive and predicated upon the surgeon's experience and technical skill. Even a dedicated microvascular surgeon often faces long operative times, and intensive postoperative monitoring.[19] Experienced centers report an overall success rate of free tissue reconstruction to be approximately 95%. Free flaps of the radial forearm, anterolateral thigh, and fibula are most widely used in the reconstruction of the RMT, and these are discussed in greater detail below.

Radial Forearm Free Flap (RFFF)

For soft tissue defects of the RMT, fasciocutaneous RFFF transfer is the most commonly utilized free tissue for reconstruction (▶ Fig. 24.2a–d).[7] The thin, pliable skin of the volar forearm provides adequate soft tissue dimensions for RMT and surrounding defects, resulting in predictable contracture with minimal atrophy (**Video 24.1**). Nearly every patient will have adequate RFFF skin to mildly overcorrect reconstruction of the RMT mucosal defect in anticipation of contracture. Despite a thin profile, some patients with obesity can have remarkably bulky skin paddles that are more difficult to contour. As with other bulky flaps, airway obstruction due to soft tissue edema should be considered, and the patient properly counseled preoperatively.

The RFFF is pedicled axially on the radial artery with accompanying venae comitantes and/or the cephalic vein, and a long pedicle facilitates many anastomotic options. Fasciocutaneous perforators arise from the pedicle and are most abundant in the distal third of the forearm. A sensate flap is possible with inclusion of the lateral antebrachial cutaneous nerve, which can be anastomosed to a transected inferior alveolar nerve. If a segmental mandibulectomy is performed, 40% of the circumference of the distal radius can be included to harvest an OC radial forearm flap. Restoration of mandibular continuity is described in more detail in Chapter 28 (Reconstruction of Mandibular Defects), and is an important consideration for ramus and angle defects to maintain proper dental occlusion in dentate patients. Dental rehabilitation per se is not a consideration for isolated RMT defects.[20]

Despite the ease of harvest and excellent soft tissue replacement of the RFFF, inadequate cosmesis of the donor site—which most commonly requires skin grafting—is often cited by surgeons, perhaps even more than by patients. With careful harvest technique, few other complications are commonly encountered—preservation of the superficial radial nerve branches and suprafascial elevation of the skin paddle minimize risk of hand numbness and restriction of wrist motion, respectively. Patients are routinely counseled that in the long term, forearm and hand function will return to normal; however certain patients—often those with manual labor occupations—may still prefer alternative donor sites, e.g., the widely used anterolateral thigh flap.[21]

Anterolateral Thigh Flap (ALT)

The ALT is also commonly utilized in the reconstruction of soft tissue RMT defects. As a fasciocutaneous flap, the

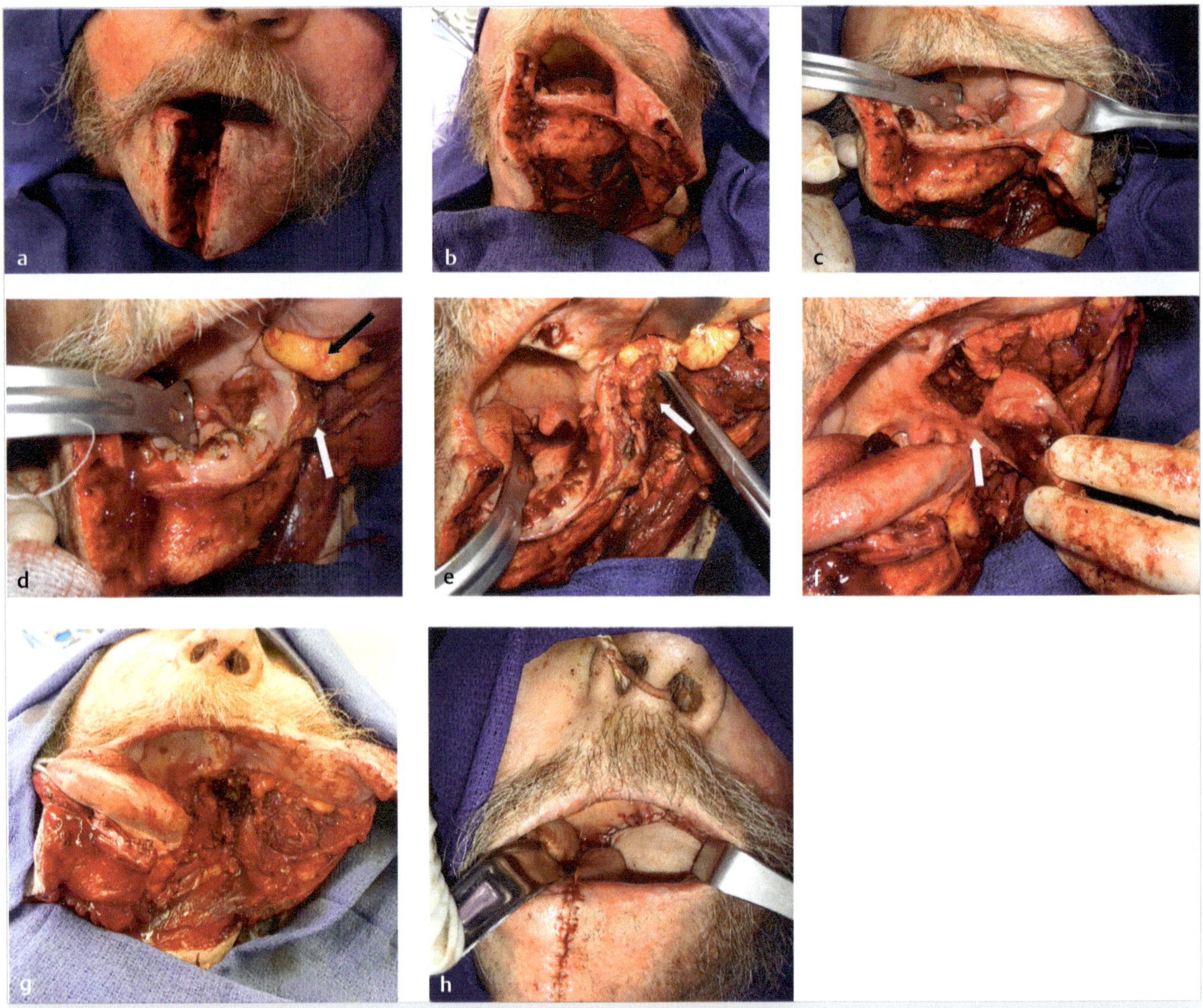

Fig. 24.1 Resection of a large retromolar trigone (RMT) squamous cell carcinoma with angle and ramus mandibulectomy, followed by pectoralis musculocutaneous flap (PMMC) soft tissue reconstruction. **(a)** For wide access to this large left RMT tumor, a lip split incision was used. **(b)** Because this patient had cortical invasion of the mandibular ramus and alveolar ridge, the mandible was maximally exposed, and the mucosa was incised close to the alveolar ridge anteriorly. **(c)** Here the RMT tumor is visualized, abutting the soft palate with extension onto the alveolar ridge and buccal mucosa. **(d)** An incision is extended through the buccal mucosa and around the lesion superiorly, leaving a 1.5 cm gross margin. Cauterized divided buccinator fibers (*white arrow*) and the buccal fat pad (*black arrow*) are visualized. **(e)** The coronoid process is identified and isolated (white arrow) and adjoining temporalis muscle fibers are divided. **(f)** The condyle has been delivered (C), medial pterygoid fibers are divided, and the specimen only remains attached via mucosa and scant muscle fibers (white arrow). **(g)** The specimen has been removed en bloc. **(h)** The appearance after inset of a PMMC in a patient who was not a candidate for microvascular osteocutaneous (OC) reconstruction.

thickness of ALT is highly customizable. Normally, a musculocutaneous or full thickness fasciocutaneous ALT is too bulky for small RMT defects. However, with dissection of the skin perforator(s), the subcutaneous fat can be thinned to as little as 3 mm thickness, while preserving a 2 cm radius of deeper adipose around the perforator(s).[22] With these modifications the ALT offers the same pliability as RFFF tissue with a pedicle of similar length.[23] Perforator dissection allows the skin paddle to have a wide range of motion over the pedicle.

This flap is based on the descending branch of the lateral circumflex femoral artery (LCFA) and associated venae comitantes. Typically, one to three septocutaneous or musculocutaneous perforators supply the anterior thigh skin. These perforators are commonly identified within a 3–5 cm radius of the midpoint between the anterior superior iliac spine (ASIS) and the lateral edge of the patella, within or just posterior to the intermuscular septum between vastus lateralis and rectus femoris muscles. The donor site is nearly always closed primarily with acceptable cosmesis and preservation of muscle function.[21]

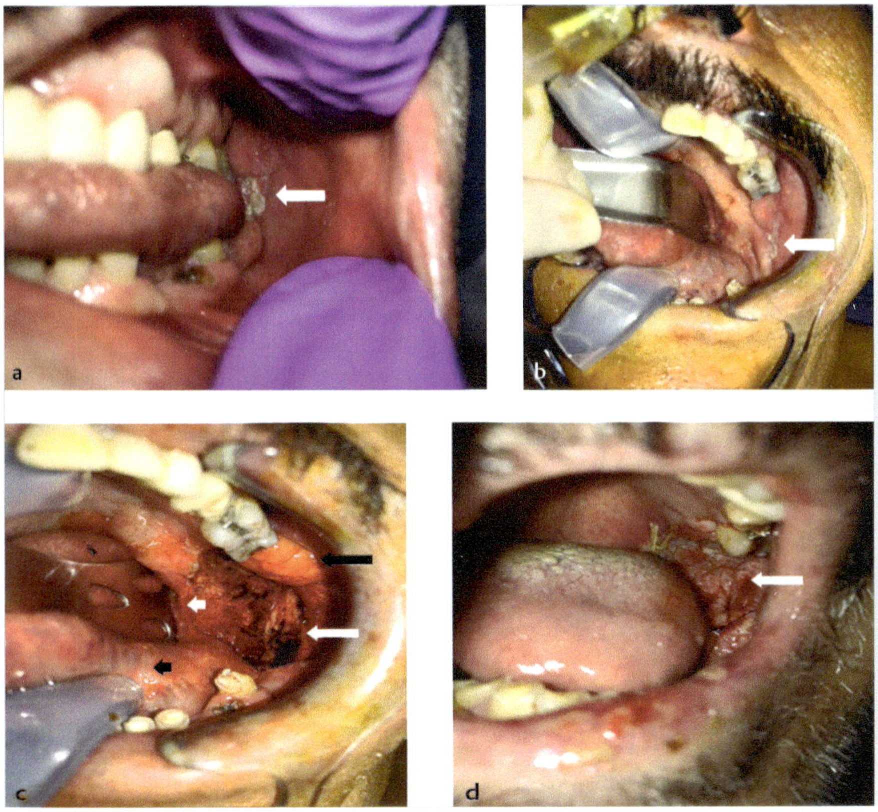

Fig. 24.2 Resection of a left retromolar trigone (RMT) squamous cell carcinoma resulting in a soft tissue defect. Reconstruction utilized a radial forearm fasciocutaneous free tissue transfer. **(a)** A small biopsy proven squamous cell carcinoma of the RMT is shown. Preoperative radiology showed no evidence of bony invasion. White arrow indicates the lesion. **(b)** Intraoperative exposure with a plastic cheek retractor and Molt oral retractor provides a wide view of the tumor, indicated by the white arrow. **(c)** The tumor has been resected with 1.5 cm gross margins. A defect of the RMT without bony disruption is shown. Long black arrow indicates the buccal fat pad. Long white arrow indicates mandibular ramus exposed bone. Short white arrow indicates the anterior tonsillar pillar. Short black arrow indicates the oral tongue. **(d)** Postoperative day one after radial forearm free tissue transfer for RMT reconstruction. Pin prick of the skin paddle elicited bright red blood. White arrow indicates the radial forearm free flap (RFFF) skin paddle.

Osteocutaneous (OC) Flaps

For RMT defects that include a segmental mandibulectomy, the decision whether to restore mandibular continuity depends upon the patient's reconstructive goals, dentition status, medical comorbidities, and extent of bone resection.[24] Mandibular reconstruction is discussed thoroughly elsewhere in this book. The skin paddles of the fibula OC and radial forearm OC flaps are thin and ideal for relining the RMT. Alternative free tissue transfers for both skin and bone replacement include the scapular, parascapular, and iliac crest-internal oblique flaps—the former two typically require repositioning of the supine patient, making it difficult to perform simultaneous cancer resection and free tissue harvest.

In the case of the fibula skin paddle, perforator dissection is possible to modestly increase pliability, although still constrained by close apposition to the fibula. The wide bone stock, multiple osteotomy options, and long available length make this a versatile OC flap for oral cavity reconstruction.[25]

24.5 Perioperative Management

Due to the small working space for maneuvering flaps into an RMT defect, meticulous flap principles are essential for successful healing. An excessively large flap may require tracheostomy for airway management, albeit temporarily. Soft tissue flaps will progressively contract, and perioperative edema will resolve. While a smaller skin/mucosal paddle may obviate the need for a tracheostomy, the surgeon must anticipate the degree and direction of contracture and avoid an undersized soft tissue reconstruction as a priority. For free tissue transfer and regional flaps, when possible, a tunnel to the neck is best placed medial to the mandible to avoid extrinsic compression and the low but true risk of facial nerve injury. If the lingual nerve was preserved during tumor resection, this can be gently medialized while tunneling along the lingual mandibular cortex into the floor of mouth. If this would create more inset and pedicle tension at the RMT site, a tunnel superficial to the mandible is absolutely feasible. Care is always taken to avoid acute twisting of the vascular pedicle. There are countless methods for actual tissue inset—ideally resulting in excellent wound eversion—e.g., with interrupted or running horizontal mattress sutures. The suturing points that most difficult to reach—often along the posterior floor of mouth—are usually completed first. Incremental delivery of a skin paddle through the tunnel may provide better visibility of the mucosal defect edges. Typically, a cheek retractor and oral opening retractor (e.g., Molt or Jennings) provide excellent exposure for transoral inset. Either securing the endotracheal tube to the opposite oral commissure or nasotracheal intubation facilitates optimal working space. Usually ischemia time of a free tissue transfer is well within limits to complete insetting prior to microvascular anastomosis. This permits removal of oral retractors and relaxation of the mandible into its resting state, which facilitates vessel exposure in the neck and anticipation of the postoperative resting position. Once the vessel anastomoses are completed, assessment of skin paddle perfusion is confirmed with both Doppler probing for pedicle or perforator signal, and pin prick or scratch of the dermis for bright red bleeding. Implantable Doppler devices placed distally to the arterial and/or venous anastomosis may also simplify monitoring of flow—but in general "end-organ" assessment with pin prick is most definitive.

Following RMT reconstruction, patients are given perioperative antibiotics for 24 hours, barring specific indications for a prolonged course (e.g., osteoradionecrosis requiring long-term parenteral antibiotics). For 5–14 days after surgery, patients should take no food or fluids by mouth to avoid disruption of the reconstruction and prevention of orocutaneous fistula formation. These patients should have a 10–12 French nasogastric tube placed during surgery, which can be removed once an oral diet is adequate for nutritional and hydration needs. If a skin graft with bolster is used for small RMT defects, overnight observation may be advisable to safely monitor the airway. Local flaps for small RMT defects typically require very little perioperative wound care, but the same oral intake precautions as free tissue transfer. Many of these patients can be discharged on the day of surgery—or their discharge is dependent upon the surgeon's preferences after neck dissection, if performed. Patients undergoing regional flap reconstruction may be best observed for a few days to ensure donor site healing, manage pain, and monitor flap perfusion.

Insetting of any flap into the RMT should anticipate potential risks for extrinsic pedicle compression. Obstruction of venous outflow due to tension during flap rotation, or twisting of a free tissue pedicle, can result in devastating loss of first-choice tissue. Poor hemostasis or a tight soft tissue tunnel to the neck can restrict venous outflow rapidly.

As a preventative measure, circumferential neck pressure, straps, or ties are best avoided for regional and free flaps with pedicles within the neck. Suspected vascular compromise is an indication for immediate operative exploration. Patients with regional flap reconstruction can typically be discharged when medically stable, after 3–4 days. Free flaps are typically monitored for 5–7 days postoperatively. The highest risk window for free tissue vascular compromise is within the first 48 hours after surgery, during which time vascular monitoring by nursing staff and physicians is most intensive. These can usually be discontinued by postoperative day five. Patients with radial and/or fibular skin donor sites should wear a splint for wrist and ankle immobilization to reduce skin graft shear, especially in the first postoperative week. Fibular free flap patients can begin toe-touch ambulation the day after surgery. All inpatients should be examined daily for operative site edema, donor site hematoma, or signs of infection. Patients who undergo surgical ablation and reconstruction of RMT defects will sometimes require an intraoperative tracheostomy tube to manage postoperative oral and pharyngeal edema, particularly if partial glossectomy is required. These patients can usually be decannulated prior to discharge.

24.6 Surgical Sequelae

The primary goals of RMT reconstruction are to maintain oral excursion and intake, expedite wound healing (compared to secondary intention), and ensure presurgical occlusion is preserved. Contracture of the RMT has a remarkably negative consequence on quality of life. Functionally significant trismus requires consideration of the RMT and buccal defects, as the potential for contracture in both of these areas needs to be addressed during reconstruction. Adherence to size and mobility limitations is essential for all flaps.[12] Methods to lengthen scar, e.g., a Z-plasty during closure of a FAMM donor site, optimize scar position.

Patients treated for cancer of the RMT can expect a level of functional impairment that correlates directly with tumor size and sacrificed oral cavity structures.[26] Postoperative pain is a major stress on patients, and should be examined carefully, both from oncologic and surgical viewpoints.[27] Analyses of quality of life metrics have reported similar outcomes compared to other oral cavity sites in the domains of cosmesis, recreational activity, employment, chewing, swallowing, speech, shoulder disability, and drooling. When patients are asked to prioritize functional goals, one study has reported in decreasing order of importance that patients value the ability to chew, produce saliva, swallow, and speak clearly.[28,29] They should be counseled clearly that improvement in speech, swallowing, and chewing progresses between weeks 3 and 20 postoperatively.[26]

Trismus is a feared consequence of RMT and buccal tumor resections. It is the main driver of reconstructive decisions. Several studies define clinically significant trismus as mouth opening < 3.5 cm—from upper to lower incisor if present. For some patients trismus can be so severe after RMT surgery as to prevent denture placement. Factors that contribute to postoperative trismus include disruption of masticatory muscles, disruption of the temporomandibular joint,[30,31] submucosal fibrosis,[8] and postoperative radiotherapy.[32] The reconstruction of an associated posterior mandible resection is selectively managed with soft tissue transfer, if this may result in less trismus than osseous reconstruction. If the RMT is reconstructed with adequate soft tissue and aggressive rehabilitation initiated, the sequelae of contracture and trismus are lessened.[16] Additionally, various devices to maintain and improve oral excursion can significantly enhance mouth opening after treatment, by repetitively disrupting scar contracture and preventing temporomandibular joint (TMJ) ankylosis.[33]

While isolated RMT surgery is not typically associated with postoperative speech deficits, loss of oral tongue sensation can result from injury to the adjacent lingual nerve along the floor of mouth.[34] If the lingual nerve can be preserved from an oncologic perspective, the reconstructive team must recognize its location during the transition to reconstruction. Interestingly, most noninnervated pedicled and free flaps will recover some degree of sensation, albeit typically modest and difficult to predict.[35]

For segmental mandibular defects of the ramus, angle, and body associated with RMT surgery, the choice of an osseous donor site is determined by both patient considerations and surgeon's experience.[36] Prospective evidence is not available to substantiate different rates of postoperative trismus and complications, despite some reports of outcomes favoring radial forearm osteocutaneous free (RFOC) tissue over fibular flaps.[37] Bony malunion can occur from flap ischemia or inadequate contact between the donor and native bones, as well as poor rigid fixation.[38] The risk of donor site radius bone fracture for RFOC flaps is mitigated by limiting harvest to 40% of the bone circumference and prophylactic plating across the marginal osteotomy.[37]

General postoperative complications include bleeding, hematoma, infection, lower face and tongue numbness, and orocutaneous fistula formation. These complications are multifactorial in origin and management, and in large part avoidable by meticulous surgical planning and technique.

Key Points

- The primary goal of RMT reconstruction is to maintain oral excursion by preventing excessively morbid wound contracture and fibrosis. Reconstructive strategies should preserve preoperative dental occlusion. A gentle discussion with the patient should clearly establish his or her personal treatment goals.
- Exposed mandibular ramus bone during RMT tumor excision should be covered by vascularized soft tissue.
- Intensive postoperative oral rehabilitation should be initiated soon after surgical wound healing has stabilized, with the goal of early return to maximal oral excursion.
- Although local pedicled flaps can provide similar tissue, shorter operative times, and potentially lower donor site morbidity, free tissue transfer is considered the gold standard in the reconstruction of the RMT. Thin regional flaps, such as the SCAIF, are also an excellent alternative.
- Postoperative complications are in large part avoidable by meticulous surgical planning and technique. Precise flap positioning must respect pedicle geometry, and achieve minimal suture line and pedicle tension. Avoidance of pedicle compression is achievable by meticulous hemostasis and soft tissue tunnels that accommodate perioperative edema.

References

[1] Montero PH, Yu C, Palmer FL, et al. Nomograms for preoperative prediction of prognosis in patients with oral cavity squamous cell carcinoma. Cancer. 2014; 120(2):214–221

[2] Faisal M, Abbas T, Khaleeq U, et al. Treatment outcomes of rare retromolar trigone squamous cell carcinoma using combined modalities. Cureus. 2017; 9 (5):e1203

[3] Genden EM, Lee BB, Urken ML. The palatal island flap for reconstruction of palatal and retromolar trigone defects revisited. Arch Otolaryngol Head Neck Surg. 2001; 127(7):837–841

[4] Horta R, Nascimento R, Silva A, Amarante J. The retromolar trigone: anatomy, cancer treatment modalities, reconstruction, and a classification system. J Craniofac Surg. 2016; 27(4):1070–1076

[5] Netter F. Atlas of Human Anatomy. 4th ed. ed: Saunders Elsevier; 2006

[6] Kuriakose MA. Contemporary Oral Oncology: Oral and Maxillofacial Reconstructive Surgery. Vol. 1st ed: Springer; 2017

[7] Rigby MH, Taylor SM. Soft tissue reconstruction of the oral cavity: a review of current options. Curr Opin Otolaryngol Head Neck Surg. 2013; 21(4):311–317

[8] Eipe N. The chewing of betel quid and oral submucous fibrosis and anesthesia. Anesth Analg. 2005; 100(4):1210–1213

[9] Rhee PH, Friedman CD, Ridge JA, Kusiak J. The use of processed allograft dermal matrix for intraoral resurfacing: an alternative to split-thickness skin grafts. Arch Otolaryngol Head Neck Surg. 1998; 124(11):1201–1204

[10] Licameli GR, Dolan R. Buccinator musculomucosal flap: applications in intraoral reconstruction. Arch Otolaryngol Head Neck Surg. 1998; 124(1):69–72

[11] Bardazzi A, Beltramini GA, Autelitano L, et al. Use of buccinator myomucosal flap in tongue reconstruction. J Craniofac Surg. 2017; 28(4):1084–1087

[12] Pribaz J, Stephens W, Crespo L, Gifford G. A new intraoral flap: facial artery musculomucosal (FAMM) flap. Plast Reconstr Surg. 1992; 90(3):421–429

[13] Squaquara R, Kim Evans KF, Spanio di Spilimbergo S, Mardini S. Intraoral reconstruction using local and regional flaps. Semin Plast Surg. 2010; 24(2): 198–211

[14] Gullane PJ, Arena S. Palatal island flap for reconstruction of oral defects. Arch Otolaryngol. 1977; 103(10):598–599

[15] Cordova A, Toia F, D'Arpa S, Giunta G, Moschella F. A new mucosal propeller flap (deep lingual artery axial propeller): the renaissance of lingual flaps. Plast Reconstr Surg. 2015; 135(3):584e–594e

[16] Cöloğlu H, Coşkun E, Uysal AC, Ataman G, Borman H. Anterior superficial temporal artery island flap: intraoral defect repair. J Craniofac Surg. 2012; 23 (6):e594–e599

[17] Alves HR, Ishida LC, Ishida LH, et al. A clinical experience of the supraclavicular flap used to reconstruct head and neck defects in late-stage cancer patients. J Plast Reconstr Aesthet Surg. 2012; 65(10):1350–1356

[18] Sandu K, Monnier P, Pasche P. Supraclavicular flap in head and neck reconstruction: experience in 50 consecutive patients. Eur Arch Otorhinolaryngol. 2012; 269(4):1261–1267

[19] Welz C, Canis M, Schwenk-Zieger S, Spiegel JL, Weiss BG, Pilavakis Y. Oral cancer reconstruction using the supraclavicular artery island flap: comparison to free radial forearm flap. J Oral Maxillofac Surg. 2017; 75(10):2261–2269

[20] Rashid M, Tamimy MS, Masroor S, et al. Mandibular reconstruction using osteocutaneous radial forearm flap. J Coll Physicians Surg Pak. 2012; 22(8):519–523

[21] Cigna E, Rizzo MI, Greco A, et al. Retromolar trigone reconstructive surgery: prospective comparative analysis between free flaps. Ann Surg Oncol. 2015; 22(1):272–278

[22] Loreti A, Di Lella G, Vetrano S, Tedaldi M, Dell'Osso A, Poladas G. Thinned anterolateral thigh cutaneous flap and radial fasciocutaneous forearm flap for reconstruction of oral defects: comparison of donor site morbidity. J Oral Maxillofac Surg. 2008; 66(6):1093–1098

[23] Wei FC, Jain V, Celik N, Chen HC, Chuang DC, Lin CH. Have we found an ideal soft-tissue flap? An experience with 672 anterolateral thigh flaps. Plast Reconstr Surg. 2002; 109(7):2219–2226, discussion 2227–2230

[24] King TW, Gallas MT, Robb GL, Lalani Z, Miller MJ. Aesthetic and functional outcomes using osseous or soft-tissue free flaps. J Reconstr Microsurg. 2002; 18(5):365–371

[25] Werle AH, Tsue TT, Toby EB, Girod DA. Osteocutaneous radial forearm free flap: its use without significant donor site morbidity. Otolaryngol Head Neck Surg. 2000; 123(6):711–717

[26] Goldie SJ, Jackson MS, Soutar DS, Shaw-Dunn J. The functional intraoral Glasgow scale (FIGS) in retromolar trigone cancer patients. J Plast Reconstr Aesthet Surg. 2006; 59(7):743–746

[27] Chang KP, Lai CS, Hsieh TY, Wu YC, Chang CH. Two-year quality of life after free flap reconstruction in tumor-site discrepancy among Taiwanese with moderately advanced oral squamous cell carcinoma. World J Surg Oncol. 2012; 10:145

[28] Li W, Xu Z, Liu F, Huang S, Dai W, Sun C. Vascularized free forearm flap versus free anterolateral thigh perforator flaps for reconstruction in patients with head and neck cancer: assessment of quality of life. Head Neck. 2013; 35(12): 1808–1813

[29] Nicoletti G, Soutar DS, Jackson MS, Wrench AA, Robertson G. Chewing and swallowing after surgical treatment for oral cancer: functional evaluation in 196 selected cases. Plast Reconstr Surg. 2004; 114(2):329–338

[30] Dhanrajani PJ, Jonaidel O. Trismus: aetiology, differential diagnosis and treatment. Dent Update. 2002; 29(2):88–92, 94

[31] Pierre CS, Dassonville O, Chamorey E, et al. Long-term functional outcomes and quality of life after oncologic surgery and microvascular reconstruction in patients with oral or oropharyngeal cancer. Acta Otolaryngol. 2014; 134 (10):1086–1093

[32] Vissink A, Jansma J, Spijkervet FK, Burlage FR, Coppes RP. Oral sequelae of head and neck radiotherapy. Crit Rev Oral Biol Med. 2003; 14(3):199–212

[33] Kamstra JI, Roodenburg JL, Beurskens CH, Reintsema H, Dijkstra PU. TheraBite exercises to treat trismus secondary to head and neck cancer. Support Care Cancer. 2013; 21(4):951–957

[34] Goldie SJ, Soutar DS, Shaw-Dunn J. The effect of surgical resection in the region of the retromolar trigone. J Plast Reconstr Aesthet Surg. 2006; 59(12): 1263–1268

[35] Lvoff G, O'Brien CJ, Cope C, Lee KK. Sensory recovery in noninnervated radial forearm free flaps in oral and oropharyngeal reconstruction. Arch Otolaryngol Head Neck Surg. 1998; 124(11):1206–1208

[36] Nishi H, Shinozaki T, Tomioka T, Maruo T, Hayashi R. Squamous cell carcinoma of the retromolar trigone: treatment outcomes. Auris Nasus Larynx. 2018; 45(2):337–342

[37] Dean NR, Wax MK, Virgin FW, Magnuson JS, Carroll WR, Rosenthal EL. Free flap reconstruction of lateral mandibular defects: indications and outcomes. Otolaryngol Head Neck Surg. 2012; 146(4):547–552

[38] Kim JH, Rosenthal EL, Ellis T, Wax MK. Radial forearm osteocutaneous free flap in maxillofacial and oromandibular reconstructions. Laryngoscope. 2005; 115(9):1697–1701

25 Squamous Cell Cancer of the Palate

Theresa Tharakan and Vikas Mehta

Summary

Squamous cell carcinoma (SCC) of the palate is rare compared to other oral cavity and oropharyngeal cancers. Due to the functional implications, primary nonsurgical therapeutic management is used for soft palate cancer which differentiates it from hard palate SCC, which is managed with primary resection. This chapter discusses the presentation, risk factors, relevant anatomy, surgical and nonsurgical treatment options, and prognosis of palate SCC.

Keywords: soft palate, hard palate, oropharynx, oropharyngeal squamous cell carcinoma

25.1 Introduction

The hard palate is a bony structure formed by the palatine processes of the maxilla and the horizontal plates of the palatine bones and bounded anterolaterally by the alveolar ridge of the maxilla. The hard palate is covered by periosteum, submucosa containing neurovasculature and minor salivary glands laterally, mucosa, and keratinized stratified squamous epithelium. The upper border of the hard palate is the floor of the nasal cavity.[1]

The soft palate is a mobile fold of tissue attached to the posterior end of the hard palate and lateral walls of the oropharynx. The posterior muscular portion hangs between the oral cavity and oropharynx and is known as the velopharynx. The velopharynx closes off the nasopharynx during speech and swallowing by approximating with the posterior pharyngeal wall. The hard and soft palates are lined with stratified squamous epithelium on the inferior oral surface and ciliated columnar epithelium on the superior nasal surface.[1]

At least two-thirds of hard palate tumors, and up to 90% of hard palate malignancies, are squamous cell carcinoma (SCC).[2,3] Other tumors of the hard palate include minor salivary gland neoplasms such as adenoid cystic carcinoma, mucoepidermoid carcinomas, and adenocarcinomas.[4] About 80% of malignancies in the soft palate are SCC (SPSCC), while the remainder are typically of minor salivary gland origin.[5–7] SPSCC is more rare than SCC at other oropharyngeal sites, such as the tonsil or base of the tongue.[5,8] The management of palate SCC is important because of its significant impact on speech, mastication, and swallowing.

25.2 Epidemiology

The estimated incidence of oral cavity and oropharyngeal cancer for 2018 is 51,540 cases.[9] Hard palate cancers account for only about 5% of all oral cavity cancers.[4] SCC of the soft palate accounts for approximately 5–12% of oropharyngeal cancers.[10] According to data from the Surveillance, Epidemiology, and End Results (SEER) database, there were 4,366 cases of SPSCC recorded from 1973 to 2015 and 1,489 cases of hard palate SCC (HPSCC) from 1973 to 2014.[11,12] The mean age of presentation of HPSCC is approximately 60–70 years old, and there is a slight female predominance.[12–14] SPSCC typically affects patients in their 6th to 7th decade and the prevalence in men is more than double that in women.[15–18] Oral cavity and oropharyngeal SCC, including palate SCC, are associated with tobacco use and alcohol consumption.[19] The carcinogenic effects of alcohol and tobacco are dose-dependent and create a synergistic effect that dramatically increases the risk of developing upper aerodigestive tract SCC.[20] HPSCC has been associated with reverse smoking practices in India and the Philippines as well as poor oral hygiene, mechanical irritation, poorly fitting dentures, and syphilis.[3]

While human papilloma virus (HPV) related oropharyngeal squamous cell carcinoma (OPSCC) has been rising at epidemic rates, high risk HPV infection rates are significantly lower in soft palate and posterior pharyngeal wall tumors than in other regions of the oropharynx with tonsillar tissue.[21,22] Gelwan et al found that the HPV-positivity rate among soft palate tumors was as low as 3.1%, compared to a 92% rate of HPV in tonsillar tumors.[21] HPV's predilection for lymphoepithelium, which has an incomplete basement membrane, explains why the infection rate of cancers in the lymphoid-rich tonsils is so much higher than in the soft palate.[21,22] HPV-mediated OPSCC do not demonstrate keratinization on histopathology and are often poorly differentated.[23] In contrast, SPSCCs are histopathologically similar to smoking-related SCCs in the oral cavity that arise from squamous dysplasia of surface epithelium and feature keratinization.[21] Therefore, SPSCC often resembles more “traditional” head and neck cancer than the base of tongue or tonsillar subsites, and is more similar to oral cavity carcinoma in its epidemiology.

25.3 Clinical Presentation

HPSCC typically presents as an ulcerating lesion, which may be asymptomatic in early stages or painful in more advanced stages.[5] Presenting symptoms also include a palatal mass, bleeding, foul odor, ill-fitting dentures, or loose teeth. A classic presentation of an occult HPSCC is when there is a sudden ill-fitting tooth with pain that does not respond to dental management. Up to 70% of lesions may extend beyond the hard palate to the soft palate, gingiva, maxillary sinus, sphenopalatine foramen, pterygopalatine fossa, and skull base.[5]

Early stage SPSCC often presents asymptomatically where the tumor is incidentally found by patients or physicians due to their visibility on routine examination.[5,7,17] Early lesions may present as leukoplakia (▶ Fig. 25.1) or erythroplakia.[24] Patients may also present with painful ulceration and odynophagia.[5,17] More advanced cancers may cause velopharyngeal insufficiency (VPI), hypernasal speech, dysphagia, referred otalgia, trismus from involvement of the pterygoid muscles, hemoptysis, or neck mass in adults.[5]

SPSCCs tend to grow submucosally and may extend laterally, anteriorly, or superiorly.[20,25] Nearly 50% of patients present with extension beyond the soft palate to sites which include, in order of frequency: the tonsil, retromolar trigone, inferior

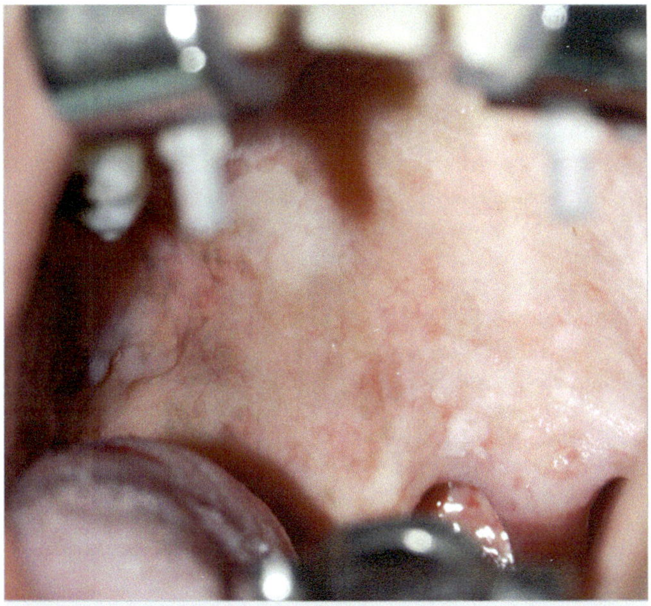

Fig. 25.1 Leukoplakia of the soft palate.

alveolar process, posterior tonsillar pillar, oropharyngeal wall, and base of the tongue.[8] Lesions that extend into the nasopharynx along the veli palatini muscles are associated with middle ear effusion.[25,26] Extension into the sphenopalatine foramen is associated with palatal swelling due to hypostasis.[26] Malignant involvement of the trigeminal nerve in the sphenopalatine foramen or pterygopalatine fossa can cause numbness of the palate.[5]

HPSCC infrequently involves neck metastases.[27] However, lymph node metastases are present in about 60% of patients with SPSCC on presentation.[25] About 25% of patients with SPSCC present with synchronous or metachronous cancers at other sites, most commonly on the floor of the mouth.[8,20]

25.4 Diagnosis and Evaluation

Evaluation of palate tumors begins with the history and physical. Physical examination should be done by inspection and palpation of the primary tumor to determine the extent of mucosal and submucosal spread.[23] Loose dentition should be evaluated for possible malignant involvement of the tooth sockets and bone.[3] Nasal endoscopy is also critical to assess for involvement of the nasal surface of the palate. Neurologic evaluation of cranial nerves should be performed due to potential involvement in advanced cancers and to assess for functional impairment.[23] An absent corneal reflex is indicative of extension to skull base through the foramen rotundum, foramen ovale, or inferior orbital fissure. Trismus, malocclusion, and pain are symptoms of invasion of the pterygoid muscles. The clinician should also assess for VPI by asking the patient about nasal regurgitation with oral intake and listening for hypernasality in the patient's voice. Nodes should be palpated and size, number, irregular shape, attachment to other nodes, and mobility should be evaluated.[23]

The primary lesion, neck nodes, and distant metastatic sites should be biopsied. Transoral biopsy of the primary lesion can be completed in the office with local anesthesia.[5] An incision through the overlying mucosa may be required for large nonulcerated lesions.[5] Excisional biopsy may be performed for small lesions.[5] Biopsy results are essential to establish the tumor etiology and determine therapeutic management since salivary gland tumors are often treated with primary surgery. A greater tumor thickness on biopsy can be predictive of cervical node metastases.[28]

Panendoscopy (direct laryngoscopy, bronchoscopy, and esophagoscopy) under anesthesia is done to map the tumor, assess margins, and rule out synchronous second primary malignancies.[5,8,29] The utility of panendoscopy for detecting synchronous cancers is greater in patients with history of tobacco use than those with no history of tobacco use.[29] Examination under anesthesia may be unnecessary in patients with very small tumors confined to the palate with all boundaries visible. In these cases, tumor mapping can be completed with flexible nasopharyngolaryngoscopy and transoral inspection and palpation.[26]

Maxillofacial and neck computed tomography (CT) with and without contrast and/or magnetic resonance imaging (MRI) provide information about primary tumor extent and nodal metastases.[3,23] Early soft palate tumors can be visualized as soft tissue swelling on imaging but can be difficult to assess radiologically until they are large.[25] However, imaging has great utility in more extensive disease and in establishing nodal stage. Coronal CT images are used to visualize bony invasion of the hard palate and extension into the nasal fossa or maxillary sinus, while axial images can reveal extension along the pterygoid plates and muscles, infratemporal fossa, and masticator space.[25,26] Tumors invading the parapharyngeal and masticator spaces may feature carotid artery encasement or superior extension to the skull base. If the tumor encases more than 270 degrees of the carotid artery on axial imaging, resection of the vessel is likely needed during tumor excision, which often makes the tumor unresectable from a staging perspective.[25] MRI can be used to assess perineural extension and dural invasion in cases of intracranial involvement.[26] MRI is useful for evaluating hard palate tumors for perineural invasion, paranasal sinus involvement, dural extension, and associated inflammation.[5]

CT is used to evaluate lymph node metastases, which are typically located in the upper and mid-jugular (levels II and III) or retropharyngeal lymph nodes (RPLNs).[23,25] Bilateral metastases are common.[23] The overall rate of RPLN metastasis in oropharyngeal cancer ranges from 14.5 to 36%, with higher rates in the soft palate and retropharyngeal wall than in base of tongue and tonsil subsites.[30] In contrast, RPLN metastasis from the hard palate and other oral cavity SCCs is uncommon. RPLNs are split into the lateral (Rouviere) and medial node chains; metastases almost always involve the lateral chains.[31] Retropharyngeal nodes may be easily overlooked because they appear isodense to the adjacent prevertebral muscles on CT unless they are cystic or necrotic.[23] If the RPLN is negative on both positron emission tomography (PET)/CT and another imaging modality, dissection of the RPLN is not needed. PET/CT is accurate at predicting RPLN disease in patients with nodal disease persistent or recurrent after chemoradiation. Chest CT/MRI is also used to evaluate for lung metastases. PET/CT can be used to evaluate metastases to lung, bone, and liver in stages III–IV disease.[23,27] Liver function tests may be sufficient to rule out liver metastases.[26]

SPSCCs are staged using the oropharyngeal SCC staging guidelines from the 8th edition of the American Joint Committee on Cancer (AJCC).[23] The AJCC recommends that all oropharyngeal cancers be tested for p16 overexpression on immunohistochemistry as a marker for HPV-mediated carcinogenesis. Tumors are classified as p16 overexpressing if they exhibit ≥+2/+3 nuclear staining intensity (with or without cytoplasmic staining) with ≥75% distribution.[23] Oropharyngeal tumors that do not meet these criteria are considered p16 negative and staged by separate criteria. Oral cavity SCCs including HPSCC are staged separately using the AJCC 8th edition, and this staging now includes depth of invasion. Oral cavity SCCs are not routinely stained for p16. Based on evidence that SPSCC is more histologically similar to SCC of the oral cavity than the other oropharyngeal sites, Gelwan et al suggest that soft palate tumors need not be routinely stained for p16. This is because in nontonsillar tumors of the oropharynx, the likelihood of detecting HPV is < 3%, the detection of HPV has no current prognostic relevance, and the positive predictive value of p16 immunohistochemical staining as a marker for HPV infection is low.[21]

25.5 Anatomic Considerations/ Relevant Anatomy

As mentioned above, the hard palate is a bony structure formed by the palatine processes of the maxilla and the horizontal plates of the palatine bones and bounded anterolaterally by the alveolar ridge of the maxilla. The hard palate is covered by periosteum, submucosa containing neurovasculature and minor salivary glands laterally, mucosa, and keratinized stratified squamous epithelium. This periosteum of the hard palate is a barrier to the spread of SCC. The hard palate is innervated by the greater and lesser palatine nerves, which contain sensory and secretomotor fibers from the maxillary branch of the trigeminal ganglion and pterygopalatine ganglion. The hard palate is supplied by descending palatine arteries from the internal maxillary artery. This neurovascular supply passes through the palatine foramen medial to the 3rd molar, which may be a conduit for the local tumor spread.[5] Additionally, the tooth sockets are not only a common site of occult disease, but can also allow for facile spread of the tumor to the maxillary sinus.

The soft palate is made up of five pairs of muscles, namely the palatopharyngeus, palatoglossus, levator veli palatini, tensor veli palatini, and uvular muscle.[32] The attachments of these muscles are shown in ▶ Table 25.1. The tensor veli palatini is innervated by the mandibular branch of the trigeminal nerve (cranial nerve V3); the other four muscles are innervated by the pharyngeal plexus of the vagus nerve (cranial nerve X).[33] All obtain their blood supply from the ascending palatine branch of the facial artery and descending palatine branch of the maxillary artery. The palatoglossus is also supplied by ascending pharyngeal arteries.[33] Due to the mucosal continuity between the soft palate and anterior tonsillar pillars and the tendency for oropharyngeal lesions to encompass more than one subsite, it may be difficult to determine if a lesion originates specifically from the soft palate.[7] Due to crossed lymphatic drainage pathways during embryonic development of the oropharynx, bilateral lymph node metastases from the soft palate are common.

There is limited data on characteristics of soft palate cancers by location. According to one study by Overton et al (2013) of the SEER database, uvular tumors tend to present in relatively lower stages of disease than tumors elsewhere in the oropharynx, likely because they are easier to visualize and manually palpate than tumors in other anatomic locations.[20,34] The same study also found that uvular tumors are less likely to have lymph node metastases. However, mortality rates were similar to those of SCC found elsewhere in the oropharynx.

25.6 Surgical Considerations and Approaches

Treatment of palate SCC is based on oral cavity SCC staging for hard palate tumors and oropharyngeal SCC staging for soft palate tumors.

For tumors that do not involve the periosteum or bone, through-and-through excision of the palate is not necessary. For these malignancies, a simple transoral excision into and including the periosteum is sufficient and the periosteum serves as the superior margin. However, these are usually rare and more often occur with nonsquamous cell carcinoma malignancies. Early hard palate lesions (T1–2, N0) are usually treated with palatectomy or radiation therapy (RT) with consideration of elective neck treatment. Surgery is preferred due to the risk of osteoradionecrosis of the maxilla with RT. cT3–4, N0 lesions are treated with surgical resection, with neck dissection and adjuvant therapy based on the pathologic features.[5]

Palatectomy of early stage SCCs involves resection of the hard palate lesion with 1 cm margins without resection of the maxillary tuberosity or anterior, lateral, or posterior walls of the

Table 25.1 Attachments and actions of soft palate muscles

Muscle	Origin	Insertion	Actions
Palatopharyngeus	Hard palate and superior palatine aponeurosis	Lateral pharyngeal wall	Tenses soft palate; pulls walls of pharynx superiorly, anteriorly, and medially during swallowing
Palatoglossus	Palatine aponeurosis	Lateral tongue	Elevates posterior tongue, depresses palate
Levator veli palatini	Temporal bone, petrous part	Palatine aponeurosis	Elevates soft palate during swallowing
Tensor veli palatini	Scaphoid fossa of medial pterygoid plate, spine of sphenoid, Eustachian tube	Palatine aponeurosis	Tenses soft palate, opens Eustachian tube during swallowing and yawning
Uvular muscle	Nasal spine, palatine aponeurosis	Mucosa of uvula	Shortens, elevates, and retracts uvula

Adapted from Atlas of Human Anatomy by Frank H. Netter.[33]

maxilla.[3,4] T2-4 cancers may require more extensive resection: type I, partial maxillectomy (resection of a single wall); type II, subtotal maxillectomy (resection of ≤ walls); type IIIA, total maxillectomy (resection of all 6 walls with preservation of the orbital contents); type IIIB, total maxillectomy and orbital exenteration (resection of all 6 walls with orbital exenteration); and type IV, orbito-maxillectomy (resection of 5 walls, orbital exenteration and preservation of the hard palate).[35] For early stage lesions, a transoral approach is often adequate. However, for those that involve the alveolar ridge or extend into the maxillary sinus or nasal cavity, a midface degloving or lateral rhinotomy approach can be considered. For further surgical considerations regarding maxillectomy approaches, please refer to Chapter 29 (Primary Malignancies of the Maxilla).

Initial treatment options for early soft palate lesions (T1–T2, N0-1) include definitive RT or transoral surgical resection of the primary with neck dissection.[27] Locoregional control and survival rates are similar for both surgery and radiotherapy.[36,37] However, primary surgery of the soft palate can cause greater impairments in speech and swallowing function if full thickness defects are necessary for resection, and therefore initial radiotherapy is often preferred.[36,37]

For more advanced stage tumors that would require extensive resection of the soft palate (▸ Fig. 25.2), primary nonsurgical therapy is often chosen due to the differences in functional outcomes between surgery and chemoradiation.[5,38,39] However, soft palate tumors with bony involvement, like primary tumors of the hard palate, are recommended to undergo primary surgery with a combined transcervical/transoral approach due to a high risk for osteoradionecrosis with primary RT. Patients with distant metastases (M1) are considered palliative and should receive primary chemotherapy.[27]

Surgical intervention is usually reserved for cases of SPSCC persistence or recurrence, or can be considered for very superficial lesions which can be removed with partial thickness resection.[37] These lesions will subsequently granulate with good functional results.[36] Additionally, tumors restricted to the uvula can be often easily removed without significant functional impairment. Nodal status should also be incorporated into the therapeutic decision-making process.

Surgical considerations for SPSCC include adequacy of margins due to tendency for submucosal spread, functional outcomes after creation of soft palate defect, and options for prosthetics and/or surgical reconstruction.[20] An advantage of surgery for advanced lesions is the ability to stratify risk of disease progression based on pathological features of the tumor such as perineural invasion, vascular embolism, presence of microscopic N2 disease, or presence of extracapsular spread.[36,40] Indications for adjuvant RT include multiple positive lymph nodes, endophytic T3 tumors, T4 tumors, perineural invasion, and lymphovascular invasion.[41] Adjuvant chemotherapy should be added in cases of extranodal extension (ENE) or positive margins.[27] Rare tumors with intracranial extension are inoperable if they infiltrate brain parenchyma.[26]

Transoral laser microsurgery (TLM) (▸ Fig. 25.3) and robotic surgery (TORS) are surgical approaches that can also be utilized to excise soft palate cancers. For success, the surgeon must be able to visualize the entire tumor and a margin of 1–2 cm, which can be determined during tumor mapping endoscopy.[5,36] Small defects at the posterior margin of the soft palate can be closed by approximating the superior and inferior mucosa.[5,42] For defects at the anterior margin of the soft palate, an advancement rotation flap from the hard palate, buccal mucosal or posterior pharyngeal wall may be used.[5] Larger defects often require the use of free tissue transfer. Reconstructive options are more extensively discussed in Chapter 26 (Reconstruction of the Palate).

Lesions that extend beyond the soft palate to the tonsil, base of tongue, or lateral pharyngeal wall may be resected using a combined transcervical/transoral "pull-through" approach.[5] After performing a neck dissection, a mucosal incision is made through the floor of the mouth and incisions are made around the tumor with 1–2 cm margin.[5] A pharyngotomy is then performed transcervically and the tumor can be removed. Care must be taken to avoid damage to the carotid vasculature and cranial nerves when performing this approach. Mandibulotomy may be necessary for T4 soft palate cancers that extend to the hard palate, lateral pharynx, tonsil, base of tongue, or mandible.[5] A mandibular swing approach involves a full thickness split of the lip, a mandibular osteotomy, a floor of the mouth

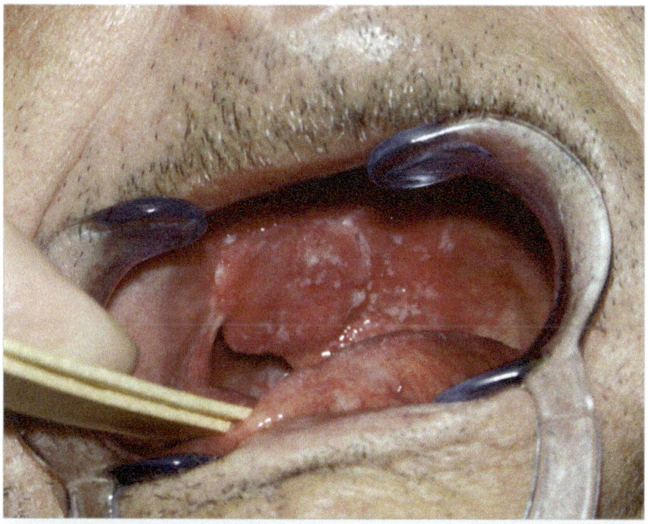

Fig. 25.2 Stage T3 soft palate squamous cell carcinoma (SPSCC).

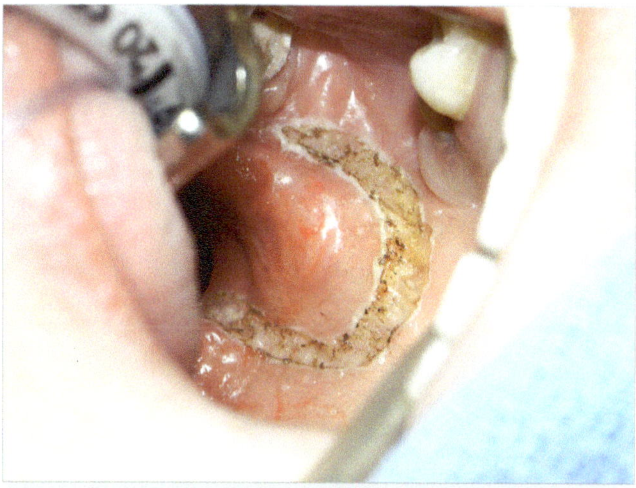

Fig. 25.3 Planned laser excision of stage T1 soft palate squamous cell carcinoma (SPSCC).

incision, and a cut of the mylohyoid to expose the tumor for resection.[5,36]

Neck management: For information regarding neck management of oral cavity SCC, including HPSCC, refer to Chapter 32 (Neck Management of Oral Malignancies).

The rate of nodal metastases at presentation of SPSCC is about 20% for T1–T2 lesions and up to 60–70% for T3 and T4 lesions.[20] Definitive treatment should address regional lymphatics for tumor of any stage. RT alone may be sufficient for patients with small tumors and N0–N1 necks. Neck dissection is used to evaluate radiographically suspicious nodes observed on CT 2–3 months after completion of RT, if they remain avid on a PET scan.[43] Elective neck dissection should be performed if primary surgery is being used for patients with clinically negative necks because the risk of occult cervical metastases in SPSCC is 20–30%.[5] In OPSCC patients with clinically negative necks, a selective neck dissection for oropharyngeal cancers would include at least lymph node levels II–IV.[27] Patients with N2-3 metastases should receive comprehensive neck dissection and postoperative RT.[27,42] Because the palate has bilateral lymphatic drainage, bilateral neck dissection is often appropriate.[27] RPLN sampling should be performed as well. The transcervical approach can be used after standard neck dissection is complete to avoid disrupting the pharynx and creating a salivary fistula if neck dissection is being performed. However, the transoral approach to the retropharyngeal space may be preferred if there is only one RPLN positive node identified on PET/CT in the recurrent setting.[30]

25.7 Surgical Sequelae

Resection of the hard palate is associated with oronasal or oroantral fistula formation and difficulty with oral alimentation. Inferior maxillary defects are associated with nasal regurgitation and midface retraction facial deformity. The anterior portion of the hard palate has plicae: irregular ridges in the mucous membrane that facilitate the movement of food backwards and assist with mastication. Additionally, the interaction between the tongue and the hard palate is essential in the formation of certain speech sounds, notably palatal consonants such as /j/ and /ɟ/. Thus, reconstruction is crucial for oral intake and speech. Reconstruction of these defects is discussed in Chapter 26 (Reconstruction of the Palate).

Primary resection of the soft palate is associated with significant functional impairment.[44] Complications include VPI, hypernasal speech, dysphagia, and middle ear effusion from scarring at the Eustachian tube opening, or loss of function of the tensor palatini muscles.[26] Among patients with small volume oropharyngeal cancers treated by TLM, patients with soft palate tumors were more likely to report problems with chewing and speech and had lower quality of life scores than patients with tumors at other oropharyngeal sites.[45] The size of the palate defect after ablative surgery is predictive of long-term speech and swallowing function.[46] Reconstruction of the soft palate with flaps and prosthetics does not restore its muscular action and therefore function is likely to be impaired.

Reported overall 5-year survival rates for HPSCC range from 33 to 86% and depend on tumor presentation and treatment modality.[12,47] A study of the SEER database found that patients treated with surgery have a higher 5-year disease-specific survival than those who were treated with RT alone (71% vs. 29%).[12] In the same study, age and higher pathologic grade were associated with worse overall survival (OS) and disease-specific survival (DSS). Most studies show that more advanced T stage is associated with worse DSS, although this is not consistent in all studies.[12,13,48,49] T2–T4 primary HPSCCs are associated with high rates of regional failure.[13] One study demonstrated that patients with clinically negative neck who underwent elective neck dissection had significantly greater OS and DSS than those who did not.[47] We argue that any T stage tumor with a clinically negative neck, except those that are extremely limited or in patients with extensive comorbidities, should undergo elective neck management with radiation, neck dissection, or sentinel lymph node biopsy due to the risk of metastases and potential for improved survival. For tumors with bony invasion, perineural invasion, ≥ 4 positive lymph nodes, extranodal extension, or positive margins, adjuvant chemoradiation is beneficial.[3]

Historical 5-year locoregional control rate, DSS, and OS for SPSCC by stage are shown in ▶ Table 25.2. Available data on SPSCC treated with RT with or without chemotherapy or neck dissection demonstrate a 5-year DSS rate of approximately 70% and 5-year OS rate of 43%.[38,39] Another study suggested that 5-year OS may be as high as 70.8% for unilateral soft palate tumors but falls to 51% for patients with tumors that cross the midline or with bilateral lesions, due to a higher incidence of regional metastasis.[20,26] In a cohort of patients treated with primary surgery (two-thirds of which used a transoral approach) with or without adjuvant RT, 5-year DSS was 71% and OS was 52%.[10] These studies did not identify significant differences in survival outcomes based on primary treatment modality.[10,38,39]

Table 25.2 Locoregional control rate, disease specific survival, and overall survival for soft palate cancers treated with radiation therapy or surgery, ± chemotherapy or neck dissection

Stage	5-year locoregional control			5-year disease specific survival			5-year overall survival		
	Erkal et al[19a]	*Chera et al*[b]	*Iyer et al*[c]	*Erkal et al*	*Chera et al*	*Iyer et al*	*Erkal et al*	*Chera et al*	*Iyer et al*
I	90%	89%	85	84%	89%	87.4	40%	52%	60.4
II	92%	88%	83.7	91%	87%	65.7	66%	61%	54.4
III	84%	96%	88.1	74%	88%	63.6	52%	56%	55.1
IV[a]	60%		53.6	48%		55.2	21%		37.2
IV-A[b]		63%			57%			31%	
IV-B[b]		43%			0%			0%	

Notes: [a]Used 1983 AJCC staging guidelines, [b]Used 2002 AJCC staging guidelines, [c]Did not specify staging guidelines.
Adapted from Erkal et al, 2001 (radiation ± neck dissection), Chera et al, 2008 (radiation ± neck dissection and/or chemotherapy), and Iyer et al, 2011 (primary surgery ± therapy).[10,38,39]

A multi-institutional study determined that OPSCC treated with TORS and adjuvant RT or chemoradiation were associated with a 2-year locoregional control rate of 91.8%, DSS of 94.5%, and OS of 91%.[50] There was no significant difference in 2-year locoregional control rates or 2-year OS for soft palate cancers when compared to other oropharyngeal subsites.[50]

Several factors may affect the prognosis of patients with SPSCC. Higher pathologic tumor volume is predictive of lower survival rates.[51] The presence of residual tumor cells in cervical lymph nodes after RT is associated with lower survival rates and is a possible marker of partial radiation failure.[52] SPSCC patients with recurrence in the neck have similar survival outcomes as patients with no recurrence, but recurrence in the parapharyngeal space has been associated with significantly lower 5-year survival.[53] The parapharyngeal space is not addressed in a transoral resection and neck dissection, but can be addressed by a transcervical or mandibulotomy approach for patients with advanced cancer and cervical lymph node involvement.[53] Poor nutritional status, depression, and overall functional performance affect quality of life and survival with oropharyngeal cancers in general, although the effects of these factors on subsites like the soft palate have not been clearly documented in the literature.[23]

Key Points

- Squamous cell carcinoma (SCC) of the palate is rare compared to other oral cancers.
- SPSCC typically presents in males in the 6th to 7th decades of life, while HPSCC has a slight female predominance.
- SCC of the palate is associated with tobacco and alcohol but not HPV.
- Initial treatment of SPSCC is usually radiation to the tumor and the neck ± chemotherapy, while HPSCCs are typically resected.
- Transoral surgical resection of the soft palate can cause VPI and is generally reserved for tumors that do not respond to chemoradiation.
- Prognosis is similar to other oral cavity SCCs and non-HPV related OPSCC.

References

[1] Standring S. Pharynx. In: Gray's Anatomy: The Anatomical Basis of Clinical Practice, Vol. 3. 41st ed. New York: Elsevier Ltd; 2016:571–585

[2] Petruzzelli GJ, Myers EN. Malignant neoplasms of the hard palate and upper alveolar ridge. Oncology (Williston Park). 1994; 8(4):43–48, discussion 50, 53

[3] Vosler PS, Myers EN. Transoral inferior maxillectomy. In: Myers EN, Snyderman CH, eds. Operative Otolaryngology. 3rd ed. 2018:227–236

[4] Truitt TO, Gleich LL, Huntress GP, Gluckman JL. Surgical management of hard palate malignancies. Otolaryngol Head Neck Surg. 1999; 121(5):548–552

[5] Sadeghi N, Panje WR. Cancer of the soft palate. In: Saclarides TJ, Millikan K, Godellas C, eds. Surgical Oncology: An Algorithmic Approach. New York: Springer-Verlag; 2003:32–39. doi:10.1007/0-387-21701-0_5

[6] Zini A, Czerninski R, Sgan-Cohen HD. Oral cancer over four decades: epidemiology, trends, histology, and survival by anatomical sites. J Oral Pathol Med. 2010; 39(4):299–305

[7] Osborne RF, Brown JJ. Carcinoma of the oral pharynx: an analysis of subsite treatment heterogeneity. Surg Oncol Clin N Am. 2004; 13(1):71–80

[8] Leemans CR, Engelbrecht WJ, Tiwari R, et al. Carcinoma of the soft palate and anterior tonsillar pillar. Laryngoscope. 1994; 104(12):1477–1481

[9] American Cancer Society. Cancer Statistics Center: Oral cavity and pharynx. 2018

[10] Iyer NG, Nixon IJ, Palmer F, et al. Surgical management of squamous cell carcinoma of the soft palate: factors predictive of outcome. Head Neck. 2011; 36 (10):1391

[11] Chan CK, Han AY, Alonso JE, et al. Squamous cell carcinoma of the soft palate in the United States: a population-based study. Otolaryngol - Head Neck Surg (United States). 2018; 159(4):662–668

[12] Alonso JE, Han AY, Kuan EC, et al. The survival impact of surgical therapy in squamous cell carcinoma of the hard palate. Laryngoscope. 2018; 128(9): 2050–2055

[13] Morris LGT, Patel SG, Shah JP, Ganly I. High rates of regional failure in squamous cell carcinoma of the hard palate and maxillary alveolus. Head Neck. 2011; 33(6):824–830

[14] Binahmed A, Nason RW, Hussain A, Abdoh AA, Sándor GKB. Treatment outcomes in squamous cell carcinoma of the maxillary alveolus and palate: a population-based study. Oral Surg Oral Med Oral Pathol Oral Radiol Endod. 2008; 105(6):750–754

[15] Russ JE, Applebaum EL, Sisson GA. Squamous cell carcinoma of the soft palate. Laryngoscope. 1977; 87(7):1151–1156

[16] Fee WE, Jr, Schoeppel SL, Rubenstein R, et al. Squamous cell carcinoma of the soft palate. Arch Otolaryngol. 1979; 105(12):710–718

[17] Evans JF, Shah JP. Epidermoid carcinoma of the palate. Am J Surg. 1981; 142 (4):451–455

[18] Chung CK, Constable WC. Squamous cell carcinoma of the soft palate and uvula. Int J Radiat Oncol Biol Phys. 1979; 5(6):845–850

[19] Forastiere A, Koch W, Trotti A, Sidransky D. Head and neck cancer. N Engl J Med. 2001; 345(26):1890–1900

[20] Cohan DM, Popat S, Kaplan SE, Rigual N, Loree T, Hicks WL, Jr. Oropharyngeal cancer: current understanding and management. Curr Opin Otolaryngol Head Neck Surg. 2009; 17(2):88–94

[21] Gelwan E, Malm IJ, Khararjian A, Fakhry C, Bishop JA, Westra WH. Nonuniform distribution of high-risk human papillomavirus in squamous cell carcinomas of the oropharynx: rethinking the anatomic boundaries of oral and oropharyngeal carcinoma from an oncologic HPV perspective. Am J Surg Pathol. 2017; 41(12):1722–1728

[22] Frandsen VL, Larsen CG, von Buchwald C. Prevalence of human papillomavirus in squamous cell carcinomas of the soft palate. J Clin Pathol. 2015; 68 (11):942–943

[23] Amin MB, Edge SB, Greene FL, et al. AJCC Cancer Staging Manual/American Joint Committee on Cancer. 8th ed. Chicago, IL: Springer; 2017

[24] El-Mofty SK, Johnson NW, Jayasekara P, et al. Squamous cell carcinoma and precursor lesions of the oral cavity: epidemiology and aetiology. Med Oral Patol Oral Cir Bucal. 2014; 5(4):19–37

[25] Tshering Vogel DW, Zbaeren P, Thoeny HC. Cancer of the oral cavity and oropharynx. Cancer Imaging. 2010; 10:62–72

[26] Sadeghi N, Meyers AD, Al-Sebeih K, Talavera F, Karen H, Calhou MAK. Malignant tumors of the palate treatment & management. Medscape. 2017:1–6

[27] Pfister DG, Spencer S, Al E. NCCN Clinical Practice Guidelines in Oncology: Head and Neck Cancers. 2017

[28] Baredes S, Leeman DJ, Chen TS, Mohit-Tabatabai MA. Significance of tumor thickness in soft palate carcinoma. Laryngoscope. 1993; 103(4 Pt 1):389–393

[29] Rodriguez-Bruno K, Ali MJ, Wang SJ. Role of panendoscopy to identify synchronous second primary malignancies in patients with oral cavity and oropharyngeal squamous cell carcinoma. Head Neck. 2011; 33(7):949–953

[30] Mehta V. Retropharyngeal neck dissection. In: Myers EN, Snyderman CH, eds. Operative Otolaryngology. 3rd ed. Pittsburgh, PA: Elsevier; 2018

[31] Harrison LB, Sessions RB, Hong WK. Head and Neck Cancer: A Multidisciplinary Approach. 3rd ed. New York, NY: LWW; 2009

[32] Cho JH, Kim JK, Lee H-Y, Yoon J-H. Surgical anatomy of human soft palate. Laryngoscope. 2013; 123(11):2900–2904

[33] Netter FH. Atlas of Human Anatomy. 6th ed. Philadelphia, PA: Saunders Elsevier; 2014

[34] Overton LJ, Fritsch VA, Lentsch EJ. Squamous cell carcinoma of the uvula: an analysis of factors affecting survival. Laryngoscope. 2013; 123(4):898–903

[35] Tirelli G, Rizzo R, Biasotto M, et al. Obturator prostheses following palatal resection: clinical cases. Acta Otorhinolaryngol Ital. 2010; 30(1):33–39

[36] Monnier Y, Simon C. Surgery versus radiotherapy for early oropharyngeal tumors: a never-ending debate. Curr Treat Options Oncol. 2015; 16(9):42

[37] Shah JP, Gil Z. Current concepts in management of oral cancer—surgery. Oral Oncol. 2009; 45(4–5):394–401

[38] Chera BS, Amdur RJ, Hinerman RW, et al. Definitive radiation therapy for squamous cell carcinoma of the soft palate. Head Neck. 2008; 30(8):1114–1119

[39] Erkal HŞ, Serin M, Amdur RJ, Villaret DB, Stringer SP, Mendenhall WM. Squamous cell carcinomas of the soft palate treated with radiation therapy alone

or followed by planned neck dissection. Int J Radiat Oncol Biol Phys. 2001; 50 (2):359–366

[40] Hinni ML, Nagel T, Howard B. Oropharyngeal cancer treatment: the role of transoral surgery. Curr Opin Otolaryngol Head Neck Surg. 2015; 23(2):132–138

[41] Weinstein GS, Quon H, Newman HJ, et al. Transoral robotic surgery alone for oropharyngeal cancer: an analysis of local control. Arch Otolaryngol Head Neck Surg. 2012; 138(7):628–634

[42] Johnson JT. Surgery of the Soft Palate. 2nd ed. (Myers EN, ed.). Elsevier; 2008

[43] Van den Wyngaert T, Helsen N, Carp L, et al. ECLYPS investigators. Fluorodeoxyglucose-positron emission tomography/computed tomography after concurrent chemoradiotherapy in locally advanced head-and-neck squamous cell cancer: The ECLYPS study. J Clin Oncol. 2017; 35(30):3458–3464

[44] Levendag P, Nijdam W, Noever I, et al. Brachytherapy versus surgery in carcinoma of tonsillar fossa and/or soft palate: late adverse sequelae and performance status: can we be more selective and obtain better tissue sparing? Int J Radiat Oncol Biol Phys. 2004; 59(3):713–724

[45] Rogers SN, Pinto RS, Lancaster J, et al. Health related quality of life following the treatment of oropharyngeal cancer by transoral laser. Eur Arch Otorhinolaryngol. 2016; 273(11):3913–3920

[46] Lv M, Shen Y, Li J, Zhang C, Zhu H, Sun J. Immediate reconstruction of soft palate defects after ablative surgery and evaluation of postoperative function: an analysis of 45 consecutive patients. J Oral Maxillofac Surg. 2014; 72(7): 1397–1406

[47] Givi B, Eskander A, Awad MI, et al. Impact of elective neck dissection on the outcome of oral squamous cell carcinomas arising in the maxillary alveolus and hard palate. Head Neck. 2016; 38 Suppl 1:E1688–E1694

[48] Eskander A, Givi B, Gullane PJ, et al. Outcome predictors in squamous cell carcinoma of the maxillary alveolus and hard palate. Laryngoscope. 2013; 123 (10):2453–2458

[49] Os AD, Karakullukcu B, Leemans CR, et al. Management of the clinically N0 neck in squamous cell carcinoma of the maxillary alveolus and hard palate. Head Neck. 2016; 38(12):1794–1798

[50] de Almeida JR, Li R, Magnuson JS, et al. Oncologic outcomes after transoral robotic surgery: a multi-institutional study. JAMA Otolaryngol Head Neck Surg. 2015; 141(12):1043–1051

[51] Nixon IJ, Palmer FL, Lakin P, Kattan MM, Lee NY, Ganly I. Pathologically determined tumor volume vs pathologic T stage in the prediction of outcome after surgical treatment of oropharyngeal squamous cell carcinoma. JAMA Otolaryngol Head Neck Surg. 2013; 139(11):1151–1155

[52] Simon C, Goepfert H, Rosenthal DI, et al. Presence of malignant tumor cells in persistent neck disease after radiotherapy for advanced squamous cell carcinoma of the oropharynx is associated with poor survival. Eur Arch Otorhinolaryngol. 2006; 263(4):313–318

[53] Douglas WG, Rigual NR, Giese W, et al. Advanced soft palate cancer: the clinical importance of the parapharyngeal space. Otolaryngol Head Neck Surg. 2005; 133(1):66–69

26 Reconstruction of the Palate

Rosh K.V. Sethi and Jeremy D. Richmon

Summary
This chapter provides an overview of soft and hard palate defects, and a discussion of management and reconstructive techniques. It is imperative that the reconstructive surgeon understand the scope of the defect, patient factors, and nuances of various reconstructive techniques outlined here.

Keywords: soft palate, hard palate, reconstruction of soft and hard palate defects

26.1 Introduction

Palatal defects following oncologic surgery can be challenging to reconstruct and profoundly impact both function and cosmesis. The reconstructive armamentarium has evolved over the past half-century allowing for more nuanced techniques, including microvascular free-tissue transfer, improving our ability to optimize phonation, alimentation, nasal function, and appearance. A comprehensive overview of these techniques and reconstructive considerations is presented in this chapter.

26.2 History

Through much of the 20th century, reconstruction of the palate was avoided in favor of leaving the defect open to maximize surveillance for residual/recurrent disease.[1] Palatal obturators have traditionally offered a convenient solution for hard and soft palate defects in this regard.[2] More definitive repairs were avoided because of difficulty encountered in obtaining appropriate bulk and adequately restoring the complex three-dimensionality when reconstructing such defects.

Multidisciplinary approaches, however, have modernized reconstruction. Hoopes and Edgerton outlined objectives for midface reconstruction in their 1966 publication, including consistently obtaining a healing wound, restoring palatal competence and function, and restoring facial contour.[3] These principles have been modified in subsequent classification schema,[4,5] and have formed the basis for modern reconstructive algorithms for midface and palatal reconstruction.

26.3 Diagnosis and Evaluation

Perhaps the most difficult decision in palatal reconstruction is determining whether to reconstruct at all. Most palatal defects are not life threatening, and the option to do nothing, obturate, or reconstruct with local or free tissue transfer requires a thorough assessment of multiple factors. These include patient age, fitness for surgery, comorbidities, dentition, access to specialist and prosthodontic care, expectations, and quality of life goals. The surgeon must also weigh factors associated with the disease process including size and functional implications of the anticipated defect, need for adjuvant therapy, and expected survival. Reconstructive decision-making, of course, is highly individualized, and will evolve with a surgeon's experience and comfort level. Furthermore, most prosthetic and dental restorations are only nominally covered by insurance plans and the patient's capacity and willingness to pay for these techniques needs to be assessed during the initial planning phase.

26.4 Anatomic Considerations/ Relevant Anatomy

In patients for whom palatal reconstruction is pursued, the primary goal is to separate the nasal and oral cavities in order to restore presurgical function including speech, deglutition, alimentation, and cosmesis. A multidisciplinary approach is paramount to successful reconstruction and rehabilitation, and includes preoperative evaluation by speech-language pathologist, prosthodontist, physical therapist, and the head and neck surgeon. A facial plastic reconstructive surgeon may also be involved if the anticipated defect is expected to significantly impact midface and/or nasal appearance. It is important to note that surgical and prosthetic methods may be utilized separately or together, guided by the size of the defect and goals of the patient and care team. To this end, classification schema may help guide reconstructive goals including closure of the palatal defect for speech and swallowing function, optimizing facial cosmesis, and permitting dental rehabilitation.[6–11]

With regards to timing, palatal reconstruction may be performed in either a primary or delayed/staged fashion; however, primary reconstruction is considered the standard of care in many institutions.[12] Staged reconstruction may be performed either shortly after the oncologic procedure or months to years later. One advantage of delaying the reconstruction several weeks is the ability to obtain definitive pathology and margin status prior to obscuring the field with mobilized tissue. This is especially helpful for the complex bony margins of the maxilla, which are challenging to assess intraoperatively. Should a positive margin result, the oncologic surgeon has a second opportunity to clear it, which may meaningfully impact overall survival. Furthermore, for those surgeons who employ three-dimensional modelling for palatal and midface reconstruction, a delay affords the opportunity to obtain a post-ablative computed tomography (CT) scan and time for precise planning and guide fabrication to optimally reconstruct the patient-specific defect. However, when reconstruction is delayed for months and defects are allowed to heal completely, they may result in muscle atrophy, soft tissue contracture, and cosmetic deformities that may be impossible to fully restore in a delayed fashion. Postoperative radiation +/– chemotherapy with subsequent fibrosis, loss of elasticity, and hypovascularity may exacerbate these functional difficulties and present additional challenges with later reconstruction.[13]

Certain reconstructive techniques are amenable to a transoral approach whereas others may require more invasive approaches, such as lip-split mandibulotomy, for adequate access to the defect and manipulation of surrounding or donor tissue. In general, the approach for reconstruction often depends on the approach taken to resect the cancer.

26.4.1 Soft Palate Considerations

The soft palate is a mucous musculoaponeurotic shelf with a central fibrous aponeurosis layer attaching to the hard palate anteriorly and suspended by attachments to palatine muscles bilaterally.[14] It serves a critical role in the velopharyngeal mechanism, and functionally can be divided into three zones. The anterior third is attached to the hard palate and is primarily fixed, the middle third is where the majority of the muscular bulk from the levator muscles lies and is primarily involved in speaking, and the posterior third elevates during deglutition and speech. Defects involving one or more of these regions may have distinct consequences for the patient and reconstructive surgeon.

The normal velopharyngeal mechanism can be markedly disrupted if the soft palate is removed in a subtotal or total fashion, resulting in rhinolalia, nasal regurgitation, and swallowing impediments.[14] The limited mucosal surface and soft tissue in the soft palate presents a challenge for the reconstructive surgeon as sufficient tissue to close a surgical defect is often not present while maintaining function.

The primary goal of soft palate reconstruction is to optimize the function of the remaining innervated soft palate. Sufficient tissue to close the velopharyngeal port during speech and swallow is critical but not always available. Greater success may be achieved in smaller unilateral and lateralized defects in which closure is possible with preservation of a patent and functional contralateral port. The contralateral side can continue to open and close to retain a nasal airway and swallow function, respectively. With larger defects this becomes increasingly difficult. One needs to consider that the choice of reconstruction, whether it be obturator or soft tissue, is usually static, and may limit the mobility of the residual soft palate. In some cases, an obturator is necessary to support a total or near total soft palate reconstruction which otherwise would be ptotic.

26.4.2 Hard Palate Considerations

The hard palate primarily serves as a means of separation between the oral and nasal cavities, permitting articulation and oral alimentation. Defects of the hard palate, if unrepaired, may result in oronasal or oroantral fistulae, cosmetic deformities with mid-facial retraction, asymmetry and loss of nasal tip support, loss of dentition, and difficulty with oral alimentation and articulation.

Optimal reconstruction is predicated on a comprehensive understanding of the extent of the maxillary defect and relevant anatomy. The maxilla is comprised of three buttresses (nasomaxillary, zygomaticomaxillary, and pterygomaxillary), and four processes (zygomatic, alveolar, palatine, and frontal) (▶ Fig. 26.1). Buttresses serve to resist the vertical forces of mastication, and the four processes function as a frame for the palate and midface.[11,12]

Classification schemes have guided approaches and algorithms to hard palate reconstruction, including the Okay palatomaxillary classification system derived from a review of 47 patients who underwent palatomaxillary reconstruction at the Mount Sinai Medical Center (▶ Table 26.1).[11] Patients were retrospectively assigned to three major classes of defects to provide a framework for reconstructive planning, taking into consideration not only the size but also the biomechanical forces that may predict success of prosthetic rehabilitation alone. While this schema has become a well-accepted approach to these defects, numerous other factors including patient comorbidities, history of prior radiation or surgery, tumor stage, and invasion into adjacent structures should be taken into account when planning definitive reconstruction.

As with soft palate reconstruction, a multidisciplinary approach is critical to provide patients with a comprehensive reconstructive and rehabilitative plan, including evaluation of benefits and disadvantages of various reconstructive strategies.

26.5 Surgical Considerations and Approaches

26.5.1 Reconstructive Techniques for Soft Palate Defects

Soft palate defects are perhaps the most challenging oral defects to reconstruct. This is due to the thin, muscular structure which is mobile and actively closes off the velopharyngeal port in speech and swallowing. Recreating the soft palate defects exactly is virtually impossible as most reconstructive options are not able to recapitulate the dynamic properties of the soft palate. Nonetheless, in the modern era of head and neck reconstruction, surgeons have an armamentarium of tools at their disposal with various local, regional, and complex free tissue transfer options, all designed with the primary goal of dynamic or static closure of the velopharyngeal port.

Injection Pharyngoplasty

The posterior pharyngeal wall may be augmented for smaller palatal defects to bring the posterior pharyngeal wall in closer proximity to the residual soft palate. Multiple augmentation techniques have been described including injectable Teflon,[15] hyaluronic acid, calcium hydroxyapatite or other injectable implants,[16] and autologous fat.[17] While straightforward to perform and often possible in the clinic setting under local anesthesia, this technique is limited in its application to smaller defects. Additionally, it may be difficult to accurately estimate how much material to inject, resulting in over- or under- correction of the defect. Overcorrection is not without risk as patients may be at higher risk for sleep apnea, hyponasality, or dysphagia.[18]

Palatal Prosthesis

Obturators may be employed in the reconstruction of soft palatal defects in an adynamic fashion. There are numerous advantages to obturation including ease of placement at the time of surgery or immediately after, minimal additional surgical time and morbidity, and ease of surveillance of the defect postoperatively. They permit immediate restoration of speech and swallowing in the postoperative setting, obviating the need for alternative means of enteral nutrition. The ability to use an obturator is often determined by the dentate status of the patient and extent of surgical resection. Edentulous patients are difficult to rehabilitate with an obturator alone due to limited anchor points for the prosthesis.

Challenges in stabilization of the prosthesis often limit the functional and rehabilitative outcomes obtained. Additionally,

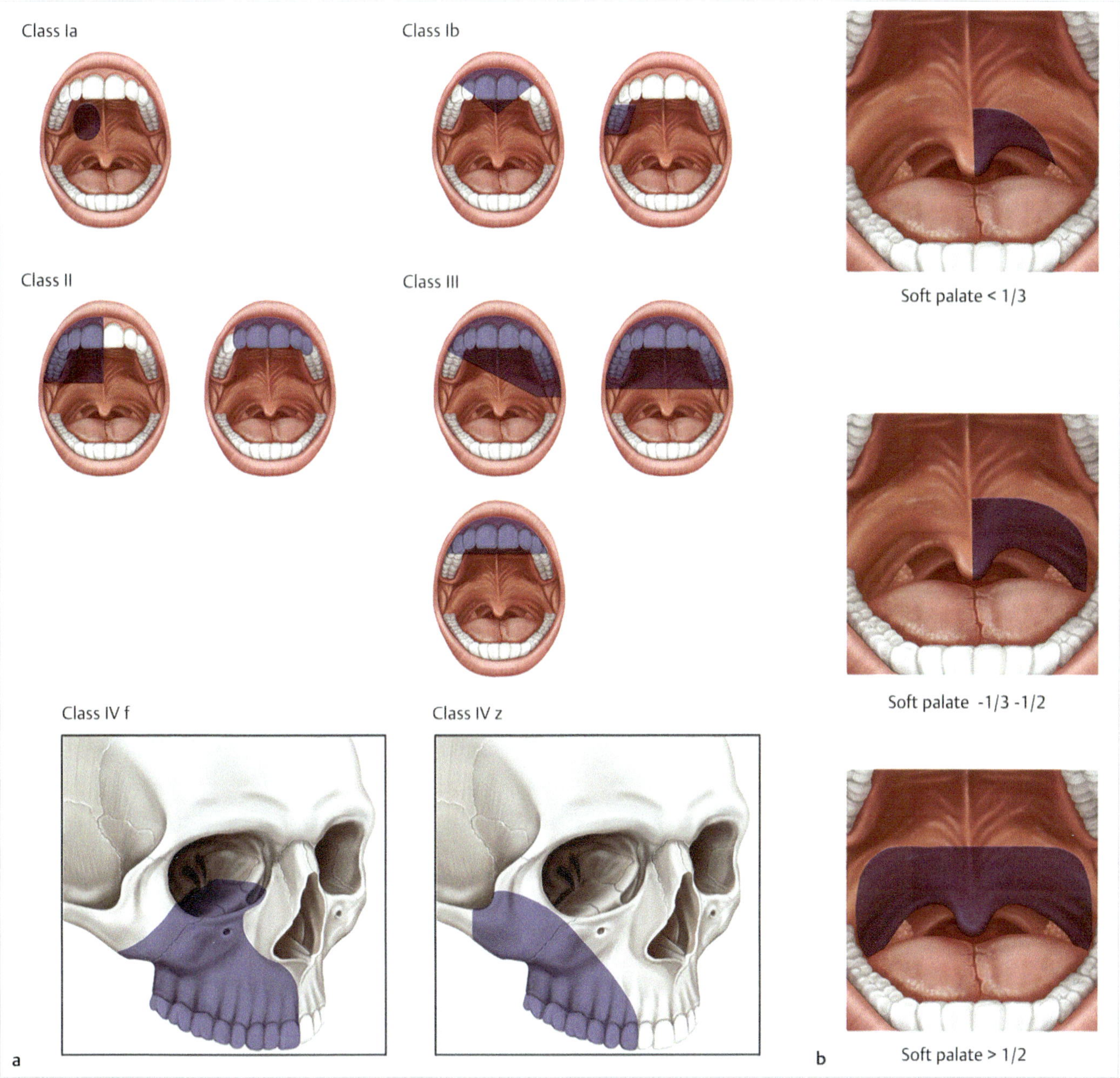

Fig. 26.1 (**a**) Okay classification scheme for hard palate defects and (**b**) illustration of soft palate defects by size.

obturators are frequently hindered by air leakage around the prosthesis and between the nasal and oral cavities resulting in unintended speech and eating difficulties. They may also cause injury to surrounding mobile mucosa and may be inconvenient and uncomfortable to wear.[14,19] Local tissue rearrangement and reconstruction may help reduce surface area of the defect and overcome challenges posed by the obturator alone.

Patients need to understand that obturators are often not worn during radiation therapy given the increased sensitivity and mucositis of the tissues, they may need multiple adjustments as tissues contract and scar tissue forms, they require regular cleaning and maintenance, and they are removed during sleep. They must be worn at times when patients desire optimal speech and swallowing function, they may cause irritation to the surrounding mucosa, and patients may have trouble with an imperfect seal resulting in undesired regurgitation or leakage.[20,21] Nonetheless, for the poor surgical candidate and/or patient looking for the easiest reconstructive option, obturators remain the optimal choice.

Local Flaps

Local flaps may be employed in the reconstruction of soft palate defects, varying in complexity and utility, including the buccal mucosal flap, palatal island rotational flap, forehead flap, palatal adhesion, uvulopalatal flap, and facial artery musculomucosal (FAMM) flap. These local options are best suited for small defects involving less than half of the soft palate.

Table 26.1 Okay classification system for palatal defects

Class	Definition
Ia	Defects involving the hard palate but not the tooth-bearing alveolus
Ib	Defects involving the pre-maxilla, or any portion of the maxillary alveolus and dentition posterior to the canines
II	Defects involving any portion of the tooth-bearing maxillary alveolus but including only one canine, and anterior transverse palatectomy defects involving less than half of the palatal surface
III	Defects involving any portion of the tooth-bearing maxillary alveolus including both canines, total palatectomy defects, and anterior transverse palatectomy involving more than half of the palatal surface
IV	Defects involving the suprastructure of the palate

The superior constrictor advancement rotation flap (SCARF) provides a dynamic closure of the choana and restoration of the velopharynx for hemi-soft palate defects. First described by Strong et al[22] in 1971, the technique allows for recreation of the sphincteric function of the velopharynx. The transected edge of the soft palate is sutured to a transected edge of the superior constrictor muscle in the posterior pharyngeal wall, thereby creating a muscular valve to recreate the velopharynx. In patients with unilateral soft palate paralysis after high vagal injuries, a similar technique in which the paralyzed hemi-soft palate is sutured to the posterior pharyngeal wall (palatal adhesion) has been described, and may be applied to smaller soft palate defects in a similar fashion.[23,24] Proponents of this technique argue that unlike other local flaps, patients achieve earlier and more dynamic restoration of velopharyngeal function with a sensate flap, they do not require wide exposure such as mandibulotomy, and they benefit from shorter hospital stay and earlier initiation of diet.[19]

The FAMM flap was first described in 1992, designed as a musculomucosal flap that combines the principles of nasolabial and buccal mucosal flaps.[25] In its original description, it can be based superiorly or inferiorly along the course of the facial artery, extending from the retromolar trigone to the level of the ipsilateral gingival labial sulcus at the level of the alar margin. The flap can be harvested with an average width of 1.5–2 cm and a length of 8–9 cm and an arc of rotation based at the retromolar trigone inferiorly or at the gingival labial sulcus superiorly. This flap can be used for hard and soft palate reconstructions.[25] In some cases, staged reconstruction may be necessary to divide the pedicle secondarily if it impedes mastication. The FAMM flap may be utilized in conjunction with bone grafts or other reconstruction options to provide a dual lining to the nasal and oral cavities.

The uvulopalatal flap, a myomucosal flap, was first described in 1998 by Zohar et al.[14] This full-thickness flap utilizes the contralateral distal soft palate posterior to the levator palatine muscle in a rotational fashion to ablate the ipsilateral defect. This technique employs principles of uvulopalatopharyngoplasty[26] and is an excellent option for small defects that do not involve the contralateral palate and in which a portion of the soft palate remains. It can be used to decrease the size of a palatal defect obviating the need for an obturator in most cases.[14,27]

While local flaps are often an excellent option, contraindications to their use include ipsilateral external carotid artery ligation, prior radiation to the palate, prior oral surgery, or any other procedure that has diminished blood supply to the intended flap.

Regional Flaps

Regional flaps may be utilized for larger defects when local flaps are insufficient.

The submental island flap was described in 1993 and may be employed in palatal reconstruction.[28] The flap is supplied by the submental artery and vein, with an average pedicle length of 6–8 cm. The skin paddle is generally determined by skin laxity in the submental region, although prior anatomic studies suggest the flap can be maximized at 18 cm by 7 cm.[29] The vascular pedicle pierces through the anterior belly of the digastric muscle, which should be harvested as part of the flap. The reconstructive surgeon must exercise caution when harvesting to avoid injury to the marginal branch of the facial nerve. The flap is located in a hair-bearing area; therefore, appropriate counseling with the patient is necessary. It is also susceptible to marginal necrosis, which can occur more frequently if the pedicle is congested due to a narrow tunnel.

The temporal muscle passes under the zygomatic arch and fans across the lateral skull and can be used to reconstruct defects of the ipsilateral maxilla and palate.[30] The vascular supply consists of the anterior deep and posterior deep temporal arteries and venae comitantes. A minor pedicle arises from the superficial temporal vessels, which frequently must be sacrificed. The flap is typically harvested as muscle only and can be grafted with skin secondarily.

The temporoparietal fascial flap was first described in 1898 and has become a versatile flap for reconstruction of a wide variety of defects in the head and neck.[31] Advantages include reliable vascular supply and minimal donor site morbidity. The reconstructive surgeon should be aware of potential pitfalls including injury to the temporal branch of the facial nerve and scar alopecia. In contrast to the temporalis muscle, this is a thin, pliable fascial flap that has greater reach and is better suited for soft palate defects that do not require much bulk.

The pectoralis major flap is a workhorse of head and neck reconstruction. The flap is supplied by the pectoral branch of the thoracoacromial artery and its venae comitantes. The flap is limited in rotation by the clavicle and can be harvested as a muscle only or musculocutaneous flap. While it can be used for defects cephalad to the oral floor, the flap is limited by size, excessive bulk, dependency, and risk of distal tip necrosis.[32] It is rarely used for soft palate reconstruction given these factors.

Free Flap Reconstruction

Soft tissue free flaps may be applied to total or subtotal soft palate defects. Proponents of this technique argue that free flap reconstruction offers multiple advantages over obturation including improved velopharyngeal competence and the ability to overcome sensory impairment with the use of innervated flaps.[33] The radial forearm free flap (RFFF) permits sensory restoration using the lateral antebranchial cutaneous nerve and offers additional benefits as a thin, pliable fasciocutaneous flap with a long pedicle that can be folded on itself if necessary (▸ Fig. 26.2 and ▸ Fig. 26.3).[33] Indeed, as with all soft tissue

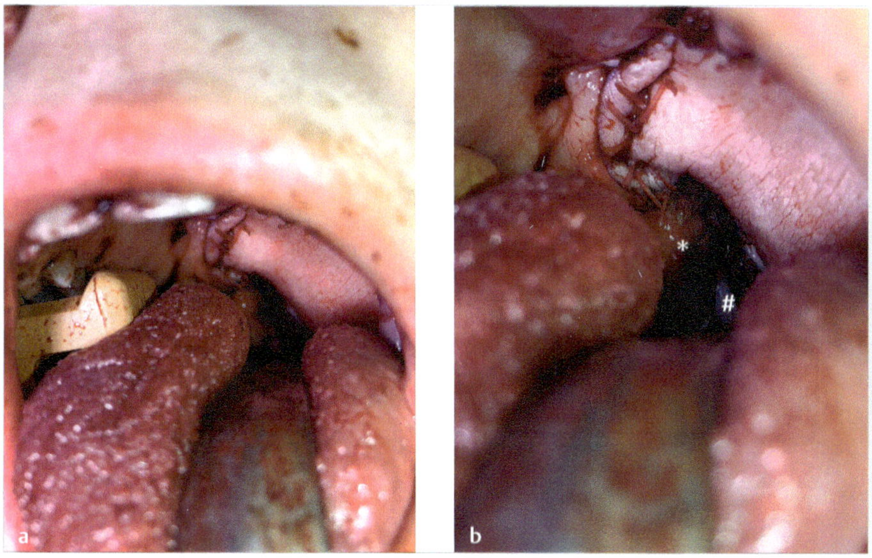

Fig. 26.2 (a, b) Three-fourths soft palate defect demonstrating ipsilateral closure of velopharyngeal port (*) and contralateral port patency (#) through which nasogastric tube is protruding.

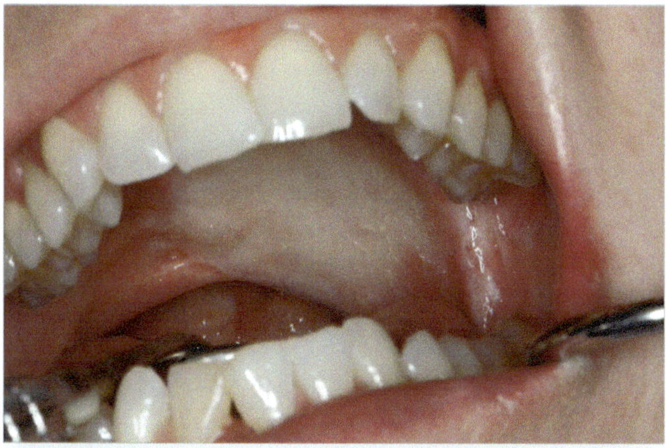

Fig. 26.3 Long-term result after reconstruction of soft palate defect with radial forearm free flap (RFFF) demonstrating patency of bilateral velopharyngeal port.

reconstructive techniques, free flap reconstruction may be combined with obturators to improve velopharyngeal function, and prior studies demonstrate improved speech outcomes when combined with RFFF for specific defects.[34] It is important to emphasize that, like other techniques described here, free tissue transfer remains an adynamic solution for soft palate reconstruction.

26.5.2 Reconstructive Algorithm for Soft Palate Defects

Soft palate defects are best assessed and reconstructed based on size criteria. We recommend the following algorithm for soft palate reconstruction.

Less than 1/3

In patients with smaller defects, the ability to restore "like with like" using a simple and safe technique is an attainable goal. Local and regional flaps have reliably demonstrated success in closure of the velopharyngeal port on the ipsilateral side with maintenance of function on the contralateral side. Therefore, our preferred reconstructive ladder for small soft palate defects includes:

- Primary closure if possible.
- Local flaps.
- Palatal obturator.

Defects 1/3 to 1/2 of the Soft Palate

Moderately sized defects involving less than 1/2 of the soft palate present additional challenges to the reconstructive surgeon as primary closure or local options may not be sufficient and unilateral velopharyngeal port closure may be difficult. Indeed, multiple techniques may be used together to optimize velopharyngeal port closure. In general, more complex reconstruction with free tissue transfer should be avoided as similar functional outcomes can be achieved with less invasive techniques. Our preference for moderately sized soft palate defects include:

- Local and regional flaps, alone or in combination.
- Palatal obturator.

Defects Greater than 1/2 of the Soft Palate

Large defects involving > 1/2 of the soft palate present significant challenges for postoperative velopharyngeal insufficiency, hypernasality, and nasal regurgitation. The two best options for reconstruction are obturation alone and free tissue transfer (▶ Fig. 26.2). Both are adynamic techniques and therefore the determination of which technique to employ is dependent upon patient and disease context.

26.5.3 Reconstruction of the Hard Palate

While soft palate reconstruction is challenging because of the complexities in reconstructing the dynamic velopharyngeal mechanism, hard palate reconstruction can be equally challenging given the three-dimensionality, bony anatomy, aesthetic implications, and dental rehabilitation concerns that must be taken into consideration. This section highlights techniques in hard palate reconstruction, spanning prosthetic devices to microvascular free flap reconstructive techniques.

Palatal Obturators

Palatal obturators have traditionally provided patients with a convenient and effective solution for hard palatal defects, offering the advantage of shorter operating room time, quicker rehabilitation, and ease of oncologic surveillance. As with soft palate defects, hard palate obturators provide an adynamic but functional restoration of speech and swallowing with an obturator bulb that can seal against the surrounding mucosa. Stability of the obturator, however, is directly correlated with size of the defect and status of the residual dentition; there is a greater risk of air and fluid leakage around the bulb and into the nasal cavity with larger defects.[35,36]

Local and Regional Flaps

Local flaps may be employed for small defects in lieu of a prosthetic obturator. Some of these flaps have been highlighted previously in the reconstruction of soft palate defects. Additional local and regional flaps have been described including forehead flaps,[37] deltopectoral flaps,[37,38] tubed flaps,[39] and nasoseptal flaps.[40]

The palatal island flap is an excellent reconstructive option for small defects and was first described in 1962 by Millard.[41] This flap is best suited for nonirriadiated patients with healthy and reliable adjacent palatal tissue. It is based on the palatine neurovascular bundle and can be raised with mucoperiosteum to separate the oral and nasal cavities. The defect from the donor site is allowed to granulate and typically heals in 3–4 weeks and patients may quickly transition to an oral diet. When the residual palate is not sufficient to close the defect, a FAMM flap is another good option for limited hard palate defects.

Advantages of local and regional techniques include immediate coverage of the defect in appropriately selected patients; however, many of these options are limited by inadequate bulk and pedicle length, difficulty in permitting eventual dental rehabilitation, and need for secondary procedures for pedicle division. Notably, calvarial bone grafts may also be used in conjunction with local soft tissue flaps.[42] However, subsequent radiation may lead to resorption and infection.

Free Flap Reconstruction

Microvascular free flap surgery has modernized the reconstructive approach to large hard palate defects. Free tissue transfer provides multiple advantages including immediate reconstruction without the need for staged procedures, substantial bulk and soft tissue density, ability to permit osseointegrated dental rehabilitation, and improved speech intelligibility and overall quality of life for larger sized defects.[20,43] Disadvantages include increased operative time, need for complex microvascular techniques and monitoring, and significant donor-site morbidity depending upon harvest site.

Multiple options for vascularized-bone free flap (VBFF) reconstruction of maxillary defects are available. One of the earliest bone flaps described was the iliac crest flaps.[44] However, criticisms of this technique include excess bulk, short pedicle length, high donor site morbidity, and decreased skin mobility around the bone.[45] The scapular osseocutaneous flap was first described by Saijo in 1978, and its use in head and neck reconstruction was popularized by Swartz et al in 1986 for use in mandibular and maxillary defects.[46] As originally described, the flap is based on the branches of the circumflex scapular artery and offers numerous advantages including multiple skin paddles on a separate vascular pedicle, thin blade of the scapula which is optimal for palatal reconstruction, and minimal donor-site morbidity.[47] The subscapular artery and vein system also permits a wide array of flaps including the latissimus dorsi musculocutaneous flap, serratus anterior with or without vascularized segment of rib, and parascapular skin flaps. A combination of these flaps may also be used for optimal reconstruction of significant defects of the oral cavity and midface.[48,49]

The scapular tip flap, based on the angular branch of the thoracodorsal artery, was first reported in 1991 and has become one of the workhorse bone flaps for maxillary reconstruction.[50,51] It offers multiple advantages over traditional scapular free flaps including longer pedicle length, favorable contour and form for maxillary and palatal reconstruction obviating the need for additional osteotomies, and excellent functional and aesthetic outcomes (▶ Fig. 26.4).[50]

The fibula free flap, osseocutaneous RFFF, and deep circumflex iliac artery free flap offer alternative options for maxillary reconstruction and may be better suited for larger maxillary defects involving additional structures beyond the maxilla and midface, if they are involved (▶ Fig. 26.5).[44,52,53] Optimal reconstruction for more extensive defects of the upper maxilla and orbit are discussed elsewhere in this book. The osseocutaneous RFFF is limited in the length and width of its bony segment and may not be suitable for larger defects.[54]

26.5.4 Hard Palate Reconstructive Algorithm

In our opinion, the optimal reconstructive algorithm for hard palate defects is based upon the Okay classification scheme. Additional criteria must be considered including anticipated use of osseointegrated implants, donor-site morbidity, and functional rehabilitation goals.[20] Our recommendations for hard palate defect reconstruction are as follows.

Okay Class I

Our preference for small defects is either obturation alone, if sufficient residual dentition is present, or local flaps. Additionally, defects with bone around all edges are optimal to obturate as they can be stably seated with excellent speech and swallow results.

Okay Class II

Larger defects may be sufficiently rehabilitated with an obturator alone; however, outcomes are less predictable based on prior studies.[43] Alternatively, local pedicled flaps and noss-

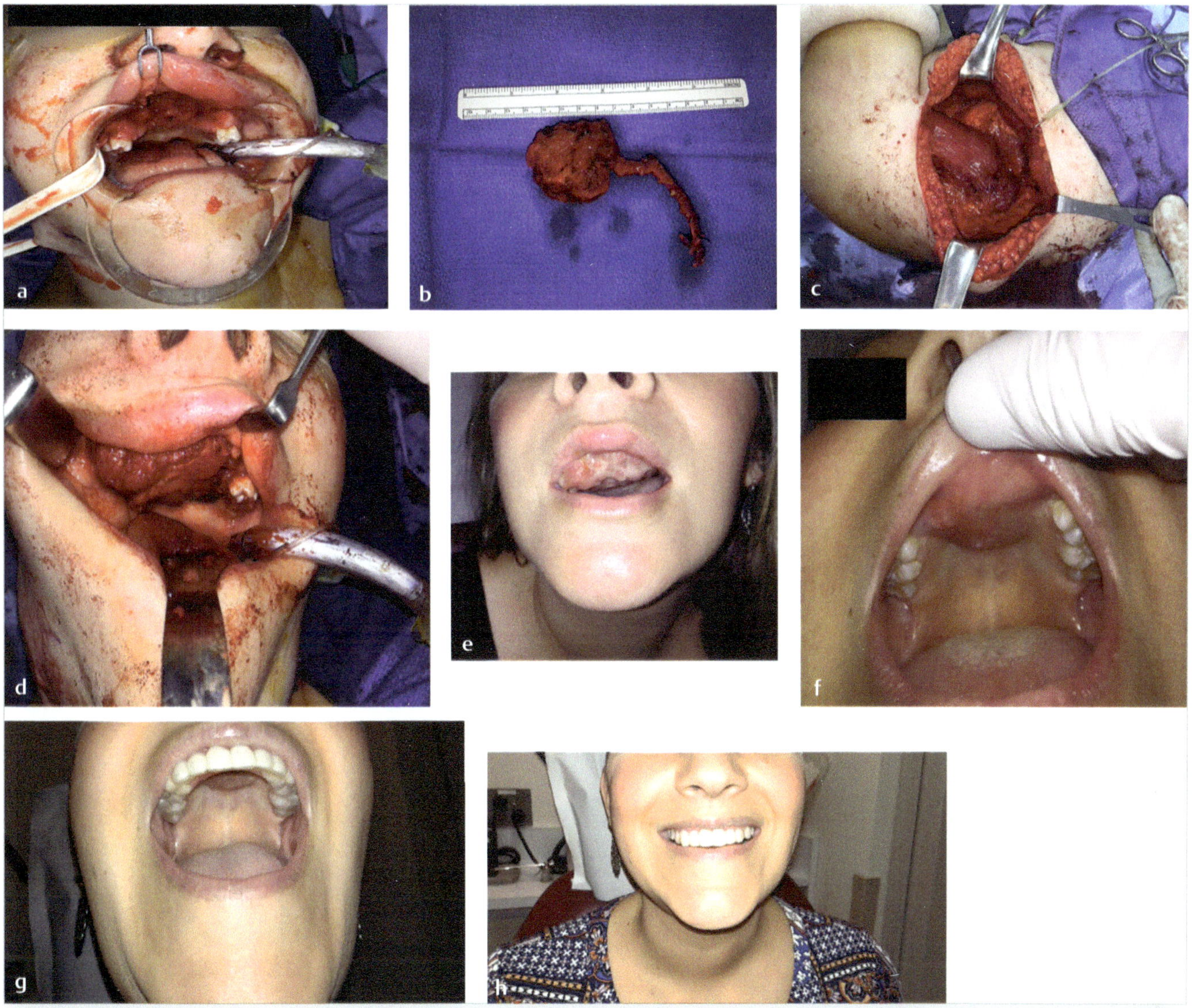

Fig. 26.4 **(a)** Premaxillary defect reconstructed with scapula tip flap. **(b, c)** Premaxillary defect after resection for osteosarcoma. **(d)** Osteomyogenous scapula tip flap used to reconstruct the defect. **(e)** Immediate postoperative appearance with muscle exposed to oral cavity. **(f, g)** Early postoperative appearance with expected muscle swelling, granulation formation, and excess bulk. **(h)** Final appearance after atrophy and remucosalization of the scapula tip flap with dental restoration.

eous flaps, including the RFFF, have also been employed for smaller hard palate defects as an alternative to obturation, but are not amenable to osseointegrated dental rehabilitation.[55] Notably, soft tissue reconstruction alone may create a flatter maxillary arch with blunted contours resulting in a "trampoline-like" surface that may impair future dental rehabilitation.[54]

Our recommendations for Okay Class II defects include:

- Palatal obturator.
- Local pedicled flaps.
- Nonosseous free flap.

Okay Class III–IV

More extensive defects (Okay Class III–IV) are not adequately reconstructed with an obturator alone given the lack of sufficient anchoring points and we therefore prefer vascularized bone containing free flaps (▶ Fig. 26.5).

26.6 Perioperative Management

Primary concerns during soft and hard palate reconstructions include anesthetic and airway considerations, and immediate postoperative care including feeding and airway management.

The oral cavity should be clear of any lines and tubes to permit optimal access during reconstruction. This can be achieved with transnasal intubation with or without subsequent tracheostomy depending on the extent of reconstruction, anticipated swelling, and patient habitus. Nasal trumpets may be utilized in the immediate postoperative setting to help maintain a patent nasal airway. Patients in whom the nasopharyngeal port is completely closed must receive close pulse oximetry monitoring, and education to the patient and care providers about their nasopharyngeal anatomy is paramount.

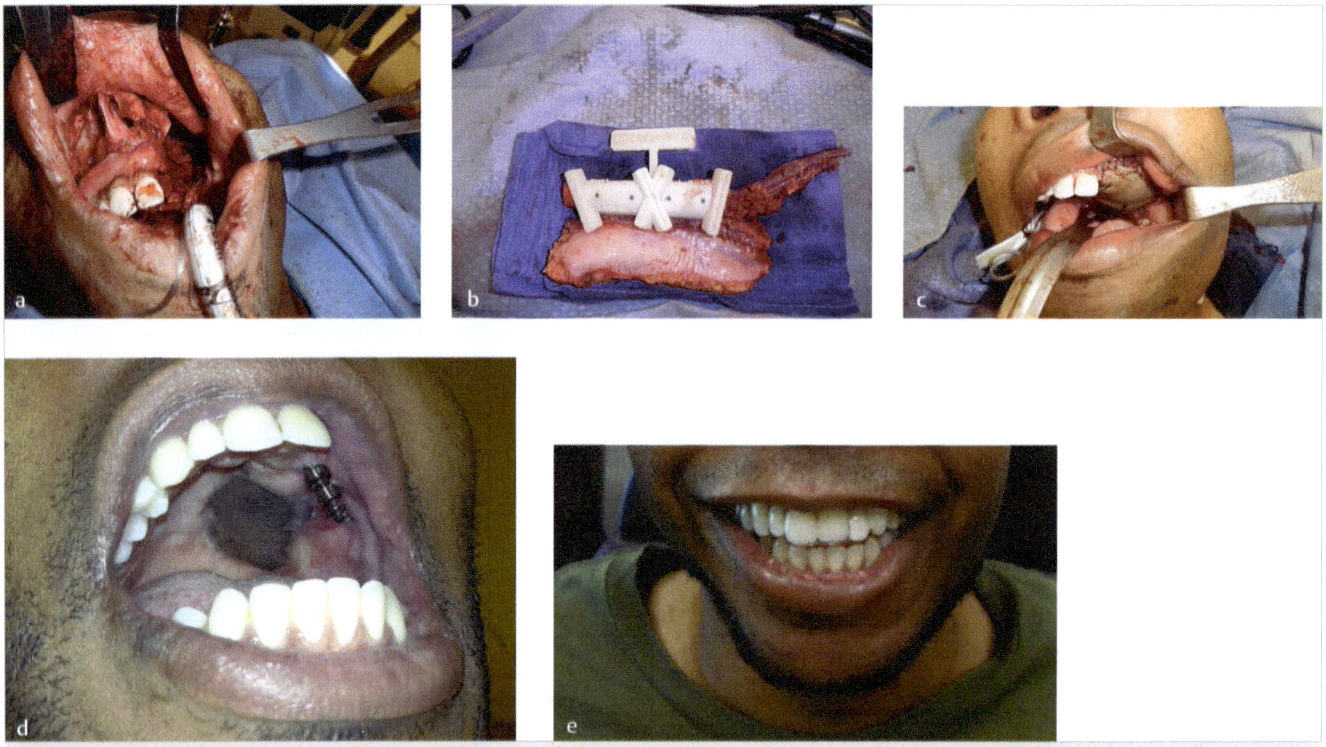

Fig. 26.5 (a) Hemi-palatal defect reconstructed with fibula free flap. (b) Hemi-palatal defect resulting from resection of ossifying fibroma. (c) Medical modeling used to create a custom cutting guide with a fibula free flap. (d) Immediate postoperative appearance. (e) Final postoperative appearance with osteointegrated implants and dental restoration.

Patients may resume oral diet immediately postoperatively if they undergo obturation or limited local reconstruction. In patients who undergo regional or free tissue transfer, oral diversion may be required to permit adequate wound healing. The duration of diversion is at the discretion of the surgeon. Several factors should be considered including the size and bulk of the reconstruction, preoperative evaluation of swallowing function, and risk of wound breakdown including history of malnutrition and radiation.

Donor-site morbidity will vary depending on the flap origin site. Similarly, the recipient site should be monitored in a routine fashion as per surgeon's preference with appropriate care depending on reconstructive choice. Overall, palatal reconstruction may be susceptible to crusting and debris formation that may require meticulous debridement and hygiene in the postoperative setting.

26.7 Surgical Sequelae

Soft and hard palate reconstructions may portend significant morbidity to a patient if they are not well planned. Reconstructive goals should be reviewed with a multidisciplinary team and the patient prior to surgery. Multidisciplinary care is necessary immediately postoperatively to help patients adapt to their new palatal lining and re-learn strategies for eating and speaking. As with any reconstruction, tissue is prone to scarring and contracture, and the dynamic nature of these changes may incur ongoing challenges for the patient and rehabilitative team. The role of the speech-language pathologist in the pre- and postoperative care of these patients cannot be understated.

Key Points

- Soft and hard palate reconstructions are perhaps the most challenging endeavor in head and neck reconstructive surgery given the inherent challenges in not only restoring a mucosal defect, but rehabilitating the patient functionally.
- The decision to reconstruct or not, followed by the type of reconstruction, is perhaps the most nuanced and challenging aspect of patient care, and requires careful review of the patient, and surgical and disease factors.
- Multidisciplinary care is imperative for patients undergoing soft or hard palate reconstruction given the immediate functional and long-term implications.
- We propose the defect size as a guiding principle for reconstructive management and highlight the strengths and weaknesses of various reconstructive options.

References

[1] Davison SP, Sherris DA, Meland NB. An algorithm for maxillectomy defect reconstruction. Laryngoscope. 1998; 108(2):215–219

[2] Gillespie CA, Kenan PD, Ferguson BJ. Hard palate reconstruction in maxillectomy. Laryngoscope. 1986; 96(4):443–444

[3] Hoopes JE, Edgerton MT. Surgical rehabilitation after radical maxillectomy and orbital exenteration. Md State Med J. 1966; 15(9):91–97

[4] Larson DL. A classification system and algorithm for reconstruction of maxillectomy and midfacial defects. Plast Reconstr Surg. 2000; 105(7): 2347–2348

[5] Cordeiro PG, Santamaria E. A classification system and algorithm for reconstruction of maxillectomy and midfacial defects. Plast Reconstr Surg. 2000; 105(7):2331–2346, discussion 2347–2348

[6] Aramany MA. Basic principles of obturator design for partially edentulous patients. Part II: Design principles. 1978 [classical article]. J Prosthet Dent. 2001; 86(6):562–568

[7] Aramany MA. Basic principles of obturator design for partially edentulous patients. Part I: Classification. 1978 [classical article]. J Prosthet Dent. 2001; 86(6):559–561

[8] Aramany MA. Basic principles of obturator design for partially edentulous patients. Part II: design principles. J Prosthet Dent. 1978; 40(6):656–662

[9] Aramany MA. Basic principles of obturator design for partially edentulous patients. Part I: classification. J Prosthet Dent. 1978; 40(5):554–557

[10] Spiro RH, Strong EW, Shah JP. Maxillectomy and its classification. Head Neck. 1997; 19(4):309–314

[11] Okay DJ, Genden E, Buchbinder D, Urken M. Prosthodontic guidelines for surgical reconstruction of the maxilla: a classification system of defects. J Prosthet Dent. 2001; 86(4):352–363

[12] Urken ML, Buchbinder D, Costantino PD, et al. Oromandibular reconstruction using microvascular composite flaps: report of 210 cases. Arch Otolaryngol Head Neck Surg. 1998; 124(1):46–55

[13] Urken ML, Buchbinder D, Weinberg H, et al. Functional evaluation following microvascular oromandibular reconstruction of the oral cancer patient: a comparative study of reconstructed and nonreconstructed patients. Laryngoscope. 2015; 125(7):1512

[14] Zohar Y, Buler N, Shvilli Y, Sabo R. Reconstruction of the soft palate by uvulopalatal flap. Laryngoscope. 1998; 108(1 Pt 1):47–50

[15] Bluestone CD, Musgrave RH, McWilliams BJ, Crozier PA. Teflon injection pharyngoplasty. Cleft Palate J. 1968; 5:19–22

[16] Brigger MT, Ashland JE, Hartnick CJ. Injection pharyngoplasty with calcium hydroxylapatite for velopharyngeal insufficiency: patient selection and technique. Arch Otolaryngol Head Neck Surg. 2010; 136(7):666–670

[17] Cao Y, Ma T, Wu D, Yin N, Zhao Z. Autologous fat injection combined with palatoplasty and pharyngoplasty for velopharyngeal insufficiency and cleft palate: preliminary experience. Otolaryngol Head Neck Surg. 2013; 149(2): 284–291

[18] Gray SD, Pinborough-zimmerman J, Catten M. Posterior wall augmentation for treatment of velopharyngeal insufficiency. Otolaryngol Head Neck Surg. 1999; 121(1):107–112

[19] Zeitels SM, Kim J. Soft-palate reconstruction with a "SCARF" superior-constrictor advancement-rotation flap. Laryngoscope. 1998; 108(8 Pt 1): 1136–1140

[20] Futran ND, Haller JR. Considerations for free-flap reconstruction of the hard palate. Arch Otolaryngol Head Neck Surg. 1999; 125(6):665–669

[21] Brown KE. Peripheral consideration in improving obturator retention. J Prosthet Dent. 1968; 20(2):176–181

[22] Strong MS, DiTroia JF, Vaughan CW. Carcinoma of the palatine arch: a review of 73 patients. Trans Am Acad Ophthalmol Otolaryngol. 1971; 75 (5):957–967

[23] Netterville JL, Fortune S, Stanziale S, Billante CR. Palatal adhesion: the treatment of unilateral palatal paralysis after high vagus nerve injury. Head Neck. 2002; 24(8):721–730

[24] Netterville JL, Vrabec JT. Unilateral palatal adhesion for paralysis after high vagal injury. Arch Otolaryngol Head Neck Surg. 1994; 120(2):218–221

[25] Pribaz J, Stephens W, Crespo L, Gifford G. A new intraoral flap: facial artery musculomucosal (FAMM) flap. Plast Reconstr Surg. 1992; 90(3): 421–429

[26] Dickson RI, Blokmanis A. Treatment of obstructive sleep apnea by uvulopalatopharyngoplasty. Laryngoscope. 1987; 97(9):1054–1059

[27] Gillespie MB, Eisele DW. The uvulopalatal flap for reconstruction of the soft palate. Laryngoscope. 2000; 110(4):612–615

[28] Martin D, Pascal JF, Baudet J, et al. The submental island flap: a new donor site. Anatomy and clinical applications as a free or pedicled flap. Plast Reconstr Surg. 1993; 92(5):867–873

[29] Chen X, Zhou H, Zhang YJ, et al. Applied anatomy of the submental island flap and its clinical application in the repair of defects following hypopharyngeal carcinoma resection. World J Otorhinolaryngol Head Neck Surg. 2015; 1(1): 44–49

[30] Clauser L, Curioni C, Spanio S. The use of the temporalis muscle flap in facial and craniofacial reconstructive surgery: a review of 182 cases. J Craniomaxillofac Surg. 1995; 23(4):203–214

[31] Mokal NJ, Ghalme AN, Kothari DS, Desai M. The use of the temporoparietal fascia flap in various clinical scenarios: a review of 71 cases. Indian J Plast Surg. 2013; 46(3):493–501

[32] Milenović A, Virag M, Uglesić V, Aljinović-Ratković N. The pectoralis major flap in head and neck reconstruction: first 500 patients. J Craniomaxillofac Surg. 2006; 34(6):340–343

[33] Lacombe V, Blackwell KE. Radial forearm free flap for soft palate reconstruction. Arch Facial Plast Surg. 1999; 1(2):130–132

[34] Yoshida H, Michi K, Yamashita Y, Ohno K. A comparison of surgical and prosthetic treatment for speech disorders attributable to surgically acquired soft palate defects. J Oral Maxillofac Surg. 1993; 51(4):361–365

[35] Shipman B. Evaluation of occlusal force in patients with obturator defects. J Prosthet Dent. 1987; 57(1):81–84

[36] Watson RM, Gray BJ. Assessing effective obturation. J Prosthet Dent. 1985; 54 (1):88–93

[37] Konno A, Togawa K, Iizuka K. Primary reconstruction after total or extended total maxillectomy for maxillary cancer. Plast Reconstr Surg. 1981; 67(4): 440–448

[38] Bakamjian V. A technique for primary reconstruction of the palate after radical maxillectomy for cancer. Plast Reconstr Surg. 1963; 31:103–117

[39] Kostrubala JG. Repair of extensive palatal defects with skin tubes. Plast Reconstr Surg (1946). 1950; 5(6):512–515

[40] Edgerton MT, Devito RV. Reconstruction of palatal defects resulting from treatment of carcinoma of palate, antrum, or gingiva. Plast Reconstr Surg Transplant Bull. 1961; 28:306–319

[41] Millard DR, Jr. Wide and/or short cleft palate. Plast Reconstr Surg Transplant Bull. 1962; 29:40–57

[42] Ewers R. Reconstruction of the maxilla with a double musculoperiosteal flap in connection with a composite calvarial bone graft. Plast Reconstr Surg. 1988; 81(3):431–436

[43] Moreno MA, Skoracki RJ, Hanna EY, Hanasono MM. Microvascular free flap reconstruction versus palatal obturation for maxillectomy defects. Head Neck. 2010; 32(7):860–868

[44] Brown JS. Deep circumflex iliac artery free flap with internal oblique muscle as a new method of immediate reconstruction of maxillectomy defect. Head Neck. 1996; 18(5):412–421

[45] Coleman JJ, III. Osseous reconstruction of the midface and orbits. Clin Plast Surg. 1994; 21(1):113–124

[46] Swartz WM, Banis JC, Newton ED, Ramasastry SS, Jones NF, Acland R. The osteocutaneous scapular flap for mandibular and maxillary reconstruction. Plast Reconstr Surg. 1986; 77(4):530–545

[47] Granick MS, Ramasastry SS, Newton ED, Solomon MP, Hanna DC, Kaltman S. Reconstruction of complex maxillectomy defects with the scapular-free flap. Head Neck. 1990; 12(5):377–385

[48] Aviv JE, Urken ML, Vickery C, Weinberg H, Buchbinder D, Biller HF. The combined latissimus dorsi-scapular free flap in head and neck reconstruction. Arch Otolaryngol Head Neck Surg. 1991; 117(11):1242–1250

[49] Valentini V, Gennaro P, Torroni A, et al. Scapula free flap for complex maxillofacial reconstruction. J Craniofac Surg. 2009; 20(4):1125–1131

[50] Choi N, Cho JK, Jang JY, Cho JK, Cho YS, Baek CH. Scapular tip free flap for head and neck reconstruction. Clin Exp Otorhinolaryngol. 2015; 8(4): 422–429

[51] Coleman JJ, III, Sultan MR. The bipedicled osteocutaneous scapula flap: a new subscapular system free flap. Plast Reconstr Surg. 1991; 87(4):682–692

[52] Shaw RJ, Brown JS. Osteomyocutaneous deep circumflex iliac artery perforator flap in the reconstruction of midface defect with facial skin loss: a case report. Microsurgery. 2009; 29(4):299–302

[53] Yim KK, Wei FC. Fibula osteoseptocutaneous free flap in maxillary reconstruction. Microsurgery. 1994; 15(5):353–357

[54] Futran ND. Retrospective case series of primary and secondary microvascular free tissue transfer reconstruction of midfacial defects. J Prosthet Dent. 2001; 86(4):369–376

[55] Funk GF, Laurenzo JF, Valentino J, McCulloch TM, Frodel JL, Hoffman HT. Free-tissue transfer reconstruction of midfacial and cranio-orbito-facial defects. Arch Otolaryngol Head Neck Surg. 1995; 121(3):293–303

27 Malignant Tumors of the Mandible

Anil D'Cruz and Richa Vaish

Summary

Malignant tumors of the mandible are a diverse group of disorders which could be either primary, secondary, or metastatic. Primary tumors could be odotogenic (tooth forming elements), nonodontogenic (from bone and cartilage), or miscellaneous (melanoma, lymphoma). Secondary tumors are the most common and are due to direct involvement from an oral cavity malignancy. Metastatic involvement is rare and is usually from primaries arising in the infraclavicular region. Thorough understanding of the anatomic considerations, blood supply, ossification centers, route of spread, in addition to biological factors specific to the type of tumor, is imperative for appropriate management of these tumors. Surgery with adequate margins is the mainstay of treatment along with adjuvant therapy in presence of high risk features. Loss of mandible is associated with functional and cosmetic morbidity and appropriate reconstruction is mandated. Various classifications of mandibular defects post surgery have been described in an attempt to standardize the optimal reconstructive procedure necessary.

Keywords: mandible, mandible anatomy and histology, mandible blood supply, mandible surgery, neoplasm, neoplasm surgery, odontogenic tumors, osteosarcoma, squamous cell carcinoma

27.1 Epidemiology: Incidence, Causes, and Clinical Characteristics

The mandible is a unique bone, important for both function and cosmesis. It is the largest and strongest part of the face and the only movable part of the facial skeleton. It provides attachments to the muscles of mastication that help in the movement of the mandible. It also gives attachment to the geniohyoid and genioglossus muscles, important for speech and swallowing. It is intimately related to the infratemporal fossa and parapharyngeal space, which are potential routes for tumor spread. Understanding the surgical anatomy, the routes of spread, and the diverse biology of tumors that involve the mandible is critical to ensure adequate oncologic clearance while maintaining function and cosmesis.

The mandible can be involved by a diverse group of malignant tumors that could be either primary, arising from tissues native to the mandible, secondary when involvement occurs from cancers in the adjacent oral cavity, or metastatic.

27.1.1 Primary

Most classification systems primarily focus on odontogenic tumors.[1] However, primary tumors can arise from other histogenetic backgrounds within the mandible in addition to those of odontogenic origin namely epithelial, osseous, glandular etc. Primary mandibular tumors are therefore best classified as odontogenic (dental origin), nonodontogenic, or miscellaneous.

Odontogenic/dental tumors can originate from epithelial, ectomesenchymal, or mesenchymal tooth forming elements. The commonly followed classification for these tumors is the WHO 4th edition (2017) (▶ Table 27.1).[1] These tumors are of relatively rare occurrence. Meanwhile, nonodontogenic tumors primarily arise from bone and cartilage and include the various types of chondrosarcomas and osteosarcomas. Osteogenic sarcoma is the most commonly encountered tumor in this group. There is also a heterogeneous group of tumors which arises from other histological origins within the mandible namely melanocytic, lymphoid, and salivary. These tumors are of very rare occurrence and behave biologically as tumors of similar origin elsewhere in the body. The latter are beyond the scope of this chapter.

Malignant Odontogenic Tumors

Malignant odontogenic tumors arise from the remnant epithelium, mesenchymal, or ectomesenchymal component of the odontogenic apparatus. These are rarely mentioned in majority of literature in the form of case reports or case series. A thorough understanding of the biological behavior and appropriate management is therefore often a challenge. The majority of odontogenic tumors are benign with only about 3% being malignant.[2] The latest WHO classification categorizes them as odontogenic carcinoma, odontogenic carcinosarcoma, and odontogenic sarcoma.[1] They can arise secondarily in the background of their benign counterparts or de novo. Presentation is usually as an expansile mass lesion, with or without pain. Neural symptoms may be present if the inferior alveolar nerve is involved.

Given the rarity of these tumors, there are no robust treatment guidelines. Malignant odontogenic tumors are therefore treated similar to other malignant tumors of the mandible with

Table 27.1 WHO classification of malignant odontogenic tumors and nonodontogenic tumors

1. Odontogenic

- Odontogenic carcinoma
  - Ameloblastic carcinoma
  - Primary intraosseous carcinoma
  - Sclerosing odontogenic carcinoma
  - Clear cell odontogenic carcinoma
  - Ghost cell odontogenic carcinoma
- Odontogenic carcinosarcoma
- Odontogenic sarcomas

2. Nonodontogenic

- Chondrosarcoma
  - G1
  - G2/3
- Mesenchymal chondrosarcoma
- Osteosarcoma, NOS
  - Intraosseous well-differentiated osteosarcoma
  - Chondroblastic osteosarcoma
  - Parosteal osteosarcoma
  - Periosteal osteosarcoma

surgery as primary modality of choice. Adjuvant radiotherapy is added in the presence of high risk factors (high grade, large tumors, extensive soft tissue component, and close or positive margins) that could predispose to recurrence.

Ameloblastic Carcinoma

This neoplasm shows areas of classical ameloblastoma along with distinct cytological features of malignancy. It may arise in the background of preexisting ameloblastoma but the majority of the cases appear to develop de novo. These lesions may or may not be associated with metastasis. There is an equal preponderance among both genders, and the lesion typically occurs in elderly. Mandible is the most common site of occurrence (~66%) with a predilection for the posterior segment. Ameloblastic carcinoma is a distinct entity from metastasizing ameloblastoma. The latter is histologically benign ameloblastoma that while maintaining characteristics of the parent tumor has the ability to metastasize. On histopathology, classical features of malignancy like pleomorphism, nuclear hyperchromasia, increased mitotic activity, and focal areas of necrosis are seen. Peripheral palisading and reverse nuclear polarization are known to be present. There may be areas of perineural and vascular invasion. Higher levels of aneuploidy and an increased proliferation index differentiates it from benign ameloblastoma.[1,3,4] Proliferation markers like Ki 67 are known to be significantly higher in ameloblastic carcinoma compared to the ameloblastoma.[4]

Primary Intraosseous Carcinoma

Primary intraosseous squamous cell carcinoma (PIOSCC) is derived from the remnant odontogenic epithelium. PIOSCC is found more often in the body and posterior mandible than in the maxilla. Most cases are asymptomatic and are incidentally discovered during routine dental evaluation. Advanced tumors may present with facial swelling and paresthesia. Mean age of occurrence is the 5–6th decade, with a male preponderance. PIOSCC must be distinguished from squamous cell carcinoma (SCC) arising from the adjoining oral mucosa that secondarily invades the mandible. This is often difficult particularly when the tumor has extraosseous spread and involves the surface epithelium. PIOSCC is also known as primary intraosseous epidermoid carcinoma. It can occur de novo or in the background of keratocystic odontogenic tumor or other odontogenic cysts.[5] The etiology of these tumors is not well understood. The most plausible explanation is an inflammatory stimulus as these areas are not exposed to carcinogens. Histologically, the tumor shows areas of squamous epithelium with features of SCC with well to moderate differentiation which can be keratinizing or nonkeratinizing.[1,3,6] The differential diagnosis includes high-grade mucoepidermoid carcinoma and metastatic lesions of mandible.

Sclerosing Odontogenic Carcinoma

This is a recent addition to the 4th edition of WHO's (2017) classification of head and neck tumors.[1] It was first reported in the literature by Koutlas et al in 2008.[7] Histologically, it shows bland cytologic features with cords and strands of cells surrounding stroma and dense sclerosis. These tumors have an aggressive pattern of growth into the local nerves and muscles. On immunohistochemistry, these are positive for cytokeratin markers, E cadherin and nuclear p63. No metastasis or disease related death has been reported with these tumors to date. There is the need for more data to properly understand the biology of this entity to guide the appropriate management algorithm.

Clear Cell Odontogenic Carcinoma

This is a rare neoplasm of odontogenic origin which usually occurs in adults in their 6th decade, with a significant female predilection. It primarily affects the mandible. The neoplasm is locally aggressive and infiltrates the surrounding medullary bone, nerves, and lymphatics. It has propensity to regional and distant metastasis. Histologically, the tumor shows a biphasic pattern characterized by a peripheral rim of hyperchromatic polygonal cells with eosinophilic cytoplasm surrounding islands of clear cells with fibrocellular stroma.[3,8] Alternatively, there may be isolated nests of clear cells. Rarely, it may be associated with an ameloblastic pattern. On immunohistochemistry, the tumor is positive for cytokeratins, p63, and epithelial membrane antigen. Recently, it has been shown that majority of the tumors show EWSR1 rearrangement commonly with AFT1.[9] This mutation is highly sensitive for clear cell odontogenic carcinoma but is not specific as it may occur in other clear cell malignancies as well. Limited intervention in form of curettage and enucleation is associated with a high rate of recurrence, and resection with clear margins is the treatment of choice. Differential diagnosis includes hyalinizing clear cell carcinoma of salivary gland.

Ghost Cell Odontogenic Carcinoma

According to WHO's description, these are rare with features of calcifying cystic odontogenic tumors or dentinogenic ghost cell tumors.[3] There is a male predilection with a peak incidence in the 4th decade. This tumor is more likely to affect maxilla, although mandibular occurrences have also been reported. The tumor can arise de novo or secondary to a benign calcifying cystic odontogenic tumor, dentinogenic ghost cell tumor, or other odontogenic cyst. Histopathologically, there are features of benign calcifying cystic odontogenic tumors with areas of malignant transformation characterized by epithelial islands in fibrous stroma with areas of mitosis. Ghost cells are present in varying amounts. The malignant component may be distinct from the benign areas or could be intermingled in a benign background. Proliferation markers Ki 67 and p53 help in differentiating the carcinoma from the benign odontogenic cysts.[10] Prognosis is variable due to the diversity of histology and biological behavior, ranging from a slow growing tumor to more aggressive variants.[11]

Odontogenic Sarcomas

These tumors are characterized by benign epithelial and malignant mesenchymal component, which include ameloblastic fibrosarcoma, ameloblastic fibrodentinosarcoma, and ameloblastic fibroodontosarcoma.[3,4] Ameloblastic fibrosarcoma may arise de novo or secondary to ameloblastic fibroma. The common presentation is in younger patients usually in the 2nd and

3rd decades, with a higher predilection for males. Mandible is commonly affected and the tumor is usually located posteriorly. Histologically, the tumor is characterized by the benign epithelial polygonal cells arranged in branching cord fashion surrounded by a hypercellular connective tissue stroma showing high mitotic rate. These tumors are highly aggressive locally but have a low propensity for distant metastasis. Ameloblastic fibrodentinosarcoma and ameloblastic fibroodontosarcoma have dysplastic dentin and/or enamel in addition to features of ameloblastic fibrosarcoma. The subclassification of odontogenic sarcoma has been deleted from the latest WHO classification.[1,12]

Odontogenic Carcinosarcoma

Initially removed from the 2005 WHO classification, odontogenic carcinosarcoma has now been reincorporated in the latest 2017 version.[1,3] The tumor is characterized by pattern similar to ameloblastic fibrosarcoma with both the epithelial and mesenchymal components showing malignant features.[1,13]

Malignant Nonodontogenic Tumors

Chondrosarcoma

Chondrosarcoma is an extremely rare tumor of the facial skeleton arising from hyaline cartilage. Only 4% of all chondrosarcomas occur in the head and neck; the mandible and maxilla are most commonly affected. Presentation is usually in the 4th decade, commonly in males. It has a predilection for the symphysis, coronoid, and condyloid processes. Visibly, these tumors are pale and glistening which on microscopy are lobulated and show round to oval cells in the background of chondroid matrix with cellularity and atypia.[3,14] IDH1 and IDH2 are the commonly encountered mutations with these tumors.[15]

Mesenchymal Chondrosarcoma

Mesenchymal chondrosarcoma is an aggressive variant that equally affects the mandible and maxilla. It commonly occurs in young adults with a female preponderance. Visibly, it appears fleshy with areas of chalky calcification. On microscopy, it shows variable amount of areas of hyaline cartilage with round to spindle cells. These cells are immunoreactive to S-100 and CD99.[3,14] HEY1-NCOA2 fusion is the common mutation which may be found in as high as 80% of cases.[16]

Osteosarcoma

Although primary osteogenic sarcoma (OS) is the commonest bony tumor of the mandible, it is relatively rare, with large centers reporting just 1–2 cases/year.[17,18] Given the rarity of this tumor, treatment guidelines are often extrapolated from extragnathic OS. OS of the mandible are however a distinct entity in that they are locally aggressive and rarely known to be associated with distant metastasis compared to the more commonly occurring tumors of the appendicular skeleton.[19,20] The majority of cases are sporadic but familial cases associated with Li Fraumeni syndrome have been described. A genetic correlation between retinoblastoma and osteosarcomas exists on the 13q14 chromosome; retinoblastoma patients are known to have a higher incidence of OS, more so if they have received radiotherapy earlier. Predisposing conditions includes Paget's disease, fibrous dysplasia, and prior radiotherapy. Radiation-induced OS occur after a median latent period of 10 or more years and are associated with an aggressive course and worse prognosis.

OS is a primary tumor of the bone, characterized by osteoid or bone formation by the tumor cells. It can be classified as low grade (parosteal or central), intermediate grade (periosteal), or high grade (conventional, telengiectasic, and small cell). Based on the predominant type of extracellular matrix produced by the tumor cell, the conventional osteosarcoma is further classified as osteoblastic, chondroblastic, and fibroblastic.[19,20] Chondroblastic OS can mimic chondrosarcoma on histology in the absence of osteoid component. Galectin 1 and ezrin help to establish the diagnosis in these cases.[1,3,14,19]

The most common presenting feature is a painless mass lesion of the jaw often mimicking benign tumors, particularly when low grade. Loosening of the teeth and radiating pain along the inferior alveolar nerve may occur. Both genders are equally affected a decade or two after long bone OS, and a typical patient presents at 30–40 years of age. The body of the mandible is most commonly involved followed by the angle and the ascending ramus. Given the anatomical constraints that preclude radical clearance, tumors are more likely to recur locally, particularly in larger lesions. Surgery is the mainstay of treatment and obtaining clear margins is of paramount importance.[19,20] Resection must be radical and there is no role for conservative procedures such as marginal mandibulectomy. A margin of 1 cm has been advocated as adequate in contrast to the 5-cm margin for long bone OS. Assessment of the extent of intramedullary involvement preoperatively by magnetic resonance imaging (MRI) helps ensure adequate bony resection. MRI is also useful for better visualization of the soft tissue extent of the tumor. The most important prognostic factor that influences outcomes is a clear margin of resection. Other factors that influence outcomes are histology and grade of the tumor (chondroblastic having better outcome than fibroblastic OS), age, advanced stage at presentation, and initial nonsurgical treatment. The role of adjuvant radiotherapy and chemotherapy has been a matter of debate for ages. Most published literature and metaanalyses reveal conflicting results primarily due to the small number of patients in each series, lack of uniformity of data, and studies being spread across long time spans.[17,18] Some of these studies are over 2 decades old making applicability to today's day and age irrelevant, given the advances in surgical technique and reconstruction. A relatively recent review article has proposed a treatment algorithm suggesting the role of radiotherapy and chemotherapy in both the adjuvant and neoadjuvant settings taking into account published literature, stage, grade, postoperative margin status, and response to chemotherapy.[19] Given that local rather than distant recurrence is the main cause of failure, most authors recommend adjuvant radiotherapy in case of close or positive margins and for tumors > 5 cm. Chemotherapy is conceptually attractive in the neoadjuvant setting in large tumors, which in the opinion of the surgeon could pose an issue in obtaining free margins, with an aim to downsize the tumors and render them operable. On one hand, Mücke et al showed adding neoadjuvant chemotherapy to osteosarcomas improves survival.[21] Adjuvant chemotherapy, on the other hand, should be considered in large and high-grade tumors where the risk of distant metastasis is theoretically higher. Hence, the decision to adjuvant chemotherapy should be individualized. Chemotherapy regimens are similar to those used for long bone OS. 5-year survival varies between 10 and 100% but is usually in the range of 60–70%.[19,20]

27.1.2 Secondary Tumors of the Mandible

This is the most common malignant involvement of the mandible which is usually from SCC of the surrounding buccal mucosa, tongue, and floor of mouth.[22] Alveolar SCC can occur but are relatively rare and form < 10% of all oral cancers.[23] This entity is similar to other oral SCC and should be distinguished from PIOSCC which is of odontogenic origin as described earlier. Mandibular involvement in oral cancers is a sign of advanced disease and is staged as T4.[24] Superficial cortical erosion by alveolar SCC, on the contrary, is not considered as T4 but is staged as per the size of the primary tumor. Though there is lack of adequate evidence, it has been postulated that medullary or inferior alveolar canal involvement has a worse prognosis when compared to the deep cortical invasion alone.[25]

27.1.3 Metastatic Tumors

The mandible may be involved by metastatic spread from primary cancers from other sites, which constitutes less than 1% of the malignant lesions of the mandible.[26] These tumors usually occur in the elderly with an equal gender predilection, although some series report slightly higher incidence in females given the high incidence associated with primary breast cancer.[27] Sarcomatous tumors from axial and appendicular skeleton metastasizing to the mandible skeleton are rare. Pediatric tumors like neuroblastoma may manifest with metastasis to the mandible.

Metastatic tumors involve the mandible approximately five times more frequently compared to maxilla.[26] These tumors are usually located in the region of the angle and posterior mandible and below the inferior alveolar nerve. The alveolar process is rarely involved by the metastatic disease. Presentation is commonly a painless diffuse bony swelling although occasionally the lesions could be circumscribed. There can be associated pain and paresthesia with the involvement of inferior alveolar nerve.[28] Radiologically, the lesions are osteolytic in the vast majority although osteoblastic and mixed lesions may occur, particularly when metastases are from the prostate and breast. Metastatic disease to the mandible usually signifies widespread disease and portends a grave prognosis with median survival of less than a year. However, when associated with biologically favorable cancers such as thyroid, prostate, and breast, prognosis is better. Metastases manifesting many years following treatment of the primary (long disease-free interval) have a better prognosis. These tumors are usually treated with systemic therapy in view of the disseminated nature of the disease. Local radiotherapy is warranted when lesions are symptomatic. In the rare occasion when mandibular metastases are the only site of disease in a biologically favorable tumor, surgery may be considered.

27.2 Clinical Presentation

Primary mandibular tumors usually present with a painless gradually increasing mass which may be associated with loosening of the teeth. The overlying skin is stretched and uninvolved except in advanced lesions. The mucosa is intact but may be breached consequent to previous biopsy attempts. In contrast, secondary invasion of the mandible is associated with mucosal ulceration, pain, and symptoms primarily located to the main cancer. There may be an associated mucosal growth that is proliferative or ulcerative. If the lesion involves the mandibular or the inferior alveolar nerve in both primary and secondary tumors, the patient may have paresthesia of the overlying skin. Trismus is a manifestation of advanced disease and is associated with invasion of the infratemporal fossa. Nodal involvement is more common with secondary lesions of the mandible. Metastatic lesions to the mandible are usually associated with symptoms related to the index cancer. Occasionally when the index cancer is silent, the manifestations are similar to primary lesions of the mandible.

27.3 Diagnosis and Evaluation

27.3.1 Biopsy

A punch biopsy from a representative area is usually adequate to establish a diagnosis. However, often this is not possible, more so with primary and metastatic lesions when the overlying mucosa is intact. Initial diagnosis of malignancy can be established by fine needle aspiration cytology (FNA) in these cases but often the material is inadequate to precisely identify the tumor type and grade. In such cases, FNA is followed by an incisional biopsy which preferably is performed intraorally. Biopsies done externally from the skin surface are to be avoided. The biopsy site on the mucosa must be excised at the time of definitive surgery. Bone lesions which do not have a soft tissue component may require a core needle biopsy using a Jamshidi (J) or other suitable needle.

27.3.2 Radiology

Appropriate imaging is important to define the extent of tumor spread as well as aid in narrowing the differential diagnosis when biopsy results are ambiguous. Conventional X-rays has been largely replaced by computed tomography (CT) scan/MRI. Panorex view is an excellent first step in the imaging of patients with a suspected pathology. CT or MRI provides detailed information with regards to the extent of mandibular involvement, extra-mandibular spread into surrounding tissues as well as metastasis to regional lymph nodes. CT scan is the investigation of choice for bony structure involvement and visualization of calcification which is pathognomonic of tumors such as osteogenic sarcoma. MRI scores over the CT scan in identifying subtle cortical erosion, medullary spread (bone marrow involvement), and extra-mandibular soft tissue extension of the tumor. Description of radiological features of each tumor is beyond the scope of this chapter but the type of bone destruction (osteolytic or osteoblastic), extent of disease (within and out of bone), periosteal/bony sclerotic reaction, medullary involvement, widening of mandibular canal, periodontal ligament space widening (Garringtons space), displacement of teeth, and pathological fracture should be noted as it may provide a clue toward possible tumor type as well as help plan appropriate surgical resection.

General rule of thumb is that benign tumors are radiolucent, often multiloculated, cystic, and expansile with scalloping edges. Benign cystic lesions are ellipsoidal, well demarcated, and radiolucent, usually unilocular with fine sclerotic rim. Malignant lesions in contrast are lytic with ill-defined margins, moth eaten, and associated with periosteal reaction.[29–31] Occasionally, malignant lesions are expansile and well demarcated. Metastatic lesions are usually lytic but at times sclerotic, more so when the primary is from breast and prostate cancers.

A lot of effort has been made to find the best imaging modality to detect mandibular invasion. A systematic review evaluating the diagnostic accuracy of common imaging modalities (CT, MRI, panoramic radiography, positron emission tomography [PET]/CT, and cone beam CT) in detecting bone invasion reported the sensitivity to be highest for MRI (94%), and specificity for CT, MRI, and cone bean CT to be uniformly high (100%).[32] In another systematic review, CT scan had reduced sensitivity (72%) and specificity (90%) in detecting mandibular invasion. However, these values improved in detection of mandibular medullary invasion with sensitivity and specificity of 81 and 85%, respectively.[33] The same group in another meta-analysis comparing the MRI and CT scan reported the MRI sensitivity to be higher and specificity to be lower.[34] Contrast-enhanced CT (CECT) underestimates bone erosion in presence of amalgam artifacts and presence of dentures leading to increase in false negatives. A recent systematic review and meta-analysis comparing CECT with MRI has shown no superiority of either modality in the detection of mandibular erosions.[35] Cone beam CT has been reported to have better sensitivity but lower specificity compared to CT and MRI for detection of bone erosion.[36] In practice, CECT is cost effective, efficient, and the first line investigation and combined with PET/CT enhances for accurate staging of advanced disease.

27.4 Anatomic Considerations/ Relevant Anatomy

The mandible consists of two parts—the body which is the horizontal curved portion and the ramus which is the perpendicular portion fused to the body at the angle. It is shaped like a bow, strongest at the center and weaker laterally at the angles. The mandible undergoes changes throughout the life of an individual. This characteristic along with its unique blood supply and ossification centers are important considerations at the time of surgery.

27.4.1 Blood Supply

The mandible has a dual blood supply. It is primarily supplied by the inferior alveolar artery which enters through the mandibular foramen and exits via the mental foramen as the mental artery. The other source of blood supply is from the overlying periosteum in addition to the nutrient vessels. The condylar region is supplied by vessels fom the temporalis muscle. Blood supply is periosteal in the body, both periosteal and endosteal at the angle and ramus, while the condyle is predominantly endosteal.[37] In elderly patients with atrophic mandible, the predominant supply is from the periosteum. While performing surgery it is advisable to preserve as much periosteum on the retained mandible as possible, more so for anterior lesions where blood supply is periosteal to prevent postoperative osteomyelitis/osteoradionecrosis. The periosteum is also a natural barrier to the spread of disease into the mandible from cancers of the adjoining oral cavity, and unnecessary sacrifice of the periosteum is best avoided.

27.4.2 Height of the Mandible and the Position of the Inferior Alveolar Nerve

The anterior mandible is higher by about 7 mm when compared to the posterior portion. The height of the alveolar bone changes throughout the life of a person, adjusting to loss of teeth which results in marked atrophy of alveolar process. A minimum of 1 cm of residual bone height is mandatory to maintain the integrity of the residual mandible following surgery as well as for placement of osseointegrated implants. Osseointegrated implants are therefore difficult following a marginal mandibulectomy. Success rates are higher with greater residual bone height.[38] Osteocutaneous fibula free flaps have been used by some in an attempt to augment the residual height of the mandible. The other option is the use of smaller (6–8 mm) implants post-marginal mandibulectomy.[39] In an atrophic mandible, the inferior alveolar nerve may be more superficial and may have to be repositioned to avoid damage by the implants. Several anatomical studies have shown that the mean distance of the mandibular canal from the lower border is about 7.6–10 mm while in edentulous mandibles it is higher by 3–6 mm.[40] The canal has also been found to be closer to the lingual aspect.

27.4.3 Ossification

The mandible is derived from Meckel's cartilage.[41] The ossification of the mandible starts early, at about the sixth to seventh week of intrauterine life. Intramembranous ossification is associated with development of the body and the ramus of the mandible. Endochondral ossification forms the symphyseal portion, condyle, coronoid process, and portion of the rami superior to the mandibular foramen. At birth the two halves of mandible are attached at the mental symphysis by a fibrous attachment which subsequently ossifies. It is important to know the location of the ossification centers. Preservation of these centers, if possible, is important to maintain normal growth of the remnant mandible when resection is necessary in the young.

27.4.4 Routes of Mandibular Involvement

Understanding the routes of spread of the cancers of the oral cavity that secondarily involves the mandible is important as it helps to offer conservative resections when feasible while ensuring oncological safety. There has been much work done in this regard over the years with seminal publications[42–45] since

Marchetta challenged the old dogma that lymphatics pass through the mandible from oral cancers and removal of the entire segment of bone was essential in every case.[42,43] The main route of spread into the mandible is now considered to be the point of abutment of the tumor with the mandible through Sharpey's fibers that are type I collagen bundles that bind the periosteum to the bone and form the potential route of spread. This usually is at the junction of the attached and reflected mucosa to the mandible. Should adequate clearance of the tumour be possible with the rim of bone for margin, conservative procedures are safe and should be considered. Large tumors where there are multiple points of abutment and post radiotherapy where periosteal integrity is compromised, opens up numerous routes of entry into the mandible making conservative procedures unsafe. In the edentulous patients where the vertical height is decreased the occlusal surface being in close proximity to the tumor is another potential route of tumor spread into the mandible. In a study focused predominantly on gingivobuccal sulcus cancers mandibular invasion was found to occur despite an intact periosteum in the dentate mandible. The potential route of spread in these cases was in all likelihood from the occlusal surface which is in contrast to invasion through the point of abutment reported for tongue and floor of mouth cancers by others.[46] Therefore, caution must be exercised in gingivobuccal sulcus tumors given this alternative route of spread into the mandible. When planning conservative procedures in these settings, occlusal surface spread of tumor must be taken into consideration. Preferential spread along the inferior alveolar nerve away from the main tumor front is rare unless the nerve is involved directly and the nerve need not be traced back to the base of the skull in patients in whom only the medullary canal is eroded by the tumor.[45] However, in adenoid cystic carcinomas this may not hold true given the preferential spread of this tumor along the nerve with skip lesions some distance away from the main tumor mass.

27.5 Surgical Considerations and Approaches

Surgery is the mainstay of treatment for malignant tumors of the mandible. There is no role for definitive radiotherapy except in cases of metastatic lesions when the aim is palliation and in the rare tumors of hemopoietic origin (leukemia, lymphoma). The extent of mandibular resection is dictated by the histology, extent of bone erosion, and soft tissue involvement of the disease.

Segmental mandibulectomy is excision of the mandibular segment in entirety. It is recommended when there is gross bone erosion or a primary tumor of the mandible. Often the soft tissue extent of the tumor necessitates resection of segment of the mandible larger than that dictated by bone erosion to ensure adequate clearance. Types of resection are based on the location of the segment resected—posterior segmental, hemimandible, extended hemimandible, arch-preserving, and middle third mandibulectomy. Multiple classification systems based on either defect created or reconstruction options have been proposed, none of which have gained universal acceptance. Jewers, Boyd (HCL), Urken, Brown, and Cordeiro are the commonly used classification systems.[47–51] Boyd HCL classification system is based on the bony defect created: lateral defect involving Hemimandible (H), Central defect (C), and Lateral defect not including condyle (L).[48] Urken classification incorporated soft tissue (mucosa, tongue, and cutaneous) and neurologic defects in addition to the bony defect.[49] Brown classification is unique in that it is based on the defect where the mandible is considered to have 4 corners, the 2 canines and 2 angles of the mandible.[50] This classification system is primarily used to help plan appropriate reconstruction. Recently Cordeiro divided the defects into three types depending upon anterior, hemimandible, and lateral segment.[51]

Conservative procedures are enucleation and marginal mandibulectomy. Enucleation is primarily performed for benign lesions and cysts of the mandible and is generally not advocated in cases of malignancy. Marginal mandibulectomy is a procedure where the portion of the mandible is removed while maintaining the continuity of the bone. It is not suitable for the primary tumors of the mandible or in the rare case of metastatic involvement where surgery is considered. It can be performed in the horizontal, vertical, or oblique planes (▶ Fig. 27.1). Horizontal marginal mandibulectomy is usually performed for buccal cancers while vertical is for tongue or floor of mouth lesions. Performing a pure vertical marginal mandibulectomy is technically difficult and the oblique marginal is a modification of the vertical procedure. Marginal mandibulectomy is usually performed to ensure adequate margins when soft tissue involvement is in close proximity to the mandible. It is not performed when the bone is involved except in the rare occasion of early superficial cortical erosion. A minimum margin of 5 mm on the bone should be aimed for to ensure oncologic safety. At least 1 cm of residual vertical height should be preserved to maintain the integrity of the mandible. Edentulous mandible (long-standing loss of dentition) and increasing age result in loss of vertical height precluding this procedure. Prior radiation makes the mandible susceptible to multiple routes of tumor entry making the procedure unsafe. Adequate clearance is difficult when inferior alveolar nerve is involved as the perineural spread can occur up to the base of skull. When paramandibular disease is present the procedure must be performed with caution as soft tissue clearance may be inadequate.

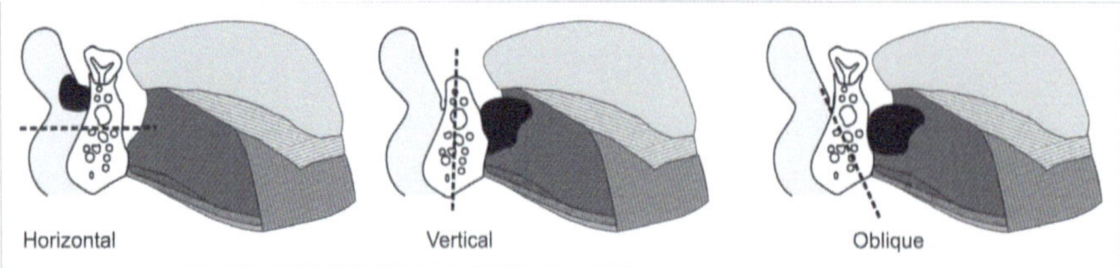

Fig. 27.1 Types of marginal mandibulectomy.

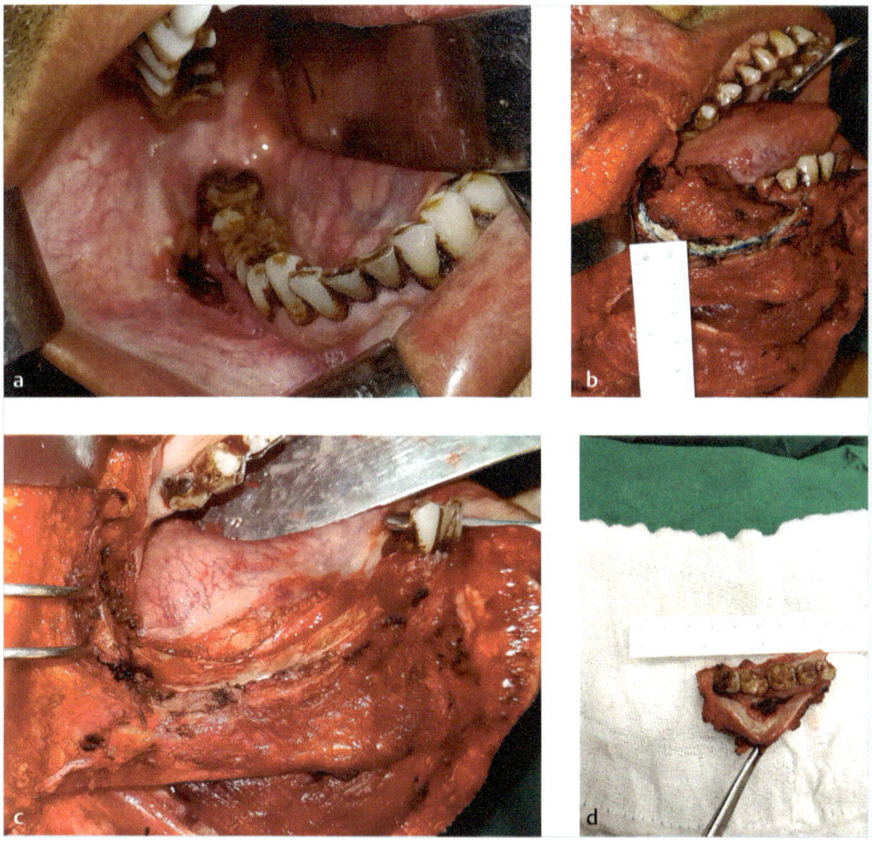

Fig. 27.2 Mandibulectomy in a gingivobuccal cancer. **(a)** Tumor juxtaposed to the mandible with no bone erosion. **(b)** The residual height of the mandible is > 1 cm. **(c)** Smooth curvilinear canoe shaped osteotomy avoiding sharp angled cuts. **(d)** Post-excision specimen with adequate soft tissue and bone margins.

Marginal mandibulectomy are usually performed via a cheek flap except for small lesions that are anteriorly placed which may be approached orally. The resection of the bone must be in a smooth curvilinear fashion, shaped like a canoe (▶ Fig. 27.2). Sharp right-angled osteotomies must be avoided as this may result in fracture due to mechanical stress of mastication. The marginal mandibulectomy can be performed involving any segment of the mandible. However, caution must be exercised for posteriorly located lesion when it is technically difficult and soft tissue clearance may be compromised.

Some authors advocate intraoperative periosteal stripping and frozen section examination in lieu of the marginal mandibulectomy procedure when the tumor is juxtaposed to the mandible with no bone erosion.[52] However, this procedure has not gained universal acceptance but may be performed in a select group of patients. Occlusal surface spread of tumor into the mandible for gingivobuccal cancers described earlier also renders this procedure oncologically unsafe.

27.5.1 Margin Assessment in Mandibular Surgery

Bone margin resection is dictated by soft tissue extension assessed intraoperatively as well as by extent of cortical and medullary bone involvement assessed via imaging. The bone needs to be decalcified before it lends itself suitable for sectioning and histopathological examination, and hence bony margin assessment in surgery by way of frozen section cannot be relied upon. During resection 1-cm margin is considered adequate. Sudden give of the bone without resistance at the time of osteotomy should prompt suspicion of bone involvement. Frozen section of curettaged bone marrow has been advocated by some as a surrogate to rule out involvement by disease.[53,54]

27.5.2 Reconstruction Principles

Microvascular surgery has revolutionized reconstruction making replacement of the entire mandible a possibility. Despite the advances, no reconstruction can match the function and cosmesis of the native mandible. Areas that are difficult to reconstruct or have implications on functional outcomes are condyle, angle, and genial complex. Others have emphasized on distinguishing between lateral and midline defects as well as the importance of canine. This highlights the fact that it is imperative to preserve as much of the mandible as possible, particularly the enumerated areas while safeguarding the oncologic principles of clearance. The other consideration that needs to be factored in while performing surgery on the mandible is that the integrity varies in different areas. The inferior border and the buccal cortex are stronger than the superior or the lingual cortex. Given that the mandible is subjected to shearing forces of mastication, this should be borne in mind when conservative procedures are performed.

It is prudent to outline areas of skin loss prior to planning incisions. The incision can then be modified to facilitate the intraoral excision as well as neck dissection. Adequate mucosal and soft tissue clearance is performed prior to establishing the bone osteotomies. As highlighted earlier, genial tubercle, angle, and condyle should be preserved if it does not compromise oncological safety. Given that bony replacement is the reconstruction choice following segmental resection the condyle and any part of ascending ramus, if saved, are useful to facilitate anchorage of the reconstructed segment. Should the condyle need to be resected the reconstructed bone is anchored in a cantilever fashion or prosthetic condyles may be used. Occasionally when free fibula flap is used the bone may be fashioned into an artificial condyle.

While performing the mandibular resection the osteotomy should be performed through the center of the tooth socket to ensure integrity and vitality of the adjoining tooth.

Appropriate mandibular reconstruction is imperative to rehabilitate patients post mandibulectomy. The goals of mandibular reconstruction are to establish the bone continuity, width, and height to restore the function and cosmesis. The reconstruction options are reviewed in depth in Chapter 28.

27.6 Surgical Sequelae

The main sequelae associated with surgery on the mandible is related to function and cosmesis. The extent to which these occur depends on the location, type of mandibular defect created, and amount of soft tissue excised.

27.6.1 Malocclusion

A common complication following surgery on the mandible is malocclusion due to loss of continuity causing the bone to deviate toward the defect. Masticatory function is compromised due to unilateral excision of muscles leading to an altered maxillomandibular relationship and loss of tooth to tooth contact. Proper alignment at reconstruction as well as the use of guide bite prosthesis postoperatively helps achieve appropriate mediolateral position and decrease the severity of this complication.

27.6.2 Aesthetic Considerations

Loss of mandibular segment is associated with severe cosmetic deformity with consequent impact on the patient's quality of life. This is encountered primarily in anterior defects compared to mandibular loss laterally and posteriorly. In anterior defects, suboptimal non-bony reconstruction would lead to the classical Andy Gump deformity. Lateral and posterior defects behind the mental foramen rarely cause disturbing cosmetic defects, but primarily result in occlusion and mastication problems.

27.6.3 Effects on Speech and Swallowing

This is apparent following middle third mandibular defects due to loss of the geniohyoid complex muscles. Loss of tongue support also affects speech, swallowing, and even oral competence at times. Excision of soft tissue or portions of the tongue compounds the problem.

27.6.4 Bone Necrosis/Orocutaneous Fistulae

Inadequate soft tissue replacement and bony coverage may lead to bone exposure, extrusion of plates, and orocutaneous fistulae. This may result in osteomyelitis of the exposed stump or in severe cases pathological fracture of the mandible.

Key Points

- Mandibular tumors can be primary from tissue native to the mandible, secondary as a consequence of invasion from surrounding oral cancer, or metastatic.
- Primary tumors that arise from the odontogenic apparatus are exceedingly rare. Osteogenic sarcoma is the commonest primary bone tumor of the mandible and is distinct from long bone OS in that these tumors are locally aggressive with low incidence of distant metastasis. Surgery with wide margins is the treatment of choice for these lesions. There is no role for conservative surgery in primary tumors of the mandible.
- Punch biopsy establishes diagnosis of secondary tumors in majority of cases as the mucosa is ulcerated. In contrast, in primary and metastatic tumors of the mandible, often submucosal and an incisional biopsy may be needed to obtain representative tissue for histology.
- CT scan is the investigation of choice to visualize cortical bone or tumor-induced bony changes. MRI is better for medullary bone visualization, nerve involvement, and soft tissue extent of the lesion.
- Surgery with tumor free margins is the treatment of choice for mandibular tumors. A margin of 1 cm is adequate for the majority of tumors. Adjuvant radiotherapy is indicated for close or positive margins, large tumors, and high-grade tumors. There is some literature to support adjuvant chemotherapy in OS but this is not backed by strong evidence and may therefore be recommended on a case by case basis.
- Microvascular free bone flap is the reconstruction of choice which can help decrease the sequelae of malocclusion, lack of cosmesis, and function as a consequence of loss of a mandibular segment.

References

[1] El-Naggar AK, Chan JKC, Grandis JR, Takata T, Slootweg PJ. WHO Classification of Head and Neck Tumours. 4th ed. Chapter 8 . 204–260 edn. Lyon: IARC; 2017

[2] Jing W, Xuan M, Lin Y, et al. Odontogenic tumours: a retrospective study of 1642 cases in a Chinese population. Int J Oral Maxillofac Surg. 2007; 36(1): 20–25

[3] Barnes L, Everson JW, Reichart P, Sidransky D, eds. World Health Organization Classification of Tumors: Pathology and Genetics of Head and Neck Tumors. Lyon: IARC Press; 2005

[4] Richardson MS, Müller S. Malignant odontogenic tumors: an update on selected tumors. Head Neck Pathol. 2014; 8(4):411–420

[5] Waldron CA, Mustoe TA. Primary intraosseous carcinoma of the mandible with probable origin in an odontogenic cyst. Oral Surg Oral Med Oral Pathol. 1989; 67(6):716–724

[6] Thomas G, Pandey M, Mathew A, et al. Primary intraosseous carcinoma of the jaw: pooled analysis of world literature and report of two new cases. Int J Oral Maxillofac Surg. 2001; 30(4):349–355

[7] Koutlas IG, Allen CM, Warnock GR, Manivel JC. Sclerosing odontogenic carcinoma: a previously unreported variant of a locally aggressive odontogenic

neoplasm without apparent metastatic potential. Am J Surg Pathol. 2008; 32 (11):1613–1619
[8] Eversole LR, Duffey DC, Powell NB. Clear cell odontogenic carcinoma: a clinicopathologic analysis. Arch Otolaryngol Head Neck Surg. 1995; 121(6): 685–689
[9] Bilodeau EA, Weinreb I, Antonescu CR, et al. Clear cell odontogenic carcinomas show EWSR1 rearrangements: a novel finding and a biological link to salivary clear cell carcinomas. Am J Surg Pathol. 2013; 37(7):1001–1005
[10] Del Corso G, Tardio ML, Gissi DB, Marchetti C, Montebugnoli L, Tarsitano A. Ki-67 and p53 expression in ghost cell odontogenic carcinoma: a case report and literature review. Oral Maxillofac Surg. 2015; 19(1):85–89
[11] Ledesma-Montes C, Gorlin RJ, Shear M, et al. International collaborative study on ghost cell odontogenic tumours: calcifying cystic odontogenic tumour, dentinogenic ghost cell tumour and ghost cell odontogenic carcinoma. J Oral Pathol Med. 2008; 37(5):302–308
[12] Soluk-Tekkeşin M, Wright JM. The World Health Organization classification of odontogenic lesions: a summary of the changes of the 2017 (4th) edition. Turk Patoloji Derg. 2018; 34(1)
[13] Kramer I, Pindborg J, Shear M. WHO International Histological Classification of Tumours: Histological Typing of Odontogenic Tumours. 2nd ed. Berlin: Springer-Verlag; 1992
[14] Stewart BD, Reith JD, Knapik JA, Chi AC. Bone- and cartilage-forming tumors and ewing sarcoma: an update with a gnathic emphasis. Head Neck Pathol. 2014; 8(4):454–462
[15] Amary MF, Bacsi K, Maggiani F, et al. IDH1 and IDH2 mutations are frequent events in central chondrosarcoma and central and periosteal chondromas but not in other mesenchymal tumours. J Pathol. 2011; 224(3):334–343
[16] Wang L, Motoi T, Khanin R, et al. Identification of a novel, recurrent HEY1-NCOA2 fusion in mesenchymal chondrosarcoma based on a genome-wide screen of exon-level expression data. Genes Chromosomes Cancer. 2012; 51 (2):127–139
[17] Kassir RR, Rassekh CH, Kinsella JB, Segas J, Carrau RL, Hokanson JA. Osteosarcoma of the head and neck: meta-analysis of nonrandomized studies. Laryngoscope. 1997; 107(1):56–61
[18] Smeele LE, Kostense PJ, van der Waal I, Snow GB. Effect of chemotherapy on survival of craniofacial osteosarcoma: a systematic review of 201 patients. J Clin Oncol. 1997; 15(1):363–367
[19] Thariat J, Julieron M, Brouchet A, et al. Osteosarcomas of the mandible: are they different from other tumor sites? Crit Rev Oncol Hematol. 2012; 82(3): 280–295
[20] Mendenhall WM, Fernandes R, Werning JW, Vaysberg M, Malyapa RS, Mendenhall NP. Head and neck osteosarcoma. Am J Otolaryngol. 2011; 32(6): 597–600
[21] Mücke T, Mitchell DA, Tannapfel A, Wolff KD, Loeffelbein DJ, Kanatas A. Effect of neoadjuvant treatment in the management of osteosarcomas of the head and neck. J Cancer Res Clin Oncol. 2014; 140(1):127–131
[22] Gilbert S, Tzadik A, Leonard G. Mandibular involvement by oral squamous cell carcinoma. Laryngoscope. 1986; 96(1):96–101
[23] Chen YK, Huang HC, Lin LM, Lin CC. Primary oral squamous cell carcinoma: an analysis of 703 cases in southern Taiwan. Oral Oncol. 1999; 35(2):173–179
[24] Amin MB, Edge SB, Greene FL, et al, eds. AJCC Cancer Staging Manual. 8th ed. New York: Springer; 2017
[25] Okura M, Yanamoto S, Umeda M, et al. Japan Oral Oncology Group. Prognostic and staging implications of mandibular canal invasion in lower gingival squamous cell carcinoma. Cancer Med. 2016; 5(12):3378–3385
[26] Zachariades N. Neoplasms metastatic to the mouth, jaws and surrounding tissues. J Craniomaxillofac Surg. 1989; 17(6):283–290
[27] Muttagi SS, Chaturvedi P, D'Cruz A, et al. Metastatic tumors to the jaw bones: retrospective analysis from an Indian tertiary referral center. Indian J Cancer. 2011; 48(2):234–239
[28] Hirshberg A, Berger R, Allon I, Kaplan I. Metastatic tumors to the jaws and mouth. Head Neck Pathol. 2014; 8(4):463–474
[29] Weber AL, Bui C, Kaneda T. Malignant tumors of the mandible and maxilla. Neuroimaging Clin N Am. 2003; 13(3):509–524
[30] Scholl RJ, Kellett HM, Neumann DP, Lurie AG. Cysts and cystic lesions of the mandible: clinical and radiologic-histopathologic review. Radiographics. 1999; 19(5):1107–1124
[31] Hofer B, Hardt N, Voegeli E, Kinser J. A diagnostic approach to lytic lesions of the mandible. Skeletal Radiol. 1985; 14(3):164–172
[32] Uribe S, Rojas LA, Rosas CF. Accuracy of imaging methods for detection of bone tissue invasion in patients with oral squamous cell carcinoma. Dentomaxillofac Radiol. 2013; 42(6):20120346
[33] Li C, Men Y, Yang W, Pan J, Sun J, Li L. Computed tomography for the diagnosis of mandibular invasion caused by head and neck cancer: a systematic review comparing contrast-enhanced and plain computed tomography. J Oral Maxillofac Surg. 2014; 72(8):1601–1615
[34] Li C, Yang W, Men Y, Wu F, Pan J, Li L. Magnetic resonance imaging for diagnosis of mandibular involvement from head and neck cancers: a systematic review and meta-analysis. PLoS One. 2014; 9(11):e112267
[35] Brandão Neto JS, Aires FT, Dedivitis RA, Matos LL, Cernea CR. Comparison between magnetic resonance and computed tomography in detecting mandibular invasion in oral cancer: a systematic review and diagnostic meta-analysis: MRI x CT in mandibular invasion. Oral Oncol. 2018; 78:114–118
[36] Linz C, Müller-Richter UD, Buck AK, et al. Performance of cone beam computed tomography in comparison to conventional imaging techniques for the detection of bone invasion in oral cancer. Int J Oral Maxillofac Surg. 2015; 44 (1):8–15
[37] Saka B, Wree A, Anders L, Gundlach KK. Experimental and comparative study of the blood supply to the mandibular cortex in Göttingen minipigs and in man. J Craniomaxillofac Surg. 2002; 30(4):219–225
[38] Juodzbalys G, Kubilius M. Clinical and radiological classification of the jawbone anatomy in endosseous dental implant treatment. J Oral Maxillofac Res. 2013; 4(2):e2
[39] Tutak M, Smektała T, Schneider K, Gołębiewska E, Sporniak-Tutak K. Short dental implants in reduced alveolar bone height: a review of the literature. Med Sci Monit. 2013; 19:1037–1042
[40] Kilic C, Kamburoğlu K, Ozen T, et al. The position of the mandibular canal and histologic feature of the inferior alveolar nerve. Clin Anat. 2010; 23(1):34–42
[41] Parada C, Chai Y. Mandible and tongue development. Curr Top Dev Biol. 2015; 115:31–58
[42] Marchetta FC, Sako K, Badillo J. Periosteal lymphatics of the mandible and intraoral carcinoma. Am J Surg. 1964; 108:505–507
[43] Marchetta FC, Sako K, Murphy JB. The periosteum of the mandible and intraoral carcinoma. Am J Surg. 1971; 122(6):711–713
[44] McGregor AD, MacDonald DG. Routes of entry of squamous cell carcinoma to the mandible. Head Neck Surg. 1988; 10(5):294–301
[45] Brown JS, Lowe D, Kalavrezos N, D'Souza J, Magennis P, Woolgar J. Patterns of invasion and routes of tumor entry into the mandible by oral squamous cell carcinoma. Head Neck. 2002; 24(4):370–383
[46] Chaukar DA, Dandekar M, Kane S, et al. Invasion of the mandible in gingivobuccal complex cancers: histopathological analysis of routes of tumour entry and correlation with preoperative assessment. Oral Oncol. 2018; 86:181–187
[47] Jewer DD, Boyd JB, Manktelow RT, et al. Orofacial and mandibular reconstruction with the iliac crest free flap: a review of 60 cases and a new method of classification. Plast Reconstr Surg. 1989; 84(3):391–403, discussion 404–405
[48] Boyd JB, Gullane PJ, Rotstein LE, Brown DH, Irish JC. Classification of mandibular defects. Plast Reconstr Surg. 1993; 92(7):1266–1275
[49] Urken ML, Weinberg H, Vickery C, Buchbinder D, Lawson W, Biller HF. Oromandibular reconstruction using microvascular composite free flaps. Report of 71 cases and a new classification scheme for bony, soft-tissue, and neurologic defects. Arch Otolaryngol Head Neck Surg. 1991; 117(7):733–744
[50] Brown JS, Barry C, Ho M, Shaw R. A new classification for mandibular defects after oncological resection. Lancet Oncol. 2016; 17(1):e23–e30
[51] Cordeiro PG, Henderson PW, Matros E. A 20-year experience with 202 segmental mandibulectomy defects: a defect classification system, algorithm for flap selection, and surgical outcomes. Plast Reconstr Surg. 2018; 141(4): 571e–581e
[52] Genden EM, Ferlito A, Silver CE, et al. Contemporary management of cancer of the oral cavity. Eur Arch Otorhinolaryngol. 2010; 267(7):1001–1017
[53] Wysluch A, Stricker I, Hölzle F, Wolff KD, Maurer P. Intraoperative evaluation of bony margins with frozen-section analysis and trephine drill extraction technique: a preliminary study. Head Neck. 2010; 32(11):1473–1478
[54] Bilodeau EA, Chiosea S. Oral squamous cell carcinoma with mandibular bone invasion: intraoperative evaluation of bone margins by routine frozen section. Head Neck Pathol. 2011; 5(3):216–220

28 Reconstruction of Mandibular Defects

Christopher Britt and Shaun C. Desai

Summary
The mandible is a horseshoe-shaped facial bone that has complex aesthetic, phonatory, masticatory, and swallowing functions. Reconstruction of the mandible is complex depending on the location of the defect, dentition of the patient, functional status, and medical status of the patient. Mandibular defects can be divided into segmental or marginal defects. Segmental defects can be divided into either anterior or lateral defects based on the mental nerve. Marginal defects are often reconstructed with soft tissue; however, segmental defects may require bony reconstruction, especially anteriorly. The most common free tissue options for bony reconstruction include fibula, scapula, iliac crest, and osteocutaneous forearm. Fibula flaps are the most commonly used flaps for mandibular reconstruction to date. When reconstructing the mandible with a bony flap, consideration should be given to plate selection, dental rehabilitation, and the need for virtual surgical planning (VSP), in select cases.

Keywords: mandible, mandibular, segemental, marginal, free tissue transfer, reconstruction, defect, bony, soft tissue, fibula, scapula, osteocutaneous

28.1 Introduction

The mandible is a horseshoe-shaped facial bone articulating with the skull that has muscular attachments corresponding to complex aesthetic, masticatory, phonatory, and swallowing functions, placing both rotational and translational forces on the bone itself.[1,2] Masticatory forces can be immense, with absolute maximal loading force of the mandible near 1,000 Newtons.[3] As a symmetric, rigid organ, the mandible needs proper alignment of bite in the dentulous patient to perform its function. In addition, the complex shape of the mandible lends itself to the framework of the shape of the lower one-third of the face and the transition of the head onto the neck. Because of the complex functional as well as aesthetic components, mandibular reconstruction is one of the most challenging in the head and neck surgery.[4]

28.2 Diagnosis and Evaluation

Discontinuities and mandibular loss are secondary to a myriad of different medical and traumatic conditions. In oral cavity cancer, the treatment of both the primary disease and sequelae may require reconstruction. Mandibular defects can be divided into partial (i.e., a marginal mandibulectomy) or segmental (**Flowchart 28.1**). In addition, the loss of mandible may include the loss of additional subsites of the oral cavity, facial skin, and/or oropharynx, with or without dental loss. A marginal mandibulectomy generally preserves a rim of bone, usually about 1 cm in vertical height.[5,6] These defects generally do not require reconstruction other than soft tissue coverage from any additional defect created. At certain centers, titanium reconstruction plates are placed to help prevent further pathologic fracture, although there is limited literature on this practice.

Segmental mandibular defects create a discontinuity of the bone with significant functional and aesthetic consequences and will be discussed herein in the rest of the chapter. Such consequences vary with the location and the size of the defect, which can be further classified as medial or lateral to the mental foramen. Defects that are medial to the mental foramen are classified as "anterior" defects, while "lateral" defects are those that are lateral to the mental foramen. Both types of segmental defects result in two independent segments that act accordingly to the remaining musculature.[7,8] Anterior defects result in the medial pterygoid pulling the remaining segments upward, posteriorly, and medially. The lip loses sensation and the tongue loses anterior support and is displaced posteriorly. These defects result in an appearance classically known as the *Andy Gump* deformity and generally require bony reconstruction for

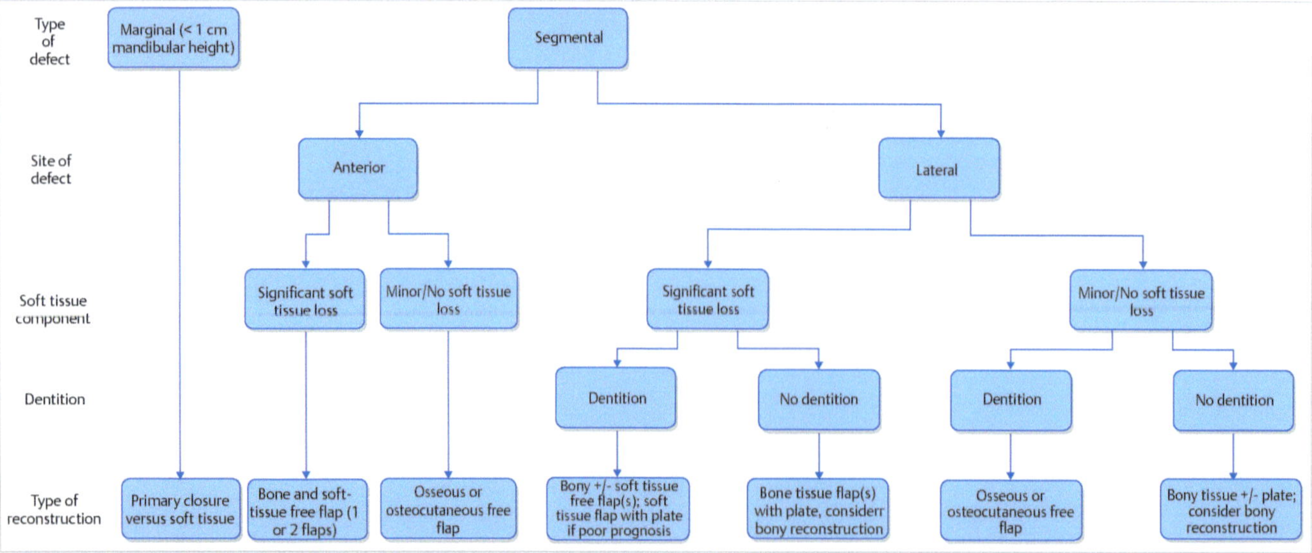

Flowchart 28.1 Algorithm for reconstruction of mandibular defects.

function and appearance. Lateral defects displace the mandible toward the site of the defect secondary to the unopposed actions of the ipsilateral muscles of mastication. Reconstruction of these defects is complex and involves considering soft tissue components of the resection, patient comorbidities and prognosis, and dental rehabilitation.[9] The current techniques for primary reconstruction of discontinuous mandibular defects will be reviewed in the following.

28.3 Anatomic Considerations/ Relevant Anatomy

The mandible itself is a continuous single bone that has two syndarthrotic joints present at each attachment in the glenoid fossa establishing a connection with the temporal bone. It consists of seven paired segments, namely, condyle, subcondyle, coronoid, ramus, angle, body, and parasymphysis, and one unpaired segment, namely, the symphysis (▶ Fig. 28.1 and ▶ Fig. 28.2). The body to the symphysis of the mandible contains two cortices with a narrow marrow space. The superior aspect of the body contains the alveolar process, which contains the dental sockets for teeth. The mandible extends toward the angle then rises to become the ramus and ends anteriorly with the coronoid and posteriorly with the condyle, the point of articulation. The mandibular notch separates the condyle and the coronoid.

The mandible derives its blood supply from the external carotid system which includes the facial artery, the lingual artery, and the inferior alveolar artery, which is a branch of the maxillary artery that enters through the mandibular foramina. The foramen also serves as the conduit for the inferior alveolar nerve, a branch of the mandibular nerve, which traverses the alveolar canal providing sensation to the lower dentition and to the chin and lower cheek through the mental nerve, which exits through the mental foramen. The mental foramen is approximately at the midway point of the mandible height and at the level of the second premolar. In an edentulous mandible, the mental foramen may be present at the upper border of the mandibular body.

Movement of the mandible is dependent on two opposing muscle groups (▶ Fig. 28.3a, b). The elevator group is composed of the masseter, medial pterygoid, and temporalis muscles. The masseter muscle inserts on the outer aspect of the ramus of the mandible, the medial pterygoid muscle inserts on the medial surface of the angle, and the temporalis muscle inserts on the coronoid. The depressor musculature consists of the geniohyoid, digastric, and mylohyoid muscles. The geniohyoid, digastric, and mylohyoid muscles all insert onto the medial aspect of

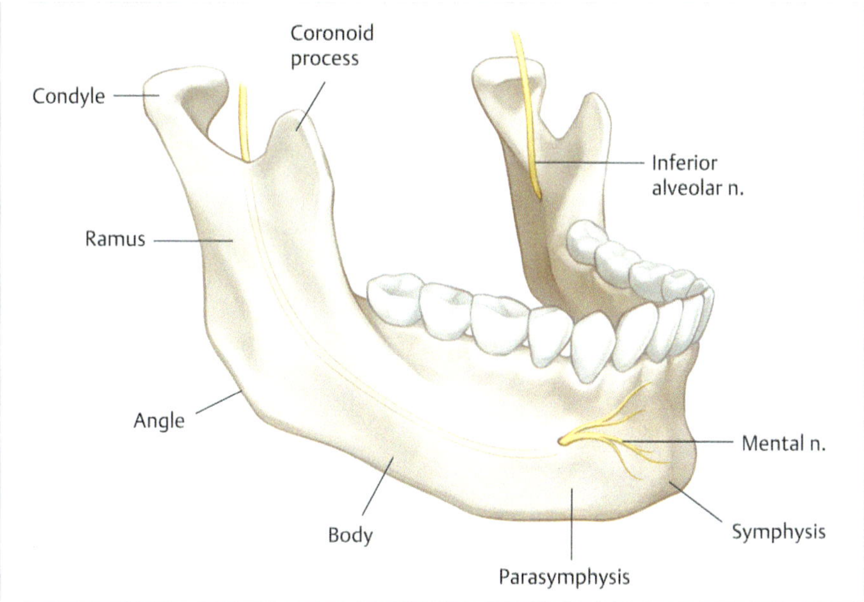

Fig. 28.1 Normal mandibular anatomy in an adult.

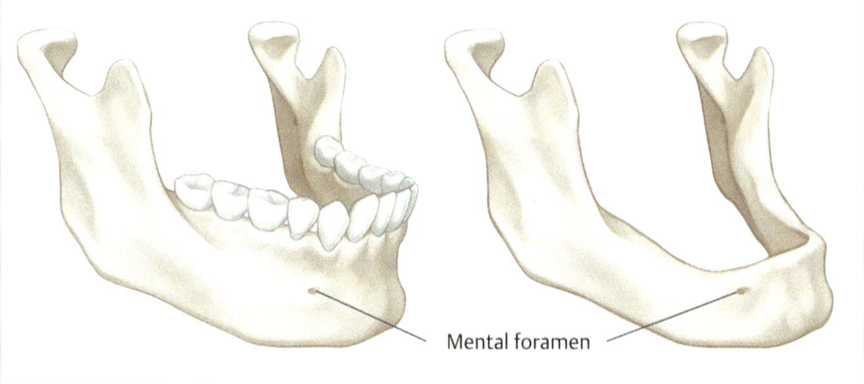

Fig. 28.2 Mandibular anatomy in the edentulous mandible.

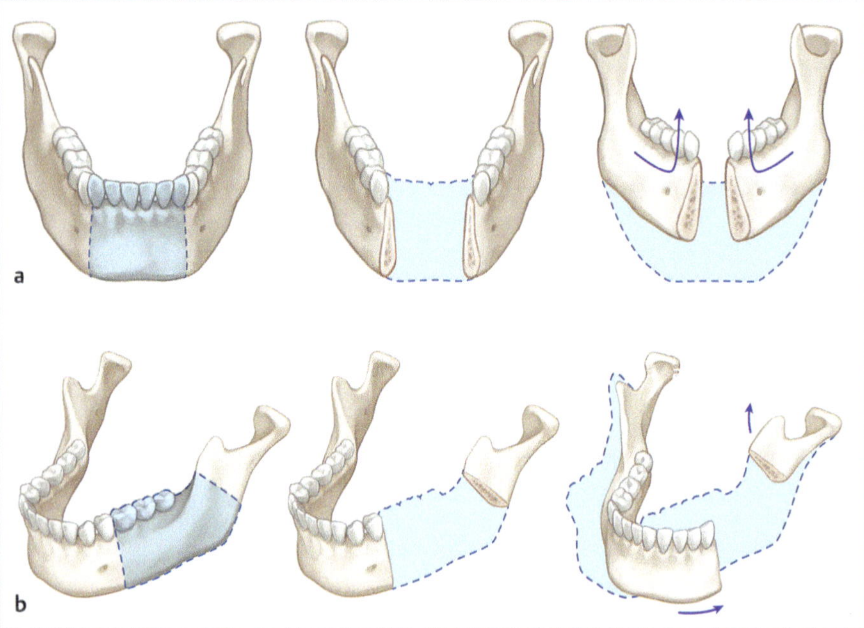

Fig. 28.3 (a, b) Muscles of mastication in anterior and lateral defects showing the various vectors of pull.

the symphyseal region onto the mylohyoid line, which extends along the internal aspect of the body. Lastly, the lateral pterygoid muscle inserts on the anterior condyle. Overall, the elevators are much stronger than the depressors and the masseter muscle is the strongest of the elevators. In the case of mandibular discontinuity, the forces of medial pterygoid muscles will dominate due to vector of force compared to other elevators.

28.4 Surgical Considerations and Approaches

As stated above, goals of reconstruction may differ depending on the extent of mandible and soft tissue envelope and concurrently resected oral cavity subsites. Defects discussed in this chapter will be limited to segmental defects and bony reconstruction. Ideally, mandibular reconstruction would allow for: (1) dental rehabilitation, and if possible, restoration of the natural occlusal relationship; (2) restoration of the natural shape of the mandible and aesthetic appearance; and (3) restoration of oral competency including sensation and motor function. As defects become more complex or as other factors, such as poor prognosis or patient health, become more prominent factors in decision-making, complete functional restoration may not be a realistic goal and thus more basic needs such as wound closure may become a higher priority. In addition, when considering the type of reconstruction, several factors must be considered including the quality of the tissue vascularization, previous surgery and/or radiation history, dental health, cancer prognosis, and general patient health.

28.5 Reconstruction Methods

Current reconstruction methods consist of five options: (1) primary closure with no plate ("letting it swing"), (2) reconstruction plate alone with no soft tissue or osseous flap, (3) reconstruction with a free bone graft and plate, (4) reconstruction with a soft tissue flap with or without plate reconstruction, or (5) reconstruction plate with an osseous free flap. Each of these strategies will be reviewed, including the advantages and disadvantages of each.

28.5.1 Bone Grafts

Mandibular reconstruction has its roots in bone grafting with the first bone graft being described as a canine xenograft in 1668 and the first autograft used in 1821.[1] Grafts became increasingly important during World War I due to the high prevalence of gunshot wounds.[10] These grafts were fixed with wire and long periods of intermaxillary fixation. The technique of free bone grafting improved in the 1970s with the use of rigid fixation using cortico-cancellous grafts from the iliac crest. Because revascularization takes place from the surrounding soft tissue, graft stability is of paramount importance. Currently, most free bone grafts are taken from the anterior or posterior iliac crest. Bone grafts as large as 5 cm can be used for mandibular reconstruction with acceptable results. Graft take is less likely with large soft tissue defects and previous radiation therapy precludes their use.[10] Free bone grafts should not be used with intraoral defects as the risk of infection, and thus graft failure, is high. For these reasons, the use of free bone grafts in cases of malignancy or postradiation osteonecrosis is limited.

28.5.2 Pedicled Flaps

Pedicled flaps were introduced in bony and soft tissue reconstruction in the 1970s. Conley reported on the use of the sternocleidomastoid flap with clavicle in 1972.[11] Demergasso and Piazza reported the first use of the trapezius osteomyocutaneous flap for mandibular reconstruction in 1979.[12] Cuono and Ariyan introduced the pectoralis major flap with the 5th or 6th rib in 1980.[13] These pedicled bone grafts have the advantage of not needing a skilled microsurgeon for reconstruction; however, their blood supply can be tenuous, and the bone quality

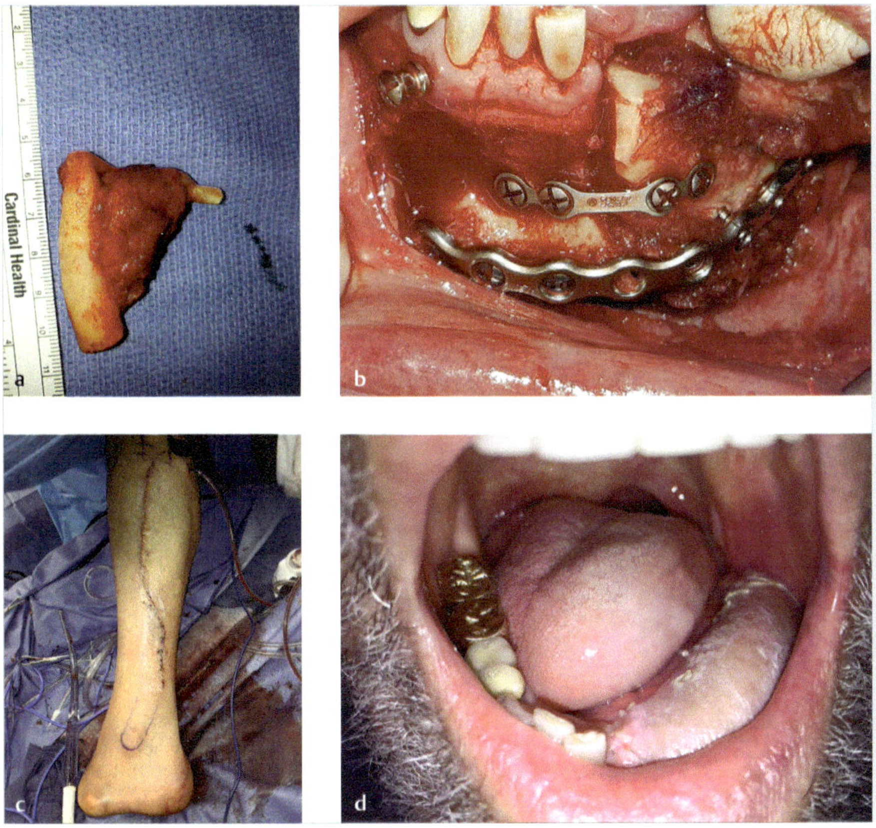

Fig. 28.4 Photo of a patient with left segmental mandibulectomy and fibula flap reconstruction. **(a)** Pathologic specimen after left segmental resection of mandible symphysis, parasymphysis, and body for squamous cell carcinoma. **(b)** Left fibula flap with angle segment 1 cm above inferior border to help improve vertical height in anticipation for dental implantation. **(c)** Left fibula flap donor site closed primarily with narrow skin paddle. **(d)** 1-month postoperative view of healthy skin paddle. Note the vertical height of the skin paddle in relation to the native teeth.

may be suboptimal. Survival of the bone graft in these instances has been reported to be as low as 50%.[14] In addition, these techniques can lead to poor cosmetic results.

Soft tissue flaps without bone are other options for reconstruction and much more commonly used. Myocutaneous pedicled flaps such as the pectoralis myocutaneous flap or the latissimus dorsi myocutaneous flap can be used with or without a plate for reconstruction of a lateral segmental defect in an edentulous patient. However, in anterior defects or in dentulous patients, soft tissue flaps with a plate are not advised given the high rate of extrusion and plate fracture, which can be as high as 38% at 10 months. In such circumstances, a vascularized osteocutaneous reconstruction is preferred. If this is not feasible, a vascularized soft tissue flap without a plate will likely lead to less complications in the segmental mandibulectomy defect in the dentulous patient as plate fracture rates are high (26.1%).[15] In an edentulous patient with poor prognosis, soft tissue reconstruction without a reconstruction plate for lateral defects is an option with rates of plate fracture at 5.9% and rates of extrusion at 8% if the soft tissue defect is overcorrected.[15]

28.5.3 Free Tissue Transfer

In the early 1990s, free tissue transfer became the dominant technique for reconstruction of segmental mandibular defects greater than 4–5 cm. Several options for reconstruction exist including a vascularized osteocutaneous fibula, osteocutaneous forearm, chimeric scapulae-based flaps, osteocutaneous anterolateral thigh flaps, and iliac crest flaps. These techniques are complex and involve the use of specialized surgeons and centers familiar with microvascular and flap monitoring techniques. However, these flaps have proven to be superior to soft tissue alone with respect to function and complication rate in particular clinical situations.[16,17]

The osteocutaneous fibula flap is the most common free tissue transfer used for mandibular reconstruction. This graft has significant bone quality, bone length up to 25 cm, excellent and reliable vascular pedicle, and minimal donor site morbidity. However, the vertical height of the bone is somewhat limited, and generally requires a technique to increase the height such as the "double-barrel" technique or placing the fibula 1 cm above the inferior mandibular border (▶ Fig. 28.4 a–d).[18–21] If this limitation cannot be satisfactorily ameliorated, then consideration of other osseous free tissue options is necessary. In addition, preoperative angiographic imaging of the lower extremities is often recommended because of anatomic variation. One such variation which exists in 5% of the population is *peronea arteria magna*, a condition where both the anterior and posterior tibial arteries are hypoplastic and a large dominant peroneal artery supplies the entire leg and foot. Another consideration for preoperative imaging is to determine if there is any vessel narrowing secondary to atherosclerotic disease in the peroneal vessels.[22,23]

Donor site morbidity in fibula free tissue can be minimized with careful consideration to a few axoms. Ankle stability is maintained on leaving at least 6 cm of bone on the distal aspect of the fibula. Plantar flexion is maintained with care to preserve the peroneus musculature and the peroneal nerve, proximally. The harvesting technique can be modified to include a skin paddle based on perforators from the peroneal artery system.

Perforators are more robust and can be more reliable when including a cuff of soleus and/or flexor hallucis longus muscle, and multiple paddles can be designed.[24,25] When harvesting a skin paddle, care should be taken to prevent compartment syndrome by closing the wound without any tension. Skin grafting can help prevent this, and Kim et al described skin grafting from the flap incision itself when used for mucosal defects to prevent secondary donor site morbidity.[26]

The iliac crest flap is based on the deep circumflex iliac artery and was initially popularized by Taylor and Urken. Advantages of this flap include an optimal vertical height to mimic native mandible and excellent bone quality for osseointegrated implantation.[27,28] However, the flap is limited by the thickness of the skin paddle, small pedicle length, and significant donor site morbidity including intractable pain, destabilization of the pelvic girdle, and abdominal herniation. While the advantages are significant, the morbidities related to this flap could be profound, limiting its popularity compared to fibula free tissue transfer.

The lateral border scapula flap is based on the circumflex scapular artery, which is part of the vasculature of the subscapular system. This flap can be harvested with several different subsystems which allows creation of a chimeric flap that can include cutaneous, muscle, and myo-osseous options making it ideal for complex defects with both intra- and extra-oral components.[29] The primary disadvantages include inadequate bone quality to support dental implants, relatively short pedicle, and difficulty in simultaneous harvest and ablation. Pedicle length can be increased using bone from the scapular tip, and modifications to harvesting technique can allow for simultaneous harvest.[30–32] Even so, limitations in bone quality and quantity make this a secondary option for many reconstructive surgeons.

The osteocutaneous radial forearm flap is another option that utilizes a well-known flap with a consistent soft tissue paddle, excellent pedicle length, and very reliable anatomy. Disadvantages of this flap include a limited quantity of thin bone of approximately 10–12 cm in total length, which portends to poor bone stock, and precludes the ability to place dental implants.[26,33,34] In addition, fracture risk of the radial bone increases with the amount of harvested bone and prophylactic plating can sometimes require specialized expertise. While this flap can be useful in edentulous patients or non-weight bearing defects such as the angle or ramus, its use for mandibular segmental reconstruction is not widespread due to the limited quantity of bone. Other options such as the anterolateral thigh osteocutaneous flap are described, but these techniques are less common and donor site morbidity such as pathologic fracture remains a serious concern.[35]

Plate Selection

Plate selection for mandibulectomy defects varies based on the type of reconstruction used. Currently, plates are constructed using titanium, a lightweight material that is rigid and stable. Complications from the use of a plate include short-term complications such as infection and exposure and long-term complications such as dehiscence, loss of fixation, fracture, and exposure.[36–38] Rates of exposure in patients with bony microvascular reconstruction are between 7 and 29% depending on the plate type used.[39–41] These complication rates will increase in patients who have a history of smoking or radiotherapy.[42]

Selection of hardware requires thorough planning and knowledge of the defect size, location, and reconstructive plan. In soft tissue reconstruction, large loadbearing plates, 2.0 mm or more, are used in reconstruction. In bony osseous free tissue reconstruction, loadbearing plates or smaller/mini-plates can be used to reconstruct gaps between osteotomies or flap and native mandible. Some advantages of smaller plates are that they are less obvious to palpation and less prone to extrusion.[39–43] Smaller plates allow the bone graft to carry the weight of the mandibular stresses, minimizing stress shielding and allowing for less bone reabsorption over time. If the patient undergoes dental implantation, smaller plates, especially mini-plates, would make planning more simplistic and can be performed even in a single stage.[43] One study demonstrated in a cadaveric model that nonlocking miniplate systems had noninferior strength compared to the strength of a single, larger plate.[44]

Dental Rehabilitation

In patients who have undergone bony reconstruction, patients oftentimes have an option for dental rehabilitation. These implants can result in improved mastication, appearance, and patient attitude, and there are few, if any, absolute contraindications.[45–47] Implants can perform well even with irradiation and succeed in 70–95% of patients.[48–51] However, implantation is costly and time consuming with average time for prosthetic rehabilitation averaging over 24 months.[52] As a result of these factors, unfortunately, few patients opt to undergo mandibular dental rehabilitation, even with bony reconstruction.

Several challenges exist related to placement of dental implants. Dental implant placement is intimately related to native dentition and placement of bony reconstruction. Currently, VSP has significantly improved implant placement and is significantly more accurate than free-hand insertion.[44,53,54] Positioning of free-tissue transfer can also make implant placement difficult. Most bony free tissue, with the exception of the iliac crest, will not have the height to cover the vertical distance of the native mandible.[55] Several techniques can correct this technique including additional bone grafting, double barreling of fibula flap, and distraction osteogenesis; however, they increase the complexity of the reconstruction.[49,50] Finally, soft tissue can create additional problems. Thickness of the surrounding soft tissue, mobility, scar contracture, and granulation around the implants can all pose problems to implant take. These require constant vigilance to avoid infection and multiple procedures are often indicated to control this soft tissue.[55,56]

Virtual Surgical Planning (VSP)

There are several challenges that exist when planning for reconstruction of a mandibular segmental defect. Generally, pre-plating of the defect is recommended prior to resection of the diseased segment to help maintain proper alignment and anatomic contour. If this is not possible secondary to large tumor burden laterally on the mandible, patients would need to be placed into mandibulomaxillary fixation (MMF) or external fixation prior to resection in order to maintain a proper dental occlusion. However, recent advances in technology now employ the use of stereolithographic modeling of the patent's mandible for reconstruction.[57] These models are created using computer-assisted design mirroring the contralateral mandible to create a model accurate to within 1 mm, which is then used to create a reconstruction plate. In addition, guides can be made to assist with creating osteotomies in the osseous free tissue to create the neomandible. While these models can save time during the operation and improve outcomes, they are expensive and require preoperative time for planning.

28.6 Perioperative Management

In preparation for surgery, it is ideal to have any patient who is to undergo reconstruction as medically optimized as possible both nutritionally and functionally; however, this is not always an option. Poor nutritional status is a significant risk factor for poor wound healing.[58,59] Preoperative imaging may also be important as in the case of the fibula free tissue transfer to ensure patency of the vasculature. In addition, speech and swallowing evaluations are necessary both pre- and postoperatively to ensure continued use of the upper digestive tract, if possible.

Intraoperatively, any intraoral communication will make bone grafting unfavorable due to infection. Consideration of reconstruction should follow the guidelines previously discussed in this chapter. If possible, plating should be done before the specimen is removed in the ablative portion of the case. When performing free tissue transfer, as much upfront preparation should be done as possible to minimize ischemia time, including the position and number of osteotomies. Chang et al found that ischemia time for fibula flaps of over 5 hours compared to all groups lead to a significantly higher chance of partial flap loss (45.5 versus 14.7%, $p = 0.02$) and complications (86 versus 56.9%, $p = 0.03$).[60]

Postoperatively, several complications can plague mandibular reconstruction. In patients undergoing free tissue transfer, elective tracheotomy is often performed to ensure airway patency during the immediate postoperative period. In select patients with isolated lateral defects, tracheotomy may be avoided in most circumstances.[61] Early postoperative complications include flap failure, wound dehiscence, infection, and donor site morbidity. Wound infection can be a devastating complication of mandibular reconstruction. Even with 48 hours of postoperative antibiotics, free tissue infection rate is around 8%.[62] Care must be taken to keep all wound dehiscence or fistulae clean with packing and antibiotics. Finally, in patients with free tissue transfer, complete flap failure is rare; however, partial flap failure is more common.[60] Diligent monitoring of the flap is required during the immediate postoperative course, and these cases should be handled in high volume centers with ancillary staff familiar with these complex cases.

28.7 Surgical Sequelae

Brown et al performed a systematic review of reports of mandibular reconstruction with vascularized bone flaps published between 1990 and 2015.[63] They identified 9,499 mandibular defects reconstructed with free tissue during this time. The most common reconstruction flap was the fibula with 6,178 (65%) flaps. Flap failure rate was highest for iliac crest at 6.2%, which was significantly different from all other flaps. This point was reiterated by Markiewicz et al who found a sevenfold higher rate of iliac crest free tissue failure compared to all other free tissue for mandibular reconstruction in a meta-analysis.[64] Osseointegrated reconstruction was significantly more common with iliac crest than with any other flap (44 versus 26%, $p < 0.001$). The analysis was somewhat limited by reporting differences. Indeed, Lonie et al found that the dental implant loss rate was three times higher for fibula flaps than iliac crest; iliac crest is recommended for body or angle defects and fibula for larger defects owing to its length.[65]

As mentioned above, there are instances where soft tissue reconstruction with a plate is preferred to bony reconstruction, which generally include poor cancer prognosis, frailty, and inadequate bony donor site. Overall, outcomes of the soft tissue reconstruction are inferior to bony reconstruction in deglutition and aesthetics, but similar in speech.[66] In patients in need of two flaps versus soft tissue and plate reconstruction alone, one study of 62 patients (31 in each group) found similar rates of plate exposure (5 years probability of 45.5 and 47.4% for the double-flap and single-flap groups, respectively, $p = 0.186$), but higher rates of wound infection and pain without bony reconstruction.[67]

Overall, patients who undergo free tissue reconstruction of the mandible have high overall functionality and acceptable quality of life scores, with one study suggesting that patients with fibula flaps may have the greatest quality of life.[68,69] However, late complications are common, with rates of osteoradionecrosis as high as 32% in patients who undergo adjuvant radiotherapy.[68] Depression is another issue which arise in patients with mandibular reconstruction. Patients with scapula flaps reconstruction have significantly higher rates of depression than patients with other reconstruction, although these patients tended to have large through-and-though defects.[69] Finally, oral rehabilitation outcomes have consistently shown that mastication is more difficult in patients who have undergone reconstruction of their mandible.[70,71] However, mastication is improved in patients with dental rehabilitation after mandibular reconstruction.[72,73]

Key Points

- The mandible is a horseshoe-shaped facial bone that has complex aesthetic, phonatory, masticatory, and swallowing functions.
- Mandibular defects can be divided into segmental or marginal defects. Segmental defects can be divided into either anterior or lateral defects based on the mental nerve.
- Reconstruction of the mandible is complex depending on the location of the defect, dentition of the patient, functional status, and medical status of the patient.
- The most common free tissue options include fibula, scapula, iliac crest, and osteocutaneous forearm. Fibula flaps are the most commonly used flaps for mandibular reconstruction to date.
- When reconstructing the mandible with a bony flap, consideration should be given to plate selection, dental rehabilitation, and the need for VSP, in select cases.

References

[1] Hjørting-Hansen E. Bone grafting to the jaws with special reference to reconstructive preprosthetic surgery: a historical review. Mund Kiefer Gesichtschir. 2002; 6(1):6–14

[2] Wong RC, Tideman H, Kin L, Merkx MA. Biomechanics of mandibular reconstruction: a review. Int J Oral Maxillofac Surg. 2010; 39(4):313–319

[3] Kuninori T, Tomonari H, Uehara S, Kitashima F, Yagi T, Miyawaki S. Influence of maximum bite force on jaw movement during gummy jelly mastication. J Oral Rehabil. 2014; 41(5):338–345

[4] Bak M, Jacobson AS, Buchbinder D, Urken ML. Contemporary reconstruction of the mandible. Oral Oncol. 2010; 46(2):71–76

[5] Barttelbort SW, Bahn SL, Ariyan SA. Rim mandibulectomy for cancer of the oral cavity. Am J Surg. 1987; 154(4):423–428

[6] Melugin MB, Oyen OJ, Indresano AT. The effect of rim mandibulectomy configuration and residual segment size on postoperative fracture risk: an in vitro study. J Oral Maxillofac Surg. 2001; 59(4):409–413, discussion 413–414

[7] Marchetta FC. Function and appearance following surgery for intraoral cancer. Clin Plast Surg. 1976; 3(3):471–479

[8] Cohen M, Schultz RC. Mandibular reconstruction. Clin Plast Surg. 1985; 12 (3):411–422

[9] Shnayder Y, Lin D, Desai SC, Nussenbaum B, Sand JP, Wax MK. Reconstruction of the lateral mandibular defect: a review and treatment algorithm. JAMA Facial Plast Surg. 2015; 17(5):367–373

[10] Goh BT, Lee S, Tideman H, Stoelinga PJ. Mandibular reconstruction in adults: a review. Int J Oral Maxillofac Surg. 2008; 37(7):597–605

[11] Conley J. Use of composite flaps containing bone for major repairs in the head and neck. Plast Reconstr Surg. 1972; 49(5):522–526

[12] Demergasso F, Piazza MV. Trapezius myocutaneous flap in reconstructive surgery for head and neck cancer: an original technique. Am J Surg. 1979; 138 (4):533–536

[13] Cuono CB, Ariyan S. Immediate reconstruction of a composite mandibular defect with a regional osteomusculocutaneous flap. Plast Reconstr Surg. 1980; 65(4):477–484

[14] Lawson W, Biller HF. Mandibular reconstruction: bone graft techniques. Otolaryngol Head Neck Surg. 1982; 90(5):589–594

[15] Chepeha DB, Teknos TN, Fung K, et al. Lateral oromandibular defect: when is it appropriate to use a bridging reconstruction plate combined with a soft tissue revascularized flap? Head Neck. 2008; 30(6):709–717

[16] Tsuchiya S, Nakatsuka T, Sakuraba M, et al. Clinical factors associated with postoperative complications and the functional outcome in mandibular reconstruction. Microsurgery. 2013; 33(5):337–341

[17] van Gemert JT, van Es RJ, Rosenberg AJ, van der Bilt A, Koole R, Van Cann EM. Free vascularized flaps for reconstruction of the mandible: complications, success, and dental rehabilitation. J Oral Maxillofac Surg. 2012; 70(7):1692–1698

[18] Wang WH, Zhu J, Deng JY, Xia B, Xu B. Three-dimensional virtual technology in reconstruction of mandibular defect including condyle using double-barrel vascularized fibula flap. J Craniomaxillofac Surg. 2013; 41(5):417–422

[19] Angiero F, Borloni R, Macchi M, Stefani M. Ameloblastic carcinoma of the maxillary sinus. Anticancer Res. 2008; 28(6B) 6b:3847–3854

[20] Gierek T, Majzel K, Slaska-Kaspera A, Gwóźdź-Jezierska M. [The results of surgical treatment of the facial nerve paralysis]. Otolaryngol Pol. 2007; 61(4): 383–386

[21] Ulkur E, Karagoz H, Kulahci Y, et al. One-and-a-half-barrel vascularized free fibular flap for the reconstruction of segmental mandibular defect. J Craniofac Surg. 2013; 24(2):e167–e169

[22] Lohan DG, Tomasian A, Krishnam M, Jonnala P, Blackwell KE, Finn JP. MR angiography of lower extremities at 3 T: presurgical planning of fibular free flap transfer for facial reconstruction. AJR Am J Roentgenol. 2008; 190(3): 770–776

[23] Rosson GD, Singh NK. Devascularizing complications of free fibula harvest: peronea arteria magna. J Reconstr Microsurg. 2005; 21(8):533–538

[24] Ghassemi A, Furkert R, Prescher A, et al. Variants of the supplying vessels of the vascularized iliac bone graft and their relationship to important surgical landmarks. Clin Anat. 2013; 26(4):509–521

[25] Thomas CV, McMillan KG, Jeynes P, Martin T, Parmar S. Use of a titanium cutting guide to assist with raising and inset of a DCIA free flap. Br J Oral Maxillofac Surg. 2013; 51(8):958–961

[26] Kim JH, Rosenthal EL, Ellis T, Wax MK. Radial forearm osteocutaneous free flap in maxillofacial and oromandibular reconstructions. Laryngoscope. 2005; 115(9):1697–1701

[27] Taylor GI, Townsend P, Corlett R. Superiority of the deep circumflex iliac vessels as the supply for free groin flaps: clinical work. Plast Reconstr Surg. 1979; 64(6):745–759

[28] Urken ML, Vickery C, Weinberg H, Buchbinder D, Lawson W, Biller HF. The internal oblique-iliac crest osseomyocutaneous free flap in oromandibular reconstruction: report of 20 cases. Arch Otolaryngol Head Neck Surg. 1989; 115(3):339–349

[29] Valentini V, Gennaro P, Torroni A, et al. Scapula free flap for complex maxillofacial reconstruction. J Craniofac Surg. 2009; 20(4):1125–1131

[30] Wagner AJ, Bayles SW. The angular branch: maximizing the scapular pedicle in head and neck reconstruction. Arch Otolaryngol Head Neck Surg. 2008; 134(11):1214–1217

[31] Clark JR, Vesely M, Gilbert R. Scapular angle osteomyogenous flap in postmaxillectomy reconstruction: defect, reconstruction, shoulder function, and harvest technique. Head Neck. 2008; 30(1):10–20

[32] Choi N, Cho J-K, Jang JY, Cho JK, Cho YS, Baek C-H. Scapular tip free flap for head and neck reconstruction. Clin Exp Otorhinolaryngol. 2015; 8(4):422–429

[33] Villaret DB, Futran NA. The indications and outcomes in the use of osteocutaneous radial forearm free flap. Head Neck. 2003; 25(6):475–481

[34] Waits CA, Toby EB, Girod DA, Tsue TT. Osteocutaneous radial forearm free flap: long-term radiographic evaluation of donor site morbidity after prophylactic plating of radius. J Reconstr Microsurg. 2007; 23(7):367–372

[35] Brody RM, Pandey NC, Bur AM, et al. Anterior lateral thigh osteomyocutaneous free flap reconstruction in the head and neck: the anterolateral thigh osteomyocutaneous femur bone flap. Head Neck. 2016; 38(12):1788–1793

[36] Maurer P, Eckert AW, Kriwalsky MS, Schubert J. Scope and limitations of methods of mandibular reconstruction: a long-term follow-up. Br J Oral Maxillofac Surg. 2010; 48(2):100–104

[37] Irish JC, Gullane PJ, Gilbert RW, Brown DH, Birt BD, Boyd JB. Primary mandibular reconstruction with the titanium hollow screw reconstruction plate: evaluation of 51 cases. Plast Reconstr Surg. 1995; 96(1):93–99

[38] Gullane PJ. Primary mandibular reconstruction: analysis of 64 cases and evaluation of interface radiation dosimetry on bridging plates. Laryngoscope. 1991; 101(6 Pt 2) Suppl 54:1–24

[39] Blackwell KE, Buchbinder D, Urken ML. Lateral mandibular reconstruction using soft-tissue free flaps and plates. Arch Otolaryngol Head Neck Surg. 1996; 122(6):672–678

[40] Klotch DW, Gal TJ, Gal RL. Assessment of plate use for mandibular reconstruction: has changing technology made a difference? Otolaryngol Head Neck Surg. 1999; 121(4):388–392

[41] Blackwell KE, Lacombe V. The bridging lateral mandibular reconstruction plate revisited. Arch Otolaryngol Head Neck Surg. 1999; 125(9): 988–993

[42] Ettl T, Driemel O, Dresp BV, Reichert TE, Reuther J, Pistner H. Feasibility of alloplastic mandibular reconstruction in patients following removal of oral squamous cell carcinoma. J Craniomaxillofac Surg. 2010; 38(5):350–354

[43] Shen YF, Rodriguez ED, Wei FC, Tsai CY, Chang YM. Aesthetic and functional mandibular reconstruction with immediate dental implants in a free fibular flap and a low-profile reconstruction plate: five-year follow-up. Ann Plast Surg. 2015; 74(4):442–446

[44] Trainotti S, Raith S, Kesting M, et al. Locking versus nonlocking plates in mandibular reconstruction with fibular graft—a biomechanical ex vivo study. Clin Oral Investig. 2014; 18(4):1291–1298

[45] Shaw RJ, Sutton AF, Cawood JI, et al. Oral rehabilitation after treatment for head and neck malignancy. Head Neck. 2005; 27(6):459–470

[46] Ferrari S, Copelli C, Bianchi B, et al. Rehabilitation with endosseous implants in fibula free-flap mandibular reconstruction: a case series of up to 10 years. J Craniomaxillofac Surg. 2013; 41(2):172–178

[47] Jacobsen C, Kruse A, Lübbers HT, et al. Is mandibular reconstruction using vascularized fibula flaps and dental implants a reasonable treatment? Clin Implant Dent Relat Res. 2014; 16(3):419–428

[48] Wu YQ, Huang W, Zhang ZY, Zhang ZY, Zhang CP, Sun J. Clinical outcome of dental implants placed in fibula-free flaps for orofacial reconstruction. Chin Med J (Engl). 2008; 121(19):1861–1865

[49] Wang F, Wu Y, Zhang C, Zhang Z. Dental implant performance in vertically distracted fibular grafts after mandibular reconstruction: a pilot series of 12 patients. Int J Oral Maxillofac Implants. 2013; 28(5):1311–1321

[50] Chenping Z, Min R, Liqun X, et al. Dental implant distractor combined with free fibular flap: a new design for simultaneous functional mandibular reconstruction. J Oral Maxillofac Surg. 2012; 70(11):2687–2700

[51] Parbo N, Murra NT, Andersen K, Buhl J, Kiil B, Nørholt SE. Outcome of partial mandibular reconstruction with fibula grafts and implant-supported prostheses. Int J Oral Maxillofac Surg. 2013; 42(11):1403–1408

[52] Adell R, Svensson B, Bågenholm T. Dental rehabilitation in 101 primarily reconstructed jaws after segmental resections—possibilities and problems: an 18-year study. J Craniomaxillofac Surg. 2008; 36(7):395–402

[53] Schepers RH, Raghoebar GM, Vissink A, et al. Fully 3-dimensional digitally planned reconstruction of a mandible with a free vascularized fibula and immediate placement of an implant-supported prosthetic construction. Head Neck. 2013; 35(4):E109–E114

[54] Nickenig HJ, Wichmann M, Hamel J, Schlegel KA, Eitner S. Evaluation of the difference in accuracy between implant placement by virtual planning data and surgical guide templates versus the conventional free-hand method—a combined in vivo-in vitro technique using cone-beam CT (Part II). J Craniomaxillofac Surg. 2010; 38(7):488–493

[55] Anne-Gaëlle B, Samuel S, Julie B, Renaud L, Pierre B. Dental implant placement after mandibular reconstruction by microvascular free fibula flap: current knowledge and remaining questions. Oral Oncol. 2011; 47(12):1099–1104

[56] Qu X, Zhang C, Yang W, Wang M. Deep circumflex iliac artery flap with osseointegrated implants for reconstruction of mandibular benign lesions: clinical experience of 33 cases. Ir J Med Sci. 2013; 182(3):493–498

[57] Zenga J, Nussenbaum B. Adjunctive use of medical modeling for head and neck reconstruction. Curr Opin Otolaryngol Head Neck Surg. 2013; 21(4): 335–343

[58] Girod DA, McCulloch TM, Tsue TT, Weymuller EA, Jr. Risk factors for complications in clean-contaminated head and neck surgical procedures. Head Neck. 1995; 17(1):7–13

[59] Arnold M, Barbul A. Nutrition and wound healing. Plast Reconstr Surg. 2006; 117(7) Suppl:42S–58S

[60] Chang SY, Huang JJ, Tsao CK, et al. Does ischemia time affect the outcome of free fibula flaps for head and neck reconstruction? A review of 116 cases. Plast Reconstr Surg. 2010; 126(6):1988–1995

[61] Lapis PN, DeLacure MD, Givi B. Factors in successful elimination of elective tracheotomy in mandibular reconstruction with microvascular tissue. JAMA Otolaryngol Head Neck Surg. 2016; 142(1):46–51

[62] Simons JP, Johnson JT, Yu VL, et al. The role of topical antibiotic prophylaxis in patients undergoing contaminated head and neck surgery with flap reconstruction. Laryngoscope. 2001; 111(2):329–335

[63] Brown JS, Lowe D, Kanatas A, Schache A. Mandibular reconstruction with vascularised bone flaps: a systematic review over 25 years. Br J Oral Maxillofac Surg. 2017; 55(2):113–126

[64] Markiewicz MR, Bell RB, Bui TG, et al. Survival of microvascular free flaps in mandibular reconstruction: a systematic review and meta-analysis. Microsurgery. 2015; 35(7):576–587

[65] Lonie S, Herle P, Paddle A, Pradhan N, Birch T, Shayan R. Mandibular reconstruction: meta-analysis of iliac- versus fibula-free flaps. ANZ J Surg. 2016; 86(5):337–342

[66] Mizukami T, Hyodo I, Fukamizu H, Mineta H. Reconstruction of lateral mandibular defect: a comparison of functional and aesthetic outcomes of bony reconstruction vs soft tissue reconstruction—long-term follow-up. Acta Otolaryngol. 2013; 133(12):1304–1310

[67] Offodile AC, II, Lin JA, Chang KP, et al. Anterolateral thigh flap combined with reconstruction plate versus double free flaps for composite mandibular reconstruction: a propensity score-matched study. Ann Surg Oncol. 2018; 25 (3):829–836

[68] Al-Hayder S, Elberg JJ, Charabi B. Clinical outcome and health-related quality-of-life following microsurgical reconstruction in patients with oral and oropharyngeal cancer. Acta Otolaryngol. 2017; 137(5):541–545

[69] Moubayed SP, L'Heureux-Lebeau B, Christopoulos A, et al. Osteocutaneous free flaps for mandibular reconstruction: systematic review of their frequency of use and a preliminary quality of life comparison. J Laryngol Otol. 2014; 128(12):1034–1043

[70] Zhu J, Yang Y, Li W. Assessment of quality of life and sociocultural aspects in patients with ameloblastoma after immediate mandibular reconstruction with a fibular free flap. Br J Oral Maxillofac Surg. 2014; 52(2):163–167

[71] Wan Q, Zwahlen RA, Cheng G, Li Z, Li Z. Influence of mandibular reconstruction on patients' health-related quality of life. J Oral Maxillofac Surg. 2011; 69 (6):1782–1791

[72] Mochizuki Y, Omura K, Harada H, Marukawa E, Shimamoto H, Tomioka H. Functional outcomes with dental prosthesis following simultaneous mandibulectomy and mandibular bone reconstruction. J Prosthodont Res. 2014; 58 (4):259–266

[73] Tang JA, Rieger JM, Wolfaardt JF. A review of functional outcomes related to prosthetic treatment after maxillary and mandibular reconstruction in patients with head and neck cancer. Int J Prosthodont. 2008; 21(4):337–354

29 Primary Malignancies of the Maxilla

Wayne Koch

Summary

Malignancies of the maxilla include squamous carcinoma and various salivary gland cancers. Various benign tumors also arise. The most common primary therapy is surgery including transoral and open approaches. Surgery of the palate impacts speech and swallowing, so treatment planning must include considerations for complete extirpation and rehabilitation. Neck node metastasis is common and must also be addressed. Multidisciplinary team approach is a key asset.

Keywords: maxillectomy, midfacial degloving, dental obturator, palatectomy

29.1 Introduction

Malignancy of the hard palate and maxillary alveolus is relatively uncommon. Several histologic types contribute to this group of patients. Surgery is the mainstay of treatment for most cancers in this area. Acceptable extirpation requires expertise in the complex anatomy, cosmetically acceptable surgical approaches, and options for reconstitution of the oral roof. Survival for early cases is good, and quality of life considerations take precedence for those individuals.

29.2 Epidemiology

Squamous carcinoma of the oral cavity roof may be associated with tobacco use, and is also more common in older individuals.[1] The minor salivary cancers have no obvious etiologic risk factors; while ameloblastoma of the maxilla is more common in women, the opposite pattern is seen in mandibular ameloblastoma.

29.3 Clinical Presentation

Squamous cancers of the oral cavity roof most frequently present as a non-healing ulceration or fungating friable carpet of mucosal irregularity (▶ Fig. 29.1). Loosened teeth may be another bellwether symptom. Slowly progressing bone distortion may be the presenting sign for ameloblastoma and other benign bony tumors of the maxilla (▶ Fig. 29.2). Minor salivary gland tumors may present as painless or painful submucosal swelling, particularly at the hard–soft palate junction near the palatine foramen. Other symptoms may include facial numbness (Vth nerve involvement) and diplopia.

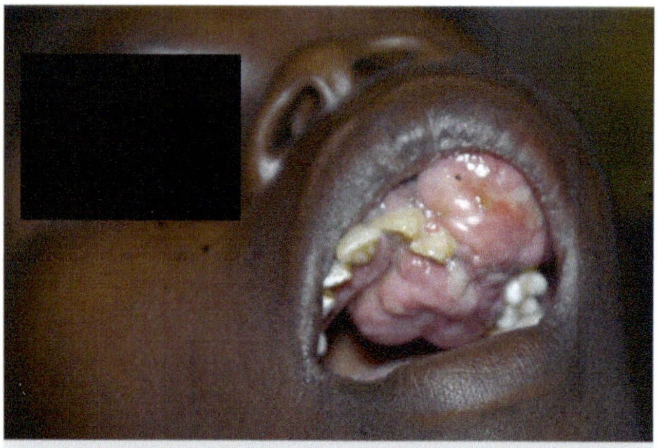

Fig. 29.1 Adenoid cystic carcinoma (ACC) of the hard palate presenting with fungating mass, loosened teeth, and pain.

29.3.1 Anatomy: Form and Function

The maxilla forms the roof of the oral cavity. Anatomically, it is a relatively simple composite structure, with mucosa covering bone with no substantial submucosal tissue, limited neurovascular structures, and no muscle. The presence of the maxillary dentition perforating the mucosa and anchored in the maxillary alveolus provides the chief topographic and functional complexity. Surfaces may be defined as bucco/labiogingival plate, vertically oriented and projecting upward from the dental structures, and intraoral plate with midline fusion ridge punctuating an otherwise smooth vault of bone. The mucosa of the buccogingival portion is "fixed" immediately above the dental crowns, and is then loose and thin above up to the sulcus of the lip/cheek. The intraoral portion of mucosa is quite thick epithelium, relatively impervious to abrasion and thermal injury by foodstuffs. Blood supply is chiefly comprised of the descending palatine artery, an end branch of the internal maxillary artery of the external carotid system. The neuronal component is purely sensory and provided by the trigeminal nerve, second division (V2). The 16 adult teeth are supplied by an alveolar branch from each side of V2 as well as an alveolar artery. Premolar and first molar teeth roots arise into the floor of the maxillary sinus skeleton, covered by the thin mucosa of the sinus. Canines and incisors are firmly embedded in cortical bone of the premaxilla and nasomaxillary buttress.

The function of the oral maxilla is principally to provide a platform for the oral preparatory phase of deglutition, holding the upper teeth firmly in place and allowing for containment of the oral bolus as it is shifted for the ongoing mastication cycle. The imperforated and bony hard palate keeps food and water out of the nasal cavity and maxillary

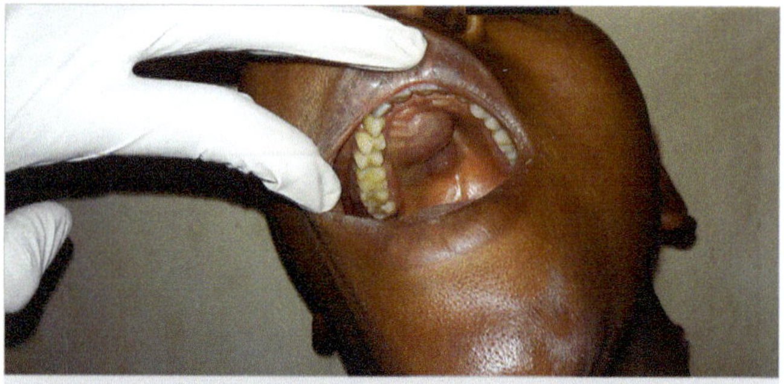

Fig. 29.2 Ameloblastoma presenting as bulging mass of hard palate without mucosal breakdown.

sinus cavity. A second -function of the hard palate is to form the roof of the oral cavity defining the resonating cavity giving voice its characteristic signature. Maintenance of the labiogingival sulcus is less important for the upper lip than the lower; however, the sulcus is important for cosmetic and dental hygiene reasons.

The maxilla can be divided into two or three structural components for the purposes of surgical and reconstructive planning: the hard palate, the maxillary alveolus, and the bucco/labial maxillary plate. Consideration of these anatomic segmentation may be useful for surgical planning.

29.3.2 Histology

Neoplasms of the oral maxilla are relatively rare, and quite eclectic in histology. While the title of this chapter indicates emphasis on malignancy, benign tumors also arise on the maxilla and present with similar treatment, surgical, and reconstructive challenges. As we have seen, the maxilla is a simple structure comprising bone, teeth, mucosa, and submucosa that contains minor salivary glands in the dense well-vascularized stroma. The neoplasms, therefore, may be of bony, dental, mucosal, and minor salivary gland origin.

Benign tumors of the maxilla include minor salivary gland pleomorphic and monomorphic adenomas, dentigerous lesions including ameloblastoma, bony lesions including fibrous dysplasia, and osteomas. The malignant neoplasms arising on the oral surfaces of the maxilla include squamous cell carcinoma (SCC), minor salivary malignancies (mucoepidermoid, adenoid cystic, adenocarcinoma), and osteosarcoma. Of these, only SCC has a well-established risk profile, being substantially more common in the setting of tobacco abuse, including such activities as inverse smoking (placing the lit end of the cigarette within the mouth). In settings where tobacco use is rare, the other cancer histologies unrelated to known risk factors may comprise a relatively higher proportion of tumors.

The rate of ameloblastoma is four times higher in the mandible than the maxilla, with 60% of maxillary ameloblastomas arising in women. It is important to properly assess the extent of the tumor and achieve complete removal with adjacent normal bone as maxillary ameloblastomas can easily recur high in the skull base and endanger vital structures. Margins of 10–15 mm of normal bone are recommended. The retromaxillary region is particularly difficult to access, requiring a lateral approach through the temporalis muscle region.[2]

Sarcomas of the head and neck are located in the maxilla and palate in 13% of cases as per the Head and Neck Sarcoma Registry.[3] Survival rates are good for chondrosarcoma and dermatofibrosarcoma, but poor (< 50% at 5 years) for osteosarcoma, angiosarcoma, and rhabdomyosarcoma. The hard palate is the most common subsite in the oral cavity for adenoid cystic carcinoma (ACC), accounting for 41% of the 1,066 ACC patients in the Surveillance, Epidemiology, and End Results (SEER) review of Dubal. (Dubal) Prognosis for ACC must take into account late recurrences after several decades. The author has followed several patients who developed a mixture of squamous carcinoma and persistent ACC coexisting in the maxillary resection bed 15–20 years after surgery followed by radiation therapy. In these cases, the squamous portion may be attributable to radiation-induced malignancy.

29.3.3 Radiographic Imaging

Documentation of bone destruction is a key goal of radiographic workup of maxillary alveolar and palatal cancers. Minor erosion of the hard palate may be difficult to ascertain with confidence as the bone of the palate has some natural irregularity. Dental films can be helpful in showing minor erosion in the bone surrounding maxillary teeth. CT imaging showing clear bone erosion is indicative of malignant disease along with extension into the pterygopalatine fossa and calcifications within the tumor.[4] The variable intensity of soft tissue demonstrable by MRI can help in distinguishing between tumor and surrounding paranasal sinus inflammation, and may help in focusing attention on certain histologic classes. ACC and B cell lymphomas are associated with homogenous signal intensity while other tumors are more heterogeneous. Post-contrast studies can help further delineate the extent of tumor infiltration.[5]

29.4 Treatment

For the vast majority of maxillary tumors, surgery is the mainstay of primary therapy. In part, this is due to the challenges of treating dental tissues directly with primary radiation therapy, particularly the maxilla with its limited soft tissue coverage. Risk of osteoradionecrosis is high when primary radiation is directed at these tissues. In addition, the relatively easy access to the oral cavity through transoral approach allows for direct surgical extirpation.

Tumor extirpation must be accomplished with adequate margins to provide the best opportunity for local control without compromise to function that cannot be managed to re-establish acceptable quality of life. The degree and approach to ablative surgery of the maxilla thus can be highly individualized based on detailed understanding of the complex three-dimensional structure to be addressed. Of course, margins are also required in all dimensions, taking into account complex saddle relationships that are difficult to conceptualize, orient, and catalogue. Exposure must also take into account the instruments such as drills and osteotomes in case they are needed to make bone cuts later. Surgical approach must permit adequate exposure of critical structures with care taken for final cosmesis after closure. The method of reconstruction that is planned will also factor into the choice of approach for extirpation. Truitt and coauthors have categorized surgical management of hard palate malignancies as consisting of alveolectomy, palatectomy, and infrastructure maxillectomy, all feasible through the oral aperature.[6]

Structures that are of cosmetic and functional importance must be considered individually to determine if sacrifice is necessary, and if so, how the loss of these will be addressed. Hard palate and dental tissues that allow for mastication and prevent sinonasal penetration can be maintained in some cases. Partial maxillectomy with preservation and primary repair of the hard palate mucosa has been described for highly select tumors of the maxilla.[7] This is most feasible for benign bony lesions and sinonasal cancers. Midface appearance is not altered by removal of bone from the canine fossa, but complete removal of the maxillary–nasal and/or maxillary–zygomatic buttresses will result in change in external contour. Sacrifice of the infraorbital nerve will result in midfacial numbness. Sacrifice of the anterior midline maxilla supporting the nasal vomer and septum can cause tip collapse. Orbital floor and rim are critical to both appearance of the orbit as well as ocular function.

Surgical approach may be divided into transoral and transfacial options and may be supplemented with endoscopic endonasal or intrasinus visualization. The midfacial degloving approach allows for maximal extension of transoral exposure (▶ Fig. 29.3, ▶ Fig. 29.4, ▶ Fig. 29.5, ▶ Fig. 29.6). A variety of facial incisions have been designed to permit exposure with maintenance of acceptable cosmesis. These incisions utilize shadows, creases and grooves, or corners to allow scar to hide or blend while preserving anatomical subunits, muscular continuity and function, and sensation as much as possible. In general, tumors that approach the orbital rim, lacrimal sac, medial canthus, or anterior ethmoid/frontal recess are likely to require a transfacial component. Facial incisions can split the upper lip in midline or along a filtrum ridge with acceptable function and appearance after repair. A group of oral maxillofacial surgeons from China recently reported satisfactory exposure and cosmesis using a lateral lip-splitting approach for access to the maxilla. They maintain that "most of the 36 patients thought their results were good or fair."[8]

The ideal of en bloc resection of the specimen (▶ Fig. 29.7 and ▶ Fig. 29.8) may not always be feasible and should not be prioritized over obtaining adequate margins with acceptable control of hemorrhage. Removal of portions of the specimen sequentially requires that the surgeon keep in mind the original and evolving relationships of tumor and normal borders so as not to miss a component of tumor, while communicating clearly with the pathologist as to the true margin edges for sampling and analysis. This approach also requires attention to integrity of thorough communication and reporting of margins between the surgeon and pathologist.

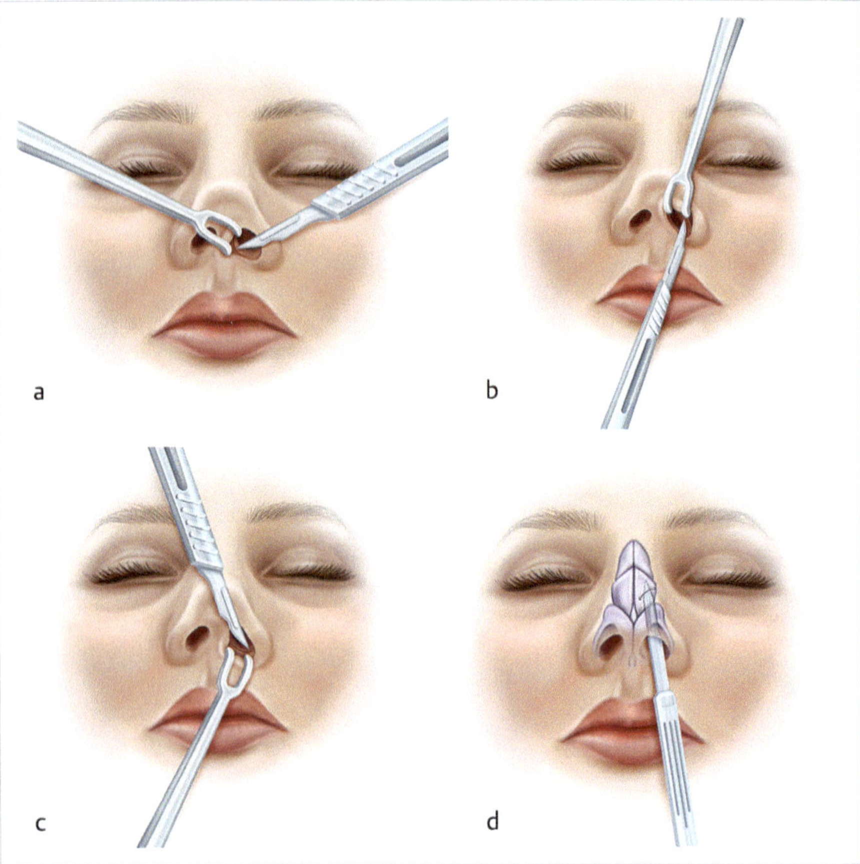

Fig. 29.3 Midfacial degloving begins with circumferential endonasal incisions and elevation of nasal dorsal soft tissue. Infiltration of lidocaine with epinephrine reduces bleeding. A transfixion incision between the lower lateral and septal cartilages **(a)** is connected to an incision just below the upper lateral cartilage **(b)** and completed with incisions in the pyriform aperture and nasal floor **(c)**. Blunt elevation of soft tissue from the nasal dorsum through the incision in the nasal dome and over the upper lateral cartilage frees the dorsal soft tissue on both sides **(d)**.

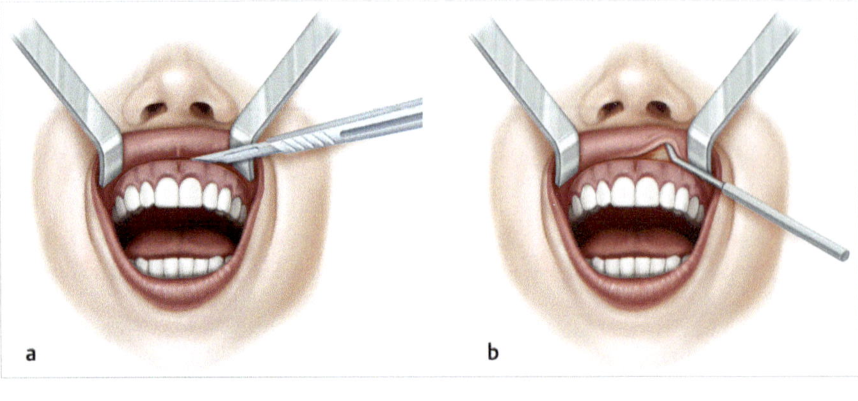

Fig. 29.4 **(a)** Midfacial degloving incisions continue with sublabial incisions above the fixed gingiva from zygoma to zygoma. **(b)** Elevation into the canine fossa and nasal floor incisions begins the elevation of cheek and nasal soft tissues as a unit.

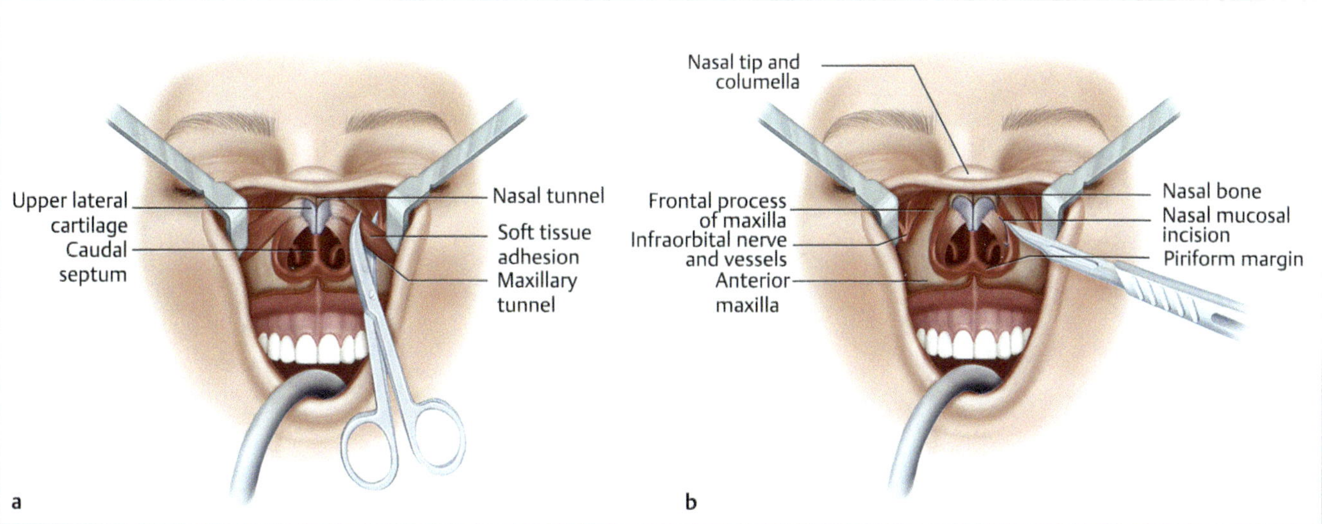

Fig. 29.5 **(a)** Midfacial degloving continues with elevation of soft tissues from canine fossa to nasal dorsum with sharp separation of muscle and cheek submucosa along pyriform incision up and over the dorsum. **(b)** This shows the full exposure of maxillary skeleton at completion of midfacial degloving approach.

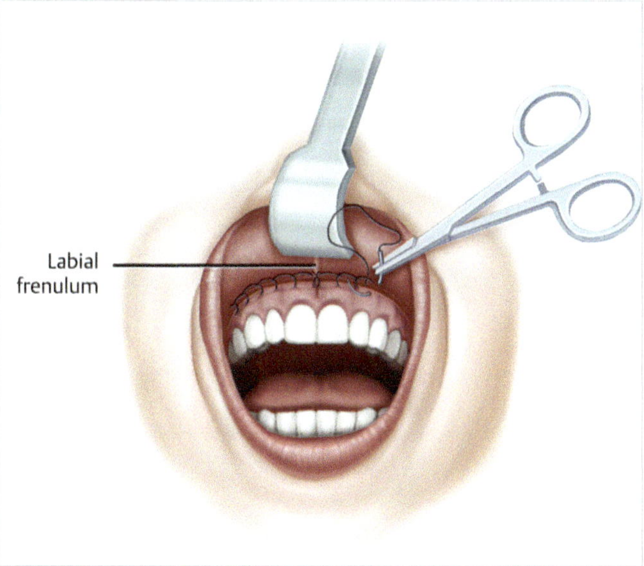

Fig. 29.6 Suture repair of midfacial degloving incisions at conclusion of resection.

Hemostasis is a challenge in maxillectomy surgery. The deep positioning of the internal maxillary artery branches necessitates that some bone cuts be made before direct ligation of the distal end is possible. The facial tissues have a very rich blood supply, and so blood loss must be anticipated and prepared for both mentally and practically with blood replacement readily available. Preparation of soft tissues where bleeding may be diminished with vasoconstrictive local injection should be undertaken as much as possible before beginning the osteotomies. Once bleeding begins deep within the bony architecture of the progressively freed maxillary box, it is best to quickly finish the bone cuts without attempts to stop all bleeding in order to attain access to the internal maxillary artery with expediency. Tying off the internal maxillary artery as it branches from the external carotid in the neck or preoperative endovascular embolization may be useful in extraordinary cases of highly vascular tumors. Local injection into the descending palatine foramen of the palate, the posterior aspect of the inferior meatus of the nose where the sphenopalatine artery is located, and in oral and nasal mucosa is also recommended.

29.4.1 Repair

After tumor has been removed, the defect between oral cavity and nose and sinus cavities must be addressed. While it is not life-threatening to experience sinonasal reflux of foods and liquids, this is uncomfortable and unlikely to be acceptable to most individuals if occurring in any quantity. Options for immediate management include gauze packing, placement of temporary obturator, or immediate flap reconstruction. The latter option is the subject of a separate chapter and will not be discussed here. Vaseline and antibiotic-impregnated gauze packing can be conformed to the sinonasal defect and suspended in place with a "spider web" of silk suture placed around the perimeter of the defect. This allows immediate oral alimentation with minimal discomfort while the packing is in place. However, packing must eventually be removed as it is a nidus for bacteria and debris accumulation. We generally leave the packing for 5 to 7 days, during which time prophylactic oral antibiotic is provided. When packing is removed, a further measure for managing the defect must be in view. A quick and inexpensive alternative to gauze packing is the use of comformable thermoplastic (Aquaplast) substance[9] which can be conformed to the remaining skeletal and dental elements, and suspended with wire to the zygoma or with suture to soft tissue. If a dental prosthodontist is part of the team, a more formal obturator may be used. The prosthesis can be fashioned before surgery by taking impressions and planning with the ablative surgeon on how much alveolus and dentition will remain for securing the obturator.

The temporary obturator is then adjusted with soft quick-setting material to fill the soft tissue defect placed

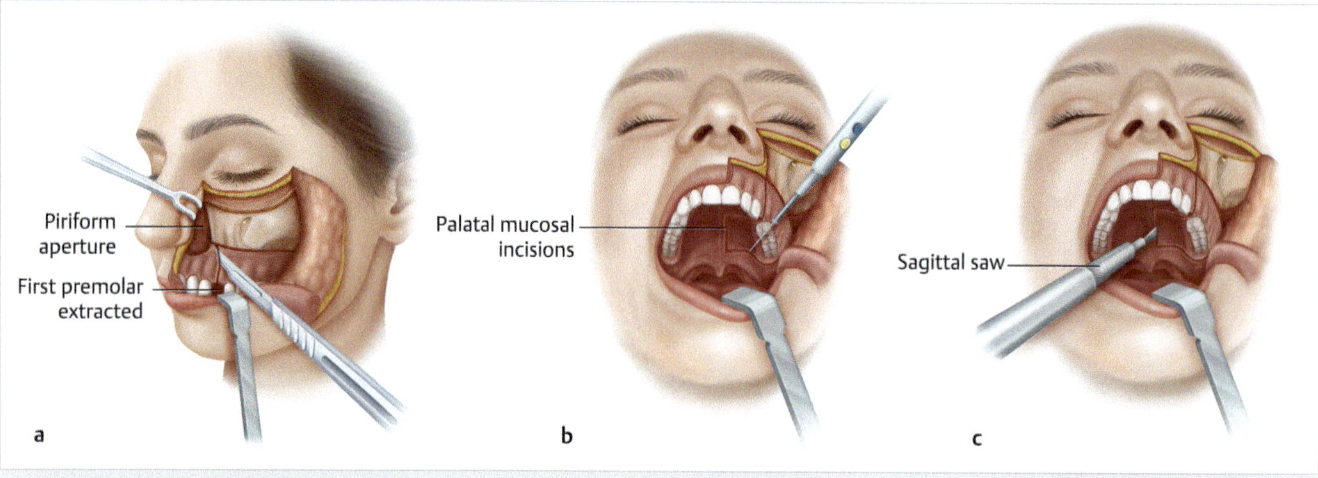

Fig. 29.7 Exposure of hemimaxilla via facial (Weber-Furgeson) incision with planned saw and bovie cuts across bony alveolus **(a)**, palate and retromaxillary soft tissues **(b)**, and palate bone cuts **(c)**.

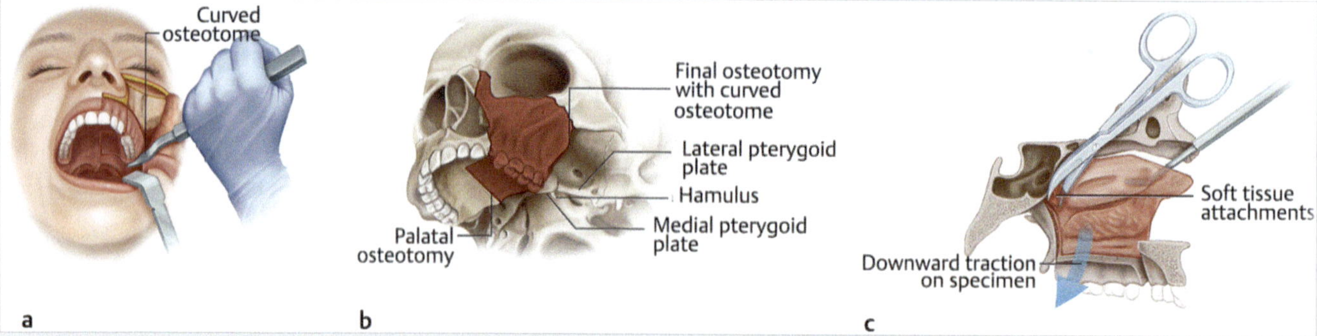

Fig. 29.8 Osteotome separation of pterygoid plate at posterior extent of hemimaxillectomy **(a)** completes the bone cuts isolating the surgical resection specimen **(b)**. Lateral nasal wall cuts can be completed with scissors through ethmoid sinus and maxillary fontanelle **(c)**.

intraoperatively. The obturator is then clipped to remaining teeth with clasps incorporated into its design. Wires to bony elements such as pterygoid plates or zygoma, or lag screws to remaining hard palate and vomer complete the fixation. After 1–2 weeks, the obturator is removed and a series of adjustments made by the prosthodontist for comfort and fixing the seal of the device. Fabrication of the final obturator is postponed until the cavity has had time to mature and reach its final endpoint of shape and size. If postoperative radiation is indicated, the fabrication of the final obturator is not recommended until at least 3 months after the completion of radiation.

Placement of a split-thickness skin graft on the raw inner surface of the cheek which remains after sublabial or transfacial incisions before placing the obturator helps prevent cheek and lip contraction with a "snarl" deformity (▶ Fig. 29.9). This also may help with patient comfort during obturator adjustment.

29.4.2 Management of Neck

Numerous articles published in the last decade make the point that nodal metastasis from SCC of the hard palate occurs stage for stage to about the same extent as occurs from other oral cavity sites. Most authors maintain that this observation is contrary to the prevailing sense of risk held by clinicians who judge metastases to be less likely to come from a roof of mouth primary. Lin and coauthors used the SEER database to analyze 715 hard palate and maxillary alveolar cancer patients and found the prevalence of nodal metastasis to be similar to other primary sites in the head and neck.[10] Since palate cancers can often be resected without an incision in the neck, there is less likelihood that neck dissection would be done regardless of T stage, as may be the case for other tumors in the oral cavity and oropharynx. Even with free flap reconstruction, the vascular anastomosis may be done using facial or superficial temporal vessels through small perifacial incisions that do not obviate concurrent neck dissection.

Os et al reported results of 114 patients with oral maxillary SCC and clinically N0 necks in the Netherlands. Of these, 26% developed neck metastases during the follow-up period. The regional metastases were operable in most (85%) cases, leading the authors to opine that "watchful waiting was feasible in this cohort."[11] Taking the alternate tack, Givi and coauthors in North America reported results for 199 clinically N0 maxillary alveolus/hard palate cancer patients. Elective neck dissection was done in 42 (21%) with cancer identified in 12 (29%). This group who had elective neck surgery experienced a lower rate of subsequent neck recurrence and better 5-year and overall survivals, leading the authors to recommend elective neck dissection at the time of primary therapy in advanced T stage cases.[12] Simental, Brown, and Koshkareva and coauthors all agree that selective neck dissection is indicated based on reports of smaller USA clinical series of maxillary oral SCC.[13–15]

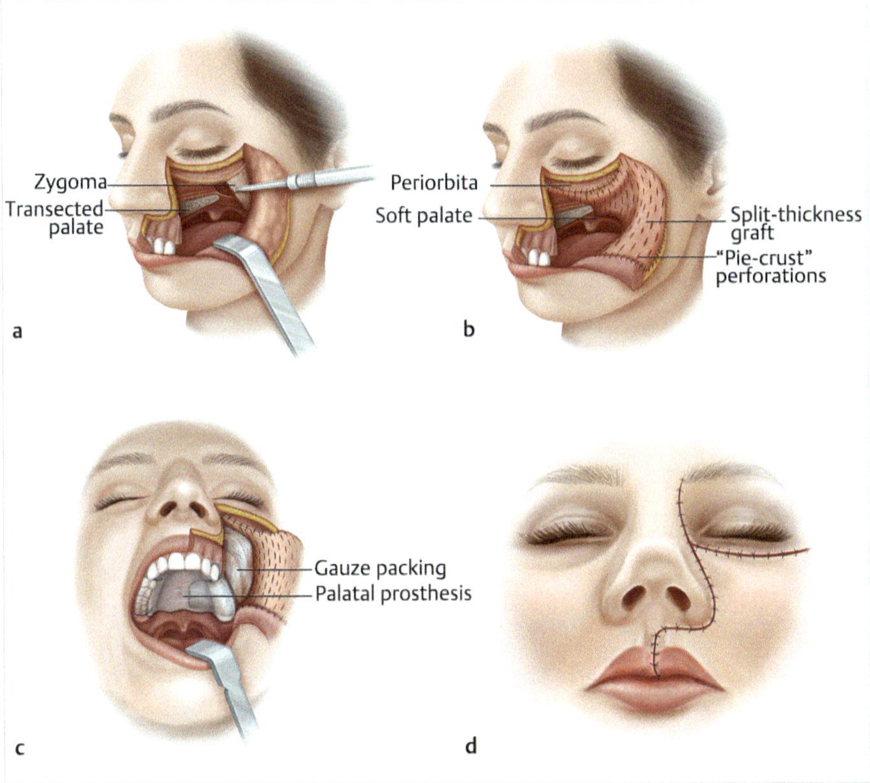

Fig. 29.9 **(a)** Closure of maxillary defect with dental obturator begins with smoothing of rough protrusive bony remnants. **(b)** A split thickness skin graft can be used to reline the inner cheek soft tissue to prevent cheek contracture. **(c)** Dental obturator in place with packing above to reduce persistent bleeding. **(d)** Closure of the facial incision.

29.5 Outcome: Survival and Quality of Life

29.5.1 Risk Factors and Survival

Many maxillary alveolar and hard palate malignancies do approach and erode palatal bone resulting in a preponderance of advanced T stage tumors in many series. As expected, early stage tumors have a relatively better likelihood of 5-year survival (50–82% T1, T2 versus 17–49% T3, T4).[16–18] A Japanese group recommended modifying the criteria for T4 upper gingival and hard palate cancers to require frank involvement of the maxillary sinus or nasal floor to warrant T4 status. Mere erosion of cortical bone would remain T3 disease. This reduced the proportion of T4 cases in their series of 43 subjects from 80% under Union for International Cancer Control (UICC) criteria to 40% using their proposed paradigm, and separated out a subset with significantly lower local control and survival.[17] Other reports include the presence of metastatic neck disease,[10,16] ulcerative features, and larger tumor volume as poor prognostic indicators.[16] Nodal status is a strong predictor of survival with a reduction from 71.3% survival at 5 years for N0 cases to 36.9% for N + cases in one large series.[19] Mean overall survival in the SEER database analysis of palatal cancers was 73.7 months for N0 cases compared to 29.8 months for N2 cases.[10] Radiation given postoperatively improves prognosis particularly for lesions that arise in the posterior aspect of the hard palate and alveolus where lymphatic drainage flows to the parapharyngeal and retropharyngeal basins.[19] Others report that the survival advantage with postoperative radiation therapy is modest (69 to 73% improvement).[18]

29.5.2 Quality of Life

While free flap reconstruction that replaces the oral roof with soft tissue, and possibly with bone, eliminates the need for a dental prosthesis, there are several published quality of life studies indicating that a prosthesis that is adjusted and fits well can provide a good functional outcome for maxillectomy patients. Both the Toronto and Memorial Sloan Kettering groups have asserted that voice quality and eating function can be quite good in this circumstance.[20,21] The best predictor of acceptable obturator function is the extent of soft palate resection and the amount of hard palate that remains. The soft palate must be able to create a seal with the prosthetic without irritation of the tissue to prevent nasal regurgitation. A longer prosthetic protruding more posteriorly is more difficult to tolerate without gagging. The presence of less than half of the hard palate causes difficulty in retention of the prosthesis during maxillary activity. Implants or wire clasps to remaining teeth can help in this regard, but without some base of support above the prosthesis on the surgically resected side, proper positioning of the obturator may be difficult to maintain.

Key Points

- Detailed knowledge of the three-dimensional anatomy of the maxilla is critical to planning and accurately executing disease extirpation.
- Rehabilitation with restoration of the roof of the mouth requires a multidisciplinary team including free tissue transfer and/or prosthodontist.

- Nodal metastasis and impacts outcome in cases of maxillary SCC are as common as in other oral cavity subsites. Therefore, addressing the at-risk nodal basins in treatment planning is critical.
- Frank tumor erosion with extension into the maxillary sinus or nasal floor identifies patients with advanced T4 disease and poorest prognosis.

References

[1] Koch WM, Patel H, Brennan J, Boyle JO, Sidransky D. Squamous cell carcinoma of the head and neck in the elderly. Arch Otolaryngol Head Neck Surg. 1995; 121(3):262–265

[2] Zwahlen RA, Grätz KW. Maxillary ameloblastomas: a review of the literature and of a 15-year database. J Craniomaxillofac Surg. 2002; 30(5):273–279

[3] Wanebo HJ, Koness RJ, MacFarlane JK, et al. Society of Head and Neck Surgeons Committee on Research. Head and neck sarcoma: report of the Head and Neck Sarcoma Registry. Head Neck. 1992; 14(1):1–7

[4] Kurabayashi T, Ida M, Yoshino N, Sasaki T, Ishii J, Ueda M. Differential diagnosis of tumours of the minor salivary glands of the palate by computed tomography. Dentomaxillofac Radiol. 1997; 26(1):16–21

[5] Ueda F, Suzuki M, Matsui O, Minato H, Furukawa M. MR findings of nine cases of palatal tumor. Magn Reson Med Sci. 2005; 4(2):61–67

[6] Truitt TO, Gleich LL, Huntress GP, Gluckman JL. Surgical management of hard palate malignancies. Otolaryngol Head Neck Surg. 1999; 121(5):548–552

[7] Molumi CP, Dubey SP, Apaio ML. Preservation of palatal mucoperiosteum for oronasal separation after total maxillectomy. Indian J Cancer. 2012; 49(2): 209–214

[8] Sun J, Shen Y, Weng Y-Q, Li J, Zhang Z-Y. Lateral lip-splitting approach for total and subtotal maxillectomy. J Oral Maxillofac Surg. 2009; 67(6):1197–1205

[9] Har-El G, Bhaya M. Intraoperative fabrication of palatal prosthesis for maxillary resection. Arch Otolaryngol Head Neck Surg. 2001; 127(7):834–836

[10] Lin HW, Bhattacharyya N. Survival impact of nodal disease in hard palate and maxillary alveolus cancer. Laryngoscope. 2009; 119(2):312–315

[11] Os AD, Karakullukcu B, Leemans CR, et al. Management of the clinically N0 neck in squamous cell carcinoma of the maxillary alveolus and hard palate. Head Neck. 2016; 38(12):1794–1798

[12] Givi B, Eskander A, Awad MI, et al. Impact of elective neck dissection on the outcome of oral squamous cell carcinomas arising in the maxillary alveolus and hard palate. Head Neck. 2016; 38 Suppl 1:E1688–E1694

[13] Simental AA, Jr, Johnson JT, Myers EN. Cervical metastasis from squamous cell carcinoma of the maxillary alveolus and hard palate. Laryngoscope. 2006; 116(9):1682–1684

[14] Brown JS, Bekiroglu F, Shaw RJ, Woolgar JA, Rogers SN. Management of the neck and regional recurrence in squamous cell carcinoma of the maxillary alveolus and hard palate compared with other sites in the oral cavity. Head Neck. 2013; 35(2):265–269

[15] Koshkareva Y, Liu JC, Lango M, Galloway T, Gaughan JP, Ridge JA. Cervical metastasis in squamous cell carcinoma of the hard palate and maxillary alveolus. Ear Nose Throat J. 2016; 95(10–11):E6–E11

[16] Wang TC, Hua CH, Lin CC, Tsou YA, Tseng HC, Tsai MH. Risk factors affect the survival outcome of hard palatal and maxillary alveolus squamous cell carcinoma: 10-year review in a tertiary referral center. Oral Surg Oral Med Oral Pathol Oral Radiol Endod. 2010; 110(1):11–17

[17] Yokoo S, Umeda M, Komatsubara H, Shibuya Y, Komori T. Evaluation of T-classifications of upper gingival and hard palate carcinomas—a proposition for new criterion of T4. Oral Oncol. 2002; 38(4):378–382

[18] Binahmed A, Nason RW, Hussain A, Abdoh AA, Sándor GKB. Treatment outcomes in squamous cell carcinoma of the maxillary alveolus and palate: a population-based study. Oral Surg Oral Med Oral Pathol Oral Radiol Endod. 2008; 105(6):750–754

[19] Yang X, Song X, Chu W, Li L, Ma L, Wu Y. Clinicopathological characteristics and outcome predictors in squamous cell carcinoma of the maxillary gingiva and hard palate. J Oral Maxillofac Surg. 2015; 73(7):1429–1436

[20] Irish J, Sandhu N, Simpson C, et al. Quality of life in patients with maxillectomy prostheses. Head Neck. 2009; 31(6):813–821

[21] Kornblith AB, Zlotolow IM, Gooen J, et al. Quality of life of maxillectomy patients using an obturator prosthesis. Head Neck. 1996; 18(4):323–334

30 Reconstruction of the Maxilla

Brittany R. Barber and Brett A. Miles

Summary
Reconstruction of the maxilla continues to pose a challenge to the head and neck oncologic surgeon due to long-term effects of adjuvant therapies, longer patient survivorship, and an increase in patient expectations regarding form and function. Multiple classification schemes have been proposed, with the aim of classifying anatomic and functional defects and guiding reconstruction strategies. Examples of defects and reconstructive approaches are described in a defect-oriented manner, and postoperative care is reviewed.

Keywords: maxilla, reconstruction, free flap, Brown classification

30.1 Introduction

The maxilla plays an integral role both in aesthesis and function of the oral cavity. It provides structural support to oral and orbital cavities, and dominates projection of the midface. Functionally, defects of the maxilla can impact speech, swallowing, and mastication. Goals of reconstruction are multifactorial, and should include: oronasal separation, maintenance of occlusion, restoration of the orbital floor, re-establishment of the load-bearing vertical buttress, patency of the nasolacrimal duct and nasal airway, support and suspension of adynamic facial soft tissue, and adequate cosmesis.[1]

Rehabilitation of both structural and functional aspects of maxillary defects can be accomplished by any of several prosthetic options or by surgical reconstruction. In the past, prosthetic rehabilitation was the predominant choice in most cases. However, in the last three decades, the advantages of surgical reconstruction have been realized through the evolution of new techniques and surgical design technology. In spite of this, appropriate selection of patients for either prosthetic or reconstructive methods remains an important point of discussion.

In light of the notorious intricacy associated with maxillary defects and their reconstruction, multiple complex classification systems have been developed to facilitate logical reconstruction strategies. However, no single classification scheme has been adopted above all others, prompting ambiguous interpretation in reconstructive results. In addition, the controversy surrounding optimal orbitomaxillary and nasomaxillary reconstruction techniques remains, particularly with respect to prevention or management of postoperative sequelae. This heterogeneity in reconstructive planning has the unfortunate effect of lack of clinical outcomes with sufficient data to drive the creation of well-accepted guidelines in this area. That being said, there is a plethora of literature supporting common principles in maxillary reconstruction, in order to achieve acceptable outcomes. This chapter will identify and discuss appropriate reconstruction strategies for the patient with a maxillary defect, perioperative considerations, and prevention and management of surgical sequelae.

30.2 Diagnosis and Evaluation

A thorough approach to assessment in maxillary reconstruction involves a complete history, physical examination, and review of biopsy and imaging results. All components warrant consideration, as they may provide insight on the most appropriate reconstructive strategy. For example, a more aggressive pathology may warrant a more aggressive resection margin, or delayed reconstruction (e.g., sinonasal undifferentiated carcinoma or sarcoma, respectively). A physical examination indicating orbital rim or floor involvement may direct the use of a different free tissue option (e.g., proptosis due to orbital floor invasion). Advanced tumor stage evident on imaging studies may portend the need for adjuvant radiation therapy, which may change the extent of soft tissue incorporated in the reconstruction.

Appropriate imaging will have significant impact on treatment planning, oncologic resection, and therefore reconstructive planning. In general, computed tomography (CT) imaging is considered a gold standard for evaluation of bony destruction. Specific structures to examine include the orbital floor, nasolacrimal duct, ethmoid sinus, posterior maxillary wall, and extent of hard palate erosion. Magnetic resonance imaging (MRI) can be considered for evaluation of the integrity of specific structures, such as the subcutaneous fat, infraorbital nerve, periorbita, extraconal fat, extraocular muscles, and optic nerve. Positron emission tomography-computed tomography (PET/CT) technology should be utilized in cases with high risk of regional or distant metastasis.

30.3 Anatomic Considerations/ Relevant Anatomy

Structural support of the midface involves both vertical and horizontal buttresses. Vertical buttresses include the nasomaxillary, zygomaticomaxillary, and pterygomaxillary buttresses.[2] These supports are vertically suspended from a thick frontal bar, and are reinforced by horizontal zygomatic, alveolar, and palatine buttresses. Regardless of the defect, regeneration of these buttresses is important to endure occlusal load, and restore facial form. In general, restoration of two of the three vertical buttresses will provide more optimal results with regards to form and function, but certainly a wide variability of reconstructive options exist with acceptable outcomes. If the goal of the reconstructive plan is eventual occlusal restoration with dental implants, then the vertical buttress construct becomes more critical in terms of the quantity and location of bone, and the increased occlusal load associated with these types of reconstructions.

While the vertical buttresses provide support for mastication, the horizontal buttresses provide support for the globe, determine the height of the occlusal plane, and contribute to aesthetic qualities of the midface. Certainly from the functional standpoint, the correct position of the globe is critical, and therefore restoration of osseous structure after ablation of the orbital rim/floor is optimal. Additional alloplastic reconstruction (i.e., titanium mesh) can supplement this osseous reconstruction. It should be noted that vascularized osseous reconstruction will help withstand the effects of radiation therapy, and provide more predictable results, when compared to non-vascularized tissue, or alloplastic-only constructs. From a functional standpoint, provided the oral cavity defect is closed, reconstruction of the osseous structure of the maxilla is critical only in cases where dental implants are planned. Careful attention to the position of osseous tissue is vital to treatment plan success in these situations.

30.4 Classification of Maxillary Defects

Classification systems can allow a defect to be succinctly deconstructed into its component parts, concentrate discussion around problem areas, focus on reconstructive options, and compare short- and long-term results. The intricacy of the anatomy and consequent defects is mirrored in the variety and number of published classification systems, none of which is universally accepted.[3–6]

Cordeiro et al[6] described a four-part classification scheme distinguishing defects based on an increasing surface area-to-volume (SA:V) ratio. Type I defects involve one or two walls of the maxilla, leaving the palate and orbital floor intact. Type II defects, or subtotal maxillectomy defects, involve resection of the maxilla, but leave the orbital floor intact. The authors subdivides Type II defects into IIA defects (involving less than 50% of the transverse palate) and Type IIB defects (involving greater than 50% of the transverse palate). Type III defects, or total maxillectomy defects, involve the entire wall of the maxilla and are subdivided into Type IIIA and Type IIIB, depending on whether the orbital contents are resected. Type IV orbitomaxillary defects involve resection of the entire orbital cavity contents, leaving dura and brain exposed. The authors produced a detailed algorithm for the type of free flap reconstruction according to defect type,[7,8] yet a significant critique of the classification scheme is the failure to consider functional dental restoration.

Okay et al[4] described a classification that illustrated maxillary defects in both horizontal and vertical planes, based on biomechanical stability for obturator retention. This was the first classification system to consider the status of the zygomatic arch and the orbital floor, and provide insight into dental restoration. In this classification, Class IA defects involve any portion of the hard palate save for the tooth-bearing alveolus. Class IB defects involve any portion of the maxilla with preservation of both canine teeth. Defects are classified as Class II if they engage only one canine or if they involve less than 50% of the hard palate. Class III defects involve resection of both canines or greater than 50% of the hard palate. Subclasses "F" and "Z" pertain to involvement of the orbital floor and zygomatic arch. The hallmark of the Okay classification is the focus on the setting necessary to accommodate effective prosthetic reconstruction. For example, Class IA and Class IB defects can be addressed with soft tissue alone, whereas Class III defects require osseous substrate to retain an obturator.

From the reconstructive standpoint, Brown and colleagues[5] perhaps introduced the most widely accepted classification which described defects according to its vertical and horizontal components. In this system the vertical component (Classes I–IV) is coupled with an appraisal of the orbit, and a horizontal component (Classes A–C). Class I defects involve resection of the alveolar ridge or palate with no oroantral defect; Class II defects involve an alveolar and antral defect but do not include the orbital floor or rim; Class III defects involve an alveolar and antral defect including the orbital floor with or without periorbita or skull base; Class IV defects involve an alveolar and antral defect including the orbital floor and orbital cavity contents with or without skull base involvement. Horizontal defects can remain on one side of the midline (Class A), cross the midline or involve the septum (Class B), or involve the entire palate (Class C). Brown and Shaw[9] expanded the existing classification system in 2010 with Class V orbitomaxillary and Class VI nasomaxillary defects. In addition, the dentoalveolar or functional side of the defect was reorganized to the following: Class A defects involving an isolated palate defect; Class B with a defect less than or equal to half of the unilateral maxilla; Class C with a defect less than or equal to half bilateral or transverse anterior maxilla; and Class D defect comprising greater than half of the maxilla. The authors reviewed 147 cases of reconstructed midface and maxillary oncologic defects reconstructed with both forearm (osteocutaneous and fasciocutaneous) and thoracodorsal angular artery (TDAA) latissimus perforator free flaps, reaching the conclusion that an obturator can be considered for Classes I, II, A, and B defects not involving the orbit, and that free flap reconstruction is recommended for more extensive defects such as Classes II, D, III–VI.

While no single classification offers a superior option for reconstructive planning, familiarity with the above three classification systems can avoid common reconstructive errors, and provide improved outcomes by preoperatively identifying critical considerations when formulating a treatment plan.

30.5 Virtual Surgical Planning (VSP)

Three-dimensional (3D) printers and medical modeling have become increasingly available, allowing for accurate measurement of both vertical and horizontal buttresses for adequate projection and improved symmetry. Previous studies have boasted both shorter ischemia and total operative time,[10,11] as well as increased accuracy and reproducibility of planned osteotomies in maxillary reconstruction.[12] Despite an increase in incurred surgical costs[11] and preoperative planning, this technology has been widely utilized in most academic centers for complex cases, and does provide an improved platform for treatment planning. It is also an excellent tool for learning and anticipating issues related to the reconstructive plan preoperatively.

30.6 Reconstructive Options

Goals of reconstruction of the maxilla include oronasal separation, restoration of structural integrity and midfacial contour, and restitution of a scaffold for suspension of soft tissues.

In short, speech, swallowing, and mastication must be re-established durably.

In the past, maxillectomy defects, regardless of the extent, were reconstructed with prosthetic obturation. The advantages of this option included partial restoration of facial contour as well as immediate dental restoration in some cases. Other advantages include accurate customization to existing anatomy and shorter operative times. However, disadvantages to this approach frequently included inadequate prosthesis–tissue seal, need for manual dexterity to manipulate the prosthesis, and chronic irritation and pain.[13] In addition, the often subsequent need for obturator revision due to maxillary cavity contraction negatively impacted patient satisfaction.[14] A study by Moreno et al[15] compared 73 obturated and 40 reconstructed patients and demonstrated that reconstruction provided better speech and swallowing outcomes, particularly in patients with defects involving a large palatal component. Even in small to medium defects, the superiority of free flaps in improving quality of life was shown by Genden et al.[16] Brown and Shaw,[9] using the 2010 classification modification, recommended obturation for Classes I, II, A, and B defects only. However, even with small defects, patient dissatisfaction with obturation has spurred the development of multiple local or pedicle flaps as substitutes.

30.6.1 Partial Hard Palate Defects

With smaller maxillary defects, cosmetic and functional deficits are less common, and the focus becomes expeditious return to function, while imparting minimal morbidity to the patient. This focus can be realized with local or regional flaps. However, careful patient selection is of the utmost importance in ensuring a good outcome, as these techniques are limited by pedicle length and soft tissue bulk.

Brown Class Ia defects, or partial defects of the hard palate, may be addressed with local, pedicled, or free flaps, depending on the size and location. Local and pedicled options may include a palatal island flap, buccal fat pad flap, temporalis muscle flap, or facial artery musculomucosal (FAMM) flaps.

The palatal island flap, based on the greater palatine vessels, may be used to resurface defects up to 15 cm^2.[17] This is commonly used for small Brown Class Ia defects, and can restore the oronasal barrier in through-and-through defects due to the thick mucosa of the hard palate. It should be noted that patients should expect moderate donor site pain during re-epithelialization which occurs within 8–12 weeks.

The buccal fat pad is situated between the masseter and buccinator muscles, and consists of a main body and four extensions: buccal, pterygoid, superficial temporal, and deep temporal. The parotid duct and zygomatic and buccal branches of the facial nerve cross the lateral surface of the pad. Its rich vascularity from the maxillary, superficial temporal, and facial arteries allows it to be used as an axial-pattern pedicled flap. Stuzin et al, who noted a mean weight and volume of 9.3 g and 9.6 mL, respectively, characterized the buccal fat pad flap in terms of its size.[18] As such, only defects less than 12 cm^2 are amenable to reconstruction with this method.[19] The utility of this flap is primarily in small posterior maxillectomy defects with no intraoral communication requiring coverage for a denture. Amin et al[20] described their experience in 24 patients with a variety of maxillary defects, wherein the buccal fat pad flap was covered with a split-thickness skin graft and an acrylic plate. Complete healing and partial dehiscence were observed within 4 weeks postoperatively in 18 and 6 patients, respectively. Of the 10 patients that underwent radiation therapy, none experienced wound breakdown.

The FAMM flap[21] can be used for lateral hard palate defects in edentulous patients. The FAMM flap is an axial flap based on the terminal branches of the facial artery as it courses deep to the buccal mucosa, lateral to the buccinator muscle, and medial to the muscles of facial expression. As such, the flap itself is composed of buccal mucosa and buccinator muscle. The flap should be designed with a wide base, and the pedicle can be identified using a Doppler probe. Careful attention to the location of the pedicle in dentate patients can prevent vascular compression and flap compromise.

Temporalis muscle flaps can be used when the maxillary defect involves more than just the palate, but only a small amount of soft tissue bulk is needed for bony coverage. For patients in whom a free flap may not be a reasonable option, a temporalis flap, with or without vascularized bone, may be used. Specifically, vascularized calvarial temporalis flaps can be used to re-contour the orbital floor or superior or anterior wall of the maxilla due to the natural curvature of the bone.[22] However, it should be noted that this requires tunneling the flap for a significant distance and/or partially resecting the zygomatic arch, necessitating identification of the frontal branch of the facial nerve. In addition, temporal hollowing, with the resultant aesthetic deformity, and postoperative trismus are donor site considerations.

For large Brown Class Ia defects spanning the entire non-tooth-bearing region of the palate, a fasciocutaneous radial forearm free flap (RFFF) can be considered.[14] This option boasts of a long, vascular pedicle, reliable anatomy, and a thin, pliable skin paddle to create a steadfast oronasal partition that will not hinder denture retention. Several other options, including myofascial free tissue transfer (i.e., serratus or vastus lateralis), may be considered in these situations.

30.6.2 Infrastructure Maxillectomy Defects

Infrastructure maxillectomy defects involve the lower alveolar and horizontal palatal shelves, with a very minor vertical defect. As such, the structural support mechanisms of the face are minimally affected. Free tissue transfer options such as the fibular free flap (FFF) and the lateral border scapular free flap (SFF) may be utilized for these predominantly horizontal defects. With a variety of options, the final decision may hinge upon the degree of vertical extension, patient-specific anatomy, and habitus as well as the prosthetic plan. Specifically, the iliac crest and SFF often provide adequate bone stock for dental implantation, yet may incorporate a thick skin paddle that precludes oral competence and may require revision. Conversely, consideration of the effect of adjuvant radiation therapy on the interposed tissue may warrant a thicker skin paddle as opposed to the FFF. With a thorough assessment of the defect, donor tissue, and anticipated adjuvant effects, an appropriate donor site may be successfully selected.

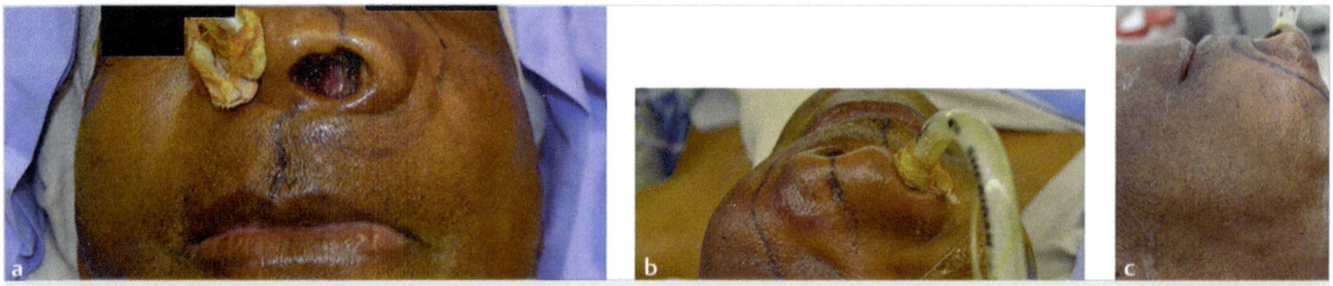

Fig. 30.1 (a–c) 63-year-old male with a T4aN2bM0 squamous cell carcinoma (SCC) of the left maxilla with erosion through the left orbital floor and extension across midline to the contralateral canine.

Fibular Free Flap

The FFF, the osseous workhorse of the head and neck reconstructive surgeon, is known for its reliable, segmented periosteal blood supply, allowing for multiple osteotomies and ability to conform to any of several complicated defects of the maxilla. The FFF is particularly well-suited for defects wherein 1–2 cm of vertical height is required with a reliable bone stock for dental implantation, and a skin paddle for resurfacing the palate. When a skin paddle is required for a mucosal defect, the fibula contralateral to the defect side should be harvested to allow for an appropriate orientation. The limitations of the FFF include a nonnegligible donor site mobility, limited soft tissue bulk for facial contouring, and the lack of three-dimensional reconstruction permitted with segmental osteotomized bone.[23,24] Therefore, the FFF is useful for Brown Class I and II defects, but becomes a secondary choice in more extensive midface defects.[25,26]

Scapular Free Flap

The scapular system, despite its now widespread use, was only described within the last three decades.[27,28] It allows for a myriad of bony and soft tissue reconstructive options, when used in the context of chimeric lateral border SFFs and scapular tip free flaps (STFFs). The SFF is based on the circumflex scapular artery (4–6 cm) and can be taken up to the axillary artery for longer pedicle length (11–14 cm)[29] and larger caliber (average 2.8 mm).[27] It can be harvested with one or two skin paddles, a 10–14 cm segment of lateral border bone, and a customizable degree of teres muscle. The selection of harvest technique between the traditional SFF and the STFF centers around the osseous and soft tissue requirements of the reconstructive plan. Illustration of an STFF with an accompanying thoracodorsal artery perforator (TDAP) flap including a skin paddle is depicted in ▶ Fig. 30.1, ▶ Fig. 30.2, ▶ Fig. 30.3, ▶ Fig. 30.4 for reconstruction of a left maxillary defect following a left total maxillectomy with orbital floor defect for maxillary squamous cell carcinoma (SCC) (▶ Fig. 30.5, ▶ Fig. 30.6, ▶ Fig. 30.7). It should be noted that the shorter pedicle of the SFF relative to the STFF may warrant a vein graft to ensure a tension-free anastomosis, although with adequate planning this is a rare occurrence in the authors' experience.

For more posterior Brown Class II defects, soft tissue-only reconstruction with a fasciocutaneous radial forearm free flap or vascularized musculofascial flap such as the serratus flap or tensor fascia lata (TFL) flap is reasonable. The serratus flap or TFL flap are the authors' primary choices given the customizable muscle bulk and long vascular pedicles, and the acceptable donor site morbidity associated with these options. The TFL mucosalizes in 4 to 6 weeks.

30.6.3 Anterior Palate Defects

Defects of the anterior palate vary in size and shape. In the past, a palatal obturator would be considered an adequate option for functional restoration. However, as the nasomaxillary buttress is ablated in this defect, excessive levering forces incurred by anterior mastication may over time destabilize any prosthesis placed.[4] In cases where obturation/prosthesis is not feasible, free tissue transfer options including the osteocutaneous radial forearm free flap (OCRFF), FFF, and STFF may be tailored to the appropriate size, and provide a firm substrate for dental implantation.

Osteocutaneous Radial Forearm Free Flap

The OCRFF provides a thin, pliable skin paddle alongside a thin strip of cortical bone with a long pedicle.[30] The bone can be oriented horizontally for arch reconstruction[31] or obliquely for zygomaticomaxillary restitution,[32] and is of sufficient quality to support a tissue-borne or implant-retained, but not implant-borne, prosthesis.[33] This option is best utilized in anterior palate defects spanning less than half the palate region (Brown Classes I, II, A, and B).[34] Pathologic donor radial bone fracture has decreased significantly with the standard of care practice of prophylactic plating, keel-shaped osteotomies, and harvesting less than 40% of the circumference of the bone. The skin paddle can be oriented to repair any existing mucosal defect or even cutaneous defects of the lip or anterior septal region. Although many reports of osseous reconstruction with this flap exist, it is not the preferred option in many situations due to the availability of adequate bone.

Scapular Tip Free Flap

When an anterior palate defect spanning greater than half the palate necessitates reconstruction, the STFF provides an adequate quantity and quality of bone.[35] The STFF is a chimeric flap capable of restoring a range of defects, from small

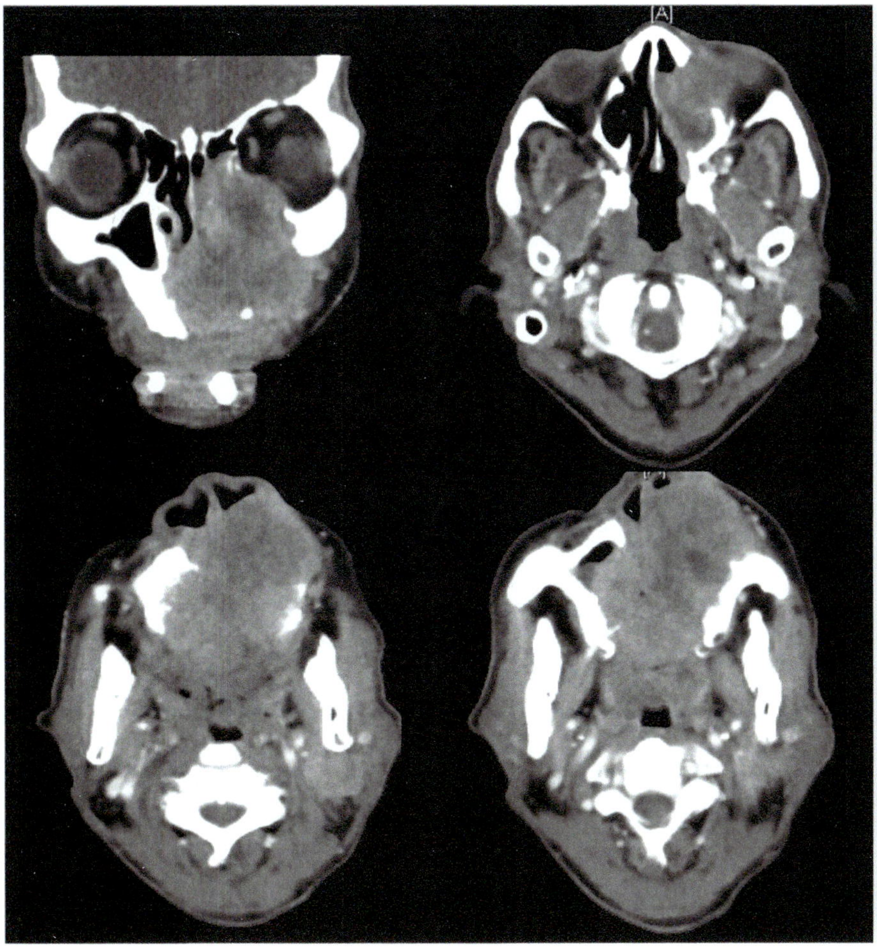

Fig. 30.2 Preoperative computed tomography (CT) imaging studies demonstrating left orbital floor involvement and extension across midline to contralateral canine, septum, and inferior maxilla.

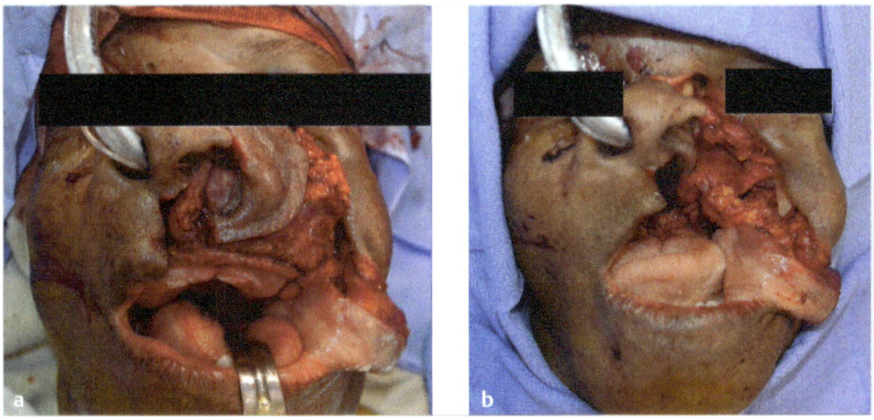

Fig. 30.3 Demonstration of the ablation margins **(a)** including a total maxillectomy, and **(b)** resection of the left orbital floor, lateral nasal wall, septum, and left ala.

premaxillary defects to more extensive defects involving the orbital floor. The STFF is harvested with the angular artery, allowing for up to 17 cm of pedicle[36] and a customizable quantity of teres muscle for palatal lining. The STFF is oriented horizontally and teres muscle is sutured to the remaining mucosa, remucosalizing over the course of several weeks. In a series of 39 patients undergoing STFF for maxillary reconstruction, all patients were able to tolerate a soft (54%) or normal (46%) diet.[37] The available bone stock is somewhat variable depending on the age and body habitus of the patient. A primary advantage of this flap is rapid mobilization postoperatively and, therefore, is an excellent choice for elderly patients.

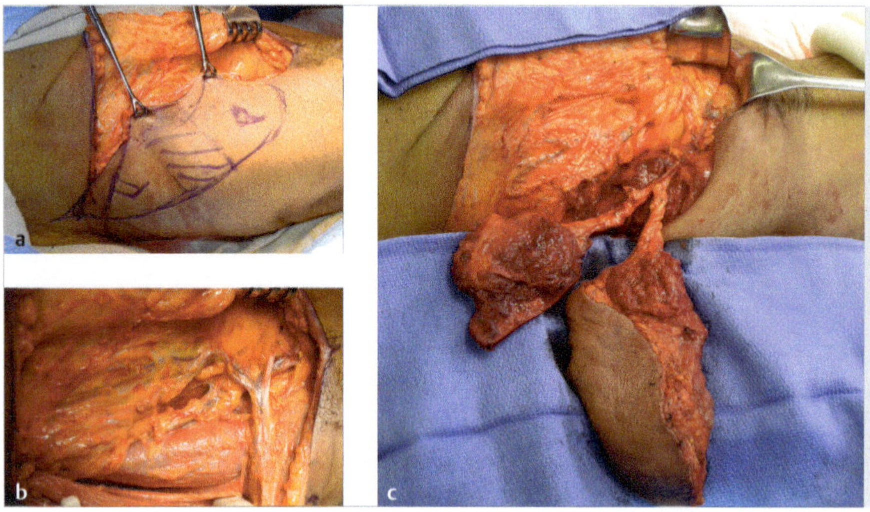

Fig. 30.4 Planned reconstruction using a scapular tip free flap (STFF) with a thoracodorsal artery perforator (TDAP) flap based on the subscapular artery. **(a)** The "F" denotes the planned external skin paddle, the "P" denotes the soft tissue hard palate coverage, and the "///" portion denotes the planned de-epithelialized portion between each to provide infranasal projection. **(b)** The angular and thoracodorsal arteries are demonstrated in red and green, respectively. **(c)** The STFF and TDAP are pedicled on the subscapular artery, prior to harvest.

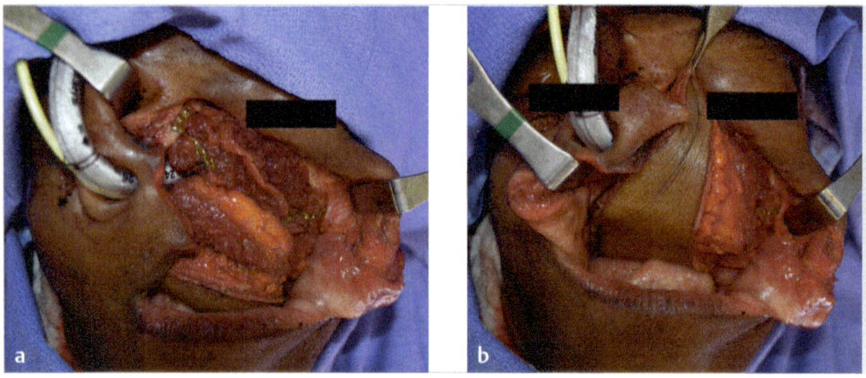

Fig. 30.5 **(a)** Inset scapular tip free flap-thoracodorsal artery perforator (STFF-TDAP) with a vertically oriented scapular tip reconstructing the left orbital rim and anterior maxilla, and the TDAP providing a soft tissue "sling" in place of the hard palate. A titanium plate was placed within the orbital floor for support. **(b)** The nasolabial skin defect is reconstructed with the distal portion of the TDAP skin paddle. The medial canthal tendon was suspended to the nasal bones using a 2–0 prolene suture.

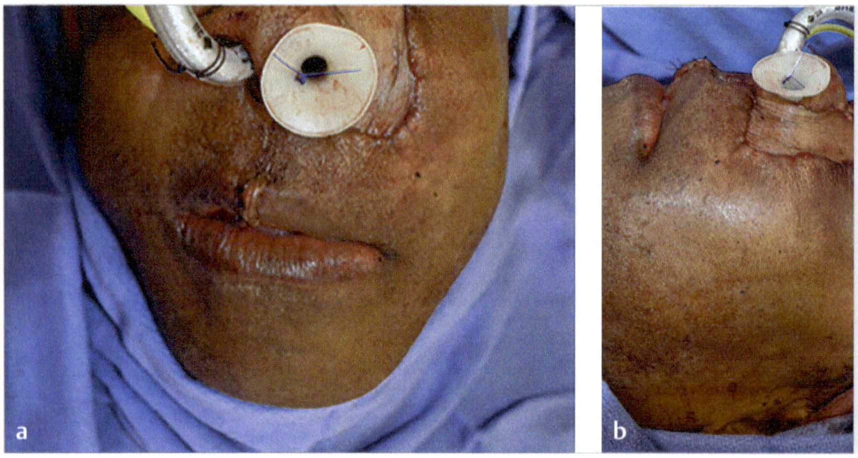

Fig. 30.6 **(a, b)** Final reconstruction and 3-week postoperative results.

30.6.4 Hemimaxillectomy

Hemimaxillectomy defects with orbital preservation can be reconstructed with any of a number of osteocutaneous free flaps, including fibula, scapular tip, or iliac crest. The decision hinges upon the vertical extension and available remaining zygoma. If the orbital rim/floor and zygoma remain intact, an FFF can be considered for its long pedicle and sculpting osteotomies. However, if a larger proportion of the anterior maxillary wall, zygoma, or orbital rim/floor has been resected, a larger volume of bone and soft tissue are necessary for facial contouring. In this case, the STFF and deep circumflex iliac artery free flap (DCIA) are excellent options.

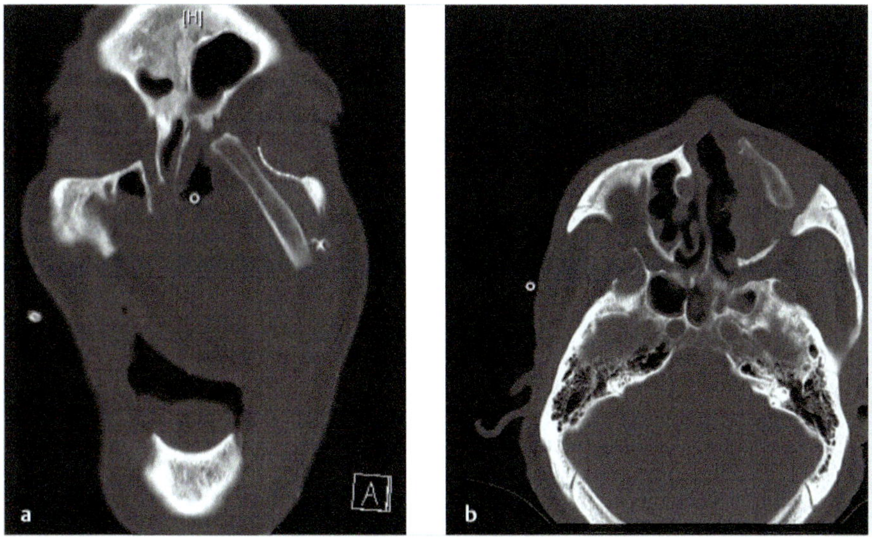

Fig. 30.7 (a, b) Postoperative imaging result at 3 weeks.

Deep Circumflex Iliac Artery Flap

The DCIA, regarding bone stock, is an excellent reconstructive option for hemimaxillectomy reconstruction when dental implantation is anticipated. The pedicle is 5–7 cm in length and approximately 2–3 mm in diameter.[38] Up to 16 cm of bone can be harvested. The modifiable degree of both soft tissue and bone allows customization to a variety of defects, from infrastructure maxillectomies to large Brown Classes III and IV defects. The inherent curvature of the bone mirrors that of the anterior maxilla, and when horizontally oriented, the bone can serve to reconstruct varying degrees of vertical bone loss, including the orbital rim. The DCIA can, alternatively, reconstruct the orbital rim and floor for prosthetic placement in patients who have undergone an orbital exenteration.[39] The flap should be harvested on the side ipsilateral to the defect and should include a healthy cuff of internal oblique muscle for palatal lining, over which mucosalization occurs rapidly. The astute surgeon may anticipate the need for a vein graft, which can be passed through tunnel medial to the mandible to the facial vessels if required.

The disadvantages of the iliac crest for Classes III and IV defects are those inherent in its design and anatomy. The short vascular pedicle, lack of soft tissue mobility, and occasionally overly-robust bone stock can limit the use of this flap in young, muscular patients.[38] Another aspect somewhat unique to this flap is the fact that the skin paddle reliability and independent rotation from the bone are inferior to other options noted. In addition, even in older patients, the incidence of hernia, chronic pain, and difficulty with mobilization in the short-term recovery period may preclude its use.[40]

Scapular Tip Free Flap

As mentioned previously, the chimeric nature of the scapular system allows for reconstructive adaptation in the maxilla. The STFF is of particular use in extensive hemimaxillectomy defects with or without orbital rim preservation given the size and thickness of the bone at the tip, pedicle length, and natural convexity of the bone. Though Seneviratne et al[41] demonstrated the length of bone supplied by the angular branch to be approximately 6 cm using injection studies, other authors have harvested up to 14 cm of lateral scapula bone base on the angular branch alone.[41] The tip can be oriented horizontally or vertically depending on correlation of the desired location of the thicker tip bone and muscle bulk and the patient's likelihood of dental restoration. Often, in order to ensure the thick tip bone is oriented inferiorly to allow for this, the scapula tip contralateral to the defect is harvested, and subsequently positioned with the tip oriented inferolaterally.[42] Osteotomies are performed to sculpt abutments with the nasal aperture, zygoma, and superior alveolus, permitting three-point fixation with 1.5 mm mini-plates. The orbital rim can be restored using vascularized scapula bone fixed with a cantilever mini-plate and/or can be further augmented by free bone grafts taken from the existing donor site if desired.[43]

The skin paddle of the traditional SFF is highly mobile for various intraoral and intranasal mucosal defects and allows for multiple skin paddles based on the scapular and parascapular branches of the circumflex scapular system. Yet, this skin can be too thick and bulky for intraoral use. As with the DCIA/internal oblique, the osteomyogenous STFF is often used with a thin layer of teres muscle to re-line the palate. Mucosalization occurs within 6 to 8 weeks in nonradiated patients.[37]

The disadvantages of the STFF include difficulty with a two-team approach, subsequent prolonged operating time, and seroma formation.[43] Despite the location of the donor site, a study by Clark et al,[43] examining the scores on the Disabilities of the Arm, Shoulder, and Hand (DASH) questionnaire, revealed an average of 10.6 in 12 patients following STFF reconstruction, all of whom demonstrated normal shoulder function at 6 months after treatment. Typically, the STFF or SFF has not been considered to be of adequate thickness for dental implantation; however, a number of authors have recently disputed this claim.[44,45] Lanzer et al performed implantation in six patients reconstructed with the SFF. However, no discussion of implant survival or long-term retention was given.[46]

30.7 Special Considerations: Total Palatomaxillary Reconstruction

A total palatomaxillary defect with limited vertical height is optimally reconstructed with either an FFF or a large horizontally oriented STFF. The FFF is osteotomized to create the neo-alveolus, and requires a large skin paddle that is de-epithelialized to reline the nasal cavity and provide skin paddle coverage over the neo-palate. As mentioned earlier, the entire scapular tip and lateral border of the scapula may be harvested based off the angular artery.[43] Pagedar et al demonstrated the radiologic congruence between a large STFF and the shape of the maxilla to within 2.04 mm in CT images of 10 patients, suggesting this to be well suited to total maxillectomy defects without a large vertical component.[47] In total palatomaxillary defects involving a significant vertical component, the DCIA is an excellent option as noted above. The limited mobility of the DCIA soft tissue is mitigated in this defect when the internal oblique muscle is used to cover the palatal area and the nasal cavity can be re-lined with the skin paddle.[5]

30.8 Special Considerations: Nasomaxillary Reconstruction

Brown Class VI defects that involve resection of dura, nasal bones, or skin require reconstruction. In nasoethmoid defects without involvement of nasal bones or skin, reconstruction is performed only for dural defects to prevent a cerebrospinal fluid leak.[48] Soft tissue coverage of bone may also be necessary if radiation therapy is planned, or in previously radiated patients undergoing an extensive ablation.[49–51] In nasomaxillary defects including skin and nasal bones, the OCRFF is an obvious choice for its long pedicle and thin, pliable skin paddle, which may be partially de-epithelialized and used to re-line the nasal cavity. In those nasomaxillary defects not involving skin or nasal bones, the vascularized TFL is an excellent option for soft tissue coverage in anticipation of radiation therapy.[52] An intraoral anastomosis may be performed if desired. In many cases, the underlying structure can be reconstructed with free tissue transfer, with a traditional paramedian forehead flap offering the optimal skin coverage. Alternatively, the entire nasal cavity can be re-lined with an RFFF or TFL flap and a nasal prosthesis can be considered.

30.9 Special Considerations: Orbitomaxillary Reconstruction

In Brown Class V defects, an orbital exenteration is necessary; yet the palate remains intact. As such, the focus becomes providing the bony and soft tissue constructs to support an orbital prosthesis. If resected, it is often necessary to reconstruct the lateral orbital wall to provide a substrate for prosthesis fixation. This can be accomplished using an OCRFF for its long pedicle, thin bone, and pliable skin paddle. For additional bulk, a beavertail modification can be applied.[53] Alternatively, a contoured serratus flap or anterolateral thigh (ALT) flap can be used to provide tailored muscle bulk to the orbital cavity. However, with this approach, the extent of muscle bulk may need to be overestimated (approximately 30%) in order to account for atrophy and the effects of radiation therapy. For smaller skin defects lacking a significant bony defect, a temporoparietal fascia flap can be considered.[54]

30.10 Perioperative Considerations and Surgical Sequelae

Given the complexity of maxillary reconstruction, the immediate and long-term management and surgical sequelae can be equally as complex. Depending on the defect, in the immediate recovery period, mastication, nasal breathing, and management of nasal secretions are concerns. Intermediately, oronasal fistulas and nasal regurgitation may be observed. In the long term, malunion/nonunion, hardware exposure, osteomyelitis, and osteoradionecrosis are concerns. Ocular complications may include enophthalmos, diplopia, lacrimal dysfunction, and ectropion.

In the short term, nasal breathing and diversion of nasal secretions can be accomplished by using appropriately placed nasal trumpets. Nasal lavage should be instituted by postoperative days 5 to 7 and even appropriate use of antibiotics can be considered in complex reconstructions with a high surface area of intranasal exposed bone. Mastication should be avoided in most patients until 4 to 6 weeks postoperatively in order to avoid shifting. Patients may remain on a liquid or soft diet during this time.

Oronasal fistula formation is common, particularly in Brown Classes III and IV defects, and often results from lack of a surgical "seal" between the muscle and the mucosa of the hard palate, in addition to exposure of the atrophying muscle to radiation therapy. In a series of 39 patients, 8 patients (21%) developed oronasal fistulas, of which 50% closed spontaneously.[37] If no spontaneous closure occurs, palatal advancement flaps and palatal obturator are options.

Hardware exposure can be avoided by judicious use of soft tissue coverage over plates, particularly in areas that have been radiated or will receive high doses of adjuvant radiation therapy.

Ocular complications are difficult to avoid and predict. Precise presurgical planning, whether using VSP or imaging measurements, is paramount to ensure symmetry in the vertical, horizontal, and sagittal planes, as well as in the residual volume in the orbital cavity. Certainly, revision surgery is the norm in cases of eyelid involvement and surgeons should prepare patients accordingly for additional procedures which are often required in this population.

30.11 Conclusion

Maxillary reconstruction continues to challenge reconstructive surgeons, despite the plethora of available techniques and recent advances in reconstructive planning. While reconstruction of critical elements to achieve the traditional goals of maxillary reconstruction is frequently possible, and often highly reliable with free tissue transfer, the sequelae of surgery and adjuvant therapy often necessitate revision procedures. The current challenges of maxillary reconstructive surgery are not the obliteration of the defect, but center around suboptimal functional and aesthetic subtleties in a large number maxillary ablative defects.

Key Points

- Review of physical examination and imaging studies, as well as consideration of the likely necessity of adjuvant radiation therapy, are paramount to appropriately plan a maxillary reconstruction.
- VSP is helpful adjunct in preoperative evaluation, and has increasing value as the complexity of the reconstructive plan increases.
- Maxillary reconstruction can involve a range of options, spanning local and pedicled flaps as well as soft tissue or composite free flaps.
- Classes I, A, and B defects may be reconstructed with local or pedicled flaps.
- Prosthetic obturation can be considered for Classes I, II, A, and B defects.
- Free tissue transfer should be strongly considered for Classes III–VI defects as it provides a range of options for restoring cosmesis, mastication, and speech.
- Surgical sequelae of maxillary reconstruction of extensive defects often results in suboptimal functional and aesthetic outcomes which require appropriate counseling and often necessitate revision procedures.

References

[1] Triana RJ, Jr, Uglesic V, Virag M, et al. Microvascular free flap reconstructive options in patients with partial and total maxillectomy defects. Arch Facial Plast Surg. 2000; 2(2):91–101

[2] Manson PN, Hoopes JE, Su CT. Structural pillars of the facial skeleton: an approach to the management of Le Fort fractures. Plast Reconstr Surg. 1980; 66(1):54–62

[3] Aramany M. Basic principles of obturator design for partially edentulous patients. Part 1: Classification. J Prosthet Dent. 1978; 40(5):554–557

[4] Okay DJ, Genden E, Buchbinder D, Urken M. Prosthodontic guidelines for surgical reconstruction of the maxilla: a classification system of defects. J Prosthet Dent. 2001; 86(4):352–363

[5] Brown JS, Rogers SN, McNally DN, Boyle M. A modified classification for the maxillectomy defect. Head Neck. 2000; 22(1):17–26

[6] Cordeiro PG, Santamaria E. A classification system and algorithm for reconstruction of maxillectomy and midfacial defects. Plast Reconstr Surg. 2000; 105(7):2331–2346, discussion 2347–2348

[7] Cordeiro PG, Chen CM. A 15-year review of midface reconstruction after total and subtotal maxillectomy: part I. Algorithm and outcomes. Plast Reconstr Surg. 2012; 129(1):124–136

[8] Cordeiro PG, Chen CM. A 15-year review of midface reconstruction after total and subtotal maxillectomy: part II. Technical modifications to maximize aesthetic and functional outcomes. Plast Reconstr Surg. 2012; 129(1):139–147

[9] Brown JS, Shaw RJ. Reconstruction of the maxilla and midface: introducing a new classification. Lancet Oncol. 2010; 11(10):1001–1008

[10] Chepeha DB, Wang SJ, Marentette LJ, et al. Restoration of the orbital aesthetic subunit in complex midface defects. Laryngoscope. 2004; 114(10): 1706–1713

[11] Moyer JS, Chepeha DB, Prince ME, Teknos TN. Microvascular reconstruction of the orbital complex. Facial Plast Surg Clin North Am. 2009; 17(2):225–237

[12] Bernstein JM, Daly MJ, Chan H, et al. Accuracy and reproducibility of virtual cutting guides and 3D-navigation for osteotomies of the mandible and maxilla. PLoS One. 2017; 12(3):e0173111

[13] Chigurupati R, Aloor N, Salas R, Schmidt BL. Quality of life after maxillectomy and prosthetic obturator rehabilitation. J Oral Maxillofac Surg. 2013; 71(8): 1471–1478

[14] Genden EM, Wallace DI, Okay D, Urken ML. Reconstruction of the hard palate using the radial forearm free flap: indications and outcomes. Head Neck. 2004; 26(9):808–814

[15] Moreno M, Skoracki R, Hanna E, Hanasono M. Microvascular free flap reconstruction versus palatal obturation for maxillectomy defects. Head Neck. 2010; 32:86:0–868

[16] Genden EM, Okay D, Stepp MT, et al. Comparison of functional and quality-of-life outcomes in patients with and without palatomaxillary reconstruction: a preliminary report. Arch Otolaryngol Head Neck Surg. 2003; 129(7): 775–780

[17] Moore BA, Magdy E, Netterville JL, Burkey BB. Palatal reconstruction with the palatal island flap. Laryngoscope. 2003; 113(6):946–951

[18] Stuzin JM, Wagstrom L, Kawamoto HK, Baker TJ, Wolfe SA. The anatomy and clinical applications of the buccal fat pad. Plast Reconstr Surg. 1990; 85(1): 29–37

[19] Arce K. Buccal fat pad in maxillary reconstruction. Atlas Oral Maxillofac Surg Clin North Am. 2007; 15(1):23–32

[20] Amin MA, Bailey BM, Swinson B, Witherow H. Use of the buccal fat pad in the reconstruction and prosthetic rehabilitation of oncological maxillary defects. Br J Oral Maxillofac Surg. 2005; 43(2):148–154

[21] Pribaz J, Stephens W, Crespo L, Gifford G. A new intraoral flap: facial artery musculomucosal (FAMM) flap. Plast Reconstr Surg. 1992; 90(3):421–429

[22] Ewers R. Reconstruction of the maxilla with a double musculoperiosteal flap in connection with a composite calvarial bone graft. Plast Reconstr Surg. 1988; 81(3):431–436

[23] Dalgorf D, Higgins K. Reconstruction of the midface and maxilla. Curr Opin Otolaryngol Head Neck Surg. 2008; 16(4):303–311

[24] Futran ND, Mendez E. Developments in reconstruction of midface and maxilla. Lancet Oncol. 2006; 7(3):249–258

[25] Futran ND, Wadsworth JT, Villaret D, Farwell DG. Midface reconstruction with the fibula free flap. Arch Otolaryngol Head Neck Surg. 2002; 128(2):161–166

[26] Kim DD, Dreher MA. The fibula free flap in maxillary reconstruction. Atlas Oral Maxillofac Surg Clin North Am. 2007; 15(1):13–22

[27] dos Santos LF. The vascular anatomy and dissection of the free scapular flap. Plast Reconstr Surg. 1984; 73(4):599–604

[28] Swartz WM, Banis JC, Newton ED, Ramasastry SS, Jones NF, Acland R. The osteocutaneous scapular flap for mandibular and maxillary reconstruction. Plast Reconstr Surg. 1986; 77(4):530–545

[29] Nassif TM, Vidal L, Bovet JL, Baudet J. The parascapular flap: a new cutaneous microsurgical free flap. Plast Reconstr Surg. 1982; 69(4):591–600

[30] Chepeha DB, Moyer JS, Bradford CR, Prince ME, Marentette L, Teknos TN. Osseocutaneous radial forearm free tissue transfer for repair of complex midfacial defects. Arch Otolaryngol Head Neck Surg. 2005; 131(6):513–517

[31] Cordeiro PG, Bacilious N, Schantz S, Spiro R. The radial forearm osteocutaneous "sandwich" free flap for reconstruction of the bilateral subtotal maxillectomy defect. Ann Plast Surg. 1998; 40(4):397–402

[32] Andrades P, Rosenthal EL, Carroll WR, Baranano CF, Peters GE. Zygomatic-maxillary buttress reconstruction of midface defects with the osteocutaneous radial forearm free flap. Head Neck. 2008; 30(10):1295–1302

[33] Funk GF, Arcuri MR, Frodel JL, Jr. Functional dental rehabilitation of massive palatomaxillary defects: cases requiring free tissue transfer and osseointegrated implants. Head Neck. 1998; 20(1):38–51

[34] Andrades P, Militsakh O, Hanasono MM, Rieger J, Rosenthal EL. Current strategies in reconstruction of maxillectomy defects. Arch Otolaryngol Head Neck Surg. 2011; 137(8):806–812

[35] Choi N, Cho JK, Jang JY, Cho JK, Cho YS, Baek CH. Scapular tip free flap for head and neck reconstruction. Clin Exp Otorhinolaryngol. 2015; 8(4):422–429

[36] Seitz A, Papp S, Papp C, Maurer H. The anatomy of the angular branch of the thoracodorsal artery. Cells Tissues Organs. 1999; 164(4):227–236

[37] Miles BA, Gilbert RW. Maxillary reconstruction with the scapular angle osteomyogenous free flap. Arch Otolaryngol Head Neck Surg. 2011; 137(11): 1130–1135

[38] Fredrickson JM, Man SC, Hayden RE. Revascularized iliac bone graft for mandibular reconstruction. Acta Otolaryngol. 1985; 99(3–4):214–223

[39] Brown JS. Deep circumflex iliac artery free flap with internal oblique muscle as a new method of immediate reconstruction of maxillectomy defect. Head Neck. 1996; 18(5):412–421

[40] Valentini V, Gennaro P, Aboh IV, Longo G, Mitro V, Ialongo C. Iliac crest flap: donor site morbidity. J Craniofac Surg. 2009; 20(4):1052–1055

[41] Seneviratne S, Duong C, Taylor GI. The angular branch of the thoracodorsal artery and its blood supply to the inferior angle of the scapula: an anatomical study. Plast Reconstr Surg. 1999; 104(1):85–88

[42] Modest MC, Moore EJ, Abel KM, et al. Scapular flap for maxillectomy defect reconstruction and preliminary results using three-dimensional modeling. Laryngoscope. 2017; 127(1):E8–E14

[43] Clark JR, Vesely M, Gilbert R. Scapular angle osteomyogenous flap in post-maxillectomy reconstruction: defect, reconstruction, shoulder function, and harvest technique. Head Neck. 2008; 30(1):10–20

[44] Frodel JL, Jr, Funk GF, Capper DT, et al. Osseointegrated implants: a comparative study of bone thickness in four vascularized bone flaps. Plast Reconstr Surg. 1993; 92(3):449–455, discussion 456–458

[45] Moscoso JF, Keller J, Genden E, et al. Vascularized bone flaps in oromandibular reconstruction: a comparative anatomic study of bone stock from various donor sites to assess suitability for enosseous dental implants. Arch Otolaryngol Head Neck Surg. 1994; 120(1):36–43

[46] Lanzer M, Gander T, Grätz K, Rostetter C, Zweifel D, Bredell M. Scapular free vascularised bone flaps for mandibular reconstruction: are dental implants possible? J Oral Maxillofac Res. 2015; 6(3):e4

[47] Pagedar NA, Gilbert RW, Chan H, Daly MJ, Irish JC, Siewerdsen JH. Maxillary reconstruction using the scapular tip free flap: a radiologic comparison of 3D morphology. Head Neck. 2012; 34(10):1377–1382

[48] Califano J, Cordeiro PG, Disa JJ, et al. Anterior cranial base reconstruction using free tissue transfer: changing trends. Head Neck. 2003; 25(2): 89–96

[49] Yeo IS, Kim SH, Park MC, Lim H, Kim JH, Lee IJ. Successful reconstruction of irradiated anterior skull base defect using the dual flap technique involving local pericranial flap and radial forearm free flap. J Craniofac Surg. 2014; 25 (4):1376–1378

[50] Ganly I, Patel SG, Singh B, et al. Complications of craniofacial resection for malignant tumors of the skull base: report of an international collaborative study. Head Neck. 2005; 27(6):445–451

[51] Disa JJ, Rodriguez VM, Cordeiro PG. Reconstruction of lateral skull base oncological defects: the role of free tissue transfer. Ann Plast Surg. 1998; 41(6): 633–639

[52] Joo YH, Cho KJ, Park JO, Kim MS. Usefulness of the anterolateral thigh flap with vascularized fascia lata for reconstruction of orbital floor and nasal surface after total maxillectomy. Laryngoscope. 2013; 123(9):2125–2130

[53] Seikaly H, Rieger J, O'Connell D, Ansari K, Alqahtani K, Harris J. Beavertail modification of the radial forearm free flap in base of tongue reconstruction: technique and functional outcomes. Head Neck. 2009; 31(2):213–219

[54] Davison SP, Mesbahi AN, Clemens MW, Picken CA. Vascularized calvarial bone flaps and midface reconstruction. Plast Reconstr Surg. 2008; 122 (1):10e–18e

31 Reconstruction of Multisite Defects

Ryan M. Smith, G. Nina Lu, and Patrick J. Byrne

Summary
The reconstruction of oral cavity defects following cancer resection can prove challenging. The close spatial relationships between distinct tissue types found in the oral cavity can allow invasive malignancies to span multiple subsites. In these cases, reconstructive strategies that restore anatomic form as well as the specialized and coordinated function of each subsite are critical for success. Patient selection, preoperative planning, operative technique, and postsurgical care all greatly influence the ultimate success of multisite reconstruction of the oral cavity. This chapter will discuss the relevant challenges and potential solutions involved in the repair of these defects.

Keywords: oral cavity, carcinoma, squamous cell carcinoma, lip, tonsil, gingiva, palate, tongue, retromolar trigone, buccal, mucosa, salivary gland, pharynx, alveolus, floor of mouth, free flap, skin graft, local flap

31.1 Introduction

Head and neck cancer has a yearly incidence of around 5%, although a disproportionate percentage of these malignancies arise within the oral cavity.[1] Dysfunction caused by oral malignancy is particularly problematic due to the high degree of coordination necessary for oral competence, digestion, swallowing, speech, and respiration. The highly specialized structures and distinct tissue types responsible for these functions are in close proximity and share tissue planes that extend across subsite boundaries. For this reason, invasive malignancies are likely to involve multiple oral cavity subsites. Surgical resection can therefore be expected to produce complicated and multifaceted defects that require careful planning and execution by the reconstructive surgeon.

The innovative architect Frank Lloyd Wright wrote in 1949 that "form and function thus become one in design and execution if the nature of materials and methods and purposes are all in unison."[2] The same is true of surgical reconstruction, where the goal of unison between form and function is achieved only after appropriate choice of replacement tissue, flap type, design, and inset. This chapter will discuss surgical considerations important in the reconstruction of multisite oral cavity defects with this goal in mind.

31.2 Diagnosis and Evaluation

31.2.1 Patient Selection

The evaluation of the patient with oral malignancy should involve the comprehensive efforts of a multidisciplinary head and neck cancer team, including the head and neck surgeon, reconstructive surgeon, pathologist, radiologist, radiation oncologist, medical oncologist, oral surgeon, prosthodontist, psychosocial oncologist, nutritionist, and speech and language pathologist.

Evaluation of the patient by the reconstructive team attempts to assess the extent of the disease, predict the anticipated defect, and create a plan for repair. The guiding principles described by Millard and Gillies "to replace like with like" and to "think of reconstruction in terms of units" are particularly relevant in cases with multisite involvement. Keeping these tenets in mind will help to sort through the various reconstructive options and present the patients with the most suitable for their specific needs. A careful conversation about all options, including a discussion of the risks and benefits inherent to each, is critical for proper informed consent. The associated donor site morbidities, the need for additional procedures, and the timeline for recovery should be outlined. It is imperative to understand the patients' goals for treatment, their motivations, and expectations. The possibility of postoperative functional and/or aesthetic deficits should be addressed so that expectations can be managed appropriately.

With the help of the head and neck cancer team, the patient's medical fitness to undergo major surgery should be determined. Consultation with other specialists for risk stratification and preoperative work-up can detect patients who should not have surgery. Ancillary testing such as angiography to assess peripheral vascularity can be considered if free tissue transfer is necessary in the setting of peripheral vascular disease.

The overall nutrition status of the patient can be assessed through history, consultation with a nutritionist, or laboratory values such as albumin and pre-albumin that can indicate malnutrition. A swallow assessment by a speech and language pathologist is important to detect dysphagia that may cause aspiration. Some patients will benefit from immediate dietary modification, nil per os (NPO) status, or prophylactic gastrostomy tube placement.[3]

A thorough history should be taken, with attention to past or current tobacco use, alcohol consumption, use of anticoagulants, prior radiation therapy, past head, neck, or extremity surgery, immunosuppression, systemic diseases such as Raynaud's disease or scleroderma, as well as current medications and allergies.

Assuming a surgical treatment is indicated and the patient is medically fit to withstand an operation, a thorough examination of the oral cavity will help to determine the best reconstructive plan. The following section will discuss considerations by oral cavity subsite.

31.2.2 Evaluation of Projected Subsite-Specific Defect

Oral cancer may present in a variety of forms, from seemingly small and superficial lesions to deeply infiltrative or submucosal masses. This variance adds to the challenge of predicting the final defect. Furthermore, the importance of obtaining negative surgical margins for oncologic control will necessarily lead to a defect larger than the size of the tumor itself. Intraoperative findings such as perineural involvement, metastatic lymphadenopathy, adherence to adjacent structures, or findings of unexpected progression can also lead to defects larger than anticipated. The concept of field cancerization represents a condition in which several tumor cells exist over a wide mucosal area, with potential segments of normal-appearing tissue in between.[4] Obtaining negative surgical margins can be difficult and may also lead to larger defects. Despite these uncertainties, "observation remains the basis of surgical diagnosis," and a systematic and careful examination of each subsite will best inform the reconstructive plan.[5]

Floor of Mouth

The floor of mouth represents a U-shaped mucosal lined space situated under the anterior ventral tongue and extending forward to the mandibular gingiva. Deep to this space, the mylohyoid muscle forms a sling which separates the floor of mouth from the submandibular and submental spaces. The sublingual frenulum bisects the floor of mouth, bordered by the paired papillae of the Wharton's ducts. Sublingual folds of redundant mucosa as well as submucosal sublingual veins are found lateral to the frenulum. The floor of mouth extends posterolaterally adjoining the inferior lateral tongue and terminating at the anterior tonsillar pillar.[6] Due to the contiguous nature of the floor of mouth, advanced tumors may invade the base of tongue or anterior mandible. Palpation of mobile mandibular segments may suggest pathologic fracture if tumor invasion of the mandible is present. Loose teeth or edentulous areas adjacent to the primary tumor or firm and fixed lesions involving the gingiva or floor of mouth mucosa along the mandible are signs for probable bony invasion. Paresthesia of the chin may suggest tumor infiltration of the inferior alveolar nerve. Palpation of the submandibular and submental spaces may detect tumor invasion through the mylohyoid sling, and inspection of the external skin for signs of ulceration or induration can detect full-thickness involvement. Because the mucosa of the anterior ventral tongue is contiguous with the floor of mouth, the junction between these two subsites is important to assess. The same is true for the posterior where the floor of mouth abuts the tongue base. Assessment of tongue mobility and direct palpation can detect extension between these subsites as well.

Buccal Mucosa

The buccal mucosa is the membranous internal lining of the cheek extending from the inner oral commissure anteriorly to the pterygomandibular raphe found just lateral to the retromolar trigone. Medially, the buccal mucosa attaches to the upper and lower alveolar ridges to create the gingivobuccal sulci. The mucosa is bordered laterally by thin layers of soft tissue including the pharyngobasilar fascia, buccinator muscle, buccal fat, facial nerve branches, superficial musculoaponeurotic system (SMAS), and cheek skin. Low resilience of these tissues to infiltrating buccal lesions can allow lateral tumor extension, which may cause facial nerve paresis, orocutaneous fistulae, or skin changes. Stensen's duct pierces the buccinator muscle and terminates at the papilla found within the buccal mucosa, creating another potential route of tumor egress. Additional routes of spread may occur in all directions to reach the alveolar ridge, retromolar trigone, ascending mandibular ramus, lateral tongue, and floor of mouth.[7]

Hard Palate and Maxilla

The hard palate creates the roof of the oral cavity and extends from the gingiva of the upper dentition to its border with the soft palate. It consists of both the primary and secondary palate, which are separated by the incisive foramen. It is covered by a thick and adherent mucosal layer. Inspection and palpation of the palate is important because although ulcerative or exophytic masses are easily seen, minor salivary gland carcinomas arise submucosally and can be covered by normal-appearing mucosa. Palatal hypoesthesia may indicate perineural invasion through the sphenopalatine or pterygopalatine fossae. Anterior midline hard palate lesions may appear isolated but lateral or posterior lesions may involve adjacent subsites including the alveolar ridges, gingiva, maxilla, or pterygoid space.[8] Due to the dense adherence of the hard palate mucosa, most lesions will be relatively fixed even in the absence of bony invasion. Diagnostic imaging is helpful to assess bony invasion. Oroantral fistulae and loose or missing dentition may be noted.

Tongue

The tongue occupies the majority of the oral cavity and consists of eight muscles covered by mucosa containing minor salivary glands, papillae, and taste buds. The tip of the tongue is the pointed anterior-most portion which is highly mobile. The body of the tongue has dorsal, ventral, and lateral surfaces and contacts the floor of mouth. The oral tongue is also divided down the midline by the fibrous lingual septum which creates the median sulcus. The base of tongue, located posterior to the circumvallate papillae, is a structure of the oropharynx. The hypoglossal nerve supplies the motor innervation to the tongue and can be assessed by tongue mobility with hypoglossal palsy causing deviation toward the ipsilateral side. The vagus nerve contributes motor innervation to the palatoglossus muscle. The mandibular division of the trigeminal nerve contributes sensation to the oral tongue, and the chorda tympani, via the facial nerve, provides taste sensation. Tumors arising within the tongue can easily extend into the floor of mouth, gingiva, and mandible.[9]

Mandible

The mandible is a horseshoe-shaped bone within the oral cavity that is covered by mucosa and gingiva and harbors the lower dentition. The muscles of mastication insert on the mandible as do the suprahyoid muscles. The bone itself is covered by a periosteal layer. The inferior alveolar nerve that enters the mandible through the mandibular foramen runs within the bone until it exits as the mental nerve through the mental foramen. The bone is subdivided into sections including the symphysis, parasymphysis, body, angle, ascending ramus, condyle, and coronoid process. The mandible has variable thickness and vertical height with both a lingual and buccal cortex. The retromolar trigone represents the region where the body of the mandible transitions to the ascending ramus and is located just posterior to the third molar. The gingiva and mucosa are tightly adherent to the bone but are contiguous with the mucosal surfaces of other subsites such as the floor of mouth and the buccal space. Inspection of the baseline occlusion is critical during the initial assessment of an oral malignancy. If the mandible is involved and requires reconstruction, restoring class I or premorbid occlusion is a major reconstructive goal. The degree of mouth opening and presence of trismus is assessed by measuring the inter-incisor distance. Tumor infiltration of the pterygoid space or pain in opening of mouth may cause severe trismus which can make airway management difficult as well as make surgery necessary.

Lips

The lips form the anterior entrance into the oral cavity and have several crucial functions including articulation of speech, facial expression and aesthetics, oral competence during eating, and sensation. The orbicularis oris muscle courses circumferentially to create the upper and lower lips which join laterally at the oral commissure. The muscle is covered by skin, vermillion mucosa, and oral mucosa. This coverage is contiguous with the gingivolabial sulci and the buccal mucosa. Motor innervation to the lips is by the facial nerve, and sensation by the second and third divisions of the trigeminal nerve. Oral competence should create a watertight seal when the mouth is closed to prevent drooling or air escape during speech. The lips can be palpated and distracted away from the jaw in order gauge mobility. For primary lip cancers, determination of the percentage of the total lip length involved is important when choosing reconstructive options microstomia is to be avoided.

31.3 Determination of Reconstructive Options

The major goals of oral cavity reconstruction include: restoring lost volume, separating the oral cavity from the neck, allowing functional speech and swallowing, maintaining tongue mobility, establishing normal occlusion, allowing normal temporomandibular function without trismus, avoiding microstomia, and providing acceptable aesthetic appearance. Defects involving multiple subsites may demand attention to all or many of these challenges.

The reconstructive ladder represents a conceptual framework useful in the assessment of any defect. It includes every surgical option starting with the simplest and least invasive and moving toward the most complicated techniques. The smallest and most superficial defects can be addressed either by healing by secondary intention or primary closure, which make up the first two rungs of the ladder. However, as this chapter focuses specifically on multisite defects, the strategies of the higher rungs including local, regional, and free tissue reconstruction will be discussed.

The size and anatomic position of the defect, involved subsites, tissue types missing, degree of volume loss, and functional deficits are all used to determine the best reconstructive option. The need for bone, soft tissue, muscle, mucosal coverage, or any combination will make certain options more suitable than others. Flaps that allow motor or sensory innervation may better address functional losses than other options. Composite flaps containing several tissue types or the use of multiple flaps may be chosen. Local and regional flaps may involve less morbidity and perhaps lower risk than free tissue transfer, but rely on the availability of adequate nearby donor tissue and limitations on pedicle rotation. Free tissue transfer involves donor site morbidity, but can reliably provide the necessary bulk, specific tissue-type required, and options for innervation. Furthermore, the large primary tumors that create multisite defects often require postoperative adjuvant radiation therapy. Vascularized free tissue can resist the effects of radiation that lead to late complications.[10] A well-designed free flap containing all necessary elements and a resilient blood supply may ultimately involve less cost and morbidity than several local or regional flaps used over time that fail to achieve their goals.

31.3.1 Diagnostic Imaging

The major imaging modalities used for the diagnosis of head and neck cancer including CT scan, MRI, and angiography can be useful in planning multisite reconstruction. CT scan is especially valuable for detecting bony invasion that may require resection of the mandible or maxilla. MRI can assess tumor invasion into adjacent soft tissue spaces, such as the tongue and floor-of-mouth or buccal space. Protocols for three-dimensional reconstruction of both CT scan and MRI images are available that may illustrate the spatial complexity of the tumor and involved tissues. The role of angiography is mainly for assessing the vascularity of potential free flap harvest sites, such as the lower leg in patients with peripheral artery disease or the forearm in patients with history of prior trauma.

Virtual surgical planning (VSP) has evolved into a useful tool in craniofacial surgery, with potential benefits of decreased operative time and increased technical precision. Pretreatment planning using CT imaging, customized plating materials, and osteotomy cutting guides can be created to exact specification (▶ Fig. 31.1). However, in oncologic surgery, tumor progression can occur between planning and treatment, and resection margins may extend further than anticipated, making VSP no longer applicable. The learning curve for efficient use of the technology is another potential challenge. A recent review of the use of VSP in craniofacial free flap surgery found that the technology was completely abandoned in 4% of cases and only partially adhered to in 11%.[11]

31.4 Surgical Considerations and Approaches

31.4.1 Tongue and Floor of Mouth

Surgical goals for reconstruction of the tongue and floor of mouth include restoring tongue mobility, avoiding tethering or contraction, providing adequate volume without excessive bulk, allowing normal submandibular gland function, and separating the floor of mouth from the neck. In order for the tongue to retain the ability to articulate speech and manipulate the food bolus, it should be separate from the floor of mouth.

Secondary intention healing or skin grafting of the floor of mouth risks contraction or scar formation; therefore flap reconstruction is optimal. The submental island flap was first described in 1993 and can provide soft tissue bulk as well as skin coverage for floor of mouth reconstruction. A skin paddle harvested from the submental region based on the submental artery, a branch of the facial artery, can be inset intra-orally (▶ Fig. 31.2). The submental flap can be used for floor of mouth

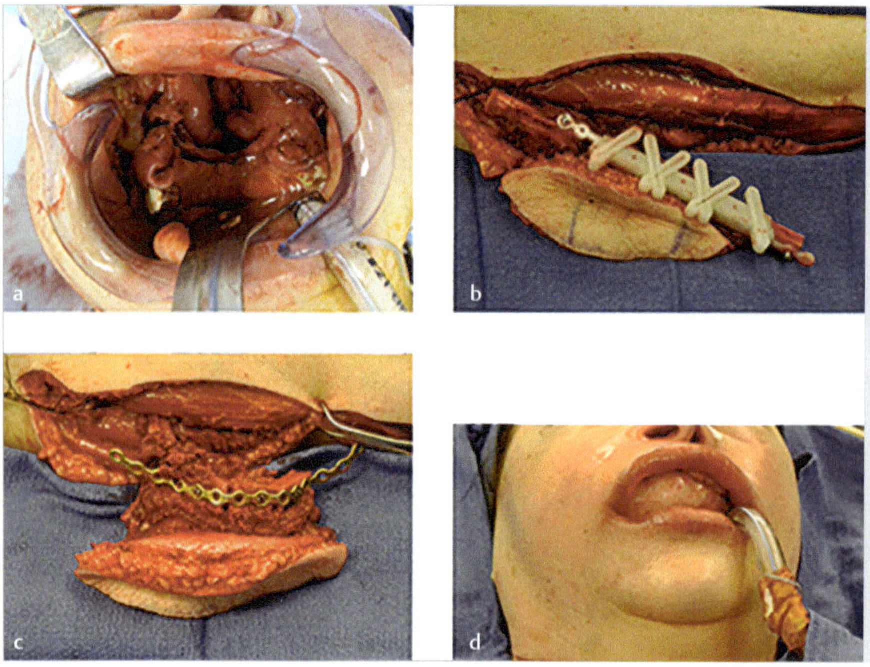

Fig. 31.1 (a–d) Osteocutaneous radial forearm free flap with utilization of cutting guides to create osteotomies for total palatal reconstruction.

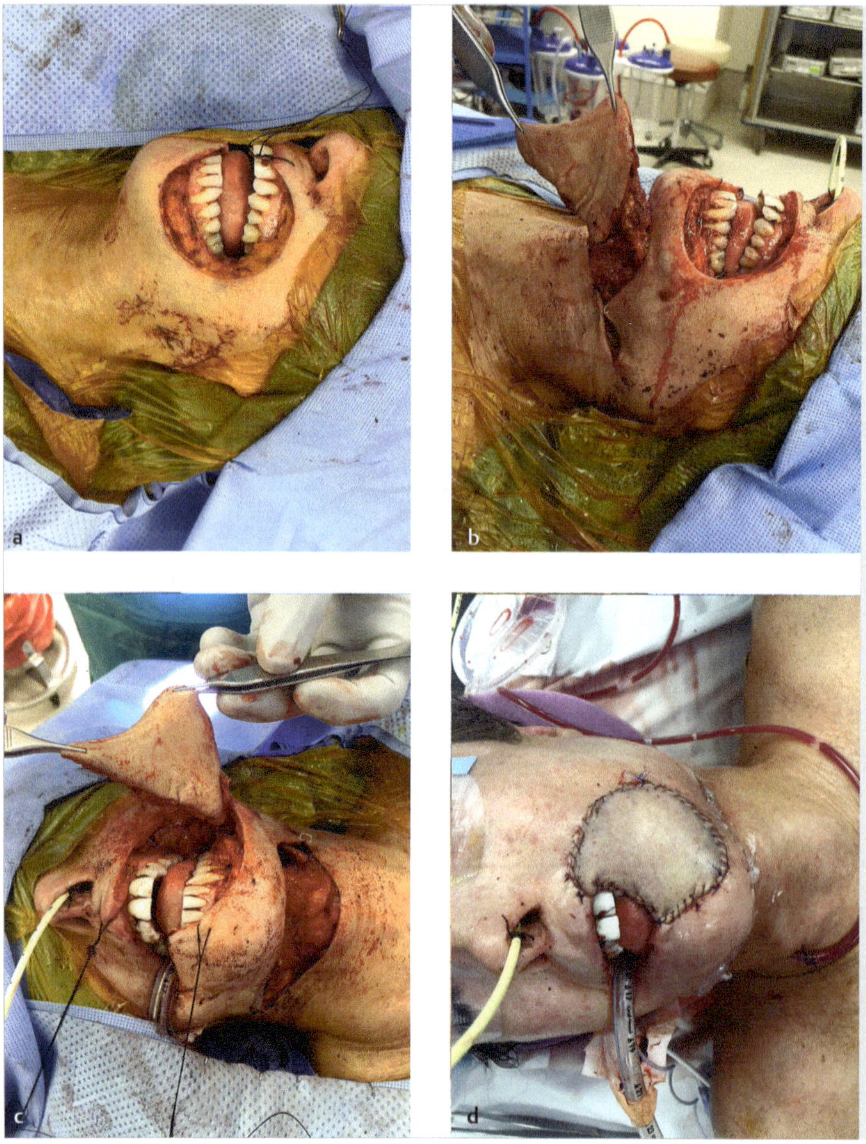

Fig. 31.2 (a–d) Through and through defect of internal and external buccal lining. Submental island flap raised based on submental artery and vein. Submental flap is tunneled subcutaneously to buccal defect and secured.

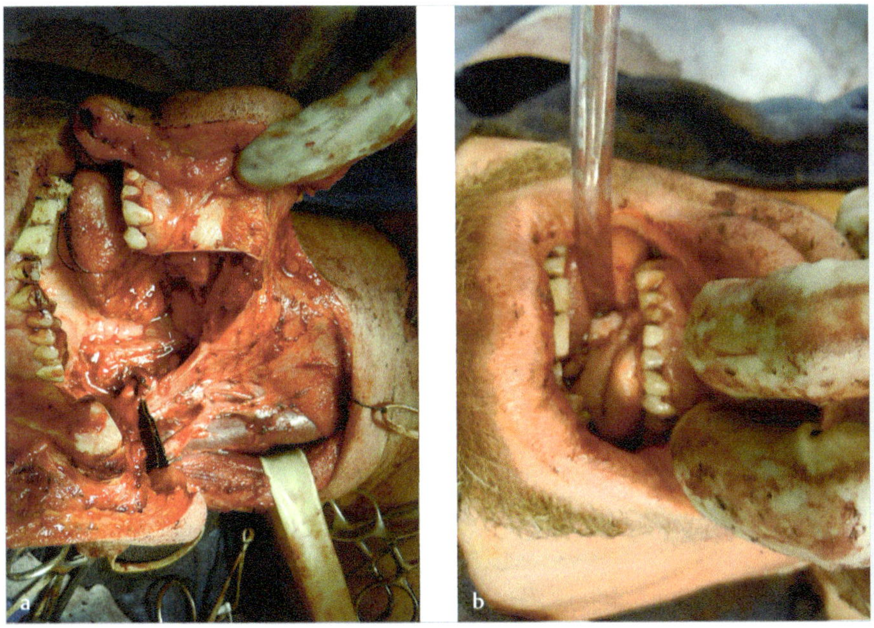

Fig. 31.3 (a, b) Right floor of mouth defect and partial glossectomy exposed through a mandibulotomy approach. Radial forearm inset to floor of mouth and tongue.

defects that extend onto the ventral anterior tongue or in combination with the radial forearm free flap for tongue reconstruction. Skin coverage of all raw surfaces is important to prevent scarring that can restrict tongue mobility. A recent retrospective review comparing the submental island flap and radial forearm free flap for floor of mouth reconstruction showed decreased hospital costs and comparable outcomes for the submental flap.[12] However, large multisite defects may be too large for the submental flap alone. The platysma flap has also been described for floor of mouth reconstruction and can be used alternatively to the submental island flap. It can be harvested as either a muscle-only or musculocutaneous flap and is based on the submental artery as well.[13]

Glossectomy defects that partially extend into the floor of mouth can be addressed with a bilobed modification of the radial forearm free flap. One lobe of the flap is used to reconstruct the shape and volume of the tongue and the second lobe is used to resurface the floor of mouth and gingiva[14] (▶ Fig. 31.3). A double bilobed design has also been described, with two bilobed flaps transposed toward the midline. This recreates the tip of the tongue and can provide adequate bulk and the depth needed to create a ventral sulcus, which maintains oral competence by collecting food and saliva.[15] Another modification of the radial forearm flap which can be used to reconstruct combined defects of the floor of mouth and tongue is the beavertail modification (▶ Fig. 31.4). In this technique, proximal fat and fascia are harvested along with the fasciocutaneous flap. The beavertail of tissue can be dissected free of the vascular pedicle and folded beneath the flap to provide more bulk or to repair adjacent floor of mouth defects.[16]

The combined use of the radial forearm free flap for glossectomy reconstruction and the facial artery musculomucosal (FAMM) flap is another option for defects involving both the tongue and floor of mouth subsites. The FAMM flap is pedicled on the facial artery and is harvested to include mucosa, submucosa, buccinator muscle, and the draining venous plexus. It can be based either superiorly or inferiorly but an inferior design with anterograde flow is best suited for floor of mouth reconstruction.[17]

The use of the buccal fat pad flap may also be considered for combined tongue and floor of mouth defects. The buccal fat is found within the masticator space between the buccinator and masseter muscles. It receives blood supply from the buccal branch of the maxillary artery and the transverse facial artery. It can quickly and easily be dissected and teased out of the masticator space or may be exposed by the surgical resection itself. The fat pad is surrounded by a thin capsule that should be preserved. Although this flap does not provide bulk, it does provide vascularized tissue that can be used to cover exposed bone or small mucosal defects that remain after adjacent subsite reconstruction. The buccal fat epithelializes by around 3 weeks and eventually is covered with mucosal lining.[18]

31.4.2 Mandible and Floor of Mouth

The goals of mandibular reconstruction include restoring continuity of the mandibular arch, establishing normal occlusion, anatomic positioning of the condyles, creation of adequate mandibular height, and avoiding trismus and oral incompetence. Combined defects of the mandible and floor of mouth require both an osseous and soft tissue component as well as lining (▶ Fig. 31.5 and ▶ Fig. 31.6). The traditional techniques for mandibular reconstruction including the fibula, scapula, and iliac crest free flaps have limited tissue available for adjacent site reconstruction. Multisite defects involving a significant portion of the lip in addition to the mandible may require a combination of free tissue transfer to adequately restore form and function of the oral sphincter (▶ Fig. 31.7).

The scapular free flap has the advantage of providing multiple fascio- and musculocutaneous paddles in addition to bone stock. Chimeric designs based on the subscapular vessel axis may include the parascapular flap, latissimus muscle, and serratus muscle. Furthermore, the bone and skin paddles have a large degree of mobility relative to one another which can

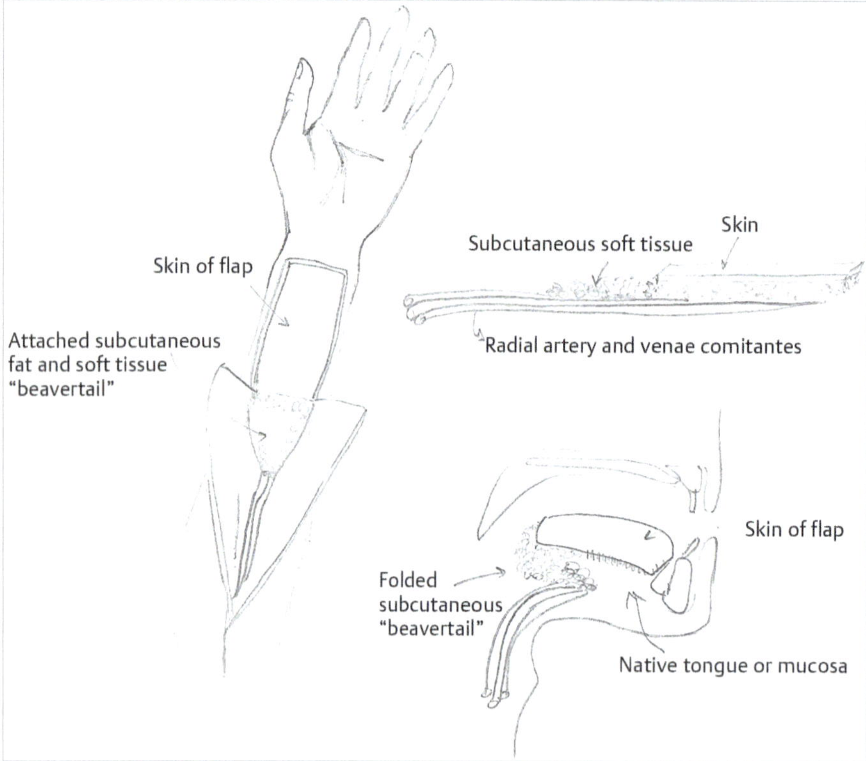

Fig. 31.4 "Beavertail" modification of radial forearm microvascular free flap includes a tail of subcutaneous tissue adjacent to area of skin harvested. This additional tail of subcutaneous tissue can be included to provide additional bulk in reconstruction.

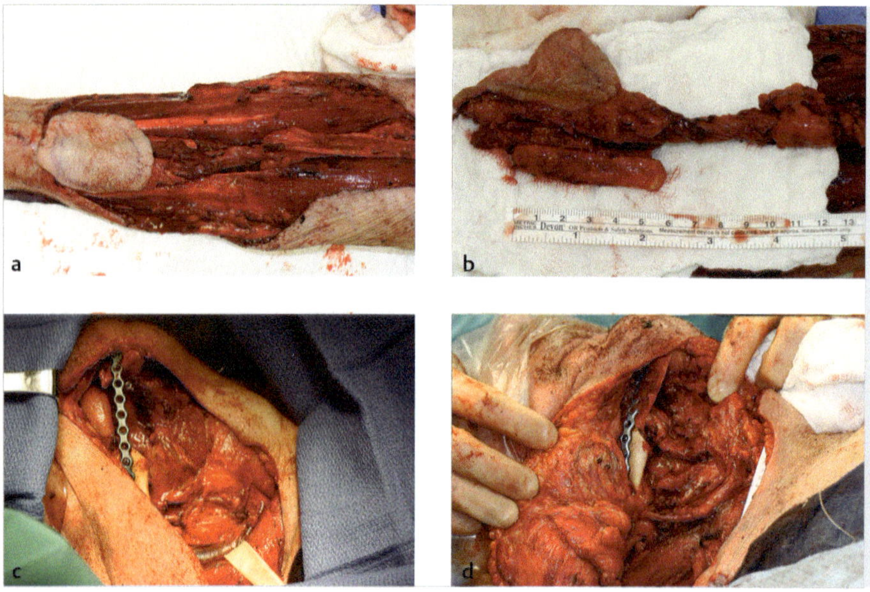

Fig. 31.5 (a–d) Right mandibular body and adjacent floor of mouth defect. Osteocutaneous radial forearm flap with 5.5 cm of bone and accompanying skin paddle used to reconstruct both mandibular bone and intraoral soft tissue defects.

facilitate inset in difficult cases involving multiple subsites.[19] The major drawback to use of the scapular flap is the need for prone positioning of the patient during harvest which can increase operative time.

Modification of the fibula free flap to incorporate two separate skin paddles supplied by the peroneal artery may allow skin coverage of both the mandibular reconstruction and floor of mouth. The second skin paddle can be raised to include perforators through the soleus muscle. A recent review of 32 procedures using the double skin paddle fibula free flap for mandibulofacial reconstruction found two partial soleus skin paddle losses and two cases of dehiscence of the second paddle causing fistulae[20,21] (▶ Fig. 31.8). In 15% of patients the proximal perforator does not arise directly from the peroneal artery in the area of dissection and requires a separate anastomosis.[20,21] Additionally, the fibula flap can be combined with cervicofacial soft tissue rotational flaps to reconstruct through and through defects (▶ Fig. 31.7). Using adjacent tissue from the head and neck also allows for better color match of external skin.

The pectoralis myocutaneous flap can be considered in addition to the options for free flap reconstruction of the mandible listed above. The large skin paddle and available muscle of this

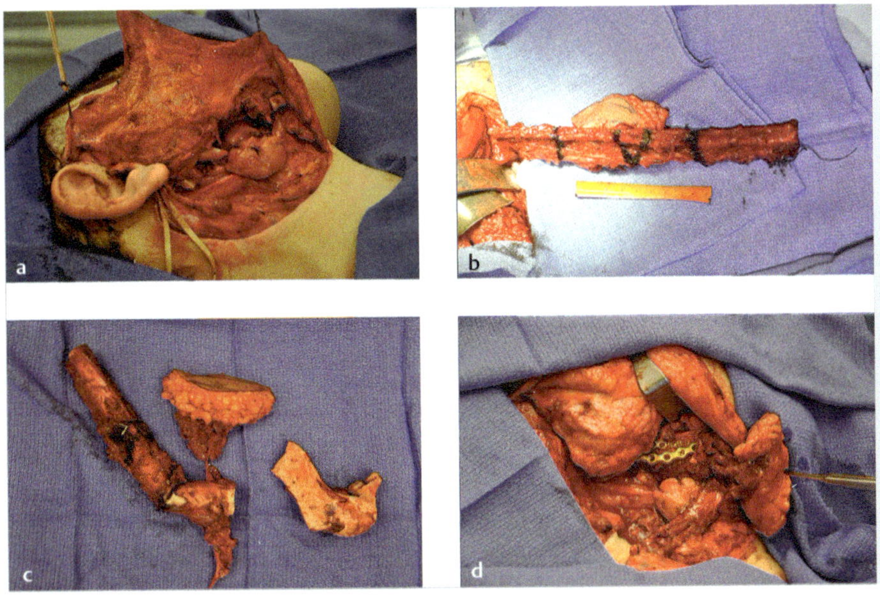

Fig. 31.6 (a–d) Right mandibular angle and floor of mouth defect. Fibula free flap design with single osteotomy. Perforator dissection of skin paddle and bony resection specimen. Inset of flap with skin paddle located intraorally and reconstruction plating.

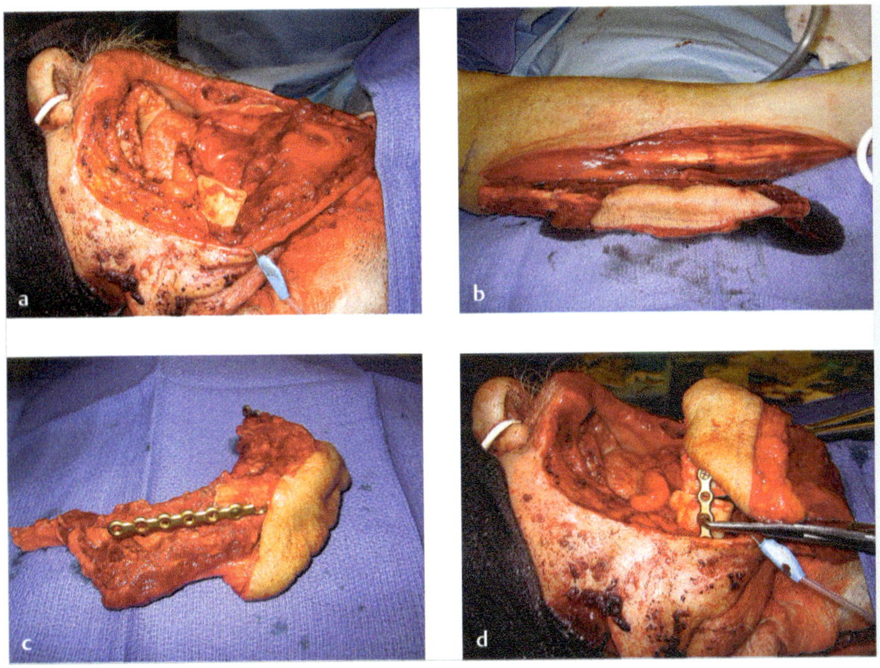

Fig. 31.7 (a–d) Defect of anterior mandibular bone, floor of mouth, and lower lip. Fibula free flap with two osteotomies. Reconstruction plate used to fixate fibula to residual mandibular body. Fibula skin paddle placed intraorally. Tensor fascia lata placed over fibula and tunneled to midline upper lip bilaterally. Anterolateral thigh skin paddle used to reconstruct external lower lip skin defect.

flap can be used for the floor of mouth, preserving the skin paddle of the osteocutaneous free flap for mandibular coverage. However, the combined use of two flaps increases donor site morbidity and is less likely to restore oral cavity function.

There is a role for skin grafting in mandibular defects that involve either the adjacent lip, floor of mouth, or buccal subsites. In these cases, the loss of an adequately deep gingivolabial, gingivobuccal, or floor of mouth sulcus can lead to oral incompetence, drooling, dysphagia, and articulation difficulties. After adequate reconstruction of the underlying soft tissue bulk using the methods previously discussed, full thickness spacer grafts can be used to recreate well-lined sulci without raw surfaces prone to contracture or areas of excessive tension.

31.4.3 Mandible and Buccal Mucosa

Buccal mucosal defects associated with lateral mandibulectomy may be closed primarily or allowed to granulate if small. However, if the buccinator muscle is involved or closure involves excess tension, trismus is likely to occur. The use of free mucosal grafts or split and full thickness skin grafts can restore lining and recreate the gingivobuccal sulcus as discussed previously. The buccal fat pad, as previously mentioned, may be used if not involved in the resection. The temporoparietal fascial flap, based on the superficial temporal system, can be rotated to provide a thin, well-vascularized fascial lining which readily accepts a skin graft.[22] The strength of the fascia makes this choice more resilient to scarring than mucosal or skin grafting

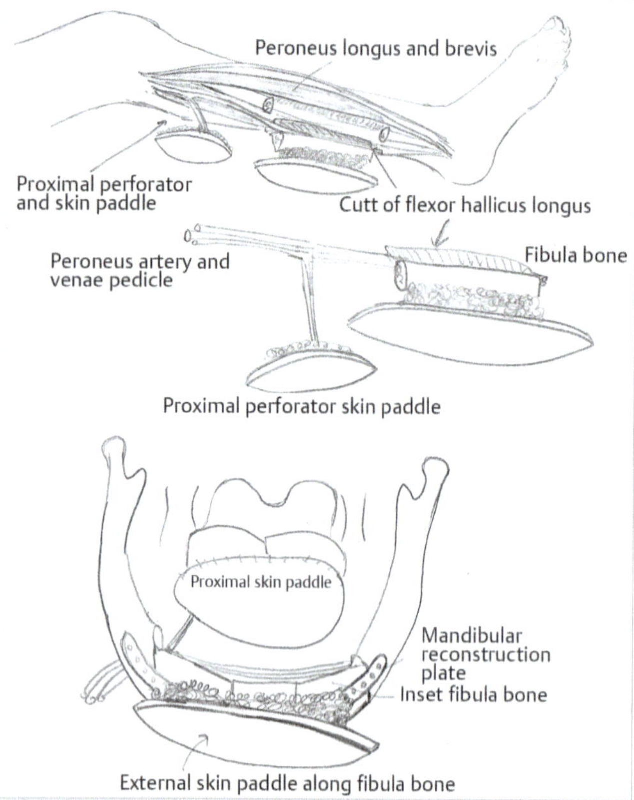

Fig. 31.8 Double paddle fibula design with a proximal skin paddle based on a proximal perforator. In majority of cases the proximal perforator joins with the peroneal pedicle but in 15% of cases an additional anastomosis is needed. The proximal perforator paddle has additional mobility that is amenable to intraoral and external defects.

alone, and the thin nature of the flap can prevent excess intraoral bulk. The temporalis muscle flap, based on the deep temporal system, can provide a 10 × 20 cm area of muscle that may be ideal for more extensive buccal defects that require more soft tissue.[23] Postoperative retraction and fibrosis can occur which can lead to trismus. The chimeric and double-skin paddle free flaps discussed above are options for combined mandible and buccal defects as well (▶ Fig. 31.8).

31.4.4 Maxilla and Hard Palate

Reconstructive goals for hard palate and maxillary defects include creating a barrier between the oral cavity and nasal cavity, establishing normal occlusion, maintaining midface projection, preserving a patent nasal cavity, and avoiding oroantral fistula. When defects are isolated to the hard palate and a majority of the maxillary alveolus is preserved, the use of obturation with a custom dental appliance provides a nonsurgical solution that some patients may prefer as an alternative to surgery. Palatal obturation is not an option for those patients that lack a stable base along the maxillary alveolus for the obturator to attach. Some patients may also prefer a permanent surgical solution over the daily maintenance, oral discomfort, and frequent modifications of their device. Defects of the hard palate and maxilla require a stable osseous component to reconstruct the maxillary arch and a soft tissue component to provide the lining of the hard palate. Through and through defects into the nasal cavity often require stenting to maintain nasal airway patency. Another challenge in extensive hard palate defects is sagging of soft tissue inferiorly into the oral cavity if not supported posteriorly. The osteocutaneous forearm, fibula, and scapular tip flaps are traditionally used for these defects as they provide an osseous component as well as thin, pliable soft tissue to recreate the oral lining (▶ Fig. 31.9, ▶ Fig. 31.10, ▶ Fig. 31.11). Fibula flaps have the advantage of possible dental implant placement in the future for dental rehabilitation.

31.5 Perioperative Management

Reconstruction of multisite oral cavity defects usually demands extensive surgery and patients should be monitored in the intensive care setting postoperatively. Specific protocols for postoperative monitoring of free flaps used for reconstruction should be implemented to identify early signs of vascular compromise. The major complications following surgery include airway compromise, bleeding, flap failure, fistulae formation, and infection. History of preoperative irradiation is a predictor of free flap complications after oral cavity reconstruction.[24,25] Diet should be managed appropriately and NPO status maintained to allow healing of incisions, epithelialization of raw surfaces, protection of flap pedicles, and prevention of orocutaneous fistulae. Furthermore, history of radiation therapy and tongue base resection are independent predictors of postsurgical aspiration.[26] Early speech and language therapy is crucial for preventing trismus, restoring the ability for oral diet, and improving speech intelligibility. Long-term management may include flap revision for debulking, release of scar tissue, creation of more effective oral sulci, or local tissue rearrangements to improve function.

31.6 Surgical Sequelae

Complex intraoral reconstruction requires long-term follow-up in order to identify functional deficits that are correctable. Scar

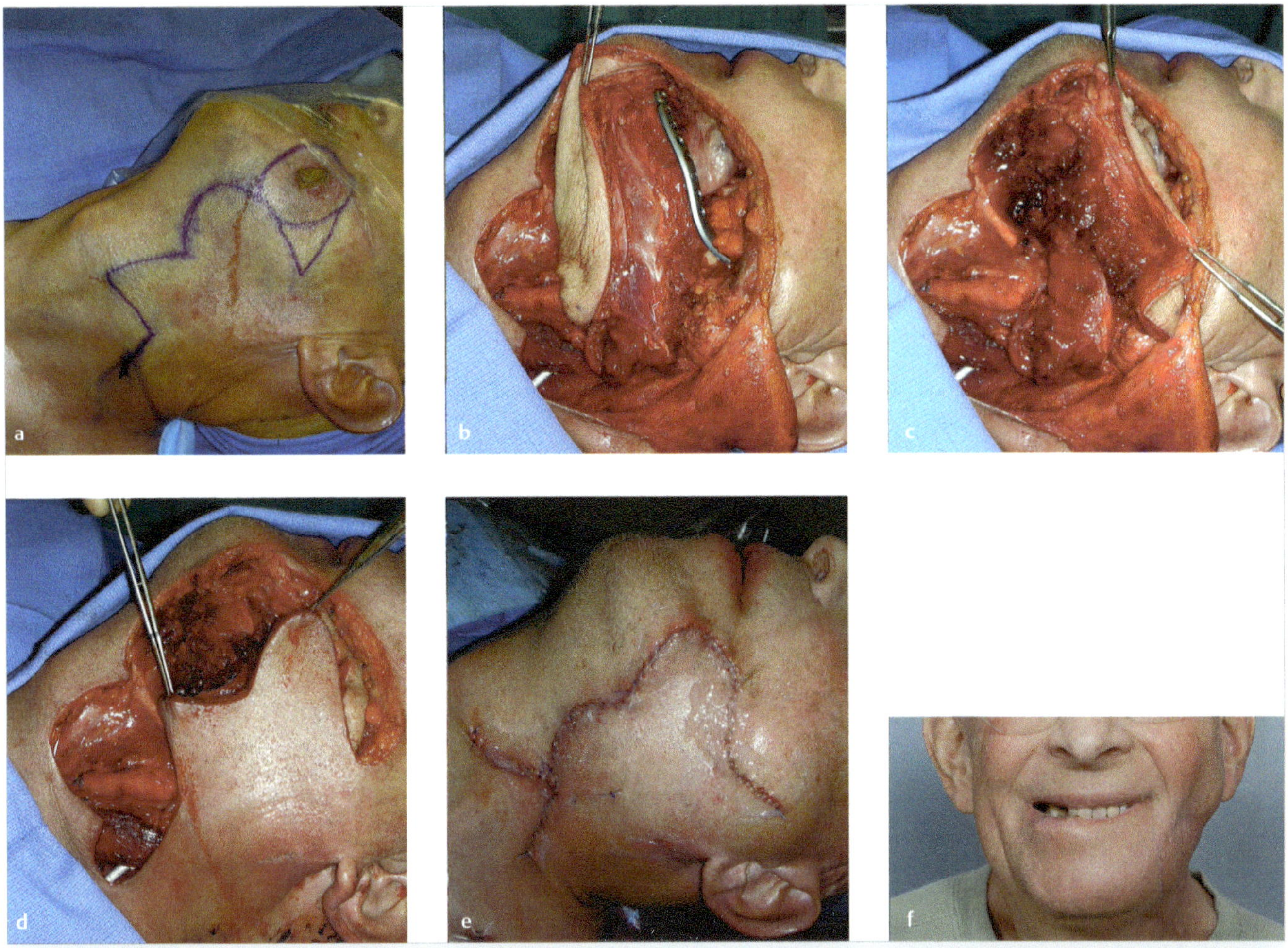

Fig. 31.9 (a–f) Bilobe flap design encompassing external skin lesion. Left mandibular angle defect with fibula flap in place. Fibula skin paddle placed intraorally. Bilobe flap rotated to cover external component.

formation between adjacent subsites may lead to immobility of structures or interference with articulation or swallowing. Serial steroid injections may have limited success but scar revision is usually required to restore function. Direct excision, z-plasty, and spacer skin grafting may all be needed. Excess soft tissue bulk may also cause speech and swallowing dysfunction. At the time of initial reconstruction, more tissue volume is generally preferred over too little, as some degree of atrophy is expected of any noninnervated flap or graft. However, revision surgery to debulk areas of excess can make significant functional improvements. Trismus is an especially problematic surgical sequelae caused by fibrosis of the temporomandibular joint (TMJ), pterygoid musculature, and buccal and masticator spaces. Aggressive physiotherapy may lead to improved mouth opening, as can steroid injection. Surgical release of fibrotic tissue or coronoidectomy may be required in severe cases. Aesthetic sequelae such as unsightly scarring, contour irregularities, or facial weakness can all be addressed after oncologic treatment and healing are complete.

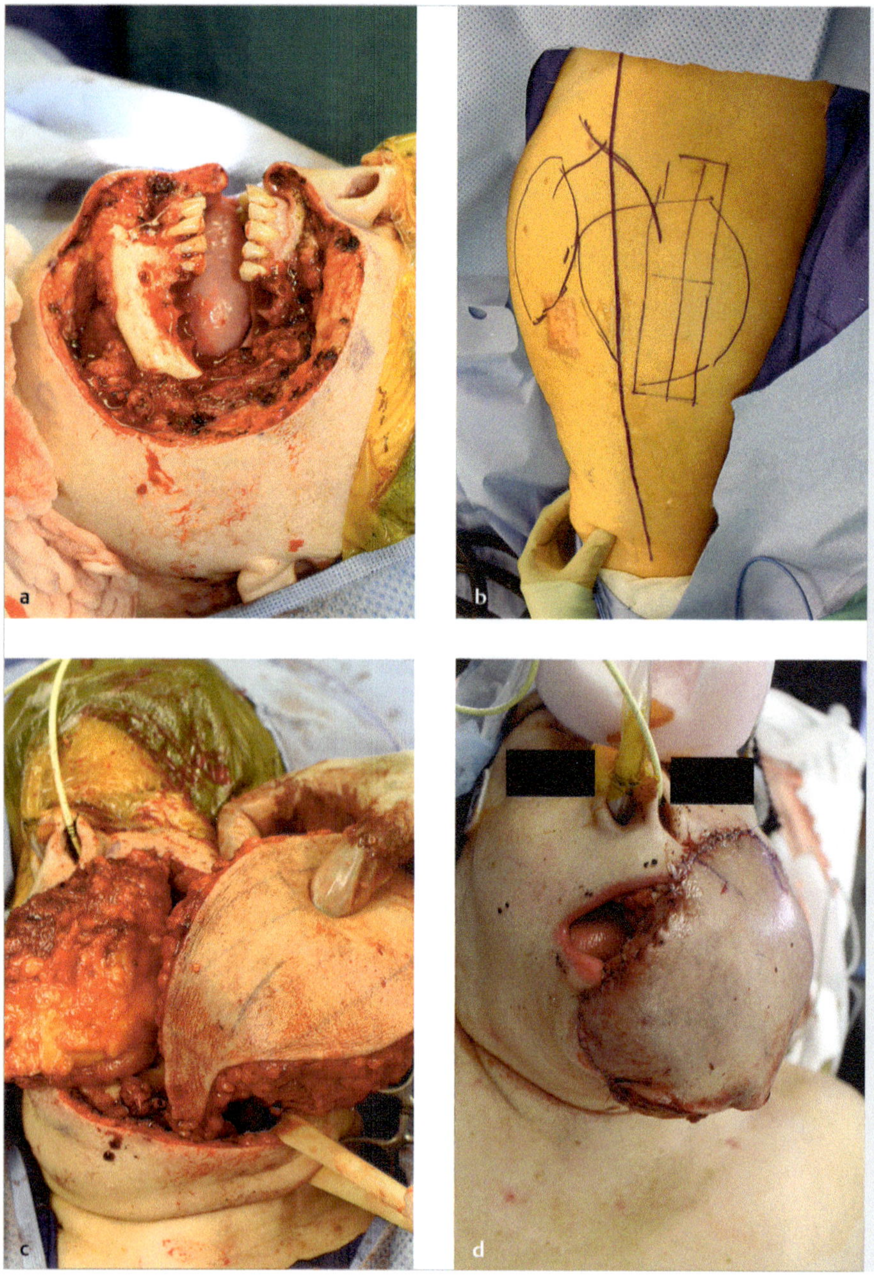

Fig. 31.10 (a–d) Through and through defect of left buccal skin and mucosa and majority of left upper and lower lip. Double paddle design to anterolateral thigh flap. Inset of intraoral and external components.

Key Points

- The close spatial relationships between distinct tissue types found in the oral cavity can allow invasive malignancies to span multiple subsites.
- Reconstruction of multisite oral cavity defects should attempt to restore both form and function including breathing, speech, swallowing, facial expression, and aesthetic appearance.
- A careful examination of all involved subsites will help predict the extent and tissues involved by the final defect.
- Multisite defects may require the use of several different techniques, modifications of a single technique, inclusion of multiple skin paddles, or chimeric flap designs.
- Identification and treatment of postoperative sequalae including trismus, intraoral scarring, excess bulk, and aesthetic deformities are important for quality of life.

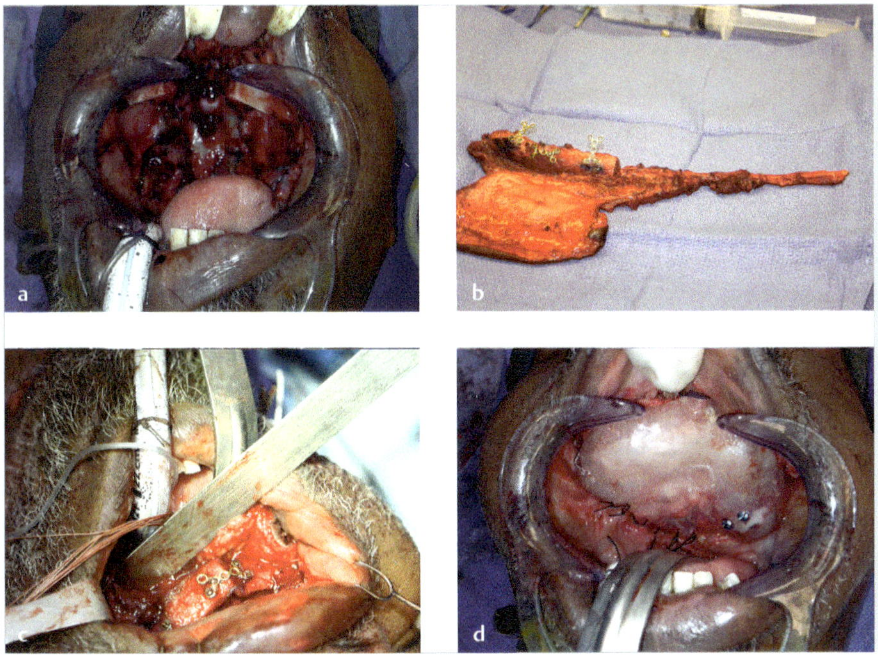

Fig. 31.11 (a–d) Defect encompassing the entire hard palate and maxillary alveolar ridge. Osteocutaneous forearm with single osteotomy. Double-Y miniplates used to fixate to anterior maxillary wall. Skin paddle secured to soft palate and left pterygoid plate.

References

[1] Vigneswaran N, Williams MD. Epidemiologic trends in head and neck cancer and aids in diagnosis. Oral Maxillofac Surg Clin North Am. 2014; 26(2):123–141

[2] Patterson T. Frank Lloyd Wright and the Meaning of Materials. 1st ed. New York, NY: Wiley; 1994

[3] Axelsson L, Silander E, Nyman J, Bove M, Johansson L, Hammerlid E. Effect of prophylactic percutaneous endoscopic gastrostomy tube on swallowing in advanced head and neck cancer: a randomized controlled study. Head Neck. 2017; 39(5):908–915

[4] Mohan M, Jagannathan N. Oral field cancerization: an update on current concepts. Oncol Rev. 2014; 8(1):244

[5] Gillies H, Millard RD. The Principles and Art of Plastic Surgery. Vol. 1. Miami, FL: Little, Brown and Co.; 1957

[6] Flint PW, Cummings CW. Cummings Otolaryngology—Head & Neck Surgery. 6th ed. Philadelphia, PA: Mosby/Elsevier; 2015

[7] Montero PH, Patel SG. Cancer of the oral cavity. Surg Oncol Clin N Am. 2015; 24(3):491–508

[8] Müller S. Update from the 4th edition of the World Health Organization of Head and Neck Tumours: Tumours of the Oral Cavity and Mobile Tongue. Head and Neck Pathology. 2017; 11(1):33–40

[9] Rana M, Iqbal A, Warraich R, Ruecker M, Eckardt AM, Gellrich N-C. Modern surgical management of tongue carcinoma—a clinical retrospective research over a 12 years period. Head Neck Oncol. 2011; 3:43

[10] Ho AS, Zumsteg ZS, Meyer A, et al. Impact of flap reconstruction on radiotoxicity after salvage surgery and reirradiation for recurrent head and neck cancer. Ann Surg Oncol. 2016; 23 Suppl 5:850–857

[11] Efanov JI, Roy A-A, Huang KN, Borsuk DE. Virtual surgical planning: the pearls and pitfalls. Plast Reconstr Surg Glob Open. 2018; 6(1):e1443

[12] Forner D, Phillips T, Rigby M, Hart R, Taylor M, Trites J. Submental island flap reconstruction reduces cost in oral cancer reconstruction compared to radial forearm free flap reconstruction: a case series and cost analysis. J Otolaryngol Head Neck Surg. 2016; 45:11

[13] Thakkur RK, Pandya SR. The posterosuperiorly based platysmal myocutaneous flap: the underutilized reconstructive option. J Maxillofac Oral Surg. 2015; 14(2):476–480

[14] Urken ML, Biller HF. A new bilobed design for the sensate radial forearm flap to preserve tongue mobility following significant glossectomy. Arch Otolaryngol Head Neck Surg. 1994; 120(1):26–31

[15] Ko AB, Lavertu P, Rezaee RP. Double bilobed radial forearm free flap for anterior tongue and floor-of-mouth reconstruction. Ear Nose Throat J. 2010; 89 (4):177–179

[16] Henry A, McCaul JA. Osseocutaneous radial forearm flap with beavertail modification; a case report of a novel, single, reconstructive free flap for the tongue, floor of mouth and mandible. Int J Surg Case Rep. 2016; 28: 270–273

[17] Pribaz J, Stephens W, Crespo L, Gifford G. A new intraoral flap: facial artery musculomucosal (FAMM) flap. Plast Reconstr Surg. 1992; 90(3):421–429

[18] Dean A, Alamillos F, García-López A, Sánchez J, Peñalba M. The buccal fat pad flap in oral reconstruction. Head Neck. 2001; 23(5):383–388

[19] Gibber MJ, Clain JB, Jacobson AS, et al. Subscapular system of flaps: an 8-year experience with 105 patients. Head Neck. 2015; 37(8):1200–1206

[20] Leclère FM, Bosc R, Temam S, et al. Reconstruction of large mandibulofacial defects with the composed double skin paddle fibula free flap: a review of 32 procedures. Laryngoscope. 2014; 124(6):1336–1343

[21] Winters HA, de Jongh GJ. Reliability of the proximal skin paddle of the osteocutaneous free fibula flap: a prospective clinical study. Plast Reconstr Surg. 1999; 103(3):846–849

[22] Squaquara R, Kim Evans KF, Spanio di Spilimbergo S, Mardini S. Intraoral reconstruction using local and regional flaps. Semin Plast Surg. 2010; 24(2): 198–211

[23] Brennan T, Tham TM, Costantino P. The temporalis muscle flap for palate reconstruction: case series and review of the literature. Int Arch Otorhinolaryngol. 2017; 21(3):259–264

[24] Lee S, Thiele C. Factors associated with free flap complications after head and neck reconstruction and the molecular basis of fibrotic tissue rearrangement in preirradiated soft tissue. J Oral Maxillofac Surg. 2010; 68(9):2169–2178

[25] Benatar MJ, Dassonville O, Chamorey E, et al. Impact of preoperative radiotherapy on head and neck free flap reconstruction: a report on 429 cases. J Plast Reconstr Aesthet Surg. 2013; 66(4):478–482

[26] Smith JE, Suh JD, Erman A, Nabili V, Chhetri DK, Blackwell KE. Risk factors predicting aspiration after free flap reconstruction of oral cavity and oropharyngeal defects. Arch Otolaryngol Head Neck Surg. 2008; 134(11):1205–1208

32 Neck Management for Oral Malignancies

Wojciech K. Mydlarz and Stephen Y. Lai

Summary

Oral cavity cancers are typically treated with surgery, and management of the regional neck lymph nodes is an important part of the initial treatment discussion. Oral cavity tumors can harbor early occult neck lymph node disease. Radiation therapy is an option for nonsurgical patients, but does not have good overall response or control rates. Patients with obvious neck disease require upfront surgical removal and potentially radiation with or without chemotherapy depending on high-risk pathologic factors. Management options of the clinically negative neck (N0) remains controversial. Elective treatment of the neck, including elective neck dissection (END) and irradiation (ENI) can play an important role and warrant careful multidisciplinary team discussion with the patient. Active investigation into the indications and timing of potential elective neck treatment will be important to guide treatment guidelines. Sentinel lymph node biopsy (SNB) may offer less invasive technique to investigate and treat the neck in oral cavity cancer patients.

Keywords: lymph node metastases, occult disease, therapeutic neck dissection, elective neck dissection, irradiation, sentinel lymph node biopsy

32.1 Introduction

Oral cavity squamous cell carcinoma (OCSCC) represents a leading form of head and neck cancer worldwide. Initial presentation varies from early manifestations of leukoplakia or erythroplakia to advanced progressively enlarging tumors involving the oral cavity and often the regional cervical lymphatics in the neck. A multidisciplinary team approach for treatment is critical for the proper evaluation, diagnosis, and management of the primary tumor site as well as the regional lymphatics that may harbor clinically apparent or occult metastatic disease. Definitive management of OCSCC at initial disease presentation offers patients the best opportunity for locoregional control and overall survival.

The 2017 National Comprehensive Cancer Network (NCCN) guidelines for cancer of the oral cavity recommend that regardless of the presentation, patients should undergo careful clinical and radiographic evaluation of the primary site as well as at least the regional lymphatics that are at risk for harboring disease. For more advanced presentations and stages of disease, evaluation should at least include imaging of the chest if not more comprehensive systemic imaging.[1] The need for careful evaluation of the neck is due to the fact that disease involvement of the regional cervical lymph nodes is the most accurate negative predictor of overall oncologic outcome other than distant metastases. Despite advances in the therapy of OCSCC and the understanding of its causes, patient outcomes remain poor and presence of cervical lymph node metastases decreases the overall patient survival by roughly 50%.[2–4] Thus, management of the neck, including appropriate staging and treatment, is critical.

Surgical management of the neck can be broken down into treatment of clinically evident cervical lymph node disease (N+) and clinically negative neck (N0) that may be at risk of harboring occult neck disease. The decision to perform neck surgery has to be carefully evaluated and all the risks and benefits need to be taken into account. Therapeutic surgical dissection of the neck is warranted in cases of N+disease, unless patients are unable to tolerate surgery or have unresectable disease.[1] Much debate still remains about whether patients with N0 disease should undergo elective neck dissections (ENDs), observation, or even elective neck radiotherapy.[5–18] A recently published large prospective clinical trial and the updated 8th edition of American Joint Committee on Cancer (AJCC) cancer staging manual on OCSCC tumor classification and staging, are influencing management of the neck in these patients.[18,19] There is increasing support for the use of END for staging and therapeutic purposes at initial OCSCC diagnosis.[13,16,18,20–22] Comprehensive evaluation and treatment recommendations must also include discussion of potential merits of adjuvant radiation therapy as well as chemotherapy.[1]

32.2 Epidemiology

Head and neck cancer is the sixth most common cancer in the world, with squamous cell carcinomas as the most prevalent form of oral malignancies (> 95%). The risk of developing cancer increases with tobacco use in a dose-dependent fashion, and alcohol consumption is synergistic when combined with tobacco use. While many advances in treatment and diagnosis have been made over time, oral cancer remains the ninth leading cause of cancer death among US males and overall survival rate has remained low.[23]

Overall in the US and Europe, the rates of oral cancer incidence and mortality have declined over time, but these declines have not been consistent in all of the population subgroups.[24] In other parts of the world such as South Asia, oral cancer is a serious and growing problem.[25] Changes in risky behaviors like decreasing tobacco and alcohol use are thought to be the main reasons for the overall decline in oral cancer incidence while increase in the use of these products in other populations has increased its incidence. Geographic location, low socioeconomic status, and lack of awareness regarding the negative effects of preventable risk factors are important variables for development of oral cancer.[25,26]

The most significant negative prognostic factor for recurrence and long-term survival is the presence of regional metastases in the cervical lymphatics. Cervical lymph node metastases diminish disease-free survival by about 50%.[5,9,27,28] Hence, the identification of neck disease is critical for appropriate multidisciplinary treatment and management discussion.

The risk of lymph node involvement increases with increasing depth of invasion and size of the tumor, making early diagnosis key for maximizing overall survival.[29] Even with negative physical examination and imaging studies, approximately 30% of all head and neck cancer patients with clinical N0 neck

Table 32.1 Frequency of occult metastases in elective RNDs in OCSCC

Study reference	pN + rate
Shah JP (1990)	34%
Byers et al (1997)	45%
Pitman et al (1997)	41%

Abbreviations: OCSCC, oral cavity squamous cell carcinoma; pN +, pathologic positive cervical metastases; RND, radical neck dissection.

may harbor occult metastases. These metastases are too small to palpate or visualize on imaging. For oral cavity subsites, the rate of occult metastatic disease may be as high as 45% (▶ Table 32.1).[9,30–32] More than two-thirds of occult metastases measure less than 10 mm, with majority measuring less than 3 mm.[33,34] There are now pathologic and clinical parameters such as depth of tumor invasion that are used to determine if the risk of neck disease is high enough to electively treat the cervical lymphatics and identify potential lymphatic metastases that are clinically unappreciable.[18,35]

32.3 Clinical Presentation

It is unusual for patients with oral cavity malignancies to present with an asymptomatic neck mass. Typically, patients first become symptomatic with suspicious mucosal changes, ulcers, or growths and the associated discomfort from the primary tumor itself. Cervical lymph node metastases are then likely identified during the initial examination or anatomic imaging evaluation. The neck masses are usually nontender, mobile, and most commonly found in the submental or submandibular region of the neck.[7,10,14] Specific attention needs to be given to the perifacial lymph nodes that are located adjacent to the mandible at the mandibular facial notch, as this is an area that may harbor neck disease. When there is presence of extracapsular extension in the lymph node, the neck mass may be less mobile or adherent to surrounding soft tissue or mandible and often becomes tender, indurated, and may have overlying skin changes or tethering.[36]

Hard palate malignancies are overall less likely to have regional neck disease given that the lymphatic drainage of this area is less robust than other subsites of the oral cavity including the floor of mouth or tongue.[37] Larger and more advanced tumors, especially in the case of delayed evaluation, are more likely to have palpable neck masses, which represent a conglomeration of involved lymph nodes, during the initial evaluation.[36,38] For early lesions, the patient may have no apparent palpable cervical lymph nodes, and we must rely on imaging to identify potential suspicious lymphadenopathy. Even when imaging does not reveal any suspicious lymph nodes, oral cavity malignancies carry significant risk of occult microscopic neck disease that needs to be considered during management of this disease.[33,34]

32.4 Diagnosis and Evaluation

Workup of oral cavity malignancies includes careful evaluation of the primary tumor site as well as the neck for possible regional disease spread into the cervical lymph nodes. Examination needs to include both careful visualization and palpation of the oral cavity and neck. Examination and palpation of the primary tumor help in providing a footprint for potential lymphatic drainage patterns and therefore understanding the at-risk nodal basins. Anatomic imaging studies are useful not only to evaluate the extent of tumor infiltration, but also to appropriately stage the neck for involved or suspicious lymphadenopathy.[1] This is especially helpful when there is no palpable cervical lymphadenopathy. A combination of physical examination and imaging has been shown to be more sensitive and specific when compared with physical examination alone for proper evaluation of the neck.[39–41] For more advanced tumors systemic evaluation for potential distant metastatic disease is also warranted as per the NCCN guidelines.[1]

High-resolution imaging usually includes computed tomography (CT), magnetic resonance imaging (MRI), ultrasound (US), and more increasingly positron emission tomography (PET). PET/CT is usually more commonly used for advanced disease.[41] There are ongoing clinical studies (ACRIN 6685) designed to determine the negative predictive value of PET/CT imaging based upon pathologic analysis of the neck lymph nodes in patients with head and neck cancer. Criteria for determining involved lymph nodes on imaging can vary among institutions; the short axis diameter must usually be at least 11–12 mm including certain features such as central necrosis, avid node enhancement with rounded appearance or rim enhancement, and potential extracapsular spread (ECS) when present.

Imaging can provide both specific location and characteristics of any involved, suspicious, or indeterminate lymph nodes which can then be further interrogated with US-guided fine needle aspiration (FNA) cytopathology or other imaging modalities, as warranted. FNA sampling is recommended for any suspicious or indeterminate lymph nodes, as this information is critical for discussion of appropriate management of the malignant disease.[36,42] Ultrasound-guided FNA is a robust technique that allows for direct sampling of lymph nodes and establishing diagnosis of metastatic disease. This is especially important when deciding on the need for cervical lymphadenectomy.

32.4.1 Anatomic Considerations

The lymphatic drainage of the mucosal surfaces of the oral cavity is directed to the lymph nodes located within the fibroadipose tissue of the neck. The cervical lymph nodes are found between the investing superficial layer of the deep cervical fascia and the visceral and prevertebral layers deeper in the neck. The lymph nodes at risk for harboring metastatic disease from oral cavity cancers are called jugulodigastric lymph nodes, and they tend to be aggregated around important neural and vascular structures including the carotid artery, transverse cervical artery, internal jugular vein, and the vagus, spinal accessory, hypoglossal and lingual cranial nerves, as well as the phrenic nerve.[37]

Recognizing the inherent complexity of the head and neck region, a uniform division and classification of the neck levels has been implemented which formally groups lymph nodes within designated anatomical boundaries into specific neck level compartments.[43,44] Development of this classification schema was important given the relatively predictable cervical lymphatic spread of oral cavity cancers (▶ Table 32.2).[30,32] With the

Table 32.2 Percentage of metastatic lymph nodes involved in elective versus therapeutic RNDs for OCSCC

Neck level	Elective RND	Therapeutic RND
I	58	61
II	51	57
III	26	44
IV	9	20
V	2	4

Adapted from Shah.[32]
Abbreviations: OCSCC, oral cavity squamous cell carcinoma; RND, radical neck dissection.

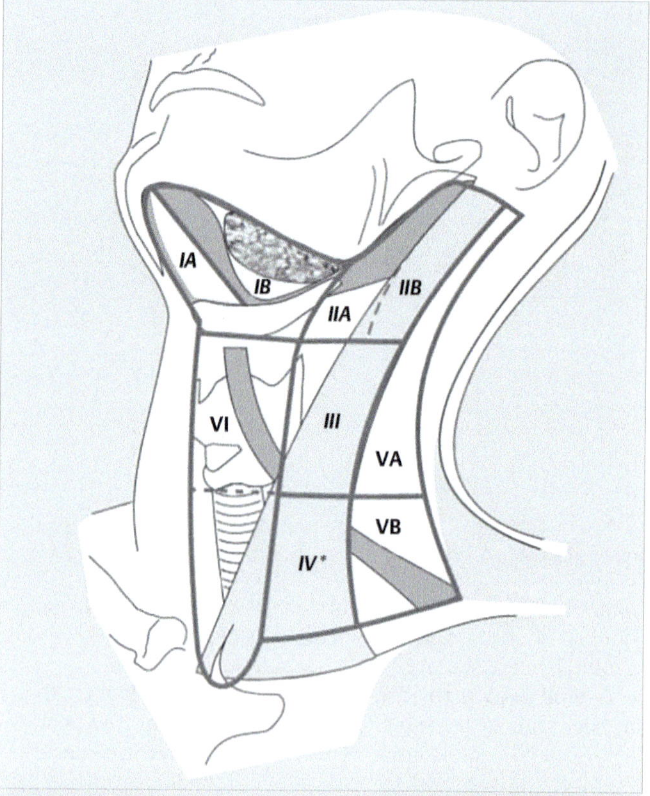

Fig. 32.1 Anatomic diagram of the neck depicting the boundaries of the neck levels and sublevels. Neck levels typically included in a selective neck dissection (SND) performed for oral cavity squamous cell carcinoma (OCSCC) are in bold.
There is variability among head and neck surgeons on whether level IV is regularly included.
Modified from Robbins et al.[44]

increasing use of more limited selective neck dissection (SND), proper identification and labeling of the nodal compartments removed are critical. SNDs are now classified by the specific neck levels dissected to remove the fibrofatty contents that contain the cervical lymph nodes.[43,44]

There are six anatomic neck levels (I–VI) in the neck but only the lateral neck compartments (I–V) are critical for evaluation of potential metastatic disease in oral cavity cancers (▶ Fig. 32.1). The anterior neck compartment level VI is unlikely to harbor any metastatic disease from these malignancies. Neck level I corresponds to the submandibular and submental nodes. Neck levels II, III, and IV are the upper, middle, and lower jugular nodes, and the posterior triangle nodes are referred to as neck level V. There are also sublevels within this classification including level IA (submental nodes), IB (submandibular nodes), IIA and IIB (separated by the spinal accessory nerve and together comprising the upper jugular nodes), VA (spinal accessory nodes), and VB (transverse cervical and supraclavicular nodes).[43,44]

32.5 Surgical Considerations and Approaches

Head and neck cancer, including oral cavity malignancies, commonly metastasize to cervical lymph nodes. When present or suspected, the cervical lymphatic metastases are typically treated with a neck dissection. Surgery usually involves removal of the fibrofatty contents of the neck while preserving the sternocleidomastoid muscle as well as critical neurovascular structures such as the carotid artery, internal jugular vein, and cranial nerves. Treatment of the neck is a key component of the management when there is obvious neck disease (N+), and it should be considered when there is significant risk of microscopic occult neck disease in the clinically N0 neck.

32.5.1 Cervical Lymph Node Metastases (N+Neck)

Surgical therapy is the mainstay of treatment of cervical lymph node metastasis in OCSCC, and therapeutic neck dissection is warranted. There are occasions when surgery may not be indicated, including patient refusal, inability to undergo surgery, or primary and/or neck disease that is unresectable. In these cases, careful multidisciplinary team approach must be adhered to for evaluation and discussion of all available treatment options, including clinical trials. When neck surgery is possible, the extent of surgery is dictated by the involved lymph nodes and the overall lymph node basins at risk for harboring occult metastatic disease.[36]

For many decades there was a debate about whether an SND targeting the lymph nodes at risk was comparable to a more comprehensive or even radical neck dissection (RND). Over time studies have shown that treatment of the neck can become less radical and more conservative, sparing the nonlymphatic structures such as the spinal accessory nerve, sternocleidomastoid muscle, and internal jugular vein. The extent of this type of modified RND has also changed and the lymphatic levels removed has also decreased to involve only those lymphatic basins that potentially harbor disease or are at risk for occult metastases and disease spread.[7,45] Many studies have shown that there is no statistically significant difference in locoregional recurrence rates between an SND and the more extensive RND in head and neck cancer, including OCSCC.[9,31]

The cervical lymph nodes at highest risk of developing metastases from OCSCC are in neck levels I, II, and III with metastatic rates to these sites of 58, 51, and 26%, respectively (▶ Table 32.2).[30,32] Follow-up studies by Byers et al noted a 15% rate of level IV skip metastasis, specifically for the oral tongue subsite and advocated that level IV should be included in SND.[31] More recently it has been demonstrated that isolated level IV lymph node metastases are less common than previously shown and that level IV can be dissected only if there are suspicious or involved nodes in that level and/or level II or III.[45] Based on surgeons' experience and practice patterns, there is great variability among head and neck surgeons and clinical centers on whether level IV is regularly included as part of the SND for OCSCC (▶ Fig. 32.1).

It is also important to note the importance of sublevels of the neck, especially levels IA and IIB, in treatment of the neck for OCSCC. Level IA dissection should be complete and include the lymph nodes in the triangle bounded by the anterior bellies of the digastric muscle due to minimal morbidity associated with this dissection and improved nodal sampling of the submental lymph nodes. There is some debate regarding the need to dissect level IIB given that this area rarely harbors occult disease, with potential involvement ranging from 1.6 to 10% of patients.[46–48] There is concern that dissection of these nodes may lead to increased stretching and trauma of the spinal accessory nerve and potential shoulder dysfunction.[49] No functional studies have been published which evaluate the potential benefits of preservation of level IIB, and given the relative ease of this dissection, it is generally recommend that level IIB nodes should be included in SND (▶ Fig. 32.1).

Overall, SND markedly reduces the postoperative morbidity of neck cancer surgery by effectively eliminating the posterior triangle neck dissection and performing targeted anterior triangle dissection.[50] This procedure has relatively low morbidity and provides pathological staging of the neck, which provides long-term prognostic information.

32.5.2 Clinically Negative Neck (N0)

Great controversy has surrounded the management of the clinically negative (N0) neck. A clinically N0 neck is defined as having no clinical evidence of cervical lymph node metastases. Determination of this is quite challenging given the potential risk of occult nodal disease but it is an important part of multidisciplinary team evaluation and discussion. Examination includes careful palpation of the neck as well as anatomic imaging. To help stage the neck, high-resolution imaging is used usually including CT, MRI, US, and increasingly PET.[41] Imaging can provide both specific location and characteristics of any suspicious or indeterminate lymph nodes which can then be further interrogated with US-guided FNA cytopathology or other imaging modalities, as warranted.[36]

Even with negative physical examination and imaging studies, approximately 30% of all head and neck cancer patients with clinical N0 neck may harbor occult metastases.[32] For oral cavity subsites, the rate of occult metastatic disease may be as high as 45% (▶ Table 32.1).[9,31,32] More than two-thirds of these occult metastases measured less than 10 mm, with majority of these measuring less than 3 mm.[33,34] The major issue is that these N0 patients may harbor lymphatic metastases that are just too small to be detected. The greatest challenge is therefore to correctly identify the subset of these patients without cervical nodal micrometastases who do not require elective neck treatment.

Given these limitations and challenges, the three management options for N0 patients are observations with therapeutic neck dissection once regional metastases become apparent, staging END, and elective neck irradiation (ENI). The debate surrounding these three options has lasted for many decades, but a recent prospective clinical trial has shed new light on the potential benefits of END, especially in treatment of tongue squamous cell carcinoma.[18]

Observation versus Elective Neck Treatment

There is a great controversy regarding the optimal therapy for clinically negative necks. The main question is whether performing an END and clearing the occult neck disease have any survival and locoregional control benefits. Most studies with only few prospective randomized studies showed that patients undergoing END have lower regional recurrence rates, but the survival advantage was not as clear with some studies showing improved survival and others no difference when comparing surgery with observation (▶ Table 32.3).[5,6,8,10,11,16,20,21]

Proponents of observation "wait and see" approach state that the morbidity of END, capability for close follow-up, and early

Table 32.3 Summary of data on elective neck dissection versus observation for N0 neck in OCSCC

Study reference	No. of patients	Elective therapy	Neck metastasis END (%)	Neck metastasis observation (%)	DFS END (%)	DFS observation (%)
Vandenbrouck et al (1980)[a]	75	RND	49	47	46	58
Fakih et al (1989)[a]	70	RND	33	58	63	53
Kligerman et al (1994)[a]	67	SND	21	42	72	49
Yuen et al (1997)	63	RND, SND	27	47	86	55
Duvvuri et al (2004)	359	SND	23	27	66	54
Smith et al (2004)	150	SND, MRND	36	20	96	92
Keski-Säntti et al (2006)	80	SND	34	24	82	81
Capote et al (2007)	154	SND, MRND	0[b]	27	93[b]	71
Mirea et al (2014)	86	SND	27	39	85[b]	62[c]

Abbreviations: DFS, disease-free survival; END, elective neck dissection; MRND, modified radical neck dissection; N0, clinically negative neck; OCSCC, oral cavity squamous cell carcinoma; RND, radical neck dissection; SND, selective neck dissection.
Notes: [a]Randomized controlled trial.
[b]Excluded patients with nodal disease found during END.
[c]Overall survival.

detection and adequate prompt treatment of lymph node metastases are good arguments for observation. Given that the occult metastatic rate to the neck from oral cavity cancer is between 30 and 40%, a significant majority of patients would be exposed to the morbidity of a potentially unnecessary END.[9,30–32] Proponents of surgery note that removal of lymph nodes can be used as an important staging procedure and as further evaluation of the pathology and any high-risk features. If there is presence of any high-risk features such as perineural invasion (PNI), lymphovascular invasion (LVI), or ECS, the patient can be considered for adjuvant therapy.[28,51,52] Specifically, in patients who were initially observed but later developed lymph node metastases requiring therapeutic neck dissection, the majority of patients had pathologically adverse findings at the time of neck dissection, including ECS, and therefore required more extensive surgery and adjuvant therapy. Additionally, overall survival rate decreased significantly in therapeutic neck dissection patients, with a much lower ability to ultimately surgically salvage the neck.[7,8,22,53] Hence, these are the arguments that support elective neck treatment in patients with N0 necks.

Few studies are available to guide the management of the N0 neck, but one study by Weiss et al proposed that observation is preferred when the probability of occult metastasis is less than 20% and elective neck treatment (radiation therapy or surgery) is preferred if the probability of occult metastasis is greater than 20%.[54] Currently, the depth of invasion and thickness of tumor seem to be the only factors to have consistently shown promise as indicators of risk for occult nodal metastasis. The recommended cutoff for considering elective neck treatment varies greatly in the literature, ranging from 1.5 to 8 mm. In the case of N0 neck with primary tumor arising from a subsite with a less than 20% occult metastatic rate, observation may be appropriate. Low rate of occult nodal spread has been observed for early T1 to T2 lip carcinomas, oral tongue carcinomas that are less than 3–4 mm thick, and floor of mouth cancers that are 1.5 mm or thinner.[29,55–59]

Recently, D'Cruz et al published a large prospective randomized trial that compared END to observation with therapeutic neck dissection ("watchful waiting"). Among 496 patients, a clear benefit was shown for the END group. Among patients with early stage OCSCC, END resulted in higher rates of overall (80 vs 67.5%) and disease-free survival (69.5 vs 45.9%) compared to the observation and therapeutic neck dissection. This study also suggested that patients with a minimal depth of invasion of the primary tumor of $\leq$ 3 mm may not benefit from END. These data are robust for oral tongue cancers, given over 85% of enrolled patients had primary tumors located in this subsite.[18] Results of this trial suggest that END at the time of resection of the primary tumor confers an overall survival benefit in patients with early-stage, clinically N0 OCSCC. However, the significant caveat here is that more patients in the END arm received adjuvant radiation therapy since the pathological status of their neck was known. Thus, early management of the neck overall appears to be more beneficial than observation.

Elective Neck Dissection versus Elective Neck Irradiation

Once the decision to treat the N0 neck has been made, the question then is whether to perform the surgical lymphadenectomy or to irradiate the neck. Several early studies showed that ENI can reduce the overall regional recurrence rate from 18% to less than 2%, and provide a 95% control rate for neck recurrences compared with 38% without ENI in early stage N0 oral tongue squamous cell carcinoma.[13,60] Overall, these early studies showed that ENI had a neck recurrence rate of around 5%, which was comparable to the regional recurrence rate of END (4 to 7%).[9,12,13,61] However, a more recent prospective study by Brennan et al that compared staged neck dissection to ENI in patients with early stage oral tongue cancers had to be terminated early because of high locoregional recurrence rate of 23%.[62] ENI is now mostly used for patients who cannot tolerate or refuse surgical treatment.[36]

The factors that influence the decision to irradiate the neck are similar to those for END. Patient's compliance with regular radiation therapy schedules and follow-up, and the morbidity and effectiveness of ENI are all important factors to consider for each patient. The modality that is chosen to treat the primary cancer should help in deciding as to how to treat the neck. If radiation therapy is used to treat the primary tumor, which is rare for OCSCC, ENI could also be performed. It is also an option for poor surgical candidates, but the likely overall decreased regional control rate needs to be addressed. If entry to the neck during surgery is necessary to treat or reconstruct the primary tumor, END can easily be performed simultaneously. Obviously, the risks of ENI and END need to be carefully considered on an individual basis for each patient in a multidisciplinary fashion.

The strongest arguments for END are the overall improved regional control of disease and the pathological staging information provided by the procedure. Pathologic evaluation of the lymph nodes can reveal key prognostic information as well as high-risk pathologic criteria that can then be used to help guide adjuvant therapy. Also, risk of developing a second primary tumor in previously treated oral cavity cancers is about 5% per year.[63] ENI, if used, will likely exclude the possibility of using radiation therapy as a treatment in the event of a second primary head and neck cancer or any future recurrence. The literature shows mixed results with regards to differences in terms of regional control and overall survival between END and ENI, although the prospective trial by Brennan et al showed a clear benefit for END and much lower regional recurrence rate. Also, END is usually better tolerated by patients than radiation therapy.[62,64,65] The most important factors in guiding this decision should be the patient's informed decision, physician and institution experience, risk of second primary occurrence in the future, and modality chosen to treat the primary cancer. Since surgery is usually the preferred treatment method for primary OCSCC, END rather than radiation therapy should be used for treatment of the N0 neck.

32.6 Future Directions

Management of the N0 neck continues to be controversial given the shortcomings of pretreatment evaluation of the neck and the real risk of occult neck disease even in early stage OCSCC. Future studies should evaluate both imaging and diagnostic technology that could help detect patients with occult neck disease. Biologic tumor staging and sentinel lymph node biopsy (SNB) are both promising techniques that may be able to accomplish this in the future.

32.6.1 Biologic Tumor Staging

Tumor thickness and more importantly depth of invasion have been shown to be predictors of occult lymph node metastases in oral cavity tumors. Most recent update in the 8th AJCC cancer staging manual showed that depth of invasion is an important prognostic marker, where even small tumors with depth of invasion > 10 mm are now classified as advanced T3 primary lesions. Pathologic predictors of occult neck metastases continue to be characterized and studied, and most likely various combinations of factors may help more accurately predict these metastases. Tumor thickness of < 3 mm has an occult metastases rate of 8% as compared to 44% for > 3 mm and 53% for > 9 mm.[29]

32.6.2 Role of Sentinel Lymph Node Biopsy

SNB offers a less invasive surgical method than END for assessing cervical nodal metastasis, while potentially decreasing patient morbidity as compared to END. This technique has been used effectively in Europe and Asia and is gaining more attention in the US and worldwide as a reliable method to sample and potentially predict occult nodal spread in the neck.

The sentinel lymph node (SLN) is the first echelon node to which a tumor will most likely metastasize via the regional lymphatics. SNB is based on the premise that lymphatic flow from the primary tumor travels sequentially to the SLN, or first-draining lymph node(s), and then on to the remaining regional lymph nodes. This technique is being studied as a staging tool for mucosal head and neck cancer, but has become the standard of care for melanoma and breast cancer.

The patient is injected at the site of the primary tumor with a radiotracer that travels along the lymphatic channels to the cervical lymph nodes. The first echelon of nodes that are localized by the radiotracer represent the lymph nodes most likely to harbor metastatic disease (▶ Fig. 32.2). Following this mapping procedure, the SLN(s) can be biopsied as part of the surgical procedure when the primary tumor is excised. Typically, a smaller incision(s) is made in the neck and less surgical manipulation is required to remove a small number of lymph nodes rather than dissect the entire lymph node basin (▶ Fig. 32.2). Pathological examination is then focused on a few nodes with the highest likelihood to harbor disease. Serial sectioning of a limited number of SLNs and immunohistochemistry studies allow for a more comprehensive examination for possible microscopic metastatic disease deposits.[66,67] With the use of new receptor-targeted radiotracer molecules (99mTc-tilmanocept/Lymphoseek™), the false negative rate was reported as 2.56%.[68]

There have been many retrospective, single-institution studies related to the efficacy of SNB.[67,69,70] Additionally, a phase II study performed in the US demonstrated feasibility and the importance of surgeon experience for SNB.[71,72] The European Organization for Research and Treatment of Cancer (EORTC) published a prospective observational study on the reliability and safety of SNB in early stage OCSCC, and showed that the sensitivity was 86% with a negative predictive value of 95%. This data showed that SNB is a reliable and safe oncological technique for staging the clinically N0 neck in patients with T1 and T2 oral cancers.[73]

SNB allows for potentially less invasive and less morbid assessment of neck disease status while focusing pathological analysis on those nodes that are most likely to harbor disease. Further prospective clinical trials comparing SNB with END should focus on establishing the standard of care for management of the neck in early stage OCSCC. Direct comparison can be performed to optimize clinical outcomes (i.e., disease-free survival, overall survival, locoregional control), while potentially improving overall quality of life and patient-reported

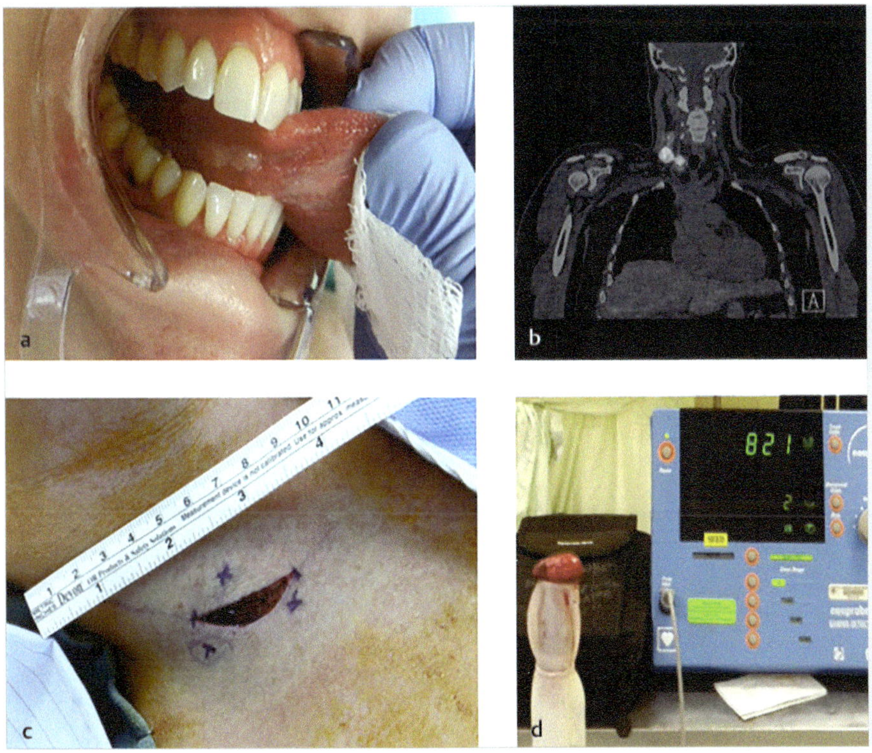

Fig. 32.2 Sentinel lymph node biopsy (SNB) technique. **(a)** T1 right lateral tongue squamous cell carcinoma just prior to injection of the radiotracer (99mTc-tilmanocept/Lymphoseek™). **(b)** Single-photon emission computerized tomography (SPECT)/CT imaging in the coronal plane demonstrating three possible sentinel lymph nodes (SLNs) localized to ipsilateral neck. **(c)** Intraoperative photo showing the skin markings of the three SLNs and the smaller incision utilized to access the SLNs within the potential incision line that could be used for an elective neck dissection (END). **(d)** Positive identification of one of the SLNs with the radioactivity level assessed *ex vivo*.

outcomes, including shoulder-related function, with less invasive neck surgery using SNB for these patients. Completion of such a study will move the field toward establishing either SNB or END as the standard of care for early-stage OCSCC and can hopefully prevent a protracted controversy such as the one that persisted between END and "watchful waiting" observation for the N0 patients for decades.

32.7 Surgical Sequelae

Medical complications can occur after any major surgical procedure and these are usually related to previous medical history and comorbidities such as hypertension, diabetes, and coronary artery disease. Others may be related to anesthesia with changes in mentation, headache, nausea, and vomiting. The use of urinary catheters and advanced age may predispose patients to urinary retention and urinary tract infections, although this is uncommon in head and neck cancer population.[74–76] Surgical complications stemming from neck dissection have been reduced as the extent and type of neck dissection performed evolved over time, especially with the use of SND. Nonetheless, patients treated surgically can develop complications, which can generally be grouped into wound, vascular, lymphatic, and nerve categories.[75]

Neck dissection is usually performed through many different variations of a transverse neck incision that is typically along relaxed skin tension lines or in a natural skin crease. This usually heals without issue and is cosmetically acceptable scar especially when tension-free, everted skin closure is performed. Scar hypertrophy can develop from increased tension at the suture line or if patient is predisposed to forming hypertrophic scars or even keloids.[77] Lymphedema and swelling of the incision and the neck soft tissues can also occur and can be worsened due to prior or postoperative radiation therapy, but this usually slowly resolves over time and with formal lymphedema therapy. Postoperative seroma is rare due to common use of suction drains that are removed after several days when the drain output is appropriately low. Infections are rare, but they can occur especially if there is a mucosal communication that introduces salivary leakage into the neck or communication with an indwelling tracheostomy tract with seeding of the neck with respiratory flora.[78,79]

Vascular complications are most commonly due to postoperative bleeding and hematoma formation. Suction drains can not only help mitigate this risk but also help identify bleeding in the neck based on the quality and volume of drainage. Bleeding is most common in the early postoperative period and usually warrants operative exploration and control of hemorrhage.[80,81] Injuries to the carotid artery and jugular vein are rare and more likely in the postradiation or chemoradiation therapy settings. The internal jugular vein may thrombose in 15–30% of cases of neck dissections, but wound complications such as infection and salivary leakage as well as radiation are known contributing factors.[82,83]

Removing the fibrofatty contents and cervical lymphatics may also cause a left-sided chyle leak given the thoracic duct usually drains into the inferior aspect of the jugular vein and subclavian vein on the left side. Chyle leaks can occur on the right side because of interruption of the right accessory lymphatic duct. There may be also a plexus of tributaries and terminal ducts, each of which can create a chylous fistula if transected or incompletely ligated during surgery. Most chyle leaks resolve with strict nonfat dietary changes, compression dressings, and suction drains, but it may require surgical or interventional radiology approaches to control if the chyle leak is high volume or persistent.[82]

Nerve injury is uncommon during neck dissection unless there is direct tumor involvement of the nerve necessitating oncologic resection to help control the disease. This is a difficult problem if the spinal accessory, hypoglossal, lingual, vagus, or phrenic nerves are involved with tumor, as resection of these nerves will cause permanent dysfunction of the involved nerve. Injury to some of these nerves (hypoglossal, vagus, phrenic) can cause significant morbidity. Shoulder disability from spinal accessory nerve injury was an expected sequela of RND but is now considered a potential complication of SND only. There can also be a temporary weakness of the marginal mandibular branch of the facial nerve, especially due to microdissection of this nerve during removal of perifacial lymph nodes in level IB, or due to compression of the nerve with retractors. If the greater auricular nerve or cervical rootlets are sacrificed, there may be persistent numbness of the ear, neck, and upper chest area, which usually have only limited recovery over time.[75,83]

Neck dissection, and more specifically SND, is overall a safe oncologic procedure with limited postoperative complications when done by an experienced surgeon. Most complications are temporary and resolve over time with adequate management and follow-up. The risks and complications of surgery are increased in the setting of advanced infiltrative disease and previous surgical and nonsurgical oncologic therapy.

32.8 Adjuvant Treatment Considerations

32.8.1 Radiation Therapy

Radiotherapy may have a very limited role in the elective treatment of the neck in OCSCC, but radiation holds a much more critical role in the postoperative therapeutic setting. Surgical management of the neck adds the benefit of pathologic evaluation and staging of the neck and identification of high-risk pathologic features. NCCN guidelines recommend that postoperative radiation therapy begin less than 6 weeks following surgery for patients with adverse features, including positive margins, extracapsular extension (ECS), T3–T4 disease, N2–N3 disease, LVI, and PNI.[1] This is based on previous studies that demonstrated locoregional recurrence rates are lowered when postoperative radiation therapy is given for multiple involved lymph nodes and high-risk pathologic factors such as perineural and lymphovascular invasion in the primary tumor.[84–87] Timing of postoperative radiation therapy is also critical with treatment delays or breaks worsening overall tumor control rate. Radiation therapy is usually started within 4 to 6 weeks after surgical therapy, as delays beyond 6 weeks have worse outcome.[38,88–90]

Currently, the NCCN guidelines recommend considering adjuvant radiation therapy for N1 disease, even in the absence of high-risk pathologic features. Postoperative radiation therapy is indicated when two or more histologically positive lymph nodes are identified.[1] At some centers, surgery alone is considered adequate treatment of a single lymph node metastasis in absence of other high-risk pathologic features. Radiation therapy has not been shown to provide additional benefit in early T1 to T2 OCSCC tumors with metastasis to a single lymph node (N1), but this is based largely on retrospective studies. There is some controversy regarding this, given studies that reported surgery only for N1 disease had regional recurrence rates from 16 to 25%. This suggest that postoperative radiation therapy may be beneficial and deserves multidisciplinary discussion.[28,51,52]

32.8.2 Chemotherapy

Multimodality treatment of surgery and radiation therapy are commonly used when dealing with advanced stages III and IV disease as recommended by the 2017 NCCN guidelines. Combination therapy certainly has improved efficacy when compared to either modality alone. Furthermore, there is also evidence that the addition of chemotherapy to radiation therapy may improve locoregional control and overall survival for these patients.[2,91] This data was based on all head and neck cancer subsites, including OCSCC, and it is not possible to extrapolate if these benefits are oral cavity tumor location specific. What is clear is that certain high-risk pathologic criteria such as positive surgical margins and lymph node ECS have poor prognosis, and the use of concomitant postoperative chemoradiation therapy was beneficial when compared to radiation therapy alone. Thus, patients with advanced bulky neck disease as well as those with microscopic disease showing lymph node ECS warrant multidisciplinary discussion for the addition of chemotherapy as part of adjuvant treatment.[36] The increased risk of complications must be weighed carefully against the potential benefit and improved disease control for each patient.

32.9 Conclusion

For patients with obvious neck involvement and metastases, surgery with therapeutic neck dissection is critical. Based on evaluation of high-risk pathologic factors, patients may also require postoperative radiation therapy if not chemotherapy. For nonsurgical patients, radiation therapy is an option, but tumor response and control rates are poor. Management of the N0 neck in OCSCC continues to be controversial, particularly the timing of elective treatment. However, because current methods to assess the risk for occult metastasis are insufficiently accurate and prone to underestimation of actual risk, limited number of studies favor elective treatment of the N0 neck due to better overall locoregional control and survival. The role of ENI can be considered, but has long-term disadvantages and worse locoregional oncologic control. END is currently the most accurate way to pathologically stage the neck, but active investigation of less invasive techniques such as SNB are being explored and hold promise for routine clinical use in the future.

Key Points

- Neck disease significantly affects overall disease-free patient survival, and appropriate evaluation and treatment are critical in oral cavity malignancies.
- Imaging evaluation of the neck should be used routinely as it can significantly help with identification of neck disease or suspicious cervical lymph nodes.
- N + neck disease requires surgical treatment with therapeutic neck dissection and potential consideration of adjuvant radiation therapy and chemotherapy based on high-risk pathologic characteristics.
- Clinical N0 neck requires careful imaging of the neck and primary tumor site evaluation for depth of invasion as END may improve disease control for deeper tumors.
- Clinical N0 ENI has worse disease control when compared to END, and should only be used in patients that are not surgical candidates or when they refuse surgical treatment.
- When neck treatment is warranted, SND can be appropriate for N + and N0 disease and needs to include all neck levels that are at risk of harboring neck disease.
- SNB is under active clinical investigation and may hold promise for less invasive evaluation and treatment of the clinically N0 neck in oral cavity malignancies.

References

[1] Pfister DG, Foote RL, Gilbert J, Gillison ML, Ridge JA, Rocco J. National Comprehensive Cancer Network. Head and neck cancers, version 2.2018. National Comprehensive Cancer Network. Head and neck cancers, version 2.2018. https://www.nccn.org/professionals/physician_gls/pdf/head-and-neck.pdf. Published 2018. Accessed November 7, 2018

[2] Bernier J, Domenge C, Ozsahin M, et al. European Organization for Research and Treatment of Cancer Trial 22931. Postoperative irradiation with or without concomitant chemotherapy for locally advanced head and neck cancer. N Engl J Med. 2004; 350(19):1945–1952

[3] Cooper JS, Pajak TF, Forastiere AA, et al. Radiation Therapy Oncology Group 9501/Intergroup. Postoperative concurrent radiotherapy and chemotherapy for high-risk squamous-cell carcinoma of the head and neck. N Engl J Med. 2004; 350(19):1937–1944

[4] Ang KK, Harris J, Wheeler R, et al. Human papillomavirus and survival of patients with oropharyngeal cancer. N Engl J Med. 2010; 363(1):24–35

[5] Vandenbrouck C, Sancho-Garnier H, Chassagne D, Saravane D, Cachin Y, Micheau C. Elective versus therapeutic radical neck dissection in epidermoid carcinoma of the oral cavity: results of a randomized clinical trial. Cancer. 1980; 46(2):386–390

[6] Fakih AR, Rao RS, Borges AM, Patel AR. Elective versus therapeutic neck dissection in early carcinoma of the oral tongue. Am J Surg. 1989; 158(4):309–313

[7] Lydiatt DD, Robbins KT, Byers RM, Wolf PF. Treatment of stage I and II oral tongue cancer. Head Neck. 1993; 15(4):308–312

[8] Kligerman J, Lima RA, Soares JR, et al. Supraomohyoid neck dissection in the treatment of T1/T2 squamous cell carcinoma of oral cavity. Am J Surg. 1994; 168(5):391–394

[9] Pitman KT, Johnson JT, Myers EN. Effectiveness of selective neck dissection for management of the clinically negative neck. Arch Otolaryngol Head Neck Surg. 1997; 123(9):917–922

[10] Smith GI, O'Brien CJ, Clark J, et al. Management of the neck in patients with T1 and T2 cancer in the mouth. Br J Oral Maxillofac Surg. 2004; 42(6):494–500

[11] Keski-Säntti H, Atula T, Törnwall J, Koivunen P, Mäkitie A. Elective neck treatment versus observation in patients with T1/T2 N0 squamous cell carcinoma of oral tongue. Oral Oncol. 2006; 42(1):96–101

[12] Ferlito A, Rinaldo A, Silver CE, et al. Elective and therapeutic selective neck dissection. Oral Oncol. 2006; 42(1):14–25

[13] Capote A, Escorial V, Muñoz-Guerra MF, Rodríguez-Campo FJ, Gamallo C, Naval L. Elective neck dissection in early-stage oral squamous cell carcinoma—does it influence recurrence and survival? Head Neck. 2007; 29(1):3–11

[14] Cheng A, Schmidt BL. Management of the N0 neck in oral squamous cell carcinoma. Oral Maxillofac Surg Clin North Am. 2008; 20(3):477–497

[15] D'Cruz AK, Siddachari RC, Walvekar RR, et al. Elective neck dissection for the management of the N0 neck in early cancer of the oral tongue: need for a randomized controlled trial. Head Neck. 2009; 31(5):618–624

[16] Mirea D, Grigore R, Safta D, et al. Elective neck dissection in patients with stage T1-T2N0 carcinoma of the anterior tongue. Hippokratia. 2014; 18(2):120–124

[17] Kelner N, Vartanian JG, Pinto CAL, Coutinho-Camillo CM, Kowalski LP. Does elective neck dissection in T1/T2 carcinoma of the oral tongue and floor of the mouth influence recurrence and survival rates? Br J Oral Maxillofac Surg. 2014; 52(7):590–597

[18] D'Cruz AK, Vaish R, Kapre N, et al. Head and Neck Disease Management Group. Elective versus therapeutic neck dissection in node-negative oral cancer. N Engl J Med. 2015; 373(6):521–529

[19] Lydiatt WM, Patel SG, O'Sullivan B, et al. Head and neck cancers—major changes in the American Joint Committee on cancer eighth edition cancer staging manual. CA Cancer J Clin. 2017; 67(2):122–137

[20] Yuen AP, Wei WI, Wong YM, Tang KC. Elective neck dissection versus observation in the treatment of early oral tongue carcinoma. Head Neck. 1997; 19 (7):583–588

[21] Duvvuri U, Simental AA, Jr, D'Angelo G, et al. Elective neck dissection and survival in patients with squamous cell carcinoma of the oral cavity and oropharynx. Laryngoscope. 2004; 114(12):2228–2234

[22] Haddadin KJ, Soutar DS, Oliver RJ, Webster MH, Robertson AG, MacDonald DG. Improved survival for patients with clinically T1/T2, N0 tongue tumors undergoing a prophylactic neck dissection. Head Neck. 1999; 21(6):517–525

[23] DeSantis CE, Lin CC, Mariotto AB, et al. Cancer treatment and survivorship statistics, 2014. CA Cancer J Clin. 2014; 64(4):252–271

[24] Kingsley K, O'Malley S, Ditmyer M, Chino M. Analysis of oral cancer epidemiology in the US reveals state-specific trends: implications for oral cancer prevention. BMC Public Health. 2008; 8:87

[25] Warnakulasuriya S. Global epidemiology of oral and oropharyngeal cancer. Oral Oncol. 2009; 45(4–5):309–316

[26] Gupta N, Gupta R, Acharya AK, et al. Changing trends in oral cancer—a global scenario. Nepal J Epidemiol. 2016; 6(4):613–619

[27] Byers RM. Modified neck dissection: a study of 967 cases from 1970 to 1980. Am J Surg. 1985; 150(4):414–421

[28] Byers RM, Clayman GL, McGill D, et al. Selective neck dissections for squamous carcinoma of the upper aerodigestive tract: patterns of regional failure. Head Neck. 1999; 21(6):499–505

[29] Po Wing Yuen A, Lam KY, Lam LK, et al. Prognostic factors of clinically stage I and II oral tongue carcinoma—a comparative study of stage, thickness, shape, growth pattern, invasive front malignancy grading, Martinez-Gimeno score, and pathologic features. Head Neck. 2002; 24(6):513–520

[30] Shah JP, Candela FC, Poddar AK. The patterns of cervical lymph node metastases from squamous carcinoma of the oral cavity. Cancer. 1990; 66(1):109–113

[31] Byers RM, Weber RS, Andrews T, McGill D, Kare R, Wolf P. Frequency and therapeutic implications of "skip metastases" in the neck from squamous carcinoma of the oral tongue. Head Neck. 1997; 19(1):14–19

[32] Shah JP. Patterns of cervical lymph node metastasis from squamous carcinomas of the upper aerodigestive tract. Am J Surg. 1990; 160(4):405–409

[33] van den Brekel MW, van der Waal I, Meijer CJ, Freeman JL, Castelijns JA, Snow GB. The incidence of micrometastases in neck dissection specimens obtained from elective neck dissections. Laryngoscope. 1996; 106(8):987–991

[34] Ferlito A, Shaha AR, Rinaldo A. The incidence of lymph node micrometastases in patients pathologically staged N0 in cancer of oral cavity and oropharynx. Oral Oncol. 2002; 38(1):3–5

[35] Sparano A, Weinstein G, Chalian A, Yodul M, Weber R. Multivariate predictors of occult neck metastasis in early oral tongue cancer. Otolaryngol Head Neck Surg. 2004; 131(4):472–476

[36] Ow TJ, Myers JN. Current management of advanced resectable oral cavity squamous cell carcinoma. Clin Exp Otorhinolaryngol. 2011; 4(1):1–10

[37] Hollingshead W. Anatomy for Surgeons: The Head and Neck. 3rd ed. Philadelphia: Lippincott Williams & Wilkins; 1982

[38] Rosenthal DI, Liu L, Lee JH, et al. Importance of the treatment package time in surgery and postoperative radiation therapy for squamous carcinoma of the head and neck. Head Neck. 2002; 24(2):115–126

[39] Curtin HD, Ishwaran H, Mancuso AA, Dalley RW, Caudry DJ, McNeil BJ. Comparison of CT and MR imaging in staging of neck metastases. Radiology. 1998; 207(1):123–130

[40] Akoğlu E, Dutipek M, Bekiş R, Değirmenci B, Ada E, Güneri A. Assessment of cervical lymph node metastasis with different imaging methods in patients with head and neck squamous cell carcinoma. J Otolaryngol. 2005; 34(6): 384–394

[41] Yoon DY, Hwang HS, Chang SK, et al. CT, MR, US,18F-FDG PET/CT, and their combined use for the assessment of cervical lymph node metastases in squamous cell carcinoma of the head and neck. Eur Radiol. 2009; 19(3):634–642

[42] Norling R, Buron BMD, Therkildsen MH, Henriksen BM, von Buchwald C, Nielsen MB. Staging of cervical lymph nodes in oral squamous cell carcinoma: adding ultrasound in clinically lymph node negative patients may improve diagnostic work-up. PLoS One. 2014; 9(3):e90360

[43] Robbins KT, Clayman G, Levine PA, et al. American Head and Neck Society, American Academy of Otolaryngology—Head and Neck Surgery. Neck dissection classification update: revisions proposed by the American Head and Neck Society and the American Academy of Otolaryngology—Head and Neck Surgery. Arch Otolaryngol Head Neck Surg. 2002; 128(7):751–758

[44] Robbins KT, Shaha AR, Medina JE, et al. Committee for Neck Dissection Classification, American Head and Neck Society. Consensus statement on the classification and terminology of neck dissection. Arch Otolaryngol Head Neck Surg. 2008; 134(5):536–538

[45] Khafif A, Lopez-Garza JR, Medina JE. Is dissection of level IV necessary in patients with T1-T3 N0 tongue cancer? Laryngoscope. 2001; 111(6):1088–1090

[46] Silverman DA, El-Hajj M, Strome S, Esclamado RM. Prevalence of nodal metastases in the submuscular recess (level IIb) during selective neck dissection. Arch Otolaryngol Head Neck Surg. 2003; 129(7):724–728

[47] Lim YC, Song MH, Kim SC, Kim KM, Choi EC. Preserving level IIb lymph nodes in elective supraomohyoid neck dissection for oral cavity squamous cell carcinoma. Arch Otolaryngol Head Neck Surg. 2004; 130(9):1088–1091

[48] Elsheikh MN, Mahfouz ME, Elsheikh E. Level IIb lymph nodes metastasis in elective supraomohyoid neck dissection for oral cavity squamous cell carcinoma: a molecular-based study. Laryngoscope. 2005; 115(9):1636–1640

[49] Cheng PT, Hao SP, Lin YH, Yeh AR. Objective comparison of shoulder dysfunction after three neck dissection techniques. Ann Otol Rhinol Laryngol. 2000; 109(8 Pt 1):761–766

[50] Terrell JE, Welsh DE, Bradford CR, et al. Pain, quality of life, and spinal accessory nerve status after neck dissection. Laryngoscope. 2000; 110(4):620–626

[51] Yuen AP, Lam KY, Chan AC, et al. Clinicopathological analysis of elective neck dissection for N0 neck of early oral tongue carcinoma. Am J Surg. 1999; 177 (1):90–92

[52] Chen MM, Harris JP, Hara W, Sirjani D, Divi V. Association of postoperative radiotherapy with survival in patients with N1 oral cavity and oropharyngeal squamous cell carcinoma. JAMA Otolaryngol Head Neck Surg. 2016; 142(12): 1224–1230

[53] Andersen PE, Cambronero E, Shaha AR, Shah JP. The extent of neck disease after regional failure during observation of the N0 neck. Am J Surg. 1996; 172 (6):689–691

[54] Weiss MH, Harrison LB, Isaacs RS. Use of decision analysis in planning a management strategy for the stage N0 neck. Arch Otolaryngol Head Neck Surg. 1994; 120(7):699–702

[55] Spiro RH, Huvos AG, Wong GY, Spiro JD, Gnecco CA, Strong EW. Predictive value of tumor thickness in squamous carcinoma confined to the tongue and floor of the mouth. Am J Surg. 1986; 152(4):345–350

[56] Mohit-Tabatabai MA, Sobel HJ, Rush BF, Mashberg A. Relation of thickness of floor of mouth stage I and II cancers to regional metastasis. Am J Surg. 1986; 152(4):351–353

[57] Jones KR, Lodge-Rigal RD, Reddick RL, Tudor GE, Shockley WW. Prognostic factors in the recurrence of stage I and II squamous cell cancer of the oral cavity. Arch Otolaryngol Head Neck Surg. 1992; 118(5):483–485

[58] O'Brien CJ, Lauer CS, Fredricks S, et al. Tumor thickness influences prognosis of T1 and T2 oral cavity cancer—but what thickness? Head Neck. 2003; 25 (11):937–945

[59] Warburton G, Nikitakis NG, Roberson P, et al. Histopathological and lymphangiogenic parameters in relation to lymph node metastasis in early stage oral squamous cell carcinoma. J Oral Maxillofac Surg. 2007; 65(3):475–484

[60] Mendenhall WM, Million RR, Cassisi NJ. Elective neck irradiation in squamous-cell carcinoma of the head and neck. Head Neck Surg. 1980; 3(1): 15–20

[61] Mendenhall WM, Million RR. Elective neck irradiation for squamous cell carcinoma of the head and neck: analysis of time-dose factors and causes of failure. Int J Radiat Oncol Biol Phys. 1986; 12(5):741–746

[62] Brennan S, Corry J, Kleid S, et al. Prospective trial to evaluate staged neck dissection or elective neck radiotherapy in patients with CT-staged T1–2 N0 squamous cell carcinoma of the oral tongue. Head Neck. 2010; 32(2):191–198

[63] Wolfensberger M, Zbaeren P, Dulguerov P, Müller W, Arnoux A, Schmid S. Surgical treatment of early oral carcinoma—results of a prospective controlled multicenter study. Head Neck. 2001; 23(7):525–530
[64] Al-Rajhi N, Khafaga Y, El-Husseiny J, et al. Early stage carcinoma of oral tongue: prognostic factors for local control and survival. Oral Oncol. 2000; 36 (6):508–514
[65] Chow JM, Levin BC, Krivit JS, Applebaum EL. Radiotherapy or surgery for subclinical cervical node metastases. Arch Otolaryngol Head Neck Surg. 1989; 115(8):981–984
[66] Amit M, Yen TC, Liao CT, et al. The origin of regional failure in oral cavity squamous cell carcinoma with pathologically negative neck metastases. JAMA Otolaryngol Head Neck Surg. 2014; 140(12):1130–1137
[67] Liu M, Wang SJ, Yang X, Peng H. Diagnostic efficacy of sentinel lymph node biopsy in early oral squamous cell carcinoma: a meta-analysis of 66 studies. PLoS One. 2017; 12(1):e0170322
[68] Agrawal A, Civantos FJ, Brumund KT, et al. [(99m)Tc]Tilmanocept accurately detects sentinel lymph nodes and predicts node pathology status in patients with oral squamous cell carcinoma of the head and neck: results of a phase III multi-institutional trial. Ann Surg Oncol. 2015; 22(11):3708–3715
[69] Broglie MA, Haerle SK, Huber GF, Haile SR, Stoeckli SJ. Occult metastases detected by sentinel node biopsy in patients with early oral and oropharyngeal squamous cell carcinomas: impact on survival. Head Neck. 2013; 35(5): 660–666
[70] Chiesa F, Mauri S, Grana C, et al. Is there a role for sentinel node biopsy in early N0 tongue tumors? Surgery. 2000; 128(1):16–21
[71] Farmer RW, McCall L, Civantos FJ, et al. Lymphatic drainage patterns in oral squamous cell carcinoma: findings of the ACOSOG Z0360 (Alliance) study. Otolaryngol Head Neck Surg. 2015; 152(4):673–677
[72] Civantos FJ, Zitsch RP, Schuller DE, et al. Sentinel lymph node biopsy accurately stages the regional lymph nodes for T1-T2 oral squamous cell carcinomas: results of a prospective multi-institutional trial. J Clin Oncol. 2010; 28 (8):1395–1400
[73] Schilling C, Stoeckli SJ, Haerle SK, et al. Sentinel European Node Trial (SENT): 3-year results of sentinel node biopsy in oral cancer. Eur J Cancer. 2015; 51 (18):2777–2784
[74] Chan JYK, Semenov YR, Gourin CG. Postoperative urinary tract infection and short-term outcomes and costs in head and neck cancer surgery. Otolaryngol Head Neck Surg. 2013; 148(4):602–610
[75] Bier-Laning C. Surgical complications of the neck. In: Flint P, Haughey B, Lund V, Niparko J, eds. Cummings Otolaryngology—Head and Neck Surgery. Philadelphia: Elsevier Mosby; 2005
[76] Shockley W, McQueen C, Postma G. Complications of neck surgery. In: Weissler M, Pillsbury H III, eds. Complications of Head and Neck Surgery. New York: Thieme; 1995
[77] Bernstein L. Incisions and excisions in elective facial surgery. Arch Otolaryngol. 1973; 97(3):238–243
[78] Deng J, Murphy BA, Dietrich MS, et al. Impact of secondary lymphedema after head and neck cancer treatment on symptoms, functional status, and quality of life. Head Neck. 2013; 35(7):1026–1035
[79] Chiu AG, Cohen JI, Burningham AR, Andersen PE, Davidson BJ. First bite syndrome: a complication of surgery involving the parapharyngeal space. Head Neck. 2002; 24(11):996–999
[80] Johnson JT, Cummings CW. Hematoma after head and neck surgery—a major complication? Otolaryngology. 1978; 86(2):ORL171–ORL175
[81] Matory YL, Spiro RH. Wound bleeding after head and neck surgery. J Surg Oncol. 1993; 53(1):17–19
[82] Delaney SW, Shi H, Shokrani A, Sinha UK. Management of chyle leak after head and neck surgery: review of current treatment strategies. Int J Otolaryngol. 2017; 2017:8362874
[83] Prim MP, De Diego JI, Verdaguer JM, Sastre N, Rabanal I. Neurological complications following functional neck dissection. Eur Arch Otorhinolaryngol. 2006; 263(5):473–476
[84] Brandwein-Gensler M, Teixeira MS, Lewis CM, et al. Oral squamous cell carcinoma: histologic risk assessment, but not margin status, is strongly predictive of local disease-free and overall survival. Am J Surg Pathol. 2005; 29(2):167–178
[85] Fan K-H, Wang H-M, Kang C-J, et al. Treatment results of postoperative radiotherapy on squamous cell carcinoma of the oral cavity: coexistence of multiple minor risk factors results in higher recurrence rates. Int J Radiat Oncol Biol Phys. 2010; 77(4):1024–1029
[86] Nair D, Mair M, Singhvi H, et al. Perineural invasion: independent prognostic factor in oral cancer that warrants adjuvant treatment. Head Neck. 2018; 40 (8):1780–1787
[87] Johnson JT, Myers EN, Bedetti CD, Barnes EL, Schramm VL, Jr, Thearle PB. Cervical lymph node metastases: incidence and implications of extracapsular carcinoma. Arch Otolaryngol. 1985; 111(8):534–537
[88] Ang KK, Trotti A, Brown BW, et al. Randomized trial addressing risk features and time factors of surgery plus radiotherapy in advanced head-and-neck cancer. Int J Radiat Oncol Biol Phys. 2001; 51(3):571–578
[89] Huang J, Barbera L, Brouwers M, Browman G, Mackillop WJ. Does delay in starting treatment affect the outcomes of radiotherapy? A systematic review. J Clin Oncol. 2003; 21(3):555–563
[90] Chen MM, Harris JP, Orosco RK, Sirjani D, Hara W, Divi V. Association of time between surgery and adjuvant therapy with survival in oral cavity cancer. Otolaryngol Head Neck Surg. 2018; 158(6):1051–1056
[91] Zorat PL, Paccagnella A, Cavaniglia G, et al. Randomized phase III trial of neoadjuvant chemotherapy in head and neck cancer: 10-year follow-up. J Natl Cancer Inst. 2004; 96(22):1714–1717

33 Definitive External Beam Radiotherapy for Oral Cavity Cancer

Zachary S. Zumsteg, Diana J. Lu, and Allen S. Ho

Summary

Oral cavity cancer is primarily treated surgically, with radiation delivered postoperatively when needed based on pathologic features. However, definitive radiation can be an important alternative modality in certain situations, such as unresectable tumors, patients that are medically inoperable, patients refusing surgery, or patients desiring organ preservation in specific situations like early stage tongue or lip cancers. This chapter summarizes the role of definitive external beam radiotherapy for oral cavity cancer.

Keywords: oral cavity cancer, radiotherapy, alveolar ridge, retromolar trigone, buccal mucosa

33.1 Introduction

Throughout the head and neck, either surgery or radiotherapy can be utilized as the primary modality for curative intent ablation of locoregional disease. Although organ-preserving definitive radiotherapy is an acceptable, and in many cases preferred, treatment for squamous cell carcinomas (SCCs) of the oropharynx, larynx, hypopharynx, and nasopharynx, the vast majority of oral cavity cancers are best managed with ablative surgery with or without adjuvant therapy. This is because (1) the oral cavity is particularly sensitive to adverse sequelae from radiotherapy at the doses required for definitive treatment, and (2) oral cavity squamous cell carcinoma (OCSCC) is considered radioresistant in comparison to SCCs of other head and neck subsites. Nevertheless, definitive radiation-based approaches can play an important role in OCSCC for a variety of reasons. In this chapter, we will focus on external beam radiotherapy (EBRT)-based approaches. Brachytherapy is discussed in Chapter 34.

33.2 Principles of Definitive External Beam Radiotherapy for Oral Cavity Cancer

Definitive radiation is a viable curative approach in select patients with early stage OCSCC (T1–2N0) to avoid functional and cosmetic defects, and is supported by National Comprehensive Cancer Network guidelines as an alternative to surgery.[1] However, several important caveats are notable. Importantly, the majority of the data showing excellent results with definitive radiation in this setting utilized either intraoral cones, a type of EBRT where a radiation source emitting either orthovoltage photons or electrons is placed inside the mouth abutting the mucosa, or brachytherapy, where radioactive sources are temporarily or permanently implanted directly into the tumor. These can be utilized either alone or in combination with standard linear accelerator-based EBRT. Unfortunately, few modern radiation oncology departments have intraoral cones available, and brachytherapy for OCSCC is also not widely used due to a relatively limited number of radiation oncologists with expertise in the delivery of brachytherapy for head and neck cancer. The most common radiation modality utilized in modern practice for head and neck cancer is, by far, linear accelerator-based EBRT. However, this modality is typically avoided for early stage OCSCC unless combined with a boost delivered via intraoral cone or brachytherapy, given that linear accelerator-based EBRT has relatively high toxicity and, potentially, relatively poor local control in comparison to other modalities for OCSCC. For example, multiple studies have suggested that EBRT without brachytherapy is associated with significantly higher local recurrence rates in early stage oral tongue SCC.[2–4] Additionally, in patients with tumors thicker than 4 mm, some type of elective neck treatment, such as neck dissection or elective neck irradiation, is typically indicated given the high risk of micrometastatic nodal spread.

For locally advanced (T3–T4 or N+) OCSCC, upfront surgical resection followed by adjuvant radiotherapy is the standard of care. Definitive radiation is typically reserved for patients with unresectable disease, those who are medically inoperable, or who refuse surgery. Multiple studies have demonstrated superior outcomes with surgery combined with pathology-directed adjuvant therapy, in comparison to definitive EBRT alone, with or without chemotherapy. For example, some of the only prospective randomized data come from a small randomized trial conducted in Singapore, where 119 patients with locally advanced head and cancer were randomized to either surgery and adjuvant radiation or definitive cisplatin and 5-FU-based concomitant chemoradiation.[5] Although in the entire cohort there was no difference in survival or locoregional control with either approach, in the subgroup of 32 patients with oral cavity primaries, there was dramatically better disease-specific survival (DSS) in patients undergoing surgery and postoperative radiation versus those receiving definitive chemoradiation (▶ Fig. 33.1, 5-year DSS: 68 vs. 12%, $P = 0.038$). There were trends toward lower locoregional relapse (approximately 30 vs. 70% at 5 years, $P = 0.355$) and distant relapse (5-year distant recurrence: 8 vs. 50%, $P = 0.05$) in the surgery arm. Only 4 out of 19 patients with oral cavity tumors undergoing definitive chemoradiation avoided surgery after completing treatment. Although this trial had multiple limitations, including limited a number of patients, early termination due to poor accrual, lack of intent-to-treat analysis, antiquated radiation techniques, somewhat lower radiation doses than used in modern practice (66 Gy in 33 fractions), and reliance on unplanned subgroup analyses, the absolute magnitude of the survival and relapse differences in the two arms are striking and suggest that definitive chemoradiation may be suboptimal for locally advanced OCSCC.

Multiple retrospective studies have also compared surgical and radiation-based approaches for oral cavity cancer (▶ Table 33.1). For example, a bi-institutional retrospective study of 104 OCSCC patients undergoing either surgery and adjuvant radiotherapy or definitive chemoradiation showed markedly worse locoregional control, DSS, and overall survival for patients undergoing definitive chemoradiation in multivariable models.[6] In addition, patients undergoing chemoradiation were more likely to require feeding tubes for at least 30 days or more after treatment (30 vs. 11%). Similarly, an analysis of 6,900 stage III–IVA OCSCC patients from the National Cancer Data Base showed vastly better survival in propensity score-matched cohorts undergoing surgery and postoperative radiation versus those undergoing chemoradiation (3-year OS: 53.9 vs. 37.8%).[7] This difference appeared to be driven by clinical stage T3–T4a tumors, whereas survival was not significantly different for those with T1–T2 disease. Similar results were observed in an analysis of the Surveillance, Epidemiology, and End Results (SEER) database[8] and a variety of smaller studies.[4,9–11]

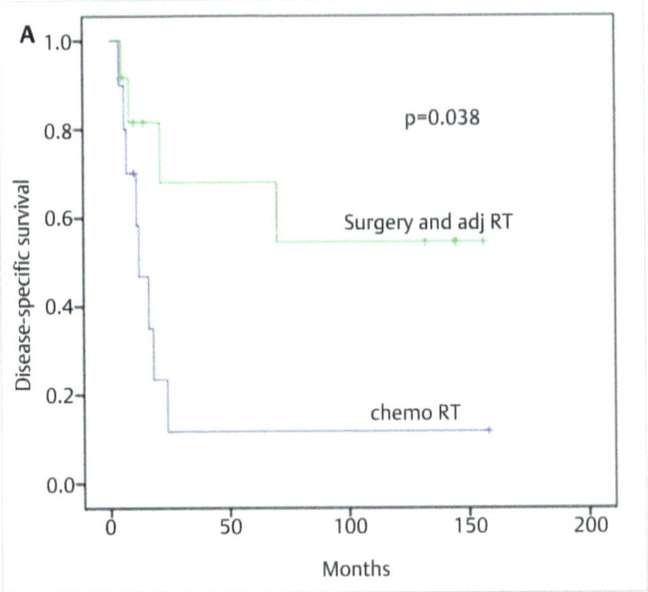

Fig. 33.1 In the subset of oral cavity squamous cell carcinoma (OCSCC) patients enrolled on a randomized controlled trial comparing definitive surgery and postoperative radiation to definitive chemoradiation, significantly better disease-specific survival (DSS) was observed for patients randomized to the surgical arm.[5]

All of these studies are limited by retrospective design and near universal imbalances in clinical and demographic features favoring the surgical cohort. Nevertheless, these studies and other noncomparative studies reporting results with definitive radiation for OCSCC (▸ Table 33.2) strongly suggest that OCSCC is relatively radioresistant. Despite this, long-term cure can be achieved in a minority of cases without surgery. Thus, some OCSCCs must have greater inherent sensitivity to radiation and chemotherapy than others. One attractive approach would be to only attempt organ preserving chemoradiation in the subset of patients with tumors that are inherently sensitive to DNA-damaging therapies. The utility of induction chemotherapy to chemo-select patients for definitive radiation has shown utility in larynx cancer,[14] but has been less well studied in oral cavity cancers. The chemo-selection paradigm hypothesizes that patients responding to chemotherapy have increased biologic sensitivity to DNA-damaging therapies, such as radiation, and likely will be better candidates for organ preservation. This was tested in a prospective single arm phase II trial at the University of Michigan.[13] Nineteen patients with stage III–IV OCSCC without bone invasion underwent 1 cycle of induction chemotherapy with cisplatin/carboplatin and 5-FU. Three weeks later,

Table 33.1 Selected series comparing surgery and postoperative radiation (S + RT) to definitive chemoradiation (CRT) in patients with locally advanced oral cavity squamous cell carcinoma (OCSCC)

Series	# OCSCC Pts (# definitive RT)	Stages	Concomitant chemotherapy with definitive RT	Local control (S + RT vs. CRT)	Disease-specific survival (S + RT vs. CRT)	Overall survival (S + RT vs. CRT)	G-tube (S + RT vs. CRT)	ORN (S + RT vs. CRT)
Iyer et al, Cancer (2015)[5]	32 (19)	III–IVA	100%	5 yr: ~70% vs. ~30%	5 yr: 68% vs. 12%	NR	NR	NR
Gore et al, Head Neck (2015)[6]	104 (50)	All stages	100%	5 yr: ~70% vs. ~35%	5 yr: ~85% vs. ~30%	5 yr: ~80% vs. ~30%	11% vs. 30%	13% vs. 12%
Spiotto et al, JAMA Otolaryngol (2017)[7]	6900 (2091)	III–IVA	100%	NR	NR	3 yr: 54% vs. 38%	NR	NR
Sher et al, IJROBP (2011)[10]	42 (12)	All stages	75%	2 yr: 91% vs. 64%	NR	2 yr: 85% vs. 63%	90% overall	5% overall
Studer et al, Radiat Onc (2012)[9]	160 (44)	All stages	68%	4 yr: 80% vs. 37%	NR	4 yr: 79% vs. 37%	NR	1% overall
Stenson et al, Laryngoscope (2010)[12]	138 (111)	"Advanced"	100%	Crude: NR vs. 89%	NR	3 yr: 63% vs. 70%	RT: 8%	RT: 18%
Daly et al, IJRBOP (2011)[11]	37 (7)	All stages	100%	3 yr: 67% vs. 60%	NR	3 yr: 60% vs. 57%	24% overall	5% overall
Chinn et al, JAMA Otolarygnol (2014)[13]	72 (19)	III–IVB	100%	5 yr: 72% vs. 26%	5 yr: 75% vs. 46%	5 yr: 65% vs. 32%	9% vs. 42%	2% vs. 16%

Abbreviations: CRT, chemoradiation; G-tube, gastrostomy tube; NR, not reported; OCSCC, oral cavity squamous cell carcinoma; ORN, osteoradionecrosis; RT, radiotherapy; S, surgery; Yr: year.

Table 33.2 Selected series reporting outcomes with definitive external beam radiotherapy for oral cavity squamous cell carcinoma

Definitive radiotherapy	*N*	Stage	Chemo	Brachy	LC	DSS	OS	ORN	G-tube
Scher et al, Oral Oncol (2015)[15]	73	I–IVB (64% T4)	67%	11%	5 yr: 37%	5 yr: 38%	5 yr: 15%	7%	Post-RT 8%
Lin et al, IJROBP (2010)[16]	115	III–IVB	83%	0%	5 yr: 23%	5 yr: 25%	5 yr: 15%	4%	NR
Turner et al, Radiother Oncol (1996)[17]	332	I–IVB (38% T4)	18%	0%	5 yr: 61%	5 yr: 55%	5 yr: 43%	9%	0%
Cohen et al, Head Neck (2009)[18]	39	T4	100%	0%	5 yr: 75%	5 yr: 67%	5 yr: 56%	18%	NR
Fuwa et al, Br J Cancer (2008)[19]	131	III–IVB	100%	31%	3 yr: 69%	NR	3 yr: 54%	NR	NR
Crombie et al, Oral Oncol (2012)[20]	54	I–IVB	98%	0%	NR	5 yr: 30%	5 yr: 29%	11% (36% of survivors)	Post-RT 54%
Fazekas et al, IJROBP (1980)[21]	146	III–IVB	0%	NR	NR	NR	5 yr: 20%	NR	NR
Leung et al, Acta Oncol (1993)[22]	117	I–IVB (27% T4)	0%	56%	10 yr: 44%	NR	10 yr: 51%	9%	NR
Dinshaw et al, Clin Oncol (2006)[23]	69	I–IVB	0%	NR	5 yr: 44%	NR	NR	NR	NR
Murthy et al, J Cancer Res Ther (2010)[24]	159	I–IVB	40%	17%	3 yr: 34%	NR	NR	NR	NR

Abbreviations: Brachy, brachytherapy; Chemo, chemotherapy; DSS, disease-specific survival; G-tube, gastrostomy-tube; LC, local control; NR, not reported; ORN, osteoradionecrosis; OS, overall survival; RT, radiotherapy; Yr, year.

patients with at least a 50% clinical response underwent definitive platinum-based chemoradiation, whereas nonresponding patients underwent surgery and postoperative radiation. The trial was stopped after meeting early stopping rules for futility. In total, 10 patients responded to induction chemotherapy and underwent definitive chemoradiation, with 30% of them having disease control at 5 years. Of the 9 nonresponding patients, 4 died before surgery could be performed. Compared to a matched group of patients treated with surgery and postoperative radiation at the same institution, patients enrolled on this trial had worse locoregional control (5-year locoregional control (LRC): 72 vs. 26%, $P<0.001$), DSS (5-year DSS: 75 vs. 46%, $P=0.001$), and overall survival (5-year overall survival [OS]: 65 vs. 32%, $P=0.01$). Moreover, gastrostomy tube (9 vs. 42%), osteoradionecrosis (2 vs. 16%), and tracheostomy tube rates (0 vs. 5%) were all higher in the cohort enrolled on this trial in comparison to the historical matched surgery cohort.

Some of the most favorable results for treating locally advanced OCSCC definitively with EBRT came from the University of Chicago. For example, in a retrospective analysis of 39 patients with T4 OCSCC enrolled on 4 prospective phase II protocols, including 16 with bone invasion, 5-year local control was 75% with definitive chemoradiation with or without induction chemotherapy, with 5-year cause-specific and overall survival of 67 and 56%, respectively.[18] Osteoradionecrosis occurred in 18% of patients, and 29% experienced severe long-term complications. A larger study of the same institution of patients with locally advanced oral cavity cancers enrolled on one of 15 clinical trials, comparing 111 patients undergoing definitive chemoradiation to 27 patients undergoing primary surgery and postoperative chemoradiation, showed no difference in overall survival or progression-free survival.[12] The rate of osteoradionecrosis was identical to what was observed in the T4 subset, and deaths from treatment complications were seen in 7%. However, it is notable that the results from the University of Chicago are difficult to extrapolate to other institutions, given that they utilize both a unique radiation regimen (75 Gy given in 1.5 Gy fraction twice daily with one week on, one week off of radiation) and a unique multi-agent radiosensitizing chemotherapy regimen (5-FU and hydroxyurea combined with either cisplatin or paclitaxel) that are rarely utilized at other centers. It is unclear if these regimens are central to the excellent results reported, as few, if any, other institutions employ them. On the other hand, an alternative explanation is that the University of Chicago preferentially treated locally advanced OCSCC with chemoradiation rather than surgery, so there may have been less selection bias against the chemoradiation patients. Another study that demonstrated fairly good results with definitive chemoradiation for stage III–IVB OCSCC was reported by Fuwa and colleagues, achieving local control in 69% of cases at 3 years.[19] Local control was 78% for T2–T3 tumors and 51% for T4 tumors. However, they used intra-arterial platinum chemotherapy, sometimes combined with systemic chemotherapy, which is rarely used at other institutions. In addition, 31% of patients received brachytherapy. Thus, these results are also difficult to extrapolate to other settings.

For those undergoing definitive EBRT with locally advanced disease, concomitant chemotherapy should be delivered in patients healthy enough to receive it. In the MACH-NC Collaborative Group meta-analysis,[25] which demonstrated improved locoregional control and overall survival with the addition of concomitant chemotherapy to radiation for head and neck cancers, 21% of patients had OCSCC. In patients unable to receive chemotherapy due to medical contraindications or refusal, hyperfractionated or accelerated radiation is an alternative treatment intensification approach that can improve both locoregional control and overall survival in head and neck cancer.[26] OCSCC made up 12.6% of patients in the MARCH meta-analysis. There is no prospective randomized data to support the use of cetuximab with definitive radiation for oral cavity cancer, given that these patients were excluded from the only trial demonstrating a benefit from this therapy with radiation.[27]

In summary, radiation is an acceptable alternative to surgery in select cases of early stage T1–2N0 OCSCC. If radiation is used in this setting, strong consideration should be given to using intraoral cones or brachytherapy either for the entire treatment or as a boost, given that the majority of historical series used these modalities. Nevertheless, surgery may be preferred in many patients with early stage OCSCC due to excellent control, favorable toxicity profile, and quicker treatment times with this modality. For those with more advanced disease, the vast majority of the data suggest that primary external beam radiation with or without chemotherapy does not result in equivalent oncologic outcomes to surgery followed by postoperative radiation. However, EBRT can still play an important role in those with unresectable disease, medical inoperability, or who refuse surgery due to morbidity or functional concerns. It is important to note that although rates of locoregional control with definitive chemoradiation are suboptimal, chemoradiation can still be curative in a subset of these patients that are either unable or unwilling to undergo surgery, and should not be withheld from patients amenable to curative-intent nonoperative therapy.

33.3 Diagnosis and Evaluation

All patients with OCSCC should undergo a detailed history and clinical exam of the head and neck. Oral cavity masses typically present in early stages as a painless lump or plaque. They can masquerade as benign lesions (e.g., papillomas, traumatic fibromas, or lichen planus), but tend to progress over time to become painful, exophytic, and friable. An index of suspicion should be raised with symptoms that involve referred otalgia, dysphagia, dysarthria, unanticipated weight loss, or associated neck lymphadenopathy. Tongue or floor of mouth fixation can imply mandibular invasion or intrinsic muscle involvement. Trismus may be suggestive of pterygoid muscle involvement or deep buccal extension. Other signs of advanced local disease include tumor immobility, loose dentition, hypoglossal nerve paralysis, or mental nerve paresthesias. In terms of clinical exam, inspection and palpation of the oral cavity are important to assess the primary tumor extent and identify any second primary tumors. Neck exam should focus on bilateral levels IA–IV. Flexible fiberoptic laryngoscopy can be helpful in patients with tumors extending into the pharynx, or in smokers to rule out second primary tumors. A punch biopsy under local anesthesia in clinic is most often preferred for diagnosis and is usually well-tolerated. Complete blood counts, comprehensive metabolic panels, and audiology testing are indicated for patients that will receive chemotherapy.

Imaging is critical for patients with OCSCC undergoing definitive EBRT, both to ensure adequate staging and for proper target delineation. Panoramic radiographs have conventionally been useful to determine bony extent, although cone beam CTs, if available, offer superior detail to three-dimensional reconstruction modeling. A CT of the neck with contrast can be useful for evaluating for pathologic lymphadenopathy and assessing for mandibular cortex involvement, but can often be suboptimal in terms of evaluation of the primary site due to poor enhancement of oral cavity tumors and dental artifacts. MRI has better soft tissue delineation and less artifact from dental hardware, and therefore is often better for visualizing oral cavity primary tumors and predicting depth of invasion. MRI is also useful for tracing retrograde perineural invasion in the oral cavity (e.g., the inferior alveolar nerve or hypoglossal nerve). Systemic imaging, such as CT of chest or PET-CT, is generally not required for patients with early stage OCSCC, but should be performed in patients with more advanced disease (e.g., stage III–IV).

Pretreatment dental evaluation is important prior to radiation for OCSCC. Patients undergoing definitive EBRT for OCSCC are at high risk for caries, primarily due to the xerostomia resulting from treatment, and more serious complications such as osteoradionecrosis, especially if extractions are performed after treatment completion. Thus, a dentist with experience in the management of head and neck cancers should evaluate the patient and perform a full cleaning. Teeth with poor prognosis should be extracted, with guidelines generally recommending 1–2 weeks for healing following extraction prior to the initiation of radiation. Fluoride trays are also often made to help prevent formation of caries.

Patients should also receive evaluations from a speech/swallowing therapist and a dietician. Supportive care and palliative medicine services can be helpful for symptom management. Many patients will require gastrostomy tube placement during treatment given that mucositis, odynophagia, phlegm, and dysgeusia can all substantially impair oral intake. Risks are highest in elderly patients and those requiring bilateral neck treatment, and prophylactic gastrostomy tube placement can be considered in these individuals.

Patients should be simulated in the supine position using a thermoplastic mask immobilizing the chin and shoulders. A custom radiation stent during simulation and treatment can be useful to physically displace uninvolved oral cavity structures from those at risk of harboring microscopic cells. For example, when treating an oral tongue cancer, a bite block can be used to physically separate the oral tongue from the palate, decreasing unnecessary radiation dose to the palate (and vice versa for hard palate cancers). Similarly, for a lateralized buccal cancer, a custom device can be used to displace the tongue away from the buccal target. All scars should be wired. For patients with extranodal extension, irradiating the skin approximately 2 cm circumferentially around the scar with bolus is often performed to prevent dermal recurrence. Fusion of the simulation CT with an MRI and/or PET/CT scan can help to better delineate the gross target volume (GTV).

33.4 Site-Specific Radiotherapy Considerations

For early stage T1–2N0 OCSCC that is ≤ 4 mm thick, intraoral cone treatment may provide less toxicity, and possibly better control, than standard linear accelerator-based EBRT (▶ Fig. 33.2). Intraoral cones need to be in constant contact with the oral mucosa, and therefore can only be used in sites that are accessible to cone placement. The tumor borders should be tattooed prior to treatment, so that the initial tumor site can be identified even if the tumor regresses. Although intraoral cones can deliver either electrons or orthovoltage photons, orthovoltage photons are typically preferred given that they deliver full dose to the surface and have less constriction of higher isodoses and bowing of lower isodoses in comparison to electrons. Intraoral cones typically cannot treat tumors larger than 3 cm. For other patients requiring more extensive definitive EBRT treatments, intensity modulated radiotherapy (IMRT) is appropriate to minimize radiation dose to uninvolved normal structures. Comprehensive IMRT can be combined with a boost to gross disease, either with an intraoral cone or brachytherapy, although many institutions lack the capabilities of delivering these treatments.

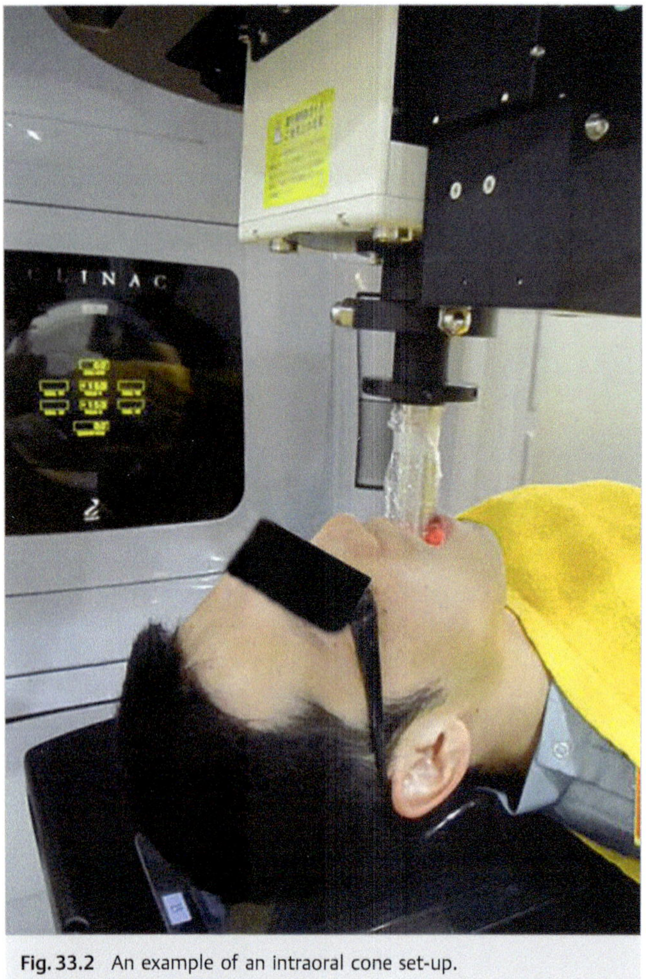

Fig. 33.2 An example of an intraoral cone set-up.

With standard fractionation using solely IMRT, the GTV is contoured. This volume is expanded to account for possible microscopic spread of cells (clinical target volume = CTV), then expanded again to account for daily set-up uncertainty (planning target volume = PTV). This PTV based on the sites of gross disease is typically prescribed 70 Gy in 35 fractions. Other areas at high risk of harboring microscopic cells are typically treated with doses between 54 and 63 Gy, and areas at lower risk are treated with 50 to 54 Gy. Specific considerations for each anatomic subsite are detailed below.

33.4.1 Lip

Definitive radiation can be considered for lip cancers involving the oral commissure, given the potential risk of oral incontinence with surgical resection (▶ Fig. 33.3). Another scenario where definitive radiation is potentially reasonable is when removal of more than half of the lower lip is necessary, given that this can be both functionally and cosmetically problematic, even with reconstruction. Some data suggest that radiation produces better preservation of sensation, intercommissural distance, elasticity, and lip seal than surgery for certain lip cancer patients.[28]

For T1 and T2 lip cancers treated with EBRT, either orthovoltage photons or electrons are effective modalities. Lead shielding can be used to minimize dose to the uninvolved oral cavity, including the teeth and gingiva. With electrons, skin surface collimation can sharpen the penumbra and reduce outward spill of lower radiation doses. Margins are typically smaller for orthovoltage irradiation (1.0–1.5 cm) than electrons (2.0–2.5 cm) due to the inward constriction of the higher isodose curves for electrons. Elective neck irradiation is usually not performed for T1 and T2 lip cancers, unless adverse risk features such as thickness > 4 mm, perineual invasion (PNI), commissure involvement, or poor differentiation are present. If needed, unilateral radiation can be employed for very well lateralized lesions.

For more locally advanced T3–T4 lesions with clinically negative necks on physical exam and imaging, elective neck irradiation should cover the bilateral cervical lymph nodes. For lower lip cancers, levels IA, IB, and II–IV should be covered. For upper lip cancers, the bilateral facial nodes and levels IB–IV should be covered. This can be accomplished with either conventional techniques (opposed lateral beams matched to a low anterior neck field with or without matched appositional electrons) or IMRT. A bite block can be used to separate the upper lips and teeth from the lower.

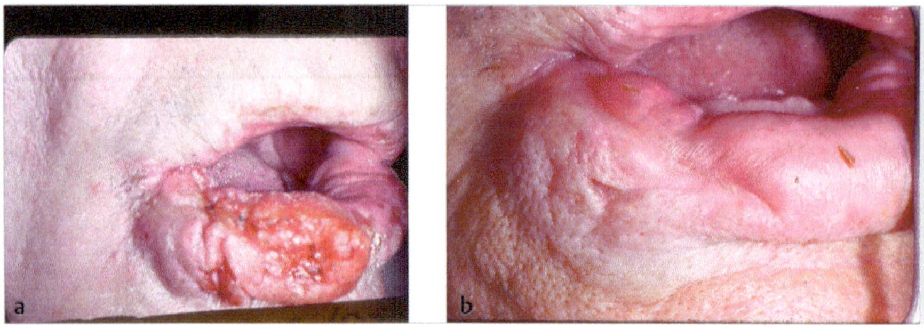

Fig. 33.3 A patient (a) before and (b) after treatment with matched electrons and photons for a cT3N0M0 squamous cell carcinoma (SCC) of the lower lip.

33.4.2 Oral Tongue

For small T1–2N0 tumors that are less than or equal to 4 mm thick, external beam techniques are usually avoided if possible, and brachytherapy is typically favored if definitive radiation is required. It is possible to treat with intraoral cones, if available, but the mobility of the tongue makes set-up reproducibility challenging. If a cone is used, wide margins (≥ 1 cm) are generally required. For thicker tumors, a combination of brachytherapy boost and external beam radiation can be used to treat both the primary and elective lymph nodes (bilateral levels IA–IV). Linear accelerator-based IMRT alone is possible, but may be suboptimal due to higher toxicity and poorer tumor control than more focal modalities.

For advanced oral tongue tumors, IMRT with or without an interstitial brachytherapy boost can be used (▶ Fig. 33.4). We include the entire oral tongue, base of tongue, and floor of mouth in the intermediate dose volume. The ipsilateral tonsil is often included, given that this is directly between the primary target and the adjacent level IIA lymph nodes. We treat bilateral levels IA–IV in all cases. Interstitial brachytherapy boost may be helpful, either planned in combination with external beam radiation or delivered to any gross residual disease after the completion of EBRT.

33.4.3 Floor of Mouth

For very early stage T1–2N0 lesions with ≤ 4 mm depth of invasion, definitive radiation utilizing either brachytherapy or intraoral cones is possible. EBRT delivered with a linear accelerator without brachytherapy or intraoral cone boost is typically avoided.

For more advanced lesions treated with IMRT, generally the entire floor of mouth is included. The ipsilateral mandibular alveolar ridge is often included as well, depending on the proximity to the tumor. Bilateral levels IA–IV should be targeted. Notably, given the proximity of the floor of mouth to the alveolar ridge, patients are at higher risk of soft tissue damage and osteoradionecrosis than some other sites of the oral cavity, especially with brachytherapy boost. Thus, the likelihood of cure without major complication is relatively low.

33.4.4 Buccal Mucosa

For definitive radiation of early stage buccal SCC, excellent results with definitive radiation have been reported by combining external beam radiation with either intraoral cone irradiation or an interstitial high dose rate (HDR) implant. We recommend treating the gross tumor with wide margins (1.5–2 cm) due to lack of anatomic barriers to spread of disease. For more advanced lesions, we recommend treating the entire ipsilateral buccal mucosa. Generally, this will extend to the inferior orbital rim superiorly and to the retromolar trigone posteriorly. If possible, the primary tumor can be boosted with either an intraoral cone or interstitial high dose rate (HDR) implant. For well-lateralized tumors, ipsilateral levels IB–IV are included. Very low rates of contralateral neck recurrence have been observed in several series.[29,30] For tumors within 1 cm of midline, invading the floor of mouth, or with bulky nodal disease potentially increasing the possibility of retrograde lymphatic flow, coverage of the contralateral neck could be considered. For anterior buccal lesions within 1 cm of the upper lip, the ipsilateral facial lymph nodes can be covered. In many cases, an intraoral stent to displace the tongue away from the buccal mucosa can be useful to reduce toxicity.

33.4.5 Alveolar Ridge/Gingiva/ Retromolar Trigone

Small lesions can be managed with combined external beam radiation and an intraoral cone. Brachytherapy is generally avoided because of the high risk of osteoradionecrosis. For larger lesions, comprehensive IMRT is generally recommended. If perineural invasion is present, the entire hemi-mandible or hemi-maxilla should be treated. In cases of invasion of a large-caliber or named nerve, the nerve should be covered to the skull base. For retromolar trigone cases specifically, the ipsilateral parapharyngeal space and pharyngeal wall up to the pterygoid plates can be covered given the potential for spread along the pterygomandibular raphe. Often, neck treatment can be confined to the ipsilateral neck (levels I–IV) unless the lesion is within 1 cm of midline, invades the floor of mouth, or there is bulky lymphadenopathy.

33.4.6 Hard Palate

SCC of the hard palate is rare, and data for definitive radiation are limited. In addition to treating the gross tumor, we recommend treating the entire hard palate in the intermediate risk CTV except for early stage lesions (T1). The bilateral necks should be treated when elective neck treatment is indicated given that most advanced palate lesions will be within 1 cm of midline.

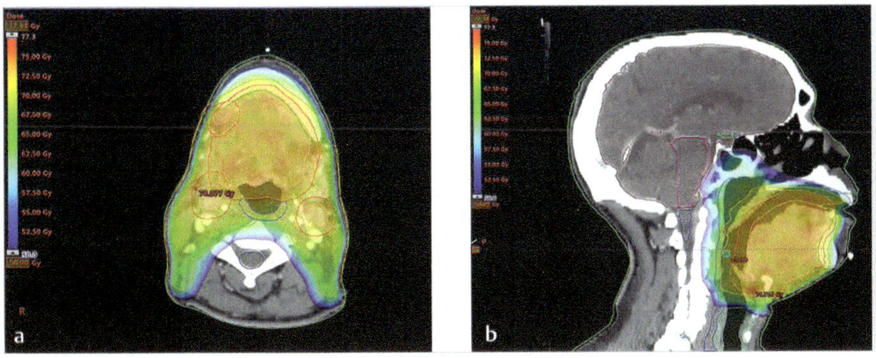

Fig. 33.4 An example of an IMRT radiation plan for a patient undergoing definitive chemoradiation after refusing total glossectomy and total laryngectomy for cT4aN2c oral tongue squamous cell carcinoma (SCC). **(a)** Axial view. **(b)** Sagittal view.

33.5 Toxicity Management

Definitive linear accelerator-based EBRT for oral cavity cancer produces some of the most significant adverse sequelae of any type of radiation treatment. Toxicity can be especially intense for patients with oral tongue and floor mouth primaries, and a vast majority will require enteral feeding and intravenous fluids to support nutrition and hydration at some point during treatment. In general, acute side effects start during the third week of treatment (although dysgeusia can start earlier, particularly for those receiving platinum-based chemotherapy), build throughout the remainder of radiation, and peak during the last week of treatment and the week following treatment. Maintaining adequate hydration and nutrition is the paramount challenge of treatment, and often requires intravenous fluid administration, gastrostomy tube feedings, or both. Side effects gradually resolve over months after treatment is completed.

Mucositis is one of the most bothersome sequelae for patients undergoing radiation to the oral cavity. This can cause severe oral pain and odynophagia, making it difficult to take food and fluids by mouth. The most effective treatment of mucositis-induced pain is narcotics, which generally need to be initiated between the third and last week of treatment. For patients requiring around-the-clock pharmaceutical pain control, utilization of long-acting narcotic formulations such as fentanyl patches can provide more consistent pain control and easier upward and downward titration of dosing. Neurontin may be a useful adjunct for pain control in certain cases, and can be used as a prophylactic medication to delay the onset of pain that requires narcotics. In addition to systemic pain control, a variety of topical agents have shown utility. Early initiation of salt water and baking soda mouth rinses can help neutralize acidity in the mouth and delay the onset of mucositis. We have patients initiate glutamine rinses and swallows early in therapy as a preventative measure.[31] Once symptomatic mucositis develops, mouth rinses are compounded with various combinations of viscous lidocaine, diphenhydramine, Maalox, and/or antifungal medicines, known collectively as "Magic Mouthwash," which can provide short-term relief from mucositis pain, generally lasting for 30–45 minutes.[32] This can be helpful prior to meals. Other topical agents, such as doxepin,[33] mucoadhesive hydrogel (MuGard),[34] and honey[35] have shown efficacy in randomized controlled trials. Gelclair can also be useful in certain cases, although clinical evidence for benefit is relatively limited.[36] Recently, GC4419, a small molecule dismutase mimetic, was granted Food and Drug Administration (FDA) breakthrough status based on a double blind, placebo randomized controlled Phase IIb trial, but this is not yet widely available. In general, topical agents have variable efficacy from patient to patient, so we generally switch to a different agent if the patient's current topical therapy is ineffective.

Thickened secretions and phlegm tend to be some of the most bothersome acute symptoms during oral cavity radiation. These mucoid secretions can be difficult to swallow and cause gagging and vomiting when eating or drinking, limiting oral intake. Almost no literature exists regarding the optimal management of this symptom, which is often not directly assessed in historical clinical trials. We recommend salt water and baking soda mouth rinses every 3 hours from the beginning of radiation. When secretions start to thicken, guaifenisin (Mucinex) can have some limited benefit. Anticholinergic medications, such as glycopyrrolate or hyoscyamine, are some of the most effective medications for reducing secretions, although they can produce dry mouth and other anticholinergic sequelae. Scopolamine patches can also have efficacy, but tend to have higher side effects than other options. Supportive measures, such as diet ginger ale gargles, meat tenderizer solution rinses, corticosteroid mouth rinses, or home suction machines can also help in certain cases.

Dysgeusia due to radiation, chemotherapy, and xerostomia is another bothersome potential sequela of oral cavity radiation.[37] This is often one of the first symptoms to develop during treatment, and also one of the slowest to recover. Although poorly characterized in the literature, clinical experience suggests that older patients, especially those aged 75 or more, are at higher risk of long-term dysgeusia after receiving high radiation doses to the oral tongue, although the majority of other patients will have near normal taste within 1 year of treatment completion. Unfortunately, there are limited options for management of dysgeusia during radiotherapy.[38] In one small randomized placebo-controlled trial performed in Iran enrolling 35 patients with head and neck cancer undergoing radiation, initiating 50 mg zinc, three times daily, taken orally at the start of radiation increased taste perception.[39] However, another larger randomized trial showed no benefit in taste recovery for head and neck cancer patients receiving zinc versus placebo.[40] In practice, dysgeusia is primarily managed through dietary counselling and selection of tolerable foods. Increased spice, if tolerated, and increased umami foods can be helpful, although this is variable.

Dermatitis is a common side effect from radiation for head and neck cancers.[41] Initially, we recommend all patients use a moisturizing lotion, such as Calendula, Eucerin, or Aquaphor, twice daily. However, lotion should not be applied within 4 hours prior to radiation treatment to avoid the possibility of a bolus effect from a layer of lotion on the skin during treatment. Tight clothing or other accessories that can mechanically irritate the skin should be avoided. Patient should also avoid sun exposure, application of skin irritants such as perfumes or alcohol-based deodorants, and scratching of the area. If pruritis develops, topical corticosteroids like mometasone 0.1% cream can be helpful. A variety of measures can be taken for patients with moist desquamation, including xeroform wraps with lidocaine cream and silvadene. Severe dermatitis, defined as skin necrosis, full dermal thickness ulceration, or spontaneous bleeding is extremely rare but may require management by a wound care specialist.

Xerostomia is perhaps the most common long-term side effect of oral cavity radiation, even though this has been substantially reduced in the modern era via widespread adoption of intensity-modulated radiotherapy.[42] Xerostomia can also cause dysphagia with dry foods such as meat, bread, and nuts, increase risk of caries, and exacerbate taste alterations. The main pharmacologic agent with established efficacy in preventing xerostomia is amifostine.[43,44] However, this is rarely used in clinical practice given that it requires daily intravenous infusion and has serious potential side effects including hypotension and nausea. Pilocarpine during radiotherapy for prevention of xerostomia has shown some efficacy in some clinical trials,[45] but results have overall been inconsistent.[46] For patients that develop xerostomia, nonpharmacologic measures include the use of oral rinses such as Biotene or NeutraSal, drinking adequate fluids, using humidifiers at night, maintaining open nasal passages to avoid mouth breathing, eating acidic food, and using sugar-free xylitol-containing candy and gum. Acupuncture has shown benefit in several randomized controlled trials.[47–49] Pharmacologic sialagogues, such as pilocarpine, bethanechol, and cevimeline, can be helpful in treating radiation-induced xerostomia in about 50% of patients.[46] However, these medications can have side effects including sweating, flushing, increased urinary frequency, nausea, and diarrhea. Rare but serious side effects include hypotension, bradycardia, and decreased night vision.

Dysphagia can be one of the most bothersome long-term side effects of radiation for OCSCC that negatively impact patient's quality of life.[50] Dysphagia has been shown to correlate with radiation dose to the pharyngeal constrictors,[51] and is significantly reduced with modern radiation techniques such as IMRT.[52] Dysphagia can be assessed with videofluoroscopy, manometry, and patient reported forms such as the MD Anderson Dysphagia Index. The etiology of dysphagia following radiation is multifactorial. Xerostomia can decrease lubrication, making it more difficult to swallow dry foods. Certain radiation fields requiring high doses to the cervical esophagus can result in esophageal stenosis, sometimes requiring dilations, although this is rare in oral cavity cancer with modern radiation planning techniques. Some studies have suggested high rates of long-term dysphagia with prophylactic G-tube placement,[53] although randomized trials have shown similar rates of long-term dependence with either prophylactic or reactive G-tubes.[54,55] Other factors, such as lower cranial nerve deficits and fibrosis of the swallowing muscles, may also play a role. Swallow therapy is a mainstay of dysphagia management. Therapists can work with patients on postural techniques, swallowing exercises, and other techniques as part of a comprehensive swallowing rehabilitation program.

Osteoradionecrosis is one of the most potentially serious long-term sequelae of oral cavity radiation, but represents a spectrum of disease from small asymptomatic bone exposures to highly symptomatic and severe destruction of the bone, most commonly involving the mandible. For mild asymptomatic osteoradionecrosis, observation with or without antibiotics is typically sufficient. Pentoxifylline 400 mg and vitamin E 400 I.U. daily may be helpful as well.[56] Conservative debridement to remove spicules of devitalized bone can be performed as well. Pain can be managed with narcotics and topical lidocaine. Hyperbaric oxygen with or without surgical debridement is also often used for severe osteoradionecrosis. However, hyperbaric oxygen can be time-consuming, often given as 30–40 treatments 5 days per week. In addition, a placebo-controlled randomized trial found potentially worse outcomes with the use of hyperbaric oxygen for osteoradionecrosis, resulting in earlier stopping of the trial at the second interim analysis,[57] although the trial's methodology and compliance have been criticized.[58,59] Segmental mandibulectomy and reconstruction may be required for severe or progressive osteoradionecrosis that is nonresponsive to conservative therapy.

Fibrosis can lead to muscle stiffness following radiation, particularly in the muscles of the neck and jaw, potentially causing neck stiffness and trismus, respectively. Unfortunately, research regarding prevention and management of fibrosis is limited. Stretching exercises are useful. Pentoxifylline and vitamin E and low-level light therapy[60] may be helpful in certain cases as well.

Key Points

- Surgery and radiation are options for definitive treatment of oral cavity cancers, with surgery being the favored modality for the vast majority of cases. This is due to the relatively greater toxicities from definitive radiation to the oral cavity, as well as the inherent radioresistance of OCSCC relative to other head and neck sites.
- Definitive radiation can be an effective option for early stage oral cavity tumors, such as T1–2N0 cancers. However, the majority of studies reporting acceptable efficacy and toxicity in this setting have used either intraoral cones or brachytherapy, alone or combined with linear accelerator-based EBRT, and these should be considered preferred modalities to linear accelerator-based EBRT alone.
- For locally advanced oral cavity cancers, definitive EBRT alone seems to offer suboptimal control and increased toxicity in comparison to surgery-based approaches in the vast majority of studies. However, cure is possible in a minority of oral cavity cancers with definitive chemoradiation, and treatment should not be withheld from patients unwilling or unable to undergo surgery. Strong consideration should be given to utilizing brachytherapy as a boost when possible.
- Potential indications for definitive radiation or chemoradiation in the locally advanced setting include unresectable disease, medical inoperability, or situations where morbidity from surgery is considered unacceptable by the patient.

References

[1] Pfister DG, Ang KK, Brizel DM, et al. National Comprehensive Cancer Network. Head and neck cancers, version 2.2013: featured updates to the NCCN guidelines. J Natl Compr Canc Netw. 2013; 11(8):917–923

[2] Gilbert EH, Goffinet DR, Bagshaw MA. Carcinoma of the oral tongue and floor of mouth: fifteen years' experience with linear acceleration therapy. Cancer. 1975; 35(6):1517–1524

[3] Ichimiya Y, Fuwa N, Kamata M, et al. Treatment results of stage I oral tongue cancer with definitive radiotherapy. Oral Oncol. 2005; 41(5):520–525

[4] Wendt CD, Peters LJ, Delclos L, et al. Primary radiotherapy in the treatment of stage I and II oral tongue cancers: importance of the proportion of therapy delivered with interstitial therapy. Int J Radiat Oncol Biol Phys. 1990; 18(6): 1287–1292

[5] Iyer NG, Tan DS, Tan VK, et al. Randomized trial comparing surgery and adjuvant radiotherapy versus concurrent chemoradiotherapy in patients with advanced, nonmetastatic squamous cell carcinoma of the head and neck: 10-year update and subset analysis. Cancer. 2015; 121(10):1599–1607

[6] Gore SM, Crombie AK, Batstone MD, Clark JR. Concurrent chemoradiotherapy compared with surgery and adjuvant radiotherapy for oral cavity squamous cell carcinoma. Head Neck. 2015; 37(4):518–523

[7] Spiotto MT, Jefferson G, Wenig B, Markiewicz M, Weichselbaum RR, Koshy M. Differences in survival with surgery and postoperative radiotherapy compared with definitive chemoradiotherapy for oral cavity cancer: a national cancer database analysis. JAMA Otolaryngol Head Neck Surg. 2017; 143(7): 691–699

[8] Cannon RB, Sowder JC, Buchmann LO, et al. Increasing use of nonsurgical therapy in advanced-stage oral cavity cancer: a population-based study. Head Neck. 2017; 39(1):82–91

[9] Studer G, Brown M, Bredell M, et al. Follow up after IMRT in oral cavity cancer: update. Radiat Oncol. 2012; 7:84

[10] Sher DJ, Thotakura V, Balboni TA, et al. Treatment of oral cavity squamous cell carcinoma with adjuvant or definitive intensity-modulated radiation therapy. Int J Radiat Oncol Biol Phys. 2011; 81(4):e215–e222
[11] Daly ME, Le QT, Kozak MM, et al. Intensity-modulated radiotherapy for oral cavity squamous cell carcinoma: patterns of failure and predictors of local control. Int J Radiat Oncol Biol Phys. 2011; 80(5):1412–1422
[12] Stenson KM, Kunnavakkam R, Cohen EE, et al. Chemoradiation for patients with advanced oral cavity cancer. Laryngoscope. 2010; 120(1):93–99
[13] Chinn SB, Spector ME, Bellile EL, et al. Efficacy of induction selection chemotherapy vs primary surgery for patients with advanced oral cavity carcinoma. JAMA Otolaryngol Head Neck Surg. 2014; 140(2):134–142
[14] Wolf GT, Fisher SG, Hong WK, et al. Department of Veterans Affairs Laryngeal Cancer Study Group. Induction chemotherapy plus radiation compared with surgery plus radiation in patients with advanced laryngeal cancer. N Engl J Med. 1991; 324(24):1685–1690
[15] Scher ED, Romesser PB, Chen C, et al. Definitive chemoradiation for primary oral cavity carcinoma: a single institution experience. Oral Oncol. 2015; 51 (7):709–715
[16] Lin CY, Wang HM, Kang CJ, et al. Primary tumor site as a predictor of treatment outcome for definitive radiotherapy of advanced-stage oral cavity cancers. Int J Radiat Oncol Biol Phys. 2010; 78(4):1011–1019
[17] Turner SL, Slevin NJ, Gupta NK, Swindell R. Radical external beam radiotherapy for 333 squamous carcinomas of the oral cavity—evaluation of late morbidity and a watch policy for the clinically negative neck. Radiother Oncol. 1996; 41(1):21–29
[18] Cohen EE, Baru J, Huo D, et al. Efficacy and safety of treating T4 oral cavity tumors with primary chemoradiotherapy. Head Neck. 2009; 31(8): 1013–1021
[19] Fuwa N, Kodaira T, Furutani K, et al. Intra-arterial chemoradiotherapy for locally advanced oral cavity cancer: analysis of therapeutic results in 134 cases. Br J Cancer. 2008; 98(6):1039–1045
[20] Crombie AK, Farah C, Tripcony L, Dickie G, Batstone MD. Primary chemoradiotherapy for oral cavity squamous cell carcinoma. Oral Oncol. 2012; 48(10): 1014–1018
[21] Fazekas JT, Sommer C, Kramer S. Adjuvant intravenous methotrexate or definitive radiotherapy alone for advanced squamous cancers of the oral cavity, oropharynx, supraglottic larynx or hypopharynx. Int J Radiat Oncol Biol Phys. 1980; 6(5):533–541
[22] Leung TW, Lee AW, Chan DK. Definitive radiotherapy for carcinoma of the oral tongue. Acta Oncol. 1993; 32(5):559–564
[23] Dinshaw KA, Agarwal JP, Ghosh-Laskar S, Gupta T, Shrivastava SK. Radical radiotherapy in head and neck squamous cell carcinoma: an analysis of prognostic and therapeutic factors. Clin Oncol (R Coll Radiol). 2006; 18(5):383–389
[24] Murthy V, Agarwal JP, Laskar SG, et al. Analysis of prognostic factors in 1180 patients with oral cavity primary cancer treated with definitive or adjuvant radiotherapy. J Cancer Res Ther. 2010; 6(3):282–289
[25] Pignon JP, le Maître A, Maillard E, Bourhis J, MACH-NC Collaborative Group. Meta-analysis of chemotherapy in head and neck cancer (MACH-NC): an update on 93 randomised trials and 17,346 patients. Radiother Oncol. 2009; 92(1):4–14
[26] Bourhis J, Overgaard J, Audry H, et al. Meta-Analysis of Radiotherapy in Carcinomas of Head and Neck (MARCH) Collaborative Group. Hyperfractionated or accelerated radiotherapy in head and neck cancer: a meta-analysis. Lancet. 2006; 368(9538):843–854
[27] Bonner JA, Harari PM, Giralt J, et al. Radiotherapy plus cetuximab for squamous-cell carcinoma of the head and neck. N Engl J Med. 2006; 354(6):567–578
[28] Stranc MF, Fogel M, Dische S. Comparison of lip function: surgery vs radiotherapy. Br J Plast Surg. 1987; 40(6):598–604
[29] Lin CS, Jen YM, Cheng MF, et al. Squamous cell carcinoma of the buccal mucosa: an aggressive cancer requiring multimodality treatment. Head Neck. 2006; 28(2):150–157
[30] Lin CS, Jen YM, Kao WY, et al. Improved outcomes in buccal squamous cell carcinoma. Head Neck. 2013; 35(1):65–71
[31] Leung HW, Chan AL. Glutamine in alleviation of radiation-induced severe oral mucositis: a meta-analysis. Nutr Cancer. 2016; 68(5):734–742
[32] Sio TT, Le-Rademacher JG, Leenstra JL, et al. Effect of Doxepin Mouthwash or Diphenhydramine-Lidocaine-Antacid Mouthwash vs Placebo on Radiotherapy-Related Oral Mucositis Pian: The Alliance A221304 Randomized Clinical Trial. JAMA. 2019; 321(15): 1481–1490
[33] Leenstra JL, Miller RC, Qin R, et al. Doxepin rinse versus placebo in the treatment of acute oral mucositis pain in patients receiving head and neck radiotherapy with or without chemotherapy: a phase III, randomized, double-blind trial (NCCTG-N09C6 [Alliance]). J Clin Oncol. 2014; 32 (15):1571–1577
[34] Allison RR, Ambrad AA, Arshoun Y, et al. Multi-institutional, randomized, double-blind, placebo-controlled trial to assess the efficacy of a mucoadhesive hydrogel (MuGard) in mitigating oral mucositis symptoms in patients being treated with chemoradiation therapy for cancers of the head and neck. Cancer. 2014; 120(9):1433–1440
[35] Co JL, Mejia MB, Que JC, Dizon JM. Effectiveness of honey on radiation-induced oral mucositis, time to mucositis, weight loss, and treatment interruptions among patients with head and neck malignancies: a meta-analysis and systematic review of literature. Head Neck. 2016; 38(7):1119–1128
[36] Barber C, Powell R, Ellis A, Hewett J. Comparing pain control and ability to eat and drink with standard therapy vs Gelclair: a preliminary, double centre, randomised controlled trial on patients with radiotherapy-induced oral mucositis. Support Care Cancer. 2007; 15(4):427–440
[37] Hovan AJ, Williams PM, Stevenson-Moore P, et al. Dysgeusia Section, Oral Care Study Group, Multinational Association of Supportive Care in Cancer (MASCC)/International Society of Oral Oncology (ISOO). A systematic review of dysgeusia induced by cancer therapies. Support Care Cancer. 2010; 18(8): 1081–1087
[38] Kumbargere Nagraj S, George RP, Shetty N, Levenson D, Ferraiolo DM, Shrestha A. Interventions for managing taste disturbances. Cochrane Database Syst Rev. 2017; 12:CD010470
[39] Najafizade N, Hemati S, Gookizade A, et al. Preventive effects of zinc sulfate on taste alterations in patients under irradiation for head and neck cancers: a randomized placebo-controlled trial. J Res Med Sci. 2013; 18(2):123–126
[40] Halyard MY, Jatoi A, Sloan JA, et al. Does zinc sulfate prevent therapy-induced taste alterations in head and neck cancer patients? Results of phase III double-blind, placebo-controlled trial from the North Central Cancer Treatment Group (N01C4). Int J Radiat Oncol Biol Phys. 2007; 67(5):1318–1322
[41] Bernier J, Bonner J, Vermorken JB, et al. Consensus guidelines for the management of radiation dermatitis and coexisting acne-like rash in patients receiving radiotherapy plus EGFR inhibitors for the treatment of squamous cell carcinoma of the head and neck. Ann Oncol. 2008; 19(1):142–149
[42] Nutting CM, Morden JP, Harrington KJ, et al. PARSPORT trial management group. Parotid-sparing intensity modulated versus conventional radiotherapy in head and neck cancer (PARSPORT): a phase 3 multicentre randomised controlled trial. Lancet Oncol. 2011; 12(2):127–136
[43] Brizel DM, Wasserman TH, Henke M, et al. Phase III randomized trial of amifostine as a radioprotector in head and neck cancer. J Clin Oncol. 2000; 18 (19):3339–3345
[44] Wasserman TH, Brizel DM, Henke M, et al. Influence of intravenous amifostine on xerostomia, tumor control, and survival after radiotherapy for head-and-neck cancer: 2-year follow-up of a prospective, randomized, phase III trial. Int J Radiat Oncol Biol Phys. 2005; 63(4):985–990
[45] Warde P, O'Sullivan B, Aslanidis J, et al. A Phase III placebo-controlled trial of oral pilocarpine in patients undergoing radiotherapy for head-and-neck cancer. Int J Radiat Oncol Biol Phys. 2002; 54(1):9–13
[46] Jensen SB, Pedersen AM, Vissink A, et al. Salivary Gland Hypofunction/Xerostomia Section, Oral Care Study Group, Multinational Association of Supportive Care in Cancer (MASCC)/International Society of Oral Oncology (ISOO). A systematic review of salivary gland hypofunction and xerostomia induced by cancer therapies: management strategies and economic impact. Support Care Cancer. 2010; 18(8):1061–1079
[47] Meng Z, Garcia MK, Hu C, et al. Randomized controlled trial of acupuncture for prevention of radiation-induced xerostomia among patients with nasopharyngeal carcinoma. Cancer. 2012; 118(13):3337–3344
[48] Meng Z, Kay Garcia M, Hu C, et al. Sham-controlled, randomised, feasibility trial of acupuncture for prevention of radiation-induced xerostomia among patients with nasopharyngeal carcinoma. Eur J Cancer. 2012; 48(11):1692–1699
[49] Wong RK, Deshmukh S, Wyatt G, et al. Acupuncture-like transcutaneous electrical nerve stimulation versus pilocarpine in treating radiation-induced xerostomia: results of RTOG 0537 phase 3 study. Int J Radiat Oncol Biol Phys. 2015; 92(2):220–227
[50] De Felice F, de Vincentiis M, Luzzi V, et al. Late radiation-associated dysphagia in head and neck cancer patients: evidence, research and management. Oral Oncol. 2018; 77:125–130
[51] Eisbruch A, Schwartz M, Rasch C, et al. Dysphagia and aspiration after chemoradiotherapy for head-and-neck cancer: which anatomic structures are affected and can they be spared by IMRT? Int J Radiat Oncol Biol Phys. 2004; 60(5):1425–1439

[52] Feng FY, Kim HM, Lyden TH, et al. Intensity-modulated chemoradiotherapy aiming to reduce dysphagia in patients with oropharyngeal cancer: clinical and functional results. J Clin Oncol. 2010; 28(16):2732–2738

[53] Chen AM, Li BQ, Lau DH, et al. Evaluating the role of prophylactic gastrostomy tube placement prior to definitive chemoradiotherapy for head and neck cancer. Int J Radiat Oncol Biol Phys. 2010; 78(4):1026–1032

[54] Axelsson L, Silander E, Nyman J, Bove M, Johansson L, Hammerlid E. Effect of prophylactic percutaneous endoscopic gastrostomy tube on swallowing in advanced head and neck cancer: a randomized controlled study. Head Neck. 2017; 39(5):908–915

[55] Brown T, Banks M, Hughes BGM, Lin C, Kenny LM, Bauer JD. Impact of early prophylactic feeding on long term tube dependency outcomes in patients with head and neck cancer. Oral Oncol. 2017; 72:17–25

[56] Okunieff P, Augustine E, Hicks JE, et al. Pentoxifylline in the treatment of radiation-induced fibrosis. J Clin Oncol. 2004; 22(11):2207–2213

[57] Annane D, Depondt J, Aubert P, et al. Hyperbaric oxygen therapy for radionecrosis of the jaw: a randomized, placebo-controlled, double-blind trial from the ORN96 study group. J Clin Oncol. 2004; 22(24): 4893–4900

[58] Laden G. Hyperbaric oxygen therapy for radionecrosis: clear advice from confusing data. J Clin Oncol. 2005; 23(19):4465–, author reply 4466–4468

[59] van Merkesteyn R, Bakker DJ. Comment on "Hyperbaric oxygen therapy for radionecrosis of the jaw: a randomized, placebo-controlled, double-blind trial from the ORN96 Study Group". J Clin Oncol. 2005; 23(19):4465–4466, author-reply 4466–4468

[60] Zecha JA, Raber-Durlacher JE, Nair RG, et al. Low level laser therapy/photobiomodulation in the management of side effects of chemoradiation therapy in head and neck cancer: part 1: mechanisms of action, dosimetric, and safety considerations. Support Care Cancer. 2016; 24(6):2781–2792

34 Brachytherapy for Oral Cavity Cancer

Sherry X. Yan, Catherine M. Concert, Glenn T. Jennings, and Kenneth S. Hu

Summary

Interstitial brachytherapy has a longstanding history of success in treating oral cavity cancers. It can be employed in the definitive setting either alone or as a boost in conjunction with external beam radiation therapy (EBRT) as an alternative to surgical approaches to preserve organ and function. The incorporation of brachytherapy to EBRT is associated with improved local disease control and survival. Brachytherapy can also be utilized adjuvantly for close or positive margins following surgical resection, or in the salvage setting in recurrent or previously treated cancers of the oropharynx. In this chapter we will cover the role of interstitial brachytherapy in treating squamous cancers of the lip, oral tongue, floor of mouth, buccal mucosa, and recurrent oral cavity squamous cell carcinoma. Brachytherapy is well tolerated, with acute mucositis that can be managed conservatively, and potential long-term complications are soft-tissue necrosis and osteoradionecrosis, which may be reduced with appropriate spacer or shielding. The development of new radioisotopes, improvement in implant technique and treatment delivery, as well as emergence of CT-based modern planning algorithms have increased safety, conformality and efficacy of brachytherapy treatment. When appropriate, patients should be referred to tertiary centers or centers of excellence with experience and expertise in brachytherapy treatment. Critical to the successful application of interstitial brachytherapy in oral cavity cancer is an experienced multi- and interdisciplinary team.

Keywords: interstitial brachytherapy, definitive radiation, adjuvant radiation, salvage therapy

34.1 Introduction

Brachytherapy plays an important role in the multidisciplinary treatment of cancers of the head and neck. It offers the unique advantage of directly delivering high doses of radiation locally to tumors while largely sparing surrounding tissues due to rapid dose fall-off. In appropriate setting, brachytherapy offers an organ and functional preservation alternative to surgical resection of oral cavity cancers. It is also a useful technique for local radiation delivery in the adjuvant or salvage settings.

34.2 Principles of Oral Cavity Brachytherapy

Marie and Pierre Curie first discovered radium and its radioactive properties, which they announced to the French Academy of Sciences in 1898. It was noted that a small amount of radium left on the skin resulted in ulceration at the site. In 1901, Danlos and Bloch treated nonmalignant skin lesions with local application of unsealed radium sources. Its oncologic application soon followed with the first reported radium treatment for cancer of the palate and pharynx in 1902 in Vienna. Alternative forms of radioactive sources such as Cs-137 and Ir-192 became available in the 1950s. These high-activity/lower energy sources require less shielding and deliver radiation at a high or low dose rate. High dose rate (HDR) brachytherapy with remotely controlled afterloading has gained popularity over the past two decades because of its primary advantage of minimal radiation exposure to hospital personnel and equivalent efficacy as low dose rate (LDR) brachytherapy. For permanent seed implants, I-125 is commonly used as it has a low energy that can safely be implanted without shielding requirements.

Brachytherapy allows dose escalation beyond the prescribed standard along with external beam radiation therapy (EBRT); yet because of the direct delivery into the implanted tumor volume, it allows for better sparing of adjacent normal tissue and higher dose conformality. It typically is utilized in a multidisciplinary setting along with external beam chemoradiation to optimize treatment of the primary site. However, for selected tumors with minimal risk of regional nodal involvement, it can be used as primary stand-alone definitive treatment such as in small tumors of the lip or tongue. It can also be utilized as an adjuvant treatment after surgical resection or as salvage therapy.

34.3 Diagnosis and Evaluation

Prior to receiving treatment, patients should undergo thorough medical evaluation and physical examination. Patients with bleeding disorders and multiple medical comorbidities are at higher risk for complications and are not ideal candidates for brachytherapy treatment. In addition, patients with altered mental status that can interfere with treatment compliance are also suboptimal candidates. The team needs to assess the patient's understanding and ability to comply with the radiation procedures and precautions associated with brachytherapy implants. Patients should be capable of self-care for the duration of brachytherapy treatment, including management of tracheostomy, percutaneous endoscopic gastrostomy or nasogastric tube, and patient-controlled analgesia, as indicated. Patients should have a dental evaluation prior to receiving brachytherapy to fabricate custom dental shields and spacers to shield the mandible from the implant.

34.4 Treatment Planning and Delivery

Brachytherapy treatments for head and neck cancer are typically delivered via interstitial implants or surface mold applicators. Interstitial brachytherapy may be delivered with radioactive sources (typically Ir-192) threaded into catheters temporarily implanted into the tumor volume. Less commonly, it is delivered with permanently implanted radioactive seeds, usually with I-125. Surface mold applicators are commonly used to treat exposed tumors located superficially. Generally, no operative procedures are required for this technique.

Brachytherapy can be delivered at different dose rates, taking into account clinical and radiobiological considerations. LDR brachytherapy has been the historic "gold standard" in treating head and neck tumors. Given at a rate of 0.4–0.5 Gy/hr over several days, LDR provides continuous radiation to the cancer cells and allows for normal tissue repair, thereby lowering the risk of late toxicity. The long duration requires patient isolation with significant staff exposure. More data have emerged demonstrating equivalent efficacy and similar late toxicity with HDR technique. Often given as twice daily treatments spaced at least 6 hours apart, HDR treatment is delivered remotely in a shielded room at more than 12 Gy/hr and allows for much shorter delivery time (minutes compared to days), enhanced dosimetry, and considerably decreased radiation exposure to medical personnel. Pulsed dose rate (PDR) brachytherapy uses similar afterloading technique as HDR but spreads delivery to hourly treatments at 0.4–0.7 Gy/hr. PDR therefore reduces radiation exposure to healthcare personnel compared to LDR and theoretically may have a normal tissue repair advantage compared to HDR given its more spread out dosing.

The technique of brachytherapy delivery has also evolved from using rigid sources of finite length like in the "Paris System" to employing flexible catheters with the afterloading technique. Paterson and Parker introduced the concept of source loading rules to a single point with the Manchester system for cervical cancer in 1934. Current brachytherapy techniques utilize CT-based planning to delineate the tumor volume and normal structures for more conformal and homogeneous radiation delivery. Inverse planning allows the planner to generate an idealized plan based on the prescription and dose constraints for the target and organs at risk. The use of geometrical, volume, and inverse optimization forms the basis of optimal planning. Fine tuning to customize clinical target volume coverage versus organ at risk of exposure can be achieved using manual tools that allow manipulation of the dose cloud by the radiation oncologist.

34.5 Supportive Care

Brachytherapy treatment is usually a coordinated multidisciplinary effort by head and neck surgeons, anesthesiologist, palliative care specialists, nutritionists, dentists, radiation oncologists, physicists, and nurses. For interstitial brachytherapy, prophylactic antibiotics are given to decrease the risk of infection at catheter insertion and surgical sites as well as pneumonia. Patient-controlled analgesia is often needed for effective pain management. Nutrition during treatment is administered with a nasogastric or gastrostomy tube. A tracheostomy may be necessary to maintain a patent airway and prevent aspiration. Tracheostomy care and suctioning of excess secretions is imperative. Patients should be monitored closely for the duration of brachytherapy treatment to ensure minimal displacement of the catheters and encouraged to ambulate to minimize risk of deep vein thrombosis. During catheter removal, the patient may develop hemorrhage, which can be controlled with bi-digital compression while the airway is protected with an inflated tracheostomy cuff. Upon removal, the insertion sites should be cleaned with iodine and saline. Patients should be discharged with adequate analgesics and appropriate education regarding oral hygiene, nutrition, and potential acute side effects, including mucositis and pain.

34.6 Site-Specific Radiotherapy Considerations

34.6.1 Squamous Cell Carcinoma of Lip

Cancer of the lip occurs most commonly as an isolated ulcer or blister on the lower lip. It can be treated by surgical excision or radiation. Radiation has the advantage of preserving lip function and cosmesis. Janeway published a series of 24 patients treated from 1915 to 1917 for lip cancer with superficial or deep tissue invasion.[1] Treatment with radium catheters embedded in dental mold in one to four sessions resulted in low failure rates. Since then, brachytherapy for lip cancer has evolved to include new techniques and technology. Brachytherapy has been employed alone or with external beam radiation as definitive treatment, adjuvantly for positive or close surgical margins, or as salvage treatment. See ▶ Table 34.1 for series of squamous cell carcinoma (SCC) of the lip treated with interstitial brachytherapy.

Low Dose Rate

LDR interstitial brachytherapy achieves excellent local control of lip cancer in single- and multi-institution studies. Jorgensen et al reported a large single-institution series of 869 cases of newly diagnosed carcinoma of the lip.[2] The majority of patients had T1–2N0 disease. Radium needles were inserted transversely and longitudinally into the lesion in the lip. Patients received a single treatment lasting for 4 hours. Five-year survival was 84% for the entire cohort. Tumors with deep invasion (T3) had a higher rate of recurrence of 24.6% at five years compared to 7.4% for T1 and 12.7% for T2 lesions, respectively. Recurrences were salvaged with surgery or further radiation treatment. The European Curietherapy Group reported the largest series of 2,363 patients treated for lip cancer from 23 centers.[3] The majority of patients had T1–2N0 disease, and 1,870 patients received brachytherapy with iridium, radium, or cesium treatments using rigid or flexible catheters delivering 60–85 Gy. Recurrence rates were 2.5, 5, and 11% for T1, T2, and T3 tumors, respectively. In this multi-institutional report, iridium was found to have improved local control of 96.6% compared to 89.1% for radium. It is thought that improved dosimetry and implant technique contributed to improved therapeutic efficacy of iridium. Beauvois et al reported outcomes of 237 patients treated with brachytherapy for SCC of the lower lip.[4] There were 158 T1, 61 T2, 17 T3, and 1 T4 lesions. Some patients were also treated with EBRT for advanced local disease. Using flexible parallel Ir-192 wires, a mean dose of 65 Gy was delivered for superficial tumors, and 68 Gy was delivered for tumors ≥ 5 mm. Five-year local control was 95%, and 5-year regional control was 91%. Increased lesion thickness ≥ 1 cm was found to be associated with a higher recurrence rate due to poorer regional control. Guibert et al reported treatment of 92 patients using iridium wires and the Paris system afterloading technique.[5] An average of 65 Gy was delivered with coplanar or multiplanar implanted wires. The authors reported 5-year local

Table 34.1 Series of squamous cell carcinoma of the lip treated with interstitial brachytherapy

First author, year	No. of patients	Dose rate	Brachy dose (Gy)	EBRT	Local control (5-yr)		Late toxicity	Cosmesis
Jorgensen, 1973	766	LDR	25–56	–	T1 T2 T3	93% 87% 75%	4%	–
Mazeron, 1984	1,870	LDR	60–70	–	T1 T2 T3	98% 97% 90%	Not reported	Unfavorable: T1, 1%; T2, 5%; T3, 9%
Beauvois, 1994	237	LDR	65–68	–	Mostly T1 T2	95%	8% G1, 3% G2, 1 ORN	92% "Good"
Guibert, 2011	92	LDR	65	–	T1 and T2	89%	6.5% G1, 8.7% G2	92% "Satisfactory"
Rio, 2013	89	LDR	58	–	Mostly T1 T2	95%	No necrosis	77% "Good" 21% "Fair" 1 "Poor"
Mukherji, 2015	7	HDR	12.5–48	40–46 Gy	T1 and T2	86% (18 mo)	No necrosis, ulcers	–
Mut, 2016	68	HDR	40–45	4 patients	T1 T2	100% 93.2%	No necrosis	–
Guinot, 2013	104	HDR	45 (alone), 40.5 (postop)	–	T1 T2 T3 T4	100% 94% - 80%	No soft tissue or bone necrosis	100% "Good/excellent"
	99	LDR	60–70 (alone), 55–60 (postop)	–	T1 T2 T3 T4	100% 87% 100% 89%	15% soft tissue necrosis One ORN	89% "Good/excellent"
Ghadjar, 2012	33	HDR	30.4–44	–	Mostly T1 T2	93%	G1: 30% G2: 12% G3: none	–
	70	LDR	48–66	–	Mostly T1 T2	93%	G1: 34% G2: 1% G3: none	–
Serkies, 2013	32	PDR	60–70	–	Mostly T1 T2	94%	G3: 3%	90% "Good/excellent"
Ayerra, 2010	100	LDR	60–70	–	Mostly T1 T2	90% (15 yr)	G3: 23% G4: 9%	–
	21	HDR	45–50	–			G3: 33% G4: 0%	

Abbreviations: EBRT, external beam radiation therapy; HDR, high dose rate; LDR, low dose rate; ORN, osteoradionecrosis; PDR, pulsed dose rate.

recurrence of 10.9%, and 8-year relapse-free survival of 75%. Patient-reported functional results were satisfactory for 99% of patients, and cosmetic results were satisfactory for 92%. Another modern single-institution series included 89 node-negative lip cancer cases, 10 after wedge-excision (6 microscopic positive margin, 4 macroscopic residual disease).[6] Patients were treated with two to five iridium wires delivering 50–62 Gy. Five-year local control rate was 95%. Five-year disease-free survival was 82% for the entire cohort, 100% for T1 and 89% for T2–T3 disease, respectively. All 61 surveyed patients reported satisfactory lip mobility and function. Patient-reported cosmesis (deformity, telangiectasia, dyspigmentation, and change in skin texture) was good for 77% of patients, fair for 21%, and one patient reported poor outcome. It was found that large tumors of > 2 cm thickness or previous surgery was associated with worse cosmesis.

High Dose Rate

HDR brachytherapy gained popularity given the shorter treatment time, widely available source, optimal treatment planning, and minimal staff exposure. Mukherji et al reported treatment of seven patients with lip cancer using HDR catheters embedded in a mold.[7] Five patients had T1N0 lesions and two patients had T2N0 lesions. The mold prepared with thermoplastic sheet and dental wax held catheters in position to the tumor surface. Using CT-based planning, 12.5–48 Gy was delivered in 2.5–3.5 Gy fractions to 80–85% isodose line. There was only one case of relapse in an ipsilateral submandibular node at 18 months after therapy. Mut et al reported outcomes of 68 patients treated with HDR for T1–T2 lip cancer.[8] Three to eight rigid needles were inserted in parallel with an external template system used for fixation. Patients received twice daily treatments (minimum 6 hours apart) of 4.5–5.5 Gy per fraction for 8–10 fractions. Eleven patients (5 T1 and 6 T2, 3 with commissural involvement) received elective cervical node treatment (four with EBRT and seven with nodal dissection). Five-year local control was 96.9% for the entire cohort, and 100 and 93.2% for T1 and T2 disease, respectively. Five-year regional control rates were 93.8 and 80.8% for T1 and T2, respectively. There were no nodal relapses in the patients who received elective nodal treatment compared to seven nodal relapses in 57 patients who did not receive neck treatment.

Several published studies reported comparable rates of effectiveness and toxicity profile between HDR and LDR treatments. Guinot et al compared 104 patients treated with HDR brachytherapy for lip cancer with a former series of 99 patients treated with LDR brachytherapy.[9] Patients were treated with definitive brachytherapy, adjuvant brachytherapy following surgery for involved margins, or salvage brachytherapy. HDR treatments consisted of nine twice daily treatments of 4.5–5 Gy per fraction prescribed to the 90% isodose line. The authors aimed to reproduce equivalent of 60–70 Gy in their previous series of patients treated with LDR. At median follow-up of 63 months for LDR and 51 months for HDR, local control rates were 94.9% for LDR versus 95.2% for HDR, and by T-stage were 100 versus 100%, 86.6 versus 94.1%, and 89.3 versus 80% for T1, T2, and T4 tumors, respectively. Overall survival and cause-specific survival were 76.7 and 95.9% for LDR and 64.4 and 94.2% for HDR, respectively. In another study comparing 33 HDR and 70 LDR cases, the two techniques demonstrated similar rates of local recurrence-free survival and similar rates of regional control of 96% at 3 years and 87% at 5 years for both groups.[10] Lastly, there is one published study using PDR brachytherapy in 32 patients with T1-4N0 lip cancer.[11] Treatment was delivered by 1 Gy/pulse every hour to a total dose of 60–70 Gy. Local control rate was 94% at 5 years.

Toxicity

Acute toxicities associated with brachytherapy for lip cancer may include desquamation, mucositis, and pain in the area being treated. Mut et al reported that severe mucositis occurred in all 68 patients treated with HDR brachytherapy, including grade 3 confluent and grade 4 hemorrhagic mucositis, which resolved within 6 weeks of topical treatment.[8] Lip mucositis with confluent ulceration or bleeding ulcer was similarly observed by Guinot et al in all 104 patients treated with HDR brachytherapy with resolution within 6 weeks of catheter removal.[9] Overall toxicities from LDR and HDR brachytherapy seem comparable. In a study comparing 100 LDR and 21 HDR brachytherapy treatments, grade 3 mucosal toxicity was observed in 23% with LDR compared to 33% with HDR; grade 4 mucosal toxicity was observed in 9% with LDR versus 0% with HDR.[12] In another study comparing 70 LDR and 33 HDR treatments, there was no difference in low grade or grade 3 acute toxicity (pain, mucositis, dermatitis) between HDR and LDR treatments ($p = 0.52$).[10]

Long-term toxicity rate is low and may include tissue atrophy, fibrosis, hypopigmentation, and pain. It was found that the rate of complications increased with treatment thickness > 1.4 cm, and treatment volume of 85% dose to ≥ 8 cm^3 in one report of LDR brachytherapy.[4] Chronic ulcer was observed in patients receiving more than one LDR brachytherapy treatment.[2] Similarly in HDR brachytherapy, toxicity may be related to the dose and volume of treated tissue, as reported by Ghadjar et al.[10] HDR brachytherapy was found to contribute to lower rates of late complications, with rates of soft tissue necrosis reported as 15.1% for LDR versus 0% for HDR, bone necrosis as 1% for LDR versus 0% for HDR, and patient-reported fair/bad cosmesis as 11.1% for LDR versus 0% for HDR.[9] However, other studies have reported similar rates of late toxicity (mucositis, pain, dermatitis, hyper/hypopigmentation, fibrosis, skin atrophy, telangiectasia) for HDR and LDR treatments.[10,12]

In order to decrease toxicity to organs near the treated lesion including the opposing lip, mandible, and oral cavity, multiple institutions put a lead wedge or plate between the lip and gingival sulcus.[3,4,8] They have noted a decrease in the rate of severe complications. Feldman et al reported a technique using catheters embedded in a customized surface mold that distances the lip from adjacent mandible or maxilla, and no osteonecrosis was observed.[13]

Lip: Case Study

For brachytherapy treatment in patient with SCC of lip refer to ▸ Fig. 34.1.

34.6.2 SCC of Oral Tongue

Oral tongue cancer is the most common cancer of the oral cavity. The standard treatment for early stage disease limited to the tongue is surgical resection. Alternatively, brachytherapy with interstitial implants can be used to achieve both organ and

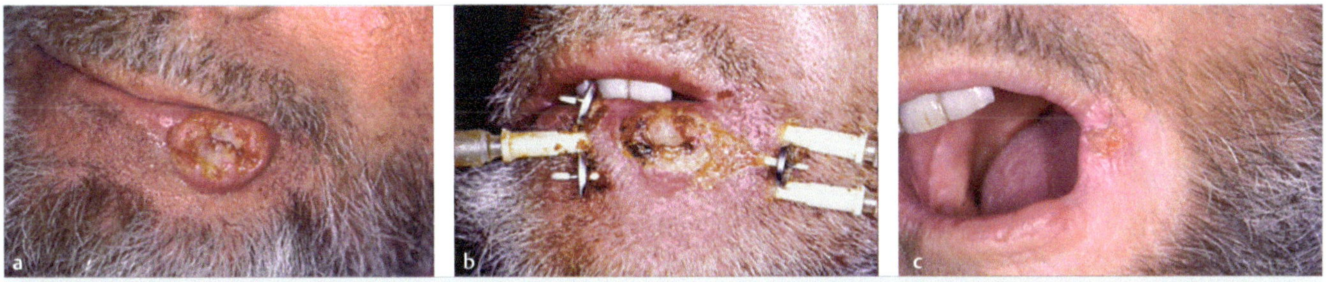

Fig. 34.1 (a-c) Brachytherapy treatment in patient with squamous cell carcinoma (SCC) of lip. Figure demonstrates before, during, and after treatment.

function preservation in combination with regional management either with neck dissection or external beam radiation. It can also be utilized after surgery if adverse pathologic risk factors indicate a need for adjuvant therapy. For locally advanced disease, brachytherapy may be added as a local boost with definitive external beam chemoradiation to achieve dose-escalation.

Definitive Brachytherapy

The two largest series reporting experience in LDR brachytherapy for oral tongue cancer were published in 1981 by Decroix et al and in 1990 by Mazeron et al.[14,15] One study included over 600 patients with T1–T3 disease treated with radium implants, and the other included 166 patients with T1–T2 disease treated with iridium implants. Local control rates were 70–80%, with higher rates of local control for smaller lesions at 85, 77, and 50% for T1, T2, and T3 tumors, respectively, comparable to historic outcomes from large surgical series such as that from the Memorial Sloan-Kettering Cancer Center.[16] Soft tissue necrosis and osteoradionecrosis are the two principal reported adverse effects that are dependent on dose rate and inter-source distance. Stannard et al reported a modern experience of LDR brachytherapy in the treatment of oral cavity and oropharyngeal cancer using I-125.[17] Brachytherapy was delivered to 72 out of 144 cases of mostly early stage tongue, soft palate, floor of mouth (FOM), and tonsil cancers. The majority of cases were treated with definitive radiation, and 47 cases were treated postoperatively. With a median number of 20 seeds and median activity of 51.6 mCi, 5-year and 10-year local control rates were 80.7 and 80%, respectively. The treatment was well tolerated, with 18.4% rate of development of mucosal ulcer. There was no observed mandibular necrosis.

More modern series have reported the experience of treating oral tongue cancers with HDR brachytherapy (see ▶ Table 34.2). In a phase III randomized trial comparing HDR and LDR treatments for early stage tongue cancer, locoregional control rates were found to be comparable between the two groups.[18] In this study including 51 patients with T1–2N0 cancers, 26 patients were treated with LDR brachytherapy (70 Gy over 4–9 days) and 25 patients were treated with HDR brachytherapy (60 Gy in 10 BID fractions). Five-year local control rates were 84 versus 87%, respectively. Similar rates of local control were reported in other nonrandomized studies.[19] Subsequently, single institutions reported their HDR experiences. Akiyama et al described the outcome of 18 patients with treated with HDR brachytherapy as monotherapy for T1–3N0 mobile tongue cancers.[20] Patients received twice a day treatments with 54 Gy in nine fractions prescribed to the 85% isodose line. Two-year local control and cause-specific survival rates were 82 and 83%, respectively. Patients with lower T stage had lower incidence of neck nodal failure after brachytherapy treatment with rates of 33, 55, and 50% for T1, T2, and T3 tumors, respectively. All patients with neck recurrence were treated with salvage neck dissection. Patients with T1–2N0 cancer also had improved cause-specific survival of 88% compared to 79% for T3N0 cancers. While there is no recommended optimal dose schedule for HDR treatment in oral tongue cancer, higher biologically equivalent doses seem to be related to local control. In a report of 92

Table 34.2 Select series of squamous cell carcinoma of the oral tongue treated with definitive brachytherapy

First author, year	No. of patients	Dose rate	EBRT dose	Brachytherapy dose (Gy)	Local control (5-year)		Late toxicity
Decroix, 1981	602	LDR	–	70 Gy (monotherapy in 52%)	T1	86%	25% STN 14% ORN
			55 Gy	20–30 Gy (25%)	T2	78%	
					T3	71%	
Mazeron, 1990	166	LDR	–	60–70 Gy	T1N0	87%	16% STN 12% ORN
					T2N0	92%	
					T1–2N +	69%	
Stannard, 2014	112 (54 oral tongue)	LDR	–	26.8–64.4 (72 monotherapy)	Mostly T1 T2	80.7%	18% STN, no ORN
			42.4–70	9.9–30.2 (42 boost)			
Inoue, 2001	59	LDR	–	70 Gy	T1–2 N0	84%	4% soft tissue ulceration No bone exposure
		HDR	–	60 Gy (10 fractions)	T1–2 N0	87%	4% soft tissue ulceration 8% bone exposure
Akiyama, 2014	18	HDR	–	54 Gy (9 fractions)	Mostly T1 T2	82% (2 yr)	28% STN and ORN
Bansal, 2016	92	HDR	–	40–52 (67% monotherapy)	T1	81.7%	Any grade 34%
					T2	56.4%	
			40 Gy	18–24 (33% boost)	T1	62.5%	Any grade 33%
					T2	51.9%	
Santos, 2017	24 (15 oral tongue)	HDR	50–60 Gy	18–24 Gy	Stage III and IV	80% (4 yr)	1 ORN

Abbreviations: EBRT, external beam radiation therapy; HDR, high dose rate; LDR, low dose rate; ORN, osteoradionecrosis; STN, soft-tissue necrosis.

patients with stages I and II oral tongue cancer treated with HDR brachytherapy alone (40–52 Gy) or in combination with EBRT (40 Gy EBRT and brachytherapy 18–24 Gy), Bansal et al found higher 5-year local control rate with brachytherapy alone (68.2%) compared to combined brachytherapy and EBRT (57.6%).[21] The authors attributed the higher local recurrence rates in the combined group to lower biologic equivalent dose (BED) achieved in this group. The authors concluded that dose escalation with brachytherapy alone and/or in combination with EBRT is needed to control primary tumors. For more advanced cases, Santos reported outcomes of 24 patients with locally advanced tongue carcinoma treated with HDR interstitial brachytherapy (18–24 Gy) as a boost to gross tumor volume following definitive chemotherapy and EBRT of 50–60 Gy to the oral cavity and cervical nodes.[22] The series included 11 patients with stage III and 13 patients with stage IV cancer, and all but one patient received chemotherapy. Brachytherapy was delivered using parallel catheters spaced 10–12 mm apart targeting residual palpable tumor and pretreatment gross tumor volume. Four-year local control, cause-specific survival, and regional control rates were 80, 68, and 76%, respectively. All patients experienced acute mucositis that resolved 4–6 weeks after treatment completion. Late complications including mucositis and dysphagia were observed in five patients, and one case of osteoradionecrosis was observed.

Oral Tongue Case Study: Definitive Radiation with EBRT and Brachytherapy Boost

A 40-year-old woman with T4N2bM0 SCC of the left oral tongue presented with progressive weight loss due to dysphagia and slurring of speech. Imaging demonstrated the mass involved the FOM, and extended across the midline to right oral tongue with involvement of bilateral tongue musculature and left base of tongue. Primary surgical approach would entail near-total glossectomy, bilateral neck dissections, and oncoplastic reconstruction, which the patient refused after multiple consultations. Multidisciplinary tumor board discussion proposed induction chemotherapy to assess response for possible definitive chemoradiation. She had an approximately 50% reduction of primary tumor after three cycles of TPF (taxotere, cisplatin, 5-FU) with improvement of speech and swallowing functions. The patient subsequently received EBRT with dose-painted intensity modulated radiation therapy (IMRT) to a dose of 54 Gy to the oral tongue, 70 Gy to involved neck nodes, and 60 Gy to the high-risk bilateral neck nodes with concurrent cisplatin. Interstitial implant was performed with six looped brachytherapy catheters placed in the entire oral tongue and left base of tongue spaced approximately 1–1.5 cm apart. A straight catheter was implanted at the tip of the tongue. Brachytherapy was delivered using Ir-192 afterloading source via 13 catheters to 16 Gy in four BID fractions. A lead mouth shield and a bite block to displace the upper palate were used. At last follow-up, 2 years from the time of implant, she had no evidence of disease (NED) with no adverse late complication and was able to teach full time as well as eat a standard diet. The patient's treatment plans and photos are shown in ▶ Fig. 34.2 and ▶ Fig. 34.3.

The incorporation of brachytherapy into multidisciplinary care for oral tongue cancer is not frequently employed in practice. In a Surveillance, Epidemiology, and End Results Program (SEER) database review of patients with SCC of the oral cavity who received definitive radiation treatment, 12% of 5,161 patients received brachytherapy.[23] The use of brachytherapy declined at a rate of 0.58% per year from 1973 to 2012. The rate of decline of brachytherapy use for tongue cancer was 1.0% per year. Nevertheless, addition of brachytherapy was associated with a decreased risk of death with hazard ratio (HR) of 0.71 on multivariate analysis. Specifically, of the 2,030 patients with tongue cancer (37% received brachytherapy alone, 56% EBRT with brachytherapy), addition of brachytherapy to EBRT was associated with a decreased risk of death with HR of 0.73 (95% confidence interval [CI]: 0.65–0.83). Similar results were found

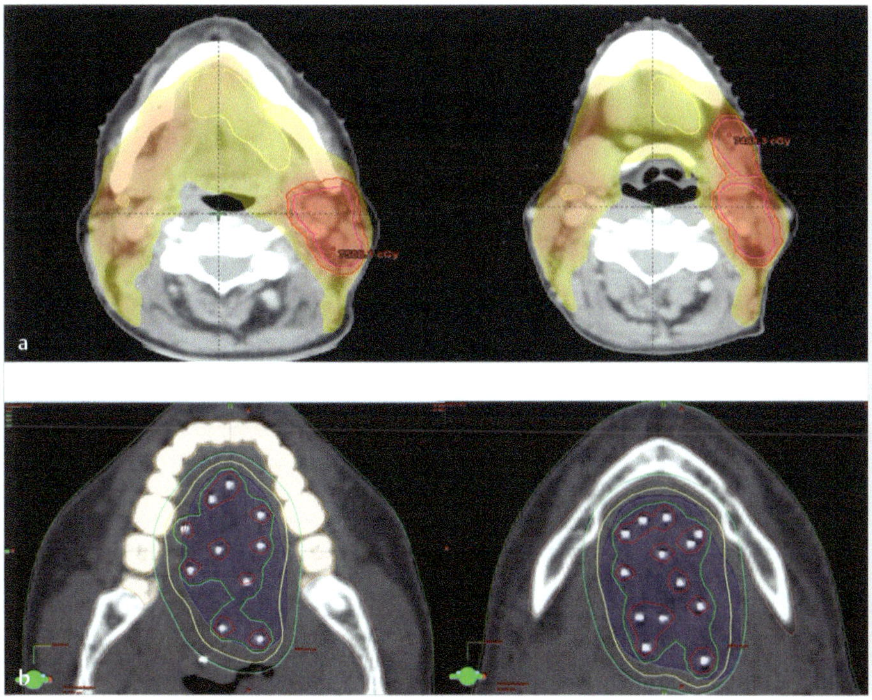

Fig. 34.2 Treatment plan from a patient treated with definitive radiation with external beam radiation therapy (EBRT) targeting the ipsilateral involved lymph nodes and high-risk lymph node regions **(a)**; with brachytherapy boost targeting the primary tumor in the oral tongue **(b)**.

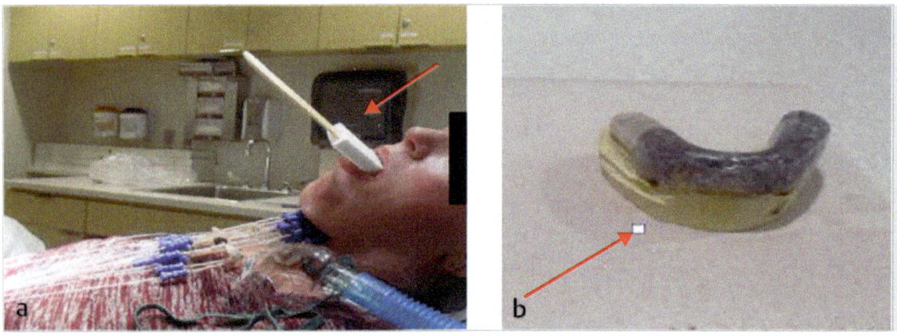

Fig. 34.3 (a, b) Interstitial brachytherapy boost after external beam radiation therapy (EBRT) in a patient with squamous cell carcinoma (SCC) of the oral tongue treated with induction chemotherapy followed by definitive chemoradiation. A customized mouth guard with lead shielding is worn during the treatment. A bite block is used to displace the soft palate away from the tongue.

Table 34.3 Select series of squamous cell carcinoma of the oral tongue treated with adjuvant brachytherapy

First author, year	No. of patients	Dose rate	EBRT dose (Gy)	Brachytherapy dose (Gy)	Local control		Late toxicity
Ange, 1975	23 (17 oral tongue)	LDR	20 (3 patients)	~50–70	T1 T2	100% (5 yr)	4 ORN, 8 STN
Lapeyre, 2000	36 (19 oral tongue)	LDR	–	50–67.4	T1 T2	88.5% (2 yr)	1 G3 ORN/STN
Mendenhall, 1989	16 (9 oral tongue)	LDR	– 30–65	56–65 (8 monotherapy) 15–35 (8 boost)	TXN0	88% (5 yr)	G1: 41% 1 requiring HO and surgery
Petera, 2015	30 (29 oral tongue)	HDR	–	66.77	T1–3	85.4 (3 yr)	1 ORN, 2 STN
Tuček, 2011	20	HDR	–	66.77	T1–2	85% (4 yr)	1 ORN, 2 STN
Chadha, 2016	39 (31 adjuvant)	LDR	54 (30–60)	10–60 (boost) 30–50 (monotherapy)	T1–4 N0–2	88% (3 yr)	N/A

Abbreviations: EBRT, external beam radiation therapy; HO, hyperbaric oxygen therapy; LDR, low dose rate; N/A, not applicable.

in another analysis of SEER data of patients with oral SCC treated with definitive or postoperative radiation.[24] In 19,343 patients with tongue (56.6%), lip (1.8%), FOM (17.4%), and gingiva (24.2%) cancers, patients who received EBRT had higher proportion of regional disease compared to those who received brachytherapy with or without EBRT, and were more likely to have undergone surgery. On multivariate analysis, brachytherapy with EBRT was associated with improved overall survival compared to EBRT alone (HR 0.61) or brachytherapy alone (HR 0.70). Size of the tumor was found to be inversely associated with survival, with an estimated 2% increase in HR for every increase in centimeter in tumor size.

Pulsed Dose Rate Brachytherapy

PDR brachytherapy has also been used for the treatment of oral cavity and oropharynx cancers. Haddad et al compared 36 patients (half of them with oral tongue cancer) treated with PDR brachytherapy to 72 match-controlled patients treated with LDR brachytherapy at their institution.[25] The majority of the patients received brachytherapy without EBRT after surgery. PDR treatment was delivered at 50–100 cGy per pulse hourly. Three-year local control rates were similar, 97% for LDR and 94% for PDR. The rates of grade 2 or higher complications were not statistically different between the two treatment groups. A large single-institution study also reported long-term results with PDR treatments for patients with head and neck cancer. Strnad described the outcome of 385 patients, 41.6% of whom had mobile tongue cancer treated with 40–70 cGy pulses delivered hourly.[26] The majority of patients (84.7%) received brachytherapy postoperatively for close or positive margins, or presence of high-risk factors on surgical pathology. Similar to the previous study, the majority of patients received brachytherapy alone to a median dose of 57 Gy. Five- and 15-year local control rates were 85.8 and 80.2%, respectively, comparable to results achieved with LDR or HDR brachytherapy. The authors reported relatively low rates of long-term toxicity with 10.2% soft tissue necrosis and 4.9% osteonecrosis.

Adjuvant Brachytherapy

Multiple single institutional studies have reported consistent excellent local control rates of 88–100% in oral tongue or FOM cancers treated with adjuvant LDR radium implants (see Table 34-3).[27–29] Chadha reported high rates of local control but highlighted the importance of combining regional management with brachytherapy treatment to the tongue in a 10-year experience using LDR Ir-192 implants.[30] Reported adverse effects included acute mucositis (15.8% in one study), soft tissue necrosis (35% in one study), long-term bone complications (46.7% in one study), and osteoradionecrosis (18% in one study). A representative LDR brachytherapy implant in a patient treated with adjuvant brachytherapy for a tongue cancer s/p glossectomy with a close margin is shown in ▶ Fig. 34.4.

More modern series have reported outcomes with adjuvant HDR brachytherapy. Petera et al reported a series including 29 patients with T1–3N0 oral tongue cancer and one patient with FOM cancer treated adjuvantly after local tumor excision.[31] Elective nodal dissection was performed in tumors with > 5 mm depth of invasion and/or presence of ulceration. Postoperative brachytherapy was given in the case of close (< 3 mm) or positive margins using HDR afterloading technique with implanted

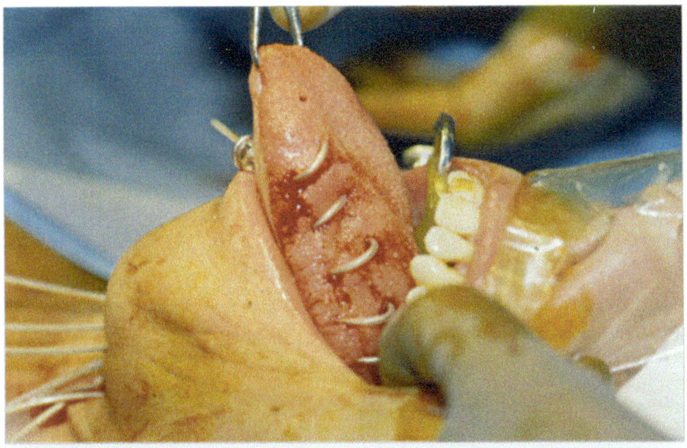

Fig. 34.4 Interstitial brachytherapy in the adjuvant setting in patient with squamous cell carcinoma (SCC) of oral tongue after surgical resection.

catheters protruding above the tongue and spaced 1 cm apart.[32] Patients were treated with twice daily fractions of 3 Gy for a total of 18 treatments with 90% of the prescription dose covering at least 90% of clinical target volume (CTV), defined as residual tumor or post-excision scar plus a 1–1.5 cm margin. Three-year local control rate and overall survival rate were 85.4 and 73.0%, respectively. On multivariate analysis, higher tumor grade was associated with local recurrence. In this series, all patients experienced grade 2 acute mucositis, which resolved completely within 8 weeks after brachytherapy treatment. Superficial osteoradionecrosis was observed in one patient treated without mandibular shielding, and soft tissue radionecrosis was observed in two patients.

Brachytherapy as Salvage Treatment

HDR brachytherapy has also been described in treatment of recurrent oral tongue cancer. A Korean study reported HDR brachytherapy outcomes in 16 patients with oral cavity cancer, of whom 13 had tongue cancer, and 5 were treated for recurrent disease after surgical resection for oral tongue primary.[33] Four patients were treated with brachytherapy alone, whereas 12 were treated with brachytherapy in combination with EBRT. In the cases of recurrent disease, HDR catheters were inserted into the gross disease. At least 95% of the gross tumor volume plus a 5 mm margin received either 50 Gy in 10 twice daily fractions in the setting of brachytherapy alone or 21 Gy in 7 twice daily fractions when combined with EBRT. Local control rate for the entire cohort was 84% at 3 years, and all 5 cases of recurrent disease were successfully salvaged.

Toxicity

Soft tissue necrosis and osteoradionecrosis are the two main long-term complications that may be seen after interstitial brachytherapy for oral tongue cancer, and these complications may be dose dependent. Mazeron et al reported 16% soft tissue ulceration and 12% bone necrosis in a series of 166 patients treated with Ir-192 LDR therapy.[15] Dose rate and inter-source spacing were found to predict the rate of necrosis on multivariate analysis, and the authors recommended an LDR of 0.4–0.5 Gy/hour or 9.6–12 Gy/day and inter-source spacing of 10–14 mm to decrease the risk of necrosis. In another study of 29 patients treated adjuvantly with HDR brachytherapy, there was one observed case of soft tissue necrosis, which the authors attributed to the large dose heterogeneity of 43% in the treated area after reviewing the treatment plan.[31] Therefore, achieving dose homogeneity may be important in reducing normal tissue injury. Many centers have employed the use of a protective spacer and shielding during HDR brachytherapy treatment in attempt to attenuate the dose to the mandible and gingiva. A lead block spacer is commonly used to increase the distance between the radiation source and the gingiva and mandible and provide additional shielding.[20,34] Murakami reported dose reduction at the mandible from 51.2% with a non-metal spacer to 40.7% with a lead spacer. Use of protective metal dentures has also been reported.[17]

34.6.3 SCC of Floor of Mouth

Surgical resection is the preferred approach for cancer of the FOM given excellent oncologic, aesthetic, and functional outcomes with modern techniques. Brachytherapy can be considered for patients who do not undergo surgical resection, such as in the setting of medical contraindication or patient refusal. It can be employed alone for T1–2N0 disease or in combination with EBRT for more advanced cases. Neck management with neck dissection or nodal irradiation should be considered even for early stage tumors, as risk of regional disease is significant.

Two large single-institution studies described outcomes of brachytherapy alone for T1–T2 FOM cancer. The gutter guide looping technique using the Paris system of non-CT based treatment planning was employed in the majority of the cases. Mazeron et al reported in a cohort of 117 patients, 5-year local control rates were 93.5, 74.5, and 65% for T1N0, T2N0, and T2 N1–3, respectively.[35] The Gustave-Roussy Institute reported excellent 5-year local control rates of 93% in T1 and 88% in T2 tumors.[36] About 40% of patients without clinically palpable lymph nodes in either series received elective neck dissection, and neck irradiation was delivered in cases with positive nodes in both series. Bone necrosis occurred in 15.5% of patients, and bone necrosis requiring hemimandibulectomy occurred in 2.5% of patients in the Mazeron study, whereas the Gustave-Roussy study reported comparable 17.9% in any grade bone complications and 7.4% with grade 3 bone complications.

Pernot et al reported on 207 patients treated with brachytherapy with or without EBRT for T1–4 N0–3 disease.[37] Five-year local control rates were 97, 72, and 51% for T1, T2, and T3 disease, respectively. On multivariate analysis, smaller tumor size was associated with improved local control. In addition, brachytherapy alone was found to result in a 5-year local control rate of 92% for T2N0 disease.

Brachytherapy boost in addition to EBRT has been found to have a survival advantage compared to EBRT alone in retrospective studies. In the previously described SEER database review of patients with SCC of the oral cavity who received definitive radiation treatment, the addition of brachytherapy to EBRT was associated with a decreased risk of death with HR of 0.87 for those patients with FOM cancer.[23] However, the use of brachytherapy for FOM cancer declined at a rate of 0.58% per year. Similar results were found in the other SEER analysis of patients with oral SCC treated with definitive or postoperative brachytherapy, with 17.4% of patients having FOM cancer.[24]

Pulsed Dose Rate Brachytherapy

Several reports of PDR brachytherapy are described above and included patients with FOM cancer. Strnad et al described the outcome of 385 patients with oral cavity and oropharynx cancers, 118 of whom had FOM cancer, with results comparable to those achieved with LDR or HDR brachytherapy.[26] Haddad et al compared 36 patients (25 with FOM cancer) treated with PDR brachytherapy to 72 match-controlled patients (21 with FOM cancer) treated with LDR brachytherapy.[25] PDR was delivered at 50–100 cGy per pulse hourly with or without EBRT. Three-year local control rates were similar, 97% for LDR and 94% for PDR. The rates of grade 2 or higher complications were not statistically different between the two treatment groups.

Toxicity

Acutely, patients may experience mucositis at the area of brachytherapy treatment, which may develop into soft tissue ulceration in up to 20% of patients. Osteoradionecrosis is a serious long-term complication occurring in up to 15% in reported series, with high-grade bone necrosis requiring surgical intervention in < 5%. In a series of 1,134 patients treated with definitive radiation for oral cavity and oropharyngeal cancers, multivariate analyses demonstrated that treatment surface area greater than 12 cm^2 and number of treatment catheters were associated with increased risk of soft tissue complications. Specifically in FOM cancers treated with brachytherapy alone, volume treated greater than 30 cc and absence of leaded protection were associated with increased risk of bone complications.[38]

34.6.4 SCC of Buccal Mucosa

For buccal cancers, brachytherapy alone can be employed as a definitive treatment option for early stage disease and has favorable cosmetic and functional outcomes. Brachytherapy may also be employed in combination with EBRT with or without concurrent chemotherapy for more advanced disease or after surgical resection as adjuvant treatment.

Definitive Radiation

The largest series of buccal mucosa cases reported by the Groupe Europeen de Curietherapie included 748 patients treated by brachytherapy alone (31%), brachytherapy in combination with EBRT (11%), EBRT alone (36%), or surgery followed by adjuvant EBRT (22%), with local control rates of 81, 65, 65, and 78%, respectively.[39] Another study by Nair et al reported outcomes of 234 patients with buccal mucosa cancer treated with definitive brachytherapy with radium brachytherapy alone (19%), EBRT alone (79.3%), or EBRT with brachytherapy (1.7%).[40] Overall disease-free survival at 3 years was 73% for T1, 47% for T2, and 42.5% for T3, and 18% for T4 disease. Brachytherapy alone resulted in 3-year disease-free survival of 75, 65, and 46% in T1, T2, and T3 disease, respectively.

Modern single-institution series have reported excellent outcome of treatment of buccal mucosa cancer with brachytherapy, with or without EBRT. Vedasoundaram et al described a series of 33 patients with early or locally advanced buccal mucosa treated with HDR brachytherapy alone or as a boost to EBRT.[41] Brachytherapy alone was performed for stage I patients at 3.5 Gy twice daily fractions for 11 fractions to 38.5 Gy. Stage II patients received EBRT to 50 Gy with brachytherapy boost of 3.5 Gy twice daily fractions for 6 fractions to 21 Gy. Stage III patients received an additional 3 doses of weekly cisplatin with concurrent EBRT. Complete response was achieved in 28 patients. Analyses of dosimetry revealed that brachytherapy treatments with more ideal coverage index and conformity index demonstrated a trend toward complete tumor response. Local control rates were 100% in stage I patients, and 84.6 and 80% in stages II and III patients. In another study of 17 patients with lip and oral cavity tumors, of whom 8 had buccal mucosa cancer, patients were treated with EBRT of 30 Gy in 15 fractions followed by HDR brachytherapy boost.[42] Brachytherapy was delivered with catheters embedded in parallel in a mold with 6 Gy fractions delivered twice daily for 2 days in 1 week to 24 Gy. Fourteen patients achieved complete response, and 5-year survival and local control rates were 68.8 and 54.1%, respectively. Two patients with buccal mucosa cancer suffered local recurrence at the planning target volume (PTV) margin at the posterior region of the buccal mucosa. The authors theorized that the decreased efficacy might be secondary to difficulty of keeping the HDR mold in place due to patients' body motion during treatment.

HDR and LDR brachytherapy treatments have been demonstrated to have comparable rates of effectiveness. Kotsuma et al compared LDR and HDR treatments in 37 cases of T1–4 N0–2 buccal mucosa cancer.[43] Thirty-one patients received EBRT with neck irradiation prophylactically or for nodal disease. For patients receiving brachytherapy, 15 received interstitial HDR treatment with median dose of 48 Gy in twice daily 6 Gy fractions, 15 received interstitial LDR treatment, and 7 received LDR mold treatment to a median dose of 70 Gy. Five-year local control rates were 82 and 72% for HDR and LDR treatments, respectively.

Adjuvant Permanent Interstitial Brachytherapy

Wu et al reported outcomes with I-125 permanent seed implant for early stage clinically nodal negative lip and buccal mucosa patients with positive or close (< 1 mm) margins.[44] The study included 27 patients, of whom 21 had buccal mucosa cancer. All patients underwent excisional biopsy or resection and brachytherapy (without EBRT) within 1 month after surgery. Permanent seed implants were placed in a single layer of the buccal mucosa via interstitial needle applicator to target residual tumor and a 1–1.5 cm margin to a peripheral dose of 9,000 cGy. Two local failures occurred in patients with buccal mucosa cancer, which resulted in a 5-year local control rate of 82.9%.

Toxicity

Patients may experience acute mucositis and dermatitis that can be managed conservatively. Late complication such as soft tissue necrosis and osteonecrosis are rare and were reported in

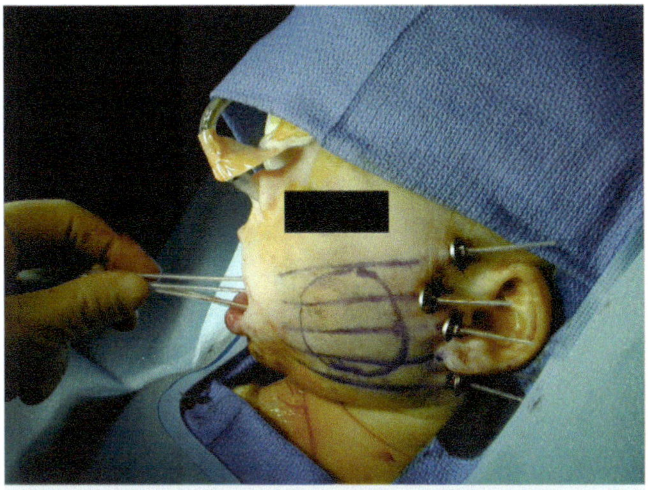

Fig. 34.5 Interstitial brachytherapy in a pediatric patient with embryonal rhabdomyosarcoma of the buccal mucosa.

less than 10% of patients in the above studies.[37,41–43] There was no significant observed difference in toxicity profile in HDR versus LDR treatments.

Buccal Mucosa: Case Study

See ▶ Fig. 34.5 for interstitial brachytherapy in a pediatric patient with embryonal rhabdomyosarcoma of the buccal mucosa.

34.7 Brachytherapy for Recurrent Oral Cavity SCC

Brachytherapy is an attractive option for salvage treatment in management of recurrent oral cavity cancer that has been previously treated with radiation. Treatment can be challenging in an area that has received extensive multimodality therapy, and retreatment with EBRT is associated with considerable toxicity such as pain, poor wound healing, osteoradionecrosis, infection, fistula, and carotid artery bleed.[45–48] Brachytherapy delivers highly conformal radiation and decreases treatment complications associated with re-irradiation. After ruling out metastatic disease, the optimal approach for salvage therapy is surgical resection combined with adjuvant brachytherapy to improve control in aggressive local disease.

For recurrent disease in the neck, adjuvant interstitial brachytherapy after neck dissection has been described. The Royal Marsden Hospital reported 74 cases of recurrent previously irradiated head and neck cancer metastatic to cervical lymph nodes treated with maximal surgical debulking and brachytherapy with Ir-192 seeds.[49] Brachytherapy afterloading tubes were placed in parallel fashion in the tumor bed at the time of surgery. Ir-192 LDR brachytherapy delivered 60 Gy to 85% isodose line of area of residual disease with a 1 cm margin. Locoregional control rates were 37% at 2 years and 23% at 5 years. Patients treated with surgical excision, brachytherapy, and reconstruction of the skin defect had the lowest rate of in-field failure (34% at 5 years) compared to brachytherapy only (100% at 2 years) and excision and brachytherapy (50% at 5 years). Reported overall major complications occurred in 15% of patients, including fistulae, hemorrhage, and wound breakdown/infection. M.D. Anderson Cancer Center reported higher 2-year locoregional control rate of 67% with similar experience in 22 patients with few complications.[50] Interstitial HDR brachytherapy has also been used after cervical neck dissection as reported by Pellizzon et al.[51] In 42 patients, 35 of whom received previous EBRT, Ir-192 HDR treatment with median dose of 24 Gy (range 12–48 Gy) was delivered with or without EBRT to a cumulative dose of 74 Gy (range 33–120 Gy). Relapse-free rates were 48.5% at 5 years and 38.1% at 8 years. Late toxicity occurred in four patients, including local wound dehiscence, ulcer, and extensive neck fibrosis.

Various reports for treating previously irradiated inoperable recurrent oral cavity and oropharyngeal cancers have been described. Older experiences with Ir-192 LDR therapy alone reported local control rates of 67–100%.[52,53] The most common complication reported was soft tissue necrosis. Puthawala et al reported outcomes of 220 patients, mostly with recurrences in the oral cavity and oropharynx, treated with Ir-192 LDR interstitial brachytherapy to a median dose of 53 Gy.[54] Patients also received interstitial hyperthermia (60%) or concurrent chemotherapy (40%). Local tumor control was 77% at 6 months, and disease-free survival rates were 60, 33, and 22% at 2, 5, and 10 years, respectively. The most common late complications were soft tissue necrosis (12.7%) and osteoradionecrosis (7.7%). A Japanese study reported repeat brachytherapy treatment for 62 patients with residual or recurrent tumors of the oral cavity.[55] Au-198 seed permanent implant was used to deliver a median of 83 Gy. The 2-year local control rate was 53%. The authors reported a low rate (8.1%) of grade 3 or 4 complications, all of which were tissue necrosis and osteoradionecrosis. The incidence of development of these toxicities was related to higher biologically effective doses delivered to the mucosa and gingiva. The Memorial Sloan-Kettering Cancer Center presented 30 patients with recurrent and previously irradiated head and neck cancers treated with HDR interstitial brachytherapy.[56] Eighteen patients received adjuvant brachytherapy after surgical resection to 34 Gy in 3.4 Gy twice daily fractions. Nine patients were treated with definitive brachytherapy alone (40 Gy in 4 Gy BID treatments), and three patients received combined EBRT (40–50 Gy) and brachytherapy (20 Gy in 4 Gy twice a day treatments). Local control rates were 80% at 1 year and 71% at 2 years. Importantly, patients who were treated with surgical resection had improved local control compared to those receiving radiation treatment alone. The use of PDR interstitial brachytherapy as salvage treatment for unresectable recurrent head and neck cancer has also been reported. In a series of 51 patients, Strnad et al treated 40 patients with PDR brachytherapy alone to mean dose of 60 Gy, and 11 patients with combination of brachytherapy (median dose 27 Gy) with EBRT (median 46 Gy).[57] Concurrent chemotherapy was administered in patients (69%) without comorbidities as a radiosensitizer. Local control rates were 71 and 57% at 2 and 5 years. The addition of concurrent chemotherapy improved local control rate at 5 years to 78.9%, compared to 38.5% without chemotherapy. The authors reported 17.7% soft tissue necrosis and 11.8% bone necrosis, of which only 2% required surgical treatment.

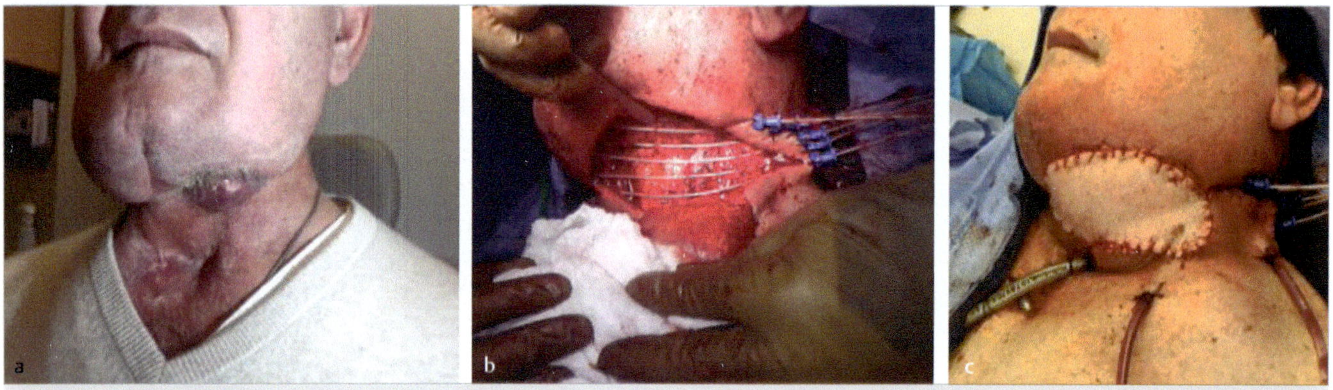

Fig. 34.6 (a–c) Salvage brachytherapy for neck recurrence. A patient with oral cavity squamous cell carcinoma (SCC) with neck recurrence treated with surgical resection, neck dissection, and interstitial high dose rate (HDR) brachytherapy. A pectoralis major flap was constructed for oncoplastic reconstruction.

34.7.1 Salvage Brachytherapy for Neck Recurrence: Case Study

A 59-year-old man with recurrent right oral tongue cancer previously treated with partial glossectomy and adjuvant chemoradiation had a local recurrence treated with partial glossectomy and neck dissection followed by proton therapy and brachytherapy boost. The patient developed osteoradionecrosis of the right mandible requiring segmental mandibulectomy. He presented with a 2nd recurrence in the left neck. After multidisciplinary tumor board discussion, the patient underwent extended left modified radical neck dissection with resection of tumor and construction of pectoralis major flap. Interstitial implant was performed at the time of neck dissection with six brachytherapy catheters placed in the left neck from the inner mandibular area along the larynx down to the cricoid cartilage. Brachytherapy was delivered using Ir-192 afterloading source to 20 Gy in five twice a day fractions. Surgical pathology demonstrated SCC with extensive extranodal spread, multifocal perineural invasion, and 1 mm resection margin. Given the high-risk pathological features, the patient subsequently received an additional course of EBRT of 4,500 cGy to the left neck, given concurrently with docetaxel and cetuximab. He tolerated the treatment without break and continued with percutaneous endoscopic gastrostomy (PEG) feeds during treatment. Nine months from the time of implant, positron emission tomography (PET) detected a hypermetabolic left retropharyngeal node suspicious for disease recurrence. The patient received stereotactic body radiation of 30 Gy in 5 fractions to the left skull base with nivolumab. At last follow-up, 2 years from the time of implant, he has no evidence of disease and remains on pembrolizumab. He developed a fistula in the reconstructed submental area that healed with conservative management. ▶ Fig. 34.6 shows the patient's neck recurrence and interstitial brachytherapy catheter placement during neck dissection.

Key Points

- In the definitive setting, brachytherapy can be employed alone or in conjunction with EBRT as an alternative to surgical approaches, achieving preservation of organ and function.
- Brachytherapy can be utilized adjuvantly after local excision of oral cavity tumors, or in the salvage setting in recurrent or previously treated cancers.
- The incorporation of brachytherapy with EBRT is associated with improved local disease control and survival in those patients treated definitively with radiation therapy.
- The development of new radioisotopes, advances in implant technique and treatment delivery, evolution from LDR to HDR delivery, and emergence of CT-based planning algorithms have increased safety, conformality, and efficacy of brachytherapy treatment.
- A multi- and interdisciplinary team approach is crucial to the successful application of brachytherapy treatment in patients with oral cavity cancers. The utilization of brachytherapy has sharply decreased. When appropriate, care can be coordinated between local specialists to deliver initial treatment whether with external beam radiation or surgery followed by brachytherapy boost delivered at tertiary centers with expertise in this highly specialized modality.

References

[1] Janeway HH. The treatment of cancer of the lip by radium: a report of twenty-four cases. JAMA. 1918; 70(15):1051–1058
[2] Jorgensen K, Elbrond O, Andersen AP. Carcinoma of the lip: a series of 869 cases. Acta Radiol Ther Phys Biol. 1973; 12(3):177–190
[3] Mazeron JJPR. Compte rendu de la XVIIIe réumon du groupe européen de ceurietherapie. Session consacrée aux cancers de la lèvre. J Eur Radiother. 1984; 5:50–56
[4] Beauvois S, Hoffstetter S, Peiffert D, et al. Brachytherapy for lower lip epidermoid cancer: tumoral and treatment factors influencing recurrences and complications. Radiother Oncol. 1994; 33(3):195–203
[5] Guibert M, David I, Vergez S, et al. Brachytherapy in lip carcinoma: long-term results. Int J Radiat Oncol Biol Phys. 2011; 81(5):e839–e843
[6] Rio E, Bardet E, Mervoyer A, Piot B, Dreno B, Malard O. Interstitial brachytherapy for lower lip carcinoma: global assessment in a retrospective study of 89 cases. Head Neck. 2013; 35(3):350–353
[7] Mukherji A, Mourougan S, Saravannan K, Vivekanandam S, Reddy KS. Dosimetric analysis and clinical outcomes in CT-based mould brachytherapy in early oral cancers in patients unfit for surgery. J Contemp Brachytherapy. 2015; 7(2):147–153
[8] Mut A, Guinot JL, Arribas L, et al. High dose rate brachytherapy in early stage squamous-cell carcinoma of the lip. Acta Otorrinolaringol Esp. 2016; 67(5):282–287
[9] Guinot JL, Arribas L, Tortajada MI, et al. From low-dose-rate to high-dose-rate brachytherapy in lip carcinoma: equivalent results but fewer complications. Brachytherapy. 2013; 12(6):528–534

[10] Ghadjar P, Bojaxhiu B, Simcock M, et al. High dose-rate versus low dose-rate brachytherapy for lip cancer. Int J Radiat Oncol Biol Phys. 2012; 83(4):1205–1212

[11] Serkies K, Ziemlewski A, Sawicki T, Kamińska J, Dziadziuszko R. Pulsed dose rate brachytherapy of lip cancer. J Contemp Brachytherapy. 2013; 5(3):144–147

[12] Ayerra AQ, Mena EP, Fabregas JP, Miguelez CG, Guedea F. HDR and LDR brachytherapy in the treatment of lip cancer: the experience of the Catalan Institute of Oncology. J Contemp Brachytherapy. 2010; 2(1):9–13

[13] Feldman J, Appelbaum L, Sela M, et al. Novel high dose rate lip brachytherapy technique to improve dose homogeneity and reduce toxicity by customized mold. Radiat Oncol. 2014; 9:271

[14] Decroix Y, Ghossein NA. Experience of the Curie Institute in treatment of cancer of the mobile tongue: I. Treatment policies and result. Cancer. 1981; 47 (3):496–502

[15] Mazeron JJ, Crook JM, Benck V, et al. Iridium 192 implantation of T1 and T2 carcinomas of the mobile tongue. Int J Radiat Oncol Biol Phys. 1990; 19(6): 1369–1376

[16] Spiro RH, Strong EW. Epidermoid carcinoma of the mobile tongue: treatment by partial glossectomy alone. Am J Surg. 1971; 122(6):707–710

[17] Stannard C, Maree G, Tovey S, Hunter A, Wetter J. Iodine-125 brachytherapy in the management of squamous cell carcinoma of the oral cavity and oropharynx. Brachytherapy. 2014; 13(4):405–412

[18] Inoue T, Inoue T, Yoshida K, et al. Phase III trial of high- vs. low-dose-rate interstitial radiotherapy for early mobile tongue cancer. Int J Radiat Oncol Biol Phys. 2001; 51(1):171–175

[19] Yamazaki H, Inoue T, Yoshida K, et al. Brachytherapy for early oral tongue cancer: low dose rate to high dose rate. J Radiat Res (Tokyo). 2003; 44(1):37–40

[20] Akiyama H, Yoshida K, Yamazaki H, et al. High-dose-rate interstitial brachytherapy for mobile tongue cancer: preliminary results of a dose reduction trial. J Contemp Brachytherapy. 2014; 6(1):10–14

[21] Bansal A, Ghoshal S, Oinam AS, Sharma SC, Dhanireddy B, Kapoor R. High-dose-rate interstitial brachytherapy in early stage oral tongue cancer—15 year experience from a tertiary care institute. J Contemp Brachytherapy. 2016; 8 (1):56–65

[22] Santos MA, Guinot JL, Tortajada MI, et al. High-dose-rate interstitial brachytherapy boost in inoperable locally advanced tongue carcinoma. Brachytherapy. 2017; 16(6):1213–1218

[23] Orton A, Boothe D, Gan M, Monroe MM, Hitchcock YJ, Lloyd S. The "decay" of brachytherapy use in tumors of the oral cavity: a population-based patterns of care and outcomes analysis from 1973 to 2012. Brachytherapy. 2016; 15 (6):851–858

[24] Agaku IT, Akinyele AO. Comparison of external beam radiation therapy and radioactive implants in the management of nonmetastatic oral squamous cell cancer: an analysis of the surveillance epidemiology and end results database. Oral Surg Oral Med Oral Pathol Oral Radiol. 2013; 115(1):38–45

[25] Haddad A, Peiffert D, Lapeyre M, Harter V, Buchheit I, Graff P. A case-control study of patients with squamous cell carcinoma of the oral cavity and oropharynx treated with pulsed-dose-rate brachytherapy. Brachytherapy. 2014; 13(6):597–602

[26] Strnad V, Lotter M, Kreppner S, Fietkau R. Interstitial pulsed-dose-rate brachytherapy for head and neck cancer—single-institution long-term results of 385 patients. Brachytherapy. 2013; 12(6):521–527

[27] Ange DW, Lindberg RD, Guillamondegui OM. Mangement of squamous cell carcinoma of the oral tongue and floor of mouth after excisional biopsy. Radiology. 1975; 116(1):143–146

[28] Lapeyre M, Hoffstetter S, Peiffert D, et al. Postoperative brachytherapy alone for T1–2 N0 squamous cell carcinomas of the oral tongue and floor of mouth with close or positive margins. Int J Radiat Oncol Biol Phys. 2000; 48(1):37–42

[29] Mendenhall WM, Parsons JT, Stringer SP, Cassisi NJ, Million RR. Radiotherapy after excisional biopsy of carcinoma of the oral tongue/floor of the mouth. Head Neck. 1989; 11(2):129–131

[30] Chadha J, Hu KS, Jacobson A, et al. The role of brachytherapy in treatment of oral tongue cancer. 2016; 94(4):890

[31] Petera J, Sirák I, Laco J, Kašaová L, Tuček L, Doležalová H. High-dose-rate brachytherapy in early oral cancer with close or positive margins. Brachytherapy. 2015; 14(1):77–83

[32] Tuček L, Petera J, Sirák I, et al. Hyperfractionated high-dose rate brachytherapy in the treatment of oral tongue cancer. Rep Pract Oncol Radiother. 2011; 16(6):243–247

[33] Lee SU, Cho KH, Moon SH, et al. Clinical outcome of high-dose-rate interstitial brachytherapy in patients with oral cavity cancer. Radiat Oncol J. 2014; 32(4): 238–246

[34] Murakami S, Verdonschot RG, Kakimoto N, et al. Preventing complications from high-dose rate brachytherapy when treating mobile tongue cancer via the application of a modular lead-lined spacer. PLoS One. 2016; 11(4):e0154226

[35] Mazeron JJ, Grimard L, Raynal M, et al. Iridium-192 curietherapy for T1 and T2 epidermoid carcinomas of the floor of mouth. Int J Radiat Oncol Biol Phys. 1990; 18(6):1299–1306

[36] Marsiglia H, Haie-Meder C, Sasso G, Mamelle G, Gerbaulet A. Brachytherapy for T1-T2 floor-of-the-mouth cancers: the Gustave-Roussy Institute experience. Int J Radiat Oncol Biol Phys. 2002; 52(5):1257–1263

[37] Pernot M, Hoffstetter S, Peiffert D, et al. Epidermoid carcinomas of the floor of mouth treated by exclusive irradiation: statistical study of a series of 207 cases. Radiother Oncol. 1995 ;35(3):177–185

[38] Pernot M, Luporsi E, Hoffstetter S, et al. Complications following definitive irradiation for cancers of the oral cavity and the oropharynx (in a series of 1134 patients). Int J Radiat Oncol Biol Phys. 1997; 37(3):577–585

[39] Gerbaulet A, Pernot M. Le carcinome epidermoide de la face interne de joue: a propos de 748 malades. J Eur Radiother. 1985; 6:1–4

[40] Nair MK, Sankaranarayanan R, Padmanabhan TK. Evaluation of the role of radiotherapy in the management of carcinoma of the buccal mucosa. Cancer. 1988; 61(7):1326–1331

[41] Vedasoundaram P, Prasanna AK, Ks R, et al. Role of high dose rate interstitial brachytherapy in early and locally advanced squamous cell carcinoma of buccal mucosa. Springerplus. 2014; 3:590

[42] Unetsubo T, Matsuzaki H, Takemoto M, et al. High-dose-rate brachytherapy using molds for lip and oral cavity tumors. Radiat Oncol. 2015; 10:81

[43] Kotsuma T, Yamazaki H, Masui K, et al. Brachytherapy for buccal cancer: from conventional low dose rate (LDR) or mold technique to high dose rate interstitial brachytherapy (HDR-ISBT). Anticancer Res. 2017; 37(12):6887–6892

[44] Wu WJ, Guo HQ, Yu GY, Zhang JG. Iodine-125 interstitial brachytherapy for pediatric desmoid-type fibromatosis of the head and neck: a case report. J Oral Maxillofac Surg. 2017; 75(4):768.e1–768.e11

[45] Langer CJ, Harris J, Horwitz EM, et al. Phase II study of low-dose paclitaxel and cisplatin in combination with split-course concomitant twice-daily reirradiation in recurrent squamous cell carcinoma of the head and neck: results of Radiation Therapy Oncology Group Protocol 9911. J Clin Oncol. 2007; 25 (30):4800–4805

[46] Lee N, Chan K, Bekelman JE, et al. Salvage re-irradiation for recurrent head and neck cancer. Int J Radiat Oncol Biol Phys. 2007; 68(3):731–740

[47] Milano MT, Vokes EE, Salama JK, et al. Twice-daily reirradiation for recurrent and second primary head-and-neck cancer with gemcitabine, paclitaxel, and 5-fluorouracil chemotherapy. Int J Radiat Oncol Biol Phys. 2005; 61(4):1096–1106

[48] Spencer SA, Harris J, Wheeler RH, et al. Final report of RTOG 9610, a multi-institutional trial of reirradiation and chemotherapy for unresectable recurrent squamous cell carcinoma of the head and neck. Head Neck. 2008; 30(3): 281–288

[49] Nutting C, Horlock N, A'Hern R, et al. Manually after-loaded 192Ir low-dose rate brachytherapy after subtotal excision and flap reconstruction of recurrent cervical lymphadenopathy from head and neck cancer. Radiother Oncol. 2006; 80(1):39–42

[50] Kupferman ME, Morrison WH, Santillan AA, et al. The role of interstitial brachytherapy with salvage surgery for the management of recurrent head and neck cancers. Cancer. 2007; 109(10):2052–2057

[51] Pellizzon AC, dos Santos Novaes PE, Conte Maia MA, et al. Interstitial high-dose-rate brachytherapy combined with cervical dissection on head and neck cancer. Head Neck. 2005; 27(12):1035–1041

[52] Mazeron JJ, Langlois D, Glaubiger D, et al. Salvage irradiation of oropharyngeal cancers using iridium 192 wire implants: 5-year results of 70 cases. Int J Radiat Oncol Biol Phys. 1987; 13(7):957–962

[53] Peiffert D, Pernot M, Malissard L, et al. Salvage irradiation by brachytherapy of velotonsillar squamous cell carcinoma in a previously irradiated field: results in 73 cases. Int J Radiat Oncol Biol Phys. 1994; 29(4):681–686

[54] Puthawala A, Nisar Syed AM, Gamie S, Chen YJ, Londrc A, Nixon V. Interstitial low-dose-rate brachytherapy as a salvage treatment for recurrent head-and-neck cancers: long-term results. Int J Radiat Oncol Biol Phys. 2001; 51(2):354–362

[55] Yoshimura R, Shibuya H, Hayashi K, et al. Repeat brachytherapy for patients with residual or recurrent tumors of oral cavity. Int J Radiat Oncol Biol Phys. 2012; 83(4):1198–1204

[56] Narayana A, Cohen GN, Zaider M, et al. High-dose-rate interstitial brachytherapy in recurrent and previously irradiated head and neck cancers—preliminary results. Brachytherapy. 2007; 6(2):157–163

[57] Strnad V, Lotter M, Kreppner S, Fietkau R. Re-irradiation with interstitial pulsed-dose-rate brachytherapy for unresectable recurrent head and neck carcinoma. Brachytherapy. 2014; 13(2):187–195

Section VI

Adjuvant Therapeutic Considerations

VI

35 Adjuvant Radiotherapy for Oral Cavity Cancer

Gregory Stachelek and Ana P. Kiess

Summary

Advanced cancers of the oral cavity often necessitate radiotherapy in addition to surgery. This chapter provides an evidence-based assessment of indications for adjuvant radiotherapy and considerations for treatment.

Keywords: adjuvant radiotherapy, radiation planning, radiation simulation

35.1 Introduction

Adjuvant (or postoperative) radiotherapy (RT) is frequently employed for patients with surgically resected oral cavity cancers who remain at high risk of locoregional failure. The goal of adjuvant treatment is to eradicate residual microscopic foci of cancer cells prior to progression to gross disease. For tumors with certain clinicopathologic features and those for which negative surgical margins cannot be attained without significant morbidity, adjuvant RT with or without concurrent systemic therapy is often indicated to decrease the probability of locoregional recurrence (LRR). This chapter provides a comprehensive overview of the indications for adjuvant RT, current clinical data underlying these recommendations, and essential considerations for delivery of adjuvant oral cavity RT including dose, targeting, techniques, and patient set-up.

35.2 Principles of Adjuvant Radiotherapy

The use of adjuvant external beam RT to improve outcomes for cancers of the head and neck has a long history. MacComb and Fletcher first described the paradigm of definitive surgery followed by RT for locally advanced head and neck cancers in 1957.[1] Fletcher and Evers later reported the results of "prophylactic irradiation" using Co-60 in 1970 in a series of 19 patients with resected head and neck cancers for whom surgical specimens did not show adequate margins.[2] On follow-up, no clinical evidence of disease was seen in 42% of patients who received adjuvant RT, versus only 11% of 147 patients who underwent salvage RT for a gross postoperative recurrence. The authors presciently concluded that, "One should not wait for a recurrence to appear in patients who are at high risk of failure after the surgical procedure. Postoperative radiotherapy should be given as soon as there is wound healing."

This fundamental tenet of adjuvant head and neck RT remained essentially unchanged over the subsequent half-century. Progress continues to be made, however, in our understanding of specific pathologic features of oral cavity squamous cell carcinomas (SCCs) that portend a high risk of recurrence, anatomic regions that warrant inclusion within the radiation field, appropriate doses for adjuvant RT, and radiosensitization with concurrent systemic therapies. Treatment of the postoperative oral cavity also presents special considerations in reproducible radiation set-up, localizing sites of potential residual disease, and minimizing risk of surgical complications and radiation toxicities in order to achieve optimal patient outcomes.

35.3 Diagnosis and Evaluation

The same principles of careful historical and physical examination detailed in Chapter 33 for definitive RT to oral cavity cancers apply in the adjuvant setting. For patients with high-risk features who are expected to undergo adjuvant RT with or without chemotherapy, the evaluation should ideally be performed by a multidisciplinary team *prior* to any surgical intervention. This is also an appropriate setting when nonsurgical management of an oral cavity cancer is being considered due to unresectable disease or for patients who are poor surgical candidates or refuse surgery.

A thorough postoperative examination including inspection and palpation of the oral cavity and neck, delineation of surgical scars and boundaries, assessment of the health of any reconstructed tissue, and dental evaluation should also be performed before initiating adjuvant RT. Care should be taken to identify and address any persistent facial edema or postoperative fluid collections so as to avoid anatomic changes during RT that may necessitate replanning. As with definitive RT, it is preferable for any necessary tooth extractions or invasive dental work to be performed prior to irradiation given the risk of osteoradionecrosis, provided that these procedures do not disrupt the surgical site or cause significant treatment delay.

35.4 Indications for Adjuvant Radiotherapy

Criteria for adjuvant RT for resected oral cavity cancers have evolved over time. Currently, the 2018 update of the National Comprehensive Cancer Network (NCCN) Clinical Practice Guidelines recommends adjuvant RT for oral cavity cancers with positive surgical margins, extranodal extension (ENE) of lymph node metastases, pT3 or pT4 primary tumor, N2 or N3 nodal disease, nodal involvement of neck levels IV and V, perineural invasion (PNI), or lymphovascular invasion (LVI).[3] For positive margins not amenable to re-resection, the NCCN provides a category 1 recommendation (reflecting uniform consensus based on high-level evidence) for the addition of concurrent systemic therapy to adjuvant RT in pT3–4 tumors and advises consideration of concurrent systemic therapy in pT1–2 tumors. Adjuvant chemoradiotherapy is a category 1 recommendation for any oral cavity cancer with ENE irrespective of T stage or margin status. The prognostic value of histopathologic grade and tumor human papillomavirus (HPV) status for postoperative recurrence in oral cavity cancers is less well established.[4–6] The above pathologic characteristics are frequently subtle. Whenever possible, it is advisable that surgical specimens be reviewed by a qualified pathologist with fellowship training in head and neck pathology or equivalent, given the implications for adjuvant treatment recommendations and prognosis.

The NCCN guidelines for adjuvant treatment of oral cavity cancers primarily reflect the best available data for LRR risk, with the clinical rationale that surgery alone is insufficient when this risk is high. There unfortunately remains a paucity of clinical trials directly comparing surgery to surgery and adjuvant RT for oral cavity cancers. Kokal and colleagues conducted an early prospective randomized trial of these modalities in stages III–IV SCCs of the oral cavity, larynx, and pharynx in the 1980s and found no benefit to locoregional control or overall survival (OS) from the addition of RT.[7] This study included only 15 oral cavity patients and utilized a relatively low RT dose of 50 Gy, however, limiting applicability to current practice. A later prospective study of 140 Indian patients with resected stages III–IV buccal mucosa SCC randomized to adjuvant RT (at doses of 58–65 Gy) or observation showed significantly improved disease-free survival (DFS) in the RT arm (68 versus 38%) as well as a trend toward improved OS (94 versus 84%).[8]

In contrast to these limited randomized trial data, nonrandomized analyses have strongly favored the use of adjuvant RT. In one retrospective matched-pair analysis by Lundahl et al of 95 patients with nodal metastases from head and neck SCC (29% arising in the oral cavity), those who underwent neck dissection alone had significantly increased relative risks of nodal recurrence in the dissected and undissected neck (relative risk [RR], 5.82 and 4.72, respectively), decreased cancer-specific survival (RR, 2.21), and decreased OS (RR, 1.67) compared to patients who received adjuvant RT.[9] The addition of radiation following surgery has therefore remained a standard of care practice for high-risk cancers of the oral cavity. In the following sections, the specific data underlying each clinicopathologic feature identified by the NCCN guidelines are discussed in detail. The presence of any of these findings differentiates oral cavity SCCs requiring adjuvant therapy from those which may be observed.

35.4.1 Positive Surgical Margins

The inability to achieve clear surgical margins after resection of SCCs of the oral cavity is a common indication for adjuvant RT. The current NCCN guidelines define a positive surgical margin as the presence of invasive carcinoma or in situ carcinoma at the specimen edge, and a close surgical margin as distance less than 5 mm from the invasive tumor front to the specimen edge. In situ carcinoma is generally not an indication for adjuvant RT, although it may be an indication for resection of additional margins. Multiple studies have shown an increased risk of local recurrence in patients for whom close or positive margins were observed.[10–13] It is important to note that these definitions have varied significantly across different clinical trials and publications. Unsurprisingly, advanced T stage is a significant predictor of positive margin status in the oral cavity,[12,14] as are high and intermediate histopathologic grades.[15] Among oral cavity subsites, retrospective analysis of greater than 20,000 patients in the National Cancer Database (NCDB) showed increased rates of positive margins for SCCs arising in the retromolar trigone (odds ratio 2.40) and buccal mucosa (odds ratio 2.06), as compared to the reference subsite of oral tongue.[15] A recent NCDB analysis of greater than 120,000 patients with oral cavity cancer demonstrated an overall positive margin rate of 12.75% across all subsites, with minimal change in rates over the study period of 1998 to 2012.[14]

It is well recognized that complete excision of gross and microscopic tumor in oral cavity cancers leads to optimal oncologic outcomes. The seminal work of Loree and Strong demonstrated a twofold increase in risk of local recurrence (36 versus 18%) in patients with positive or close margins compared to those with clear margins.[12] Further, the presence of positive surgical margins has been demonstrated to decrease overall and disease-specific survival across multiple subsites of the oral cavity.[13,16,17] The combination of adjuvant radiation and systemic therapy is often indicated in head and neck tumors with positive margins given the results of the Radiation Therapy Oncology Group (RTOG) 9501 and European Organisation for Research and Treatment of Cancer (EORTC) 22931 randomized phase III clinical trials,[18,19] in which approximately one-quarter of enrolled patients had oral cavity cancers. The addition of concurrent cisplatin chemotherapy to adjuvant RT significantly improved rates of LRR (in both trials), DFS (in both trials), and OS (in EORTC 22931 only) on initial analysis as compared to adjuvant RT alone. 10-year follow-up showed continued benefit of chemoradiotherapy for LRR (21 versus 33.1%) and DFS (18.4 versus 12.3%), but not OS, in the subset of tumors with positive margins or ENE.[20] It is important to note that the definition of positive margins differed slightly in each trial: tumor within 5 mm of the specimen edge for EORTC 22931 and microscopically involved resection margins for RTOG 9501.

Several recent studies have attempted to scrutinize the 5 mm cutoff as designating "close margins" in predicting LRR of resected oral cavity cancers. A retrospective analysis of 382 patients at Memorial Sloan Kettering Cancer Center (MSKCC) with oral tongue SCC demonstrated that margin cutoffs of > 2.2 mm (invasive carcinoma to inked edge) were not predictive of increased LRR.[21] Similarly, Tasche et al retrospectively stratified 432 patients with oral cavity SCC by margin distance and found no significant increase in LRR for any distance > 1 mm.[22] Earlier, Dutch and Australian studies had also found no difference in LRR or disease-specific survival for patients with oral cavity SCCs with close margins (< 3 or < 5 mm, respectively) who underwent observation, compared to those with negative margins.[23,24] Together, these data provide a provocative argument for observation in resected oral cavity cancers with close margins but no other risk factors for LRR. However, it should be noted that the studies were not designed or powered to specifically test the impact of RT in these patients. Further prospective analysis will be necessary to fully elucidate the long-term oncologic outcomes of this approach.

35.4.2 Extranodal Extension

Metastasis to cervical lymph nodes is seen in approximately half of all oral cavity SCCs.[25] While the size, number, and nodal station of lymph nodes all have prognostic significance in oral cavity cancers, the presence or absence of ENE has perhaps the greatest impact on recurrence risk and treatment outcomes. ENE (alternately extracapsular extension, extracapsular spread, extranodal spread) refers to perforation of the lymph node capsule and invasion of perinodal tissue by tumor. This comprises microscopic extension detected on pathologic examination of resected lymph nodes as well as macroscopic extension which may be suspected on clinical examination or preoperative radiology studies. The American Joint Committee on Cancer (AJCC) now includes ENE as a component of N stage for the oral cavity in the 8th Edition staging guidelines, a change from the previous edition. Clinically, overt ENE is designated cN3b while ENE in surgical specimens is designated pN2a for a single positive lymph node of ≤ 3 cm in dimension and pN3b for all other cases.[26]

Clinically, the poor prognosis of ENE-positive oral cavity SCCs is a consequence of increased rates of both LRR and distant metastases. Analysis of a UK cohort of 400 patients who underwent neck dissection for oral cavity SCC demonstrated ENE incidence of 25%, and these patients showed a two- to threefold increase in risk of local, regional, and distant failure relative to node-negative patients or node-positive patients without ENE.[27] Five-year OS was 23% for patients with ENE versus 61.6% for patients without ENE, with a similar disparity in cancer-specific survival. A recent MSKCC retrospective study also reported a significant difference in rates of 5-year cancer-specific survival (25% for patients with ENE versus 57.8% for patients without ENE).[28] Rates of ENE did not appear to vary significantly by oral cavity subsite in either study. There is again a lack of clinical trials directly comparing surgery alone to surgery with adjuvant RT in the setting of ENE. Among the most compelling data are those from a series of 441 patients with head and neck cancer treated at the Medical College of Virginia by different surgical groups with variable referral patterns for adjuvant RT.[29] Three-year local control for patients with ENE who underwent surgery alone was significantly inferior to those who received adjuvant RT, at 31 versus 66%. In patients with both ENE and positive surgical margins, the difference in 3-year local control with and without adjuvant RT was even more striking, at 68 versus 0%.

There exists an ongoing debate regarding the relative prognostic implication of microscopic versus macroscopic ENE in oral cavity SCCs. While macroscopic ENE is almost universally acknowledged to be an adverse clinicopathologic finding, there is no such consensus for microscopic extension. As detailed above, the NCCN considers the presence of ENE (whether macroscopic or microscopic) to be a category 1 indication for adjuvant RT with concurrent systemic therapy regardless of other favorable tumor characteristics, given the short- and long-term outcomes of the RTOG 9501 and EORTC 22931 trials.[18–20] A 2002 analysis showed a significant long-term survival decrement associated with both microscopic and macroscopic ENE in a cohort of 173 patients who underwent resection and neck dissection for oral cavity (83%) or oropharyngeal (17%) SCC, as compared to patients with no ENE.[30] Similarly, Greenberg and colleagues identified equally poor long-term survival outcomes in patients with oral tongue cancer who had ≤ 2 or > 2 mm of ENE.[31]

Conversely, more recent studies in varying patient populations have demonstrated similar DFS outcomes in patients with microscopic ENE compared to patients with no ENE,[28,32] calling into question the necessity of adjuvant chemoradiation in this setting. Broader interpretation of these data is difficult: the MSKCC analysis compared no ENE to any ENE < 1.7 mm based on receiver-operator curve analysis,[28] while Prabhu et al compared no ENE to any degree of "microscopic" ENE without overt obliteration of nodal tissue architecture.[32] Given this uncertainty and the current absence of prospective evidence, it has remained our practice to recommend adjuvant RT with concurrent chemotherapy to all patients with resected oral cavity SCCs where operative pathology shows any degree of ENE, as long as they have no contraindications and are expected to tolerate treatment.

35.4.3 Pathologic T Stage

Clinical and pathologic evaluation of the T stage of oral cavity cancers is an essential consideration in selecting appropriate treatment paradigms. The primary extent of tumors may not be fully apparent prior to resection, necessitating pathologic upstaging and adjuvant therapy. Currently, the AJCC 8th Edition staging criteria for pT3 and pT4 tumors of the oral cavity are greatest tumor dimension of > 4 cm *or* depth of invasion (DOI) of > 10 mm (pT3), or locally advanced disease (pT4).[26] The pT4 classification is divided into pT4a and pT4b classifications based on extent of invasion, with the latter generally being considered unresectable. pT4a comprises tumors invading through the cortical bone, the skin of the face, or into the maxillary sinus; or, for lip SCCs, invasion of the inferior alveolar nerve or floor of mouth. pT4b represents very advanced disease with invasion into the masticator space, pterygoid plates, or skull base; or tumors encasing the internal carotid artery. DOI is measured from the basement membrane to the deepest point of invasive tumor and should not be confused with tumor thickness, which measures from the tumor surface to the deepest point of invasion. Large, exophytic lesions may therefore still have a shallow DOI. Though pT3–4 status increases the risk of additional adverse pathologic findings such as inability to obtain clear surgical margins, as described previously, advanced T stage is also an independent negative prognostic factor in SCCs of the oral cavity.

Increasing primary tumor size and involvement of nearby critical structures often reflect delayed diagnosis or aggressive tumor biology and are associated with poorer outcomes in essentially all malignancies and anatomic sites. The significance of DOI, however, has been increasingly appreciated for tumors arising in the oral cavity. The AJCC 8th Edition head and neck staging guidelines are the first iteration of the manual to incorporate DOI as a modifier of the T stage in oral cavity cancers.[33] This important change reflects the extensive body of work that has emerged over the last several decades demonstrating that increasing pathologic DOI within the oral cavity is associated with increased rates of locoregional failure,[34,35] increased rates of cervical lymph node metastases,[36–38] and worsened survival outcomes.[39–42] With this revision to the prior T stage criteria, any oral cavity tumor with DOI > 10 mm is an indication for adjuvant RT by current NCCN clinical practice guidelines, independent of its maximal dimension. Indeed, many institutions, including ours, had already incorporated DOI into clinical practice as a potential indication for adjuvant RT, and several studies suggest benefit of RT for patients with this risk factor.[38,43]

35.4.4 Pathologic N Stage

As noted above, cervical lymph node involvement is a common finding in oral cavity SCCs.[25] Nodal metastasis is a significant adverse prognostic factor and is often an indication for adjuvant RT even in the setting of a small, completely resected primary lesion, given the frequency with which it is seen. The AJCC 8th Edition staging criteria for clinical and pathologic nodal disease in the oral cavity have been modified from the 7th Edition to include ENE, as noted above. The AJCC group staging has not changed and any node-positive cancer of the oral cavity is still at least stage III, reflecting the prognostic importance of nodal dissemination.

The poor survival of patients with oral cavity SCC with lymph node metastases has been appreciated for decades.[44–46] Neck dissection with pathologic evaluation is the most sensitive means of nodal staging given high rates of occult disease in clinically node-negative patients.[47] Further, mortality risk escalates continuously with increasing burden of metastatic lymph nodes.[48] There is clear benefit from adjuvant neck irradiation in the setting of node-positive head and neck cancer. Analysis of 8,795 patients with node-positive disease (27% with oral cavity cancer) in the Surveillance, Epidemiology, and End Results (SEER) database treated with either surgery or surgery followed by adjuvant radiation demonstrated absolute OS increases of 10.5% at 3 years and 9.8% at 5 years for patients who underwent RT.[49] A separate SEER analysis by Shrime et al of 1,539 patients with resected early-stage SCCs of the oral cavity and a single positive lymph node (T1–2N1) found that the addition of adjuvant RT significantly improved 5-year OS (48.8 versus 32.5%) and 5-year disease-specific survival (69.5 versus 57.0%) for T2N1 disease.[50] For these reasons, the NCCN recommends adjuvant RT for any N2/N3 disease and advises consideration of adjuvant RT even in the setting of N1 disease. Given that the presence of metastasis in level IV/V lymph nodes is independently predictive of decreased disease-specific survival in oral cavity cancers,[39] adjuvant RT is also recommended for isolated lymph node metastases in these nodal levels.

For adjuvant RT for oral cavity SCCs, the decisions regarding which lymph node levels warrant inclusion in the radiation field and what cumulative doses they should receive may be challenging. Please refer *Site-Specific Adjuvant Radiotherapy Considerations* later in this chapter for a detailed discussion.

35.4.5 Perineural Invasion and Lymphovascular Invasion

PNI refers to the presence of tumor cells within the perineural space or nerve sheath, while LVI is defined by the presence of tumor cells or tumor emboli within the local microvasculature or lymphatic endothelium. Direct extension along nerves as well as distant dissemination via blood vessels or lymphatics are well recognized routes of spread in a variety of malignancies, including cancers of the oral cavity. Thus, despite not being encompassed within the current AJCC TNM staging system, the presence of PNI and/or LVI has been recognized as an adverse pathologic finding and is an indication for adjuvant RT by current NCCN guidelines. The College of American Pathologists now considers assessment of PNI and LVI a required element of pathologic reporting for all cancers of the oral cavity.[51]

There is considerable variation in the reported incidence of PNI and LVI in oral cavity SCCs in the literature. An analysis using immunohistochemical staining to enhance detection found PNI and LVI rates of 82 and 42%, respectively,[52] although other studies have described far lower incidences.[53] This may reflect epidemiological differences in study populations. Stratification by subsite has identified the oral tongue as having the highest relative rates of PNI and LVI.[54] Conversely, PNI was observed least frequently in hard palate lesions and rates of LVI were lowest in the lip.[54] Retrospective analyses of pathologic specimens from patients who had undergone definitive surgery for SCCs of the oral tongue and floor of mouth demonstrated that PNI was associated with increased locoregional failure and decreased OS.[55,56] In a series of 239 head and neck SCC patients at the Royal Marsden Hospital (more than 1/3 arising in the oral cavity), 5-year OS rates were 16% for PNI-positive tumors and 44% for PNI-negative tumors.[57] Subsequent work has essentially recapitulated the negative prognostic findings associated with PNI in both small and large nerves.[58,59] LVI in oral cavity cancer is less well studied but multiple analyses have demonstrated an association between the presence of LVI and decreased OS,[60–62] implicating LVI as a surrogate for the risk of developing distant metastases. In one retrospective study of consecutive patients with resected floor of mouth SCC, the addition of adjuvant RT conferred a significant OS benefit when PNI or LVI was identified.[62]

Contradictory evidence does exist for the negative prognostic implications of PNI and LVI in early-stage (AJCC group stage I or II) oral cavity SCC. Retrospective analysis of a Taiwanese cohort of 442 patients with early stage disease showed no significant difference in 5-year DFS or OS between patients with LVI and/or PNI as compared to those without either feature,[63] even when no adjuvant RT was given. A recent meta-analysis of 325 patients across six studies of adjuvant RT in the oral cavity found no evidence to support improved outcomes with RT for patients with histologic risk factors (PNI, LVI, or high grade) but otherwise low-risk disease.[64] However, this study may not be generalizable owing to selection bias and limited ability to control for confounding risk factors. It has therefore remained our practice to recommend adjuvant RT for most patients with PNI or LVI based on the existing NCCN guidelines.

35.5 General Treatment Considerations

For oral cavity cancers, NCCN guidelines recommend that adjuvant RT be initiated within 6 weeks of surgery. Extended duration of the "treatment package" from surgery to the completion of RT has been associated with inferior outcomes.[65] Total radiation dose to the primary site in the adjuvant setting is typically dictated by surgical margin status: approximately 60 Gy for negative margins, 66 Gy for microscopic positive margins, and 70 Gy for gross residual disease, in fractional doses of 2.0 Gy (▶ Fig. 35.1). Other high-risk areas including sites of ENE should also be treated to approximately 66 Gy. Whether using a sequential boost technique or a simultaneous integrated boost, we prefer the use of intensity-modulated radiotherapy (IMRT)-based dose painting for treatment in the head and neck, as this allows for more effective sparing of the parotid glands, uninvolved oral mucosa, larynx, and in some cases the contralateral submandibular gland. Use of brachytherapy or intraoral cone RT for adjuvant treatment may also be considered, but these

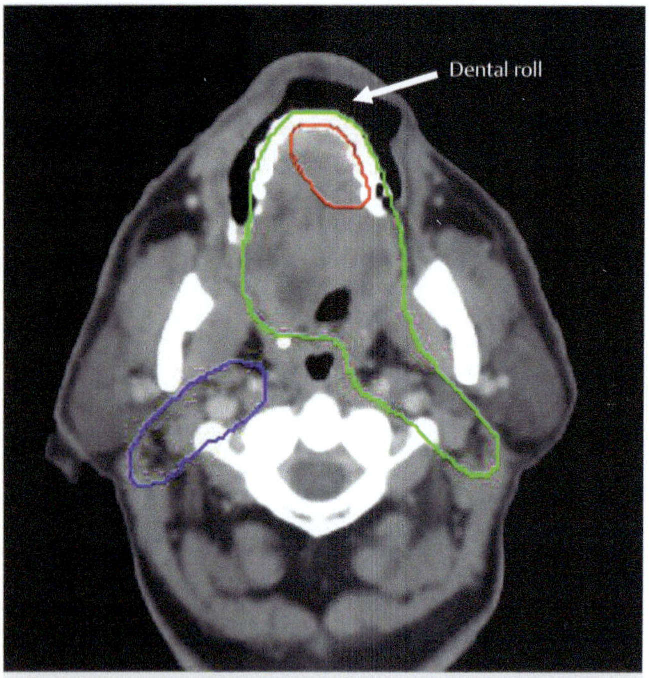

Fig. 35.1 Axial computed tomography (CT) simulation image from a 56-year-old man with stage pT2N2bM0 left floor of mouth cancer extending to the ventral tongue with a close margin anteriorly. A dental roll was used to displace the lip anteriorly away from the high-risk clinical target volume (red, clinical target volume [CTV] 66 Gy). The CTV 60 Gy (green) and CTV 54 Gy (blue) are also shown.

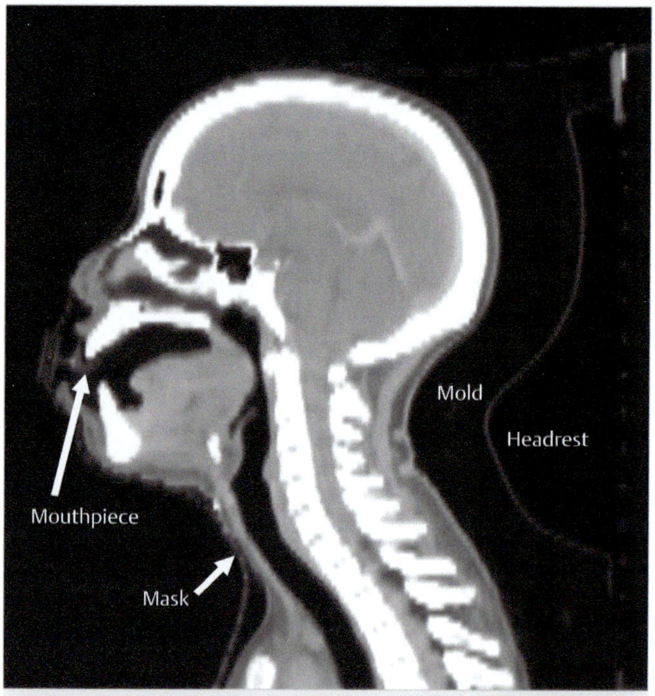

Fig. 35.2 Sagittal computed tomography (CT) simulation image from a 47-year-old woman with stage pT2N1 oral tongue cancer. She was positioned supine and immobilized with a headrest, mold, and thermoplastic mask. A mouthpiece is attached to the mask with a tongue depressor to displace the tongue from the palate and maxilla.

techniques are often not widely available. Adjuvant brachytherapy techniques are described in detail in Chapter 34 and are particularly recommended in the setting of reirradiation.

Simulation is performed with the patient supine and immobilized using a large thermoplastic mask extending to the shoulders (▶ Fig. 35.2). It is important to assess for edema or fluid collections that may shift and result in poor mask fitting during treatment. External surgical scars should be delineated with nonmetallic wire, and bolus may be considered to increase surface dose over the neck scar in patients with ENE. When possible, we often displace uninvolved oral cavity structures away from the anticipated radiation field to minimize treatment-related toxicity. For example, we often use a bite block or mouthpiece to decrease dose to the maxilla and palate (▶ Fig. 35.2). For lateralized tumors, we have had success in using a customized mouthpiece to keep the tongue comfortably situated on the contralateral side. In patients with intact dentition, dental rolls are an effective means to displace the lips anteriorly or laterally in order to reduce radiation dose to the lip mucosa (▶ Fig. 35.1). For adjuvant RT in the oral cavity and neck, it is generally our practice to obtain a simulation computed tomography (CT) scan with intravenous contrast given 30 to 40 seconds prior to image acquisition. Preoperative imaging may also be fused to the simulation CT to guide targeting.

We encourage the early involvement of an interdisciplinary team for all patients undergoing multimodality therapy for oral cavity cancers, with continued evaluation throughout the course of treatment. This comprises speech and language pathologists, clinical dieticians, dentists, and physical therapists, among others. Other chapters of this book address in detail the roles of these important team members in the evaluation and management of patients with oral cavity cancers. In the adjuvant RT setting, this interdisciplinary approach is invaluable to anticipate and mitigate potential short- and long-term sequelae of oral cavity and neck radiation including weight loss, speech and swallowing dysfunction, muscle fibrosis, aspiration pneumonia, and osteoradionecrosis. Further, it may reduce dependence on enteral feeding tubes for nutritional support during and after RT.

35.6 Site-Specific Adjuvant Radiotherapy Considerations

The oral cavity comprises a diverse group of anatomic subsites that present unique challenges to the safe and effective delivery of adjuvant radiation. In addition to the broader treatment considerations above, here we offer specific recommendations for adjuvant RT target volumes, reproducible patient set-up, and mitigation of treatment toxicities. Unless noted otherwise, we treat the postoperative oral cavity with once per day IMRT with daily image guidance. Our preference is to utilize daily cone beam CT imaging guidance during treatment, to improve reproducibility and allow for decreased treatment volumes. Twice per day fractionation should be considered in the adjuvant setting when the patient has undergone prior RT in the region of the treatment field.

The primary site target volumes noted below for each subsite represent sites of highest risk for involvement and should be treated to radiation doses of at least 60 Gy, as noted above. Neck lymph node levels I and II represent the primary lymphatic drainage of the oral cavity, but levels III through V are often also at risk. Lower risk clinical target volumes may be treated to a lower dose of approximately 54 Gy. Level V should be included for patients with node-positive disease. For early stage disease, the omission of nodal irradiation can be considered at the physician's discretion. For lesions originating in one subsite but which have invaded adjacent oral cavity sites, coverage should be extended to incorporate the recommended target volumes from all involved sites. In general, radiation target volumes should include the entire surgical scar and the entire flap if reconstructed.

35.6.1 SCC of Lip

The lip is a relatively uncommon site for adjuvant RT except in more advanced lesions. Lip SCC usually involves the lower lip. Bolus may be necessary to ensure adequate dose is delivered to the surface of the resection site. A mouth block can be used to isolate and reduce radiation dose to the opposing uninvolved lip. Target volumes include the tumor bed and the levels IA–IV lymph nodes (omission of level IA can be considered for cancers of the upper lip). For small and well-lateralized lip lesions it is reasonable to cover only the ipsilateral lymphatics, but in most cases bilateral neck irradiation will be warranted.

35.6.2 SCC of Oral Tongue

The majority of SCCs of the oral tongue arise in the lateral or ventral aspects of the tongue, and those lesions requiring adjuvant RT are frequently in the middle third or posterior third of the tongue. Lesions may extend laterally to the floor of mouth or posteriorly to the tonsillar pillars, retromolar trigone, or base of tongue. These regions have decreased mobility relative to the anterior third of the tongue, but reproducible positioning is always an essential consideration when treating the oral tongue using external beam RT. As noted above, during simulation and treatments we often use a mouthpiece or bite block to reduce the radiation dose to the superior oral cavity. We instruct the patient to extend the tongue under the bite block with the tip touching the back of the lower incisors. Dental rolls may be used to displace the lips for patients with anterior target volumes. Target volumes include the entire oral tongue, flap (if reconstructed), and bilateral levels IA–IV lymph nodes. The contralateral lymph nodes should routinely be included.[38] For patients with nerve involvement, we recommend coverage of the involved nerve within the RT field anterograde and retrograde to the skull base.

35.6.3 SCC of Floor of Mouth

The floor of mouth is anatomically compact and tumors (and resection cavities) may frequently involve the oral tongue or mandibular alveolar ridge. Target volumes include the entire floor of mouth and adjacent oral cavity subsites, flap (if reconstructed), and bilateral levels IA–IV lymph nodes. As with lesions of the oral tongue, a bite block may be used to minimize dose to the superior oral cavity. The contralateral lymph nodes should be included to subclinical doses.

35.6.4 SCC of Buccal Mucosa

Buccal cancer resections may be extensive owing to the lack of anatomic barriers to submucosal spread, and tumors can extend to involve many other sites within the oral cavity, in particular the retromolar trigone and alveolar ridge. Target volumes include the entirety of the tumor bed with wide margins, the flap (if reconstructed), and the ipsilateral levels I–IV lymph nodes. Bilateral cervical lymph node metastases are rare, but irradiation of the contralateral neck should be considered for advanced primary tumors, extension of the tumor within 1 cm of midline, or extensive lymph node involvement. For deeply invasive lesions involving the skin, use of external bolus may be necessary to achieve satisfactory dosage to the full resection cavity. In cases of clinical or pathologic nerve involvement, we recommend coverage of the involved nerve within the RT field anterograde and retrograde to the skull base. In some patients, the oral tongue may be displaced away from the radiation field with a custom mouthpiece.

35.6.5 SCC of Alveolar Ridge

The mandibular and maxillary alveolar ridges are anatomically distinct and warrant individual consideration. Adjuvant RT for cancers arising in the mandibular alveolar ridge is generally analogous to that for cancers of the floor of mouth, with the same general recommendations detailed above. However, alveolar ridge SCCs are frequently bone-invasive and patients may have undergone segmental or marginal mandibulectomy. Ipsilateral nodal irradiation may be considered for well-lateralized lesions.

Cancers arising in the maxillary alveolar ridge may invade directly into the maxilla, buccal mucosa, or posteriorly into the hard palate. For these lesions, a mouthpiece or bite block may also be utilized to facilitate sparing of the tongue and inferior oral cavity from receiving full radiation dose. Target volumes include the tumor bed with a wide margin, flap (if reconstructed), adjacent bone, and the levels I–IV lymph nodes. Ipsilateral nodal irradiation may be considered for well-lateralized lesions.

35.6.6 SCC of Retromolar Trigone

As seen in cancers of the alveolar ridges, tumors of the retromolar trigone are often bone-invasive and patients may have undergone segmental or marginal mandibulectomy. Lesions can also extend along the contiguous buccal mucosa. Trismus is frequently associated with invasion of the medial pterygoid muscle. Target volumes include the tumor bed, flap (if reconstructed), and the levels I–IV lymph nodes, as well as the involved mandibular segment for bone invasion. For lesions that do not invade toward the midline, it is reasonable to omit contralateral nodal irradiation. In cases of pterygoid invasion, the pterygomandibular space should be covered. PNI necessitates coverage of the involved nerves anterograde and retrograde to the skull base.

35.6.7 SCC of Hard Palate

Primary SCCs of the hard palate are uncommon, although invasion from adjacent sites may be seen. Patients with more extensive lesions who have undergone palatectomy or maxillectomy may have a palatal obturator or flap reconstruction. The obturator may be left during simulation or recreated using dental wax to improve interfraction reproducibility of set-up and oral cavity airspace as well as increase superficial dose via bolus effect. Again, a mouthpiece with attached tongue depressor may be used to displace the tongue and mandible away from the radiation field. Primary target volumes include the tumor bed and the levels I–IV lymph nodes.

35.7 Toxicity Management

General toxicities of RT for oral cavity cancer are addressed in Chapter 41, including mucositis, xerostomia, osteoradionecrosis, dysphagia, odynophagia, dysgeusia, dental complications, and trismus. In patients who undergo adjuvant RT, there are also specific risks of fistula, impaired wound healing, flap failure, flap contraction/fibrosis, and lymphedema. In a series of 100 patients undergoing fibular free flap reconstruction of the mandible, rates of mild and severe complications with adjuvant RT were 46 and 25%, respectively, with no statistical difference from patients undergoing neoadjuvant RT or no RT.[66] No complete flap failures were observed with adjuvant RT, and partial flap loss and fistula formation were seen in only two patients each (6%). The rate of mild dehiscence owing to poor wound healing was 14% in patients receiving adjuvant RT, again no significant change from surgery alone. However, these risks are significantly higher in patients with a history of prior radiation due to chronic microvascular damage.

While rates of radiation-induced postoperative complications are generally low, it is well established that several risk factors for the development of oral cavity SCC are also risk factors for surgical complications, including smoking and alcohol use.[67,68] A retrospective analysis by Schwam and colleagues found 30-day complication and mortality rates of 20.3 and 1.0%, respectively, for cancers of oral cavity.[67] Therefore, treatment teams will be often faced with the difficult decision of when to begin adjuvant RT in patients with existing postoperative complications. While physicians may be tempted to delay RT in order to allow for further wound healing, this places the patient at higher risk of recurrence.[65] In instances of mild dehiscence, we generally initiate RT within 6 weeks of surgery as recommended by the NCCN, given the data show frequent spontaneous wound closure and low rates of serious complications.[69] Even for feared complications such as open fistulous tracts, adjuvant RT can often be delivered in a timely fashion. A U.C. Davis case series examined 17 postoperative patients with orocutaneous or pharyngocutaneous fistula who underwent adjuvant RT, with a median of 39 days between surgery and first fraction of RT.[70] Only four (24%) of these patients developed serious complications and there was no associated mortality.

While care should be always taken to carefully assess each patient's unique comorbidities, overall prognosis, and expected radiation fields when evaluating for potential toxicity, the above data suggest that adjuvant RT may not need to be significantly delayed in the setting of some postoperative complications. Multidisciplinary discussions about the timing of therapy and the relative risks are essential in order to ensure optimal patient outcomes.

Key Points

- DOI of tumor is now a component of AJCC T staging for oral cavity lesions, reflecting its importance as a risk factor; any DOI > 10 mm should warrant adjuvant RT.
- Adjuvant RT should be initiated within 6 weeks of the date of surgery whenever possible.
- The presence of pathologic lymph node metastases from oral cavity SCC is nearly always an indication for adjuvant RT.
- Sites of positive margins or ENE should be treated as high-risk areas when considering radiation dose and target volumes. Concurrent chemotherapy should also be recommended for patients with positive margins or ENE.
- RT fields should be customized for each patient according to the site, laterality, and extent of disease.

References

[1] MacComb WS, Fletcher GH. Planned combination of surgery and radiation in treatment of advanced primary head and neck cancers. Am J Roentgenol Radium Ther Nucl Med. 1957; 77(3):397–414

[2] Fletcher GH, Evers WT. Radiotherapeutic management of surgical recurrences and postoperative residuals in tumors of the head and neck. Radiology. 1970; 95(1):185–8

[3] National Comprehensive Cancer Network. Head and Neck Cancers. (Version 1.2014). http://www.nccn.org/professionals/physician_gls/pdf/head-and-neck.pdf. Accessed June 18, 2018

[4] Hasegawa T, Tanakura M, Takeda D, et al. Risk factors associated with distant metastasis in patients with oral squamous cell carcinoma. Otolaryngol Head Neck Surg. 2015; 152(6):1053–1060

[5] Hosni A, Huang SH, Xu W, et al. Distant metastases following postoperative intensity-modulated radiotherapy for oral cavity squamous cell carcinoma. JAMA Otolaryngol Head Neck Surg. 2017; 143(4):368–375

[6] Lee L-A, Huang C-G, Liao C-T, et al. Human papillomavirus-16 infection in advanced oral cavity cancer patients is related to an increased risk of distant metastases and poor survival. PLoS One. 2012; 7(7):e40767

[7] Kokal WA, Neifeld JP, Eisert D, et al. Postoperative radiation as adjuvant treatment for carcinoma of the oral cavity, larynx, and pharynx: preliminary report of a prospective randomized trial. J Surg Oncol. 1988; 38(2):71–76

[8] Mishra RC, Singh DN, Mishra TK. Post-operative radiotherapy in carcinoma of buccal mucosa, a prospective randomized trial. Eur J Surg Oncol. 1996; 22(5): 502–504

[9] Lundahl RE, Foote RL, Bonner JA, et al. Combined neck dissection and post-operative radiation therapy in the management of the high-risk neck: a matched-pair analysis. Int J Radiat Oncol Biol Phys. 1998; 40(3):529–534

[10] Looser KG, Shah JP, Strong EW. The significance of "positive" margins in surgically resected epidermoid carcinomas. Head Neck Surg. 1978; 1(2):107–111

[11] Chen TY, Emrich LJ, Driscoll DL. The clinical significance of pathological findings in surgically resected margins of the primary tumor in head and neck carcinoma. Int J Radiat Oncol Biol Phys. 1987; 13(6):833–837

[12] Loree TR, Strong EW. Significance of positive margins in oral cavity squamous carcinoma. Am J Surg. 1990; 160(4):410–414

[13] Buchakjian MR, Tasche KK, Robinson RA, Pagedar NA, Sperry SM. Association of main specimen and tumor bed margin status with local recurrence and survival in oral cancer surgery. JAMA Otolaryngol Head Neck Surg. 2016; 142 (12):1191–1198

[14] Orosco RK, Tapia VJ, Califano JA, et al. Positive surgical margins in the 10 most common solid cancers. Sci Rep. 2018; 8(1):5686

[15] Luryi AL, Chen MM, Mehra S, Roman SA, Sosa JA, Judson BL. Positive surgical margins in early stage oral cavity cancer: an analysis of 20,602 cases. Otolaryngol Head Neck Surg. 2014; 151(6):984–990

[16] Sessions DG, Spector GJ, Lenox J, et al. Analysis of treatment results for floor-of-mouth cancer. Laryngoscope. 2000; 110(10 Pt 1):1764–1772

[17] Haque R, Contreras R, McNicoll MP, Eckberg EC, Petitti DB. Surgical margins and survival after head and neck cancer surgery. BMC Ear Nose Throat Disord. 2006; 6:2

[18] Cooper JS, Pajak TF, Forastiere AA, et al. Radiation Therapy Oncology Group 9501/Intergroup. Postoperative concurrent radiotherapy and chemotherapy

for high-risk squamous-cell carcinoma of the head and neck. N Engl J Med. 2004; 350(19):1937–1944

[19] Bernier J, Domenge C, Ozsahin M, et al. European Organization for Research and Treatment of Cancer Trial 22931. Postoperative irradiation with or without concomitant chemotherapy for locally advanced head and neck cancer. N Engl J Med. 2004; 350(19):1945–1952

[20] Cooper JS, Zhang Q, Pajak TF, et al. Long-term follow-up of the RTOG 9501/intergroup phase III trial: postoperative concurrent radiation therapy and chemotherapy in high-risk squamous cell carcinoma of the head and neck. Int J Radiat Oncol Biol Phys. 2012; 84(5):1198–1205

[21] Zanoni DK, Migliacci JC, Xu B, et al. A proposal to redefine close surgical margins in squamous cell carcinoma of the oral tongue. JAMA Otolaryngol Head Neck Surg. 2017; 143(6):555–560

[22] Tasche KK, Buchakjian MR, Pagedar NA, Sperry SM. Definition of "close margin" in oral cancer surgery and association of margin distance with local recurrence rate. JAMA Otolaryngol Head Neck Surg. 2017; 143(12):1166–1172

[23] Dik EA, Willems SM, Ipenburg NA, Adriaansens SO, Rosenberg AJ, van Es RJ. Resection of early oral squamous cell carcinoma with positive or close margins: relevance of adjuvant treatment in relation to local recurrence: margins of 3 mm as safe as 5 mm. Oral Oncol. 2014; 50(6):611–615

[24] Ch'ng S, Corbett-Burns S, Stanton N, et al. Close margin alone does not warrant postoperative adjuvant radiotherapy in oral squamous cell carcinoma. Cancer. 2013; 119(13):2427–2437

[25] Shah JP, Candela FC, Poddar AK. The patterns of cervical lymph node metastases from squamous carcinoma of the oral cavity. Cancer. 1990; 66(1): 109–113

[26] Amin MB, Edge S, Greene F, et al (Eds.). AJCC Cancer Staging Manual (8th edition). Springer International Publishing: American Joint Commission on Cancer; 2017

[27] Shaw RJ, Lowe D, Woolgar JA, et al. Extracapsular spread in oral squamous cell carcinoma. Head Neck. 2010; 32(6):714–722

[28] Wreesmann VB, Katabi N, Palmer FL, et al. Influence of extracapsular nodal spread extent on prognosis of oral squamous cell carcinoma. Head Neck. 2016; 38 Suppl 1:E1192–E1199

[29] Huang DT, Johnson CR, Schmidt-Ullrich R, Grimes M. Postoperative radiotherapy in head and neck carcinoma with extracapsular lymph node extension and/or positive resection margins: a comparative study. Int J Radiat Oncol Biol Phys. 1992; 23(4):737–742

[30] Woolgar JA, Rogers SN, Lowe D, Brown JS, Vaughan ED. Cervical lymph node metastasis in oral cancer: the importance of even microscopic extracapsular spread. Oral Oncol. 2003; 39(2):130–137

[31] Greenberg JS, Fowler R, Gomez J, et al. Extent of extracapsular spread: a critical prognosticator in oral tongue cancer. Cancer. 2003; 97(6):1464–1470

[32] Prabhu RS, Hanasoge S, Magliocca KR, et al. Extent of pathologic extracapsular extension and outcomes in patients with nonoropharyngeal head and neck cancer treated with initial surgical resection. Cancer. 2014; 120(10): 1499–1506

[33] Lydiatt WM, Patel SG, O'Sullivan B, et al. Head and neck cancers—major changes in the American Joint Committee on Cancer Eighth Edition Cancer Staging Manual. CA Cancer J Clin. 2017; 67:122–37

[34] Mishra RC, Parida G, Mishra TK, Mohanty S. Tumour thickness and relationship to locoregional failure in cancer of the buccal mucosa. Eur J Surg Oncol. 1999; 25(2):186–189

[35] Yuen AP, Lam KY, Wei WI, et al. A comparison of the prognostic significance of tumor diameter, length, width, thickness, area, volume, and clinicopathological features of oral tongue carcinoma. Am J Surg. 2000; 180(2):139–143

[36] Clark JR, Naranjo N, Franklin JH, de Almeida J, Gullane PJ. Established prognostic variables in N0 oral carcinoma. Otolaryngol Head Neck Surg. 2006; 135 (5):748–753

[37] Huang SH, Hwang D, Lockwood G, Goldstein DP, O'Sullivan B. Predictive value of tumor thickness for cervical lymph-node involvement in squamous cell carcinoma of the oral cavity: a meta-analysis of reported studies. Cancer. 2009; 115(7):1489–1497

[38] Ganly I, Goldstein D, Carlson DL, et al. Long-term regional control and survival in patients with "low-risk," early stage oral tongue cancer managed by partial glossectomy and neck dissection without postoperative radiation: the importance of tumor thickness. Cancer. 2013; 119(6):1168–1176

[39] Kang CJ, Liao CT, Hsueh C, et al. Outcome analysis of patients with well-differentiated oral cavity squamous cell carcinoma. Oral Oncol. 2011; 47(11): 1085–10-9–1

[40] Liao CT, Lin CY, Fan KH, et al. Identification of a high-risk group among patients with oral cavity squamous cell carcinoma and pT1–2N0 disease. Int J Radiat Oncol Biol Phys. 2012; 82(1):284–290

[41] Tan WJ, Chia CS, Tan HK, Soo KC, Iyer NG. Prognostic significance of invasion depth in oral tongue squamous cell carcinoma. ORL J Otorhinolaryngol Relat Spec. 2012; 74(5):264–270

[42] Ebrahimi A, Gil Z, Amit M, et al. International Consortium for Outcome Research (ICOR) in Head and Neck Cancer. Primary tumor staging for oral cancer and a proposed modification incorporating depth of invasion: an international multicenter retrospective study. JAMA Otolaryngol Head Neck Surg. 2014; 140(12):1138–1148

[43] Shim SJ, Cha J, Koom WS, et al. Clinical outcomes for T1–2N0–1 oral tongue cancer patients underwent surgery with and without postoperative radiotherapy. Radiat Oncol. 2010; 5:43

[44] Kalnins IK, Leonard AG, Sako K, Razack MS, Shedd DP. Correlation between prognosis and degree of lymph node involvement in carcinoma of the oral cavity. Am J Surg. 1977; 134(4):450–454

[45] Schuller DE, McGuirt WF, McCabe BF, Young D. The prognostic significance of metastatic cervical lymph nodes. Laryngoscope. 1980; 90(4):557–570

[46] Grandi C, Alloisio M, Moglia D, et al. Prognostic significance of lymphatic spread in head and neck carcinomas: therapeutic implications. Head Neck Surg. 1985; 8(2):67–73

[47] Greenberg JS, El Naggar AK, Mo V, Roberts D, Myers JN. Disparity in pathologic and clinical lymph node staging in oral tongue carcinoma: implication for therapeutic decision making. Cancer. 2003; 98(3):508–515

[48] Ho AS, Kim S, Tighiouart M, et al. Metastatic lymph node burden and survival in oral cavity cancer. J Clin Oncol. 2017; 35(31):3601–3609

[49] Lavaf A, Genden EM, Cesaretti JA, Packer S, Kao J. Adjuvant radiotherapy improves overall survival for patients with lymph node-positive head and neck squamous cell carcinoma. Cancer. 2008; 112(3):535–543

[50] Shrime MG, Gullane PJ, Dawson L, et al. The impact of adjuvant radiotherapy on survival in T1–2N1 squamous cell carcinoma of the oral cavity. Arch Otolaryngol Head Neck Surg. 2010; 136(3):225–228

[51] Seethala RR, Martin JM, Carlson DL, et al. Protocol for the Examination of Specimens from Patients with Cancers of the Lip and Oral Cavity. Version 4.0.0.0. June 2017

[52] Kurtz KA, Hoffman HT, Zimmerman MB, Robinson RA. Perineural and vascular invasion in oral cavity squamous carcinoma: increased incidence on re-review of slides and by using immunohistochemical enhancement. Arch Pathol Lab Med. 2005; 129(3):354–359

[53] Lin YT, Chien CY, Lu CT, et al. Triple-positive pathologic findings in oral cavity cancer are related to a dismal prognosis. Laryngoscope. 2015; 125(9):E300–E305

[54] Liu S-A, Wang CC, Jiang R-S, Lee FY, Lin WJ, Lin JC. Pathological features and their prognostic impacts on oral cavity cancer patients among different subsites—a singe institute's experience in Taiwan. Sci Rep. 2017; 7(1):7451

[55] O'Brien CJ, Lahr CJ, Soong SJ, et al. Surgical treatment of early-stage carcinoma of the oral tongue—would adjuvant treatment be beneficial? Head Neck Surg. 1986; 8(6):8401–8408

[56] Brown B, Barnes L, Mazariegos J, Taylor F, Johnson J, Wagner RL. Prognostic factors in mobile tongue and floor of mouth carcinoma. Cancer. 1989; 64(6): 1195–1202

[57] Soo K-C, Carter RL, O'Brien CJ, Barr L, Bliss JM, Shaw HJ. Prognostic implications of perineural spread in squamous carcinomas of the head and neck. Laryngoscope. 1986; 96(10):1145–1148

[58] Fagan JJ, Collins B, Barnes L, D'Amico F, Myers EN, Johnson JT. Perineural invasion in squamous cell carcinoma of the head and neck. Arch Otolaryngol Head Neck Surg. 1998; 124(6):637–640

[59] Brandwein-Gensler M, Teixeira MS, Lewis CM, et al. Oral squamous cell carcinoma: histologic risk assessment, but not margin status, is strongly predictive of local disease-free and overall survival. Am J Surg Pathol. 2005; 29(2): 167–178

[60] Jones HB, Sykes A, Bayman N, et al. The impact of lymphovascular invasion on survival in oral carcinoma. Oral Oncol. 2009; 45(1):10–15

[61] Jardim JF, Francisco AL, Gondak R, Damascena A, Kowalski LP. Prognostic impact of perineural invasion and lymphovascular invasion in advanced stage oral squamous cell carcinoma. Int J Oral Maxillofac Surg. 2015; 44(1):23–28

[62] Fives C, Feeley L, O'Leary G, Sheahan P. Importance of lymphovascular invasion and invasive front on survival in floor of mouth cancer. Head Neck. 2016; 38 Suppl 1:E1528–E1534

[63] Chen TC, Wang CP, Ko JY, et al. The impact of perineural invasion and/or lymphovascular invasion on the survival of early-stage oral squamous cell carcinoma patients. Ann Surg Oncol. 2013; 20(7):2388–2395

[64] Liu T, Chua B, Batstone M. Postoperative radiotherapy for oral squamous cell carcinoma with histologic risk factors: are we over-treating? J Oral Maxillofac Surg. 2018; 76(7):1565–1570. pii: S0278-2391(18) 30080-6
[65] Ang KK, Trotti A, Brown BW, et al. Randomized trial addressing risk features and time factors of surgery plus radiotherapy in advanced head-and-neck cancer. Int J Radiat Oncol Biol Phys. 2001; 51(3):571–578
[66] Choi S, Schwartz DL, Farwell DG, Austin-Seymour M, Futran N. Radiation therapy does not impact local complication rates after free flap reconstruction for head and neck cancer. Arch Otolaryngol Head Neck Surg. 2004; 130 (11):1308–1312
[67] Schwam ZG, Sosa JA, Roman S, Judson BL. Complications and mortality following surgery for oral cavity cancer: analysis of 408 cases. Laryngoscope. 2015; 125(8):1869–1873
[68] Eliasen M, Grønkjær M, Skov-Ettrup LS, et al. Preoperative alcohol consumption and postoperative complications: a systematic review and meta-analysis. Ann Surg. 2013; 258(6):930–942
[69] Isaacs JH, Jr, Thompson WB, Cassisi NJ, Million RR. Postoperative radiation of open head and neck wounds. Laryngoscope. 1987; 97(3 Pt 1):267–270
[70] Lau V, Chen LM, Farwell DG, Luu Q, Donald P, Chen AM. Postoperative radiation therapy for head and neck cancer in the setting of orocutaneous and pharyngocutaneous fistula. Am J Clin Oncol. 2011; 34(3):276–280

36 Adjuvant Chemotherapy/Novel Therapeutics

Ranee Mehra and Karim Boudadi

Summary

This chapter will provide an overview of risk factors for recurrence in oral cavity cancers, current standard treatment options, and the current state of clinical trials.

Keywords: adjuvant, epidermal growth factor receptor, PD-1 inhibitor

36.1 Introduction

Despite adequate surgical resection, the risk of recurrence of locally advanced oral cavity cancers is still high. Treatment decisions regarding the optimal adjuvant treatment are often multidisciplinary, with input from head and neck surgery, radiation oncology, and medical oncology. Factors to consider include clinical and pathological risk factors for recurrence, potential toxicity, and patient performance status. In addition, an assessment of concomitant comorbidities is essential.

The Meta-Analysis of Chemotherapy on Head and Neck Cancer (MACH-NC), which was updated in 2009, pooled individual patient data from 93 trials and 16,485 patients with resectable or unresectable oral cavity, oropharyngeal, hypopharyngeal, and laryngeal cancers. In all trials, patients were randomly assigned to definitive locoregional therapy alone (surgery and/or radiation) or definitive locoregional therapy in combination with chemotherapy (induction, concurrent, or sequential). Concurrent chemotherapy was assessed in 50 trials that included 9605 patients, with mean follow-up 5.6 years. Concurrent chemotherapy significantly decreased the risk of death compared with definitive local therapy alone (hazard ratio [HR] = 0.81, 95% CI: 0.78–0.86). This corresponded to a 6.5% absolute decrease in 5-year mortality. The MACH-NC meta-analysis found a greater benefit for platinum-based chemotherapy regimen as compared with other chemotherapy regimens, although the various chemotherapy regimens have not been directly compared with each other in adequately powered, randomized trials.[1] There is a modest benefit with adjuvant chemoradiation, at the expense of engendering increased toxicity, illustrating the importance of assessing risk factors and patient selection to determine who would have maximal benefit due to the addition of adjuvant cytotoxic therapy.

36.2 Prognostic Risk Factors for Recurrence

Retrospective series have indicated high-risk prognostic characteristics for recurrence of oral head and neck cancers that include margin status, presence of extranodal extension (ENE), tumor thickness, perineural invasion, and lymphovascular invasion.[2–6] A clear margin is defined as at least 5-mm distance from invasive tumor, although this can vary based on the primary site and anatomy.[7] Assessment of margin status often requires close communication between the head and neck surgeon and pathologist to ensure that the orientation of the specimen and association with landmarks is understood.

Extranodal extension of lymph node metastases is another known risk factor for locoregional recurrence of oral cavity cancers.[8–11] Prognostically, among ENE patients, macroscopic ENE patients had a 5-year overall survival of 19% compared to 31% in patients with microscopic ENE.[10] In another series, extension of ENE beyond 1.7 mm was associated with an inferior disease-specific survival.[12] However, currently the degree of ENE does not impact current recommendations for adjuvant treatment of oral cavity cancer.

36.2.1 Molecular Markers of Prognosis

Analysis of surgical margins has yielded some potential prognostic markers relevant to locoregional recurrence risk. Nathan et al hypothesized that mammalian target of rapamycin (mTOR) signaling was relevant to the natural history of squamous cell carcinoma of the head and neck (SCCHN) and found that eIF4E-binding protein-1 (4E-BP1), which inhibits cap dependent translation, is overexpressed in a subset of head and neck surgical margins, and is associated with mTOR/Akt signaling.[13] This prompted the study of mTOR inhibition in FaDu cell lines of head and neck squamous cell carcinoma (HNSCC), and xenografts including a minimal residual disease model in which there was significantly less tumor growth among the cohort that was treated with the mTOR inhibitor CCI-779.[14]

In another analysis, investigators from Johns Hopkins looked at the disrupted p53 status of resected head and neck tumors. TP53 mutations were detected in 53% of tumors; of these, 40% of the total patients were found to have disruptive mutations. In a multivariate analysis, there was an inferior survival among the patients with the disruptive TP53 mutation (HR = 1.7, $p = 0.003$).[15] This data has prompted the ongoing ECOG-ACRIN trial (EA3132, NCT02734537) in which patients with resected head and neck tumors, who lack the risk factors of + margin status and + ENE, are stratified by p53 status and randomized to radiation monotherapy versus cisplatin and radiation.[15]

Given the known critical role of DNA damage and repair with regards to platinum and radiation sensitivity, biomarkers related to DNA repair have been another relevant area of study. ERCC1, which is a key component of the nucleotide repair pathway that typically repairs cisplatin-induced DNA adduct formation, has been assayed in head and neck cancers with immunohistochemistry (IHC) techniques. Specimens from 107 patients with SCCHN who had received cisplatin-based induction therapy were analyzed by IHC for ERCC1 levels; patients with low ERCC1 level had a four-fold greater odds of achieving an objective response to platinum-based chemotherapy.[16] A series published from Fox Chase Cancer Center, which consisted of surgically resected tumors from patients who then received adjuvant radiation or chemoradiation, utilized the ERCC1-specific antibody HPA029773. A longer median survival was observed in ERCC1-low versus ERCC1-high tumors (64 vs. 29 months; $p = 0.02$).[17]

Additional biomarkers were studied in this human papilloma virus (HPV)-negative series, including the *KRAS* variant, a single nucleotide polymorphism in let-7 complementary site 6 (LCS-6) of the *KRAS* 3'UTR, which has been associated with platinum resistance,[18] and phosphorylated Rb. Among 99 available tumors cases from the Fox Chase series, 27% were noted to have the *KRAS* variant alteration. There was a non-significant trend toward increased overall survival among the *KRAS*-variant treated with surgery and adjuvant radiation ($p = 0.08$).[19]

It is now known that dysregulation of the cell cycle pathway is of relevance in the pathogenesis of HPV-negative head and neck cancers.[20] In The Cancer Genome Atlas (TCGA) analysis, amplification of cyclin D1 was identified and associated with a worse prognosis.[21,22] In order to study these pathways further, expression of epidermal growth factor receptor (EGFR) and inactivated phospho-T356 Rb was also quantified in 99 patients from the Fox Chase TMA. An improvement in survival was noted among the patients with low phospho-Rb.[21] In addition, an inverse relationship was noted between phospho-Rb and EGFR expression.[23] While these biomarkers were associated with survival among HPV-negative patients who were treated with adjuvant radiation/chemoradiation, incorporation of these markers into therapeutic trials remains to be a question for the future.

36.3 Standard Treatment Considerations and Approaches

Definitive local therapy (surgery and/or radiation therapy [RT]) is the mainstay of treatment for stage I and II squamous cell cancer (SCC) of the oral cavity. There is currently no evidence to support the use of chemotherapy for early stage disease. Locally advanced (stage III and IV) SCC of the oral cavity is associated with high rates of locoregional and distant recurrence and often requires a multimodal approach involving chemotherapy. For patients with unfavorable pathological features (ENE, positive resection margins, N2 or N3 nodal disease, nodal disease in levels IV or V, perineural invasion, or vascular invasion), postoperative concurrent chemoradiation has been shown to improve locoregional control (LRC) and survival in several landmark clinical trials. Targeted therapies can also be combined with concurrent RT, and combined RT plus checkpoint inhibitor immunotherapy is currently under active investigation. These treatment approaches will be discussed here.

36.3.1 Platinum-based Chemotherapy

The use of cytotoxic therapy, in particular cisplatin, had been incorporated with radiation in the setting of definitive treatment for curative intent. The mechanism of action of platinum involves induction of DNA damage via platinum–DNA adduct formation, resulting in inhibition of DNA replication and increased apoptosis. Preclinical data has demonstrated synergy with radiation, which results in single and double stranded DNA breaks, and cisplatin. This process is dependent on the presence of a functional nonhomologous end joining (NHEJ) DNA repair pathway which typically is involved in the repair of double strand breaks.[24]

For definitive treatment of SCCHN, results from the Radiation Therapy Oncology Group (RTOG) 91-11 trial demonstrated high rates of acute severe (grade 3 and 4) adverse events, specifically 47% hematologic side effects, 43% stomatitis, 35% dysphagia or odynophagia, and 20% nausea or vomiting.[25] Only 120 of 172 patients (70%) treated with this regimen completed all three cycles of cisplatin. In the RTOG 0129 trial, once-daily fractionation RT for 7 weeks, in combination with three cycles of cisplatin (100 mg/m^2 on days 1, 22, and 43), was compared with accelerated boost RT (42 fractions given over 6 weeks) with two cycles of cisplatin (100 mg/m^2 on days 1 and 22). There was no statistically significant difference in overall survival when patients receiving two cycles of cisplatin with once-daily fractionation were compared with those receiving three cycles plus once-daily fractionation, although only a small number of patients received two cycles.[26]

Concurrent chemoradiotherapy with a platinum-based agent, such as cisplatin, has also become the standard for adjuvant chemotherapy. High-dose bolus cisplatin (100 mg/m^2 every 21 days) is often considered the preferred concurrent regimen, although it is associated with severe acute and late toxicities. As such, it is typically reserved for patients with excellent performance status and minimal comorbidities.[27] Two randomized trials have established the efficacy of cisplatin with radiation in the adjuvant setting. The European Organization Research and Treatment of Cancer (EORTC) 22931 study randomized patients to radiation alone versus bolus dosing cisplatin and radiation.[28] Eligibility criteria included pT3/pT4 stage with positive nodes, or an early stage tumor with N2/3 disease, extranodal spread, positive resection margins, or perineural involvement. The combined modality therapy with chemotherapy resulted in a statistically significant improvement in progression-free survival (PFS), LRC, and overall survival (HR = 0.70, $p = 0.02$). A similar study conducted in North America, RTOG 9501, included patients with high-risk features of two or more lymph nodes, ENE of nodal disease, and microscopically involved margins. Disease-free survival (DFS) favored the combined modality group, but there was not a significant benefit in overall survival (HR = 0.84, $p = 0.19$).[29] A meta-analysis of these two studies confirmed the benefit of adjuvant chemoradiation among patients who had either ENE or positive margins.[30]

Alternative cisplatin dosing schedules (30–40 mg/m^2 weekly) are sometimes used because of improved patient tolerance. However, data comparing high-dose cisplatin with alternative regimens is limited. In a randomized phase III trial which included 87% oral cavity cancers, cisplatin, 30 mg/m^2 given weekly, resulted in significantly worse LRC compared with cisplatin 100 mg/m^2 every 3 weeks (2-year control rate 58.5 vs. 73.1%, HR = 1.76, 95% CI: 1.11–2.79).[31] However, there was no significant difference in overall survival with 22-month follow-up (median 39.5 vs. not reached, HR = 1.14, 95% CI: 0.79–1.65). This trial had several limitations and used a lower dose of cisplatin than is generally used (35–40 mg/m^2 weekly).

In another large phase III trial of patients in India with locally advanced oral cavity cancer, 900 patients with predominantly gingival or buccal carcinoma were randomly assigned following surgery to RT alone, accelerated RT, or concurrent chemoradiation with cisplatin 30 mg/m^2 weekly. For the entire study population, there was no difference in locoregional tumor control, DFS, or overall survival. However, in a post hoc analysis, there was significant improvement in all three outcomes, particularly overall survival, for high-risk patients (T3-T4, N2/

N3, ENE) and for patients treated with concurrent cisplatin 30 mg/m^2 weekly.[32]

Concurrent chemoradiation using carboplatin has also been studied. Carboplatin is more acutely myelosuppressive than cisplatin but results in less nephrotoxicity, neurotoxicity, and nausea and vomiting. Whether carboplatin is as effective as cisplatin as a radiation sensitizer is unclear, as head-to-head randomized trials have not been conducted. At least one trial suggested that every 3 week carboplatin is not as effective as high-dose cisplatin.[33] However, for patients with renal disease, or limited performance status, or for those unable to tolerate large fluid volumes, weekly carboplatin (AUC 1.5 to 2) remains an alternative to cisplatin. The combination of carboplatin plus fluorouracil may also represent another option when cisplatin is not feasible, although with potential greater toxicity.[34]

Overall, it is known that platinum-based therapy with radiation results in increased acute toxicity with an exacerbation of mucositis, increased nausea, and myelosuppression. In addition, cisplatin often results in increased risk of ototoxicity, renal insufficiency, and electrolyte abnormalities.[35]

36.3.2 Cetuximab

The EGFR is highly overexpressed in HNSCC and is associated with a poor prognosis. EGFR activation facilitates tumor growth by promoting angiogenesis and proliferation and metastasis by increasing motility and adhesion of tumor cells.

Cetuximab is a chimeric monoclonal antibody (65% human and 35% murine) constructed on an immunoglobulin (Ig) G1 framework, which targets an extracellular epitope in the EGFR ligand-binding domain.[36] Cetuximab blockade of the EGFR results in inhibition of tumor growth, metastasis, DNA damage repair, and angiogenesis.[37,38]

Several mechanisms that contribute to the antitumor activity of cetuximab have been identified. One is interference by cetuximab with the binding of natural ligands to the receptor itself, thereby disrupting EGFR signaling pathways.[39] Another mechanism involves depletion of the targeted receptors from the cell surface via induction of receptor endocytosis.[40] Finally, cetuximab's construction on an IgG1 framework potentially allows this agent to mediate antibody-dependent cell-mediated cytotoxicity (ADCC) via recruitment of natural killer cells and macrophages.[41,42]

Preclinical studies have shown that EGFR inhibition sensitizes HNSCC to the effects of ionizing radiation.[43–46] In mouse A431 xenografts of HNSCC, the combination of cetuximab and cisplatin led to greater growth inhibition than that achieved with either agent alone.[47]

For the definitive treatment of locally advance disease, it was evaluated in a large international trial of 424 patients with locally advanced HNSCC randomly assigned to RT with or without concurrent weekly cetuximab.[46] Median follow-up was 54 months. Overall survival was significantly better for the cetuximab-treated group compared to RT alone (3-year survival 55 vs. 45%, HR = 0.73), as was LRC (50 vs. 41%). It is important to note that this trial compared concurrent cetuximab with RT alone, which is no longer considered a standard approach for locally advanced disease.

For some time, it was not known whether cetuximab and radiation was equivalent to cisplatin and radiation. A retrospective analysis from MSKCC compared the outcome of 125 patients who received cisplatin (100 mg/m^2 every 3 weeks) with radiation to 50 patients who received cetuximab (400 mg/m^2 loading dose and 250 mg/m^2 weekly) with radiation.[48] Recognizing that these were two different patient populations, a multivariate analysis to address prognostic imbalances was performed. Despite this adjustment, results for local failure, DFS, and overall survival all favored the cisplatin arm ($p < 0.0001$ for LF and DFS, $p = 0.0017$ for OS). A randomized phase II trial that compared concurrent cetuximab plus RT with weekly cisplatin plus RT suggested that cetuximab was associated with more acute toxicity (mucositis, dermatitis, weight loss, and requirements for enteral feeding), more radiation treatment interruptions, and a trend toward worse survival outcomes.[49] However, the trial was terminated early and was underpowered to draw definitive conclusions. Given these results though, it is not possible to make assumptions about its role in the adjuvant setting.

RTOG 1016, a large phase III effort which randomized HPV + oropharyngeal cancer patients to cetuximab/radiation versus bolus cisplatin/radiation recently confirmed the survival superiority of the platinum-based regimen, calling into question the future role of cetuximab.[50] Additional ongoing studies with cetuximab are discussed below.

36.4 Current Areas of Investigation

36.4.1 Current Trials of Adjuvant Cetuximab and Taxanes

The cooperative groups have looked at the question of non-platinum therapies in the adjuvant setting. In addition to cetuximab, the study of taxanes has been of interest. These agents have a long standing role in the treatment of a variety of solid tumors, and function by stabilizing microtubules. The resulting disruption of cell cycle progression promotes apoptosis.[51] In RTOG 0234, 238 patients were enrolled and randomized to cetuximab, weekly cisplatin with 60-Gy radiation or cetuximab, weekly docetaxel and 60-Gy radiation. Two-year overall survival and 2-year DFS both favored the group treated with docetaxel (79 and 66% respectively).[52] A follow-up study, RTOG 1216 (NCT01810913) was designed to further study the role of adjuvant docetaxel among patients with ENE or positive margins. In this ongoing phase II/III effort, patients have been randomized to adjuvant radiation with cisplatin, docetaxel, or docetaxel plus cetuximab.

While many adjuvant studies select patients with the known poor prognostic risk factors of ENE and positive margins, it remains to be seen if there is a role for the addition of systemic therapy for tumors with intermediate risk factors including lymphovascular invasion, perineural invasion, close margins, and > /= 2 nodes. RTOG 0920 (NCT00956007) was designed to answer this question and it randomized patients to 60-Gy radiation versus 60-Gy radiation plus cetuximab with analysis of EGFR expression as an alternative.

36.4.2 Small Molecular Inhibitors

Beyond monoclonal antibodies, small molecule agents targeting EGFR have been studied in HNSCC. Afatinib, an oral anilinoquinazoline derivative, differs from the first-generation EGFR small molecule inhibitors, erlotinib and gefitinib, in that it binds irreversibly to EGFR and has activity against HER2 and ErbB4 receptors.[53–55] This allows for longer suppression of ErbB signaling and more complete blockade of EGFR signaling pathways.[56] The toxicity profile of afatinib and the other irreversible tyrosine kinase inhibitors appears to be similar to first-generation iterations, with rash and diarrhea remaining the most common adverse effects.[57] In patients with advanced, platinum-resistant SCCHN, a randomized, phase II study showed comparable efficacy for afatinib and cetuximab, with a trend toward improved disease control rate and overall response rate with afatinib.[58] Afatinib was compared to placebo in the adjuvant setting in a phase III trial of 617 patients with locoregionally advanced intermediate-to-high-risk HNSCC who had been rendered disease free with chemoradiotherapy. The primary endpoint of the study was DFS.[59] After a planned interim analysis, there was no difference in DFS between the afatinib group (median 43.4 months) and placebo (not reached) (HR = 1.15, 95% CI: 0.81–1.57), and the trial was stopped for futility.[60]

WEE1 has been implicated as a potential therapeutic target for HNSCC, with increased DNA damage noted with the WEE1 inhibitor AZD1775, in particular in p53 mutated HNSCC cell lines.[61] An ongoing phase I study has combined AZD1775 with weekly cisplatin and radiation in the adjuvant setting (NCT03028766).

36.4.3 Novel Therapeutics—Adjuvant Immunotherapy

With the Food and Drug Administration approval of two immune checkpoint programmed death-1 (PD-1) inhibitors for recurrent/metastatic head and neck cancer, study of these agents in the adjuvant setting is a logical progression of investigation. Recently, two anti-PD-1 antibodies nivolumab (Opdivo, Bristol-Myers Squibb) and pembrolizumab (Keytruda, Merck)] have been approved to treat patients with advanced SCCHN. These drugs target receptors which provide inhibitory signals to T-cells, thus amplifying T-cell activity in an attempt to generate antitumor immune response. SCCHN is thought to be an immune responsiveness disease, based on evidence of PDL-1 expression, as well as a relatively high tumor mutation burden compared to other solid tumors.[62–64] In addition, suppressive regulatory T cells (Tregs) have been linked to SCCHN tumor progression.[53]

Immune checkpoint inhibitors offer promise as a novel therapeutic approach for-SCCHN. Keynote-012 was a phase 1b study of pembrolizumab in SCCHN patients with recurrent/metastatic SCCHN. A total of 192 patients were treated in two cohorts with differing doses. It was previously shown that the activity was similar between the weight based and fixed dose schedule.[54,55] The combined analysis resulted in a response rate of 18%; a small group of patients did complete 2 years of planned therapy without progression.[65] A single-arm phase II study of pembrolizumab, an anti-PD1 antibody, in SCCHN patients who had failed platinum and cetuximab, pembrolizumab also showed an ORR of 18%,[56] and it was the combined data of these two studies led to approval of this agent in platinum refractory RM-SCCHN patients.

In a large randomized double blinded phase III clinical trial, nivolumab, almost doubled 1-year overall survival and showed a response rate of 13% in patients with recurrent/metastatic SCCHN.[57] Given these successes of immune checkpoint inhibitors in RM-SCCHN, there is enthusiasm to bring these agents in earlier stage of SCCHN.

One challenge to incorporate PD-1 inhibitors for adjuvant treatment is the relatively modest response rate of both nivolumab and pembrolizumab among unselected patients with recurrent disease who had platinum previously. In addition, while the risk of serious immune-mediated toxicity is low, myocarditis, diabetes type I, endocrinopathies, colitis, and pneumonitis have been reported.[58,66–68] The risk of these potential toxicities cannot be minimized in an otherwise asymptomatic group of patients who are clinically free of disease. However, this field is encouraged by the positive results of the phase III Pacific study which studied the role of adjuvant durvalumab after platinum-based chemoradiation for stage III non-small-cell lung cancer.[69] In this study, the median PFS strongly favored durvalumab at 16.8 months versus 5.6 months in the group who received placebo. There are ongoing studies in HNSCC with immunotherapy either combined with RT or after the completion of RT (▶ Table 36.1). Patient selection with regards to

Table 36.1 Current adjuvant immunotherapy trials for head and neck cancer

Brief title	Phase	Number of patients	Agent(s)	NCT number
Phase II Study of Adjuvant Pembrolizumab vs. Placebo in HNSCC at High Risk for Recurrence—The PATHWay Study	II	100	Pembrolizumab versus placebo	NCT02841748
Adjuvant Nivolumab After Salvage Resection in Head and Neck Cancer Patients Previously Treated With Definitive Therapy	II	24	Nivolumab	NCT03355560
Phase II Trial of Adjuvant Cisplatin and Radiation With Pembrolizumab in Resected Head and Neck Squamous Cell Carcinoma	II	80	Pembrolizumab Radiation Cisplatin (high risk features)	NCT02641093
Durvalumab and Tremelimumab With Radiotherapy for Adjuvant Treatment of Intermediate Risk SCCHN	I	24	Durvalumab Tremelimumab Radiation	NCT03529422
A Study of Atezolizumab (Anti–Pd-L1 Antibody) as Adjuvant Therapy After Definitive Local Therapy in Patients With High-Risk Locally Advanced HNSCC	III	400	Atezolizumab	NCT03452137
Adjuvant Nivolumab and Lirilumab in Patients With Relapsed, Resectable Squamous Cell Carcinoma of the Head and Neck	II	58	Nivolumab Lirilumab	NCT03341936
NRG-HN003: A Phase I and Expansion Cohort Study of Adjuvant Cisplatin, Intensity-Modulated Radiotherapy, and Pembrolizumab in High-Risk HNSCC	I	56	Pembrolizumab Cisplatin Radiation	NCT02775812

identifying those who have a high risk of recurrence as well as those with an increased chance of benefit to checkpoint inhibitors will be important factors to consider as data matures and is analyzed.

Currently, the role of immunotherapy relevant biomarkers is an active area of study for SCCHN. Recently, results of Keynote-048 were reported.[70] This phase III study randomized patients to pembrolizumab, pembrolizumab plus platinum double therapy, and the platinum doublet plus cetuximab EXTREME regimen. Among tumors that had a PDL1 tumor and immune cell combined positive score (CPS) of > 20% and > 1%, patients who were treated with pembrolizumab had an improved overall survival compared to those treated with the EXTREME regimen. This trial not only is practice changing in the first-line setting for recurrent/metastatic disease, but also provides data for a biomarker which could be incorporated in future studies.

36.5 Conclusion

Current clinical factors to identify an indication for adjuvant platinum-based chemoradiotherapy remain to be positive margins and positive ENE. Given the risk of recurrence associated with many oral cavity cancers, it is important that new biomarkers for recurrence are identified. Similarly, novel systemic agents are now being studied in the adjuvant space, although it may take years before a new standard of care can be adopted. In the interim, support of ongoing studies will be essential to advance the field.

Key Points

- Adjuvant cisplatin with radiation is the standard postoperative treatment for oral cavity patients with positive surgical margins and extranodal extension.
- Disease specific risk biomarkers to study included disrupted p53.
- Novel agents in the adjuvant setting, such as immunotherapy, are investigational at this time.

References

[1] Pignon JP, le Maître A, Maillard E, Bourhis J, MACH-NC Collaborative Group. Meta-analysis of chemotherapy in head and neck cancer (MACH-NC): an update on 93 randomised trials and 17,346 patients. Radiother Oncol. 2009; 92(1):4–14

[2] Looser KG, Shah JP, Strong EW. The significance of "positive" margins in surgically resected epidermoid carcinomas. Head Neck Surg. 1978; 1(2):107–111

[3] Warburton G, Nikitakis NG, Roberson P, et al. Histopathological and lymphangiogenic parameters in relation to lymph node metastasis in early stage oral squamous cell carcinoma. J Oral Maxillofac Surg. 2007; 65(3):475–484

[4] Salesiotis AN, Cullen KJ. Molecular markers predictive of response and prognosis in the patient with advanced squamous cell carcinoma of the head and neck: evolution of a model beyond TNM staging. Curr Opin Oncol. 2000; 12 (3):229–239

[5] Valente G, Mamo C, Bena A, et al. Prognostic significance of microvessel density and vascular endothelial growth factor expression in sinonasal carcinomas. Hum Pathol. 2006; 37(4):391–400

[6] Olsen KD, Caruso M, Foote RL, et al. Primary head and neck cancer. Histopathologic predictors of recurrence after neck dissection in patients with lymph node involvement. Arch Otolaryngol Head Neck Surg. 1994; 120(12):1370–1374

[7] Williams MD. Determining adequate margins in head and neck cancers: practice and continued challenges. Curr Oncol Rep. 2016; 18(9):54

[8] Mamelle G, Pampurik J, Luboinski B, Lancar R, Lusinchi A, Bosq J. Lymph node prognostic factors in head and neck squamous cell carcinomas. Am J Surg. 1994; 168(5):494–498

[9] Snow GB, Annyas AA, van Slooten EA, Bartelink H, Hart AA. Prognostic factors of neck node metastasis. Clin Otolaryngol Allied Sci. 1982; 7(3):185–192

[10] Shaw RJ, Lowe D, Woolgar JA, et al. Extracapsular spread in oral squamous cell carcinoma. Head Neck. 2010; 32(6):714–722

[11] Myers JN, Greenberg JS, Mo V, Roberts D. Extracapsular spread. A significant predictor of treatment failure in patients with squamous cell carcinoma of the tongue. Cancer. 2001; 92(12):3030–3036

[12] Wreesmann VB, Katabi N, Palmer FL, et al. Influence of extracapsular nodal spread extent on prognosis of oral squamous cell carcinoma. Head Neck. 2016; 38 Suppl 1:E1192–E1199

[13] Nathan CO, Amirghahari N, Abreo F, et al. Overexpressed eIF4E is functionally active in surgical margins of head and neck cancer patients via activation of the Akt/mammalian target of rapamycin pathway. Clin Cancer Res. 2004; 10 (17):5820–5827

[14] Nathan CO, Amirghahari N, Rong X, et al. Mammalian target of rapamycin inhibitors as possible adjuvant therapy for microscopic residual disease in head and neck squamous cell cancer. Cancer Res. 2007; 67(5):2160–2168

[15] Poeta ML, Manola J, Goldwasser MA, et al. TP53 mutations and survival in squamous-cell carcinoma of the head and neck. N Engl J Med. 2007; 357(25): 2552–2561

[16] Handra-Luca A, Hernandez J, Mountzios G, et al. Excision repair cross complementation group 1 immunohistochemical expression predicts objective response and cancer-specific survival in patients treated by Cisplatin-based induction chemotherapy for locally advanced head and neck squamous cell carcinoma. Clin Cancer Res. 2007; 13:3855–3859

[17] Mehra R, Zhu F, Yang D-H, et al. Quantification of excision repair cross-complementing group 1 and survival in p16-negative squamous cell head and neck cancers. Clin Cancer Res. 2013; 19:6633–6643

[18] Chung CH, Lee JW, Slebos RJ, et al. A 3'-UTR KRAS-variant is associated with cisplatin resistance in patients with recurrent and/or metastatic head and neck squamous cell carcinoma. Ann Oncol. 2014; 25(11):2230–2236

[19] Mufson J, Handorf E, Weidhaas J, et al. Analysis of KRAS variant in a cohort of resected HPV negative HNSCC [abstract]. In: Proceedings of the American Association for Cancer Research Annual Meeting 2017; 2017 Apr 1-5; Washington, DC. Philadelphia (PA): AACR; Cancer Res 2017;77(13 Suppl):Abstract nr 4732. doi:10.1158/1538-7445.AM2017-4732

[20] Ai L, Stephenson KK, Ling W, et al. The p16 (CDKN2a/INK4a) tumor-suppressor gene in head and neck squamous cell carcinoma: a promoter methylation and protein expression study in 100 cases. Mod Pathol. 2003; 16 (9):944–950

[21] Beck TN, Kaczmar J, Handorf E, et al. Phospho-T356RB1 predicts survival in HPV-negative squamous cell carcinoma of the head and neck. Oncotarget. 2015; 6(22):18863–18874

[22] Cancer Genome Atlas N, Cancer Genome Atlas Network. Comprehensive genomic characterization of head and neck squamous cell carcinomas. Nature. 2015; 517(7536):576–582

[23] Beck TN, Georgopoulos R, Shagisultanova EI, et al. EGFR and RB1 as dual biomarkers in HPV-negative head and neck cancer. Mol Cancer Ther. 2016; 15 (10):2486–2497

[24] Boeckman HJ, Trego KS, Turchi JJ. Cisplatin sensitizes cancer cells to ionizing radiation via inhibition of nonhomologous end joining. Mol Cancer Res. 2005; 3(5):277–285

[25] Forastiere AA, Goepfert H, Maor M, et al. Concurrent chemotherapy and radiotherapy for organ preservation in advanced laryngeal cancer. N Engl J Med. 2003; 349(22):2091–2098

[26] Ang KK, Harris J, Wheeler R, et al. Human papillomavirus and survival of patients with oropharyngeal cancer. N Engl J Med. 2010; 363(1):24–35

[27] Adelstein DJ, Li Y, Adams GL, et al. An intergroup phase III comparison of standard radiation therapy and two schedules of concurrent chemoradiotherapy in patients with unresectable squamous cell head and neck cancer. J Clin Oncol. 2003; 21(1):92–98

[28] Bernier J, Domenge C, Ozsahin M, et al. European Organization for Research and Treatment of Cancer Trial 22931. Postoperative irradiation with or without concomitant chemotherapy for locally advanced head and neck cancer. N Engl J Med. 2004; 350(19):1945–1952

[29] Cooper JS, Pajak TF, Forastiere AA, et al. Radiation Therapy Oncology Group 9501/Intergroup. Postoperative concurrent radiotherapy and chemotherapy for high-risk squamous-cell carcinoma of the head and neck. N Engl J Med. 2004; 350(19):1937–1944

[30] Bernier J, Cooper JS, Pajak TF, et al. Defining risk levels in locally advanced head and neck cancers: a comparative analysis of concurrent postoperative radiation plus chemotherapy trials of the EORTC (#22931) and RTOG (# 9501). Head Neck. 2005; 27(10):843–850

[31] Noronha V, Joshi A, Patil VM, et al. Once-a-week versus once-every-3-weeks cisplatin chemoradiation for locally advanced head and neck cancer: a phase III randomized noninferiority trial. J Clin Oncol. 2018; 36(11):1064–1072

[32] Lasker S, Chaukar D, Deshpande M, et al. Phase III randomized trial of surgery followed by conventional radiotherapy (5 fr/Wk) (Arm A) vs concurrent chemoradiotherapy (Arm B) vs accelerated radiotherapy (6fr/Wk) (Arm C) in locally advanced, stage III and IV, resectable, squamous cell carcinoma of oral cavity- oral cavity adjuvant therapy (OCAT): Final results (NCT00193843). J Clin Oncol. 2016; 34:6004

[33] Fountzilas G, Ciuleanu E, Dafni U, et al. Concomitant radiochemotherapy vs radiotherapy alone in patients with head and neck cancer: a Hellenic Cooperative Oncology Group Phase III Study. Med Oncol. 2004; 21(2):95–107

[34] Denis F, Garaud P, Bardet E, et al. Final results of the 94-01 French Head and Neck Oncology and Radiotherapy Group randomized trial comparing radiotherapy alone with concomitant radiochemotherapy in advanced-stage oropharynx carcinoma. J Clin Oncol. 2004; 22(1):69–76

[35] Trotti A, Pajak TF, Gwede CK, et al. TAME: development of a new method for summarising adverse events of cancer treatment by the Radiation Therapy Oncology Group. Lancet Oncol. 2007; 8(7):613–624

[36] Goldstein NI, Prewett M, Zuklys K, Rockwell P, Mendelsohn J. Biological efficacy of a chimeric antibody to the epidermal growth factor receptor in a human tumor xenograft model. Clin Cancer Res. 1995; 1(11):1311–1318

[37] Baselga J. The EGFR as a target for anticancer therapy—focus on cetuximab. Eur J Cancer. 2001; 37 Suppl 4:S16–S22

[38] Ciardiello F, Tortora G. A novel approach in the treatment of cancer: targeting the epidermal growth factor receptor. Clin Cancer Res. 2001; 7(10):2958–2970

[39] Li S, Schmitz KR, Jeffrey PD, Wiltzius JJ, Kussie P, Ferguson KM. Structural basis for inhibition of the epidermal growth factor receptor by cetuximab. Cancer Cell. 2005; 7(4):301–311

[40] Sigismund S, Woelk T, Puri C, et al. Clathrin-independent endocytosis of ubiquitinated cargos. Proc Natl Acad Sci U S A. 2005; 102(8):2760–2765

[41] López-Albaitero A, Ferris RL. Immune activation by epidermal growth factor receptor specific monoclonal antibody therapy for head and neck cancer. Arch Otolaryngol Head Neck Surg. 2007; 133(12):1277–1281

[42] Kurai J, Chikumi H, Hashimoto K, et al. Antibody-dependent cellular cytotoxicity mediated by cetuximab against lung cancer cell lines. Clin Cancer Res. 2007; 13(5):1552–1561

[43] Harari PM, Huang SM. Head and neck cancer as a clinical model for molecular targeting of therapy: combining EGFR blockade with radiation. Int J Radiat Oncol Biol Phys. 2001; 49(2):427–433

[44] Huang SM, Bock JM, Harari PM. Epidermal growth factor receptor blockade with C225 modulates proliferation, apoptosis, and radiosensitivity in squamous cell carcinomas of the head and neck. Cancer Res. 1999; 59(8):1935–1940

[45] Feng FY, Lopez CA, Normolle DP, et al. Effect of epidermal growth factor receptor inhibitor class in the treatment of head and neck cancer with concurrent radiochemotherapy in vivo. Clin Cancer Res. 2007; 13(8):2512–2518

[46] Bonner JA, Harari PM, Giralt J, et al. Radiotherapy plus cetuximab for squamous-cell carcinoma of the head and neck. N Engl J Med. 2006; 354(6):567–578

[47] Fan Z, Baselga J, Masui H, Mendelsohn J. Antitumor effect of anti-epidermal growth factor receptor monoclonal antibodies plus cis-diamminedichloroplatinum on well established A431 cell xenografts. Cancer Res. 1993; 53(19):4637–4642

[48] Riaz N, Sherman E, Koutcher L, et al. Concurrent chemoradiotherapy with cisplatin versus cetuximab for squamous cell carcinoma of the head and neck. Am J Clin Oncol.2016; 39(1):27–31

[49] Magrini SM, Buglione M, Corvò R, et al. Cetuximab and radiotherapy versus cisplatin and radiotherapy for locally advanced head and neck cancer: a randomized phase II trial. J Clin Oncol. 2016; 34(5):427–435

[50] Gillison ML, Trotti AM, Harris J, et al. Radiotherapy plus cetuximab or cisplatin for human papillomavirus (HPV)-positive oropharyngeal cancer: a randomized, multicenter, non-inferiority clinical trial. Lancet. 2019; 393 (10166): 40–50

[51] Abal M, Andreu JM, Barasoain I. Taxanes: microtubule and centrosome targets, and cell cycle dependent mechanisms of action. Curr Cancer Drug Targets. 2003; 3(3):193–203

[52] Harari PM, Harris J, Kies MS, et al. Postoperative chemoradiotherapy and cetuximab for high-risk squamous cell carcinoma of the head and neck: Radiation Therapy Oncology Group RTOG-0234. J Clin Oncol. 2014; 32(23): 2486–2495

[53] Ferris RL. Immunology and immunotherapy of head and neck cancer. J Clin Oncol. 2015; 33(29):3293–3304

[54] Chow LQM, Haddad R, Gupta S, et al. Antitumor activity of pembrolizumab in biomarker-unselected patients with recurrent and/or metastatic head and neck squamous cell carcinoma: results from the Phase Ib KEYNOTE-012 Expansion Cohort. J Clin Oncol. 2016; 34(32):3838–3845

[55] Seiwert TY, Burtness B, Mehra R, et al. Safety and clinical activity of pembrolizumab for treatment of recurrent or metastatic squamous cell carcinoma of the head and neck (KEYNOTE-012): an open-label, multicentre, phase 1b trial. Lancet Oncol. 2016; 17(7):956–965

[56] Bauml J, Seiwert TY, Pfister DG, et al. Pembrolizumab for platinum- and cetuximab-refractory head and neck cancer: results from a single-arm, phase II study. J Clin Oncol. 2017; 35(14):1542–1549

[57] Ferris RL, Blumenschein G, Jr, Fayette J, et al. Nivolumab for recurrent squamous-cell carcinoma of the head and neck. N Engl J Med. 2016; 375(19): 1856–1867

[58] Naidoo J, Page DB, Li BT, et al. Toxicities of the anti-PD-1 and anti-PD-L1 immune checkpoint antibodies. Ann Oncol. 2016; 27(7):1362

[59] Burtness B, Bourhis JP, Vermorken JB, Harrington KJ, Cohen EE. Afatinib versus placebo as adjuvant therapy after chemoradiation in a double-blind, phase III study (LUX-Head & Neck 2) in patients with primary unresected, clinically intermediate-to-high-risk head and neck cancer: study protocol for a randomized controlled trial. Trials. 2014; 15:469

[60] Burtness B, Haddad RI, Dinis J, et al. LUX-head and neck 2: Randomized, double-blind, placebo-controlled, phase III tiral of afatinib as adjuvant therapy after chemoradiation (CRT) in primary unresected, high/intermediate-risk, squamous cell cancer of the head and neck (HNSCC) patients (pts). *J Clin Oncol.* 2017;35(suppl; abstr 6001)

[61] Kao M, Green C, Sidorova J, Méndez E. Strategies for targeted therapy in head and neck squamous cell carcinoma using WEE1 inhibitor AZD1775. JAMA Otolaryngol Head Neck Surg. 2017; 143(6):631–633

[62] Lyford-Pike S, Peng S, Young GD, et al. Evidence for a role of the PD-1:PD-L1 pathway in immune resistance of HPV-associated head and neck squamous cell carcinoma. Cancer Res. 2013; 73(6):1733–1741

[63] Alexandrov LB, Nik-Zainal S, Wedge DC, et al. Australian Pancreatic Cancer Genome Initiative, ICGC Breast Cancer Consortium, ICGC MMML-Seq Consortium, ICGC PedBrain. Signatures of mutational processes in human cancer. Nature. 2013; 500(7463):415–421

[64] Topalian SL, Taube JM, Anders RA, Pardoll DM. Mechanism-driven biomarkers to guide immune checkpoint blockade in cancer therapy. Nat Rev Cancer. 2016; 16(5):275–287

[65] Mehra R, Seiwert TY, Gupta S, et al. Efficacy and safety of pembrolizumab in recurrent/metastatic head and neck squamous cell carcinoma: pooled analyses after long-term follow-up in KEYNOTE-012. Br J Cancer. 2018; 119(2): 153–159

[66] Godwin JL, Jaggi S, Sirisena I, et al. Nivolumab-induced autoimmune diabetes mellitus presenting as diabetic ketoacidosis in a patient with metastatic lung cancer. J Immunother Cancer. 2017; 5:40

[67] Naidoo J, Wang X, Woo KM, et al. Pneumonitis in patients treated with anti-programmed death-1/programmed death ligand 1 therapy. J Clin Oncol. 2017; 35(7):709–717

[68] Neilan TG, Rothenberg ML, Amiri-Kordestani L, et al. Checkpoint Inhibitor Safety Working Group. Myocarditis associated with immune checkpoint inhibitors: an expert consensus on data gaps and a call to action. Oncologist. 2018; 23(8):874–878

[69] Antonia SJ, Villegas A, Daniel D, et al. PACIFIC Investigators. Durvalumab after chemoradiotherapy in stage III non-small-cell lung cancer. N Engl J Med. 2017; 377(20):1919–1929

[70] Burtness B, Harrington KJ, Greil R, Soulières D, et al. Pembrolizumab alone or with chemotherapy versus cetuximab with chemotherapy for recurrent or metastatic squamous cell carcinoma of the head and neck (KEYNOTE-048): a randomised, open-label, phase 3 study. Lancet. 2019; 394(10212):1915–1928

Section VII

Management of Nonsquamous Cell Cancers of the Oral Cavity

VII

37 Oral Cavity Salivary Gland Malignancies (Sublingual and Minor)

Eleni M. Rettig and David W. Eisele

Summary
Oral cavity minor salivary gland malignancies are relatively rare, but exhibit diverse histopathology. Mucoepidermoid carcinoma and adenoid cystic carcinoma are the most common types; adenoid cystic carcinoma is notable for its high rates of perineural invasion and late distant metastases. Surgical resection, with postoperative radiation for high-risk tumors, is the mainstay of treatment. Prognosis is generally good for early-stage and low-grade tumors, but tumors that are high-grade, large, and associated with cervical lymph node or distant metastases typically have poor outcomes.

Keywords: minor salivary gland malignancy, adenoid cystic carcinoma, mucoepidermoid carcinoma, genetic translocations, hard palate, magnetic resonance imaging, surgical resection, radiation therapy

37.1 Introduction

Minor salivary gland neoplasms are rare and exhibit a remarkable histologic diversity.[1,2] Although minor salivary gland neoplasms are less common than those of major glands, representing just 9 to 23% of all salivary gland tumors,[3] they are more likely to be malignant. Approximately 40 to 75% of minor salivary gland neoplasms are malignant, compared with 20% of major salivary gland neoplasms.[3,4,56] The oral cavity harbors more minor salivary glands than other anatomic sites, comprising approximately 90% of the 450 to 1000 minor salivary glands that line the upper aerodigestive tract, and, therefore, is the most common site of minor salivary gland neoplasms.[7,8] Within the oral cavity, the most common tumor types are mucoepidermoid carcinoma and adenoid cystic carcinoma.[3] Despite the diversity of minor salivary gland malignancies, their management almost always involves surgical resection for operable disease, with or without adjuvant radiation therapy.

This chapter will describe the epidemiology, clinical presentation, evaluation, and management of minor salivary gland malignancies in the oral cavity, with a focus on the most common histopathologic tumor types. Although sublingual glands are considered major salivary glands, the contents of this chapter are considered applicable to these neoplasms as well, due to their location in the oral cavity. For more detailed histopathologic information see Chapter 9 (Pathology: Oral Cavity Salivary Gland Malignancies).

37.2 Epidemiology

The rarity of minor salivary gland malignancies and ongoing changes to the World Health Organization's histologic classification schema[2,9] make epidemiologic studies challenging, so that much of what is known thus far is extrapolated from individual case series.

The estimated incidence of salivary gland malignancies is 4 to 135 cases per million per year, accounting for just 3% of head and neck cancers overall[10]; among salivary gland malignancies, 10 to 25% arise from minor salivary glands.[7,11] The oral cavity is the predominant site of origin for minor salivary gland cancers, accounting for 55 to 70% of cases (▶ Fig. 37.1).[12,13] Among oral cavity minor salivary gland malignancies, up to 50 to 75% occur on the hard palate, which is the most common primary site in most series (▶ Fig. 37.2a).[7,14] The posterior hard palate at the junction with the soft palate is a particularly common location for minor salivary gland tumors.[3,12]

37.2.1 Risk Factors

Etiologic risk factors for salivary gland malignancies are not well understood due to paucity of robust studies, but several risk factors have been suggested. Some occupational exposures[15,16] and dietary factors have been implicated.[17] A history of radiation to the head and neck, for example, exposure to nuclear fallout among atomic bomb survivors, has been associated with increased risk of mucoepidermoid carcinoma in particular.[16,18,19] Radioiodine for the treatment of well-differentiated thyroid carcinoma[20] and chemotherapy for childhood cancers have also been suggested to increase the risk of mucoepidermoid carcinoma.[1] Despite these reported associations, most salivary gland malignancies cannot be attributed to a specific etiology.

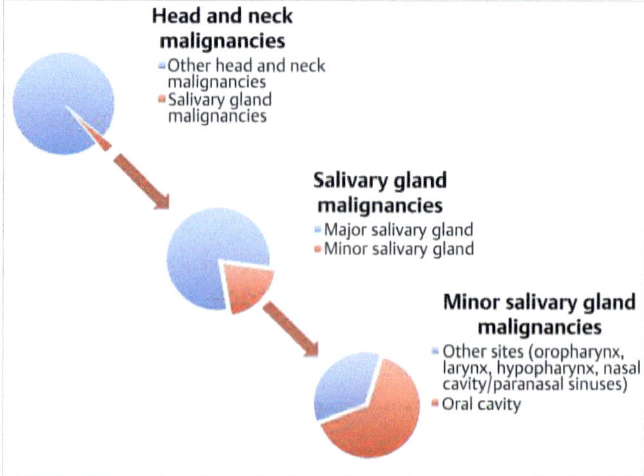

Fig. 37.1 Distribution of minor salivary gland malignancies. Salivary gland malignancies comprise just 3% of head and neck malignancies; of these, minor salivary gland malignancies account for 10–25%. The oral cavity is the most common site of minor salivary gland malignancies (55–70% of cases), and 50–75% of these arise from the hard palate.

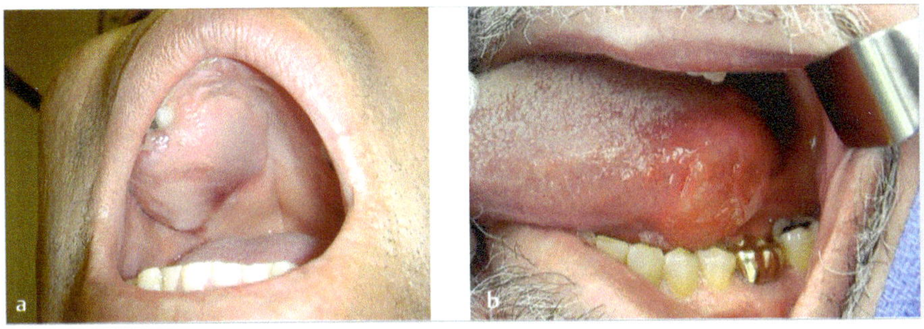

Fig. 37.2 Presentation of oral cavity minor salivary gland malignancies. (a) Typical presentation of intraoral minor salivary gland tumor as painless bulge of hard palate. Biopsy showed adenoid cystic carcinoma. (b) Left lateral oral tongue adenocarcinoma, NOS.

37.2.2 Patient Population

Most minor salivary gland malignant neoplasms affect individuals in their fifth and sixth decades of life and have a slight female predominance with female-to-male ratios of approximately 1.5 to 1.[1,7,8,11,12] Minor salivary gland malignancies can also rarely affect children, with mucoepidermoid carcinoma the most common subtype, followed by adenoid cystic carcinoma, and adenocarcinoma. Similar to adults, the most common anatomic location for malignancies in children is the oral cavity, in particular the hard palate.[21] Pediatric malignancies are rarely high-grade, and often require only complete surgical resection.[21] Most series report favorable long-term outcomes with a low risk of recurrence.[21–23]

37.2.3 Classification

There are a number of different histopathologic tumor types observed among malignancies of the minor salivary glands. The World Health Organization recently released a new classification schema in its 2017 4th edition guideline which identifies 22 malignant and 11 benign entities (▶ Table 37.1).[1] The two most frequently encountered malignancies in the oral cavity are mucoepidermoid carcinoma (15–59%) and adenoid cystic carcinoma (26–60%), with a lower prevalence of polymorphous adenocarcinoma (previously known as polymorphous low-grade adenocarcinoma) (15–26%),[1,2] adenocarcinoma, NOS (7–22%), and acinic cell carcinoma (2–3%).[7,8,24–27]

37.2.4 Clinical Presentation

Minor salivary gland malignancies typically present as a slow-growing firm or soft mass (▶ Fig. 37.2), often on the hard palate. The mass is usually covered with intact mucosa but sometimes may exhibit bleeding or ulceration. Most masses are asymptomatic. In edentulous patients, difficulty wearing dentures may be the initial presenting symptom. A small subset of tumors present with pain, which is more commonly associated with malignant compared with benign tumors.[5,28] Adenoid cystic carcinoma in particular has a propensity for perineural invasion, and thus may present with nerve-related symptoms such as numbness or weakness in addition to pain.[29] It is generally not possible to definitively distinguish malignant from benign tumors on physical examination alone.

37.3 Diagnosis and Evaluation

In cases of a suspected intraoral minor salivary gland malignancy, workup includes a full history and thorough head and

Table 37.1 World Health Organization 2017 classification of salivary gland tumors with ICD-O codes

Malignant:

- Mucoepidermoid carcinoma
- Adenoid cystic carcinoma
- Acinic cell carcinoma
- Polymorphous adenocarcinoma[a]
- Clear cell carcinoma
- Basal cell adenocarcinoma
- Intraductal carcinoma
- Adenocarcinoma, NOS
- Salivary duct carcinoma
- Myoepithelial carcinoma
- Epithelial-myoepithelial carcinoma
- Carcinoma ex pleomorphic adenoma
- Secretory carcinoma
- Sebaceous adenocarcinoma
- Carcinosarcoma
- Poorly differentiated carcinoma
  - Undifferentiated carcinoma
  - Large-cell neuroendocrine carcinoma
  - Small-cell neuroendocrine carcinoma
- Lymphoepithelial carcinoma
- Squamous cell carcinoma
- Oncocytic carcinoma
- *Uncertain malignant potential*: Sialoblastoma

Benign tumors:

- Pleomorphic adenoma
- Myoepithelioma
- Basal cell adenoma
- Warthin's tumor
- Oncocytoma
- Lymphadenoma
- Cystadenoma
- Sialadenoma papilliferum
- Ductal papillomas
- Sebaceous adenoma
- Canalicular adenoma and other ductal adenomas

Nonneoplastic epithelial lesions:

- Sclerosing polycystic adenosis
- Nodular oncocytic hyperplasia
- Lymphoepithelial sialadenitis
- Intercalated duct hyperplasia

Benign soft-tissue lesions:

- Hemangioma
- Lipoma/sialolipoma
- Nodular fasciitis

Hematolymphoid tumors:

- Extranodal marginal zone lymphoma of mucosa-associated lymphoid tissue (MALT lymphoma)

(Adapted from: Tumours of Salivary Glands. In: El-Naggar A, Chan JKC, Grandis JR, Takata T, Slootweg PJ, eds. WHO Classification of Head and Neck Tumors, 2017:159–202.)

[a]Formerly known as "polymorphous low-grade adenocarcinoma."

neck physical examination, with special attention to any signs of local invasion or regional spread. Imaging studies and pathologic evaluation are critical for further assessment and treatment planning.

37.3.1 Differential Diagnosis

The differential diagnosis for oral cavity lesions includes a wide array of benign and inflammatory processes such as mucoceles, fibromas, granulomas, etc. as well as benign minor salivary gland lesions, the most common of which is pleomorphic adenoma (▸ Table 37.1).[3] Other malignant neoplasms include the more common mucosal squamous cell carcinoma, and rarely, lymphoma, metastases from other primary tumors, or mesenchymal malignant tumors, such as malignant schwannoma, malignant fibrous histiocytoma, and rhabdomyosarcoma.[30]

37.3.2 Considerations for Biopsy of Suspected Malignancy

The role of biopsy in the workup of intraoral salivary gland neoplasms is to (1) establish the tissue of origin (e.g., salivary gland versus mucosal lesion or lymphoma), and (2) determine whether the tumor is benign or malignant in order to guide surgical planning and patient counseling. Although it is useful for the surgeon to know the histologic subtype and grade of malignancy, this is not always possible if tissue sampling is limited. A small biopsy specimen may preclude evaluation of important pathological features such as infiltrative growth and tissue architecture that are necessary to differentiate tumor types.[31] Many salivary gland tumors have heterogenous growth patterns, and histologic features may be shared amongst several tumor types, thus increasing diagnostic complexity. A possible exception is mucoepidermoid carcinoma, which can often be diagnosed even with a scant tissue sample.[31]

Core needle, punch, and incisional biopsies provide more tissue for pathologic evaluation than fine-needle aspiration cytology (FNAC),[32] and for salivary gland neoplasms arising in the oral cavity, these biopsies are often readily attainable. Whereas incisional biopsy is rarely recommended for major salivary gland tumors given their proximity to important neural structures, and risk of tumor spillage for pleomorphic adenomas in particular; there is typically less risk associated with such biopsies for intraoral minor salivary gland neoplasms due to their location. Ultrasound guidance, which is often useful for major gland masses, is rarely necessary for oral cavity neoplasms. Although there is a concern for tumor seeding in cases of pleomorphic adenoma that may give pause to clinicians considering biopsy of a suspected salivary gland neoplasm, there are very few such reported cases attributed to FNAC or core needle biopsies.[32,33] Excisional biopsy is not recommended due to high rates of positive margins and increased difficulty of planning or undertaking the definitive resection.[7]

37.3.3 Imaging Studies and Extent of Disease Evaluation

Imaging studies are indicated to evaluate the local extent of the tumor with regard to surgical resectability, and for extent of disease evaluation, for example, to assess for cervical lymphadenopathy and/or distant metastases.

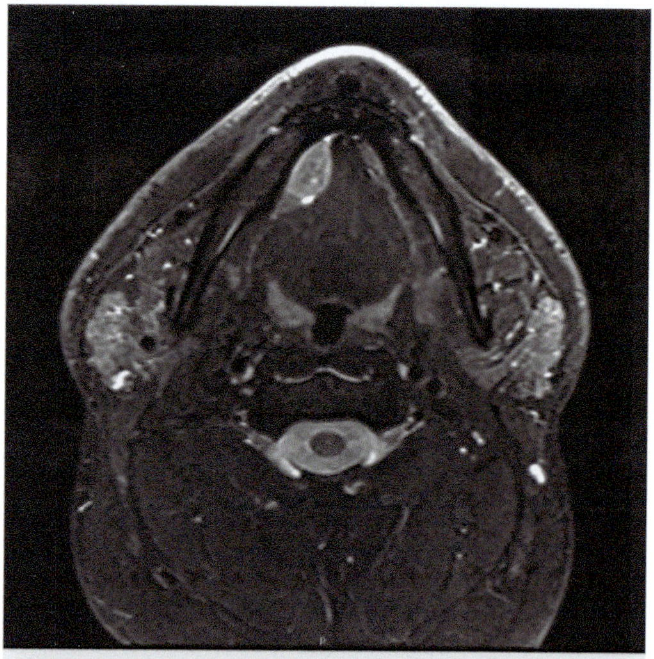

Fig. 37.3 Magnetic resonance image of right sublingual gland low-grade malignancy in an asymptomatic 27-year-old man, noted incidentally during dental examination.

Magnetic resonance imaging (MRI) with gadolinium contrast enhancement is the imaging modality of choice for evaluation of salivary gland tumors and provides valuable information regarding local tumor spread and perineural invasion (▸ Fig. 37.3). Characteristics that suggest a high-grade salivary malignancy include invasion of adjacent structures, irregular or poorly defined borders, low signal on T2 images, heterogeneous enhancement, and central tumor necrosis.[30]

In addition to tumor characteristics observable on standard MRI, evolving MRI techniques have allowed for increasingly accurate prediction of tumor biology. Apparent diffusion coefficients (ADC) on diffusion-weighted imaging (DWI) can give valuable clues as to whether a tumor is benign or malignant, and it can even suggest a specific histology and grade. Multiple studies have reported a lower ADC for malignant tumors compared with benign tumors. Lower ADC is attributed to the restricted diffusion of water protons through tumors with cytotoxic edema and high cellularity compared with normal tissues and vasogenic edema.[34,35] The sensitivity, specificity, and positive and negative predictive values of DWI for identifying malignant versus benign salivary gland tumors have been reported at 91 to 100%.[34,36] Dynamic contrast-enhanced (DCE) MRI is another technique that measures tumor enhancement over time and gives additional parameters that can help distinguish malignant from benign tumors.[30] It is recommended that DWI and DCE be added to MRI with contrast in the workup of intraoral minor salivary gland tumors whenever possible.

A limitation of MRI is its ability to evaluate bony detail. Computed tomography (CT) scanning provides excellent bony resolution, therefore a CT scan can be a valuable adjunct to MRI in cases of questionable bone involvement (▸ Fig. 37.4a). Contrast-

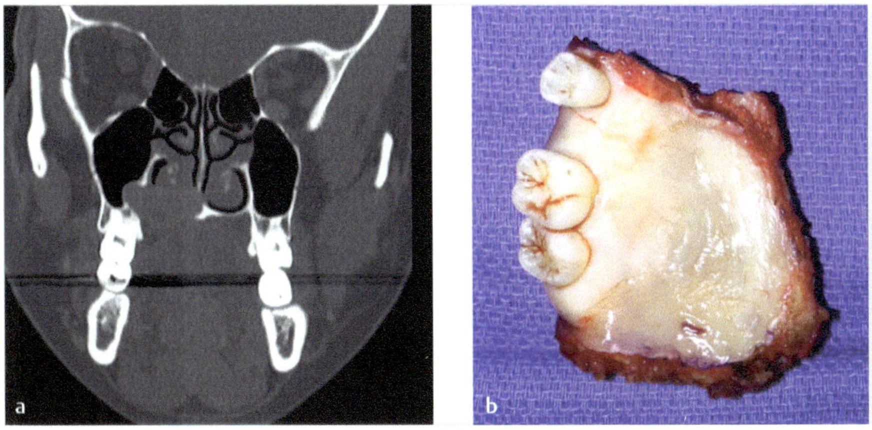

Fig. 37.4 Polymorphous adenocarcinoma variant noted incidentally in a 53-year-old woman. **(a)** Computed tomography image showing bone erosion into right maxillary sinus. **(b)** Composite resection of maxillary alveolus and hard palate.

enhanced CT scan can also provide soft tissue evaluation in patients with contraindications to MRI, such as those with pacemakers or other implants. ^{18}fluorodeoxyglucose (FDG) positron emission tomography (PET)-CT is not always useful for distinguishing benign versus malignant salivary gland diseases because some benign tumors may demonstrate PET avidity.[30]

Approximately 15% of patients with minor salivary gland malignancies have cervical lymph node metastases.[11,26,37] The cervical lymph nodes should be included in any head and neck imaging study so that the neck is evaluated for possible regional nodal involvement. Distant metastases are not uncommon in certain minor salivary gland malignancies and develop in 15 to 30% of patients, with the highest risk among those with high-grade tumors and with clinically positive cervical lymph nodes.[38,39] The lungs are the most common site for distant metastasis, and should be evaluated as part of the initial workup with a noncontrast chest CT scan or chest radiograph, or other imaging modality.[30] Adenoid cystic carcinoma, in particular, has a well-described propensity for lung metastases that may develop in > 50% of patients[1] even in the absence of involved neck lymph nodes.[38,40]

Other less common sites of distant metastases are the liver, bone, and distant lymph nodes.[38] Additional evaluation for distant metastatic disease outside of the lungs and in the absence of symptoms, however, is not standard. ^{18}FDG PET-CT has been shown in recent studies to change management for a subset of patients (15–40% of reported cohorts) with salivary gland malignancies in whom distant metastatic disease is identified using this imaging modality. Most of these cases represented a transition in the goals of management from curative to palliative intent with the discovery of distant metastases (see later discussion of distant metastases).[18,41–44] FDG PET-CT is not yet routinely recommended as part of initial staging, but may become so in the future if it is consistently shown both to change management and be cost-effective.

37.3.4 Molecular Alterations

Recent advances in molecular testing offer an unprecedented understanding of the genetic alterations that underlie salivary gland malignancies, holding promise for increased diagnostic accuracy as well as therapeutic targeting and improved prognostic information. In particular, a number of salivary gland malignancies harbor specific genetic translocations (▶ Table 37.2). Up to 80% of adenoid cystic carcinomas have a t(6;9)(q22–23;p23–24) rearrangement resulting in a *MYB-NFIB* fusion gene, which is a useful ancillary diagnostic test. Approximately 40 to 80% of mucoepidermoid carcinomas have t(11;19)(q21;p13) rearrangement resulting in *CRTC1-MAML2* fusion gene that may be associated with less aggressive disease and improved prognosis in both low- and high-grade mucoepidermoid carcinomas. Nearly all mammary analogue secretory carcinomas harbor t(12;15)(p13;q25) rearrangement with *ETV6-NTRK3* fusion. Although these genetic alterations are currently useful primarily for diagnostic purposes, future research may shed light on their potential roles as therapeutic targets.[45]

37.3.5 Staging, Grading and Prognosis

Malignant minor salivary gland neoplasms have a generally favorable prognosis with mean survival of over 10 years, but there are aggressive exceptions such as high-grade mucoepidermoid carcinoma and adenocarcinoma.[1,8] Expected survival related to specific tumor type is displayed in ▶ Table 37.2.

Minor salivary gland malignancies are staged according to the American Joint Committee on Cancer (AJCC) TNM guidelines for squamous cell carcinoma corresponding to their site of origin;[49] for example, the oral cavity staging guideline is used for the intraoral tumors considered in this chapter.[1] AJCC staging has consistently been shown to be strongly prognostic in multivariate models,[7,8,12,37,39] and in most studies is a more robust predictor of prognosis than histologic subtype or grade.

Although staging remains the most reliable prognostic factor overall, tumor grading is also relevant for select histopathologic tumor types, most notably mucoepidermoid carcinoma and adenocarcinoma, NOS.[11] Both histologies are categorized into low, intermediate, and high grade.[1] High-grade mucoepidermoid carcinoma has been shown to have worse prognosis than low- and intermediate-grade tumors, with 5-year overall survival rates of 56% compared with 94 and 91%, respectively. This survival difference persists even after adjustment for other factors including clinical stage.[12] Adenocarcinoma NOS has reported 15-year survival rates of 54, 31 and 3% for low-, intermediate-, and high-grade tumors, respectively.[1] For both histologies, tumor grade is also a significant predictor of lymph node metastases.[11]

Table 37.2 Characteristics of common intraoral minor salivary malignancies.[1,7,8,12,24–27,45–48]

Characteristic	Mucoepidermoid carcinoma	Adenoid cystic carcinoma	Polymorphous adenocarcinoma	Adenocarcinoma, NOS	Acinic cell carcinoma
General	Low- and intermediate-grade indolent; high-grade aggressive with poor prognosis	Slow-growing but relentless and locally aggressive, tendency for perineural invasion and distant metastases	Previously known as polymorphous low-grade adenocarcinoma (PLGA); name changed because some can exhibit aggressive clinical behavior, although considered indolent	Epithelial carcinomas not otherwise categorized; includes former cystadenocarcinoma. High grade with worse prognosis	More common in parotid gland. Subset recently reclassified as secretory carcinoma. Typically not aggressive
Percentage of intraoral minor salivary gland malignancies	Up to 60%	Up to 60%	15–26%	7–22%	2–3%
Epidemiology	F:M = 1.5:1 Median age 52 years Most common salivary gland malignancy in children	F:M = 1.5:1 Median age 57 years	F:M = 2:1 Mean age 59 years	Mean age 58 years	F:M = 1.5:1 Mean age 50 years Second most common salivary gland malignancy in children
Clinically relevant histopathologic features	Low, intermediate, and high grade	Solid, cribriform, and tubular growth patterns; > 30% solid growth pattern more aggressive. Perineural invasion common. Rare high-grade transformation	Perineural invasion common. High-grade transformation associated with shorter survival	Low, intermediate, and high grade based on degree of cellular atypia	High-grade transformation associated with shorter survival
Genetic alterations	t(11;19)(q21;p13) translocation and *CRTC1-MAML2* gene fusion in 40–80%	t(6;9) or t(8;9) translocations resulting in fusions of *MYB or MYBL1* oncogenes with transcription factor *NFIB* in > 80%	Hotspot activating point mutations of *PRKD1* (73%)		
Prognosis	10-year OS: low-grade 90%, intermediate-grade 70%, high-grade 25%	10-year OS: 50–70%, 20-year OS: 30–50% Regional mets uncommon. High risk of distant mets (> 50% of cases), usually to the lungs, and may occur many years after treatment	10-year OS: 73%, DSS: 96–99%, RFS: 83%. Regional and distant mets uncommon (9–15% and 4.3%)	15-year OS: 54% for low grade, 31% for intermediate grade, and 3% for high grade	20-year OS: 90%

Abbreviations: DSS, disease-specific survival; OS, overall survival; RFS, recurrence-free survival.

In the case of adenoid cystic carcinoma, histologic pattern is indicative of tumor aggressiveness and outcome. Adenoid cystic carcinomas with tubular and cribriform growth patterns tend to be less aggressive than those with a component of solid growth pattern. Typically more than one-third of solid growth pattern is necessary to classify a tumor as having a solid growth pattern, but this may vary by report.[1,7,50] Whether histologic pattern adds significant prognostic information to tumor stage is unclear.[50,51]

Multiple other prognostic factors have been identified for minor salivary gland malignancies. A recent large study of 639 oral cavity minor salivary gland cancers included in the Surveillance, Epidemiology, and End Results (SEER) database from 1988 to 2005 with mean overall survival of 139 months found that N stage was the most robust predictor of survival, followed by T stage, advanced age, and male gender.[8] Other reported adverse prognostic features include positive surgical margins, perineural invasion, and vascular invasion.[7] The way tumor histology contributes to independent prognostic information, after adjustment for other factors, varies among published series. Although several large studies did not find significant survival differences,[8,52] other analyses have demonstrated worse overall or recurrence-free survival for specific tumor histologies, most notably adenoid cystic carcinoma.[26,53]

37.4 Anatomic Considerations

Minor salivary glands are composed of unencapsulated acinar units with serous and/or mucinous cells, with a short duct. These glands line the entire oral cavity including the hard palate, buccal mucosa, floor of mouth, and tongue. The sublingual glands are considered major salivary glands but are often categorized together with minor salivary glands. Most minor salivary glands are mixed serous and mucinous, with the exception of some purely mucinous hard palate glands and the purely serous Von Ebner's glands that are located near the circumvallate papilla.[54] The posterior hard palate harbors the highest concentration of minor salivary glands, which is congruent with the fact that it is the most common site of minor salivary gland malignancies.[55]

There are important anatomical considerations when managing minor salivary gland malignancies of the oral cavity due to the variety of proximate structures and their functional significance in speaking, swallowing, and maintaining airway patency. Tumors of the hard palate can require through-and-through resection of oral mucosa, bone, and sinonasal mucosa resulting in communication between the oral cavity and nasal cavity or paranasal sinuses. The resultant defect may be managed with either a reconstructive surgical procedure or obturation with a prosthesis (▸ Fig. 37.4 and ▸ Fig. 37.5). Tumors that require soft palate excision increase the risk of velopharyngeal insufficiency. Tumors involving the tongue can result in significant difficulties with the oral phase of swallowing and with articulation, depending on the extent of tongue resection required. The floor of mouth and lateral tongue contain important neurovascular structures including the lingual and hypoglossal nerves and the lingual artery with its branches. The not only mandible has the obvious functional role of bearing teeth for chewing, but also is critical for maintaining airway patency through suspension of the tongue and floor of mouth soft tissues. Reconstructive surgeons should be consulted and rehabilitative services provided as indicated (see chapters on reconstruction and rehabilitation).

An understanding of the neural anatomy of the oral cavity is particularly important when treating adenoid cystic carcinoma, with its propensity for perineural spread. For example, adenoid cystic carcinomas of the hard palate may follow the greater palatine nerve superiorly through the greater palatine foramen into the nasal cavity toward the pterygopalatine ganglion; those of the posterior mandible or retromolar trigone may involve the inferior alveolar nerve; and tumors of the lateral floor of mouth may invade the lingual nerve.[56] Preoperative MRI is useful in evaluating perineural spread, and a CT scan may show enlarged neural foramina.[56] Surgeons may need to follow nerves further than expected to achieve complete surgical resection of the tumor. Frozen section pathology is useful intraoperatively to assess perineural spread and to achieve negative surgical margins.

37.5 Management

The treatment of choice for oral cavity minor salivary gland tumors of all histologies is complete surgical resection, with the assumption that postoperative radiation therapy will be given to select patients who have tumors with adverse features. This recommendation is based on heterogenous studies that generally include an array of tumor histologies, stages, and sites. The rarity of minor salivary gland malignancies unfortunately has precluded rigorous randomized controlled trials.[57] Radiation therapy alone, or with chemotherapy, may be used for unresectable tumors or for palliative therapy. Neck dissection is indicated for clinically N-positive necks and the neck may also be treated in other situations, depending on the characteristics of the primary tumor.

37.5.1 Tumor Excision

Tumor resectability to clear surgical margins is guided by clinical features, preoperative imaging studies, and intraoperative findings. There are no universally agreed upon, ideal surgical margins for minor salivary gland tumors due to a lack of large case series, and therefore, the surgeon must exercise sound judgment for each individual tumor. In general, surgical management should be balanced, aggressive enough to obtain clear surgical margins but not overly morbid when all gross disease has been removed. High-grade tumors such as mucoepidermoid carcinoma or adenocarcinoma NOS are often treated similar to mucosal squamous cell carcinomas, with a goal of a 1-cm surgical margin where possible. Adenoid cystic carcinoma is an exception and may require a wider margin of 1.5 cm due to its propensity for perineural spread, with frozen section evaluation of any involved named nerves. Some authors recommend wider margins, up to 2 to 3 cm.[26] Less than 5 mm margins on final pathology are often considered "close."[58] Unfortunately, negative margins can be difficult to achieve in some minor salivary gland tumors, particularly in the case of adenoid cystic carcinomas due to perineural spread, and case series report rates of positive surgical margins up to 40 to 64%.[13,52,59] The presence of positive surgical margins has been reported as a negative prognostic factor,[12,27,60,61] indicative of aggressive disease. Reoperation should be considered for

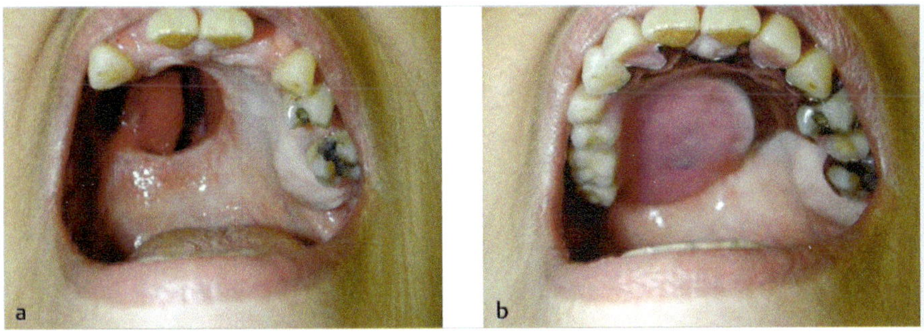

Fig. 37.5 **(a)** Through-and-through composite resection of a hard palate tumor resulting in communication with the sinonasal cavity. **(b)** Obturator in place to separate sinonasal and oral cavities.

positive margins. For close margins, postoperative radiation therapy may be recommended.[62]

37.5.2 Bone Resection

Deep margins in the oral cavity often involve bone of the hard palate or mandibular or maxillary alveolus, which may be approached differently depending on tumor histology. Bone resection can carry significant functional consequences. There are no well-described guidelines for bone resection. Tumor stage and histology should be taken into account, and in situations with little historical data to guide treatment decisions, paradigms developed for mucosal squamous cell carcinoma are often adapted, that is, the presence of bone invasion should be treated with composite resection of a margin of bone with the soft tissue (▶ Fig. 37.4).[62]

An exception to this general rule may be low-grade mucoepidermoid carcinoma, which is relatively indolent with low rates of perineural spread and local recurrence.[57] Several case series have described soft tissue and periosteum excision, leaving hard palate bone intact in cases of low- and intermediate-grade mucoepidermoid carcinomas where there is no radiographic or intraoperative visual evidence of bony erosion,[63,64] with recurrence rates approaching 0% in these series.[58]

Adenoid cystic carcinoma of the hard palate, in contrast, is very difficult to control locally given its propensity to spread along periosteum and nerves, with a high local recurrence rate of 23%.[65] Therefore, consideration should be given to resection of bone even when not grossly involved with tumor.[57,58] Polymorphous adenocarcinoma (formerly polymorphous low-grade adenocarcinoma) also has a relatively high local recurrence rate of 19% in a large series of 456 cases, 60% of which originated on the palate,[66] prompting the recommendation for bone resection in these cases.[58]

37.5.3 Sublingual Gland Neoplasms

Sublingual gland neoplasms should be resected completely. For small neoplasms, a transoral approach is usually sufficient. Larger tumors may require a combined external approach or a mandibulotomy for surgical access. Resection may require lingual nerve resection, partial glossectomy, submandibular gland resection, or segmental mandibulectomy. If the submandibular gland is preserved, a submandibular duct sialodochoplasty should be performed. Defect reconstruction is variable depending on the size and nature of the defect. Options include split thickness skin graft, platysma flap, and free tissue transfer.

37.5.4 Management of Cervical Lymph Nodes

Clinical metastases to the cervical lymph nodes are uncommon in oral cavity minor salivary gland malignancies and are present in approximately 15% of cases. Their presence is associated with poor prognosis.[8,11] A SEER analysis of 2,667 minor salivary gland malignancies in oral cavity and other sites found that independent predictors of nodal metastases included T3-T4 stage, male gender, and high-grade adenocarcinoma or high-grade mucoepidermoid carcinoma histologies. Grade was not predictive of N stage for other histologic types.[11] Similarly, an analysis of 530 mucoepidermoid carcinomas in the National Cancer Database found that predictors of occult nodal disease were high tumor grade and T stage of T3–T4, both of which were associated with approximately six-fold increased risk of occult nodal disease compared with low grade or T1–T2 tumors.[12]

Cervical lymph node metastases are generally regarded as uncommon in adenoid cystic carcinoma, but occult nodal disease has been detected in up to 15% of cases, leading some to recommend consideration of elective neck dissection in certain instances.[67,68] It is not known whether elective neck dissection in adenoid cystic carcinoma improves survival compared with the more commonly accepted strategy of planned postoperative radiation therapy to the cervical lymph nodes.[68]

Based on the available evidence, reasonable recommendations for management of the neck seem to be the following. Comprehensive neck dissection is indicated in case of clinically evident cervical lymph node metastases. Elective neck treatment for possible occult metastases should be considered in T3–T4 or high-grade tumors. This may consist of either selective neck dissection or postoperative radiation therapy, particularly in cases where high-grade features may not be evident until the final pathologic evaluation, and should address levels I–III of the neck. Either observation or elective neck treatment is reasonable in cases of small T1–T2 tumors that are of low grade.[57]

37.5.5 Radiation Therapy

Although postoperative radiation therapy has not been evaluated in a randomized, controlled trial, the data from retrospective cohorts studies and data extrapolated from major salivary gland studies support the use of radiation therapy in patients with high-risk tumors.[13,24,52,69] According to the National Comprehensive Cancer Network Guidelines (NCCN; Version 1.2018), postoperative radiation therapy is indicated as adjuvant treatment after surgical excision of minor salivary gland tumors in cases of high- or intermediate-grade tumors, adenoid cystic carcinoma, positive or close margins, lymph node metastases, perineural or lymphovascular invasion, and T3–T4 tumors.[62]

Most available cohort studies demonstrate control rates of surgery with postoperative radiation therapy among high-risk patients that are comparable to those for surgery alone in low-risk patients. A study of 103 patients with minor salivary gland carcinoma of the hard palate reported 5-year recurrence-free survival of 64% versus 67.5% for patients undergoing surgery alone (low-risk tumors) versus surgery plus radiation therapy (high-risk tumors; $p = 0.76$).[24] Importantly, in a recent analysis of 2,222 minor salivary gland tumors of all sites that are included in the SEER database from 1988 to 2008, 58% of which originated in the oral cavity, one-third (724, 33%) of patients underwent postoperative radiation therapy. After adjustment for other prognostic factors, treatment with radiation therapy was associated with a 24% decreased risk of death; propensity matched scoring revealed that radiation therapy only conferred a survival benefit for high-risk patients, for example, those with T3/T4 disease, positive cervical lymph nodes, and adenoid cystic carcinoma histology.[53]

Radiation therapy doses are typically 60 to 70 Gy to the postoperative primary site, with 54 to 60 Gy to the cervical lymph nodes.[13,69] Although radiation therapy sequelae, such as mucositis and dermatitis, occur in over two-thirds of patients, toxicities have decreased with the introduction of intensity-modulated radiation therapy.[52]

There is no proven role for systemic therapy in minor salivary gland malignancy treatment; however, chemotherapy may be considered along with radiation therapy for unresectable or very high-risk disease, or for patients with distant metastases (see next section on distant metastases).[62] The impact on survival of adding cisplatin to radiation therapy alone is currently under investigation in a randomized clinical trial (RTOG 1008).

37.5.6 Distant Metastases

The presence of distant metastases portends a poor prognosis for most minor salivary gland malignancies. Patients with distant metastases from mucoepidermoid carcinomas have just a 9% 5-year overall survival, compared with 88% for those without distant metastases.[12] Adenoid cystic carcinoma, which accounts for 60% of distant metastatic salivary gland malignancies, can be an exception.[70] Some patients with distant adenoid cystic carcinoma metastases, which are most often found in the lungs, can live for 10 years or more. Still, approximately one-third of these patients die of disease within 2 years of developing metastases, with a median survival of 3 years.[71] Therefore, the approach to patients with distant metastatic disease must be individualized.

The detection of distant metastases from nonadenoid cystic carcinoma histologies generally signals a transition from curative to palliative intent of treatment. Systemic therapy is commonly offered at the time of diagnosis in these cases, although there is scant evidence from small and heterogenous studies to guide agent choice for individual histologies.[70] If tumors are symptomatic and causing significant pain or disfigurement, surgery and/or radiation therapy to the primary site may also be offered at the discretion of the treating team if symptom palliation is thought to be likely.

In contrast, when adenoid cystic carcinoma distant metastases are diagnosed, initial observation is often favored rather than immediate systemic therapy, due to the typically indolent progression of metastases and the toxicities associated with chemotherapy. Lung metastases seem to exhibit slower disease progression than metastases at other sites. Surgery with radiation therapy for primary disease control and symptom palliation is frequently offered in these cases despite the presence of distant metastases, as patients may survive for many years. Consideration of systemic therapy is reserved for cases of rapidly progressive or symptomatic distant metastatic disease, with variable results. Systemic therapy for adenoid cystic carcinoma remains unsatisfactory with low response rates and no proven increase in survival or quality of life despite reports of symptom relief.[70,71] Although adenoid cystic carcinoma has been studied more extensively than other histologies, there are still limited data to guide agent choice, with a lack of phase III randomized trials.[70] The most commonly used combination based on available data is cisplatin and anthracycline.[70,71] Metastasectomy or local radiation therapy can also be considered for amenable isolated metastases.

In summary, the management of patients with distant metastases from minor salivary gland malignancies should take into account the tumor histology, disease-related symptoms, treatment toxicities, and patient factors such as preferences, comorbidities, and performance status. Importantly, efforts should be made to enroll patients with distant metastatic disease into clinical trials, especially as the fields of targeted therapeutics and immunotherapy evolve.[62,72,73]

37.5.7 Posttreatment Follow-up

Although prognosis is generally favorable after treatment for minor salivary gland malignancies, locoregional and distant recurrences can occur many years after the primary treatment. Adenoid cystic carcinoma in particular is known for its tendency to recur long after treatment, with falling survival rates 10, 20, and even 30 years posttreatment. Recurrence often manifests as distant metastases to the lungs, leading many to consider adenoid cystic carcinoma an essentially incurable disease.[68] For these reasons, it is emphasized that patients with minor salivary gland malignancies should undergo history and physical examination at least yearly for the rest of their lives, in addition to the standard NCCN head and neck cancer follow-up recommendations.[62]

37.6 Treatment Sequelae

The sequelae of treatment for minor salivary gland malignancies are widely variable depending on the extent and location of surgery, and whether adjuvant radiation therapy was given. Complications in the postoperative period can include wound infection and orocutaneous fistulas. Severe soft tissue edema after large resections with free tissue transfer can cause airway obstruction, such that a tracheostomy should be considered at the time of surgery in select patients. Iatrogenic communications between the oral cavity and sinonasal cavity can cause swallowing and speech deficits, and require either obturation or surgical reconstruction (▸ Fig. 37.5). In the longer term, extensive resections can result in significant swallowing difficulties due to impaired tongue mobility and tethering, and decreased sensation if the lingual or glossopharyngeal nerves were resected. Speech articulation may be affected for the same reasons, and velopharyngeal insufficiency can result from soft palate resection.[74]

Postoperative radiation therapy is associated with both short- and long-term toxicities. In the short term, mucositis and dermatitis contribute to odynophagia. In the long term, xerostomia and taste impairment are common complaints.[7] Fibrosis of the pharyngeal constrictors and tongue musculature as well as trismus can further impair swallow function. Speech-language pathologists should be involved in the care of such patients.[75] Osteoradionecrosis (ORN) of the mandible is a rare but serious late sequela of radiation therapy to the oral cavity. ORN can cause pathologic fractures and chronic pain. It is usually treated conservatively with hyperbaric oxygen therapy; however, surgical resection with reconstruction may be required. Post-radiation therapy patients are also at risk for dental caries and periodontal disease, and should be routinely evaluated by dental providers familiar with radiation therapy-related dental sequelae.[76,77]

37.7 Conclusion

Minor salivary gland malignancies of the oral cavity are most commonly mucoepidermoid carcinoma or adenoid cystic carcinoma, but may also include a wide variety of less common histologic types. Tumor stage is by far the most important prognostic factor. Recommended treatment is complete surgical resection, followed by radiation therapy for all but small low-grade tumors. Patients should be closely followed for life after treatment. Advances in molecular genetics have greatly enhanced our understanding of salivary gland tumor biology, and hold future promise for improved diagnostic accuracy and the development of targeted therapeutics and other novel treatments.

Key Points

- Oral cavity salivary gland malignancies are rare and include a remarkable diversity of histopathologic tumor types.
- Mucoepidermoid carcinoma and adenoid cystic carcinoma are the most common histopathologic types of minor salivary gland malignancies in the oral cavity.
- MRI is the imaging study of choice for salivary gland tumors. CT images are useful for assessing bone involvement.
- Oral cavity minor salivary gland tumors are staged according to the AJCC staging system for oral cavity squamous cell carcinomas.
- Stage is the strongest prognostic factor for minor salivary gland tumors.
- The treatment for oral cavity salivary gland malignancies is surgical resection with postoperative radiation for high-risk tumors.
- Neck dissection is indicated for clinically evident cervical lymph node metastases. Elective neck treatment with either neck dissection or radiation therapy may be considered for high-risk tumors.
- High-risk features of minor salivary gland malignancies include high- or intermediate-grade tumors, adenoid cystic carcinoma histopathology, positive or close surgical margins, lymph node metastases, perineural or lymphovascular invasion, and T3–T4 tumors.

References

[1] Tumours of salivary glands. In: El-Naggar A, Chan JKC, Grandis JR, Takata T, Slootweg PJ, eds. WHO Classification of Head and Neck Tumors. 4th ed. 2017:159–202

[2] Seethala RR. Update from the 4th Edition of the World Health Organization Classification of Head and Neck Tumours: Preface. Head and Neck Pathology. 2017; 11(1):1–2

[3] Pires FR, Pringle GA, de Almeida OP, Chen SY. Intra-oral minor salivary gland tumors: a clinicopathological study of 546 cases. Oral Oncol. 2007; 43(5): 463–470

[4] Oh YS, Russell MS, Eisele DW. Salivary Gland Neoplasms. In: Johnson JT, Rosen CA, eds. Bailey's Head and Neck Surgery: Otolaryngology 2014

[5] Renehan A, Gleave EN, Hancock BD, Smith P, McGurk M. Long-term follow-up of over 1000 patients with salivary gland tumours treated in a single centre. Br J Surg. 1996; 83(12):1750–1754

[6] Oh YS, Russell MS, Eisele D. Salivary gland neoplasms. In: Johnson JT, Rosen CA, eds. Bailey's Head and Neck Surgery: Otolaryngology. Vol Two. Philadelphia, PA: Lippincott Williams & Wilkins; 2014

[7] Vander Poorten V, Hunt J, Bradley PJ, et al. Recent trends in the management of minor salivary gland carcinoma. Head Neck. 2014; 36(3):444–455

[8] Kakarala K, Bhattacharyya N. Survival in oral cavity minor salivary gland carcinoma. Otolaryngol Head Neck Surg. 2010; 143(1):122–126

[9] Seethala RR. An update on grading of salivary gland carcinomas. Head Neck Pathol. 2009; 3(1):69–77

[10] Spitz MR, Batsakis JG. Major salivary gland carcinoma. Descriptive epidemiology and survival of 498 patients. Arch Otolaryngol. 1984; 110(1): 45–49

[11] Lloyd S, Yu JB, Ross DA, Wilson LD, Decker RH. A prognostic index for predicting lymph node metastasis in minor salivary gland cancer. Int J Radiat Oncol Biol Phys. 2010; 76(1):169–175

[12] Ellis MA, Graboyes EM, Day TA, Neskey DM. Prognostic factors and occult nodal disease in mucoepidermoid carcinoma of the oral cavity and oropharynx: An analysis of the National Cancer Database. Oral Oncol. 2017; 72:174–178

[13] Garden AS, Weber RS, Ang KK, Morrison WH, Matre J, Peters LJ. Postoperative radiation therapy for malignant tumors of minor salivary glands. Outcome and patterns of failure. Cancer. 1994; 73(10):2563–2569

[14] Sarmento DJ, Morais ML, Costa AL, Silveira EJ. Minor intraoral salivary gland tumors: a clinical-pathological study. Einstein (Sao Paulo). 2016; 14(4):508–512

[15] Swanson GM, Burns PB. Cancers of the salivary gland: workplace risks among women and men. Ann Epidemiol. 1997; 7(6):369–374

[16] Horn-Ross PL, Ljung BM, Morrow M. Environmental factors and the risk of salivary gland cancer. Epidemiology. 1997; 8(4):414–419

[17] Zheng W, Shu XO, Ji BT, Gao YT. Diet and other risk factors for cancer of the salivary glands:a population-based case-control study. Int J Cancer. 1996; 67 (2):194–198

[18] Land CE, Saku T, Hayashi Y, et al. Incidence of salivary gland tumors among atomic bomb survivors, 1950–1987. Evaluation of radiation-related risk. Radiat Res. 1996; 146(1):28–36

[19] Beal KP, Singh B, Kraus D, Yahalom J, Portlock C, Wolden SL. Radiation-induced salivary gland tumors: a report of 18 cases and a review of the literature. Cancer J. 2003; 9(6):467–471

[20] Saluja K, Butler RT, Pytynia KB, et al. Mucoepidermoid carcinoma post-radioactive iodine treatment of papillary thyroid carcinoma: unique presentation and putative etiologic association. Hum Pathol. 2017; 68:189–192

[21] Galer C, Santillan AA, Chelius D, et al. Minor salivary gland malignancies in the pediatric population. Head Neck. 2012; 34(11):1648–1651

[22] Cockerill CC, Gross BC, Contag S, et al. Pediatric malignant salivary gland tumors: 60 year follow up. Int J Pediatr Otorhinolaryngol. 2016; 88:1–6

[23] Ritwik P, Cordell KG, Brannon RB. Minor salivary gland mucoepidermoid carcinoma in children and adolescents: a case series and review of the literature. J Med Case Reports. 2012; 6:182

[24] Li Q, Zhang XR, Liu XK, et al. Long-term treatment outcome of minor salivary gland carcinoma of the hard palate. Oral Oncol. 2012; 48(5):456–462

[25] Jaber MA. Intraoral minor salivary gland tumors: a review of 75 cases in a Libyan population. Int J Oral Maxillofac Surg. 2006; 35(2):150–154

[26] Lopes MA, Santos GC, Kowalski LP. Multivariate survival analysis of 128 cases of oral cavity minor salivary gland carcinomas. Head Neck. 1998; 20(8):699–706

[27] Mücke T, Robitzky LK, Kesting MR, et al. Advanced malignant minor salivary glands tumors of the oral cavity. Oral Surg Oral Med Oral Pathol Oral Radiol Endod. 2009; 108(1):81–89

[28] Spiro RH. Salivary neoplasms: overview of a 35-year experience with 2,807 patients. Head Neck Surg. 1986; 8(3):177–184

[29] Spiro RH, Huvos AG, Strong EW. Adenoid cystic carcinoma of salivary origin. A clinicopathologic study of 242 cases. Am J Surg. 1974; 128(4): 512–520

[30] Freling N, Crippa F, Maroldi R. Staging and follow-up of high-grade malignant salivary gland tumours: The role of traditional versus functional imaging approaches—A review. Oral Oncol. 2016; 60:157–166

[31] Turk AT, Wenig BM. Pitfalls in the biopsy diagnosis of intraoral minor salivary gland neoplasms: diagnostic considerations and recommended approach. Adv Anat Pathol. 2014; 21(1):1–11

[32] Douville NJ, Bradford CR. Comparison of ultrasound-guided core biopsy versus fine-needle aspiration biopsy in the evaluation of salivary gland lesions. Head Neck. 2013; 35(11):1657–1661

[33] Witt BL, Schmidt RL. Ultrasound-guided core needle biopsy of salivary gland lesions: a systematic review and meta-analysis. Laryngoscope. 2014; 124(3): 695–700

[34] Milad P, Elbegiermy M, Shokry T, et al. The added value of pretreatment DW MRI in characterization of salivary glands pathologies. Am J Otolaryngol. 2017; 38(1):13–20
[35] Habermann CR, Gossrau P, Graessner J, et al. Diffusion-weighted echo-planar MRI: a valuable tool for differentiating primary parotid gland tumors? RoFo Fortschr Geb Rontgenstr Nuklearmed. 2005; 177(7):940–945
[36] Celebi I, Mahmutoglu AS, Ucgul A, Ulusay SM, Basak T, Basak M. Quantitative diffusion-weighted magnetic resonance imaging in the evaluation of parotid gland masses: a study with histopathological correlation. Clin Imaging. 2013; 37(2):232–238
[37] Vander Poorten VL, Balm AJ, Hilgers FJ, Tan IB, Keus RB, Hart AA. Stage as major long term outcome predictor in minor salivary gland carcinoma. Cancer. 2000; 89(6):1195–1204
[38] Bradley PJ. Distant metastases from salivary glands cancer. ORL J Otorhinolaryngol Relat Spec. 2001; 63(4):233–242
[39] Spiro RH, Thaler HT, Hicks WF, Kher UA, Huvos AH, Strong EW. The importance of clinical staging of minor salivary gland carcinoma. Am J Surg. 1991; 162(4):330–336
[40] Spiro RH. Distant metastasis in adenoid cystic carcinoma of salivary origin. Am J Surg. 1997; 174(5):495–498
[41] Park MJ, Oh JS, Roh JL, et al. 18F-FDG PET/CT Versus Contrast-Enhanced CT for Staging and Prognostic Prediction in Patients With Salivary Gland Carcinomas. Clin Nucl Med. 2017; 42(3):e149–e156
[42] Razfar A, Heron DE, Branstetter BF, IV, Seethala RR, Ferris RL. Positron emission tomography-computed tomography adds to the management of salivary gland malignancies. Laryngoscope. 2010; 120(4):734–738
[43] Park HL, Yoo IeR, Lee N, et al. The value of F-18 FDG PET for planning treatment and detecting recurrence in malignant salivary gland tumors: comparison with conventional imaging studies. Nucl Med Mol Imaging. 2013; 47(4): 242–248
[44] Jeong HS, Chung MK, Son YI, et al. Role of 18F-FDG PET/CT in management of high-grade salivary gland malignancies. J Nucl Med. 2007; 48(8):1237–1244
[45] Skálová A, Stenman G, Simpson RHW, et al. The role of molecular testing in the differential diagnosis of salivary gland carcinomas. Am J Surg Pathol. 2018; 42(2):e11–e27
[46] Weinreb I, Piscuoglio S, Martelotto LG, et al. Hotspot activating PRKD1 somatic mutations in polymorphous low-grade adenocarcinomas of the salivary glands. Nat Genet. 2014; 46(11):1166–1169
[47] Elhakim MT, Breinholt H, Godballe C, et al. Polymorphous low-grade adenocarcinoma: a Danish national study. Oral Oncol. 2016; 55:6–10
[48] Patel TD, Vazquez A, Marchiano E, Park RC, Baredes S, Eloy JA. Polymorphous low-grade adenocarcinoma of the head and neck: a population-based study of 460 cases. Laryngoscope. 2015; 125(7):1644–1649
[49] AJCC Cancer Staging Manual 8th edition. 2017
[50] van Weert S, van der Waal I, Witte BI, Leemans CR, Bloemena E. Histopathological grading of adenoid cystic carcinoma of the head and neck: analysis of currently used grading systems and proposal for a simplified grading scheme. Oral Oncol. 2015; 51(1):71–76
[51] Spiro RH, Huvos AG. Stage means more than grade in adenoid cystic carcinoma. Am J Surg. 1992; 164(6):623–628
[52] Zeidan YH, Shultz DB, Murphy JD, et al. Long-term outcomes of surgery followed by radiation therapy for minor salivary gland carcinomas. Laryngoscope. 2013; 123(11):2675–2680
[53] Zeidan YH, Pekelis L, An Y, et al. Survival benefit for adjuvant radiation therapy in minor salivary gland cancers. Oral Oncol. 2015; 51(5):438–445
[54] Hellquist H, Skalova A. Histopathology of the Salivary Glands. Springer; 2014
[55] Myers EN, Ferris RL. Salivary Gland Disorders. Springer Science & Business Media; 2007
[56] Paes FM, Singer AD, Checkver AN, Palmquist RA, De La Vega G, Sidani C. Perineural spread in head and neck malignancies: clinical significance and evaluation with 18F-FDG PET/CT. Radiographics. 2013; 33(6):1717–1736
[57] Lombardi D, McGurk M, Vander Poorten V, et al. Surgical treatment of salivary malignant tumors. Oral Oncol. 2017; 65:102–113
[58] Ord RA, Ghazali N. Margin analysis: malignant salivary gland neoplasms of the head and neck. Oral Maxillofac Surg Clin North Am. 2017; 29(3):315–324
[59] Le QT, Birdwell S, Terris DJ, et al. Postoperative irradiation of minor salivary gland malignancies of the head and neck. Radiother Oncol. 1999; 52 (2):165–171
[60] Li F, Lai ZP, Lin JK, Zhu G, Feng H. Radical treatment strategies improve the long-term outcome of recurrent atypical meningiomas. Chin Med J (Engl). 2011; 124(15):2387–2391
[61] Bjørndal K, Krogdahl A, Therkildsen MH, et al. Salivary gland carcinoma in Denmark 1990–2005: outcome and prognostic factors. Results of the Danish Head and Neck Cancer Group (DAHANCA). Oral Oncol. 2012; 48(2):179–185
[62] Network NCC. Head and Neck Cancers (Version 1.2018). NCCN Clinical Practice Guidelines in Oncology (NCCN Guidelines(R)) https://www.nccn.org/professionals/physician_gls/PDF/head-and-neck.pdf. Accessed March 29, 2018
[63] Eversole LR, Rovin S, Sabes WR. Mucoepidermoid carcinoma of minor salivary glands: report of 17 cases with follow-up. J Oral Surg. 1972; 30(2):107–112
[64] Ord RA, Salama AR. Is it necessary to resect bone for low-grade mucoepidermoid carcinoma of the palate? Br J Oral Maxillofac Surg. 2012; 50(8):712–714
[65] Tran L, Sadeghi A, Hanson D, Ellerbroek N, Calcaterra TC, Parker RG. Salivary gland tumors of the palate: the UCLA experience. Laryngoscope. 1987; 97 (11):1343–1345
[66] Kimple AJ, Austin GK, Shah RN, et al. Polymorphous low-grade adenocarcinoma: a case series and determination of recurrence. Laryngoscope. 2014; 124(12):2714–2719
[67] Lee SY, Kim BH, Choi EC. Nineteen-year oncologic outcomes and the benefit of elective neck dissection in salivary gland adenoid cystic carcinoma. Head Neck. 2014; 36(12):1796–1801
[68] Coca-Pelaz A, Rodrigo JP, Bradley PJ, et al. Adenoid cystic carcinoma of the head and neck—an update. Oral Oncol. 2015; 51(7):652–661
[69] Salgado LR, Spratt DE, Riaz N, et al. Radiation therapy in the treatment of minor salivary gland tumors. Am J Clin Oncol. 2014; 37(5):492–497
[70] Alfieri S, Granata R, Bergamini C, et al. Systemic therapy in metastatic salivary gland carcinomas: a pathology-driven paradigm? Oral Oncol. 2017; 66:58–63
[71] Laurie SA, Ho AL, Fury MG, Sherman E, Pfister DG. Systemic therapy in the management of metastatic or locally recurrent adenoid cystic carcinoma of the salivary glands: a systematic review. Lancet Oncol. 2011; 12(8):815–824
[72] Chang H, Kim JS, Choi YJ, et al. Overexpression of PD-L2 is associated with shorter relapse-free survival in patients with malignant salivary gland tumors. OncoTargets Ther. 2017; 10:2983–2992
[73] Schmitt NC, Kang H, Sharma A. Salivary duct carcinoma: an aggressive salivary gland malignancy with opportunities for targeted therapy. Oral Oncol. 2017; 74:40–48
[74] Zuydam AC, Lowe D, Brown JS, Vaughan ED, Rogers SN. Predictors of speech and swallowing function following primary surgery for oral and oropharyngeal cancer. Clin Otolaryngol. 2005; 30(5):428–437
[75] Murphy BA, Gilbert J. Dysphagia in head and neck cancer patients treated with radiation: assessment, sequelae, and rehabilitation. Semin Radiat Oncol. 2009; 19(1):35–42
[76] Jawad H, Hodson NA, Nixon PJ. A review of dental treatment of head and neck cancer patients, before, during and after radiotherapy: part 2. Br Dent J. 2015; 218(2):69–74
[77] Jawad H, Hodson NA, Nixon PJ. A review of dental treatment of head and neck cancer patients, before, during and after radiotherapy: part 1. Br Dent J. 2015; 218(2):65–68

38 Uncommon Oral Cavity Malignancies

Nicole C. Schmitt

Summary

In addition to squamous cell carcinoma, several other rare tumors can arise in the oral cavity. Detection of these other tumors often requires a high index of suspicion and careful pathologic review. Treatment is tailored to the tumor type but often consists of surgical resection.

Keywords: oral melanoma, sarcoma, lymphoma, Kaposi's sarcoma

38.1 Introduction

Although squamous cell carcinoma and salivary gland carcinomas are by far more common tumors, other malignant tumors including melanoma, sarcomas, and lymphomas can also arise in the oral cavity. These tumors are rare and can often be mistaken for squamous cell carcinoma, so a proper pathologic diagnosis is critical. Most of these uncommon malignancies are treated with comprehensive surgical resection, except for lymphomas and some sarcomas.

38.2 Epidemiology

Given its rarity, epidemiologic data on oral mucosal melanoma (OMM) have been compiled primarily from small case series, database searches, and systematic reviews of the literature. Primary melanoma of the oral cavity is estimated to represent less than 1% of all melanoma cases[1–3] and 0.26% of oral cavity tumors.[4] It is more common in certain geographic areas and ethnic groups, with the highest incidence in Asia and lower incidence in North America and Europe.[4–6] OMM is usually noted in patients in their fourth to sixth decades of life and is exceedingly rare in younger patients.[3,5–7] The etiology of OMM is unclear. Some of these lesions arise de novo, but evolution of a benign pigmented lesion into a melanoma has also been reported.[3,4,8] No environmental risk factors have been identified, though OMM appears to be slightly more common in smokers.[3,7] A variety of genomic alterations have been identified in OMM including mutations in *p53, p16, bcl-2,* and *NRAS*.[3,7] The biology of mucosal melanoma is different in many ways from cutaneous melanoma. OMMs are more likely to have mutations in *c-KIT* and less likely to have mutations in *BRAF*.[3,6,7] There is no definite gender predominance,[1,2,5,6,8] though men with this disease appear more likely to develop distant metastases.[1]

The vast majority of patients will develop distant metastatic disease even when good local control is achieved, and the prognosis is poor.[4,6,7] The 5-year overall survival for OMM is approximately 20%[2] with a range of 13 to 40% in the literature.[3,4,7] Age greater than 55 to 60 years; stage; thickness, ulceration, and mitotic rate of the tumor; positive surgical margins; and nonsurgical therapy are associated with worse survival in OMM.[1–3,5,7] As with other oral cavity lesions, lymphovascular and perineural invasions are also adverse prognostic features in OMM.[7]

Sarcomas of the oral cavity are also relatively rare. Osteosarcoma and rhabdomyosarcoma are seen more frequently, but a number of sarcoma types have been reported to arise in the oral cavity, including Ewing's sarcoma, angiosarcoma, granulocytic sarcoma, leiomyosarcoma, liposarcoma, myeloid sarcoma, malignant fibrous histiocytoma, fibrosarcoma, synovial sarcoma, spindle cell sarcoma, and malignant peripheral nerve sheath tumor.[9–21] These sarcomas can arise in the bone of the mandible/maxilla, temporomandibular joint, muscles, mucosa of the oral cavity, or salivary glands.[22] Osteosarcoma that arises de novo is most frequently seen in patients in their third or fourth decade of life.[20] Rhabdomyosarcoma and Ewing's sarcoma are more common in children or adolescents and rarely seen in adults.[11,23] Characteristics of several sarcoma types previously reported to arise in the oral cavity are listed in ▶ Table 38.1.

Prior radiation is one known risk factor for oral cavity sarcoma, most commonly osteosarcoma. The latency period between radiation and development of osteosarcoma of the mandible is usually 10 years or more.[20,24] Kaposi's sarcoma may be noted in association with human immunodeficiency virus (HIV) infection, though cases in patients without HIV infection have also been reported.[25–28]

While extranodal lymphoma of the head and neck arises most commonly in the lymphoid tissue of Waldeyer's ring, it can also arise in the oral cavity. Intraoral lymphomas are found in patients of all ages,[29–31] though the mean age was 71 years in one series.[32] There is no clear gender predominance.[30,32] Most are B cell lymphomas with aggressive clinical behavior, most commonly diffuse large B cell lymphoma (DLBCL).[32] A particularly aggressive subtype of DLBCL, plasmablastic lymphoma, is most often seen in patients with a history of HIV infection.[33–35] Burkitt's lymphoma may also arise in the oral cavity in endemic areas of Africa or patients with HIV.[32] Less commonly, oral Hodgkin's lymphoma, T cell or NK/T cell lymphomas may develop.[32,36–38] Patients with a history of Sjogren's syndrome may also be at risk for development of oral cavity lymphomas, though these lesions usually arise in the major salivary glands.[39] Sjogren's-associated lymphoma is most commonly mucosa-associated lymphoid tissue (MALT) lymphoma, but this can transform into a more aggressive DLBCL.[39] Given the lymphoma risk, a biopsy should be performed on any solid oral cavity or salivary gland mass in patients with a history of Sjogren's syndrome. Finally, patients who have had bone marrow or solid organ transplants can, on rare occasion, develop posttransplant lymphoproliferative disease (PTLD) of the oral cavity.[40]

38.3 Clinical Presentation

As can be expected, mucosal melanoma of the oral cavity usually presents as a painless, pigmented lesion (▶ Fig. 38.1), though they do often ulcerate and bleed when more advanced.[2,3,5,7,8] The pigment may be black, brown, grey, red or purple, and in some cases the lesions are nonpigmented.[2–4] This may be related to lower levels of pigment production in melanocytes of oral mucosa versus melanocytes of the skin.[5] Similar

Table 38.1 Sarcoma types reported in the oral cavity.[9–21,23–27]

Histology	Typical age at presentation	OC subsites	Risk factors	Behavior	Recommended treatment modalities
Osteosarcoma	3rd/4th decade (de novo), 5th decade (radiation induced)	Mandible, maxilla	Prior radiation	Varies according to histologic grade	Surgery, adjuvant RT or chemotherapy
Rhabdomyosarcoma	Pediatric	Varies	Prior radiation	Aggressive	Surgery, adjuvant RT and/or chemotherapy
Ewing's sarcoma	Adolescence	Mandible, maxilla	Unknown	Aggressive	Chemotherapy followed by surgery; adjuvant RT and/or chemotherapy
Kaposi's sarcoma	Varies	Palate, gingiva, dorsal tongue	HIV infection, immuno-suppression, prior radiation	Varies	Systemic or intralesional chemotherapy, RT
Chondrosarcoma	Varies	Maxilla, TMJ	Maffucci syndrome, Ollier disease	Varies according to histologic grade	Surgery, adjuvant RT
Malignant fibrous histiocytoma/ fibrosarcoma/spindle cell sarcoma	Varies	Varies	Prior radiation	Aggressive	Surgery, adjuvant RT and/or chemotherapy
MPNST	Varies	Mandible, maxilla, lip or buccal mucosa	Prior radiation, NF1	Aggressive	Surgery, adjuvant RT
Liposarcoma	Bimodal (3rd/4th vs. 7th decade)	Buccal mucosa, tongue	Unknown	Indolent	Surgery
Leiomyosarcoma	Varies	Varies	Unknown	Aggressive	Surgery
Angiosarcoma	Varies	Tongue, gingiva	Unknown	Aggressive	Surgery, adjuvant RT and/or chemotherapy
Synovial sarcoma	Varies	Varies	Unknown	Aggressive	Surgery, adjuvant RT and/or chemotherapy
Myeloid sarcoma	Fourth decade	Mandible, maxilla, gingiva, palate	Leukemia or other hematologic malignancies	Aggressive	Systemic therapy
Granulocytic sarcoma	Fourth decade	Varies	History of leukemia	Varies	Systemic therapy for underlying leukemia

Abbreviations: MPNST, malignant peripheral nerve sheath tumor; NF1, neurofibromatosis type 1; RT, radiation therapy; TMJ, temporomandibular joint.

to cutaneous melanomas, OMMs exhibit asymmetry, indistinct borders, and satellite lesions.[5] Because it causes few other symptoms, primary melanoma of the oral cavity often presents at advanced stage.[1] The most common subsites of the oral cavity involved by OMM are the hard palate and gingiva, but other sites including the tongue, floor of mouth, and buccal mucosa may also be involved in rare cases.[1–6,8] Invasion of surrounding soft tissue and bony structures is also common.[3] Mucosal melanomas of the oral cavity are more likely to metastasize to the neck than melanomas of the paranasal sinuses, with rates of nodal metastasis estimated to be 25 to 43%.[3,8] Over half of OMM patients will have regional metastatic disease in the neck upon presentation, while distant metastases are not usually detected until later.[2,8] Common sites of distant metastasis include the lungs, brain, bone, and liver.[5]

Sarcomas of the oral cavity are often rapidly growing lesions, though some may have more indolent behavior.[16] They often present as a painless mass or swelling.[14,15,17,20] Osteosarcomas may present as new mass in a prior radiation field and may be mistaken for osteoradionecrosis.[20,24,41] Other lesions may be mistaken for squamous cell carcinoma, which is far more common. Sarcomas involving the mandible or maxilla may present with loss or mobility of teeth.[20]

Extranodal lymphomas of the oral cavity often arise as a swelling or ulceration in the gingiva, spreading to the mandible, maxilla, or zygoma where they can cause pain and bony destruction,[29–32] as shown in ▶ Fig. 38.2. These lesions can progress rapidly.[29] Lymphomas of the oral cavity are often solitary lesions with no involvement elsewhere; however, many patients will have other bony lesions or disseminated disease.[31]

38.4 Diagnosis and Evaluation

A thorough head and neck examination and biopsy should be done for any suspicious pigmented lesion of the oral cavity to rule out OMM. Immunohistochemical staining for S-100, vimentin, HMB45, and melan-A are important for diagnosis, especially for nonpigmented melanomas that can be mistaken for squamous cell carcinomas.[5–8] As with cutaneous melanoma, tumor thickness appears to be prognostic in OMM and thus should be evaluated when feasible.[5] Magnetic resonance imaging can be quite helpful for delineating the extent of the primary tumor, and computed tomography scan is helpful for imaging the neck. As discussed above, OMM frequently metastasizes to the neck and to distant sites. While most oral melanomas are primary lesions, they can also metastasize to the oral cavity from other sites.[5,42] For both reasons, a positron emission tomography scan to rule out distant disease is crucial. Staging for OMM using traditional staging systems for cutaneous melanoma has been contested, since mucosal melanoma tends to be more aggressive. Thus, cutaneous staging systems may not accurately reflect prognosis in OMM.[3] Various alternative staging systems have been proposed for mucosal melanoma, but none have been widely adopted for this rare disease.[3]

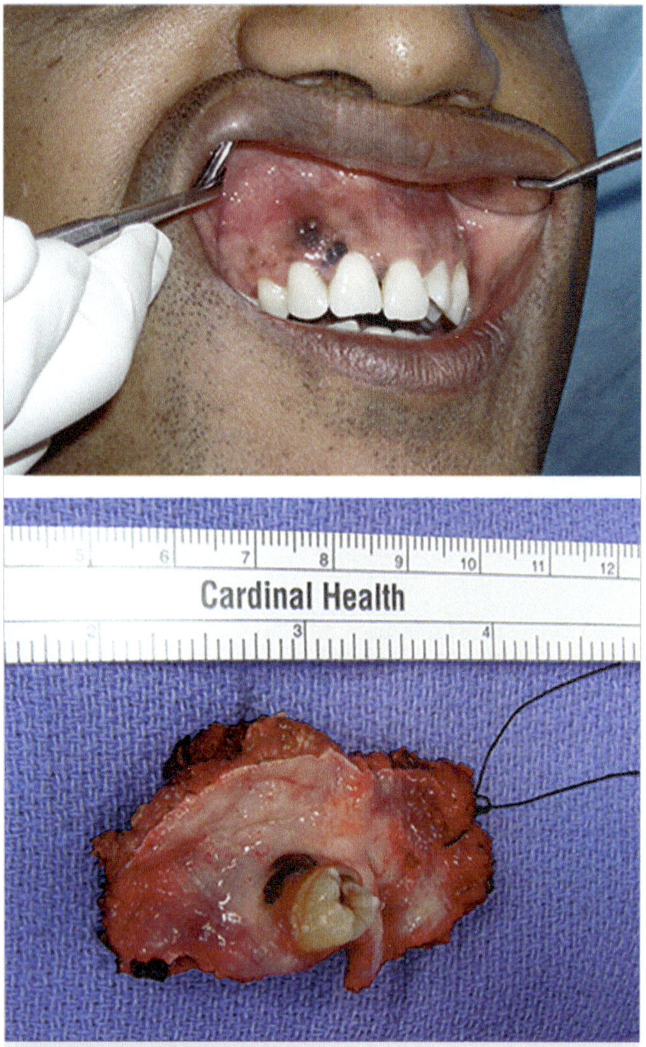

Fig. 38.1 Examples of oral melanoma.

Patients with sarcoma of the oral cavity should have a thorough evaluation for disease elsewhere, as these tumors can metastasize to the oral cavity from other sites and vice versa. Similarly, patients with oral lymphomas may have a solitary oral lesion or disseminated disease, requiring extensive imaging and bone marrow biopsy for staging.[31] Patients with a history of hematologic malignancy can also develop rare sarcomas of the oral cavity.[9,21]

Unusual lesions of the oral cavity may be noted in patients with a history of HIV infection, which may go undiagnosed. In addition to rare and aggressive fungal and bacterial infections of the oral cavity, patients with HIV may develop Kaposi's sarcoma or non-Hodgkin's lymphoma (NHL) in this area.[26,27] These lesions are more common in patients who are not treated with highly active antiretroviral therapy (HAART).[26,27] Intraoral Kaposi's sarcoma can affect a variety of oral cavity subsites and often presents initially as a red or purple macule that grows over time (▶ Fig. 38.3); NHL on the other hand is more often firm, nodular, raised, or ulcerated.[26] Oral Kaposi's sarcoma is sometimes seen in patients with iatrogenic immunosuppression and rarely in patients with normal immune systems.[28]

38.5 Anatomic Considerations/ Relevant Anatomy

The anatomic subsite of OMM may be an important factor, as palate lesions are associated with worse survival than lesions of the gingiva and other oral cavity subsites.[7] Oral cavity sarcomas and lymphomas can affect virtually any subsite of the oral cavity. For lesions involving the maxilla or mandible with bony destruction noted on imaging, osteosarcoma and lymphoma should be in the differential diagnosis. These lesions can have similar appearances on imaging studies[43] (▶ Fig. 38.2).

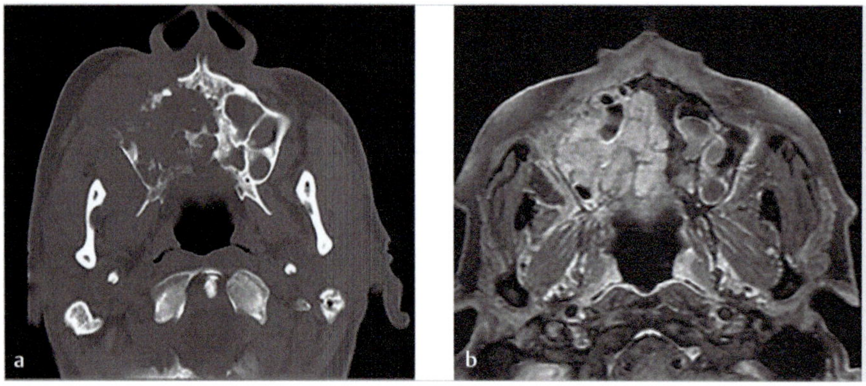

Fig. 38.2 Imaging showing bony destruction by a patient with intraoral diffuse large B cell lymphoma. **(a)** Axial CT scan; **(b)** axial postcontrast T1-weighted magnetic resonance image from the same patient.

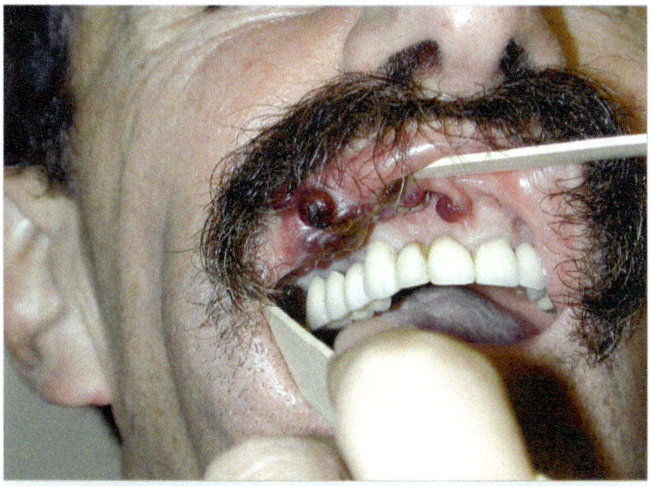

Fig. 38.3 Example of oral Kaposi's sarcoma in a patient with human immunodeficiency virus.

38.6 Treatment Considerations and Approaches

As with other anatomic sites, the mainstay of therapy for melanoma and sarcoma of the oral cavity is surgery. In contrast, lymphoma of the oral cavity is generally treated with chemotherapy, often followed by consolidative radiation therapy.

38.6.1 Surgical Options and Approaches

For OMM, the primary lesion should be surgically resected with generous margins when feasible. Though data are not available to determine the optimal extent of surgical margins for OMM, gross margins of 1.5 to 2 cm are generally recommended.[5,7,8] Given that the most common sites of OMM are the hard palate and maxillary gingiva, this often involves a partial or total maxillectomy. Maxillectomy is discussed in detail in Chapter 29.

Like squamous cell carcinoma of the oral cavity, oral melanoma tends to metastasize to levels Ib to III of the neck, and less commonly to levels IV and V.[2,3] Nodal metastases may be more common for primary tumors with more than 5 mm depth of invasion and for tumors with a more nodular (versus macular) growth pattern.[3,44] Given the relatively high rate of occult metastases on presentation, elective neck dissection of these areas should be considered for both therapeutic and staging purposes.[2,3,6,7] However, there is no definitive evidence that elective neck dissection improves survival in OMM,[5,6] and thus elective neck dissection remains somewhat controversial. In cases where the neck will be accessed for microvascular reconstruction of the primary site, a neck dissection adds little additional morbidity. Sentinel node biopsy may be an alternative but has not been extensively studied in mucosal melanoma.[3,6]

The mainstay of treatment for most sarcomas of the oral cavity is surgery with wide margins when feasible.[20] Neck dissection is often recommended for some more aggressive sarcomas, such as angiosarcoma or leiomyosarcoma, though dissection of the N0 neck is controversial for most sarcoma types.[16,19]

Surgery is not generally recommended for most oral lymphomas, other than to obtain adequate tissue for diagnosis. However, reconstructive surgery may be necessary in cases where lymphoma has caused substantial destruction of bone.[29]

38.6.2 Radiation Therapy

Mucosal melanoma is generally resistant to radiation therapy as primary therapy, and therefore primary radiation therapy should be reserved for unresectable tumors or other situations where surgery is not feasible.[3,6,8] Following surgery for OMM, adjuvant radiotherapy should be strongly considered for most patients with positive nodal disease to improve locoregional control.[5,7,8] Data on mucosal melanoma of the nasal cavity, paranasal sinuses, and oral cavity suggest that adjuvant radiation therapy does not increase overall survival.[6,8] The role of elective neck radiation therapy for the cN0 neck is controversial, with limited data to support its benefit.[6]

Radiation therapy has also been used in the neoadjuvant or adjuvant setting for oral sarcomas, especially in cases with positive margins, though it is unclear whether this has any impact on survival.[10,20] Radiation therapy with concurrent chemotherapy is often used as the primary treatment modality for rhabdomyosarcoma of the head and neck, though accessible lesions of the oral cavity are often treated with a combination of surgery, radiation therapy, and chemotherapy.[11,23]

38.6.3 Medical/Rehabilitative Options

Historically, systemic treatment with cytokines, such as interleukin-2 and interferon alpha, has been used for treatment of oral melanoma with some success especially when used as an adjuvant to surgery.[2,6,8] Chemotherapy may be used for OMM as adjuvant therapy or alone when surgery or radiation therapy are not feasible, with few studies showing any benefit.[2,3,5-8] Results from one study suggest that chemotherapy may be more useful than high-dose interferon as adjuvant therapy following surgery for mucosal melanoma.[45] The tyrosine kinase inhibitor imatinib and other KIT inhibitors may be useful in some cases with *c-KIT* mutations.[3,6] Inhibitors of BRAF may also be used,[3] though these may be less useful given the infrequent *BRAF* mutations in mucosal melanoma.

The treatment of metastatic melanoma has advanced dramatically with the use of antibodies blocking immune checkpoints, including the programmed cell death-1 (PD-1) pathway and cytotoxic T lymphocyte-associated antigen 4 (CTLA-4). Clinical trials using the CTLA-4 inhibitor ipilimumab and including mucosal melanoma have shown some good responses, though the overall response rate has been low.[3] Studies of anti-PD-1 antibodies, used alone or in combination with ipilimumab, have not usually included subgroup analyses of mucosal melanoma but have shown encouraging responses for metastatic melanoma overall.[3]

For oral sarcomas, chemotherapy may be used in the neoadjuvant or adjuvant setting with surgery,[20,24] depending on the histologic subtype. Oral Kaposi's sarcoma is treated primarily with systemic chemotherapy and immunomodulating agents[25] but has also been successfully treated by intralesional injection with vinblastine.[26]

Intraoral lymphoma, including HIV-associated NHL, is treated with multiagent systemic chemotherapy.[25] Though they can behave aggressively, oral lymphomas generally do respond well to chemotherapy.[32] In many cases of oral lymphoma, consolidative radiation therapy is also used following chemotherapy.[31]

Key Points

- Mucosal melanoma of the oral cavity is a rare malignancy with poor prognosis.
- Sarcomas of the oral cavity are rare. They may arise de novo, metastasize from other sites, or develop in prior radiation fields.
- Sarcomas of the oral cavity affect patients of all ages. Most are aggressive, but some forms are indolent.
- Patients with a history of HIV infection, other forms of immunosuppression, hematologic malignancies, and Sjogren's syndrome are at risk of developing sarcomas or lymphomas of the oral cavity.
- As with squamous cell carcinoma of the oral cavity, surgery is the preferred primary treatment modality for oral melanoma and most types of oral sarcoma.
- Lymphomas of the oral cavity are usually treated with systemic chemotherapy, often followed by consolidative radiation therapy.
- Immunotherapy has dramatically changed treatment for metastatic melanoma, though studies including oral melanomas specifically are limited.

References

[1] Wushou A, Zhao YJ. The management and site-specific prognostic factors of primary oral mucosal malignant melanoma. J Craniofac Surg. 2015; 26(2): 430–434

[2] Sun CZ, Chen YF, Jiang YE, Hu ZD, Yang AK, Song M. Treatment and prognosis of oral mucosal melanoma. Oral Oncol. 2012; 48(7):647–652

[3] Ascierto PA, Accorona R, Botti G, et al. Mucosal melanoma of the head and neck. Crit Rev Oncol Hematol. 2017; 112:136–152

[4] Sortino-Rachou AM, Cancela MdeC, Voti L, Curado MP. Primary oral melanoma: population-based incidence. Oral Oncol. 2009; 45(3):254–258

[5] Mohan M, Sukhadia VY, Pai D, Bhat S. Oral malignant melanoma: systematic review of literature and report of two cases. Oral Surg Oral Med Oral Pathol Oral Radiol. 2013; 116(4):e247–e254

[6] Green B, Elhamshary A, Gomez R, Rahimi S, Brennan PA. An update on the current management of head and neck mucosal melanoma. J Oral Pathol Med. 2017; 46(7):475–479

[7] Chatzistefanou I, Kolokythas A, Vahtsevanos K, Antoniades K. Primary mucosal melanoma of the oral cavity: current therapy and future directions. Oral Surg Oral Med Oral Pathol Oral Radiol. 2016; 122(1):17–27

[8] Breik O, Sim F, Wong T, Nastri A, Iseli TA, Wiesenfeld D. Survival outcomes of mucosal melanoma in the head and neck: case series and review of current treatment guidelines. J Oral Maxillofac Surg. 2016; 74(9):1859–1871

[9] de Andrade BA, Farneze RB, Agostini M, et al. Myeloid sarcoma of the oral cavity: a case report and review of 89 cases from the literature. J Clin Exp Dent. 2017; 9(9):e1167–e1171

[10] do Amaral TL, Valiati R, de Andrade BA, et al. Malignant peripheral nerve sheath tumor of the lower labial mucosa: case report and literature review. Oral Surg Oral Med Oral Pathol Oral Radiol. 2016; 122(2):e64–e68

[11] França CM, Caran EM, Alves MT, Barreto AD, Lopes NN. Rhabdomyosarcoma of the oral tissues—two new cases and literature review. Med Oral Patol Oral Cir Bucal. 2006; 11(2):E136–E140

[12] Giorgione C, Passali FM, Varakliotis T, Sibilia M, Ottaviani F. Temporo-mandibular joint chondrosarcoma: case report and review of the literature. Acta Otorhinolaryngol Ital. 2015; 35(3):208–211

[13] Kim YB, Leem DH, Baek JA, Ko SO. Atypical lipomatous tumor/well-differentiated liposarcoma of the gingiva: a case report and review of literature. J Oral Maxillofac Surg. 2014; 72(2):431–439

[14] Margaix-Muñoz M, Bagán J, Poveda-Roda R. Ewing sarcoma of the oral cavity. A review. J Clin Exp Dent. 2017; 9(2):e294–e301

[15] Meer S, Coleman H, Altini M. Oral synovial sarcoma: a report of 2 cases and a review of the literature. Oral Surg Oral Med Oral Pathol Oral Radiol Endod. 2003; 96(3):306–315

[16] Nagata M, Yoshitake Y, Nakayama H, et al. Angiosarcoma of the oral cavity: a clinicopathological study and a review of the literature. Int J Oral Maxillofac Surg. 2014; 43(8):917–923

[17] Piperi E, Tosios KI, Nikitakis NG, et al. Well-differentiated liposarcoma/atypical lipomatous tumor of the oral cavity: report of three cases and review of the literature. Head Neck Pathol. 2012; 6(3):354–363

[18] Reddy SS, Sharma S, Mysorekar V, Sharma P, Kaur A. Oral spindle cell sarcoma: a rare case report and review of literature. J Clin Diagn Res. 2017; 11 (4):ZD23–ZD25

[19] Schütz A, Smeets R, Driemel O, et al. Primary and secondary leiomyosarcoma of the oral and perioral region: clinicopathological and immunohistochemical analysis of a rare entity with a review of the literature. J Oral Maxillofac Surg. 2013; 71(6):1132–1142

[20] Thariat J, Julieron M, Brouchet A, et al. Osteosarcomas of the mandible: are they different from other tumor sites? Crit Rev Oncol Hematol. 2012; 82(3): 280–295

[21] Xie Z, Zhang F, Song E, Ge W, Zhu F, Hu J. Intraoral granulocytic sarcoma presenting as multiple maxillary and mandibular masses: a case report and literature review. Oral Surg Oral Med Oral Pathol Oral Radiol Endod. 2007; 103 (6):e44–e48

[22] Cockerill CC, Daram S, El-Naggar AK, Hanna EY, Weber RS, Kupferman ME. Primary sarcomas of the salivary glands: case series and literature review. Head Neck. 2013; 35(11):1551–1557

[23] Chigurupati R, Alfatooni A, Myall RW, Hawkins D, Oda D. Orofacial rhabdomyosarcoma in neonates and young children: a review of literature and management of four cases. Oral Oncol. 2002; 38(5):508–515

[24] Zhu W, Hu F, Zhao T, Wang C, Tao Q. Clinical characteristics of radiation-induced sarcoma of the head and neck: review of 15 cases and 323 cases in the literature. J Oral Maxillofac Surg. 2016; 74(2):283–291

[25] Patton LL. Oral lesions associated with human immunodeficiency virus disease. Dent Clin North Am. 2013; 57(4):673–698

[26] Fatahzadeh M, Schwartz RA. Oral Kaposi's sarcoma: a review and update. Int J Dermatol. 2013; 52(6):666–672

[27] Patton LL. Current strategies for prevention of oral manifestations of human immunodeficiency virus. Oral Surg Oral Med Oral Pathol Oral Radiol. 2016; 121(1):29–38

[28] Bottler T, Kuttenberger J, Hardt N, Oehen HP, Baltensperger M. Non-HIV-associated Kaposi's sarcoma of the tongue. Case report and review of the literature. Int J Oral Maxillofac Surg. 2007; 36(12):1218–1220

[29] Matsuzaki H, Katase N, Hara M, et al. Primary extranodal lymphoma of the maxilla: a case report with imaging features and dynamic data analysis of magnetic resonance imaging. Oral Surg Oral Med Oral Pathol Oral Radiol Endod. 2011; 112(3):e59–e69

[30] Guevara-Canales JO, Morales-Vadillo R, de Faria PE, Sacsaquispe-Contreras SJ, Leite FP, Chaves MG. Systematic review of lymphoma in oral cavity and maxillofacial region. Acta Odontol Latinoam. 2011; 24(3):245–250

[31] Pazoki A, Jansisyanont P, Ord RA. Primary non-Hodgkin's lymphoma of the jaws: report of 4 cases and review of the literature. J Oral Maxillofac Surg. 2003; 61(1):112–117

[32] Kemp S, Gallagher G, Kabani S, Noonan V, O'Hara C. Oral non-Hodgkin's lymphoma: review of the literature and World Health Organization classification with reference to 40 cases. Oral Surg Oral Med Oral Pathol Oral Radiol Endod. 2008; 105(2):194–201

[33] Bibas M, Castillo JJ. Current knowledge on HIV-associated plasmablastic lymphoma. Mediterr J Hematol Infect Dis. 2014; 6(1):e2014064

[34] Choi SY, Cho YA, Hong SD, Lee JI, Hong SP, Yoon HJ. Plasmablastic lymphoma of the oral cavity in a human immunodeficiency virus-negative patient: a case report with literature review. Oral Surg Oral Med Oral Pathol Oral Radiol. 2014; 117(2):e115–e120

[35] Scheper MA, Nikitakis NG, Fernandes R, Gocke CD, Ord RA, Sauk JJ. Oral plasmablastic lymphoma in an HIV-negative patient: a case report and review of the literature. Oral Surg Oral Med Oral Pathol Oral Radiol Endod. 2005; 100 (2):198–206

[36] Matsumoto N, Ohki H, Mukae S, et al. Anaplastic large cell lymphoma in gingiva: case report and literature review. Oral Surg Oral Med Oral Pathol Oral Radiol Endod. 2008; 106(4):e29–e34
[37] Meng W, Zhou Y, Zhang H, et al. Nasal-type NK/T-cell lymphoma with palatal ulcer as the earliest clinical manifestation: a case report with literature review. Pathol Oncol Res. 2010; 16(1):133–137
[38] Whitt JC, Dunlap CL, Martin KF. Oral Hodgkin lymphoma: a wolf in wolf's clothing. Oral Surg Oral Med Oral Pathol Oral Radiol Endod. 2007; 104(5): e45–e51
[39] Turner MD. Salivary gland disease in Sjögren's syndrome: sialoadenitis to lymphoma. Oral Maxillofac Surg Clin North Am. 2014; 26(1):75–81
[40] Ojha J, Islam N, Cohen DM, Marshal D, Reavis MR, Bhattacharyya I. Post-transplant lymphoproliferative disorders of oral cavity. Oral Surg Oral Med Oral Pathol Oral Radiol Endod. 2008; 105(5):589–596
[41] Wood J, Ver Halen J, Samant S, Florendo N. Radiation-induced sarcoma masquerading as osteoradionecrosis: case report and literature review. J Laryngol Otol. 2015; 129(3):279–282
[42] Mifsud M, Padhya TA. Metastatic melanoma to the upper aerodigestive tract: a systematic review of the literature. Laryngoscope. 2014; 124(5):1143–1149
[43] Buchanan A, Kalathingal S, Capes J, Kurago Z. Unusual presentation of extranodal diffuse large B-cell lymphoma in the head and neck: description of a case with emphasis on radiographic features and review of the literature. Dentomaxillofac Radiol. 2015; 44(3):20140288
[44] Wu Y, Zhong Y, Li C, Song H, Guo W, Ren G. Neck dissection for oral mucosal melanoma: caution of nodular lesion. Oral Oncol. 2014; 50(4):319–324
[45] Lian B, Si L, Cui C, et al. Phase II randomized trial comparing high-dose IFN-α2b with temozolomide plus cisplatin as systemic adjuvant therapy for resected mucosal melanoma. Clin Cancer Res. 2013; 19(16):4488–4498

Section VIII

Posttreatment Considerations

VIII

39 Oral Rehabilitation

Lauren M. Bolding and Ghassan G. Sinada

Summary

This chapter reviews the necessary steps and timeline for prosthetic reconstruction following surgical resection and/or reconstruction for head and neck cancer. Close communication between members of a patient's oncologic team is necessary in order to deliver the best postsurgical results to the patient. The ultimate goal is to restore form and function as close as possible to presurgical conditions.

Keywords: obturator, prosthesis, dentition, impressions

39.1 Introduction

Maxillofacial prosthetics is a subspecialty of prosthodontics which focuses on rehabilitation of those patients with defects or dysfunction resulting from disease, such as cancer, trauma, or congenital malformations. In restoring the oral cancer patient, it is the goal of the maxillofacial prosthodontist to achieve form and function as close to the pre-disease state as possible. In these patients, problems with swallowing, chewing, speaking, and lip function are common, depending on the size and location of the tumor.

At present, there exist two options for restoring form and function to those patients having undergone a maxillectomy. Prosthetic treatment consists of construction of removable obturator prosthesis to fill the remaining void after total or partial resection of the osseous and soft tissues of the maxilla. Surgical reconstruction of the defect using a microvascular free flap, often containing bone, is another alternative.[1]

Reconstruction with an obturator prosthesis reduces surgical time and offers the immediate restoration of form and function. Having a removable obturator allows for evaluation of the surgical site thereby allowing recurrence to be detected at an early stage and without relying solely on serial imaging. Conversely, a malfunctioning obturator may result in speech deficits, improper mastication, dysphagia, or facial disfigurement.[2–5]

39.2 Surgical Obturator

39.2.1 Presurgical Visit

About 2 weeks prior to the planned surgical procedure, it is important to make preliminary impressions. The impressions are needed of both arches and can be made with irreversible hydrocolloid. Making two maxillary impressions allows for utilization of one cast for the surgical obturator and keeping an unmodified cast for fabrication of the interim obturator. This is important in the event that positive margins dictate the need for further resection than originally planned. It is necessary to extend the impression posteriorly in order to capture the area of the hard and/or soft palate which will be resected.

The stone model should then be marked by the surgeon to indicate the planned extent of the resection, including any teeth which will be removed along with the resection. A surgical obturator will then be designed and fabricated out of polymethyl methacrylate resin in the laboratory for insertion immediately following the resection. In these instances, it is always helpful to maintain remaining dentition in which to anchor the surgical obturator, whether by clasps or by wiring around the teeth. The number of wire clasps to retain the obturator should be increased in order to account for any additional teeth that may be needed to be removed with the resection that were not foreseen. Should no teeth be available for clasping, it is always possible to wire the surgical obturator in place through residual maxillary alveolus.

It is prudent to fabricate surgical obturators without any denture teeth replacing missing dentition due to the lack of ability for adjustments and try-ins prior to or during the surgical procedure. In order to not create any occlusal interferences, it is best to leave the surgical obturator out of the occlusal plane. If the patient is losing teeth in a highly esthetic area or the patient is not having any opposing dentition, it is possible to fabricate the surgical prosthesis with denture teeth. The surgical obturator should return from the laboratory finely polished and ready for insertion (▶ Fig. 39.1 and ▶ Fig. 39.2).

39.2.2 Time of Surgery

The surgical obturator can be inserted by the surgeon following the resection or by a dental team member, namely the maxillofacial prosthodontist. The surgical obturator is installed following placement of surgical dressing and will remain in place for 7 to 10 days following the surgery. The surgical obturator will allow the patient to speak and swallow normally immediately postoperatively. It also has many psychological benefits as well, as it allows the patient to wake up from surgery without feeling the extent of their surgical defect. Once the surgery is completed, the second stone cast can be modified to indicate the

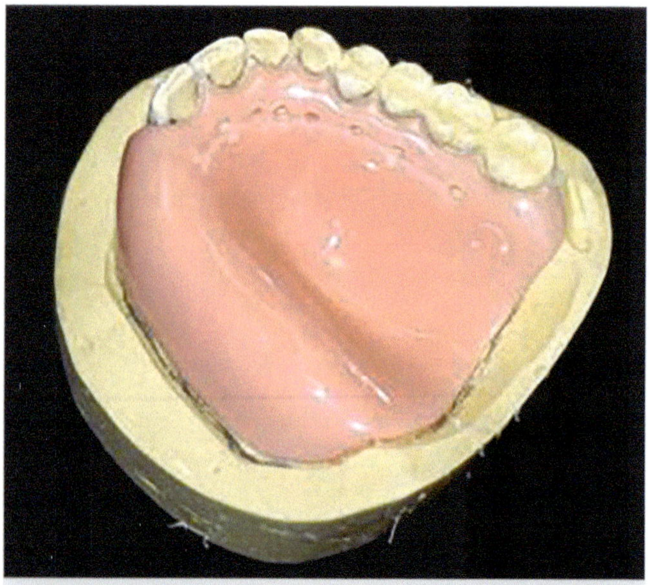

Fig. 39.1 Maxillary surgical obturator to be retained by wires around remaining dentition.

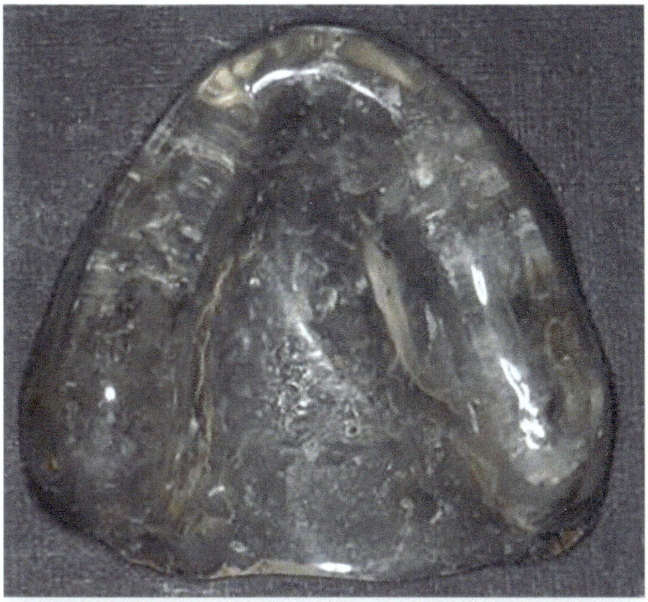

Fig. 39.2 Maxillary surgical obturator for edentulous patient to be retained by palatal screw.

teeth removed during surgery. This cast is then sent to the laboratory for fabrication of an interim obturator which will also include denture teeth to replace the missing dentition.

39.2.3 Postsurgical Visit

After 7 to 10 days of healing, the surgical obturator and surgical dressing is removed by the dental team member. This is generally performed without any local anesthetic; although, when wiring through the residual alveolus is performed, some topical or local anesthetic may decrease patient discomfort. If the surgical obturator is fixated to the teeth or alveolus, the wires are cut and removed with a quick pulling motion, followed by the removal of the surgical obturator. If no fixation of the obturator was performed, the surgical obturator is removed, revealing the surgical dressing. The surgical dressing is then removed, and the defect is evaluated for any debris, signs of infection, or bleeding. Suction is used to remove any debris and the defect is now prepared for insertion of the interim obturator prosthesis.

39.3 Interim Obturator

An interim maxillary obturator, generally replacing most or all teeth within the defect, is made after surgical resection and inserted once initial healing is completed to restore functions such as speech, mastication, and deglutition. This prosthesis also plays an important role in preventing collapse of facial soft tissues in the area of the defect and irritation to the surgical site.[6] Once the surgical obturator is removed and the surgical defect is cleaned, the interim obturator is tried in. A resilient silicon liner is used to mold the obturator to the surgical defect. The material is allowed to set while the patient performs some head motions, such as chin-to-chest and chin-to-shoulder, as well as neck circles in order to capture movements of the surrounding tissue. When the material has fully set, the interim obturator is removed and excess material is trimmed, making certain not to remove too much material from the posterior and lateral aspects of the obturator which would compromise the seal of the prosthesis.

The obturator seal is then tested by having the patient insert the prosthesis and drink water without having any nasal leakage of the water. Speech is also tested and hyponasality or hypernasality, if present, are identified. The goal is to have the speech just slightly hyponasal in order to minimize the chance of air escape and nasal leakage quickly once the patient starts healing. If the patient's voice is too hyponasal, breathing through his/her nose will be difficult and modifications must be made to the bulb portion of the obturator which is likely occluding the nasal passages. If the patient's voice is hypernasal, more resilient liner may need to be added to the area of suspected air escape, typically at the posterior aspect of the obturator prosthesis.

For the first 1 to 2 months of healing post surgery, the patient should be evaluated every 2 to 4 weeks for nasal leakage of fluids, hypernasality, or sore areas caused by the obturator prosthesis. At these visits, silicon liner may need to be added to certain areas of the obturator in order to recreate the seal of the prosthesis. If sore areas develop, the obturator can be adjusted to provide relief there. Postsurgical chemotherapy or radiation therapy will lengthen healing time following surgery and predispose the patient to developing more irritation from the obturator. With these patients, frequent follow-up of 1 to 2 weeks is sometimes necessary in order to provide relief of the prosthesis.

Typically, about 3 months, following surgical resection in an otherwise healthy patient without chemotherapy or radiation therapy, is adequate time for complete healing. In patients with delayed healing, such as diabetics, waiting 4 to 6 months for complete healing is recommended. For a patient who has received chemotherapy or radiation therapy following surgical resection, it is recommended to wait at least 3 months following completion of chemotherapy or radiation therapy to start planning for a definitive restoration.

39.4 Definitive Obturator

39.4.1 Partially Edentulous

Restoring a patient who has had a maxillectomy and still has intact supporting dentition is one of the more favorable circumstances in maxillofacial prosthetics. It is of utmost importance to determine the survivability of the remaining dentition prior to designing an obturator framework (▶ Fig. 39.3, ▶ Fig. 39.4, and ▶ Fig. 39.5).

Following are some key points to consider:

- What is the patient's dental history? For example, do they seek routine dental care? Do they practice good oral hygiene? This is very important in determining which teeth, if any, should be utilized for supporting a prosthesis.
- Does the patient have a history of head and neck radiation? If so, what was the dose to the area of the dentition? Postradiation patients are highly susceptible to developing dental caries at a much faster rate than nonirradiated patients; however, the dentition must be carefully examined and restored prior to fabricating any definitive prosthesis.
- Are any teeth actively diseased? If so, these teeth need to be treated appropriately prior to fabricating any definitive restoration.

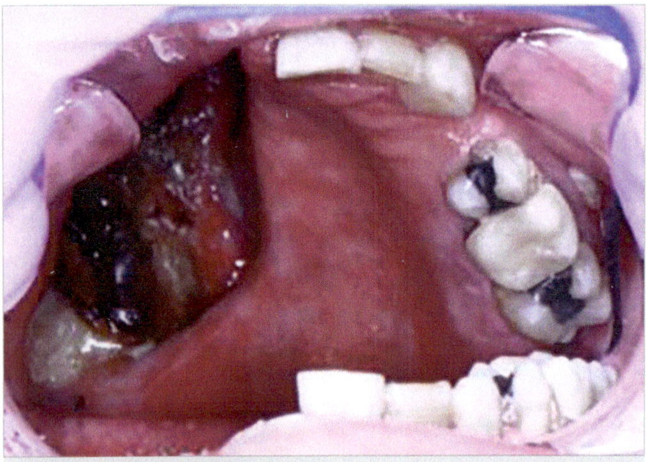

Fig. 39.3 Right partial maxillectomy defect.

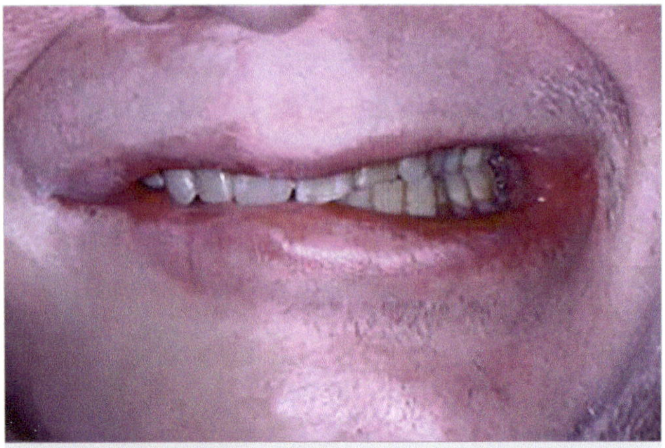

Fig. 39.4 Maxillary interim obturator in place.

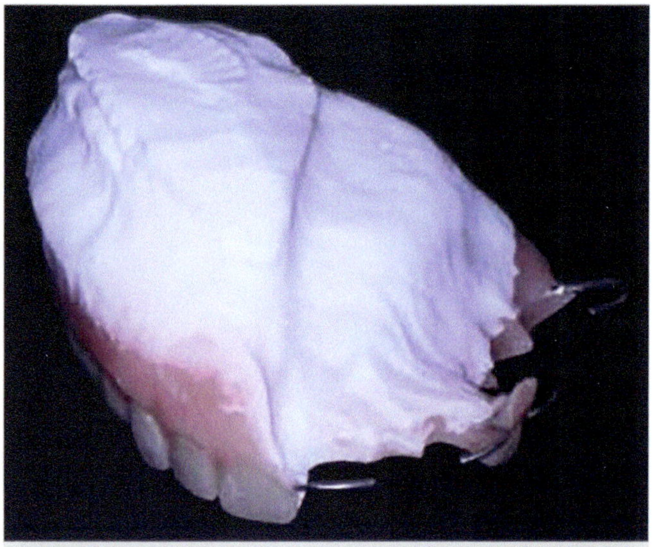

Fig. 39.5 Maxillary interim obturator with wrought wire clasps, relined with soft liner material.

The prosthesis framework should be designed so as to distribute forces among the strongest remaining teeth while spreading out the forces as much as possible throughout the arch. It is important not to place too much pressure on any one tooth which could cause it to loosen prematurely, resulting in loss of a strategic tooth in the obturator design. Upon presentation following healing from surgery and radiation, preliminary impressions are made in order to evaluate the remaining dentition and design an appropriate obturator framework.

At a subsequent visit, selected teeth are prepared slightly in order to accept a metal framework. The framework itself is mostly tooth supported, which allows for less pressure to the underlying mucosa. The framework resting on the dentition allows for less movement of the obturator prosthesis during function. Once the teeth are modified accordingly, a final impression is made and a stone cast is poured. A metal framework, typically made of Cr-Co or Ni-Cr, is fabricated and subsequently tried in the patient's mouth. The framework should have a passive fit and not put excessive pressure on any particular area. Slight adjustments can be made in order to achieve a passive fit of the metal framework.

Once the metal framework is completed, wax is placed in the edentulous areas in order to capture an occlusal relationship between the maxillary and mandibular dentition. This allows for prosthetic tooth placement corresponding to the patient's existing dentition. Measurements are also made to determine the correct size and shape of the prosthetic teeth as well as the midline, if necessary, and occlusal plane. A shade is also selected in order to match the remaining dentition.

The next step is try-in of the metal framework with denture teeth set in wax to restore the edentulous areas. This is an important step for testing speech, esthetics, and occlusion prior to finalization of the prosthesis. Any changes to the teeth position, shape, size, or shade should be made while the teeth are still placed in wax. Once the wax set-up is acceptable to both the patient and the clinician, the prosthesis should be processed into acrylic resin at the laboratory. This process is done under heat and pressure to ensure a dense material which is more resistant to forces placed on the prosthesis by the opposing dentition.

The final processed prosthesis is then tried in and adjusted for areas of excess pressure on the tissue surface of the obturator. Pressure indicating paste is used to establish these areas and a bur is used to reduce the acrylic in the corresponding areas. The occlusion is also checked and adjusted as well as the tightness of any of the clasps incorporated in the prosthesis. The patient is then evaluated for speech and nasal leakage of fluids, just as in prior steps. It is important for the patient to be able to insert and remove the prosthesis without difficulty but also to have enough retention so that the obturator does not move while speaking and eating. The patient should also be given proper home care instructions for the prosthesis. It is important to keep the prosthesis clean and to not sleep with the prosthesis, as fungal infections can develop if the obturator is not removed for enough time during a 24-hour period. Follow-up adjustments are necessary, as with any new prosthesis, it can take some time to adapt to the new contours of the obturator. Generally, the first visit about 2 weeks following insertion of the definitive obturator is indicated, then every 2 to 4 weeks until the patient is comfortable (▶ Fig. 39.6, ▶ Fig. 39.7, and ▶ Fig. 39.8).

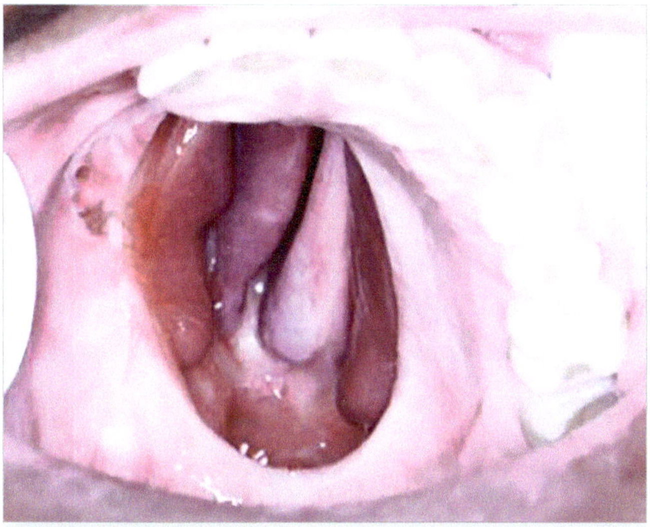

Fig. 39.6 Right partial maxillectomy defect.

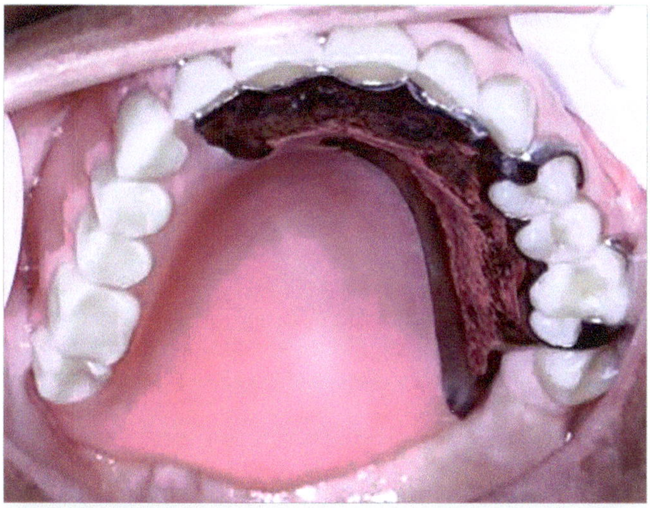

Fig. 39.7 Maxillary definitive obturator in place.

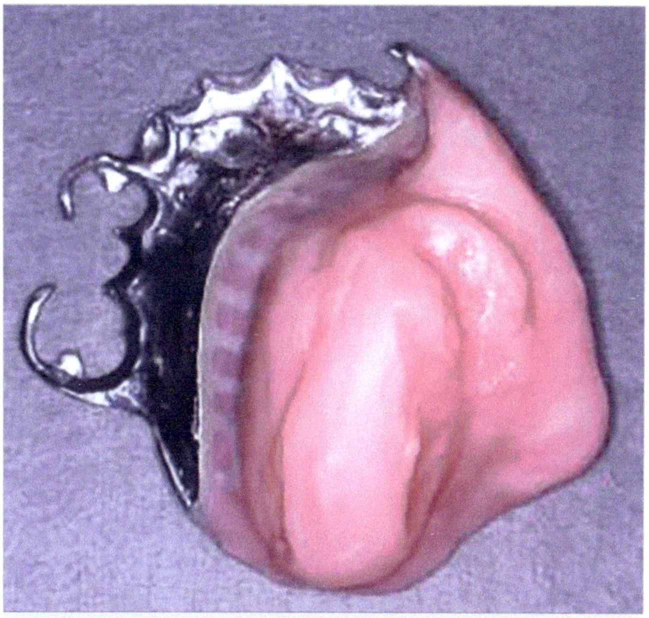

Fig. 39.8 Tissue surface of maxillary definitive obturator.

39.4.2 Completely Edentulous Without Implants

In less favorable presentations, a patient may present either completely edentulous with a partial maxillectomy or with a total maxillectomy. In either scenario, there are no remaining teeth to support or retain the obturator prosthesis; therefore, the retention of the prosthesis relies on anatomical undercuts and the peripheral seal of the prosthesis, when possible. These prostheses are generally tougher for patients to adapt, due to the increased movement of the prosthesis during speaking and eating, as compared to a conventional denture or an obturator supported and retained by teeth.

Following complete healing after surgery and any adjunctive therapy, preliminary impressions are made, and a custom impression tray is fabricated. The defect area is carefully molded with a stiff material and the rest of the tray is filled with a less viscous material in order to capture the details of the surrounding soft tissues. From this final impression, a master stone cast is created upon which the prosthesis is built. Occlusal records are obtained, and the prosthesis is tried in and viewed in wax prior to finalization. The prosthesis is processed into an acrylic resin material. The material is left highly polished so as to not create additional friction against the more easily injured soft tissue of the defect site.

At the insertion visit, pressure spots and occlusion are marked and adjusted, as described previously. Speech and nasal leakage of fluids are checked, and material is added as needed to create a better seal against the leakage of fluids or to provide additional retention if necessary. The patient is instructed in home care and asked to report back for follow-up and adjustments every 2 to 4 weeks, until the patient is comfortable with the prosthesis (▸ Fig. 39.9 and ▸ Fig. 39.10).

39.4.3 Completely Edentulous with Implants

When a patient has previously placed endosteal implants, or they are a good candidate for pre- or postsurgical implant placement, this adds additional support and retention to any obturator. Implants are especially helpful in situations where no teeth are left to support an obturator. An attachment system deemed best for the patient is chosen by the clinician and installed onto the endosteal implants. During the final impression phase of the obturator fabrication, impression copings are utilized to capture the location of the implants. Subsequent try-in steps are thus made easier due to being able to utilize the retention and support of the implants.

Steps in fabrication of the actual prosthesis are the same as in a completely edentulous obturator without implants, until the day of insertion of the prosthesis. Once the obturator is relieved of any

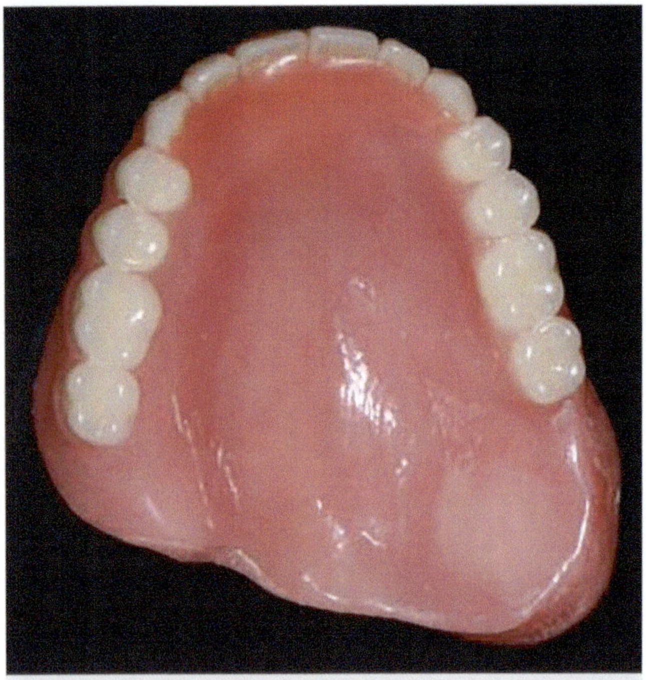

Fig. 39.9 Polished surface of definitive obturator for edentulous patient.

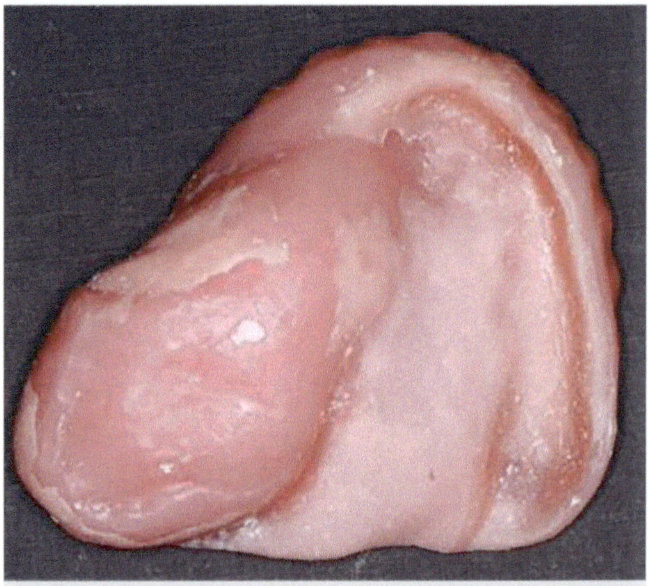

Fig. 39.10 Tissue surface of definitive obturator for edentulous patient.

anticipated pressure areas and occlusion is adjusted, the tissue surface of the prosthesis is relieved in order to capture the matching component of the implant attachment assembly. These components are incorporated into the obturator chairside utilizing an autopolymerizing acrylic resin and allowed to set fully. Excess material is then trimmed. This results in a more retentive, more stable prosthesis than one without any supporting dentition.

39.5 Palatal Augmentation Prosthesis (Also Known as a Palatal Drop Prosthesis)

A palatal augmentation prosthesis is most often fabricated for a patient with a partial glossectomy who still has some mobility of the residual tongue. The purpose of a palatal augmentation prosthesis is to create a prosthetic palate which will be in reach of the resected tongue in order to facilitate swallowing and speech. The tongue–palate interaction is very important in both swallowing and speech. During normal swallowing, the anterior tongue surface first contacts the hard palate just behind the maxillary incisors. The area of contact between the tongue and palate expands gradually, moving backward, as the masticated food is squeezed back along the palate to the oropharynx.[2] After a partial glossectomy, the configuration and volume of the vocal tract changes which alters the resonance and articulation produced by the patient, which in turn has a large effect on the patient's speech intelligibility.[7] In speech, the tongue–palate interaction is crucial for forming linguoalveolar sounds such as "d, t, l, and n." This interaction is also present in sounds like "s." If the residual tongue is unable to contact the palate, these sounds cannot be formed intelligibly. A palatal augmentation prosthesis will sit on the natural palate and drop to a level where the residual tongue can make contact.

39.5.1 Dentate Patient

Assuming a stable remaining dentition, whether complete or partial, preliminary impressions are made from irreversible hydrocolloid. A resin-based palatal plate is then fabricated at the laboratory on these casts and is retained by wrought wire clasps. At a subsequent visit, this plate is tried in and adjusted for comfort. A silicon liner is then added to the surface of the prosthesis that contacts the tongue and is inserted into the patient's mouth. The patient is then asked to speak certain words which include the sounds mentioned above. The set material will conform to touch the resected tongue in these movements. Excess material is then trimmed away, and the patient is asked to wear the prosthesis throughout the day to assist with swallowing and speaking.

After an adaptation period of weeks to months, and once the patient feels the palatal augmentation prosthesis is making a positive impact on speech and/or swallowing, a definitive prosthesis is fabricated. A metal framework is designed to rest on strong remaining dentition and to be retained with clasps by select teeth. This planning is generally performed on a stone cast made of the patient's existing dentition. Tooth preparations are then made and an impression is made for fabrication of the metal framework. Once the framework is tried in and exhibits retention while still being passive on the remaining dentition, the palatal augmentation portion of the prosthesis is formed utilizing the same materials and methods as in the interim

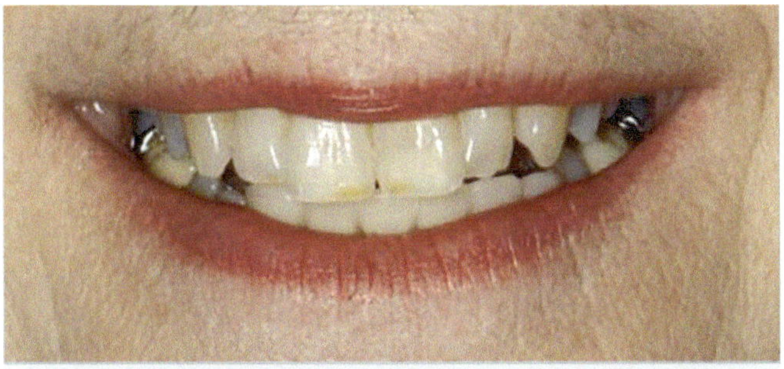

Fig. 39.11 Mandibular resection prosthesis in place—frontal smile view.

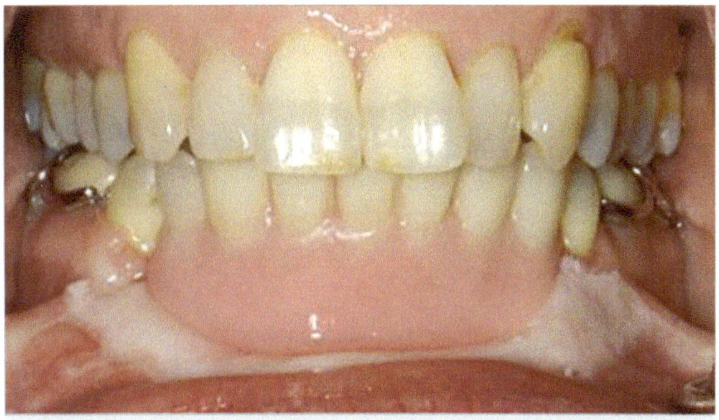

Fig. 39.12 Mandibular resection prosthesis in place—frontal retracted view.

prosthesis. This is then sent to the laboratory and the soft lining material is converted to a hard acrylic resin which is then finely polished. There will likely be a period of adjustments following insertion of the definitive prosthesis but if the interim prosthesis is used as a guide for the formation of the definitive prosthesis, the adjustment period should be shortened.

39.5.2 Edentulous Patient

In an edentulous patient in need of a palatal augmentation prosthesis, two scenarios exist. The patient may already have a well-fitting complete denture or it might not be the case. If the patient has a well-fitting denture with which they are satisfied, the palatal aspect of the denture can be modified to conform to the patient's restricted tongue movements. The initial modification is performed in a soft silicon liner and once the patient has adapted well and adjustments have decreased in frequency, the liner is then converted in the laboratory to a heat and pressure processed hard acrylic resin which is highly polished. Should the patient initially present without a complete denture, a new, well-fitting, retentive denture should be fabricated which includes the palatal augmentation aspect. The augmentation can be done before final processing of the denture in order to minimize laboratory time and number of visits for the patient.

39.6 Mandibular Resection Prosthesis

A removable mandibular resection prosthesis is often fabricated for patients having undergone marginal mandibulectomy to restore lost dentition. They are planned and fabricated in much the same way as a removable partial denture or an obturator in a patient who is partially edentulous; however, close attention must be paid to the depth of the lingual and buccal vestibules. In addition, scar tissue of the buccal mucosa will restrict the restorative space allowed for the prosthetic dentition, often leading to cheek biting, chronic irritation, or dislodging of the prosthesis. As with obturator prostheses, incorporation of endosteal implants to retain the removable prosthesis will enhance retention and chewing capabilities. These prostheses must be carefully planned and designed to minimize problems for the patient.

In the scenario where a patient has had a segmental mandibulectomy, attention must be paid to the patient's postoperative occlusion. If reconstructed, the prosthetic occlusion should be made to favor maximum contacts for improved chewing function in the newly edentulous area. If nonreconstructed, the mandibular resection prosthesis can be fabricated with a guide flange which will utilize the maxillary dentition in order to guide the patient's mandible into proper alignment; however, among clinicians, there is not agreement whether prosthetically guiding mandibular closure is desirable or necessary (▶ Fig. 39.11 and ▶ Fig. 39.12).[8]

39.7 Fixed Implant Supported Prosthesis

When a patient has enough native bone remaining, or is reconstructed with bone following a mandibular resection surgery, endosteal implants can be placed in order to restore form and function with a fixed prosthesis. Guided implant planning is often utilized by an oral and maxillofacial surgeon in order to optimize size and location of the implants. Once the implants are healed and ready to be restored, a provisional prosthesis is often first fabricated in order to test the placement of the prosthetic dentition. Since the patient will have become accustomed to not having a stable dentition during the healing time following implants, things like cheek and tongue biting, speech accommodation, and potential muscle tightness and discomfort can be problematic. For this reason, it is wise to test these new prosthetic teeth first with a provisional, make necessary adjustments, and then mimic the accepted provisionals in the final restoration.

The final restoration may be fabricated from precious metal and porcelain, titanium and acrylic or zirconia. The opposing dentition and the vertical and horizontal span of the restoration are important factors in choosing a restorative material (▶ Fig. 39.13, ▶ Fig. 39.14, ▶ Fig. 39.15, and ▶ Fig. 39.16).[9–12]

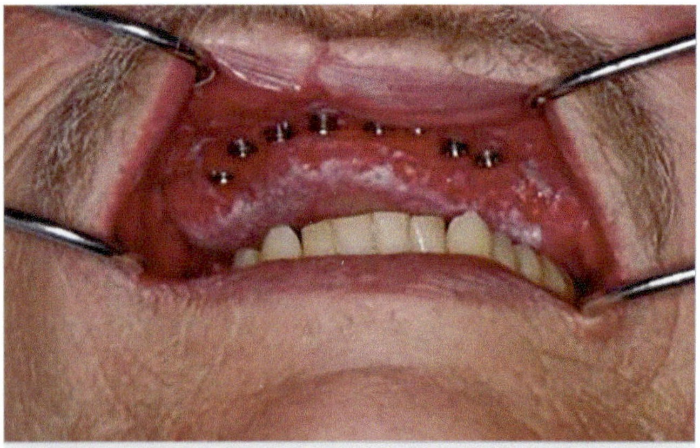

Fig. 39.13 Endosteal implants placed in reconstructed maxilla. (This image is provided courtesy of Dr. Carl Driscoll.)

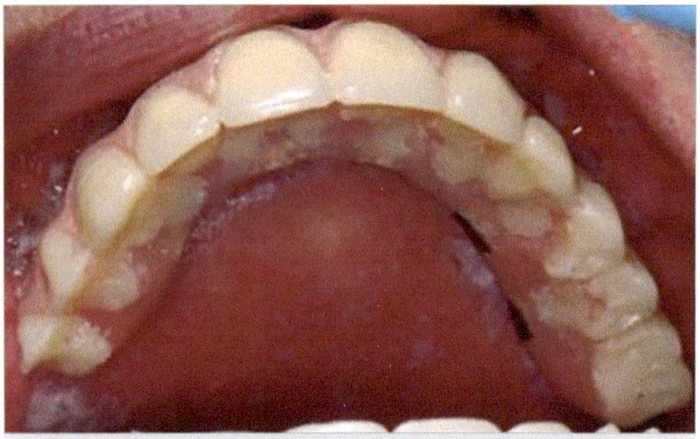

Fig. 39.14 Fixed implant provisional placed in reconstructed maxilla—occlusal view. (This image is provided courtesy of Dr. Carl Driscoll.)

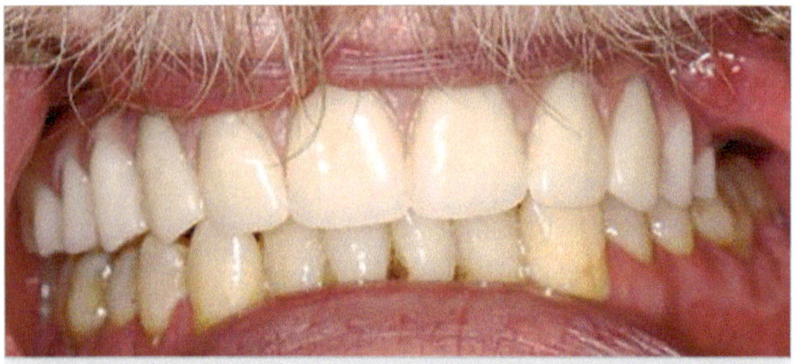

Fig. 39.15 Fixed implant provisional placed in reconstructed maxilla—frontal view. (This image is provided courtesy of Dr. Carl Driscoll.)

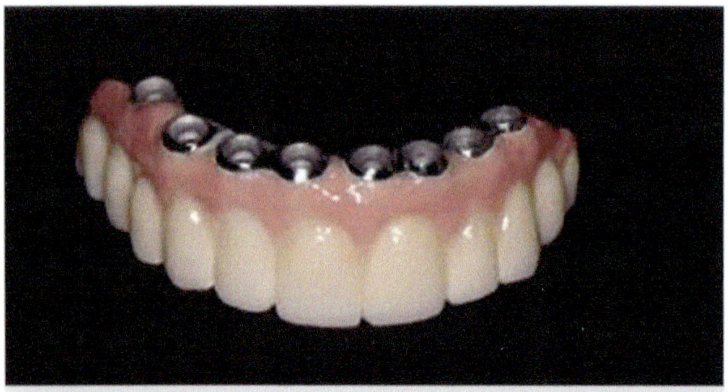

Fig. 39.16 Final porcelain fused to metal fixed implant prosthesis. (This image is provided courtesy of Dr. Carl Driscoll.)

Key Points

- Oral cancer patients often present with defects or lack of function which compromises the ability to chew, speak, and swallow.
- Restoration of the oral cancer patient is routinely done with fixed and/or removable prosthetics, often in conjunction with surgical reconstruction.
- There are many factors which should be considered in planning the type and design of prosthetics for oral cancer patients.
- The appropriate surgical and prosthetic reconstruction of the oral cancer patient relies on thorough planning and communication between various members of the patient's medical team.

References

[1] Rieger JM, Tang JAL, Wolfaardt J, Harris J, Seikaly H. Comparison of speech and aesthetic outcomes in patients with maxillary reconstruction versus maxillary obturators after maxillectomy. J Otolaryngol Head Neck Surg. 2011; 40(1):40–47

[2] Matsuo K, Palmer JB. Anatomy and physiology of feeding and swallowing: normal and abnormal. Phys Med Rehabil Clin N Am. 2008; 19(4):691–707, vii

[3] Borlase G. Use of obturators in rehabilitation of maxillectomy defects. Ann R Australas Coll Dent Surg. 2000; 15:75–79

[4] Kornblith AB, Zlotolow IM, Gooen J, et al. Quality of life of maxillectomy patients using an obturator prosthesis. Head Neck. 1996; 18(4):323–334

[5] Matsuyama M, Tsukiyama Y, Tomioka M, Koyano K. Clinical assessment of chewing function of obturator prosthesis wearers by objective measurement of masticatory performance and maximum occlusal force. Int J Prosthodont. 2006; 19(3):253–257

[6] Choudhury M, Shanmuganathan N, Padmanabhan TV, Swarup S, Grover M, Arumugam M. Rehabilitation of post surgical maxillectomy defects using interim obturators: a case series. Indian J Surg Oncol. 2014; 5(4):315–320

[7] Davis JW, Lazarus C, Logemann J, Hurst PS. Effect of a maxillary glossectomy prosthesis on articulation and swallowing. J Prosthet Dent. 1987; 57(6):715–719

[8] Schneider RL, Taylor TD. Mandibular resection guidance prostheses: a literature review. J Prosthet Dent. 1986; 55(1):84–86

[9] Logemann JA. CCC-SLP, BRS-S. Oral Tongue vs. Base of Tongue in Normal Swallow Function. 2012

[10] Kumar P, Alvi HA, Rao J, et al. Assessment of the quality of life in maxillectomy patients: a longitudinal study. J Adv Prosthodont. 2013; 5(1):29–35

[11] Martin JW, King GE, Kramer DC, Rambach SC. Use of an interim obturator for definitive prosthesis fabrication. J Prosthet Dent. 1984; 51(4):527–528

[12] Wolfaardt JF. Modifying a surgical obturator prosthesis into an interim obturator prosthesis. A clinical report. J Prosthet Dent. 1989; 62(6):619–621

40 Complications of Oral Cancer Surgery

Mary Jue Xu and William R. Ryan

Summary

Surgery for oral cavity carcinoma is a delicate balance between oncologic control and functional preservation. For each procedure, intraoperative awareness of anatomy and careful clinical observation postoperatively helps prevent, identify, and effectively manage complications. Though some complications are expected as sequelae of surgery, comprehensive knowledge of all possible consequences improves how physicians communicate postsurgical expectations with patients and manage complications when they arise.

Keywords: complications, oral cavity cancer, surgery, reconstruction, sequela

40.1 Introduction

Nearly one-third of head and neck cancers occur in the oral cavity.[1,2] Surgery is the preferred initial treatment over radiation for oral cavity cancers.[3] Analysis of the Surveillance, Epidemiology, and End Results (SEER) database supports the improved overall survival and disease-specific survival of primary surgery over radiotherapy for both early- and late-stage tumors.[4,5] Each oral cavity cancer resection and reconstruction is a delicate balance between disease eradication, functional restoration, and expected sequelae, with the risks of possible complications. Complications may include bleeding, hematoma, inadvertent trauma, seroma, infection, wound dehiscence, mucocele, ranula, submandibular and parotid duct iatrogenic stenosis with sialadenitis, unsatisfactory scar, inadvertent or expected temporary or permanent nerve injury, tooth injury or loss, dysarthria, dysgeusia, dysphagia (with difficulty chewing and/or difficulty swallowing), oral or facial sensory loss, xerostomia, thickened saliva, salivary fistula, oral cutaneous fistulae, oral-sinonasal fistulae, skin graft loss, failure of pedicled flap or free flap, facial cosmetic alteration, osteoradionecrosis (ORN) of the mandible or maxilla, infected or extruded hardware, anesthesia-related cardiopulmonary problems, or even death in rare cases. In this chapter, we discuss the sequelae and complications associated with oral cavity cancer resection and reconstruction. The expected sequelae, varying with the extent of the resection and degree of reconstruction, may include nerve injuries, tooth loss, functional impairment, sensory loss, dry mouth, and/or cosmetic changes. Going forward, such sequelae will be referred to as complications for the purpose of this discussion.

40.2 Epidemiology

40.2.1 Incidence

Fully determining complication rates for any surgical procedure is a challenge given varied studies with heterogeneous reporting and differing definitions of complications. Although in experienced hands morbidity can be fairly low, complication rates for oral cavity carcinoma surgery have been reported to be as high as 20 to 50%.[6,7] Complications are likely less common in lower-stage cancers for which less extensive operations are generally indicated. ▶ Table 40.1 lists incidence rates reported by various studies of complications following oral cavity cancer surgery.

Initiatives such as the American College of Surgeons (ACS) National Surgical Quality Improvement Program (NSQIP) and the American Academy of Otolaryngology—Head and Neck Surgery's Reg-ent, clinical data registries, both aim to standardize the frequency and manner in which postoperative complications are reported. Based on the ACS-NSQIP database, an analysis of 408 oral cavity cancer patients, treated between 2005 and 2010, showed the short-term complication rate within 30-days of surgery was 20.3%.[8] No tumor staging information was provided by this database. The most common complications were the need for reoperation (9.6%), infections including pneumonia, urinary tract infections, and sepsis (6.6%), respiratory problems (5.2%), and surgical site infections and/or dehiscence (4.7%). The majority of complications occurred from 2 to 10 days following surgery and, when present, extended the mean length of hospital stay from 3 to 15 days.

Oral cavity resections with complex reconstruction generally have a higher risk of complications. Lodder et al[7] reported complication rates at a single institution following oral cavity composite ablative surgery and free flap reconstruction. For their 184 patients who underwent 189 composite resections and free flaps, the complication rate was 40.2%. The most common surgical complications were flap related (6.9%, 13 patients), wound infection (8.5%, 16 patients), and donor site complications

Table 40.1 The incidence of complications following surgery of oral cavity cancers

Complication	Rate	Reference
Reoperation	9.6%	Schwam et al (2015)[8]
Infection	22.7% 8.5% 6.6%	de Melo et al (2001)[6] Lodder et al (2015)[7] Schwam et al (2015)[8]
Surgical site	4.7%	Schwam et al (2015)[8]
Dehiscence	20.9% 1.6%	de Melo et al (2001)[6] Lodder et al (2015)[7]
Flap failure	2.2%	Schwam et al (2015)[8]
Hematoma	3.7% 3.7%	de Melo et al (2001)[6] Lodder et al (2015)[7]
Poor osteotomy site healing	7%	Nam et al (2006)[9]
Exposed/infected hardware	3.2%	Lodder et al (2015)[7]
Osteoradionecrosis of mandible	5–15%	Balough et al (1989)[10]
Orocutaneous fistula	4.2%	Awad et al (2015)[11]
Chylous fistula	1.8%	de Melo et al (2001)[6]
Mortality	3.6% 1.6% 1% 0.8%	de Melo et al (2001)[6] Lodder et al (2015)[7] Schwam et al (2015)[8] Awad et al (2015)[11]

(5.3%, 10 patients). Twenty-one patients (11.1%) required a return to the operating room and corrective surgery.

40.2.2 Causes/Risk Factors

Comorbidities, cancer-related characteristics, and surgical factors all contribute to complications. The presence of comorbidities in the head and neck cancer population are associated with worse survival and complication rates. A prospective study of comorbidities in cancer patients treated at academic teaching hospitals showed that an estimated 21% of head and neck cancer patients had moderate-to-severe comorbidities with the severity associated with poorer overall survival.[12] In a retrospective review of 110 patients with tongue and floor of mouth tumors, Ribiero et al[13] found that survival within each tumor stage could be further stratified by medical comorbidities. Moreover, tobacco and alcohol use, common risk factors for head and neck malignancies, along with malnutrition and diabetes are known to impair wound healing and increase risk of healing-related complications.[8,14]

Cancer-related risk factors such as advanced staged disease and certain critical tumor locations can result in more extensive and/or impactful surgical resections with more consequential sequelae and rehabilitation needs. Furthermore, patients who require adjuvant radiation or have a history of radiation are more prone to breakdown due to radiation-induced damage to the extracellular matrix, stromal cells, and microvasculature.[15]

Surgical risk factors include the extent of surgery such as the inclusion of neck dissections, choice of reconstruction, duration of surgery, time under anesthesia, and presence and extent of prophylactic antibiotics. For example, Schwam et al[8] reported a correlation between the addition of neck dissections and surgical site and infection-related complications. Higher complication rates are generally found in oral cavity cancer patients who undergo resection with free flap surgery as shown above. These cases are also associated with longer anesthesia time and blood transfusions.[7]

While disease-related risk factors cannot be modified, patient-related and surgical risk factors can influence the surgical plan and the nature of counseling with patients, given the expectation for certain complications. For example, in an elderly, malnourished patient with cardiac comorbidities, nutritional supplementation can be initiated preoperatively; also, the choice of reconstruction following tumor resection may favor a shorter operative duration. Additional modifiable risk factors will be discussed later in this chapter.

40.3 Clinical Presentation

Many complications overlap in presentation. Pain, swelling, signs of infection, fever, salivary leakage, changes in drain content, neurologic dysfunction, and poorly healing surgical sites can signal the development of a complication. Immediately following surgery, monitoring for hematoma, seroma, signs of infection, and malunion following mandibulotomies or mandibulectomies should be performed. Paresthesias and paresis can indicate nerve injury. Nonhealing surgical incisions or open cutaneous wounds can indicate an oral-cutaneous fistula. Delayed complications such as ORN can present as trismus, exposed bone, bony necrosis, and pain.

Free flap reconstruction carries its own subset of complications. Commonly assessed problems include, but are not limited to, loss of blood flow to the flap (due to thrombosis, vessel compression, or anastomotic leak), reconstruction break down with salivary fistula or functional impairment, donor site infections, donor site sensory or motor nerve injury, and donor site distal ischemia. Monitoring of the free flap may reveal venous congestion in the case of venous thromboses or a pale cool flap in the setting of arterial thromboses. The clinical exam may also include pricking the flap with a needle away from the vascular pedicles during which bright brisk bleeding indicates a healthy flap while dark blood indicates venous congestion. Additional tools to supplement the clinical exam include Doppler probes to measure pulse, implantable Doppler probes placed near the draining vein useful in buried flaps, temperature probes, pulse oximeter probes, and near-infrared spectroscopy.[16] Additional resources highlight these nuances specific to free tissue reconstruction.[17,18]

40.4 Diagnosis and Evaluation

Most complications can be diagnosed by physical exam. Close assessment of the surgical site and a thorough head and neck exam may reveal erythema, edema, drainage, or dehiscence suggesting reconstruction breakdown or brewing infections. Surgical drains may show fresh blood indicative of a hematoma, pus indicative of an abscess or salivary fistula, saliva or food/drink/tube feeds suggestive of a salivary fistula, or cloudy fluid suggestive of a chylous fistula. Following radiation, patients should be monitored for trismus due to radiation-induced tissue changes and exposed hardware from poorly vascularized tissue. Assessing occlusion, loose teeth, and motion of the temporomandibular joint can help identify malunion, loose hardware, or developing ORN.

Labs, pathology, and imaging support but do not replace clinical findings. Leukocytosis can indicate infection or presence of tumor. A decrease in hemoglobin may signal a hematoma. Fluid from surgical drains can be tested for triglycerides if there is a concern for a chyle leak. In the setting of poor wound healing, labs such as thyroid-stimulating hormone, albumin, and erythrocyte sedimentation rate can be sent to assess for degree of malnutrition. In addition, any surgical sites with concern for infection should be cultured for culture-directed antibiotic treatment.

Biopsy should be considered if there is a concern for recurrence. In cases of advanced disease following surgery, patients may present with what appears as an infection: draining purulent wounds, leukocytosis, and rim-enhancing fluid collections on imaging (▶ Fig. 40.1). While infection is a clear differential diagnosis, persistent or recurrent cancer may also be a differential diagnosis and fine-needle aspiration or open biopsy should be performed.

Imaging bolsters the clinical exam by better assessing deep tissue structures. Computed tomography (CT) with contrast is an important modality to assess for rim-enhancing fluid collections or phlegmon representing infection, possible recurrence, and bone quality signaling ORN or postsurgical fractures. Magnetic resonance imaging (MRI) is valuable following free tissue reconstruction to further delineate soft tissue changes.

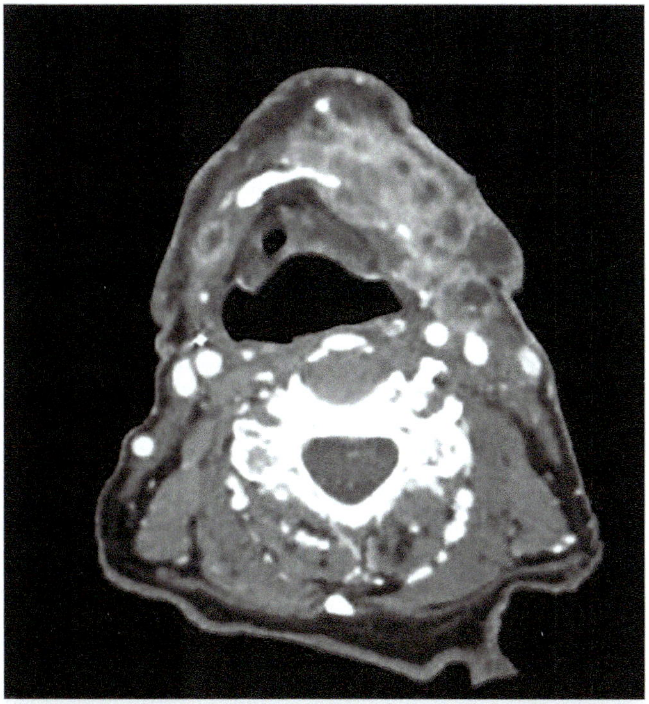

Fig. 40.1 Rim-enhancing fluid collections in the neck with externally draining purulence concerning for infection or recurrent tumor. This patient initially presented with late stage tongue carcinoma and underwent resection and free flap reconstruction. After delays to his radiation appointments, he presented 2 months following his surgical date with fevers, leukocytosis, and purulent drainage from an open neck wound. Clinical presentation and imaging suggested an infection but concern about recurrence is critical. Fine-needle aspiration cytology for this patient returned squamous cell carcinoma.

40.5 Anatomic Considerations/ Relevant Anatomy

The oral cavity is a compact area of intricate anatomic structures that can be divided into tissue components including muscles, nerves, salivary ducts/glands, teeth, blood vessels, and bone, or anatomic regions including the tongue, floor of mouth, buccal regions, upper alveolar ridge, lower alveolar ridge, retromolar trigone, and hard palate. Functional categories of the oral cavity include breathing, speech, taste, chewing, drinking, swallowing, intimacy, singing, and even playing a musical instrument. Unfortunately, surgery can inevitably alter or harm these aspects and functions.

40.5.1 Muscle and Soft Tissue

Muscle and soft tissue are inherent in the function of the mouth and form of the face. There are areas of the oral cavity where tissue redundancy allows for primary closure with minimal functional or cosmetic impact, particularly with small resections of the tongue, floor of mouth, and buccal regions. However, larger resections and others areas of the mouth often need tissue advanced from nearby regions or added from afar for proper reconstruction. Some areas need special attention to maintain function and cosmesis. For instance, following a segmental mandibulectomy, the orbicularis oris should be reapproximated to prevent oral incompetence.[19] Moreover, injury to structures outside of the oral cavity can lead to consequences within the mouth; violation of the pterygoid musculature can result in trismus, which impairs eating and oral hygiene, and complicates airway management.

40.5.2 Nerves

Oral cavity surgery can require the surgeon to manage the following nerves: lingual, hypoglossal, inferior alveolar/mental, and marginal mandibular. During surgery, nerves may be deliberately sacrificed for oncologic control to achieve an adequate surgical margin or if infiltrated by cancer. Given this possibility, a thorough informed consent is essential with each patient. ▶ Table 40.2 shows a list of the nerves at risk during surgery. If transection of a nerve is identified intraoperatively, repair should be performed if possible. With primary neurorrhaphy or cable grafts, return of function, at least for motor nerves, can range from months to a year.[20,21]

40.5.3 Bone

Bone remodeling is a balance between osteogenesis and resorption, both of which affect the healing rates of osteotomy sites, postsurgical fractures, and the evolution of ORN. New bone formation develops over approximately 4 to 6 months.[22] Nonunion following osteotomies can lead to instability of the bone and associated pain, malocclusion, cosmetic asymmetry, chewing dysfunction, hardware extrusion, and possible infection.[9]

To prevent postsurgical fractures of the mandible, the tension and sheering forces of bone need to be managed with proper presurgical planning and intraoperative adjustments to the plating system. Fractures can occur if an inadequate amount of bone is left along the inferior border of the mandible. The poor bone substrate of edentulous mandibles in which the alveolar ridge is absorbed and of irradiated mandibles are both more prone to fractures.[23]

For tumors of the hard palate, the priority of surgical reconstruction is to recreate the oronasal barrier relying on dentition for prosthesis attachment or the addition of free tissue to separate the mouth and the nose. Unless just a superficial upper alveolar ridge resection is performed, a maxillectomy inherently results in an oronasal fistula. If poorly repaired or replaced by an inadequate prosthesis, the following functional impairments can ensue: nasal regurgitation, poor swallowing from difficulty moving a food bolus, and hypernasal speech. The choice of prostheses or free tissue transfer with or without dental implants for maxillectomy defects depends on patient choice, the degree of patient frailty, the defect size, the nature of the dentition, and the remaining bone quality. Inadequate remaining teeth or poor dentition can result in a poorly fitting prosthetic obturator. Attenuated bone may be inadequate for dental implants. Larger defects when over half of the palate is resected are often associated with improved outcomes following free flap reconstruction.[24]

40.5.4 Teeth

Teeth can be injured in multiple ways during oral surgery. Tooth roots can be injured from bone cuts as well as from bone

Table 40.2 The nerves of the oral cavity and modalities for injury during surgery

Nerve	Function	Anatomy	Risk of injury
Lingual	Provides sensation and taste function to anterior two-third of the tongue	From the mandibular division of the trigeminal nerve, this nerve runs medial to the third molar, crosses lateral to deep and then medial to the submandibular duct at the first or second molar and branches into the tongue	During mandibulotomy, glossectomy, floor of mouth resection, and during the closure of floor of mouth incisions
Mental	Sensation to the lower lip and chin	From the mandibular division of the trigeminal nerve, this nerve travels through the mental foramen to the lower lip and chin mucosa and skin	During incision or exposure for mandibulotomy or mandibulectomies
Inferior alveolar	Sensation to lower teeth	From the mandibular division of the trigeminal nerve The nerve is high and medial in the posterior part of the mandible Near midline, the inferior alveolar nerve and canal runs anterior and inferior along with inferior alveolar artery Branches of the inferior alveolar nerve include the mylohyoid and mental branches	During marginal or segmental mandibulectomies
Marginal mandibular	Lowers ipsilateral lower lip	Branch of the facial nerve Superficial to the facial artery and vein	Neck skin flap elevation, external mandible exposure, and buccal resections
Hypoglossal	Motor innervation of muscles of the tongue except palatoglossus	Runs deep to the posterior belly of the digastric muscle, crosses the lingual artery at the level of the hyoid bone, and travels between the mylohyoid and hyoglossus muscles	Glossectomy and floor of mouth resection, and neck dissection for any oral cavity resection case

resorption at the edge of osteotomy sites. To prevent these injuries, careful attention to the sites of the tooth roots is important. Furthermore, ostomy sites should be made in the middle of the tooth sockets following the extraction to maximize the residual bone stock around the remaining teeth and offset the expected postsurgical bony resorption that can lead to dental destabilization.[19] In patients who will be undergoing postoperative radiation, decayed teeth should be extracted.

40.5.5 Airway

The airway remains the priority following surgery of the oral cavity. Postoperatively, a loss of airway can occur when an unexpected amount of upper airway edema or hemorrhage develops. A prophylactic tracheostomy may be indicated in certain resections and reconstructions when there are risks of compromising the oral air passage way. Preoperatively, baseline risks such as trismus or impaired cervical mobility due to cervical arthritis can increase the difficulty of intubation. An airway that is difficult to access can be exacerbated by procedures such as maxillary mandibular fixation and free tissue reconstruction. These are some of the influences that factor into the use of awake fiberoptic-guided intubation, transnasal intubation, and awake tracheostomy.

40.5.6 Salivary Glands

During oral cavity cancer resections, injury to the salivary ducts and glands may lead to salivary duct obstruction, sialadenitis, sialoceles, and ranulas. If damage of the parotid and or submandibular ducts occurs intraoperatively, primary repair, sialodochoplasty, placement of a stent, or marsupialization are possible solutions. To prevent ranula, at times, with the loss of the overlying mucosa and duct of Rivinus, a sublingual gland excision may be necessary along with the tumor resection. Postoperatively, revision sialendoscopic-assisted ductal dilation or sialodocoplasty, salivary gland suppression with botulinum toxin, and needle aspiration of salivomas can be used in addition to possible gland excision.

40.5.7 Orbit

Awareness of lacrimal duct anatomy can help avoid iatrogenic stenoses, epiphora, and abscesses following maxillectomy. When lacrimal duct violation is necessary, dacyrocystorhinostomy stent placements are helpful.

40.6 Treatment Considerations and Approaches

40.6.1 Medical/Rehabilitative Options

The postoperative care period provides opportunities to promote healing and lessen complications. Diet, rehabilitation therapy, antibiotics, and hyperbaric oxygen (HBO) are modifiable factors that can influence postsurgical outcomes.

With many complications involving wound healing, diet and nutrition are critical perioperatively. An estimated 75 to 80% of head and neck cancer patients lose weight during treatment with some patients losing up to 15to 20%.[25,26] Nutritional optimization in head and neck cancer patients has been associated with improved symptoms and quality of life metrics following treatment.[27] Options include nutritional supplements if swallowing function is intact, enteral tube feeds if swallow function has been compromised, and rarely, parenteral nutrition, which is accompanied by increased risk of infection.[28] Postoperatively, pureed or soft diets can to promote healing. Diets are often slowly advanced particularly after free flaps in coordination with swallow evaluation.

Speech and swallow rehabilitation can help foster return of function of the oral cavity and improve overall conditioning. Speech language pathologists are critical components of the multidisciplinary head and neck treatment team. Therapy provided can promote the use of the following muscles: the muscles of mastication to reduce trismus, the tongue musculature to reduce dysarthria, and tongue and the swallowing muscles to reduce dysphagia. For overall conditioning, even following free flap reconstruction, early mobilization is encouraged.[29]

Antibiotics are commonly used for perioperative prophylaxis, infection, and ORN. Clean-contaminated head and neck surgeries have reported infection rates ranging from 24 to 87% without antibiotics.[30,31] Perioperative antibiotics should cover oral flora and anaerobes;[32] thus, common regimens include either ampicillin/sulbactam or clindamycin. Multiple randomized control trials have shown that prolonged courses of antibiotics do not offer definite additional benefits in comparison to shorter courses.[29,33,34] In a meta-analysis of four randomized controlled trials assessing the duration following oral cavity cancer resection with some trials including free flap reconstruction, there was no appreciable difference between a 1- or 5-day course of postoperative antibiotics.[34,35] Antibiotics also serve as a main component of treatment for mucocutaneous fistulas and ORN.

The individual studies on the benefit of HBO for ORN in head and neck cancer patients are varied. However, a 2016 Cochrane review of 753 participants in 14 trials found that HBO therapy significantly improved mucosal coverage of ORN, decreased risk of wound breakdown following surgery, and improved healing following dental extractions of radiated sites.[36] HBO can also help assist in prolonged postsurgical poor wound healing cases.

40.6.2 Surgical Options and Approaches

Common operations of the oral cavity include partial glossectomy, marginal and segmental mandibulectomy, partial maxillectomy, and buccal resections. These approaches and strategies for optimizing outcomes and reconstruction have been presented in prior chapters with a summary of key points for each procedure (▸ Table 40.3).

Complications that are common across multiple surgical approaches are critical to recognize and have specific treatments including the following: exposed or infected hardware, ORN, and oral-cutaneous fistula.

Exposed or Infected Hardware

To prevent hardware infection and exposure, adequate tissue coverage during the initial surgery promotes thorough vascularization and healing of the surgical site. This is especially important if adjuvant radiation is planned given expected atrophy and microvascular injury. Once hardware is exposed or infected, strong consideration should be given for removal. If supportive plating is removed before adequate osteogenesis, external fixation or intermaxillary fixation are the options. The exposed site should also be covered with vascularized tissue in the form of a local or free tissue flap.

Osteoradionecrosis

An estimated 4 to 6% of all head and neck cancer patients who undergo primary radiation or adjuvant radiation experience ORN.[40,41] Risk can be minimized preoperatively with a thorough dental evaluation and planned dental extractions to minimize the need for extractions following radiation.[10] Improving the blood supply with vascularized tissue can improve the condition of the bone. If presenting early, medical management with pentoxifylline, vitamin E, and long-term antibiotics and use of HBO may be sufficient to avoid surgery. Surgical debridement can at times avoid full osseous free flap reconstruction. Also, in select cases coverage of an exposed bone segment with a soft tissue free flap can restore blood flow to the area, preserve the bone, and avoid the need for an osseous free flap.

Orocutaneous Fistula

Orocutaneous fistulas can occur after oral cavity resections and reconstruction.[19] Dehiscent neck skin wounds should be opened up to allow for drainage of pus with cultures taken for species-directed antibiotics. Drains can be kept in place if present. Adequate prophylaxis often includes ampicillin/sulbactam or amoxicillin/clavulanic acid. After the wound is cleaned, gauze packing and removal 2 to 3 times a day will help develop granulation tissue for wound tract closure. Eventually as the wound heals, the amount of packing needed decreases. This process can take days to even months, depending on the size of the fistula. The patient should also not take any food by mouth until the fistula fully heals. There are cases in which the fistula tract crosses or abuts the carotid artery or other large-caliber vasculature. If the fistula is not properly drained in this situation, there is a risk for the amylase and oral flora-related inflammation and infection to spread to the blood vessels possibly leading to rupture.[42] In these cases, surgical tissue coverage with a rotational or free flap may be warranted.[43]

Table 40.3 Summary of common surgical procedures in the oral cavity, related complications, and surgical considerations

Procedure	Complications	Strategies for prevention and treatment
Glossectomy	• Aspiration • Dysarthria • Dysgeusia • Dysphagia	• Palatal prostheses can be used to drop the hard palate down for better contact with a depressed tongue dorsum • Speech and swallowing therapy exercises to increase neuromuscular coordination and strength and to break scar tissue
	• Scarring and tethering of the tongue to the floor of mouth	• Use of split-thickness skin grafts or free flap (radial forearm or anterolateral thigh) to prevent scarring and tethering to floor of mouth • Posterolateral tongue defects can be left for secondary intention healing to reduce risk of tethering • Reconstruction with adequate soft-tissue bulk for dorsum to reach hard palate
	• Submandibular duct obstruction	• Sialodochoplasty of submandibular duct
	• Ducts of Rivinus obstruction (ranula)	• Sublingual gland excision during glossectomy
Mandibulotomy and mandibulectomy	• Misaligned mastication • Malunion • Iatrogenic fractures	• For mandibulotomy, step osteotomy approach allows mastication forces to drive the osteomy site together • Preplating the mandible prior to resection helps maintain contour and occlusion • In cases where there is sparse remaining ascending ramus that cannot undergo plating, consider resecting the remaining ramus and condyle to prevent pain[19]
	• Trismus	• Coronoidectomy can reduce postoperative and postradiation trismus[37]
	• Tooth injury	• For mandibulotomy, when possible the incision should be between the lateral incisor and the canine where tooth roots are pointed away from each other[38,39] • Bony cuts made in the middle of a tooth socket after tooth extraction is safer than between tooth sockets to prevent tooth root injury and account to bony resorption[19] • Use of a thin blade for the osteomies • Irrigation to prevent heat injury during cuts
	• Exposed or infected hardware	• Tissue coverage with adequate vascular supply during the initial surgery as a preventative measure, especially if adjuvant radiation is planned • Hardware removal • Consider external fixation or intermaxillary fixation if support needed
Maxillectomy	• Oral-sinonasal fistula	• Adequate prosthesis seal of defect • Use of adequate tissue bulk if using tissue reconstruction
	• Epistaxis	• Adequate packing/limiting unnecessary mucosal lacerations
	• Nasal tip drop	• Prosthesis/free flap septal base support
	• Epiphora	• Maintain patency of the nasolacrimal duct by marsupialization or stent placement if encountered
	• Corneal abrasion	• Temporary tarsorrhaphy • Corneal shield
	• Numbness of the cheek	• Preservation of the infraorbital nerve if uninvolved
Buccal resection	• Scar contracture causing cheek skin dimpling	• Split-thickness skin grafts or free flap reconstruction of wider buccal defects
	• Parotid duct obstruction (from scarring or reconstruction graft coverage	• Parotid duct sialodochoplasty and or stent placement
	• Trismus from scar contracture	• Postoperative jaw stretching exercises and rehabilitation
	• Facial nerve injury	• Use of nerve monitors to identify and avoid iatrogenic nerve damage

Key Points

- Patient must be counseled about expected sequelae and possible complications of oncologic resections of the oral cavity for cancer.
- The most common complications include systemic infections and surgical site infections and/or dehiscence.
- Medical factors that can be modified include perioperative nutrition, prophylactic antibiotics, and rehabilitative therapy.

Key considerations of surgical approaches include:

- Avoid unnecessary nerve injury.
- Ensure well-vascularized tissue at the site of resection and bony reconstruction.
- Mandibulectomy osteotomies should be made in the middle of an extracted tooth socket with account for bony resorption at the osteotomy site.
- Coronoidectomy can reduce postoperative and postradiation trismus.
- Plan for adequate tissue bulk following glossectomy.
- Manage fistulas more aggressively if vasculature may be involved.
- Repair any iatrogenic injury to salivary ducts by stent placement, marsupialization, or salivary gland excision.

References

[1] Siegel RL, Miller KD, Jemal A. Cancer statistics, 2015. CA Cancer J Clin. 2015; 65(1):5–29

[2] Vigneswaran N, Williams MD. Epidemiologic trends in head and neck cancer and aids in diagnosis. Oral Maxillofac Surg Clin North Am. 2014; 26(2):123–141

[3] Network NCC. Head and Neck Cancers Version 1.2018. 2018; https://www.nccn.org/professionals/physician_gls/pdf/head-and-neck.pdf. Accessed Feb 20, 2018

[4] Sowder JC, Cannon RB, Buchmann LO, et al. Treatment-related determinants of survival in early-stage (T1-2N0M0) oral cavity cancer: a population-based study. Head Neck. 2017; 39(5):876–880

[5] Cannon RB, Sowder JC, Buchmann LO, et al. Increasing use of nonsurgical therapy in advanced-stage oral cavity cancer: a population-based study. Head Neck. 2017; 39(1):82–91

[6] de Melo GM, Ribeiro KC, Kowalski LP, Deheinzelin D. Risk factors for postoperative complications in oral cancer and their prognostic implications. Arch Otolaryngol Head Neck Surg. 2001; 127(7):828–833

[7] Lodders JN, Parmar S, Stienen NL, et al. Incidence and types of complications after ablative oral cancer surgery with primary microvascular free flap reconstruction. Med Oral Patol Oral Cir Bucal. 2015; 20(6):e744–e750

[8] Schwam ZG, Sosa JA, Roman S, Judson BL. Complications and mortality following surgery for oral cavity cancer: analysis of 408 cases. Laryngoscope. 2015; 125(8):1869–1873

[9] Nam W, Kim HJ, Choi EC, Kim MK, Lee EW, Cha IH. Contributing factors to mandibulotomy complications: a retrospective study. Oral Surg Oral Med Oral Pathol Oral Radiol Endod. 2006; 101(3):e65–e70

[10] Balogh JM, Sutherland SE. Osteoradionecrosis of the mandible: a review. J Otolaryngol. 1989; 18(5):245–250

[11] Awad MI, Shuman AG, Montero PH, Palmer FL, Shah JP, Patel SG. Accuracy of administrative and clinical registry data in reporting postoperative complications after surgery for oral cavity squamous cell carcinoma. Head Neck. 2015; 37(6):851–861

[12] Piccirillo JF. Importance of comorbidity in head and neck cancer. Laryngoscope. 2000; 110(4):593–602

[13] Ribeiro KC, Kowalski LP, Latorre MR. Impact of comorbidity, symptoms, and patients' characteristics on the prognosis of oral carcinomas. Arch Otolaryngol Head Neck Surg. 2000; 126(9):1079–1085

[14] Shigeishi H, Ohta K, Takechi M. Risk factors for postoperative complications following oral surgery. J Appl Oral Sci. 2015; 23(4):419–423

[15] Haubner F, Ohmann E, Pohl F, Strutz J, Gassner HG. Wound healing after radiation therapy: review of the literature. Radiat Oncol. 2012; 7:162

[16] Salgado CJ, Chim H, Schoenoff S, Mardini S. Postoperative care and monitoring of the reconstructed head and neck patient. Semin Plast Surg. 2010; 24 (3):281–287

[17] Urken MLCM, Blackwell KE, Harris JR, Hadlock TA, Futran N. Regional and Free Flaps for Head and Neck Reconstruction. 2nd ed. Baltimore: Lippincott Williams & Wilkins; 2012

[18] Forget FG, Tabet P, Rahal A, et al. Free versus pedicled flaps for reconstruction of head and neck cancer fefects: a systematic review. J Otolaryngol Head Neck Surg. 2019; 48 (1):13

[19] Boyle JORV. Complications of surgery of the oral cavity. In: David W. Eisele RVS, ed. Complications in Head and Neck Surgery. 2nd ed. Philadelphia: Mosby 2009:257–266

[20] Burnett MG, Zager EL. Pathophysiology of peripheral nerve injury: a brief review. Neurosurg Focus. 2004; 16(5):E1

[21] Menorca RM, Fussell TS, Elfar JC. Nerve physiology: mechanisms of injury and recovery. Hand Clin. 2013; 29(3):317–330

[22] Clarke B. Normal bone anatomy and physiology. Clin J Am Soc Nephrol. 2008; 3 Suppl 3:S131–S139

[23] Song CS, Har-El G. Marginal mandibulectomy: Oncologic and nononcologic outcome. Am J Otolaryngol. 2003; 24(1):61–63

[24] Moreno MA, Skoracki RJ, Hanna EY, Hanasono MM. Microvascular free flap reconstruction versus palatal obturation for maxillectomy defects. Head Neck. 2010; 32(7):860–868

[25] Nugent B, Lewis S, O'Sullivan JM. Enteral feeding methods for nutritional management in patients with head and neck cancers being treated with radiotherapy and/or chemotherapy. Cochrane Database Syst Rev. 2013(1): CD007904

[26] Jager-Wittenaar H, Dijkstra PU, Vissink A, van der Laan BF, van Oort RP, Roodenburg JL. Critical weight loss in head and neck cancer—prevalence and risk factors at diagnosis: an explorative study. Support Care Cancer. 2007; 15 (9):1045–1050

[27] Ravasco P, Monteiro-Grillo I, Marques Vidal P, Camilo ME. Impact of nutrition on outcome: a prospective randomized controlled trial in patients with head and neck cancer undergoing radiotherapy. Head Neck. 2005; 27(8):659–668

[28] Dissanaike S, Shelton M, Warner K, O'Keefe GE. The risk for bloodstream infections is associated with increased parenteral caloric intake in patients receiving parenteral nutrition. Crit Care. 2007; 11(5):R114

[29] Dort JC, Farwell DG, Findlay M, et al. Optimal perioperative care in major head and neck cancer surgery with free flap reconstruction: a consensus review and recommendations from the Enhanced Recovery After Surgery Society. JAMA Otolaryngol Head Neck Surg. 2017; 143(3):292–303

[30] Weber RS, Callender DL. Antibiotic prophylaxis in clean-contaminated head and neck oncologic surgery. Ann Otol Rhinol Laryngol Suppl. 1992; 155:16–20

[31] Dor P, Klastersky J. Prophylactic antibiotics in oral, pharyngeal and laryngeal surgery for cancer: (a double-blind study). Laryngoscope. 1973; 83(12): 1992–1998

[32] Johnson JT, Yu VL. Antibiotic use during major head and neck surgery. Ann Surg. 1988; 207(1):108–111

[33] Veve MP, Davis SL, Williams AM, McKinnon JE, Ghanem TA. Considerations for antibiotic prophylaxis in head and neck cancer surgery. Oral Oncol. 2017; 74:181–187

[34] Vila PM, Zenga J, Jackson RS. Antibiotic prophylaxis in clean-contaminated head and neck surgery: a systematic review and meta-analysis. Otolaryngol Head Neck Surg. 2017; 157(4):580–588

[35] Carroll WR, Rosenstiel D, Fix JR, et al. Three-dose vs extended-course clindamycin prophylaxis for free-flap reconstruction of the head and neck. Arch Otolaryngol Head Neck Surg. 2003; 129(7):771–774

[36] Bennett MH, Feldmeier J, Hampson NB, Smee R, Milross C. Hyperbaric oxygen therapy for late radiation tissue injury. Cochrane Database Syst Rev. 2016; 4: CD005005

[37] Bhrany AD, Izzard M, Wood AJ, Futran ND. Coronoidectomy for the treatment of trismus in head and neck cancer patients. Laryngoscope. 2007; 117(11): 1952–1956

[38] Dai TS, Hao SP, Chang KP, Pan WL, Yeh HC, Tsang NM. Complications of mandibulotomy: midline versus paramidline. Otolaryngol Head Neck Surg. 2003; 128(1):137–141

[39] Pan WL, Hao SP, Lin YS, Chang KP, Su JL. The anatomical basis for mandibulotomy: midline versus paramidline. Laryngoscope. 2003; 113(2):377–380

[40] Owosho AA, Tsai CJ, Lee RS, et al. The prevalence and risk factors associated with osteoradionecrosis of the jaw in oral and oropharyngeal cancer patients treated with intensity-modulated radiation therapy (IMRT): The Memorial Sloan Kettering Cancer Center experience. Oral Oncol. 2017; 64:44–51

[41] Kuhnt T, Stang A, Wienke A, Vordermark D, Schweyen R, Hey J. Potential risk factors for jaw osteoradionecrosis after radiotherapy for head and neck cancer. Radiat Oncol. 2016; 11:101

[42] Upile T, Triaridis S, Kirkland P, et al. The management of carotid artery rupture. Eur Arch Otorhinolaryngol. 2005; 262(7):555–560

[43] Hillerman BL, Kennedy TL. Carotid rupture and tissue coverage. Laryngoscope. 1982; 92(9 Pt 1):985–988

41 Radiotherapy Related Side Effects in the Treatment of Oral Cavity Malignancies

Matthew P. Deek, Brandi R. Page, and Harry Quon

Summary
Radiation therapy is an integral part of the management in those with oral cavity cancer. However, its benefits come with the risk of numerous acute and long term toxicities. A strong understanding of the pathogenesis and management of these toxicities is necessary to avoid serious complications and guide a patient through a course of therapy. This chapter therefore details these possible complications and how to treat them when they arise.

Keywords: toxicity, radiation therapy, oral cavity

41.1 Principles of Radiation Toxicity

Adjuvant radiotherapy is a mainstay in the management of oral cavity cancers as its use decreases the risk of cancer recurrence.[1,2] However, these benefits come at the cost of various side effects. Similar to surgical procedures, radiotherapy is a locally directed therapy and most (though not all) related sequelae are anatomically directed and dependent on the volumes a radiation oncologist decides to treat. Therefore, deciding what to treat and what not to treat is a crucial part of radiotherapy design. Advances in technology such as the development of intensity-modulated radiotherapy (IMRT), which is standard of care for most head and neck cancers,[3] allows for tighter treatment margins resulting in better sparing of normal tissues.[4] Despite this, toxicity still remains significant and impacts the quality of life.[5] Key research goals include anatomically guiding which normal tissues can be safely spared and identifying what are the meaningful radiotherapy dose volume constraints to the normal tissues.

Side effects of radiotherapy can be viewed as a continuum of acute (during radiotherapy and several weeks after recovery), intermediate (within several months post radiotherapy), and late term (1 year or later) effects in their manifestation. Acute-term effects start at a delayed rate (about 2 weeks into the course). In the oral cavity, these may include progressively worsening oral mucositis or ulceration, thickened saliva, radiation dermatitis, which may result in desquamation at its peak, dysgeusia or ageusia (dysfunction in taste), lymphedema, cosmetic alteration in skin and tissue integrity, and overgrowth of opportunistic pathogens, such as candida, or soft-tissue infections.[6] The underlying pathophysiology of these side effects are thought to reflect direct target cell injury[7] and loss of function followed by the expected inflammatory response for wound healing.

Late manifesting complications in the neck include skin and muscle and fibrovascular tissue fibrosis, fistula formation, chronic orofacial/neck pain, and decreased range of mobility in the neck. Endocrinopathies in the thyroid and/or pituitary can also occur. In the oral cavity and oropharynx, complications include xerostomia, osteoradionecrosis (ORN), scarring in the tongue/soft tissues worsening speech quality and swallow ability potentially resulting in risk of aspiration or feeding tube dependence, trismus which can make speech and chewing difficult, and risk of dental complications including dental caries.[8,9] The pathophysiology of late manifesting complications is less clear, but believed to reflect a progressive local fibroproliferative process and possibly the effectiveness of stem cells from the bone marrow or local microenvironment. Management is largely symptom directed at this time and requires significant hands-on counseling by the radiation oncologist in conjunction with a multidisciplinary team including surgeons, medical oncologists, nurses, speech language pathologists (SLPs), and physical therapists. This chapter will focus on identifying and effectively managing many of these radiation side effects in order to optimize efficacy of cancer-related treatments while minimizing their impact on a patient's overall quality of life. The future directions of reducing and managing radiation toxicities will also be addressed.

41.2 Diagnosis and Evaluation

The first step in assessing radiation-associated side effects is proper evaluation of the patient, beginning with a history and physical examination. Evaluation of the oral cavity can reveal dry mucous membranes, loss of enamel, or tooth decay suggesting xerostomia. Ulceration of the mucosa represents mucositis and if necrotic bone is exposed it could be indicative of ORN. Thrush can be diagnosed clinically as a white covering on the tongue. Externally, lymphedema can be characterized by painless swelling of soft-tissue structures, while radiation fibrosis presents with reduced tissue elasticity and flexibility and reduced range of motion, usually of the neck.

Visualization of structures further along the aerordigestive tract, including those of the larynx and pharynx, can be done using a rhinolaryngoscope allowing for assessment of anatomic integrity. Complementary to an anatomic assessment is a functional assessment often done by an SLP through a fiberoptic endoscopic evaluation of swallowing (FEES). FEES allows the clinician to evaluate an individual's management of secretions, spontaneous swallow, and physiologic swallow through presentation of food and liquid while the rhinolaryngoscope is still in place.[10] Physiologic evaluation of swallow function is also done with a modified barium swallow (MBS). During a MBS, the patient is given liquid with radio-opaque barium, which is swallowed while taking fluoroscopic images allowing for visualization of the liquid as it moves through the upper digestive tract. A particular strength of the MBS is the ability to identify penetration and potential aspiration of the swallow bolus. A penetration aspiration score can then be assigned to denote its severity. Emerging strategies to quantify swallow function include the use of high-resolution manometry and impedance that has been traditionally limited to the esophagus. Recent investigations have demonstrated that the pressure and flow data that is also measured in the pharyngeal portion of a manometry study is not only reproducible, but can yield swallow function variables that robustly describe swallow dysfunction and the risk of aspiration.[11–14]

Evaluation of the severity of toxicities can be done by either the clinician or patient. Clinician-driven evaluations are usually through qualitative and semi-quantitative grading systems such as the common terminology criteria for adverse events (CTCAE), which typically grades side effects on a scale of 1 to 5 using a combination of history, physical examination, and laboratory data. The second approach is the use of patient-reported outcomes (PROs) typically through the completion of paper-based validated instruments, which offer the benefit of understanding symptoms from a patient's perspective.[15] It is important to recognize that PROs are not necessarily synonymous with quality of life assessments which further reflect additional dimensions such as a patient's expectations and potentially their coping skills. For example, dysphagia is often assessed with the M. D. Anderson Dysphagia Inventory (MDADI) which was developed to assess patient perspective views of their swallowing ability and its effects on quality of life.[16] In contrast, the Sydney Swallow Questionnaire (SSQ) was developed to measure patient-reported oral-pharyngeal swallow function.[17] Coadministration of these two instruments has demonstrated that while correlated, they also provide complementary information with the SSQ scores separating patients by swallow function and the MDADI providing insight into the impact the dysphagia had on their quality of life.[18,19]

41.3 Mucositis

Mucositis describes an inflammatory state that reflects a complex interplay of repeated mucosal injury, subsequent inflammatory response, and the effects of a wound healing response that can be incomplete after a given radiation treatment. As such, progressive clinically evident mucosal injury can be observed as fractionated radiotherapy progresses. As with head and neck carcinomas[20,21] the proliferative kinetics of the normal mucosa can also increase with increasing radiation doses leading also to accelerated wound healing (▶ Fig. 41.1).[22]

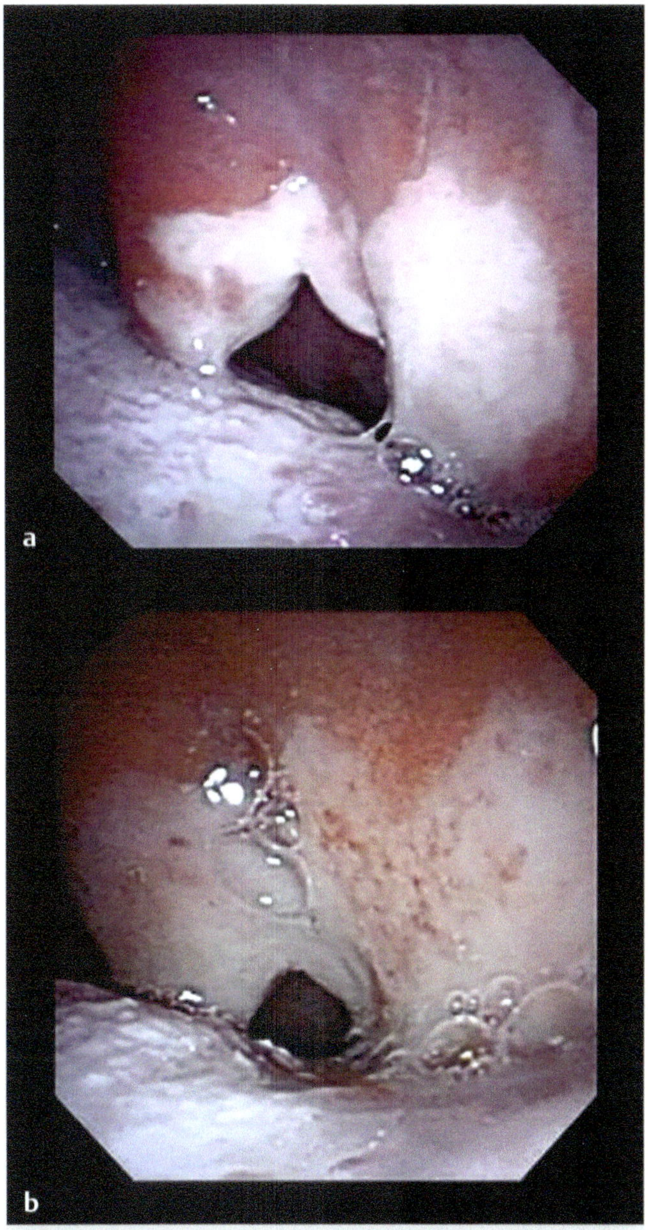

Fig. 41.1 Development of mucositis during a course of radiotherapy as seen during evaluation at 4400 cGy **(a)** and expected proliferation and expansion by 6380 cGy **(b)**.

Studies have demonstrated the importance of the dose delivered during each fraction of radiation (and likely to how large of a volume of mucosa) and the complex interplay with net healing occurring during weekends when treatment is not administered. If insufficient healing of mucosal injury during treatment should occur, persistent mucositis leading to chronic mucosal ulceration has been described as seen in randomized studies evaluating the benefit of continuous daily irradiation including weekend days.[23,24] Similarly, prolonged interruptions in the delivery of radiotherapy can impact tumor control rates due to accelerated tumor repopulation in response to the mucosal injury. For daily fractionation (i.e., conventional fractionation) the peak of the mucosal injury typically occurs during the latter half of the course of the radiotherapy. For more accelerated radiotherapy schedules involving multiple fractions per day, depending on the size of the radiotherapy fraction, the peak of the injury can occur after completion of the course of the radiotherapy. These considerations may be relevant in the scheduling of care for patients receiving radiotherapy and offer insights into the management of acute mucositis and reducing the risk of late consequential mucosal ulceration.

In the upper aerodigestive tract, mucositis typically is associated with functional effects on swallow, speech, and taste. The severity of mucositis is often qualitatively scored using the CTCAE, graded from 1 to 5 representing mild, moderate, severe, life threatening, and death due to toxicity and is based on pain, dietary alterations, extent/confluence, and depth of the mucositis.

The risk of developing oral mucositis increases as the radiation dose to the oral cavity increases. Narayan et al[25] found that oral mucositis could be limited to mild (grade 1 or less) and short term (one week or less) when point doses to the oral cavity were kept less than 32 Gy. Rosenthal et al[26] similarly found maximum point dose of 33.5 Gy or higher to the anterior

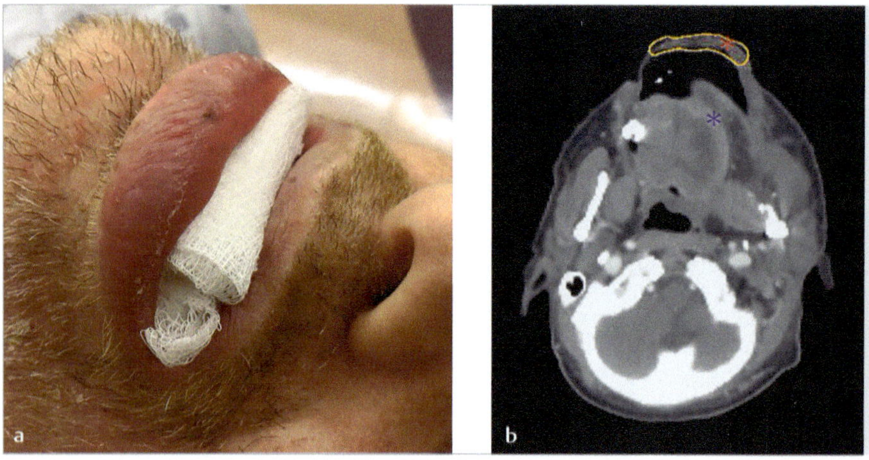

Fig. 41.2 (a, b) Lower lip dental roll placed at the time of the radiotherapy simulation and immobilization, effectively separating the lower lip (*red**) from the adjacent surgical bed (*blue star*).

mandible was associated with the development of grade ≥ 1 oral mucositis. As dose to the oral cavity rises, so does the risk of higher-grade mucositis. Narayan et al found more moderate (grade 2) and longer lasting (3 weeks or longer) mucositis was associated with oral cavity point doses of 39.1 Gy or higher, and Bhide et al[27] reported mean dose of ≥ 51 Gy to the oral cavity was correlated with the development of grade 3 oral cavity mucositis. In addition to the impact of radiotherapy dose, the volume of mucosa irradiated is also an important factor in the development of mucositis. Higher ratios of involved to normal mucosa, indicating a large primary tumor, places an individual at higher risk for severe (grade 3) mucositis.[28]

Though multimodality therapy with concurrent chemotherapy (CRT) improves cancer survival outcomes, it also significantly increases toxicity. Individually, chemotherapy and RT are known independent risk factors for the development of mucositis. However, when combined they act synergistically to increase the risk of severe mucositis in a multiplicative rather than additive fashion.[29] Rates of mucositis were significantly higher in the combination CRT of GORTEC 94–01 (71 vs 39%) as were rates of severe (grade ≥ 3) mucositis in the combination CRT arm of the intergroup study (43 vs. 32%).[30,31] There was optimism that replacing traditional chemotherapeutics with targeted agents (e.g., cetuximab) might result in equally efficacious oncologic outcomes while reducing toxicity.[32] However, RTOG 1016, a trial of over 800 patients randomized to cetuximab versus cisplatin with concurrent accelerated fractionated radiotherapy, has demonstrated that oncologic outcomes for human papillomavirus-associated oropharyngeal carcinomas are inferior when patients are treated with concurrent cetuximab.[33] It is also noteworthy that an incompletely accrued phase II study randomizing patients with head and neck squamous cell carcinoma including oral cavity carcinomas to cisplatin versus cetuximab with concurrent radiotherapy raised concerns that patients receiving cetuximab demonstrated a higher rate of acute toxicities necessitating enteral support, raising caution regarding its use as a potentially less toxic radiosensitizer.[34]

The first step in managing mucositis is minimizing the impact of any mucositis that would be expected based on the radiotherapy dosimetry. In the oral cavity, radiotherapy target volumes that approximate the lips present unique challenges to reduce the impact of mucositis. Where significant mucositis may be expected, the use of dental rolls or spacers placed at the time of radiotherapy simulation and immobilization allows for the displacement of the lips, offering an opportunity to reduce the severity of mucositis on the lips (▶ Fig. 41.2). Similarly, the introduction of a mouth piece with a spacer displacing the palate from the tongue can be beneficial to reduce the risk of mucositis on the palate. This is a particularly beneficial strategy for oral cavity/tongue malignancies where the tongue may be more immobilized due to the effects of surgery limiting its movement and ensuring its position is reproducible with each radiotherapy fraction. However, in patients with a mobile tongue and where it is part of the target volume, judgment is recommended as to whether the benefits with the introduction of a mouth piece displacing it from the palate may be offset by the risk of day-to-day variability in the tongue position due to the presence of the mouth piece.

During radiotherapy, ongoing close surveillance of the oral cavity mucosa to identify areas of mucositis is beneficial for several reasons. It not only ensures additional quality assurance of the delivery of the radiotherapy plan, but also allows for several interventions that can reduce its impact on oral cavity function. Mucosal injury arising from bite-line trauma offers opportunities for dental solutions to minimize the damage. Often, it is the secondary mucosal edema that may be exacerbated by the prior oncologic surgery that contributes to the risk of developing dental trauma and requires ongoing evaluation. In addition, dental amalgam can create scatter beta-radiation contributing to premature mucositis beyond what is expected based on the planned dosimetry. In the oral cavity, the buccal and oral tongue mucosa are particularly sensitive to this given the proximity to the teeth and their movement in the oral swallow phase preparing the food bolus. Identifying these areas offers opportunities to either replace the amalgam or to introduce a spacer with either a dental roll or wax, provided this does not alter the reproducibility of the target volumes.

Lastly, ongoing surveillance of areas of mucosal ulceration is important to determine if sufficient normal tissue repair response is occurring based on the severity of the acute mucositis. This is important as it has been demonstrated that severe acute mucosal ulceration in the setting of insufficient normal mucosal repair during the radiotherapy can lead to an increased risk of consequential late mucosal side effects[24,35] due to injury to the mucosal stem cell population.[36] Reducing the severity of the acute injury has been proposed as a strategy to reduce this risk.[37] Minimizing trauma, replanning of radiotherapy dosimetry, and judicious use of treatment interruptions are potential strategies to consider.

Maintaining oral hygiene is imperative to reduce microbial overgrowth that can lead to an aggravation of mucositis.[38] Salt and baking soda rinses can be used several times a day and if microbial overgrowth is suspected, appropriate antimicrobial agents (Nystatin for yeast) should be prescribed. Pain control is essential for patients to maintain nutrition, engage the muscles to reduce the risk of late swallowing complications,[39,40] and avoid treatment breaks. Topical anesthetics, such as lidocaine, can be used alone or in combination with diphenhydramine solution and simethicone-based antacid products for initial pain management. High-dose gabapentin (900 mg TID) can be slowly titrated up prior to beginning treatment and maintained for the duration of radiotherapy. Its role in the management of mucositis pain remains an active area of investigation and one with significant promise as it has been associated with decreased narcotic use and treatment breaks.[41] As treatment progresses, additional pharmacologic interventions can be used as pain dictates typically with the introduction of short-acting opioids (i.e., oxycodone, hydrocodone) titrated to maintain pain control. Long-acting narcotics can be used as well, but with extreme caution if short-acting narcotics are still to be titrated up given the risk of respiratory depression and sedation these agents can cause. Several other drugs, including amifostine[42,43] and granulocyte macrophage stimulating factor[44,45] have demonstrated mixed results.

41.4 Xerostomia

Xerostomia is the subjective feeling of dry mouth as well as an objective decline in salivary flow, which when caused by radiotherapy is due to damage to the major and minor salivary glands. Beyond a perceived feeling of discomfort, xerostomia can also result in pain, dental caries, changes in voice quality, and swallowing dysfunction.

A mean dose of 10 to 15 Gy to the parotid typically results in minimal impairment of gland function. However, as mean RT dose increases to 20 to 40 Gy, gland function reduces and at doses of > 40 Gy severe (> 75%) reduction in gland function is observed.[46,47] IMRT is now frequently used in order to spare the contralateral parotid with the hopes of avoiding long-term xerostomia. Quantitative Analyses of Normal Tissue Effects in the Clinic (QUANTEC) guidelines recommend sparing at least one parotid gland to a mean dose of < 20 Gy or both parotids to a mean dose of < 25 Gy in order to avoid long-term severe (< 25% of baseline) salivary dysfunction[48] and a study by Portaluri et al observed that a mean dose of < 30 Gy to the contralateral parotid was associated with only mild subjective xerostomia.[49] These investigations typically summarized the parotid dosimetry as the average dose and assumes that the spatial function of the parotid gland is uniform. However, evidence in both animal models and more recently in humans supports the conclusion that parotid gland function is not uniform and offers unique opportunities to develop new strategies to further reduce this complication. Rat xerostomia models have demonstrated that irradiation of only the cranial half of the parotid glands results more permanent xerostomia compared to the caudal half where recovery was observed (▶ Fig. 41.3).[50] Further preclinical studies have identified stem cells which are speculated to be responsible for the improvement in the xerostomia.[51] Investigations by our group using a growing clinical big data inventory of National Cancer Institute (NCI) CTCAE grading of xerostomia further supports not only improvement in the irradiated head and neck cancer patient with time, but has also demonstrated the importance of parotid sub-volumes that are more at risk of injury and are associated with the severity of xerostomia at 3 to 6 months after completion of radiotherapy (▶ Fig. 41.4).[52,53]

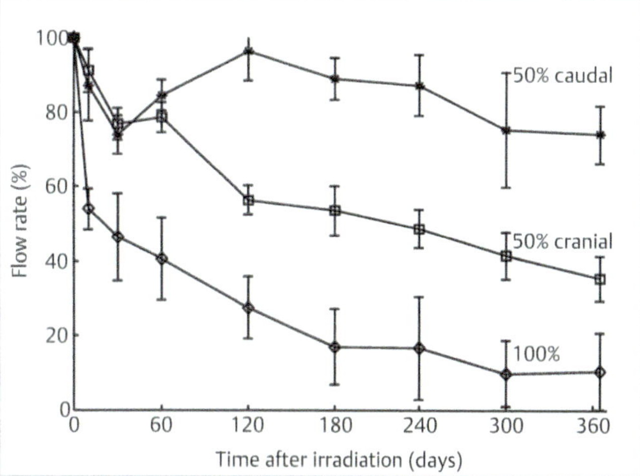

Fig. 41.3 Rat xerostomia models demonstrating more permanent xerostomia with irradiation of only the cranial half of the parotid glands compared to the caudal half.

Applying a data science approach to understand which factors are associated and predictive of the risk of severe xerostomia (CTCAE grade ≥ 2) at different time points (i.e., 3–6 months vs. 18 months or greater) following radiotherapy has further demonstrated that the risk of severe xerostomia is also dependent on the dosimetry to sub-volumes in the parotid glands. The importance of the dosimetry to these parotid sub-volumes offers the potential to develop future radiotherapy strategies to further reduce this risk. While it is clear that the parotid dosimetry to these sub-volumes (especially the cranial portions) dictates a great deal of the risk of severe xerostomia, patient factors along with the dosimetry to the oral cavity minor salivary glands[54,55] and submandibular glands[56] appear to be secondarily modifying this risk. For example, the application of radiomic analysis of parotid and submandibular glands based on the baseline computed tomography (CT) images used for radiotherapy planning allows one to quantify the "health state" of the glands. In doing so, our group has demonstrated that these salivary gland radiomic features further add to the accuracy of xerostomia prediction models suggesting that they may reflect baseline salivary gland function or regions at greater risk for RT-injury.[53]

Symptomatic xerostomia is often managed with salivary substitutes, which can provide temporary hydration and lubrication of the oral cavity and be used several times per day. Lozenges with acidic, bitter, or sweet flavors can be used as

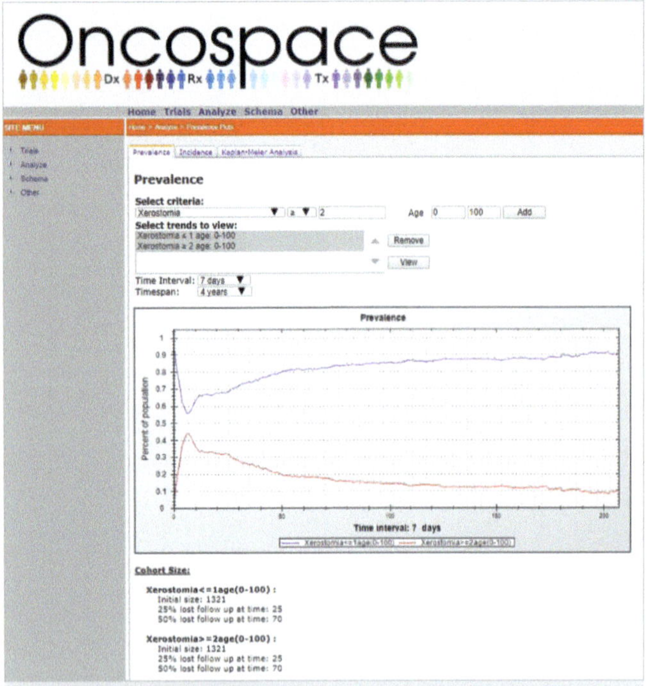

Fig. 41.4 Prevalence of National Cancer Institute-Common Terminology Criteria for Adverse Events (NCI-CTCAE) xerostomia grades in irradiated head and neck cancer patients ($n = 1321$) captured within the Oncospace learning health system. CTCAE xerostomia grading is captured at each patient encounter leading to a growing inventory of xerostomia grades that allow for the natural history of radiation-induced xerostomia to be characterized and studied.

gustatory salivary stimulants of saliva production. Pharmacologic salivary stimulants, such as pilocarpine or cevimeline, can also be used in symptom management. Pilocarpine has been evaluated in randomized studies and when compared to placebo in patients treated with historic non-parotid sparing radiotherapy techniques, 5 mg of pilocarpine three times per day improved symptomatic oral dryness (44 vs. 25%) with similar results seen with 10 mg three times per day.[57] Side effects seen with pilocarpine are typically anticholinergic (sweating, flushing, nausea, headache, diarrhea) and were moderate enough to cause 5 and 20% of patients on the 5 mg and 10 mg TID arms respectively to stop treatment.

Acupuncture-like transcutaneous nerve stimulation in the treatment of xerostomia was recently compared to pilocarpine treatment in a randomized fashion.[58] Both demonstrated subjective improvements in xerostomia-related quality of life, though no assessment could be made in terms of superiority. Acupuncture has also been studied in the prevention of radiation-induced xerostomia. When administered three times per week concurrently with radiotherapy, acupuncture improved both subjective xerostomia as well as objective salivary flow rates.[59] Finally, the use of submandibular gland transfer to the submental space has been explored in nasopharyngeal carcinoma with success; however, the dosimetric benefit for oral cavity cancer is not as clear given the physical limitations to which the submandibular gland can be transferred relative to the radiotherapy doses that are typically prescribed for oral cavity malignancies.[60]

41.5 Osteoradionecrosis

ORN[61] is a serious complication of radiotherapy resulting in nonhealing and possibly devitalized bone. Affected tissues can become hypovascular, hypocellular, and hypoxic reducing the chances of future healing.[62] Rates of ORN have declined from 11.8% before 1968 to 5.4% from 1968 to 1992 to less than 3% today with improvements in radiation dose conformality as well as dental care.[63–65]

Radiation dose to the mandible is a strong risk factor for ORN and ideally the maximum dose is kept below 66 to 70 Gy (RTOG 0225, RTOG 1016) as doses greater than 70 Gy increase the risk of developing ORN.[66] However, the volume of mandible receiving slightly lower doses of radiation (40–60 Gy) is also strongly correlated with risk of developing ORN. In a matched cohort of patients, each percentage increase in the volume of the mandible receiving 50 Gy resulted in a 9% increased risk of ORN (odds ratio: 1.09, $p = 0.02$).[67] Underlying dental health is another probable risk factor, with individuals requiring dental extractions prior to radiotherapy and those already edentulous prior to treatment are at higher risk of developing ORN.[67] The importance of dental health is highlighted by the higher than expected rates of ORN in clinical trials such as RTOG 0022[68] where there was not rigorous use of prophylactic dental care. This is in contrast to published series where stringent dental evaluation was required, including extractions of decaying or nonrestorable teeth prior to therapy and daily topical fluoride use where no cases of ORN were observed.[64] Other noted risk factors include a history of smoking and alcohol use, which is often associated with poor baseline dental health, as well as larger primary tumors, likely a surrogate for larger volumes of the mandible receiving radiation[67] and the addition of a brachytherapy boost.[66] Whether it is necessary to remove healthy teeth that could require future extractions prior to radiotherapy is not clear at this time.

Management of ORN is often based on its severity. Conservative management includes local irrigation (with saline, bicarbonate, or chlorhexidine), avoidance of irritants such as smoking and alcohol, and continued maintenance of oral hygiene.[69] Pharmacologic interventions include the antitumor necrosis factor agent pentoxifylline (400 mg BID) and the antioxidant tocopherol (1,000 IU daily) also known as vitamin E.[70] The PENTACLO regimen, consisting of 800 mg pentoxifylline, 1,000 IU vitamin E, and 1,600 mg clodronate 5 days per week alternating with 20 mg prednisone and 1,000 mg ciprofloxacin 2 days per week has proven safe and effective in the treatment of ORN.[71] The use of hyperbaric oxygen in patients with ORN is controversial. The only randomized placebo controlled trial conducted on the subject did not show any benefit to its use, though the study of often criticized for its design and definition of ORN. Surgical management is the most invasive intervention, but has benefited from technological advancements. Myocutaneous flaps and the use of microvascular free bone replaces dead bone with a vascularized bone-containing flap, allowing for reconstruction of the mandible and transposition of nonirradiated soft tissue with intact blood supply to help the healing process.[69] A general rule of thumb is the more extensive the ORN, the less likely conservative measures will be effective. For example, Notani et al reported that 70% of patients with ORN confined to the alveolar and/or mandible above the level of the alveolar canal healed with conservative therapy alone. However, only 10% of the patients with ORN that extended to the mandible below the level of the alveolar canal, ORN with a skin fistula, or pathologic fracture healed with conservative therapy, but 40% of those were salvaged by surgery.[72]

Poor dental health after radiotherapy requiring tooth extraction or major work is difficult situation in follow-up. Hyperbaric oxygen has been suggested as a prophylactic measure to decrease the risk of ORN in these situations. Marx et al performed a randomized trial comparing the use of prophylactic hyperbaric oxygen to penicillin and found the use of hyperbaric oxygen decreased the risk of ORN (5 vs. 30%).[73] However, the generalizability of this study has been questioned given the very high rate of ORN in the penicillin arm. A pooled analysis of studies since 1986 by Wahl demonstrated a rate of ORN of only 3.5% without hyperbaric oxygen[65] and therefore the utility of prophylactic hyperbaric oxygen is not clear. Whether there are specific doses to the mandible, above which would preclude tooth extraction due to untenably high ORN risk, is not well established either. Several authors posit that doses of > 50 to 60 Gy to the area undergoing extraction puts an individual at a > 10% risk for development of ORN; however, in one of the largest experiences of 528 in-field tooth extractions, only 4 developed ORN.[63,74,75]

41.6 Dysphagia

Dysphagia in the setting of radiotherapy or chemoradiotherapy is the result of a complex interplay of structural, mechanical, and neurologic systems that affect one or both of the oral and pharyngeal phases of a normal swallow. Dysphagia is often divided into three time courses: acute (< 3 months), subacute (3–6 months), and chronic (> 6 months). Acute and subacute dysphagia is often caused by cell death from radiation with a subsequent inflammatory response, while the chronic state is due to damage to the surrounding vasculature and connective tissue resulting in and from fibrosis.[40] Patients may often endorse dysphagia secondary to mucositis or xerostomia, which are topics discussed in detail in preceding sections. However, cancer treatment with both surgery and radiation therapy not only can affect the oral phase but the pharyngeal phase of swallow. The latter can result due to the role the suprahyoid muscles play in laryngeal elevation and the safe passage of the swallow bolus in its pharyngeal transit.[76,77] It can also occur due to the challenges in radiotherapy target delineation especially for oral cavity malignancies with posterior extension and the need to anatomically distinguish the adjacent oropharynx and larynx that do not need irradiation from the adjacent floor of mouth muscles and cervical neck that do. Identifying these structures allows for the use of avoidance volumes that can effectively reduce the risk of acute and potentially late dysphagia complications (▶ Fig. 41.5).

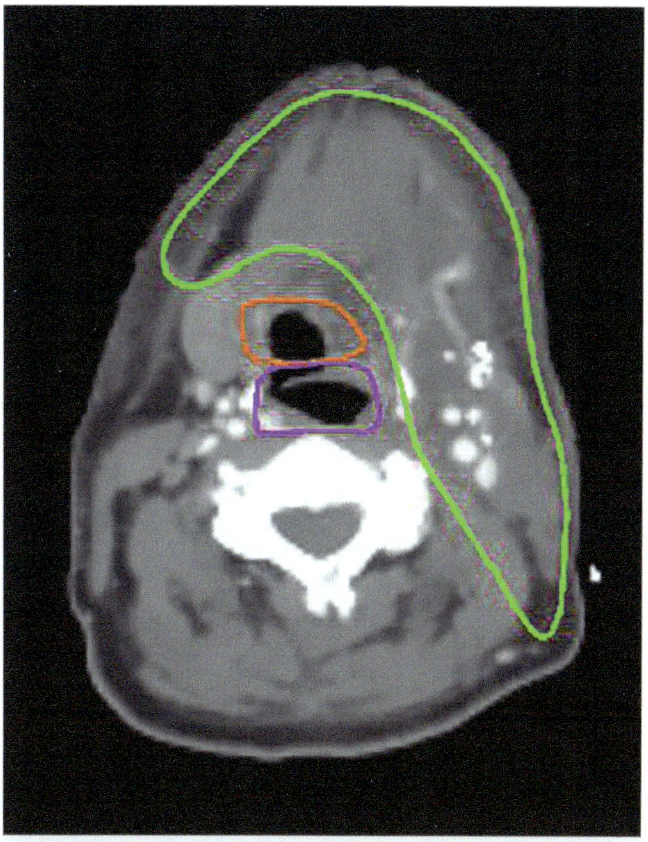

Fig. 41.5 Planning target volume treating the floor of mouth muscles and adjacent cervical nodes. Avoidance volumes encompassing the adjacent tongue base and epiglottis are drawn to reduce the dose to these structures that are not at risk of cancer involvement.

Posttreatment dysphagia is a significant problem in individuals treated for oral cavity cancer. Long-term dysphagia causing pain and an inability to tolerate solids following chemoradiation or surgery and postoperative radiation can be as high as 15%, even when utilizing advanced techniques such as IMRT.[5,78] Dysphagia is a significant driver of quality of life following treatment and also has a significant impact on morbidity and mortality.[79,80] Long-term results from RTOG 91-11 showed the CRT group had the lowest risk of laryngeal cancer death; however, this group also had a high proportion of patients who died due to reasons unrelated to laryngeal cancer, raising concerns about fatal treatment-related episodes due to late effects such as weight loss, esophageal strictures, airway obstruction, and pneumonia (possibly aspiration related), all of which are associated with long-term dysphagia.[81–83] Though these observations occurred in larynx cancer patients, it is noteworthy that similar observations have been made in oral cavity malignancies where late mortality due specifically to aspiration pneumonia was associated with the radiotherapy dosimetry in the cricopharyngeus muscle of the upper esophageal sphincter.[84] Similar relationships between this pattern of esophageal dysphagia and the risk of aspiration pneumonia mortality are seen in frail patients who have unsensed penetration of the food bolus. Interestingly, in a study of over 2,600 MBS studies, traditional strategies of nothing by mouth or the use of modified food consistencies did not reduce the aspiration mortality risk compared to full diet recommendations.[85] Collectively, reducing the risk of late pharyngeal dysphagia and aspiration mortality risks from radiotherapy should involve careful radiotherapy treatment planning with careful consideration of the radiotherapy dose to the upper esophageal sphincter/cricopharyngeus and the upper esophagus.

Management of dysphagia should be centered on efforts to promote and maintain the use of the swallow muscles starting from the initiation of treatment.[86] Prolonged disuse of the swallowing apparatus can lead to weakness and atrophy of these muscles and dysphagia in itself.[87] In the acute setting, the first step to facilitate continued oral intake is adequate analgesic control similar to the paradigm used for mucositis. Patients should be seen and evaluated by SLP before and throughout treatment. Prophylactic swallowing exercises should be started at the initiation of treatment and have demonstrated improved constrictor muscles maintenance and swallowing function when studied in a prospective randomized fashion.[88,89] Transcutaneous neuromuscular electrical stimulation, which involves transmission of low voltage current via the skin surface causing muscle contraction, can also be used as an adjunct to swallowing exercises and appears to improve long-term dysphagia-related outcomes.[90]

In the past, prophylactic percutaneous endoscopic gastrostomy (PEG) tubes were often placed prior to beginning radiotherapy; however, we advise that routine prophylactic placement of PEG should be avoided if possible.[86] While they may result in improved early enteral nutrition and rates of malnutrition, long-term detriments in nourishment or weight maintenance are not observed without them and their use has been associated with poorer long-term swallowing outcomes as described above.[87] Partial oral intake with aggressive use of nutritional supplements is preferred to maintain use of the pharyngeal apparatus. If necessary, a nasogastric tube may be placed as this can provide nutritional supplementation while still allowing patients to have oral intake during and after treatment. Decisions on which individuals warrant placement of a nasogastric tube can be based on both subjective and objective indicators. Validated PROs including the MDADI and SSQ provide an excellent means of tracking individuals with decompensated swallowing function during and after treatment.[16,18] Laboratory values also provide a means of monitoring patients; weight loss of 10% or more of pretreatment values often is a trigger for nasogastric tube placement. These same metrics can be used to monitor patients once a nasogastric tube is placed to determine when it can be removed.

41.7 Radiation Fibrosis

Radiation fibrosis is an abnormally excessive host reaction to radiotherapy-induced cellular damage associated with aberrant stromal tissue remodeling and eventual tissue contraction. Clinically, this often presents in patients as reduced tissue flexibility and mobility.[91] The normal wound healing process can broadly be categorized into three phases: inflammation, tissue formation, and remodeling. While not completely understood at a molecular level, macroscopic radiation fibrosis is thought to be due to an overactive remodeling phase. Histologically, this is characterized by persistence of myofibroblasts, which are key cells regulating extracellular components, such as collagen, resulting in fibrosis.[92] In addition, damage to vascular tissue also likely plays a role through hypoxia-mediated recruitment of inflammatory cells with subsequent release of profibrotic factors such as transforming growth factor beta 1.[93]

There are several factors associated with a higher risk of radiation fibrosis. Treatment-related factors include total dose, dose per fraction, volume of tissue treated, treatment time, and concurrent chemotherapy. As expected, higher dose and volume treated increase the risk of radiation-induced fibrosis. Hypofractionated regimens, with higher doses per fraction, and the use of concurrent chemotherapy are also risk factors for radiation fibrosis.[94–96] Patient-related risk factors include increasing age and coexistent connective tissue diseases such as scleroderma or systemic lupus erythematosus.[94,97] Finally, the important role genetics plays in radiation fibrosis is beginning to be better understood. Mutations in multiple genes including ataxia-telangiectasia mutated gene, superoxide dismutase 2, X-ray repair cross-complementing proteins 1 and 3, and transforming growth factor beta 1 are now known to be associated with radiation-induced fibrosis.[98–101]

Assessment of radiation-induced fibrosis should begin with a thorough physical examination of all areas within the radiation field. Further quantitative characterization of fibrosis can be done through ultrasound imaging but routine strategies remain limited to the use of CTCAE grading schemas.[102] Other assessment tools are available but require further validation.[103,104]

The first step in management of radiation-induced fibrosis is to avoid any factors that could potentially lead to further injury including fibrogenic chemotherapeutics or local trauma to the area (additional surgical procedures). Anti-inflammatories such as corticosteroids or nonsteroidal anti-inflammatories can be used to reduce acute inflammation associated with fibrosis, though no evidence exists for their efficacy in individuals with established radiation-induced fibrosis.[105] Pentoxifylline is a methylxanthine derivative with several effects including increase in blood flow, inhibition of coagulation, fibroblast and collagen proliferation, and reduction in immunologic and inflammatory reactions that theoretically would make it ideal for treating radiation-induced fibrosis. Okunieff et al demonstrated functional improvements including active and passive range of motion, muscle strength, and limb edema at 8 weeks with the use of 1,200 mg daily; however, there was loss of these improvements after stopping pentoxifylline.[106] It appears that 1,200 mg daily is the threshold dose necessary to see these improvements as studies using lower doses (800 mg/daily) did not show any benefit.[107] Alpha-tocopherol (vitamin E) has also been examined given its ability to scavenge radical oxygen species as an antioxidant. Thus far studies investigating its use have shown mixed results in terms of efficacy as a single agent treatment.[107] While neither pentoxifylline nor vitamin E alone has shown convincing effectiveness at maintaining long-term symptom control, the combination of the two does appear to have some benefit. Delanian et al showed the combination of 800 mg daily of pentoxifylline and 1,000 IU/day of vitamin E taken daily for 6 months substantially reduced the surface area of radiation-induced fibrosis in head and neck and breast cancer patients.[108] A follow-up trial randomizing individuals to pentoxifylline + vitamin E, single agent + placebo, or double agent placebo confirmed the efficacy of the combination of pentoxifylline + vitamin E in reducing superficial radiation-induced fibrosis.[107]

41.8 Lymphedema

Lymphedema is a common side effect seen following head and neck radiotherapy with documented rates of up to 75 to 80%.[109,110] It is especially a challenge in the oral cavity patient where neck dissection can impact its development and resolution after a course of radiotherapy. Clinically, patients will often present with painless swelling of external soft tissues in the head and neck. However, lymphedema can also occur in internal structures such as the mucous membranes of the aerodigestive tract, which can lead to difficulty swallowing or breathing. Lymphedema is caused by impairment of the normal lymphatic drainage pathways and can be due to trauma secondary to surgical manipulation and removal of lymph nodes, impaired lymph vessel contractility due to surgery or radiation, and recurrent infections such as cellulitis.[111] Without adequate efforts at prevention and treatment, long-term lymphedema can result in poor cosmesis and functional impairment in swallowing and phonation. Several risk factors exist for development of lymphedema including increasing radiation dose, use of multimodality therapy (i.e., surgery with postop radiation), especially following neck dissection,[112] and location of primary tumor (pharyngeal being high risk).[110]

A diagnosis of lymphedema can be made clinically through history and physical examination. Several classification systems are available to evaluate and stage lymphedema once diagnosed including the M. D. Anderson head and neck lymphedema rating scale which stages on a scale from 0 to 3.[103,113] Stage 0 represents lymphedema without visible edema but a sensation of tissue heaviness; stage 1a shows soft visible edema without pitting that is reversible; stage 1b demonstrates soft pitting edema that still remains reversible; stage 2 displays firm pitting edema that is irreversible but lacks tissue changes; and stage 3 lymphedema shows irreversible tissue changes such as hyperkeratosis or papillomatosis.

Initial treatment typically begins with manual lymph drainage performed several times per week for a month on an outpatient basis by a certified lymphedema therapist. This is combined with the use of compressive bandages on the affected area, careful skin care, and physical exercises of the head and neck to form what is known as complete decongestive therapy. Compressive bandages are typically placed immediately after a manual lymph drainage session in order to promote continued lymphatic drainage. Manual lymph drainage techniques are eventually transition to the home setting through self-techniques involving gentle circular motion massaging affected areas in order to increase lymphatic drainage; however, these home techniques can also be done concurrently with outpatient therapy. Manual lymph drainage techniques should be tailored for each patient based on their treatment regimen and pattern of scarring and may require assistance from a second person. With the use of these techniques, greater than 50% of patients can experience improvement in their lymphedema. Factors typically associated with better response rates are higher levels of adherence to treatment protocols and outpatient sessions with certified lymphedema therapists.[111]

41.9 Dysgeusia

Sensory changes during (chemo)radiation in head and neck cancer patients occur frequently. Dysgeusia, defined as distortion of the sense of taste, can mildly or severely impact patients' quality of life along a spectrum of complete (ageusia) or partial (hypogeusia) loss of the sense of taste. During radiotherapy, dysgeusia is typically one of the first side effects (followed by mucositis, dermatitis, thickened saliva) and progresses with increasing radiotherapy dose.[114] The ability to taste is an important aspect in enjoying food, and impacts one's ability to take in nutrition and enjoy social interactions and activities focused around food. Dysgeusia can therefore contribute to mood changes, decreased nutritional intake, and the risk of malnutrition. Malnourished patients are at a higher risk for poor wound healing due to decreases in cellular and humoral immunity, hospitalization for failure to thrive, and instrumentation with nasogastric tube or gastrostomy tube.[115,116]

Causes of dysgeusia are likely multifactorial and incompletely understood possibly due to limitations as developing an effective and robust measure of taste changes during radiotherapy.[117,118] Dysgeusia has been preliminarily associated with high doses to the oral cavity where RT has a known cytotoxic effect leading to loss of taste buds.[114,119] Surgical therapy results in direct severing of nerves and removal of taste buds within resected tissue. Cytotoxic chemotherapy targets rapidly dividing cells, and the widely used concurrent head and neck cancer chemotherapies, cisplatin and carboplatin are known to be associated with dysgeusia.[120]

While taste buds are often thought to be on the oral tongue, they are also located in the posterior pharyngeal wall, floor of mouth, base of tongue, buccal mucosa, soft palate, and upper esophagus, areas also often included in the radiation field.[114] Due to the late healing and return of taste function, some have postulated RT damages the neural component.[121] RT-induced inflammation of the afferent nerves that supply the taste buds, direct damage to differentiated taste cells, and eradication of proliferating progenitors prevent renewal of the short-lived taste cells.[118] Studies of epithelial, stromal, and glandular changes in the oral cavity in patients receiving RT have shown diverse pathological effects to include fibrosis, necrosis, atrophy, and vascular damage. Furthermore, radiotherapy produces a wide spectrum of DNA changes which includes nuclear base damage, single and double strand breaks of various complexity, and DNA cross links. These altered cells undergo repair, which if effective results in functionally normal cells.[122]

There is no known proven therapy for treatment of dysgeusia. Treatment of other competing factors for malnourishment, such as nausea, fatigue, oral hygiene, and pain secondary to mucositis, is recommended. More studies are necessary to further characterize the impact and measurement of taste function and possible therapeutic interventions.

41.10 Trismus

A detailed discussion of trismus can be found in Chapter 47. This section will focus on the subject from a radiation oncologist's viewpoint. In patients presenting for initial evaluation of head and neck cancer, trismus is usually caused by malignant invasion into the muscles of mastication (masseter and pterygoid muscles), neural structures innervating these muscles, the temporomandibular joint (TMJ), or other supportive tissues.

Treatment of oral cavity cancer, through surgical manipulation of the TMJ and muscles of mastication or through radiation therapy can also result in trismus. Radiation-induced trismus is likely due to damage and fibrosis of the muscles of mastication and TMJ[123] with higher doses to the ipsilateral masseter,[124] medial pterygoid,[125] and TMJ most associated with its development.[126] The hypomobility from radiation-induced fibrosis can ultimately lead to atrophy of the muscles and TMJ and when not used, these structures will rapidly degenerate causing worsening of symptoms.[127,128] While treatment-related effects are often the cause, when an individual presents with trismus following definitive cancer management, tumor recurrence must also be ruled out.

Early intervention in treating trismus is key factor as disuse atrophy can rapidly set in. Exercise therapy is one of the most important modes of intervention. This includes active jaw opening using objects such as tongue depressors or finger stretching. Jaw opening devices can also be used.[129] If conservative measures such as these fail, surgical intervention with a coronoidectomy (removal of the coronoid process of the mandible) can be considered.[130,131]

41.11 The Oncospace Project

To date, insights into the development and prevention of radiation complications in the head and neck cancers have been based on retrospective institutional reviews. These analyses have typically analyzed the dose–volume histogram (DVH) which summarizes the radiotherapy dose to organs contoured during the radiotherapy planning process and related these to toxicity endpoints. Often, these toxicity assessments are retrospectively abstracted from clinical documentation where the absence of toxicity grading often leads to missing data limiting not only the statistical assessments, but the potential introduction of biases typically toward severe complications. Moreover, the study of radiotherapy toxicities has largely been limited to the use of semiquantitative scales such as the NCI CTCAE grading scales. The output of these assessment scales often limit the ability to understand important relationships with lesser degrees of treatment complication that offer insight into the natural history of the complications and strategies for its prevention. Lastly, the use of the DVH as a summary of the radiotherapy makes a fundamental assumption that each volume of the normal organ is equally at risk of radiation injury. Evidence suggests that if resident stem cells are important for an organ's function and recovery from radiotherapy injury,[51] spatial analysis of the radiotherapy dosimetry is important and that the use of traditional statistical summaries such as the mean dose may not be adequate.

In 2007, the Oncospace project was initiated at the Johns Hopkins University. This project sought to leverage the intrinsic database and imaging platforms that are inherent to the quality care delivery process of modern radiotherapy to create a learning health system. The informatics infrastructure created seeks to curate a comprehensive and growing dataset of patients treated with radiotherapy whereby each treated patient's experience would incrementally add cumulative insights accelerating changes in clinical care (▶ Fig. 41.4). An early focus of this project has been but not limited to the evaluation of radiotherapy toxicities. Collected oncologic outcomes as they mature will broaden the scope of clinical questions that can be addressed. By curating the radiotherapy dosimetry as a series of analyzable relational tables whereby the spatial orientation of the dose is preserved, even to the level defined by the CT voxels used to plan the radiotherapy (i.e., dosomics), our group has demonstrated that the spatial analysis of the radiotherapy dosimetry is not only feasible but particularly relevant. As described above, the application of advanced algorithmic modeling has identified spatially dependent dosimetric relationships identifying the importance of key sub-volumes in the parotid glands especially in the recovery from radiation-induced xerostomia. It is also clear that the heterogeneity in patients and their organ function further complicates the prediction and our ability to reduce the risk of radiation toxicities. As such, the early findings that texture analysis of the parotid glands offer a strategy to quantify baseline parotid sub-volumes at risk for injury is an attractive and important future research strategy to advance in our pursuit of personalizing radiotherapy for the head and neck cancer patient. As radiation injury represents a complex wound, developing more effective and granular tools of radiation toxicity will only help to further complement and facilitate the translational potential of an informatics infrastructure such as Oncospace. Lastly, Oncospace was developed based on the vision of a federated data research network whereby data sharing between institutions can be safely operationalized while ensuring patient confidentiality. Such a network of data enclaves will allow for the generalizability of observations to be tested, accelerating the advancement of new strategies to reduce radiation toxicities.

Key Points

- Effective management of radiation-associated side effects begins with an understanding of the dosimetric implications of each individual patient's treatment plan in order to predict subsequent symptom development. This necessitates a multidisciplinary knowledge base and approach including input from radiation oncologist, surgeons, medical oncologists, nurses, SLPs, nutritionists, and physical therapists.
- Management of radiation mucositis requires ongoing close surveillance during treatment to allow early identification and subsequent interventions (i.e., reducing bite trauma) and effective pain management ranging from topical anesthetics (lidocaine) to oral narcotics (oxycodone, hydrocodone).
- Avoiding long-term xerostomia begins with the radiation planning process by choosing treatment volumes that allow dose reduction to salivary glands while maintaining appropriate target coverage. The optimal salivary gland radiotherapy planning dose constraints remain an active area of investigation with the spatial localization of the radiotherapy emerging as an important concept to minimize the risk of severe xerostomia. Symptomatic xerostomia can be managed with salivary substitutes that provide temporary hydration and lubrication or stimulants including lozenges and pharmacologic agents such as pilocarpine and cevimeline.
- Dysphagia represents a potentially serious source of morbidity and mortality following radiation therapy. It is best avoided by minimizing disuse atrophy of the swallow muscles through appropriate pain control and the use of prophylactic swallowing exercises during and after treatment regardless of whether or not a prophylactic PEG tube is placed. For patients who need supplemental nutrition during and shortly after treatment placement, a nasogastric tube may be considered.

- Postradiation lymphedema can result in poor cosmesis and functional impairment in swallowing and phonation. Individuals who develop lymphedema can be referred to a certified lymphedema therapist for manual lymph drainage and should be educated on these techniques for self-use.

References

[1] Mishra RC, Singh DN, Mishra TK. Post-operative radiotherapy in carcinoma of buccal mucosa, a prospective randomized trial. Eur J Surg Oncol. 1996; 22 (5):502–504

[2] Ang KK, Trotti A, Brown BW, et al. Randomized trial addressing risk features and time factors of surgery plus radiotherapy in advanced head-and-neck cancer. Int J Radiat Oncol Biol Phys. 2001; 51(3):571–578

[3] Hartford AC, Palisca MG, Eichler TJ, et al. American Society for Therapeutic Radiology and Oncology, American College of Radiology. American Society for Therapeutic Radiology and Oncology (ASTRO) and American College of Radiology (ACR) Practice Guidelines for Intensity-Modulated Radiation Therapy (IMRT). Int J Radiat Oncol Biol Phys. 2009; 73(1):9–14

[4] Chen AM, Daly ME, Farwell DG, et al. Quality of life among long-term survivors of head and neck cancer treated by intensity-modulated radiotherapy. JAMA Otolaryngol Head Neck Surg. 2014; 140(2):129–133

[5] Chen WC, Hwang TZ, Wang WH, et al. Comparison between conventional and intensity-modulated post-operative radiotherapy for stage III and IV oral cavity cancer in terms of treatment results and toxicity. Oral Oncol. 2009; 45(6):505–510

[6] Fogh S, Yom SS. Symptom management during the radiation oncology treatment course: a practical guide for the oncology clinician. Semin Oncol. 2014; 41(6):764–775

[7] Puck TT, Marcus PI. Action of X-rays on mammalian cells. J Exp Med. 1956; 103(5):653–666

[8] Xu B, Boero IJ, Hwang L, et al. Aspiration pneumonia after concurrent chemoradiotherapy for head and neck cancer. Cancer. 2015; 121(8):1303–1311

[9] Garcia-Serra A, Amdur RJ, Morris CG, Mazzaferri E, Mendenhall WM. Thyroid function should be monitored following radiotherapy to the low neck. Am J Clin Oncol. 2005; 28(3):255–258

[10] Leder SB, Murray JT. Fiberoptic endoscopic evaluation of swallowing. Phys Med Rehabil Clin N Am. 2008; 19(4):787–801, viii–ix

[11] Cook IJ. Combined pharyngeal impedance-manometry: has it finally come of age? Clin Gastroenterol Hepatol. 2011; 9(10):813–815

[12] Omari TI, Papathanasopoulos A, Dejaeger E, et al. Reproducibility and agreement of pharyngeal automated impedance manometry with videofluoroscopy. Clin Gastroenterol Hepatol. 2011; 9(10):862–867

[13] Hoffman MR, Ciucci MR, Mielens JD, Jiang JJ, McCulloch TM. Pharyngeal swallow adaptations to bolus volume measured with high-resolution manometry. Laryngoscope. 2010; 120(12):2367–2373

[14] Mielens JD, Hoffman MR, Ciucci MR, Jiang JJ, McCulloch TM. Automated analysis of pharyngeal pressure data obtained with high-resolution manometry. Dysphagia. 2011; 26(1):3–12

[15] Neben-Wittich MA, Atherton PJ, Schwartz DJ, et al. Comparison of provider-assessed and patient-reported outcome measures of acute skin toxicity during a phase III trial of mometasone cream versus placebo during breast radiotherapy: the North Central Cancer Treatment Group (N06C4). Int J Radiat Oncol Biol Phys. 2011; 81(2):397–402

[16] Chen AY, Frankowski R, Bishop-Leone J, et al. The development and validation of a dysphagia-specific quality-of-life questionnaire for patients with head and neck cancer: the M. D. Anderson dysphagia inventory. Arch Otolaryngol Head Neck Surg. 2001; 127(7):870–876

[17] Szczesniak MM, Maclean J, Zhang T, Liu R, Cook IJ. The normative range for and age and gender effects on the Sydney Swallow Questionnaire (SSQ). Dysphagia. 2014; 29(5):535–538

[18] Quon H, Hui X, Cheng Z, et al. Quantitative evaluation of head and neck cancer treatment-related dysphagia in the development of a personalized treatment deintensification paradigm. Int J Radiat Oncol Biol Phys. 2017; 99(5): 1271–1278

[19] Peng LC, Hui X, Cheng Z, et al. Prospective evaluation of patient reported swallow function with the Functional Assessment of Cancer Therapy (FACT), MD Anderson Dysphagia Inventory (MDADI) and the Sydney Swallow Questionnaire (SSQ) in head and neck cancer patients. Oral Oncol. 2018; 84: 25–30

[20] Withers HR, Taylor JM, Maciejewski B. The hazard of accelerated tumor clonogen repopulation during radiotherapy. Acta Oncol. 1988; 27(2):131–146

[21] Maciejewski B, Withers HR, Taylor JM, Hliniak A. Dose fractionation and regeneration in radiotherapy for cancer of the oral cavity and oropharynx: tumor dose-response and repopulation. Int J Radiat Oncol Biol Phys. 1989; 16(3):831–843

[22] Fenwick JD, Pardo-Montero J, Nahum AE, Malik ZI. Impact of schedule duration on head and neck radiotherapy: accelerated tumor repopulation versus compensatory mucosal proliferation. Int J Radiat Oncol Biol Phys. 2012; 82 (2):1021–1030

[23] Suwinski R, Bankowska-Wozniak M, Majewski W, et al. Randomized clinical trial on continuous 7-days-a-week postoperative radiotherapy for high-risk squamous cell head-and-neck cancer: a report on acute normal tissue reactions. Radiother Oncol. 2005; 77(1):58–64

[24] Maciejewski B, Skladowski K, Pilecki B, et al. Randomized clinical trial on accelerated 7 days per week fractionation in radiotherapy for head and neck cancer. Preliminary report on acute toxicity. Radiother Oncol. 1996; 40(2): 137–145

[25] Narayan S, Lehmann J, Coleman MA, et al. Prospective evaluation to establish a dose response for clinical oral mucositis in patients undergoing head-and-neck conformal radiotherapy. Int J Radiat Oncol Biol Phys. 2008; 72(3):756–762

[26] Rosenthal DI, Chambers MS, Fuller CD, et al. Beam path toxicities to non-target structures during intensity-modulated radiation therapy for head and neck cancer. Int J Radiat Oncol Biol Phys. 2008; 72(3):747–755

[27] Bhide SA, Gulliford S, Schick U, et al. Dose-response analysis of acute oral mucositis and pharyngeal dysphagia in patients receiving induction chemotherapy followed by concomitant chemo-IMRT for head and neck cancer. Radiother Oncol. 2012; 103(1):88–91

[28] Mazzola R, Ricchetti F, Fersino S, et al. Predictors of mucositis in oropharyngeal and oral cavity cancer in patients treated with volumetric modulated radiation treatment: a dose-volume analysis. Head Neck. 2016; 38 Suppl 1: E815–E819

[29] Sanguineti G, Sormani MP, Marur S, et al. Effect of radiotherapy and chemotherapy on the risk of mucositis during intensity-modulated radiation therapy for oropharyngeal cancer. Int J Radiat Oncol Biol Phys. 2012; 83(1):235–242

[30] Adelstein DJ, Li Y, Adams GL, et al. An intergroup phase III comparison of standard radiation therapy and two schedules of concurrent chemoradiotherapy in patients with unresectable squamous cell head and neck cancer. J Clin Oncol. 2003; 21(1):92–98

[31] Calais G, Alfonsi M, Bardet E, et al. Randomized trial of radiation therapy versus concomitant chemotherapy and radiation therapy for advanced-stage oropharynx carcinoma. J Natl Cancer Inst. 1999; 91(24):2081–2086

[32] Bonner JA, Harari PM, Giralt J, et al. Radiotherapy plus cetuximab for squamous-cell carcinoma of the head and neck. N Engl J Med. 2006; 354(6):567–578

[33] National Institutes of Health. Cetuximab with radiation found to be inferior to standard treatment in HPV-positive oropharyngeal cancer. 2018

[34] Magrini SM, Buglione M, Corvò R, et al. Cetuximab and radiotherapy versus cisplatin and radiotherapy for locally advanced head and neck cancer: a randomized phase II trial. J Clin Oncol. 2016; 34(5):427–435

[35] Peters LJ, Ang KK, Thames HD, Jr. Accelerated fractionation in the radiation treatment of head and neck cancer. A critical comparison of different strategies. Acta Oncol. 1988; 27(2):185–194

[36] Dörr W. Three A's of repopulation during fractionated irradiation of squamous epithelia: asymmetry loss, acceleration of stem-cell divisions and abortive divisions. Int J Radiat Biol. 1997; 72(6):635–643

[37] Dörr W, Hendry JH. Consequential late effects in normal tissues. Radiother Oncol. 2001; 61(3):223–231

[38] Folwaczny M, Hickel R. Control of bacterial infection for effective treatment of oral mucositis. Lancet. 2002; 360(9332):574

[39] Delanian S, Lefaix JL. The radiation-induced fibroatrophic process: therapeutic perspective via the antioxidant pathway. Radiother Oncol. 2004; 73(2): 119–131

[40] King SN, Dunlap NE, Tennant PA, Pitts T. Pathophysiology of radiation-induced dysphagia in head and neck cancer. Dysphagia. 2016; 31(3):339–351

[41] Bar Ad V, Weinstein G, Dutta PR, et al. Gabapentin for the treatment of pain syndrome related to radiation-induced mucositis in patients with head and neck cancer treated with concurrent chemoradiotherapy. Cancer. 2010; 116 (17):4206–4213

[42] Brizel DM, Wasserman TH, Henke M, et al. Phase III randomized trial of amifostine as a radioprotector in head and neck cancer. J Clin Oncol. 2000; 18 (19):3339–3345

[43] Antonadou D, Pepelassi M, Synodinou M, Puglisi M, Throuvalas N. Prophylactic use of amifostine to prevent radiochemotherapy-induced mucositis and xerostomia in head-and-neck cancer. Int J Radiat Oncol Biol Phys. 2002; 52 (3):739–747

[44] Su YB, Vickers AJ, Zelefsky MJ, et al. Double-blind, placebo-controlled, randomized trial of granulocyte-colony stimulating factor during postoperative radiotherapy for squamous head and neck cancer. Cancer J. 2006; 12(3): 182–188

[45] Makkonen TA, Minn H, Jekunen A, Vilja P, Tuominen J, Joensuu H. Granulocyte macrophage-colony stimulating factor (GM-CSF) and sucralfate in prevention of radiation-induced mucositis: a prospective randomized study. Int J Radiat Oncol Biol Phys. 2000; 46(3):525–534

[46] Chao KS, Deasy JO, Markman J, et al. A prospective study of salivary function sparing in patients with head-and-neck cancers receiving intensity-modulated or three-dimensional radiation therapy: initial results. Int J Radiat Oncol Biol Phys. 2001; 49(4):907–916

[47] Blanco AI, Chao KS, El Naqa I, et al. Dose-volume modeling of salivary function in patients with head-and-neck cancer receiving radiotherapy. Int J Radiat Oncol Biol Phys. 2005; 62(4):1055–1069

[48] Deasy JO, Moiseenko V, Marks L, Chao KS, Nam J, Eisbruch A. Radiotherapy dose-volume effects on salivary gland function. Int J Radiat Oncol Biol Phys. 2010; 76(3) Suppl:S58–S63

[49] Portaluri M, Fucilli FI, Castagna R, et al. Three-dimensional conformal radiotherapy for locally advanced (Stage II and worse) head-and-neck cancer: dosimetric and clinical evaluation. Int J Radiat Oncol Biol Phys. 2006; 66(4): 1036–1043

[50] Konings AW, Coppes RP, Vissink A. On the mechanism of salivary gland radiosensitivity. Int J Radiat Oncol Biol Phys. 2005; 62(4):1187–1194

[51] van Luijk P, Pringle S, Deasy JO, et al. Sparing the region of the salivary gland containing stem cells preserves saliva production after radiotherapy for head and neck cancer. Sci Transl Med. 2015; 7(305):305ra147

[52] Robertson SP, Quon H, Kiess AP, et al. A data-mining framework for large scale analysis of dose-outcome relationships in a database of irradiated head and neck cancer patients. Med Phys. 2015; 42(7):4329–4337

[53] Nakatsugawa M, Cheng Z, Goatman KA, et al. Radiomic analysis of salivary glands and its role for predicting xerostomia in irradiated head and neck cancer patients. Int J Radiat Oncol Biol Phys. 2016; 96(2):Supplement, Page S217

[54] Eisbruch A, Kim HM, Terrell JE, Marsh LH, Dawson LA, Ship JA. Xerostomia and its predictors following parotid-sparing irradiation of head-and-neck cancer. Int J Radiat Oncol Biol Phys. 2001; 50(3):695–704

[55] Little M, Schipper M, Feng FY, et al. Reducing xerostomia after chemo-IMRT for head-and-neck cancer: beyond sparing the parotid glands. Int J Radiat Oncol Biol Phys. 2012; 83(3):1007–1014

[56] Wang ZH, Yan C, Zhang ZY, et al. Impact of salivary gland dosimetry on post-IMRT recovery of saliva output and xerostomia grade for head-and-neck cancer patients treated with or without contralateral submandibular gland sparing: a longitudinal study. Int J Radiat Oncol Biol Phys. 2011; 81(5):1479–1487

[57] Johnson JT, Ferretti GA, Nethery WJ, et al. Oral pilocarpine for post-irradiation xerostomia in patients with head and neck cancer. N Engl J Med. 1993; 329(6):390–395

[58] Wong RK, Deshmukh S, Wyatt G, et al. Acupuncture-like transcutaneous electrical nerve stimulation versus pilocarpine in treating radiation-induced xerostomia: results of RTOG 0537 phase 3 study. Int J Radiat Oncol Biol Phys. 2015; 92(2):220–227

[59] Meng Z, Garcia MK, Hu C, et al. Randomized controlled trial of acupuncture for prevention of radiation-induced xerostomia among patients with nasopharyngeal carcinoma. Cancer. 2012; 118(13):3337–3344

[60] Zhang X, Liu F, Lan X, et al. Clinical observation of submandibular gland transfer for the prevention of xerostomia after radiotherapy for nasopharyngeal carcinoma: a prospective randomized controlled study of 32 cases. Radiat Oncol. 2014; 9:62

[61] Tamhankar MA, Biousse V, Ying GS, et al. Isolated third, fourth, and sixth cranial nerve palsies from presumed microvascular versus other causes: a prospective study. Ophthalmology. 2013; 120(11):2264–2269

[62] O'Dell K, Sinha U. Osteoradionecrosis. Oral Maxillofac Surg Clin North Am. 2011; 23(3):455–464

[63] Gomez DR, Estilo CL, Wolden SL, et al. Correlation of osteoradionecrosis and dental events with dosimetric parameters in intensity-modulated radiation therapy for head-and-neck cancer. Int J Radiat Oncol Biol Phys. 2011; 81(4): e207–e213

[64] Ben-David MA, Diamante M, Radawski JD, et al. Lack of osteoradionecrosis of the mandible after intensity-modulated radiotherapy for head and neck cancer: likely contributions of both dental care and improved dose distributions. Int J Radiat Oncol Biol Phys. 2007; 68(2):396–402

[65] Wahl MJ. Osteoradionecrosis prevention myths. Int J Radiat Oncol Biol Phys. 2006; 64(3):661–669

[66] Chang DT, Sandow PR, Morris CG, et al. Do pre-irradiation dental extractions reduce the risk of osteoradionecrosis of the mandible? Head Neck. 2007; 29 (6):528–536

[67] Tsai CJ, Hofstede TM, Sturgis EM, et al. Osteoradionecrosis and radiation dose to the mandible in patients with oropharyngeal cancer. Int J Radiat Oncol Biol Phys. 2013; 85(2):415–420

[68] Eisbruch A, Harris J, Garden AS, et al. Multi-institutional trial of accelerated hypofractionated intensity-modulated radiation therapy for early-stage oropharyngeal cancer (RTOG 00-22). Int J Radiat Oncol Biol Phys. 2010; 76(5): 1333–1338

[69] Nadella KR, Kodali RM, Guttikonda LK, Jonnalagadda A. Osteoradionecrosis of the jaws: clinico-therapeutic management: a literature review and update. J Maxillofac Oral Surg. 2015; 14(4):891–901

[70] Beech N, Robinson S, Porceddu S, Batstone M. Dental management of patients irradiated for head and neck cancer. Aust Dent J. 2014; 59(1):20–28

[71] Delanian S, Chatel C, Porcher R, Depondt J, Lefaix JL. Complete restoration of refractory mandibular osteoradionecrosis by prolonged treatment with a pentoxifylline-tocopherol-clodronate combination (PENTOCLO): a phase II trial. Int J Radiat Oncol Biol Phys. 2011; 80(3):832–839

[72] Notani K, Yamazaki Y, Kitada H, et al. Management of mandibular osteoradionecrosis corresponding to the severity of osteoradionecrosis and the method of radiotherapy. Head Neck. 2003; 25(3):181–186

[73] Marx RE, Johnson RP, Kline SN. Prevention of osteoradionecrosis: a randomized prospective clinical trial of hyperbaric oxygen versus penicillin. J Am Dent Assoc. 1985; 111(1):49–54

[74] Nabil S, Samman N. Incidence and prevention of osteoradionecrosis after dental extraction in irradiated patients: a systematic review. Int J Oral Maxillofac Surg. 2011; 40(3):229–243

[75] Sulaiman F, Huryn JM, Zlotolow IM. Dental extractions in the irradiated head and neck patient: a retrospective analysis of Memorial Sloan-Kettering Cancer Center protocols, criteria, and end results. J Oral Maxillofac Surg. 2003; 61(10):1123–1131

[76] Pearson WG, Jr, Langmore SE, Yu LB, Zumwalt AC. Structural analysis of muscles elevating the hyolaryngeal complex. Dysphagia. 2012; 27(4):445–451

[77] Kumar R, Madanikia S, Starmer H, et al. Radiation dose to the floor of mouth muscles predicts swallowing complications following chemoradiation in oropharyngeal squamous cell carcinoma. Oral Oncol. 2014; 50(1):65–70

[78] Scher ED, Romesser PB, Chen C, et al. Definitive chemoradiation for primary oral cavity carcinoma: A single institution experience. Oral Oncol. 2015; 51 (7):709–715

[79] Hunter KU, Schipper M, Feng FY, et al. Toxicities affecting quality of life after chemo-IMRT of oropharyngeal cancer: prospective study of patient-reported, observer-rated, and objective outcomes. Int J Radiat Oncol Biol Phys. 2013; 85(4):935–940

[80] Nguyen NP, Frank C, Moltz CC, et al. Impact of dysphagia on quality of life after treatment of head-and-neck cancer. Int J Radiat Oncol Biol Phys. 2005; 61(3):772–778

[81] Gourin CG, Starmer HM, Herbert RJ, et al. Short- and long-term outcomes of laryngeal cancer care in the elderly. Laryngoscope. 2015; 125 (4):924–933

[82] Forastiere AA, Zhang Q, Weber RS, et al. Long-term results of RTOG 91-11: a comparison of three nonsurgical treatment strategies to preserve the larynx in patients with locally advanced larynx cancer. J Clin Oncol. 2013; 31(7): 845–852

[83] Nguyen NP, Frank C, Moltz CC, et al. Aspiration rate following chemoradiation for head and neck cancer: an underreported occurrence. Radiother Oncol. 2006; 80(3):302–306

[84] O'Hare J, Maclean J, Szczesniak M, et al. Laryngeal tumours and radiotherapy dose to the cricopharyngeus are predictive of death from aspiration pneumonia. Oral Oncol. 2017; 64:9–14

[85] Bock JM, Varadarajan V, Brawley MC, Blumin JH. Evaluation of the natural history of patients who aspirate. Laryngoscope. 2017; 127 Suppl 8:S1–S10

[86] Hutcheson KA, Bhayani MK, Beadle BM, et al. Eat and exercise during radiotherapy or chemoradiotherapy for pharyngeal cancers: use it or lose it. JAMA Otolaryngol Head Neck Surg. 2013; 139(11):1127–1134

[87] Langmore S, Krisciunas GP, Miloro KV, Evans SR, Cheng DM. Does PEG use cause dysphagia in head and neck cancer patients? Dysphagia. 2012; 27(2): 251–259

[88] Carnaby-Mann G, Crary MA, Schmalfuss I, Amdur R. "Pharyngocise": randomized controlled trial of preventative exercises to maintain muscle structure and swallowing function during head-and-neck chemoradiotherapy. Int J Radiat Oncol Biol Phys. 2012; 83(1):210–219

[89] Kotz T, Federman AD, Kao J, et al. Prophylactic swallowing exercises in patients with head and neck cancer undergoing chemoradiation: a randomized trial. Arch Otolaryngol Head Neck Surg. 2012; 138(4):376–382

[90] Bhatt AD, Goodwin N, Cash E, et al. Impact of transcutaneous neuromuscular electrical stimulation on dysphagia in patients with head and neck cancer treated with definitive chemoradiation. Head Neck. 2015; 37(7):1051–1056

[91] Moloney EC, Brunner M, Alexander AJ, Clark J. Quantifying fibrosis in head and neck cancer treatment: An overview. Head Neck. 2015; 37(8):1225–1231

[92] Westbury CB, Yarnold JR. Radiation fibrosis: current clinical and therapeutic perspectives. Clin Oncol (R Coll Radiol). 2012; 24(10):657–672

[93] Rabbani ZN, Mi J, Zhang Y, et al. Hypoxia inducible factor 1alpha signaling in fractionated radiation-induced lung injury: role of oxidative stress and tissue hypoxia. Radiat Res. 2010; 173(2):165–174

[94] Borger JH, Kemperman H, Smitt HS, et al. Dose and volume effects on fibrosis after breast conservation therapy. Int J Radiat Oncol Biol Phys. 1994; 30 (5):1073–1081

[95] Johansson S, Svensson H, Denekamp J. Dose response and latency for radiation-induced fibrosis, edema, and neuropathy in breast cancer patients. Int J Radiat Oncol Biol Phys. 2002; 52(5):1207–1219

[96] Toledano A, Garaud P, Serin D, et al. Concurrent administration of adjuvant chemotherapy and radiotherapy after breast-conserving surgery enhances late toxicities: long-term results of the ARCOSEIN multicenter randomized study. Int J Radiat Oncol Biol Phys. 2006; 65(2):324–332

[97] Gold DG, Miller RC, Petersen IA, Osborn TG. Radiotherapy for malignancy in patients with scleroderma: The Mayo Clinic experience. Int J Radiat Oncol Biol Phys. 2007; 67(2):559–567

[98] Straub JM, New J, Hamilton CD, Lominska C, Shnayder Y, Thomas SM. Radiation-induced fibrosis: mechanisms and implications for therapy. J Cancer Res Clin Oncol. 2015; 141(11):1985–1994

[99] Cheuk IW, Yip SP, Kwong DL, Wu VW. Association of XRCC1 and XRCC3 gene haplotypes with the development of radiation-induced fibrosis in patients with nasopharyngeal carcinoma. Mol Clin Oncol. 2014; 2(4):553–558

[100] Azria D, Ozsahin M, Kramar A, et al. Single nucleotide polymorphisms, apoptosis, and the development of severe late adverse effects after radiotherapy. Clin Cancer Res. 2008; 14(19):6284–6288

[101] Azria D, Gourgou S, Sozzi WJ, et al. Concomitant use of tamoxifen with radiotherapy enhances subcutaneous breast fibrosis in hypersensitive patients. Br J Cancer. 2004; 91(7):1251–1260

[102] Yang X, Yoshida E, Cassidy RJ, et al. Quantitative ultrasonic Nakagami imaging of neck fibrosis after head and neck radiation therapy. Int J Radiat Oncol Biol Phys. 2015; 92(2):407–414

[103] Deng J, Dietrich MS, Ridner SH, Fleischer AC, Wells N, Murphy BA. Preliminary evaluation of reliability and validity of head and neck external lymphedema and fibrosis assessment criteria. Eur J Oncol Nurs. 2016; 22:63–70

[104] Shaw SM, Skoretz SA, O'Sullivan B, Hope A, Liu LW, Martino R. Valid and reliable techniques for measuring fibrosis in patients with head and neck cancer postradiotherapy: a systematic review. Head Neck. 2016; 38 Suppl 1:E2322–E2334

[105] Delanian S, Lefaix JL. Current management for late normal tissue injury: radiation-induced fibrosis and necrosis. Semin Radiat Oncol. 2007; 17(2): 99–107

[106] Okunieff P, Augustine E, Hicks JE, et al. Pentoxifylline in the treatment of radiation-induced fibrosis. J Clin Oncol. 2004; 22(11):2207–2213

[107] Delanian S, Porcher R, Balla-Mekias S, Lefaix JL. Randomized, placebo-controlled trial of combined pentoxifylline and tocopherol for regression of superficial radiation-induced fibrosis. J Clin Oncol. 2003; 21(13):2545–2550

[108] Delanian S, Balla-Mekias S, Lefaix JL. Striking regression of chronic radiotherapy damage in a clinical trial of combined pentoxifylline and tocopherol. J Clin Oncol. 1999; 17(10):3283–3290

[109] Deng J, Ridner SH, Dietrich MS, et al. Prevalence of secondary lymphedema in patients with head and neck cancer. J Pain Symptom Manage. 2012; 43 (2):244–252

[110] Deng J, Ridner SH, Dietrich MS, et al. Factors associated with external and internal lymphedema in patients with head-and-neck cancer. Int J Radiat Oncol Biol Phys. 2012; 84(3):e319–e328

[111] Smith BG, Hutcheson KA, Little LG, et al. Lymphedema outcomes in patients with head and neck cancer. Otolaryngol Head Neck Surg. 2015; 152(2):284–291

[112] Ahlberg A, Nikolaidis P, Engström T, et al. Morbidity of supraomohyoidal and modified radical neck dissection combined with radiotherapy for head and neck cancer: a prospective longitudinal study. Head Neck. 2012; 34(1):66–72

[113] Smith BG, Lewin JS. Lymphedema management in head and neck cancer. Curr Opin Otolaryngol Head Neck Surg. 2010; 18(3):153–158

[114] Irune E, Dwivedi RC, Nutting CM, Harrington KJ. Treatment-related dysgeusia in head and neck cancer patients. Cancer Treat Rev. 2014; 40(9):1106–1117

[115] Zhang FF, Liu S, John EM, Must A, Demark-Wahnefried W. Diet quality of cancer survivors and noncancer individuals: Results from a national survey. Cancer. 2015; 121(23):4212–4221

[116] Zabernigg A, Gamper EM, Giesinger JM, et al. Taste alterations in cancer patients receiving chemotherapy: a neglected side effect? Oncologist. 2010; 15(8):913–920

[117] Murtaza B, Hichami A, Khan AS, Ghiringhelli F, Khan NA. Alteration in taste perception in cancer: causes and strategies of treatment. Front Physiol. 2017; 8:134

[118] Nguyen HM, Reyland ME, Barlow LA. Mechanisms of taste bud cell loss after head and neck irradiation. J Neurosci. 2012; 32(10):3474–3484

[119] Sapir E, Tao Y, Feng F, et al. Predictors of dysgeusia in patients with oropharyngeal cancer treated with chemotherapy and intensity modulated radiation therapy. Int J Radiat Oncol Biol Phys. 2016; 96(2):354–361

[120] Wickham RS, Rehwaldt M, Kefer C, et al. Taste changes experienced by patients receiving chemotherapy. Oncol Nurs Forum. 1999; 26(4):697–706

[121] Mossman KL. Gustatory tissue injury in man: radiation dose response relationships and mechanisms of taste loss. Br J Cancer Suppl. 1986; 7:9–11

[122] Pandya JA, Srikant N, Boaz K, Manaktala N, Kapila SN, Yinti SR. Post-radiation changes in oral tissues: an analysis of cancer irradiation cases. South Asian J Cancer. 2014; 3(3):159–162

[123] Wang CJ, Huang EY, Hsu HC, Chen HC, Fang FM, Hsiung CY. The degree and time-course assessment of radiation-induced trismus occurring after radiotherapy for nasopharyngeal cancer. Laryngoscope. 2005; 115(8):1458–1460

[124] Gebre-Medhin M, Haghanegi M, Robért L, Kjellén E, Nilsson P. Dose-volume analysis of radiation-induced trismus in head and neck cancer patients. Acta Oncol. 2016; 55(11):1313–1317

[125] Rao SD, Saleh ZH, Setton J, et al. Dose-volume factors correlating with trismus following chemoradiation for head and neck cancer. Acta Oncol. 2016; 55(1):99–104

[126] Chen YY, Zhao C, Wang J, et al. Intensity-modulated radiation therapy reduces radiation-induced trismus in patients with nasopharyngeal carcinoma: a prospective study with > 5 years of follow-up. Cancer. 2011; 117 (13):2910–2916

[127] Bensadoun RJ, Riesenbeck D, Lockhart PB, Elting LS, Spijkervet FK, Brennan MT, Trismus Section, Oral Care Study Group, Multinational Association for Supportive Care in Cancer (MASCC)/International Society of Oral Oncology (ISOO). A systematic review of trismus induced by cancer therapies in head and neck cancer patients. Support Care Cancer. 2010; 18(8):1033–1038

[128] Rapidis AD, Dijkstra PU, Roodenburg JL, et al. Trismus in patients with head and neck cancer: etiopathogenesis, diagnosis and management. Clin Otolaryngol. 2015; 40(6):516–526

[129] Cohen EG, Deschler DG, Walsh K, Hayden RE. Early use of a mechanical stretching device to improve mandibular mobility after composite resection: a pilot study. Arch Phys Med Rehabil. 2005; 86(7):1416–1419

[130] Bhrany AD, Izzard M, Wood AJ, Futran ND. Coronoidectomy for the treatment of trismus in head and neck cancer patients. Laryngoscope. 2007; 117 (11):1952–1956

[131] Mardini S, Chang YM, Tsai CY, Coskunfirat OK, Wei FC. Release and free flap reconstruction for trismus that develops after previous intraoral reconstruction. Plast Reconstr Surg. 2006; 118(1):102–107

42 Psychosocial Rehabilitation of Oral Cancer Patients

Amy Williams

Summary

Treatment for oral cavity malignancies has the potential to interfere with the most fundamental activities of daily function, such as eating, drinking, speaking, and breathing. These impairments in fundamental daily functions are related to the physical changes and effects of treatment, as discussed in earlier chapters of this book. However, these changes have a dynamic relationship with quality of life and psychosocial function in survivorship. Psychosocial survivorship includes areas of social functioning (i.e., employment, finances, insurance, social interactions, and cognitive impairment) and psychological functioning (i.e., depression/anxiety, substance use, fear of recurrence, body image, and stigma). The caregiver should also be included in the supportive care of the patient with head and neck cancer (HNC). Psychosocial interventions for patients and caregivers exist. However, given the limited access to behavioral health specialists (BHS) with experience in HNC, stepped care is followed in which all patients receive common low-intensity treatment (e.g., patient education) and only those with additional need are "stepped up" to more intensive treatment from a BHS. Those medical providers who treat HNC are encouraged to develop knowledge of the BHS/psych-oncology specialists in their hospital and community so that they can have the expertise to work with HNC patients and their caregivers. Larger tertiary specialty care centers that treat HNC are encouraged to integrate BHS/psych-oncology specialists, such as clinical health psychologists, into their multidisciplinary approach to aid in treating the more complex and advanced stage HNC patients that these centers typically treat.

Keywords: psychosocial assessment, distress, tobacco cessation, psychosocial intervention, financial toxicity

42.1 Introduction

Head and neck cancer (HNC) survivors account for 3% of all cancer survivors in the United States,[1] and treatment for HNC impacts the most visible aspects of the body. This impact has the potential to interfere with the most fundamental activities of daily function, such as eating, drinking, speaking, and breathing, particularly with oral cavity malignancies. Improvements in treatment have resulted in more patients surviving HNC for longer span of time.[2] These impairments in fundamental daily functions are related to the physical changes and effects of treatment, as discussed in earlier chapters of this book. However, these changes have a dynamic relationship with quality of life (QoL) and psychosocial function in survivorship. Psychosocial survivorship includes areas of social functioning such as employment, finances, insurance, social interactions, and psychological functioning, including symptoms of depression and anxiety, substance use, fear of recurrence, body image, and stigma.

The American Cancer Society Head and Neck Cancer Survivorship Care Guidelines include recommendations for assessment and management of long-term psychosocial effects of HNC and health promotion.[3] In addition, LIVESTRONG Essential Elements of Survivorship Care identifies psychosocial elements of psychosocial assessment, such as symptom screening through systematic evaluation of psychosocial distress through survivorship continuum, and care, including access to psychoeducational materials on stress management, support groups, appropriate referrals within the institution or community. Moreover, family/caregiver support, such as spousal support and/or education groups, bereavement groups, psychoeducational materials, appropriate referrals, as well as health promotion education and counseling for practical issues, such as finances, insurance, and employment—both education and appropriate referrals, are included in these essential elements.[4]

Previous research has consistently demonstrated that QoL improves, returning approximately to baseline, by a year post treatment, after the greatest decrease in QoL seen at 3 to 4 weeks into adjuvant radiotherapy.[5] Psychosocial functioning has been associated with patient's QoL, adherence to medical recommendations, and overall morbidity and mortality.[6] Other research has demonstrated that psychosocial function is an area that can be influenced by identification and intervention, thus improving QoL in survivorship, adherence, and possibly disease-free survival.[7] Additionally, though not often considered part of survivorship care of the patient, the psychosocial functioning of their family or caregivers has also been shown to impact patient's QoL, adherence, and overall morbidity.[8] The subsequent subsections of this chapter will review the various psychosocial considerations in oral cancer survivorship, some of which is common across cancer in general.

42.2 Primary Psychosocial Issues in Survivorship

42.2.1 Socioeconomic Considerations and Disparities

As highlighted in the Institute of Medicine publication "Unequal Treatment," those from lower socioeconomic groups or who are medically underserved are more likely to be diagnosed at later stages, and these people have worse treatment outcomes and experience shortened survivorship.[9] Internationally, minority groups are more likely to be poor, have lower education levels, lack health insurance coverage or have poorer insurance coverage, and have no source of primary care.[9] These treatment disparities result in more frequent cancer recurrence, shorter disease-free survival periods, and higher mortality.[9] Low-income individuals tend to experience more chronic stress related to job insecurity, financial strain, greater environmental exposures to toxins at work and home, less social support, and have more behavioral risk factors associated with poor health, such as alcohol use, smoking, sedentary lifestyle, and poor nutrition.[10] Moreover, even in countries where insurance is less of a barrier, delays in care are common among lower socioeconomic status (SES), such as diagnosis at later stage, longer intervals between onset of symptoms, surgical referral, and hospital admission, access to comprehensive cancer treatment at regional center rather than local hospital, palliative care and appropriate pain management, new technologies that allow for a prognostic assessment and prediction of response to certain treatments.[10] Overall, the impact of cancer is greater for individuals with poorer living conditions and lower SES.

The burden of cancer mortality disproportionately falls on lower SES due to disparities in psychosocial factors (i.e., coping, stress, and social support), health behaviors, comorbidities, access to care, screening, and treatment, and access to and understanding of clinical trials.[10] Further, the late effects of treatment are also more pronounced in patients of lower SES. Lower SES tends to be associated with lower QoL after cancer treatment, less chances of return to work, slower re-employment, involuntary unemployment, and greater chances of early retirement.[10] Difficulties with re-employment or retirement result in income reductions that can contribute to decreased access to resources to maintain health, such as surveillance and insurance for preventative care. The Institute of Medicine report "From cancer patient to cancer survivor: Lost in transition" makes recommendations for survivorship plans to include information on legal protections regarding employment and access to health insurance.[11]

A newly recognized area of psychosocial concern in survivorship is financial toxicity, or the problems that patients face that are related to the cost of their medical care. Financial toxicity includes cost of treatment (co-pays, spend downs, out of pocket costs for DMEs), cost of rehabilitation (physical/occupational therapy, dentistry/dental reconstruction, speech language pathologist, RD), lost income for diagnostic and treatment appointments (often both patient and caregiver), travel costs for many with tertiary centers providing specialized care, disability due to treatment making it difficult or impossible to return to prior employment, limited flexibility in employers to offer accommodations on the job, difficulty obtaining insurance in future, and ongoing surveillance toxicity (often requiring appointments with each oncology provider).[10] In addition, often patients do not return to work, decisions about moving, selling off cars, discontinuing health insurance may need to made in order to cover costs of basic needs.[12]

42.2.2 Behavioral Risk: Tobacco Use and Cessation

The main behavioral risk factors associated with HNC are tobacco use, which has been linked to 85% of squamous cell carcinoma HNC, alcohol abuse, and betel nut chewing, which is common in southeast Asia and associated with oral cavity malignancies, and sexual activity and number of sexual partners, which is associated with risk of human papilloma virus (HPV).[13] Throughout treatment, the main focus for behavioral interventions historically has been on tobacco cessation due to its effects on treatment efficacy, worsening treatment side effects, and higher rates of recurrence.[14]

Tobacco use is influenced by physical dependence on nicotine, operant and classical conditioning, environmental and social factors, cognitive expectations, active depression, and active substance abuse. Physical dependence refers to the level of nicotine dependence, typically related to the amount smoked daily and how soon after waking one has the first cigarette.[15] Environmental and social factors highlight the importance of involving family members in cessation education because often family members also smoke and can influence cessation attempts.[10,16] Cognitive expectations include beliefs about the benefits of smoking, fatalistic debriefs (e.g., "I've already got cancer"), self-efficacy and motivation to quit, fear of recurrence, and decreased risk perceptions associated with smoking.[17,18] Active depression is associated with decreased motivation to quit and cessation relapse is more likely to occur with active depression.[19] Finally, active alcohol abuse is commonly linked with tobacco use, and continuing alcohol use has been associated with difficulties in tobacco cessation and being less likely to enroll in tobacco cessation programs.[20]

With up to 48% of oral cavity and pharynx cancer related deaths being attributable to tobacco use,[21] tobacco cessation at diagnosis is important. Prior research has demonstrated that continued smoking after cancer diagnosis has known impacts on overall survival, decreased treatment effects of radiation therapy, chemotherapy, and surgery, increased occurrence of treatment complications (i.e., infection, poor wound healing, exacerbated side effects of treatment like mucositis), exacerbation of immune function due to nicotine's suppressive effect, increased weight loss due to suppression of appetite, increased risk of depression/anxiety following cancer treatment, decreased QoL in survivorship, and increased risk of recurrence and second primaries.[10]

Unfortunately, 14 to 58% of patients have been reported to continue to smoke in survivorship in a 3-year follow up, with the percentage smoking remaining fairly stable across this period. Similar to the general population, relapse after cessation occurs in up to 60% patients.[22,23] However, unlike general population who relapse in first week after cessation, patients with cancer tend to relapse in the first few months following quit attempt, typically after active treatment ends.[24] Tobacco cessation is most likely to happen in patients with more severe disease or more invasive treatment; thus patients with earlier stage disease or tumors of oral cavity compared to larynx with total laryngectomy are more likely to continue smoking.[24] Furthermore, older patients are typically heavier smokers and have more difficulty with quitting.[25] Of note, white patients are more likely to participate in smoking cessation programs, although black patients have higher self-efficacy for quitting and are more interested in cessation services.[26]

It is important to note that patients are also highly motivated to quit with many making quit attempts at diagnosis, thus making time between diagnosis and end of active treatment an optimal window for provision of smoking cessation interventions.[27] Research shows that for patients with cancer, the optimal window for cessation intervention is in the preoperative period.

Brief tobacco interventions provided by the patient's medical provider can have a large impact. The "5 As" from medical providers, a brief 3-minute intervention, has been proven beneficial in oncology.[28] The 5 As include: ask about tobacco use, advise to quit using a clear and personalized message, assess willingness to quit, assist to quit, and arrange follow-up and

Table 42.1 Pharmacotherapy for tobacco cessation

Medication	OTC/RX	Dosing	Notes
NRT gum	OTC	> 25 PPD: 4 mg, < 25 PPD: 2 mg	Use up to 12 weeks
NRT lozenge	OTC	2–4 mg, up to 20 lozenges/day	Use up to 12 weeks
NRT patch	OTC	21 mg × 4 weeks, 14 mg × 2 weeks, 7 mg × 2 weeks	Use up to 12 weeks, consistent dose across the day, slower bioavailability
NRT nasal spray	RX	1–2 sprays/hr, up to 40 sprays/day	Use 3–6 months, reaches peak concentration rapidly
NRT inhaler	RX	6–16 cartridges/day	Use up to 6 months, reaches peak concentration rapidly
Bupropion SR	RX	150 mg/day for 3 days, then 150 mg BID	Up to 6 months
Varenicline	RX	0.5 mg/day for 3 days, 0.5 mg BID for 4 days, 1 mg BID	Up to 3 months

Abbreviations: NRT, nicotine replacement therapy; OTC, over the counter.

support.[29] When providing assistance in quitting, research has shown that single treatment approaches have limited success and long-term outcomes are best seen with multimodal treatment.[29]

It is recommended that pharmacotherapy be routinely offered to smokers attempting to quit.[30] Pharmacotherapy with common dosage is shown in ▶ Table 42.1. All forms of nicotine replacement therapy (NRT) are relatively equivalent with a 6-month abstinence of 20 to 25% with single modality.[30] All but the transdermal patch is contraindicated in oral malignancies.[10] NRT is typically used during the first 8 to 12 weeks after cessation, when nicotine withdrawal symptoms are strongest. There are specific considerations with NRT in cancer treatment, namely evidence that nicotine may accelerate tumor growth, inhibit apoptosis induced by several chemotherapies, negative response to radiotherapy, and issues with cardiovascular effects following microvascular free flap surgeries.[10] Bupropion SR (Wellbutrin ®/Zyban ®) is a selective serotonin-norepinephrine reuptake inhibitor that attenuates nicotine withdrawal and cravings and reduces post cessation weight gain. It appears to inhibit neuronal uptake of dopamine and norepinephrine (neurotransmitters involved in maintenance of nicotine dependence) and may also have antagonistic effect on nicotine receptors (decreasing perceived satisfaction with smoking).[30] Bupropion has demonstrated abstinence rates double that compared to placebo, with a 6-month abstinent rate of 24%. Bupropion is recommended to be started 1 week prior to planned quit date to achieve steady-state blood levels. Bupropion is contraindicated in those with history of seizure disorder or factors that increase seizure risk (e.g., alcoholism, serious head trauma) and those using monoamine oxidase inhibitors.[10] Varenicline (Chantix ®) is a partial antagonist of nicotinic acetylcholine receptors, thus appears to reduce cravings and withdrawal symptoms related to nicotine, as well as decreasing the reinforcing effects of smoking (including perceived satisfaction). Varenicline typically outperforms bupropion, with triple the abstinence compared to placebo, and a 6-month abstinence of 33%.[30] Varenicline is recommended to be started 1 to 4 weeks prior to the planned quit date to achieve steady-state blood levels. Common side effects include mild/moderate nausea, agitation, and changes in behavior that are not typical for the person. There is also some evidence that varenicline may increase the risk of a major cardiovascular event.[10] As single-modality treatment is not as effective as multimodal therapy for tobacco cessation, there are recommendations to combine long-acting, relatively stable medication (i.e., NRT patch) with shorter-acting medication as needed (i.e., NRT gum, nasal spray, lozenge, or inhaler) or combining the NRT patch with bupropion SR for improved abstinence rates.[30]

In addition to pharmacotherapy for tobacco cessation, behavioral treatments are recommended adjuvants.[30] Key recommendations combine counseling and medication, as it is more effective approach than either alone in producing abstinence, with highest rates of abstinence seen in pharmacotherapy with intensive counseling (33% abstinence).[30] The higher abstinence with combination therapy is thought to be due to pharmacotherapy reducing withdrawal symptoms and craving, while behavioral treatments (i.e., counseling) teaching cognitive and behavioral coping strategies and providing valuable social support. Behavioral treatments include self-help materials, telephone quit lines, and both brief and intensive counseling interventions. Self-help materials (e.g., pamphlets, booklets, videos) have been found ineffective in initial quit attempts, though these can be helpful for preventing smoking relapse when provided shortly after quitting smoking.[30] Telephone quit lines, such as 1-800-QUIT-NOW, provide a central access point to state and federal quit lines. Telephone counseling can provide personalized and intensive help and can have greater therapeutic reach than face-to-face counseling, as it is more readily available, and has a 6-month abstinence rate of 3 to 5% if used as a single modality.[30]

Brief interventions are typically provided by medical providers. Appropriately provided physician advice increases abstinence by 2.3 to 2.5%.[10] There is a dose response with brief interventions, with minimal counseling (< 3 minutes) yielding 13.4% 6-month abstinence, low-intensity counseling (3–10 minutes) yielding 16%, and higher-intensity counseling (> 10 minutes) yielding 22.1% 6-month abstinence.[23] Six-month abstinence rates also increase with the number of counseling meetings and/or the number of clinician types delivering the cessation message to the patient. Intensive interventions are empirically supported, multisession, typically offered through smoking cessation clinics or BHSs, either in group or individual format. The interventions typically include patient education regarding nicotine dependence and withdrawal, identifying triggers to use nicotine, teaching and practicing both cognitive and behavioral responses for coping with urges and stressors, discussing long-term risk factors, and teaching how to respond to a relapse. When used as a single-modality treatment, intensive interventions have a 6-month abstinence rate of 16.2%.[23,30]

42.3 Psychological Distress and Risk Factors

Screening for psychosocial distress during cancer care is mandated by American College of Surgeons Commission on Cancer.[31] This screening has been proven to be well tolerated in HNC.[32] Prior research has demonstrated that QoL in those with oral cancer malignancies returns to the levels found in the general population by 5 years post treatment.[33] Health-related quality of life (HRQoL) is often restored to pretreatment levels by the end of the first year post treatment; however, it remains unclear if this represents a return to premorbid function, a response shift or changes in expectations of what represents HRQoL, or a posttraumatic growth.[34] There does not appear to be gender differences in HRQoL at the end of treatment except in role functioning, with women perceiving lower role functioning, which may be due to the younger age of women with HNC.[35] Despite these positive long-term QoL outcomes, patients face the immediate and latent physical effects of treatment and facial disfigurement. These many effects of treatment may lead to shame, social avoidance, depression, anxiety, and decreased QoL.[10]

42.3.1 Disfigurement and Body Image

Typically attributed to surgery, disfigurement is the most disturbing stressor associated with HNC.[10] Treatment for HNC is often associated with changes in swallowing, chewing, eating, speaking. These functions are important to one's sense of self, interpersonal relationships, communication, and social function (e.g., eating in public, speaking in groups). Fifty percent of patients report posttreatment speech problems.[36] Dysfunction in any of these areas may contribute to social avoidance and depression.[37]

Fingeret et al demonstrated that 75% of patients treated for HNC reported "concerns or embarrassment" due to their treatment-related body changes.[38] In this sample, 50% of patients reported frequent thoughts about appearance changes.[38] Further, 38% of patients reported avoidance of social activities and social disruption was reported in 80% of patients.[39] Of particular importance to the treating medical team, 69% reported dissatisfaction with information regarding body image provided by their medical providers, with previous research indicating that patients prefer information about what to expect with body image changes and how to cope with these changes prior to treatment.[38] Other research has found that body dissatisfaction increases after initial surgical intervention and remains elevated for 1 year post surgery.[10] Individual factors were found to moderate the effect of disfigurement and body image, including age (younger more dissatisfied), social support, social self-efficacy or the belief that one can exercise control over the reactions and openness of other people, illness intrusiveness, and stigma associated with diagnosis.[10] Of note, oral cavity malignancies are associated with higher body image concerns, particularly with eating and speaking as compared to skin or other mid face cancers, with stage of survivorship having little effect on QoL from pretreatment to 1-year post treatment.[38]

42.3.2 Stigma

Those cancers whose etiologies are associated with one's actions (e.g., tobacco, alcohol, sexual behaviors) are highly stigmatized (e.g., lung cancer, HNC). Through successful public education campaigns by national health organizations, the risks/contributors to HNC are more widely known and HNC is more often being associated with risk behaviors that are seen as "under one's control." Thus HNC, regardless of whether associated with one's actions or not, is associated with more self-blame and the patient is more likely to encounter rejection or stigma because the disease and/or treatment effects and disfigurement are more visible to the outside world.[37] This cancer-related stigma is negatively associated with psychosocial well-being, interpersonal relationships, financial opportunities, and delayed treatment seeking.[40]

42.3.3 Coping Strategies

Coping strategies and personality traits have long been examined in relation to disease. Similar to the general literature, the personality trait of neuroticism, or the trait of being predisposed to the experience of negative emotional states, such as anxiety, depression, anger, envy, is associated with poorer QoL and head and neck function at 3 years post treatment.[10] Also, avoidant coping, such as choosing behavior based on avoidance or escape of unpleasant thoughts/feelings (e.g., behavioral disengagement/withdrawal, substance abuse), and problem-solving coping, or the attempts to change or eliminate the source of stress, are related to poorer QoL, increased incidence of substance use, and lower head and neck function.[41] In cancer research in general, younger patients tended to use active coping strategies, such as behavioral and psychological strategies that are aimed at control, tolerate, reduce, or minimize stressful events, both before and after treatment, while older patients were more likely to use avoidant strategies.[42] It is recommended that psychosocial interventions should be aimed at discouraging the maladaptive coping strategies by providing alternatives, such as relaxation techniques, mindfulness, and cognitive restructuring.

42.3.4 Anxiety and Depression

Throughout active treatment, 71% of patients report depressive symptoms[39] and 30 to 40% of patients experience clinically significant anxiety or depression at some point during cancer trajectory.[32,43] Furthermore, psychological distress is negatively associated with QoL, treatment adherence, satisfaction with care, and overall survival in HNC.[43] Thus, it is recommended that patients be screened for depression and anxiety using validated screening tools at 3 months post treatment and at least annually thereafter. It is also recommended that oncology providers refer to BHSs based on these screenings.[3] Of note, given the possibility of treatment effects mimicking depression and anxiety, it is important to include evaluation of thyroid function, anemia, and nutritional status as part of the evaluation for depressive and anxious disorders.

Depression

As per the patient reports, the first month post treatment tends to be the most difficult. Patients report "feeling abandoned" as they have transitioned from the "job" of active treatment with regular contact with medical team (with the assurances and security that comes with that) to sudden lack of that support and "nothing but time" to think about treatment and current dysfunction and worry for future. Contrary to the general population, depression does not often accompany the diagnosis of cancer, but rather reflects a cumulative, delayed response to multiple stressors/burdens associated with cancer and treatment; thus depression symptoms typically peak at 3 months post treatment.[44,45]

Across studies examining depression in patients with cancer, the rates of major depressive disorder (i.e., clinical depression) are typically 10 to 25%, which is four times higher than the general population.[46] Depressive symptoms are associated with advanced disease, uncontrolled pain, and other physical impairments or symptoms.[46] However, in HNC 15 to 50% of patients report significant depressive symptoms,[47] with previous reports of 40% of patients becoming clinically depressed in the first year after treatment.[48] Within HNC, severe physical distress and dysfunction (particularly loss of sense taste, speech, libido, dry mouth, and weight loss), social support, low spiritual well-being, young age, tumor stage, pretreatment depression, avoidant coping, and premorbid alcohol and tobacco use were predictive of depressive symptoms in survivorship.[49] Depression prior to treatment has also been found to predict survival and nutritional status in HNC,[50] as well as completion of adjuvant treatment, higher narcotic dependence, more functional impairment, and lower QoL at 12 months—independent of demographics, tumor variables, surgery type, adjuvant treatment, or medical comorbidities,[51] poorer swallow outcomes, and continued tobacco use.[4] Depression prior to treatment is also predictive of HRQoL in speech, eating, aesthetics, and social disruption at 3 and 12 months.[52] Conversely, remaining abstinent from tobacco post treatment is associated with lower depressive symptoms.[10]

Anxiety

Anxiety is common in cancer, with 50% of all patients with a cancer diagnosis endorsing anxiety.[47] Anxiety typically peaks at diagnosis[44,45] and is related to transitions from active treatment to follow-up, with predictable increases in anxiety preceding and following surveillance scans until results are known. Across the survivorship trajectory, worries about latent effects of treatment, uncertainty or heightened sense of vulnerability, psychosocial reorientation, and finances are common.[53] In addition, prior research has demonstrated that 22% of patients treated for HNC met criteria posttraumatic stress disorder (PTSD) at 6 months post diagnosis, with 14% meeting criteria for PTSD at 1 year post diagnosis. These rates of PTSD are similar to those found in other cancer literature.[54]

Fear of recurrence (FoR) or the persistent anxiety associated with cancer, is often described as "waiting for the other shoe to drop." FoR is associated with difficulties in planning for the future (e.g., return to work, retirement, vacations, etc.) and lower HRQoL.[55] Within general cancer populations, FoR and distress prior to treatment predicts both FoR and distress post treatment.[56] Also, FoR tends to be high prior to treatment and can remain relatively stable across time.[57]

Suicide

Rates of suicide are elevated across all cancers and are highest in HNC.[58] Oral cavity cancer is in the top four cancer populations with highest rate of suicide.[59] Risk factors for suicide in HNC include advanced disease, low social or cultural support, limited treatment options, pain, disability, body image issues, psychosocial function, anxiety, psychological distress, and depression.[7,60] Across cancer, the risk of suicide peaks in the first few years after diagnosis and the risk of suicide remains elevated throughout the course of survivor's life.[61] Given this elevated risk, it is recommended that routine screening using psychometrically sound, self-report instruments occurs and that these screenings are integrated into clinical practice with follow-up and appropriate referral to BHSs.[3]

42.4 Psychosocial Outcomes

42.4.1 Cognitive Impairment

Cognitive impairment post treatment has been reported in the cancer literature, with up to 75% of patients reporting cognitive difficulties during treatment.[62] These impairments can interfere in functioning at work, educational pursuits, and QoL. Within HNC, cognitive impairments have been identified in almost half of patients prior to treatment at a tertiary care center[63] and are associated with QoL.[64] In addition, recent research has demonstrated that cognitive impairments may increase across treatment and up to 2 years post treatment in patients treated with primary chemoradiotherapy or radiation therapy.[65] When patients report cognitive changes, a referral to a neuropsychologist for evaluation and recommendations should be made. Moreover, confounding factors such as anemia, vitamin deficiencies, endocrine or metabolic dysfunction, and medical side effects should be addressed. A referral to behavioral health for pharmacotherapy (i.e., stimulants, cognition-enhancing medications, or antidepressants) or psychotherapy (i.e., cognitive rehabilitation and cognitive training) can be helpful. Behavioral recommendations, such as good sleep and nutrition, cognitive activity (e.g., crosswords, Sudoku), physical activity, use of compensatory strategies (e.g., day planner, To-Do lists, notes), and following routines, as well as avoiding substances known to interfere in cognition (e.g., alcohol, illicit drugs, certain medications including sedatives) have been helpful in managing cognitive impairment.

42.4.2 Fatigue

Posttreatment fatigue is common, even years after treatment. If fatigue is a problem, it is important to rule out anemia, thyroid dysfunction, cardiac dysfunction, sleep disturbance, mood disorders, and pain in survivors.[3] There exists good evidence that physical activity interventions have both short- and long-term benefits to patients with fatigue, and can also aid in sleep, mood upliftment (anxiety/depression), health, and well-being.[66] Common recommendations in survivorship include avoidance of inactivity and a return to normal daily activities as soon as possible after treatment, if not maintained through treatment. Patients should aim for 150 minutes of moderate or 75 minutes of vigorous aerobic exercise per week and should also include strength training at least 2 days per week.[3] Cognitive behavioral therapy (CBT) is also beneficial not just for mood disorders but also for fatigue, sleep disturbance, pain, and exercise adherence.[10]

42.4.3 Pain

Posttreatment pain is addressed elsewhere in this book. However, it should be noted that posttreatment pain is associated with discontinued employment pain after treatment,[67] increased psychological distress, and poor long-term HRQoL.[39] CBT for pain has been shown to aid in the patient's sense of control over pain experience, thus influencing their overall experience of pain.[68]

42.5 Caregivers

John Donne wrote "No man is an island, entire of itself; every man is a piece of a continent, a part of the main." Such is also the patient with cancer as cancer treatment affects the whole system in which the patient exists—partner/spouse, children, parents, siblings, friends, and work colleagues. The primary caregivers through cancer treatment represent an area in need of support from the medical team.

Through cancer treatment both patient and partner are required to suspend personal pursuits and assume the role of caregiver/patient. Often these changes occur in relationships in which the partners have been performing their precancer roles for years and have not spent a good portion of each day together at any point in their relationship. In addition to increased contact between patient and caregiver, the changes in roles and physical demands of treatment can lead to increased conflict between patient and caregiver. Indeed, 83% of couples reported an increase in conflict during HNC treatment.[69] Marital couples demonstrated that the couple had unmet needs of understanding the severity of the physical effects of treatment, timeline for recovery, and managing their own and each other's emotional reactions to treatment.[69] These spouses wanted information about balancing competing roles/responsibilities, time for self-care, and ways to encourage patient self-care.[69]

Caregiver perceptions of patient illness matters, as does the congruence between patient and caregiver perceptions of illness.[70] Caregiver perceptions can impact QoL and HRQoL scores depending on congruence with patient perceptions, with incongruence being associated with decreased social, functional QoL and congruence being associated with improved social and functional well-being for the patient.[70] Of note, 20% of caregivers report FoR in long-term follow-up at 5 to 10 years.[71] Caregiver research in cancer has found that FoR is often higher in caregivers than patients and this FoR in caregivers predicts caregiver QoL at long-term survivorship more than patient's QoL or FoR.[72] In addition, caregivers also tend to perceive treatment as less helpful and are more likely to see treatment as having a longer timeline compared to patients.[70]

Caregivers require but often do not receive respite, their own health care, psychosocial, and financial assistance while they provide care for patient. Moreover, they carry the patient's psychosocial burden as well.[53] Indeed, 20% of caregivers had clinically significant psychological distress, often when the patient is not reporting distress.[73] Compared to men with HNC, their female partners report greater distress and more frequent anxiety disorders. Caregivers were also at increased risk of developing PTSD after their partner receives a HNC diagnosis.[74]

Since a cancer diagnosis can impact the caregiver's perceptions and coping and thus can impact patient outcomes, interventions need to be aimed at both patients and caregivers. These interventions should target individual perceptions about the disease making sure that both hold accurate perceptions about what to expect from HNC treatment, including consequences, duration, identity, and emotional impact, and that these perceptions are appropriate and congruent with one another.[70] Greater clinical support in the form of practical assistance and information is required for those who care for patients with HNC.[75] It is important to provide individualized information that can improve understanding, especially in caregivers, who typically see treatment as having greater emotional impact, perceived worse consequences, longer timeline, and treatment less helpful than patients.[70]

42.6 Psychosocial Interventions

Multidisciplinary HNC care is becoming recognized as the gold standard of care. This multidisciplinary care should include oncology (medical, radiation, surgical), SLP, registered diet, occupational/physical therapy, dentistry, and psychosocial care (i.e., social work and BHSs/psych-oncology specialists). Given all the information previously presented, psychological support should be provided along with physical and functional care for the best outcomes in QoL, adjustment, and survival in HNC.

Within HNC, many intervention studies have focused on tobacco cessation, given the importance of cessation to treatment, QoL, and survival. Those recommendations are indicated above in the *Tobacco Use and Cessation* section. This section will provide a review of some of the published research on psychosocial interventions in HNC.

One of the widely available psychosocial interventions in HNC is providing tailored patient education materials. These materials include patient booklet with medical information, interactive computer programs with detailed information about site, stage, and details specific to patient's disease and treatment, computer animation, online videos regarding HNC care, and database to capture specific patient information to facilitate patient/provider communication (e.g., regular distress screening across survivorship). An online resource table is at the end of this chapter for materials and referrals for patients (▶ Table 42.2). Patient education materials have been found to be associated with decreased anxiety and depressive symptoms at 3 and 6 months post treatment.[10] Brief pre-/posttreatment supportive contact with trained nurse, who provides both verbal and written psychoeducational information regarding HNC has been found to reduced distress and increase knowledge, as well as increase satisfaction with appearance post treatment.[10]

Interventions that go beyond disease information provision have included brief didactic information about effective communication, problem-solving, goal-setting, and engaging social supports for improvements in coping have been associated with improvements in depression, psychosocial functioning, and HRQoL at 3-month follow-up.[10] CBT interventions have involved problem-focused strategies in which the patient identifies three problem areas (e.g., appearance, eating/drinking, distress, speech issues etc.) and works with cognitive and behavioral strategies for addressing these. CBT has been associated with decreased distress and social impairment and better HRQoL.[7] There exist CBT interventions for disfigurement focused on exposure-based techniques and cognitive restructuring, as well as telephonic

Table 42.2 Online resources for patients with head and neck cancer

Website	Description
www.cancercare.org	One-on-one counseling, group therapy, information, and education—available by telephone and via internet 800–813-HOPE
www.cancer.org	ACS I Can Cope program—series of classes for practical coping skills, online peer support and information, 800–4-CANCER
www.livestrong.org	Information and education online or via telephone
www.oralcancerfoundation.org	Online support group, information and education
www.ahns.info/patient-information	Information and education, survivorship issues, online
www.gildasclub.org	Local support groups and programming for patient, family/caregivers, online support groups and education
www.thewellnesscommunity.org	Online information and support groups, local offices in 22 states for nutrition/exercise/wellness programs
www.cancerhopenetwork.org	One-on-one peer support via telephone

interventions for stress management.[10] Both of which have demonstrated reductions in depression, anxiety, and patient satisfaction with the programs. However, given the limited access to behavioral health providers with experience in HNC, stepped care is followed, in which all patients receive common low-intensity treatment (e.g., patient education materials and education) and only those who do not sufficiently benefit are "stepped up" to more intensive treatment from a BHS.[76,77] Those medical providers who treat HNC are encouraged to develop knowledge of the BHSs/psych-oncology specialists in their hospital and community who have the expertise to work with patients with HNC and their caregivers. Larger tertiary specialty care centers that treat HNC are encouraged to integrate BHSs/psych-oncology specialists, such as clinical health psychologists, into their multidisciplinary approach to aid in treating the more complex and advanced stage patients with HNC that these centers typically treat.

Key Points

- Psychosocial survivorship includes areas of social functioning such as employment, finances, insurance, social interactions, and psychological functioning, including symptoms of depression and anxiety, substance use, fear of recurrence, body image, stigma.
- Psychosocial functioning has been associated with patient's QoL, adherence to medical recommendations, and overall morbidity and mortality. Psychosocial function can be influenced by identification and intervention, thus improving QoL in survivorship, adherence, and possibly disease-free survival.
- Tobacco cessation and abstinence remains important in survivorship as up to 60% of patients return to tobacco use after treatment. Providers are encouraged to consistently use the 5 As: ask about tobacco use, advise to quit using a clear and personalized message, assess willingness to quit, assist to quit, and arrange follow-up and support. When providing assistance in quitting, single-treatment approaches have limited success and long-term outcomes are best seen with multimodal treatment (i.e., medication, NRT, behavioral intervention).
- While rates of survival in oral cavity cancer tend to be good, patients face the immediate and latent physical effects of treatment and facial disfigurement. The effects of treatment may lead to shame, social avoidance, depression, anxiety, and decreased QoL. Screening and appropriate referral for these psychosocial risks and outcomes should occur regularly across survivorship. Familiarity with local behavioral health resources with expertise in treating those with cancer, and the integration of BHSs/psych-oncology specialists into the multidisciplinary treatment teams, particularly in large tertiary treatment centers, are strongly encouraged.

References

[1] DeSantis CE, Lin CC, Mariotto AB, et al. Cancer treatment and survivorship statistics, 2014. CA Cancer J Clin. 2014; 64(4):252–271

[2] SEER Cancer Statistics Review, 1975–2013. Bethesda, MD: National Cancer Institute; 2016

[3] Cohen EEW, LaMonte SJ, Erb NL, et al. American Cancer Society Head and Neck Cancer Survivorship Care Guideline. CA Cancer J Clin. 2016; 66(3):203–239

[4] Arvey SR, Rechis R. The LIVESTRONG essential elements of survivorship care: advancing quality survivorship care in clinical care settings. J Clin Oncol. 2012; 30(34_suppl):155–155

[5] Chawla S, Mohanti BK, Rakshak M, Saxena S, Rath GK, Bahadur S. Temporal assessment of quality of life of head and neck cancer patients receiving radical radiotherapy. Qual Life Res. 1999; 8(1–2):73–78

[6] Østhus AA, Aarstad AKH, Olofsson J, Aarstad HJ. Prediction of 5 year survival from level of perceived distress in newly diagnosed head and neck squamous cell carcinoma patients. Oral Oncol. 2013; 49(9):964–969

[7] Semple C, Parahoo K, Norman A, McCaughan E, Humphris G, Mills M. Psychosocial interventions for patients with head and neck cancer. Cochrane Database of Systematic Reviews. 2013(7):CD009441

[8] Sterba KR, Zapka J, Cranos C, Laursen A, Day TA. Quality of life in head and neck cancer patient-caregiver dyads: a systematic review. Cancer Nurs. 2016; 39(3):238–250

[9] Smedley BD, Stith AY, Nelson AR. Unequal Treatment: Confronting Racial and Ethnic Disparities in Health Care. Washington, DC, US: National Academies Press; 2003

[10] Devins GM, Otto KJ, Irish JC, Rodin G. Head and neck cancer. In: Holland JC, Breitbart WS, Butow PN, et al., eds. Psycho-oncology. New York, NY, US: Oxford University Press; 2015:92–97

[11] Hewitt MGS, Stovall E. From Cancer Patient to Cancer Survivor: Lost in Transition. Washington DC: National Academies Press; 2006

[12] Balfe M, Butow P, O'Sullivan E, Gooberman-Hill R, Timmons A, Sharp L. The financial impact of head and neck cancer caregiving: a qualitative study. Psychooncology. 2016; 25(12):1441–1447

[13] Ekramuddaula FM, Siddique BH, Islam MR, Kabir MS, Alam MS. Evaluation of risk factors of oral cancer. Mymensingh Med J. 2011; 20(3):412–418

[14] Chen AM, Chen LM, Vaughan A, et al. Tobacco smoking during radiation therapy for head-and-neck cancer is associated with unfavorable outcome. Int J Radiat Oncol Biol Phys. 2011; 79(2):414–419

[15] Fidler JA, Shahab L, West R. Strength of urges to smoke as a measure of severity of cigarette dependence: comparison with the Fagerström Test for Nicotine Dependence and its components. Addiction. 2011; 106(3):631–638
[16] Schnoll RA, Wileyto EP, Leone FT, Langer C, Lackman R, Evans T. Is a cancer diagnosis a teachable moment for the patient's relative who smokes? Cancer Causes Control. 2013; 24(7):1339–1346
[17] Schnoll RA, Subramanian S, Martinez E, Engstrom PF. Correlates of continued tobacco use and intention to quit smoking among Russian cancer patients. Int J Behav Med. 2011; 18(4):325–332
[18] Schnoll RA, Hitsman B, Blazekovic S, et al. Longitudinal changes in smoking abstinence symptoms and alternative reinforcers predict long-term smoking cessation outcomes. Drug Alcohol Depend. 2016; 165:245–252
[19] Epstein JF, Induni M, Wilson T. Patterns of clinically significant symptoms of depression among heavy users of alcohol and cigarettes. Prev Chronic Dis. 2009; 6(1):A09
[20] Piasecki TM, McCarthy DE, Fiore MC, Baker TB. Alcohol consumption, smoking urge, and the reinforcing effects of cigarettes: an ecological study. Psychol Addict Behav. 2008; 22(2):230–239
[21] Siegel RL, Jacobs EJ, Newton CC, et al. Deaths due to cigarette smoking for 12 smoking-related cancers in the United States. JAMA Intern Med. 2015; 175 (9):1574–1576
[22] Ehrenzeller MF, Mayer DK, Goldstein A. Smoking prevalence and management among cancer survivors. Oncol Nurs Forum. 2018; 45(1):55–68
[23] Nayan S, Gupta MK, Strychowsky JE, Sommer DD. Smoking cessation interventions and cessation rates in the oncology population: an updated systematic review and meta-analysis. Otolaryngol Head Neck Surg. 2013; 149(2):200–211
[24] Ostroff JS, Jacobsen PB, Moadel AB, et al. Prevalence and predictors of continued tobacco use after treatment of patients with head and neck cancer. Cancer. 1995; 75(2):569–576
[25] Messer K, Trinidad DR, Al-Delaimy WK, Pierce JP. Smoking cessation rates in the United States: a comparison of young adult and older smokers. Am J Public Health. 2008; 98(2):317–322
[26] Stevens VJ, Solberg LI, Bailey SR, et al. Assessing trends in tobacco cessation in diverse patient populations. Nicotine Tob Res. 2016; 18(3):275–280
[27] Chen AM, Vazquez E, Courquin J, Donald PJ, Farwell DG. Tobacco use among long-term survivors of head and neck cancer treated with radiation therapy. Psychooncology. 2014; 23(2):190–194
[28] Simmons VN, Litvin EB, Patel RD, et al. Patient-provider communication and perspectives on smoking cessation and relapse in the oncology setting. Patient Educ Couns. 2009; 77(3):398–403
[29] Fucito LM, Czabafy S, Hendricks PS, Kotsen C, Richardson D, Toll BA. Pairing smoking-cessation services with lung cancer screening: a clinical guideline from the Association for the Treatment of Tobacco Use and Dependence and the Society for Research on Nicotine and Tobacco. Cancer. 2016; 122(8): 1150–1159
[30] Siu AL, U.S. Preventive Services Task Force. Behavioral and pharmacotherapy interventions for tobacco smoking cessation in adults, including pregnant women: U.S. Preventive Services Task Force Recommendation Statement. Ann Intern Med. 2015; 163(8):622–634
[31] Wagner LI, Spiegel D, Pearman T. Using the science of psychosocial care to implement the new American College of Surgeons Commission on cancer distress screening standard. J Natl Compr Canc Netw. 2013; 11(2):214–221
[32] Katz MR, Kopek N, Waldron J, Devins GM, Tomlinson G. Screening for depression in head and neck cancer. Psychooncology. 2004; 13(4):269–280
[33] Herce Lopez J, Rollon Mayordomo A, Lozano Rosado R, Salazar Fernandez CI, Gallana S. Quality of life in long-term oral cancer survivors: a comparison with Spanish general population norms. J Oral Maxillofac Surg. 2009; 67(8): 1607–1614
[34] Sim BY, Lee YW, Kim H, Kim SH. Post-traumatic growth in stomach cancer survivors: prevalence, correlates and relationship with health-related quality of life. Eur J Oncol Nurs. 2015; 19(3):230–236
[35] Egestad H, Emaus N. Changes in health related quality of life in women and men undergoing radiation treatment for head and neck cancer and the impact of smoking status in the radiation treatment period. Eur J Oncol Nurs. 2014; 18(4):339–346
[36] Rinkel RN, Verdonck-de Leeuw IM, Doornaert P, et al. Prevalence of swallowing and speech problems in daily life after chemoradiation for head and neck cancer based on cut-off scores of the patient-reported outcome measures SWAL-QOL and SHI. European Archives Of Oto-Rhino-Laryngology. 2016; 273(7):1849–1855
[37] Lang H, France E, Williams B, Humphris G, Wells M. The psychological experience of living with head and neck cancer: a systematic review and meta-synthesis. Psychooncology. 2013; 22(12):2648–2663
[38] Fingeret MC, Yuan Y, Urbauer D, Weston J, Nipomnick S, Weber R. The nature and extent of body image concerns among surgically treated patients with head and neck cancer. Psychooncology. 2012; 21(8):836–844
[39] Funk GF, Karnell LH, Christensen AJ. Long-term health-related quality of life in survivors of head and neck cancer. Arch Otolaryngol Head Neck Surg. 2012; 138(2):123–133
[40] Lebel S, Castonguay M, Mackness G, Irish J, Bezjak A, Devins GM. The psychosocial impact of stigma in people with head and neck or lung cancer. Psychooncology. 2013; 22(1):140–152
[41] Dunne S, Mooney O, Coffey L, et al. Psychological variables associated with quality of life following primary treatment for head and neck cancer: a systematic review of the literature from 2004 to 2015. Psychooncology. 2017; 26 (2):149–160
[42] Aarstad AK, Aarstad HJ, Olofsson J. Personality and choice of coping predict quality of life in head and neck cancer patients during follow-up. Acta Oncol. 2008; 47(5):879–890
[43] Kanatas A, Ghazali N, Lowe D, Rogers SN. The identification of mood and anxiety concerns using the patients concerns inventory following head and neck cancer. Int J Oral Maxillofac Surg. 2012; 41(4):429–436
[44] Nordgren M, Hammerlid E, Bjordal K, Ahlner-Elmqvist M, Boysen M, Jannert M. Quality of life in oral carcinoma: a 5-year prospective study. Head Neck. 2008; 30(4):461–470
[45] Kohda R, Otsubo T, Kuwakado Y, et al. Prospective studies on mental status and quality of life in patients with head and neck cancer treated by radiation. Psychooncology. 2005; 14(4):331–336
[46] Caruso R, Nanni MG, Riba M, et al. Depressive spectrum disorders in cancer: prevalence, risk factors and screening for depression: a critical review. Acta Oncol. 2017; 56(2):146–155
[47] Buchmann L, Conlee J, Hunt J, Agarwal J, White S. Psychosocial distress is prevalent in head and neck cancer patients. Laryngoscope. 2013; 123(6): 1424–1429
[48] Sehlen S, Lenk M, Herschbach P, et al. Depressive symptoms during and after radiotherapy for head and neck cancer. Head Neck. 2003; 25(12):1004–1018
[49] Wu Y-S, Lin P-Y, Chien C-Y, et al. Anxiety and depression in patients with head and neck cancer: 6-month follow-up study. Neuropsychiatr Dis Treat. 2016; 12:1029–1036
[50] Kim S-A, Roh JL, Lee SA, et al. Pretreatment depression as a prognostic indicator of survival and nutritional status in patients with head and neck cancer. Cancer. 2016; 122(1):131–140
[51] Barber B, Dergousoff J, Nesbitt M, et al. Depression as a predictor of postoperative functional performance status (PFPS) and treatment adherence in head and neck cancer patients: a prospective study. J Otolaryngol Head Neck Surg. 2015; 44(1):38
[52] Howren MB, Christensen AJ, Karnell LH, Funk GF. Health-related quality of life in head and neck cancer survivors: impact of pretreatment depressive symptoms. Health Psychol. 2010; 29(1):65–71
[53] Ganz PA. Late effects of cancer and its treatment. Semin Oncol Nurs. 2001; 17 (4):241–248
[54] Kangas M, Henry JL, Bryant RA. Predictors of posttraumatic stress disorder following cancer. Health Psychol. 2005; 24(6):579–585
[55] Humphris GM, Rogers S, McNally D, Lee-Jones C, Brown J, Vaughan D. Fear of recurrence and possible cases of anxiety and depression in orofacial cancer patients. Int J Oral Maxillofac Surg. 2003; 32(5):486–491
[56] Lee-Jones C, Humphris G, Dixon R, Hatcher MB. Fear of cancer recurrence: a literature review and proposed cognitive formulation to explain exacerbation of recurrence fears. Psychooncology. 1997; 6(2):95–105
[57] Mehta SS, Lubeck D, Pasta DJ, Litwin MS. Fear of cancer recurrence in patients undergoing definitive treatment for prostate cancer: results from CaPSURE. J Urol. 2003; 170(5):1931–1933
[58] Kam D, Salib A, Gorgy G, et al. Incidence of suicide in patients with head and neck cancer. JAMA Otolaryngol Head Neck Surg. 2015; 141(12): 1075–1081
[59] Misono S, Weiss NS, Fann JR, Redman M, Yueh B. Incidence of suicide in persons with cancer. J Clin Oncol. 2008; 26(29):4731–4738
[60] Walker J, Waters RA, Murray G, et al. Better off dead: suicidal thoughts in cancer patients. J Clin Oncol. 2008; 26(29):4725–4730
[61] Epstein JB, Thariat J, Bensadoun RJ, et al. Oral complications of cancer and cancer therapy: from cancer treatment to survivorship. CA Cancer J Clin. 2012; 62(6):400–422
[62] Jean-Pierre P, Winters PC, Ahles TA, et al. Prevalence of self-reported memory problems in adult cancer survivors: a national cross-sectional study. J Oncol Pract. 2012; 8(1):30–34

[63] Williams AM, Lindholm J, Siddiqui F, Ghanem TA, Chang SS. Clinical assessment of cognitive function in patients with head and neck cancer: prevalence and correlates. Otolaryngol Head Neck Surg. 2017; 157(5): 808–815
[64] Williams AM, Lindholm J, Cook D, Siddiqui F, Ghanem TA, Chang SS. Association between cognitive function and quality of life in patients with head and neck cancer. JAMA Otolaryngol Head Neck Surg. 2017; 143(12): 1228–1235
[65] Zer A, Pond GR, Razak ARA, et al. Association of neurocognitive deficits with radiotherapy or chemoradiotherapy for patients with head and neck cancer. JAMA Otolaryngol Head Neck Surg. 2018; 144(1):71–79
[66] Buffart LM, Ros WJG, Chinapaw MJM, et al. Mediators of physical exercise for improvement in cancer survivors' quality of life. Psychooncology. 2014; 23 (3):330–338
[67] Buckwalter AE, Karnell LH, Smith RB, Christensen AJ, Funk GF. Patient-reported factors associated with discontinuing employment following head and neck cancer treatment. Arch Otolaryngol Head Neck Surg. 2007; 133(5): 464–470
[68] Breitbart WS, Park J, Katz AM. Pain. In: Holland JC, Breitbart WS, Jacobsen PB, et al., eds. Psycho-oncology. New York, NY, US: Oxford University Press; 2010:215–228
[69] Badr H, Yeung C, Lewis MA, Milbury K, Redd WH. An observational study of social control, mood, and self-efficacy in couples during treatment for head and neck cancer. Psychol Health. 2015; 30(7):783–802
[70] Richardson AE, Morton R, Broadbent E. Caregivers' illness perceptions contribute to quality of life in head and neck cancer patients at diagnosis. J Psychosoc Oncol. 2015; 33(4):414–432
[71] Balfe M, O'Brien K, Timmons A, et al. The unmet supportive care needs of long-term head and neck cancer caregivers in the extended survivorship period. J Clin Nurs. 2016; 25(11–12):1576–1586
[72] Mellon S, Kershaw TS, Northouse LL, Freeman-Gibb L. A family-based model to predict fear of recurrence for cancer survivors and their caregivers. Psychooncology. 2007; 16(3):214–223
[73] Boele FW, van Uden-Kraan CF, Hilverda K, et al. Attitudes and preferences toward monitoring symptoms, distress, and quality of life in glioma patients and their informal caregivers. Support Care Cancer. 2016; 24(7):3011–3022
[74] Posluszny DM, Dougall AL, Johnson JT, et al. Posttraumatic stress disorder symptoms in newly diagnosed patients with head and neck cancer and their partners. Head Neck. 2015; 37(9):1282–1289
[75] Ross S, Mosher CE, Ronis-Tobin V, Hermele S, Ostroff JS. Psychosocial adjustment of family caregivers of head and neck cancer survivors. Support Care Cancer. 2010; 18(2):171–178
[76] Jansen F, Krebber AMH, Coupé VMH, et al. Cost-utility of stepped care targeting psychological distress in patients with head and neck or lung cancer. J Clin Oncol. 2017; 35(3):314–324
[77] Krebber A-MH, Leemans CR, de Bree R, et al. Stepped care targeting psychological distress in head and neck and lung cancer patients: a randomized clinical trial. BMC Cancer. 2012; 12(1):173–173

43 Posttreatment Surveillance

Carole Fakhry and Christopher Britt

Summary
Posttreatment surveillance schedules in oral cavity cancer are multifaceted and incorporate patient demographics, stage, treatment, treatment-related sequelae, and quality of life in their construction. These schedules should be agreed upon by both patient and physician and should incorporate both clinical examination and functional outcomes. In addition to clinical examination, posttreatment locoregional imaging is essential in establishing a baseline for monitoring for recurrence, especially in advanced disease. Imaging is also important in monitoring for distant metastases. Finally, patients undergoing all forms of radiotherapy should have biannual dental evaluations and annual thyroid function testing. Each evaluation should be complete and comprehensive.

Keywords: oral cavity cancer, posttreatment, surveillance, thyroid function testing

43.1 Epidemiology: Incidence, Causes, and Clinical Characteristics

Oral cavity cancer (OCC) represents a heterogenous group of malignancies with variable etiologies, histologies, and natural histories. Consistent with the Institute of Medicine definition of survivorship, the latter begins at diagnosis and continues until one expires.[1] Therefore, treatment hopefully represents the initial phase of the survivorship period and the immediate posttreatment recovery period to assess nutritional and rehabilitative goals. The remainder of survivorship entails posttreatment surveillance (PTS).

Rationale for PTS involves the identification of pathologic as well as toxicity-related issues that may arise in the survivorship period. Disease recurrence rates for OCC range from 10 to 48%.[2–4] Local and regional recurrences account for 90% of all treatment failures.[5,6] In patients with OCC that recur, 86% of all recurrences will appear within 2 years and the median time to recurrence is 7.5 to 15 months after treatment end.[4,7–10] Not unexpectedly, overall survival rates at 2 years and at 5 years in patients with recurring OCC are significantly lower than those who remain without evidence of malignancy (67.6 vs. 88.0%, 31.8 vs. 79.9%, $p < 0.001$).[4] Detection of recurrence is critical as early detection of locoregional recurrence can result in curative salvage and improvements in current techniques, and new therapies, such as immunotherapy, may extend survival and improve quality of life (QoL) measures for patients with distant disease.[11–13]

Risk of recurrence is associated with a host of factors including social and demographic characteristics, and tumor histopathology. Male gender, advancing age, and non-white race have each been found to have an association with increased risk of recurrence, but the poor prognostic role is weak relative to histopathologic features of tumor or lymph node.[14] These factors include tumor differentiation, perineural invasion, lymphatic invasion, bone invasion, tumor subsite, invasion depth, and proximity of margins.[15] The presence of multiple risk factors contributes additively to increase the risk of recurrence.[15] Lymph node metastasis, extracapsular extension of disease, and positive surgical margins are the greatest risk factors for recurrence.[9,16,17]

PTS is also useful to assess for second primaries. Rates of new tumors in OCC patients vary from 10 to 20% in the lungs and esophagus.[18,19] One study examining 72 patients with OCC over a 10-year period showed a 27.8% rate of second primaries independent of the initial tumor at a median of 32 months.[20] Seventy-five percent of second primaries discovered were in the oral cavity and 80% developed within 5 years.[20] These results mirror a larger study of 1,609 head and neck cancer (HNC) patients of which 1,153 had OCC.[21] In this subgroup, there was a second primary rate of 20%. In both studies, patients with second primaries had significantly worse survival than patients without second primaries.

Continued use of tobacco is recognized as a risk factor for recurrence. Approximately 20 to 30% of HNC patients continue to smoke after treatment.[22] Indeed, in a study that evaluated tobacco use across HNC sites, only 35.8% of OCC survivors stopped smoking, the lowest rate of all HNC sites.[23] Risk of recurrence in this population is unclear. A matched pair study of 66 never smokers, ever smokers, and current smokers showed that recurrence-free survival ($p = 0.006$) and disease-specific survival ($p = 0.027$) were significantly worse for ever smokers as compared with never smokers.[24] However, there was no difference between ever smokers, the ones who had quit at least 1 year before presentation, and current smokers.[24] Regardless, smoking increases the risk of second primaries in other organs and increases risks for other long-term health complications and therefore cessation remains advisable.

Continued alcohol use may also pose a higher risk of recurrence for OCC patients. In a study of 264 HNC patients with median follow-up of 51 months after treatment, patients who continued drinking (average of 2.3 drinks per day) had significantly increased risk of recurrence (relative risk (RR) = 2.7, 95% CI: 1.2–6.1).[25] Indeed, the patient group that drank most after diagnosis or patients who consumed more than five alcoholic drinks per day had an increased risk of mortality (RR = 4.9, 95% CI: 1.5–16.3).[25] Continued consumption of alcohol after diagnosis of HNC impacts the survival. Increased awareness of this coupled with encouragement of abstention should be incorporated into survivorship care.

Finally, sequelae of treatments and disease, both physical and mental, should be monitored. Late toxicity of OCC treatment may include osteoradionecrosis (ORN) of the mandible, pain, numbness, mucositis, dysphagia, dysgeusia, xerostomia, trismus, infection, fistula, gastric tube dependence, or even death.[26] Rates of complications are broad ranging depending on the condition of interest. For example, chronic periodontitis is observed in approximately 70% of patients post radiation therapy while ORN, a relatively rare complication, occurs in up to 5% of patients.[26–28] These sequelae can cause significant morbidity and decrease in QoL; this highlights the importance of prevention, when possible, and recognition of early clinical signs that must be prevented, if possible, or recognized early.

43.2 Clinical Presentation

Recurrent OCC can be much more difficult to detect. While in the primary setting symptoms and anatomy may be more clinically apparent, after-treatment symptoms may be attributed to the preceding therapy and possible distorted anatomy thus making detection more challenging.[29] In a study of 101 HNC patients with 30 recurrences, pain (Odds ratio (OR) = 16.07, 95% CI: 5.94–43.51, $p < .001$), odynophagia (OR = 11.20, 95% CI: 3.13–40.04, $p < .001$), and dysphonia (OR = 5.90, 95% CI: 1.77–17.28, $p = .003$) were all found to be associated with recurrence whereas dysphagia, xerostomia, and dyspnea were not.[29] Of note, 27% of patients with recurrence in this study were asymptomatic.[29] There was another study with 278 OCC patients, of which 54 had recurrent disease (21 local, 22 regional, 6 locoregional, and 6 distant) with the most common presentation of a lump ($n = 35$, 64%).[29] The remainder had an ulcer ($n = 7$, 13%) or were completely asymptomatic ($n = 6$, 11%).[30] These studies emphasize that recurrent symptoms may not be as recognizable to the patient as compared to primary tumors.

43.3 Diagnosis and Evaluation

Several guideline recommendations are available for OCC (▶ Table 43.1). These guidelines provide recommendations for clinical follow-up and some, but not all, provide additional recommendations for imaging, smoking cessation, swallowing rehabilitation, and for other treatment and tumor sequelae.[31] Surveillance guidelines address several issues including duration, frequency and intensity of follow-up visits, the role of imaging, symptom versus protocol-driven follow-up routine, and how to assess QoL.

Table 43.1 Various head and neck surveillance guidelines

	Posttreatment year	Follow-up schedule
National Comprehensive Cancer Network[31] 2018	1 2 3–5 >5	1–3 months 2–6 months 4–8 months Yearly
British Association of Head and Neck Oncologists[32] 2016	1–2 3–5	At least every 2 months 3–6 months Minimum of 5 years total
European Society for Medical Oncology[33] 2010	No specific recommendations	

43.3.1 Surveillance Schedule

In the literature, there is significant variation regarding recommendations for PTS schedule for both clinical and radiologic evaluations for OCC. The initial question of management is whether follow-up should be symptom driven or schedule driven. Some contend that regular follow-up is laborious and costly while others argue that a decrease in follow-up leads to delays in detection of recurrence.[10,34–37] In addition, patients have low compliance with follow-up appointments, with one study indicating 11% of patients followed up consistently during the first 3 years of PTS.[38] Nevertheless, a survey of 400 members of the American Head and Neck Society showed that the vast majority of surgeons recommended routine, long-term follow-up.[39] When examining surveillance for OCC, the optimal intensity, duration, and methods of surveillance should be considered.

Given that the median time to recurrence is between 7.5 and 15 months after initial treatment,[4,8,10] and events of recurrence decline after 2 years (▶ Table 43.2),[2,10,36,37,40,41] surveillance intensity in the National Comprehensive Cancer Network (NCCN) guidelines is highest in the initial years after treatment and tapers off after the first 2 to 3 years. In a representative study, approximately half of recurrences were detected during regularly scheduled visits (every 2–3 months for the first 2 years then every 4 months for the third year) and the other half had their recurrences detected through symptom-directed visits.[2] Presumably, earlier detection by regularly scheduled visits appears to be associated with a survival advantage. For example, among 428 patients with HNC, 154 recurrences were identified and median survival after diagnosis of recurrence for patients undergoing routine PTS was 58 months compared to 32 months for symptom-driven self-referral.[37] This suggests that increased surveillance identified asymptomatic tumors at an earlier time than symptom-driven, thus leading to improved survival.

While many guidelines recommend life-long surveillance, albeit at lower intensity than the first 2 years, the available data question its utility, especially for early-stage disease. For early-stage OCC, the risk of recurrence appears to be drastically reduced after 4 years. In a study of 102 patients with early-stage OCC with 10-year regular follow-up, no recurrences were detected after year 4.[10] However, in the same study, nine of the second primaries occurred after year 4, six of which were iden-

Table 43.2 Cumulative percent recurrence rates for various follow-up studies

Author	Patient population	No. of Patients	Percent recurrences at 1 year	Cumulative percent recurrences at 2 years	Cumulative percent recurrences at 3 years
Boysen et al[40]	All HNC	661	n/a	76	87
Merkx et al[9]	Early-stage OCC	102	60	90	90
Cooney et al[1]	All HNC	302	50	n/a	89
Wensing et al[36]	OCC	197	n/a	83	90
Ohkubo et al[41]	OCC and lip	113	73	n/a	96
De Visscher et al[37]	All HNC	428	47	69	76

Abbreviations: HNC, head and neck cancer; OCC, oral cavity cancer.

tified in routine follow-up.[9] While detection of recurrences drops off after 3 years, many a times second primaries are also detected in the follow-up period.[39,41] Therefore, routine surveillance for recurrence is necessary 3 years after completion of therapy, and thereafter long-term surveillance may be useful to monitor for second primaries in a high-risk population.

In keeping with the available literature, NCCN guidelines are broad and recommend 4 to 12 visits the first year, 2 to 6 visits the second year, and 3 to 9 visits in the following 3 years.[31] In addition, they recommend annual follow-up after 5 years. The important caveat is that patients are encouraged to schedule an appointment earlier than follow-up if they develop symptoms. In addition, visits with the multidisciplinary team are encouraged.[31]

43.3.2 Clinical Surveillance

Physical examination remains the cornerstone of surveillance for OCC.[42–44] For local recurrence, physical examination is reliable.[45] In addition, skilled mirror examination or flexible fiberoptic endoscopy, should be utilized for a comprehensive head and neck evaluation.[46] Narrow-band imaging has also been reported as a potential aid in detection of OCC.[47] A standardized checklist during surveillance, which includes measuring functional outcomes such as weight, pain, swallowing, and voice has been proposed to ensure a comprehensive evaluation.[48] We recommend a comprehensive head and neck examination at each clinical visit with attention to the site of the primary malignancy as well as other mucosal sites at risk for second primary.

43.3.3 Imaging Surveillance

Imaging surveillance for local recurrence in the oral cavity can be difficult secondary to the dental anatomy, changes in postsurgical or postradiation anatomy secondary to reconstruction or edema, and the inherent limitations of imaging and visualization of the oral cavity. However, regional recurrences of the neck and metastatic recurrences may not easily be identified with physical examination and may instead require imaging. Multiple imaging modalities are useful to assess locoregional recurrence, including ultrasound (US), computed tomography (CT), magnetic resonance imaging (MRI), and positron emission computed tomography (PET/CT). In addition, chest X-ray (CXR), PET/CT, and CT are used for identification of metastatic lesions which will be discussed separately.

CT and MRI are often used in PTS either for asymptomatic surveillance or for identification of the extent of a lesion identified on physical examination or for correlation of a symptom. CT is generally easier to tolerate for a patient than the MRI, cheaper, and allows for better bony evaluation, whereas MRI allows for better soft tissue evaluation, tumor extension, and neural involvement. Baseline imaging is typically performed after therapy and may consist of either CT, MRI, or PET/CT. Typically, it is recommended that baseline imaging be performed 3 to 6 months after completion of primary treatment.[31,49] Most authors recommend not performing PET/CT until at least 12 weeks after treatment to decrease false positives.[50,51] The 2018 NCCN guidelines recommend posttreatment imaging within 6 months of treatment and further reimaging as necessary based on symptoms, smoking history, or areas inaccessible to clinical exam.[31]

US is a noninvasive, radiation-free imaging modality traditionally used for evaluation of nodal metastases that can be used in conjunction with biopsy, and is of lower cost than other imaging modalities.[52–55] In early staged, untreated OCC, neck US can be used to detect occult metastasis at the time of diagnosis and longitudinally.[53] Yuasa et al showed US has a high specificity (96%, 95% CI: 82–99%), sensitivity (100%, 95% CI: 70–100%), and positive predictive value (92%, 95% CI: 62–100%) in untreated necks; however, this study was limited by low number.[52] US can also be combined with fine-needle aspiration (FNA) which may hasten time to diagnosis of recurrence to salvage surgery.[56,57] Ultrasound-guided FNA (USFNA) may be used routinely in some clinical situations, alternatively to help guide management of suspicious nodes identified on physical examination or with other imaging modalities. In addition to nodal evaluation, US can be used to evaluate the primary oral cavity site.[58,59] Intraoral US can more accurately delineate tumor thickness in oral tongue cancer and may be more suited for evaluation of tumors less than 5 mm in size; however, exam is limited by trismus.[58,59]

Longitudinal posttreatment imaging concomitant with clinical surveillance for locoregional recurrence has been evaluated. Atula et al directly compared N0 necks on clinical exam with CT, MRI, US, and with USFNA when necessary for HNC patients.[60] They found that CT was superior to MRI for detection of small pathologic lymph nodes; however, the MRI used was less than 3 Tesla. They also observed that USFNA can identify malignancy within small lymph nodes not deemed suspicious by either CT or MRI. When US, USFNA, CT, and MRI were compared in a meta-analysis, USFNA had the highest accuracy for detection of metastasis.[61] The value of long-term MRI surveillance in asymptomatic OCC greater than 6 months post treatment appears to be low. Among 46 patients, only 1 true recurrence was found with 10 false positives which suggests that MRI may be costly and unnecessary after 6 months post treatment in the absence of symptoms.[62] It is unclear from these studies if there is any long-term value for CT or MRI for locoregional asymptomatic surveillance.

PET/CT can detect relatively small lymph nodes (> 5 mm size) and is highly sensitive for the detection of distant metastasis.[63–65] In the surveillance setting, a strength of PET/CT is a high negative predictive value.[64] A prospective study of 278 patients over at least 2 years compared imaging surveillance for PET/CT and CT or MRI with chest CT. PET/CT showed statistically superior sensitivity and specificity for detection of recurrence over conventional imaging and clinical examination.[65] A negative PET/CT was associated with higher 2-year disease-specific and overall survival.[66,67] Lin et al examined the use of PET/CT as a surveillance tool by comparing overall and disease-specific survival for 111 asymptomatic HNC patients who either received PET/CT routine surveillance or symptom-based surveillance. Survival was significantly higher in the PET/CT surveillance group.[68] In a similar study of 143 patients, the PET/CT group had a higher detection rate of recurrence compared to clinical evaluation.[69] However, other studies have failed to reproduce such results. Ho et al examined 175 patients with surveillance PET/CT at 1 year and 2 years.[70] They saw no difference in overall or disease-specific survival between patients who had PET/CT and those who did not. They concluded that patients who had negative scans at 3 months did not derive benefit from subsequent scans.[70] PET/CT is commonly used post chemoradiotherapy at 3 months, but not generally used for subsequent surveillance. Contrast-enhanced CT neck and noncontrast low-dose chest CT is likely sufficient.

43.4 Anatomic Considerations/ Relevant Anatomy

The NCCN follow-up guidelines do not differentiate between anatomic subsites of the oral cavity for posttreatment clinical examination.[31] Those patients who have undergone radiation or chemoradiation should have a clinical evaluation of the neck at 4 to 8 weeks after completion of treatment. If there is progression of the disease, additional imaging can be considered and surgical intervention may be warranted.[31]

43.4.1 Surveillance for Non-head and Neck Primaries

The lungs represent the most common site for metastasis in HNC and primary metachronous lung cancer accounts for 23% of all second primaries in HNC patients.[71–73] NCCN guidelines recommend yearly CT for patients who have had HNC, are more than 50 years of age, and have a more than 20 pack per year smoking history.[31] In a large study reviewing the use of annual low-dose CT for lung cancer screening in high-risk patients versus chest radiograph, low-dose CT screening saw a relative reduction of 20% in mortality (95% CI: 6.8–26.7) and a 7% (95% CI: 1.2–13.6) reduction in all-cause mortality.[74] While there is a subset of OCC patients who are nonsmokers, no evidence exists that these patients should undergo routine chest imaging.

43.4.2 Thyroid Surveillance

When treatment of OCC includes neck irradiation, there will be incidental exposure to surrounding tissues. Using conventional radiation techniques, approximately 50% of patients will experience hypothyroidism at 44 Gy.[75] Sinard et al showed that half of patients who will develop hypothyroidism will do so in the first 5 years, with the highest incidence at 3 years.[76] Patients who receive radiation therapy to the neck should be monitored annually for thyroid-stimulating hormone by the head and neck surgeon or primary care physician.[31]

43.5 Treatment Considerations and Approaches

43.5.1 Quality of Life Surveillance

QoL is an important aspect of PTS in HNC patients. In a Surveillance, Epidemiology, and End Results study, QoL was found to decrease to a nadir 13 months post treatment with slow recovery toward baseline between 2 and 5 years. Radiotherapy and advanced stage were associated with greater declines in health-related QoL during diagnosis and treatment ($p < .001$). Higher pre-diagnosis health-related QoL was independently associated with improved overall survival (adjusted hazard ratio for 10-point increase = 0.91, 95% CI: 0.85–0.97).[77] In patients who had radiotherapy or free tissue transfer, QoL related to emotional functioning, social functioning, swallowing, speech, taste/smell, dry mouth, sticky saliva, and coughing may never fully recover to base line, even 8 to 11 years post treatment.[78] These issues are critical not only to the patient, but have implications for the health care system also.

Posttreatment QoL can be measured both by physical metrics related to the sequelae of the disease and its treatment, and psychological metrics related to the mental trauma of the treatment, burden of the diagnosis, and dramatic life changes. In one study, approximately 41% of patients had high level of psychological distress in the first year after treatment.[79] Sammut et al showed that patients who remained physically active post treatment had an improved QoL ($p > .001$) but that there was a significant reduction in physical activity after diagnosis in HNC patients ($p > .001$).[73] Finally, HNC survivors' families often lack the support they need to care for these patients. Breen et al concluded that treatment programs for HNC survivors and their families to promote psychological resilience and improved QoL may be necessary.[80] Clearly, QoL is not only a factor in well-being of the mind and body of the patient, but also for the patient's loved ones.

Mobility concerns should be addressed at follow-up directly with the patient. A questionnaire-based study by van Nieuwenhuizen et al showed that higher levels of physical activity are significantly associated with higher QoL.[81] It is known that HNC survivors are at risk for low physical activity levels.[73,82] Van Nieuwenhuizen et al stressed that most physical activity comes from household work and thus survivors should be questioned about their household routine, not just work or leisure.[81] In addition, exercise does improve QoL and patient function in all cancer patients.[83] Specific concerns addressing treatment-related mobility issues must also be addressed. Patients who underwent neck dissection would have higher rates of shoulder dysfunction than those who did not and rates can be as high as 10 to 100% in patients undergoing radical neck dissection.[84] These patients should be screened and set up with the appropriate physical therapy early to ameliorate loss of function.

Head and neck treatment-related morbidities should also be discussed. Dysphagia and hoarseness are shown to depress QoL in HNC population.[85] Pain should be addressed at every visit, as well. Terkawi et al found that 30% of HNC survivors had chronic pain, and that 42% of postsurgical patients had chronic pain. These patients had overall lower QoL scores, decreased mood, decreased activity, and poor sleep.[86] Finally, continued tobacco use must be addressed after treatment of cancer as not only does it lead to the potential for long-term and short-term ill effects, it also decreases the patients' QoL.[87]

43.6 Surgical Sequelae (Short and Long Term)

Surgical resection of OCC can disrupt the oral preparatory phase of swallowing and articulation of speech by impairing the coordination of the oral cavity substructures. Fibrosis and scaring from surgery further impair speech and swallowing as time progresses requiring a relationship with speech-language pathology to decrease or avoid gastric tube dependence, recurrent aspiration, and difficulties with communication.[88–90] In addition to mechanical complications, limitation of the interincisal opening of the oral aperture, or trismus, may impair eating and is a common sequelae of both oral cavity surgery and adjuvant therapy. Management consists of early mobilization using exercise or mouth opening assisting devices; however, if not employed early, limited improvement may be gained by such therapies.[91–94]

Both motor and sensory nerves are at risk during surgery of the oral cavity and of the associated neck. Peri-incisional numbness is frequent after neck dissection and tumors involving the mandible or lip may result in damage to the inferior alveolar or mental nerves. Anesthesia from a mental nerve injury will improve, but not completely, in these patients if the lip was not sacrificed.[95] The spinal accessory nerve, phrenic nerve, sympathetic trunk, and vagus nerve can all be injured during the neck dissection. While these injuries are not directly related to oral cavity function, care must be taken during the surgical procedure and postoperatively to limit sequelae of injury or sacrifice. The lingual nerve and/or hypoglossal nerve may be impacted. Injury or sacrifice can lead to impaired taste, poor food bolus preparation, accidental tongue biting, and dysarthria. In the case of bilateral hypoglossal injury, the airway can be compromised through posterior positioning of the tongue in the supine position. Long-term management involves speech and language therapy rehabilitation for patients with unilateral, clinical injury and potentially surgical airway management with bilateral hypoglossal injury.[96,97] Finally, the marginal mandibular branch of the facial nerve is at risk during both primary resection of oral cavity masses and during the neck dissection. Injury to this nerve can impair oral liquid consumption, contribute to drooling, and may result in impaired cosmesis of the lower lip. Rehabilitation may consist of contralateral chemical denervation if cosmetic or lip wedge resection functional concerns are present.

Patients who undergo radiation therapy have significantly decreased salivary gland function and subsequent xerostomia making them increasingly susceptible to dental caries. Radiation-related dental caries can appear within 3 months post radiation.[98,99] NCCN guidelines recommend frequent dental evaluations to detect dental disease, dietary counseling, and long-term high-potency topical floride.[31] Refer to Chapter 45, Posttreatment Dental Considerations, for a more in-depth review of posttreatment dental management.

Key Points

- PTS in OCC is complex and depends on a variety of factors including patient demographics, stage, treatment, cancer and treatment-related sequelae, and QoL.
- Having an agreed upon schedule with the patient is paramount. Clinical examination and assessment of functional outcomes is necessary at each visit.
- Posttreatment imaging is useful to establish a baseline after treatment and for monitoring distant metastasis overtime.
- Patients who undergo radiation therapy should have thyroid function checked at least annually and have biannual dental evaluations.
- Comprehensive evaluation is paramount.

References

[1] Grant M, Economou D, Ferrell B, Uman G. Educating health care professionals to provide institutional changes in cancer survivorship care. J Cancer Educ. 2012; 27(2):226–232

[2] Cooney TR, Poulsen MG. Is routine follow-up useful after combined-modality therapy for advanced head and neck cancer? Arch Otolaryngol Head Neck Surg. 1999; 125(4):379–382

[3] Virgo KS, Paniello RC, Johnson FE. Costs of posttreatment surveillance for patients with upper aerodigestive tract cancer. Arch Otolaryngol Head Neck Surg. 1998; 124(5):564–572

[4] Wang B, Zhang S, Yue K, Wang XD. The recurrence and survival of oral squamous cell carcinoma: a report of 275 cases. Chin J Cancer. 2013; 32(11):614–618

[5] Leemans CR, Tiwari R, Nauta JJ, van der Waal I, Snow GB. Recurrence at the primary site in head and neck cancer and the significance of neck lymph node metastases as a prognostic factor. Cancer. 1994; 73(1):187–190

[6] Agra IM, Filho JG, Martins EP, Kowalski LP. Second salvage surgery for re-recurrent oral cavity and oropharynx carcinoma. Head Neck. 2010; 32(8): 997–1002

[7] Carvalho AL, Kowalski LP, Agra IM, Pontes E, Campos OD, Pellizzon AC. Treatment results on advanced neck metastasis (N3) from head and neck squamous carcinoma. Otolaryngol Head Neck Surg. 2005; 132(6):862–868

[8] Kowalski LP, Carvalho AL, Martins Priante AV, Magrin J. Predictive factors for distant metastasis from oral and oropharyngeal squamous cell carcinoma. Oral Oncol. 2005; 41(5):534–541

[9] Fan S, Tang QL, Lin YJ, et al. A review of clinical and histological parameters associated with contralateral neck metastases in oral squamous cell carcinoma. Int J Oral Sci. 2011; 3(4):180–191

[10] Merkx MA, van Gulick JJ, Marres HA, et al. Effectiveness of routine follow-up of patients treated for T1–2N0 oral squamous cell carcinomas of the floor of mouth and tongue. Head Neck. 2006; 28(1):1–7

[11] Ridge JA. Squamous cancer of the head and neck: surgical treatment of local and regional recurrence. Semin Oncol. 1993; 20(5):419–429

[12] Machiels JP, Haddad RI, Fayette J, et al. LUX-H&N 1 investigators. Afatinib versus methotrexate as second-line treatment in patients with recurrent or metastatic squamous-cell carcinoma of the head and neck progressing on or after platinum-based therapy (LUX-Head & Neck 1): an open-label, randomised phase 3 trial. Lancet Oncol. 2015; 16(5):583–594

[13] Soulières D, Faivre S, Mesía R, et al. Buparlisib and paclitaxel in patients with platinum-pretreated recurrent or metastatic squamous cell carcinoma of the head and neck (BERIL-1): a randomised, double-blind, placebo-controlled phase 2 trial. Lancet Oncol. 2017; 18(3):323–335

[14] Woolgar JA. Histopathological prognosticators in oral and oropharyngeal squamous cell carcinoma. Oral Oncol. 2006; 42(3):229–239

[15] Camisasca DR, Silami MA, Honorato J, Dias FL, de Faria PA, Lourenço SdeQ. Oral squamous cell carcinoma: clinicopathological features in patients with and without recurrence. ORL J Otorhinolaryngol Relat Spec. 2011; 73(3):170–176

[16] Warnakulasuriya S. Global epidemiology of oral and oropharyngeal cancer. Oral Oncol. 2009; 45(4–5):309–316

[17] Campana JP, Meyers AD. The surgical management of oral cancer. Otolaryngol Clin North Am. 2006; 39(2):331–348

[18] Schwartz LH, Ozsahin M, Zhang GN, et al. Synchronous and metachronous head and neck carcinomas. Cancer. 1994; 74(7):1933–1938

[19] Sturgis EM, Miller RH. Second primary malignancies in the head and neck cancer patient. Ann Otol Rhinol Laryngol. 1995; 104(12):946–954

[20] Liu CH, Chen HJ, Wang PC, Chen HS, Chang YL. Patterns of recurrence and second primary tumors in oral squamous cell carcinoma treated with surgery alone. Kaohsiung J Med Sci. 2013; 29(10):554–559

[21] Yamamoto E, Shibuya H, Yoshimura R, Miura M. Site specific dependency of second primary cancer in early stage head and neck squamous cell carcinoma. Cancer. 2002; 94(7):2007–2014

[22] Nayan S, Gupta MK, Strychowsky JE, Sommer DD. Smoking cessation interventions and cessation rates in the oncology population: an updated systematic review and meta-analysis. Otolaryngol Head Neck Surg. 2013; 149(2): 200–211

[23] Chan Y, Irish JC, Wood SJ, et al. Smoking cessation in patients diagnosed with head and neck cancer. J Otolaryngol. 2004; 33(2):75–81

[24] Fang QG, Shi S, Liu FY, Sun CF. Squamous cell carcinoma of the oral cavity in ever smokers: a matched-pair analysis of survival. J Craniofac Surg. 2014; 25 (3):934–937

[25] Mayne ST, Cartmel B, Kirsh V, Goodwin WJ, Jr. Alcohol and tobacco use prediagnosis and postdiagnosis, and survival in a cohort of patients with early stage cancers of the oral cavity, pharynx, and larynx. Cancer Epidemiol Biomarkers Prev. 2009; 18(12):3368–3374

[26] Epstein JB, Corbett T, Galler C, Stevenson-Moore P. Surgical periodontal treatment in the radiotherapy-treated head and neck cancer patient. Spec Care Dentist. 1994; 14(5):182–187

[27] Marques MA, Dib LL. Periodontal changes in patients undergoing radiotherapy. J Periodontol. 2004; 75(9):1178–1187

[28] Marx RE. Osteoradionecrosis: a new concept of its pathophysiology. J Oral Maxillofac Surg. 1983; 41(5):283–288

[29] Nisa L, La Macchia R, Boujelbene N, Sandu K, Khanfir K, Giger R. Correlation between subjective evaluation of symptoms and objective findings in early recurrent head and neck squamous cell carcinoma. JAMA Otolaryngol Head Neck Surg. 2013; 139(7):687–693

[30] Kissun D, Magennis P, Lowe D, Brown JS, Vaughan ED, Rogers SN. Timing and presentation of recurrent oral and oropharyngeal squamous cell carcinoma and awareness in the outpatient clinic. Br J Oral Maxillofac Surg. 2006; 44(5): 371–376

[31] Members NGVP. NCCN Clinical Practice Guidelines in Oncology: Head and Neck Cancers. 2018

[32] Simo R, Homer J, Clarke P, et al. Follow-up after treatment for head and neck cancer: United Kingdom National Multidisciplinary Guidelines. J Laryngol Otol. 2016; 130 S2:S208–S211

[33] Grégoire V, Lefebvre JL, Licitra L, Felip E, EHNS-ESMO-ESTRO Guidelines Working Group. Squamous cell carcinoma of the head and neck: EHNS-ESMO-ESTRO Clinical Practice Guidelines for diagnosis, treatment and follow-up. Ann Oncol. 2010; 21 Suppl 5:v184–v186

[34] Boysen M. Value of follow-up in patients treated for squamous cell carcinomas of the oral cavity and oropharynx. Recent Results Cancer Res. 1994; 134: 205–214

[35] Rivelli V, Luebbers HT, Weber FE, Cordella C, Grätz KW, Kruse AL. Screening recurrence and lymph node metastases in head and neck cancer: the role of computer tomography in follow-up. Head Neck Oncol. 2011; 3:18

[36] Wensing BM, Merkx MA, Krabbe PF, Marres HA, Van den Hoogen FJ. Oral squamous cell carcinoma and a clinically negative neck: the value of follow-up. Head Neck. 2011; 33(10):1400–1405

[37] de Visscher AV, Manni JJ. Routine long-term follow-up in patients treated with curative intent for squamous cell carcinoma of the larynx, pharynx, and oral cavity. Does it make sense? Arch Otolaryngol Head Neck Surg. 1994; 120 (9):934–939

[38] Gellrich NC, Schramm A, Böckmann R, Kugler J. Follow-up in patients with oral cancer. J Oral Maxillofac Surg. 2002; 60(4):380–386, discussion 387–388

[39] Marchant FE, Lowry LD, Moffitt JJ, Sabbagh R. Current national trends in the posttreatment follow-up of patients with squamous cell carcinoma of the head and neck. Am J Otolaryngol. 1993; 14(2):88–93

[40] Boysen M, Lövdal O, Tausjö J, Winther F. The value of follow-up in patients treated for squamous cell carcinoma of the head and neck. Eur J Cancer. 1992; 28(2–3):426–430

[41] Ohkubo H, Maeda T, Hirano M, Kurita S, Mihashi S. Carcinoma of the lip and oral cavity: a retrospective investigation of 113 patients. Kurume Med J. 1982; 29 Suppl:S61–S78

[42] Johnson F, Johnson M, Virgo K. Current follow-up strategies after potentially curative resection of upper aerodigestive tract epidermoid carcinoma. Int J Oncol. 1997; 10(5):927–931

[43] Paniello RC, Virgo KS, Johnson MH, Clemente MF, Johnson FE. Practice patterns and clinical guidelines for posttreatment follow-up of head and neck cancers: a comparison of 2 professional societies. Arch Otolaryngol Head Neck Surg. 1999; 125(3):309–313

[44] Manikantan K, Khode S, Dwivedi RC, et al. Making sense of post-treatment surveillance in head and neck cancer: when and what of follow-up. Cancer Treat Rev. 2009; 35(8):744–753

[45] Daisne JF, Duprez T, Weynand B, et al. Tumor volume in pharyngolaryngeal squamous cell carcinoma: comparison at CT, MR imaging, and FDG PET and validation with surgical specimen. Radiology. 2004; 233(1):93–100

[46] British Association of Head and Neck Oncologists. Practice care guidance for clinicians participating in the management of head and neck cancer patients in the UK. Drawn up by a Consensus Group of Practising Clinicians. Eur J Surg Oncol. 2001; 27 Suppl A:S1–S17

[47] Chu PY, Tsai TL, Tai SK, Chang SY. Effectiveness of narrow band imaging in patients with oral squamous cell carcinoma after treatment. Head Neck. 2012; 34(2):155–161

[48] Digonnet A, Hamoir M, Andry G, et al. Post-therapeutic surveillance strategies in head and neck squamous cell carcinoma. European Archives of Otorhinolaryngology. 2013; 270(5):1569–1580

[49] de Bree R, Haigentz M, Jr, Silver CE, et al. Distant metastases from head and neck squamous cell carcinoma. Part II. Diagnosis. Oral Oncol. 2012; 48(9): 780–786

[50] Yao M, Smith RB, Graham MM, et al. The role of FDG PET in management of neck metastasis from head-and-neck cancer after definitive radiation treatment. Int J Radiat Oncol Biol Phys. 2005; 63(4):991–999

[51] Porceddu SV, Jarmolowski E, Hicks RJ, et al. Utility of positron emission tomography for the detection of disease in residual neck nodes after (chemo) radiotherapy in head and neck cancer. Head Neck. 2005; 27(3):175–181

[52] Yuasa K, Kawazu T, Kunitake N, et al. Sonography for the detection of cervical lymph node metastases among patients with tongue cancer: criteria for early detection and assessment of follow-up examination intervals. AJNR Am J Neuroradiol. 2000; 21(6):1127–1132

[53] Snow GB. Follow-up in patients treated for head and neck cancer: how frequent, how thorough and for how long? Eur J Cancer. 1992; 28(2–3):315–316

[54] Baatenburg de Jong RJ, Rongen RJ, Laméris JS, Harthoorn M, Verwoerd CD, Knegt P. Metastatic neck disease. Palpation vs. ultrasound examination. Arch Otolaryngol Head Neck Surg. 1989; 115(6):689–690

[55] Fruehwald FX. Clinical examination, CT and US in tongue cancer staging. Eur J Radiol. 1988; 8(4):236–241

[56] van den Brekel MW, Reitsma LC, Quak JJ, et al. Sonographically guided aspiration cytology of neck nodes for selection of treatment and follow-up in patients with N0 head and neck cancer. AJNR Am J Neuroradiol. 1999; 20(9): 1727–1731

[57] Nieuwenhuis EJ, Castelijns JA, Pijpers R, et al. Wait-and-see policy for the N0 neck in early-stage oral and oropharyngeal squamous cell carcinoma using ultrasonography-guided cytology: is there a role for identification of the sentinel node? Head Neck. 2002; 24(3):282–289

[58] Lodder WL, Teertstra HJ, Tan IB, et al. Tumour thickness in oral cancer using an intra-oral ultrasound probe. Eur Radiol. 2011; 21(1):98–106

[59] Shintani S, Yoshihama Y, Ueyama Y, et al. The usefulness of intraoral ultrasonography in the evaluation of oral cancer. Int J Oral Maxillofac Surg. 2001; 30 (2):139–143

[60] Atula TS, Varpula MJ, Kurki TJ, Klemi PJ, Grénman R. Assessment of cervical lymph node status in head and neck cancer patients: palpation, computed tomography and low field magnetic resonance imaging compared with ultrasound-guided fine-needle aspiration cytology. Eur J Radiol. 1997; 25(2):152–161

[61] de Bondt RB, Nelemans PJ, Hofman PA, et al. Detection of lymph node metastases in head and neck cancer: a meta-analysis comparing US, USgFNAC, CT and MR imaging. Eur J Radiol. 2007; 64(2):266–272

[62] Al-Shwaiheen FA, Wang SJ, Uzelac A, Yom SS, Ryan WR. The advantages and drawbacks of routine magnetic resonance imaging for long-term post-treatment locoregional surveillance of oral cavity squamous cell carcinoma. Am J Otolaryngol. 2015; 36(3):415–423

[63] Evangelista L, Cervino AR, Chondrogiannis S, et al. Comparison between anatomical cross-sectional imaging and 18F-FDG PET/CT in the staging, restaging, treatment response, and long-term surveillance of squamous cell head and neck cancer: a systematic literature overview. Nucl Med Commun. 2014; 35(2):123–134

[64] Connell CA, Corry J, Milner AD, et al. Clinical impact of, and prognostic stratification by, F-18 FDG PET/CT in head and neck mucosal squamous cell carcinoma. Head Neck. 2007; 29(11):986–995

[65] Kim SA, Roh JL, Kim JS, et al. 18F-FDG PET/CT surveillance for the detection of recurrence in patients with head and neck cancer. Eur J Cancer. 2017; 72:62–70

[66] Lee P, de Bree R, Brokx HA, Leemans CR, Postmus PE, Sutedja TG. Primary lung cancer after treatment of head and neck cancer without lymph node metastasis: is there a role for autofluorescence bronchoscopy? Lung Cancer. 2008; 62(3):309–315

[67] Kao J, Vu HL, Genden EM, et al. The diagnostic and prognostic utility of positron emission tomography/computed tomography-based follow-up after radiotherapy for head and neck cancer. Cancer. 2009; 115(19):4586–4594

[68] Lin HC, Kang CJ, Huang SF, et al. Clinical impact of PET/CT imaging after adjuvant therapy in patients with oral cavity squamous cell carcinoma. Eur J Nucl Med Mol Imaging. 2017; 44(10):1702–1711

[69] Kim JW, Roh JL, Kim JS, et al. (18)F-FDG PET/CT surveillance at 3–6 and 12 months for detection of recurrence and second primary cancer in patients with head and neck squamous cell carcinoma. Br J Cancer. 2013; 109(12): 2973–2979

[70] Ho AS, Tsao GJ, Chen FW, et al. Impact of positron emission tomography/computed tomography surveillance at 12 and 24 months for detecting head and neck cancer recurrence. Cancer. 2013; 119(7):1349–1356
[71] Ferlito A, Shaha AR, Rinaldo A, Pellitteri PK, Mondin V, Byers RM. "Skip metastases" from head and neck cancers. Acta Otolaryngol. 2002; 122(7):788–791
[72] León X, Quer M, Orús C, del Prado Venegas M, López M. Distant metastases in head and neck cancer patients who achieved loco-regional control. Head Neck. 2000; 22(7):680–686
[73] Sammut L, Fraser LR, Ward MJ, Singh T, Patel NN. Participation in sport and physical activity in head and neck cancer survivors: associations with quality of life. Clin Otolaryngol. 2016; 41(3):241–248
[74] Aberle DR, Adams AM, Berg CD, et al. National Lung Screening Trial Research Team. Reduced lung-cancer mortality with low-dose computed tomographic screening. N Engl J Med. 2011; 365(5):395–409
[75] Bakhshandeh M, Hashemi B, Mahdavi SR, Nikoofar A, Vasheghani M, Kazemnejad A. Normal tissue complication probability modeling of radiation-induced hypothyroidism after head-and-neck radiation therapy. Int J Radiat Oncol Biol Phys. 2013; 85(2):514–521
[76] Sinard RJ, Tobin EJ, Mazzaferri EL, et al. Hypothyroidism after treatment for nonthyroid head and neck cancer. Arch Otolaryngol Head Neck Surg. 2000; 126(5):652–657
[77] Rettig EM, D'Souza G, Thompson CB, Koch WM, Eisele DW, Fakhry C. Health-related quality of life before and after head and neck squamous cell carcinoma: Analysis of the Surveillance, Epidemiology, and End Results-Medicare Health Outcomes Survey linkage. Cancer. 2016; 122(12):1861–1870
[78] Oskam IM, Verdonck-de Leeuw IM, Aaronson NK, et al. Prospective evaluation of health-related quality of life in long-term oral and oropharyngeal cancer survivors and the perceived need for supportive care. Oral Oncol. 2013; 49 (5):443–448
[79] Ninu MB, Miccinesi G, Bulli F, et al. Psychological distress and health-related quality of life among head and neck cancer patients during the first year after treatment. Tumori. 2016; 102(1):96–102
[80] Breen LJ, O'Connor M, Calder S, Tai V, Cartwright J, Beilby JM. The health professionals' perspectives of support needs of adult head and neck cancer survivors and their families: a Delphi study. Support Care Cancer. 2017; 25(8): 2413–2420
[81] van Nieuwenhuizen AJ, Buffart LM, van Uden-Kraan CF, et al. Patient-reported physical activity and the association with health-related quality of life in head and neck cancer survivors. Support Care Cancer. 2018; 26(4):1087–1095
[82] Rogers LQ, Courneya KS, Robbins KT, et al. Physical activity and quality of life in head and neck cancer survivors. Support Care Cancer. 2006; 14(10): 1012–1019
[83] Buffart LM, Kalter J, Sweegers MG, et al. Effects and moderators of exercise on quality of life and physical function in patients with cancer: an individual patient data meta-analysis of 34 RCTs. Cancer Treat Rev. 2017; 52:91–104
[84] Gane EM, Michaleff ZA, Cottrell MA, et al. Prevalence, incidence, and risk factors for shoulder and neck dysfunction after neck dissection: a systematic review. Eur J Surg Oncol. 2017; 43(7):1199–1218
[85] Daugaard R, Kjaer T, Johansen C, et al. Association between late effects assessed by physicians and quality of life reported by head-and-neck cancer survivors. Acta Oncol. 2017; 56(2):342–347
[86] Terkawi AS, Tsang S, Alshehri AS, Mulafikh DS, Alghulikah AA, AlDhahri SF. The burden of chronic pain after major head and neck tumor therapy. Saudi J Anaesth. 2017; 11 Suppl 1:S71–S79
[87] Reeve BB, Cai J, Zhang H, et al. Factors that impact health-related quality of life over time for individuals with head and neck cancer. Laryngoscope. 2016; 126(12):2718–2725
[88] LaBlance GR, Kraus K, Steckol KF. Rehabilitation of swallowing and communication following glossectomy. Rehabil Nurs. 1991; 16(5):266–270
[89] Pauloski BR, Logemann JA, Rademaker AW, et al. Speech and swallowing function after anterior tongue and floor of mouth resection with distal flap reconstruction. J Speech Hear Res. 1993; 36(2):267–276
[90] Rentschler GJ, Mann MB. The effects of glossectomy on intelligibility of speech and oral perceptual discrimination. J Oral Surg. 1980; 38(5):348–354
[91] Buchbinder D, Currivan RB, Kaplan AJ, Urken ML. Mobilization regimens for the prevention of jaw hypomobility in the radiated patient: a comparison of three techniques. J Oral Maxillofac Surg. 1993; 51(8):863–867
[92] Dijkstra PU, Kalk WW, Roodenburg JL. Trismus in head and neck oncology: a systematic review. Oral Oncol. 2004; 40(9):879–889
[93] Ichimura K, Tanaka T. Trismus in patients with malignant tumours in the head and neck. J Laryngol Otol. 1993; 107(11):1017–1020
[94] Dijkstra PU, Huisman PM, Roodenburg JL. Criteria for trismus in head and neck oncology. Int J Oral Maxillofac Surg. 2006; 35(4):337–342
[95] Robinson PP. Observations on the recovery of sensation following inferior alveolar nerve injuries. Br J Oral Maxillofac Surg. 1988; 26(3):177–189
[96] Kim DD, Ord RA. Complications in the treatment of head and neck cancer. Oral Maxillofac Surg Clin North Am. 2003; 15(2):213–227
[97] Schauber MD, Fontenelle LJ, Solomon JW, Hanson TL. Cranial/cervical nerve dysfunction after carotid endarterectomy. J Vasc Surg. 1997; 25(3):481–487
[98] Epstein JB, Thariat J, Bensadoun RJ, et al. Oral complications of cancer and cancer therapy: from cancer treatment to survivorship. CA Cancer J Clin. 2012; 62(6):400–422
[99] Murdoch-Kinch CA, Zwetchkenbaum S. Dental management of the head and neck cancer patient treated with radiation therapy. J Mich Dent Assoc. 2011; 93(7):28–37

44 Posttreatment Speech-language Pathology

Heather M. Starmer

Summary
Rehabilitation of speech and swallowing function is a critical aspect of recovery from oral cavity cancer. Functional outcomes are impacted by tumor characteristics, treatment characteristics, and therapeutic intervention. These issues will be discussed in this chapter on posttreatment rehabilitation.

Keywords: dysphagia, speech changes, rehabilitation, oral cancer

44.1 Introduction

The oral cavity serves as an important conduit for important functions such as speech and oral intake. Cancers arising in the oral cavity are typically initially managed with surgical resection leading to alteration of structure and function. In this chapter, we will review functional changes to speech and swallowing associated with treatment for oral cavity cancer, how to best evaluate the functional impact of oncologic treatments, and rehabilitative treatments that may be employed to manage them.

44.2 Epidemiology of Dysphagia in Oral Cavity Cancer

Description of the epidemiology of dysphagia in patients following treatment for oral cavity cancer is challenging due to the heterogeneous nature of this population. Surgical resection may be simple or complex and may include primary closure, locoregional or flap reconstruction. Further, some patients will require adjuvant treatment following surgical resection. Hence, there is great variability of functional outcomes in this population. A systematic review completed by Kao et al (2016)[1] provides some composite information regarding patients treated surgically for oral cavity and oropharyngeal cancers. Their report cites a posttreatment aspiration prevalence of 15.22%, gastrostomy tube (G-tube) dependence rate of 8%, and tracheostomy dependency in less than 1% of patients treated for oral and oropharyngeal squamous cell cancers. Patients requiring postoperative radiation/chemoradiation were at elevated risk for posttreatment dysphagia. In addition, radiation toxicities such as fibrosis, edema, trismus, and xerostomia further impacted patients' perceived swallowing quality of life. In general, higher tumor stages are associated with poorer functional outcomes.[2] While these trends provide an important starting point in the understanding of dysphagia following oral cavity cancer treatment, consideration of particular regions of resection may help provide more insight and expectations of posttreatment function.

44.3 Clinical Presentation

Functional ramifications of oral cavity cancer treatment can be divided into three categories: anatomic, physiologic, and a combination of the two. Changes in the oral cavity, as a result of surgical and adjuvant treatment, will potentially impact the muscles and nerves as well as the vascular and lymphatic systems. Anatomic changes are more commonly associated with surgical resection while physiologic changes are commonly associated with nonoperative treatment modalities; however in the era of combined modality treatment, most patients will experience both anatomic and physiologic changes that may influence speech and swallowing outcomes. It is important to consider each of these types of changes as each may require different interventions. While many patients may present with intelligible speech after oral cavity resection, it is important to acknowledge that atypical speech characteristics may persist, which may draw attention to the speaker and influence communication in a variety of settings.[3]

Specific functional deficits are strongly correlated with tumor site and extent of the surgical procedure. In addition, regions of the oral cavity resected may provide some prediction of functional outcomes. Schache and colleagues described the "oral subsites concept" in their 2009 publication.[4] They divided oral cavity defects as lateral, central, anterior, and oropharyngeal, and concluded that resections leading to central defects were more likely to yield poor functional outcomes. Each specific anatomic structure and region will be considered individually throughout this chapter, though in reality, surgical resections are commonly more complex and involve more than one structure.

44.4 Glossectomies

When considering the impact of glossectomy on speech and swallowing, it is important to consider not only the extent (partial [< 50%], hemi [50%], subtotal [> 50% but < 90%], or total [> 90%] of oral and tongue base), but also the region of the tongue resected. The major functional regions of the tongue include the tongue tip, tongue body, and tongue base.

The tongue serves as the primary articulator of both vowel and consonants. Resections of different regions of the tongue will lead to variable alteration in sound production.[5] From a speech perspective, surgeries involving the tongue tip are likely to impact articulatory precision and speech clarity. Sounds frequently impacted by tongue tip resection include t, d, n, l, r, s, z, and "th." Resection of the lateral tongue will frequently impact intelligibility to a lesser degree; however, particular sounds such as s, z, and "sh" tend to be problematic for patients. If surgery extends to the tongue base, issues with production of velar plosives (k, g) may be observed. In considering relative intelligibility by extent of resection, Fletcher reported near 100% of word/syllable intelligibility in a patient with 10% tongue volume reduction, 30 to 50% intelligibility in an individual with ~40% tongue resection, and 15 to 40% intelligibility for an individual with ~75% tongue resection.[6]

From a swallowing perspective, different regions of resection may be associated with predicted swallowing difficulties as well. Surgeries involving the tongue tip are likely to result in oral stage difficulties with bolus containment, mastication, and oral clearance while surgeries including the body of the tongue will result in issues with bolus containment and posterior propulsion. Resection of the lateral tongue is likely to result in difficulty with bolus lateralization for mastication as well as clearance of the oral cavity on the resected side. Aspiration is a common finding following subtotal and total glossectomy due to reduced bolus clearance and reduced hyolaryngeal excursion due to removal of the suprahyoid muscles.[7] Aspiration rates have been reported as high as 40% one year following surgical resection including the oral tongue.[2] Gastrostomy dependency at 12 months post total glossectomy with free flap reconstruction is estimated at 24% based on a systematic review of the literature.[8]

In addition to considering the extent of resection, we also must consider the surgical approach and type of reconstruction after completion of the ablative procedure. Patients requiring mandibulotomy have higher risk of functional deficits than patients whose tumors can be approached transorally.[9] The primary functional purpose of reconstruction following glossectomy is to provide bulk within the oral cavity to assist with speech and swallowing function. Contact between the palate and the remnant tongue/reconstruction provides benefit in regards to both speech and swallowing.[10] If the degree of resection is limited, the surgical field is typically closed through primary closure. Research has demonstrated functional superiority of primary closure compared to tissue transfer when the extent of surgical resection is limited to less than 25% of the tongue.[11] More extensive excisions may require reconstruction using skin grafts or tissue transfer. Skin flaps involve transportation of skin and underlying subcutaneous tissue from one region to another while maintaining a pedicle to the original site. Myocutaneous flaps also include underlying muscle and are used for more extensive reconstructions. Examples of myocutaneous flaps include the pectoralis major flap and the platysma flap. Microvascular advances permit the transfer of muscle and tissue from a remote area of the body to the surgical site by ability anastomosis of distant and regional blood supplies to maintain the viability of the tissue. A primary advantage of this type of flap is the ability to be more selective about the amount of tissue harvested/transplanted. This prevents both inadequate and excessive bulk, both of which may negatively impact speech and swallowing outcomes. In addition, anastomosis of nerves in the graft to regional nerves may allow for sensory innervation of flaps. There is evidence that patients undergoing hemi- and subtotal glossectomy have more favorable swallowing outcomes if they receive innervated flaps.[12] These "free flaps" are commonly utilized for reconstruction of larger tongue resections. Examples of free flaps include the radial forearm free flap and the anterolateral thigh flap. There is no clear evidence of superiority of the different types of free flaps on swallow or speech function.

44.4.1 Oral Composite Resections

Composite resections involve removal of more than one component structure of the oral cavity and may include excision of the floor of mouth, mandible, maxilla, and tongue. As with glossectomy, the amount and location of resection have significant implications for function. Resection of the floor of mouth will commonly result in anchoring or tethering of the anterior tongue leading to issues with anterior bolus loss, bolus manipulation for mastication, and oral clearance. From a speech perspective, speech sounds requiring elevation of the tongue tip (such as /t, d, l, r, n/) may have reduced precision. Floor of mouth and alveolar ridge resection will also commonly lead to removal of dentition, impacting bite and mastication. Laryngeal elevation may be impacted due to removal of suprahyoid musculature, thus increasing risk of aspiration due to reduced closure of the laryngeal vestibule. With extended mandibular resection, reconstruction plays a significant role in preserving function. Osseocutaneous flaps have been shown to improve speech and swallowing outcomes after mandibular resection.[13]

44.4.2 Maxillary Resections

Tumors arising from the palate will result in resection of the maxilla and potentially the soft palate as well. As the palate serves as the barrier between the oral and nasal cavities, the primary concern with maxillary resection is the potential for hypernasality and nasal regurgitation. In addition, if velopharyngeal incompetence results from palatal resection, the ability to generate intraoral pressure may lead to reduced speech clarity and poor pharyngeal clearance due to lack of driving pressure behind the bolus. Finally, loss of maxillary teeth can impact both speech and mastication.

44.5 Diagnosis and Evaluation of Speech and Dysphagia in Patients with Oral Cavity Cancer

Assessment of speech after oral cavity resection may include measures of articulator mobility and strength, specific sound generation, communicative intelligibility, and patient perceived communication function. While there are no "gold standard" tests to assess speech outcomes, many clinical tools have been validated for use in this population. Lazarus and colleagues[14] described a range of motion measurement scale to be used to quantify restriction in tongue mobility as a way to predict function. This tool has been shown to correlate with speech and swallowing outcomes, performance status, and patient-rated quality of life. Maintenance of tongue strength has also been associated with more favorable patient reported outcomes with 30 kPa reflecting a predictive cutoff for anticipating outcomes.[15] Precision of consonant and vowel production can be estimated by a skilled speech language pathologist (SLP) both in isolation and in variable phonetic contexts. Similarly, intelligibility can be rated at the single word, passage, and conversation level using tests such as the Speech Intelligibility Test,[16] the Assessment of Intelligibility of Dysarthric Speech,[17] and the Frenchay Dysarthria Assessment.[18] Patient-reported quality of life measures that may be used to quantify speech-related disability include the Speech Handicap Index[19] and the speech domains of the Performance Status Scale, Head and Neck.[20]

The measurement of dysphagia is a multidimensional construct and there is limited consensus in the literature about the most appropriate measures to quantify and describe dysphagia in the head and neck population. Diagnosis of dysphagia in head and neck cancer patients should consider anatomic and physiologic changes as measured during instrumental swallowing assessments, impact on oral diet, tube feeding reliance, and patient-perceived swallowing function/quality of life. This global assessment will provide the most comprehensive picture of how the patient is experiencing swallowing.

Due to the elevated risk of silent dysphagia in head and neck cancer, instrumental assessment is essential following oral cavity resection, particularly for those individuals who are at highest risk for dysfunction.[21] A recent investigation of the ability of clinical evaluations to predict aspiration following head and neck cancer surgery demonstrated poor predictive value of clinical findings such as tongue weakness, tongue immobility, and wet voice.[22] These findings suggest the importance of instrumental assessment for detection of dysphagia and aspiration following surgical resection. Untreated dysphagia may lead to adverse outcomes such as aspiration pneumonia, dehydration, and malnutrition. Such events may compromise healing following surgical procedures, oncologic outcomes due to treatment breaks, and may place the patient at elevated risk for long-term health consequences including death. Determining aspiration risk following treatment may assist in ensuring optimal intervention by the SLP through application of compensatory maneuvers, dietary modifications, and rehabilitative interventions.

Instrumental swallowing evaluation can be accomplished through videofluoroscopic swallowing studies (VFSS) or fiberoptic endoscopic evaluation of swallowing (FEES). These tools are complimentary and both play a valuable role in the assessment of dysphagia in patients with head and neck cancer. VFSS is generally considered the gold standard for assessment of oropharyngeal disorders due to its ability to provide visualization of the coordinated stages of swallowing as well as specific physiology (**Video 44.1**). In addition, use of VFSS allows for evaluation of the oral and esophageal aspects of swallowing which are not visualized on endoscopic examination. In contrast, FEES provides the benefits of avoiding radiation exposure, a flexible service delivery model, and direct visualization of relevant anatomy (**Video 44.2**). Investigation of the comparability of these tools has revealed high levels of agreement, sensitivity, specificity, and positive and negative predictive values.[23] A thorough FEES evaluation conducted by an experienced SLP can provide anatomic and physiologic information, assessment of swallowing safety/efficiency across viscosities and textures, and implementation of compensatory postures and strategies when dysfunction is identified. It can be implemented in the early recovery period to establish safety to initiate first oral intake. Despite the fact that both tools have high levels of utility, in the oral cancer population, VFSS is typically the preferred method for assessing swallow function as it allows for full visualization of the oral cavity and the transition between the oral and pharyngeal phases of swallowing. Based upon a systematic review of the literature, Mylnarek and colleagues[24] proposed that instrumental swallowing evaluation, assessment of speech intelligibility, supplemental speech evaluation when indicated, and patient reported swallowing outcomes should be measured prior to, during, and following treatment for oral and oropharyngeal cancers.

44.6 Treatment Considerations and Approaches

Speech therapy is a critical aspect of recovery following oral cavity cancer treatment. The primary goal of the SLP should be to optimize functional communication according to the needs of the individual client. Ideally, needs assessment will be performed by the SLP prior to surgery to determine what the patient's communicative needs may be. Following surgery, the SLP treatment recommendations should be made based upon functional impairments measured during assessment procedures and patient goals. The SLP will provide the patient with education regarding typical speech production and articulatory contacts and will provide guidance on how to achieve alternative articulatory contacts based on remaining structures. These alternative articulatory contacts should first be established in isolation and then extended to syllable, word, phrase, and sentence level stimuli. The long-term goal should be establishing new articulatory strategies in functional contexts to optimize intelligibility and speech naturalness to the greatest degree possible.

Management of dysphagia arising from surgical treatments is heavily influenced by the type and extent of the surgical procedure performed. In general, rehabilitation may encompass use of compensatory strategies, dietary modifications, range of motion, and strengthening exercises. The goal of intervention should be to facilitate a safe and efficient swallow with the least restrictions or adaptations required. When possible, adaptations should be selected to mimic more normal eating behaviors so that the patient will be more apt to adhere to in social settings. Compensatory maneuvers have been shown to eliminate aspiration in up to 81% of patients following head and neck surgery.[25]

Resections limited to the oral cavity primarily impact bolus control, propulsion, and clearance. Thus strategies should be chosen to optimize each. Anterior bolus loss due to facial palsy can often be overcome by tilting the head to the uninvolved side during mastication and by use of a straw placed on the intact side during drinking. When patients experience issues with bolus containment due to intraoral resections, strategies such as a head tilt to the unaffected side or a head tilt back may allow for better bolus control. Patients with oral bolus control issues typically do best with thicker viscosities. Preferential bolus placement to the posterior aspect of the better side paired with a head tilt back may be of benefit when patients have difficulty with posterior bolus propulsion.[26] For patients with posterior bolus spillage, a chin tuck may be beneficial for bolus containment.[27] If a significant portion of the tongue has been resected, a palatal drop prosthesis may provide additional benefit by narrowing the oral cavity, thus resulting in an easier target for the tongue to oppose against.[28] Poor oral bolus clearance resulting from restricted propulsion may be compensated for thorough use of a liquid wash. In general, patients experiencing issues with bolus propulsion and clearance do better with thinner viscosities. For patients with inability to propel the bolus due to subtotal/total glossectomy, gavage feeding can be used to bypass the oral phase, particularly in the early stages of recovery. A red-rubber catheter can be affixed to a syringe and liquids and thinner purees can be piped directly into the pharynx. The SLP should take care to ensure adequate patient preparation and airway protection prior to using this technique. Patients undergoing maxillary resection without primary reconstruction may experience hypernasality and nasal regurgitation. A palatal obturator can be fashioned by a maxillofacial prosthodontist to fill the defect leading to more favorable speech and swallowing outcomes.[29] Therapeutic exercises for oral resection may include range of motion and strengthening exercises. Range-of-motion exercises applied for the first 3 months following surgery result in better long-term outcomes.[30]

Trismus, or restricted mouth opening, can create significant issues with oral intake including inability to bite something like a sandwich and difficulty inserting utensils into the mouth. Use of shallow dish spoons (e.g., infant spoons) can help with oral bolus delivery, though in severe cases a straw may be the only useful implement for oral bolus delivery. Cutting foods into smaller bites may help facilitate consumption of solid foods. Jaw stretches and use of a Therabite trismus device can contribute to improved oral aperture.[31,32]

Direct exercises to work on range of motion and strength typically require clearance by the surgeon and these do not begin until ~2 weeks following surgery. This allows ample time for healing for most patients, though for patients with complex reconstructions or delayed healing, exercises may be deferred for a greater duration. Exercises should target intact musculature to improve the safety and efficiency of swallowing. Swallowing therapy often also includes diet progression from least to most difficult using appropriate strategies, as outlined above. It is important to note that patients frequently have complicated resections involving one or more of the regions discussed above. In addition, patients frequently receive a combination of therapies (e.g., chemoradiation followed by salvage surgery), thus may require a combination of strategies to achieve safe and efficient swallowing.

44.7 Short- and Long-term Sequelae

The ability to communicate is the key to human interaction and sense of self. As a result, a change in a person's ability to communicate can have both short-term and long-term consequences. In the short term, patients have high communication needs during hospitalization. The inability to communicate with staff and family may make them vulnerable to poor pain management and psychological distress such as depression and anxiety.[33–35] Implementation of simple alternative communication options such as communication boards and technological communication aids may help to mitigate distress in patients during hospitalization.[36,37] Long-term communication changes may result in lack of participation in meaningful life activities impacting return to work as well as social interactions.[38]

Similar to communication issues, patients with dysphagia may suffer from psychosocial challenges as well as medical sequela. Head and neck cancer survivors cite dysphagia as a primary factor impacting feelings of physical, social, and emotional loss.[39] In the early stages of recovery, anxiety and fear of eating/choking may be common; while in the later stages of recovery, depression may be more common.[40] Dysphagia may also lead to medical complications including but not limited to feeding tube dependence, tracheostomy dependence, malnutrition, dehydration, and pulmonary consequences of chronic aspiration.[41] Such complications may increase risk of mortality.[42] Hence, consideration of functional outcomes and rehabilitation of patients with oral cavity cancer is of utmost importance.

44.8 Conclusion

Communication and swallowing function can be changed markedly following oncologic treatment of oral cavity cancer. The region and extent of the resection will have direct bearing on communication and oral intake. The SLP plays an important role in evaluating communication and swallowing following treatment and in developing a comprehensive rehabilitation plan. Such rehabilitation has the potential for far-reaching impact on patient function, quality of life, and health status.

Key Points

- Communication and swallowing challenges are common after treatment for oral cavity cancer.
- Extent and region of resection has a direct impact on the degree of dysfunction.
- Rehabilitation is a multidisciplinary endeavor and includes aspects of surgical ablation, reconstruction, prosthetic management of tissue defects, and speech and swallowing rehabilitation provided by SLPs.
- Failure to address rehabilitative needs may increase potential for health and psychosocial difficulties both in the short and long term.

References

[1] Kao SS, Peters MDJ, Krishnan SG, Ooi EH. Swallowing outcomes following primary surgical resection and primary free flap reconstruction for oral and oropharyngeal squamous cell carcinomas: a systematic review. Laryngoscope. 2016; 126(7):1572–1580

[2] Borggreven PA, Verdonck-de Leeuw I, Rinkel RN, et al. Swallowing after major surgery of the oral cavity or oropharynx: a prospective and longitudinal assessment of patients treated by microvascular soft tissue reconstruction. Head Neck. 2007; 29(7):638–647

[3] Kreeft AM, van der Molen L, Hilgers FJ, Balm AJ. Speech and swallowing after surgical treatment of advanced oral and oropharyngeal carcinoma: a systematic review of the literature. Eur Arch Otorhinolaryngol. 2009; 266(11):1687–1698

[4] Schache AG, Lieger O, Rogers P, Kelly A, Newman L, Kalavrezos N. Predictors of swallowing outcome in patients treated with surgery and radiotherapy for advanced oral and oropharyngeal cancer. Oral Oncol. 2009; 45(9):803–808

[5] Matsui Y, Shirota T, Yamashita Y, Ohno K. Analyses of speech intelligibility in patients after glossectomy and reconstruction with fasciocutaneous/myocutaneous flaps. Int J Oral Maxillofac Surg. 2009; 38(4):339–345

[6] Fletcher SG. Speech production following partial glossectomy. J Speech Hear Disord. 1988; 53(3):232–238

[7] Hirano M, Kuroiwa Y, Tanaka S, Matsuoka H, Sato K, Yoshida T. Dysphagia following various degrees of surgical resection for oral cancer. Ann Otol Rhinol Laryngol. 1992; 101(2 Pt 1):138–141

[8] Dziegielewski PT, Ho ML, Rieger J, et al. Total glossectomy with laryngeal preservation and free flap reconstruction: objective functional outcomes and systematic review of the literature. Laryngoscope. 2013; 123(1):140–145

[9] O'Malley BW, Jr, Weinstein GS, Snyder W, Hockstein NG. Transoral robotic surgery (TORS) for base of tongue neoplasms. Laryngoscope. 2006; 116(8):1465–1472

[10] Hsiao HT, Leu YS, Chang SH, Lee JT. Swallowing function in patients who underwent hemiglossectomy: comparison of primary closure and free radial

forearm flap reconstruction with videofluoroscopy. Ann Plast Surg. 2003; 50 (5):450–455
[11] McConnel FM, Pauloski BR, Logemann JA, et al. Functional results of primary closure vs flaps in oropharyngeal reconstruction: a prospective study of speech and swallowing. Arch Otolaryngol Head Neck Surg. 1998; 124(6):625–630
[12] Chang EI, Yu P, Skoracki RJ, Liu J, Hanasono MM. Comprehensive analysis of functional outcomes and survival after microvascular reconstruction of glossectomy defects. Ann Surg Oncol. 2015; 22(9):3061–3069
[13] Buchbinder D, Urken ML, Vickery C, Weinberg H, Sheiner A, Biller H. Functional mandibular reconstruction of patients with oral cancer. Oral Surg Oral Med Oral Pathol. 1989; 68(4 Pt 2):499–503, discussion 503–504
[14] Lazarus CL, Husaini H, Jacobson AS, et al. Development of a new lingual range-of-motion assessment scale: normative data in surgically treated oral cancer patients. Dysphagia. 2014; 29(4):489–499
[15] Lazarus CL, Husaini H, Anand SM, et al. Tongue strength as a predictor of functional outcomes and quality of life after tongue cancer surgery. Ann Otol Rhinol Laryngol. 2013; 122(6):386–397
[16] Yorkston KM, Beukelman DR, Hakel M. Speech intelligibility test (computer software). 1996. Nebraska: Communication Disorders Software
[17] Yorkston KM, Beukelman DR. Assessment of Intelligibilty of Dysarthric Speech. Austin: Pro Ed.; 1984
[18] Enderby P, Palmer R. Frenchay Dysarthria Assessment. Austin: Pro Ed.; 2008
[19] Rinkel RN, Verdonck-de Leeuw IM, van Reij EJ, Aaronson NK, Leemans CR. Speech Handicap Index in patients with oral and pharyngeal cancer: better understanding of patients' complaints. Head Neck. 2008; 30(7):868–874
[20] List MA, Ritter-Sterr C, Lansky SB. A performance status scale for head and neck cancer patients. Cancer. 1990; 66(3):564–569
[21] Simental AA, Carrau RL. Assessment of swallowing function in patients with head and neck cancer. Curr Oncol Rep. 2004; 6(2):162–165
[22] Hey C, Lange BP, Aere C, et al. Predictability of oral and laryngopharyngeal function for aspiration and limitation of oral intake in patients after surgery for head and neck cancer. Anticancer Res. 2013; 33(8):3347–3353
[23] Langmore SE, Schatz K, Olson N. Endoscopic and videofluoroscopic evaluations of swallowing and aspiration. Ann Otol Rhinol Laryngol. 1991; 100(8): 678–681
[24] Mlynarek AM, Rieger JM, Harris JR, et al. Methods of functional outcomes assessment following treatment of oral and oropharyngeal cancer: review of the literature. J Otolaryngol Head Neck Surg. 2008; 37(1):2–10
[25] Logemann JA, Rademaker AW, Pauloski BR, Kahrilas PJ. Effects of postural change on aspiration in head and neck surgical patients. Otolaryngol Head Neck Surg. 1994; 110(2):222–227
[26] Furia CL, Carrara-de Angelis E, Martins NM, Barros AP, Carneiro B, Kowalski LP. Video fluoroscopic evaluation after glossectomy. Arch Otolaryngol Head Neck Surg. 2000; 126(3):378–383
[27] Welch MV, Logemann JA, Rademaker AW, Kahrilas PJ. Changes in pharyngeal dimensions effected by chin tuck. Arch Phys Med Rehabil. 1993; 74(2):178–181
[28] Toyoshita Y, Koshino H, Hirai T, Matsumi T. Effect of wearing a palatal plate on swallowing function. J Prosthodont Res. 2009; 53(4):172–175
[29] Hertrampf K, Wenz HJ, Lehmann KM, Lorenz W, Koller M. Quality of life of patients with maxillofacial defects after treatment for malignancy. Int J Prosthodont. 2004; 17(6):657–665
[30] Logemann JA, Pauloski BR, Rademaker AW, Colangelo LA. Speech and swallowing rehabilitation for head and neck cancer patients. Oncology (Williston Park). 1997; 11(5):651–656, 659, discussion 659, 663–664
[31] Kamstra JI, Roodenburg JL, Beurskens CH, Reintsema H, Dijkstra PU. TheraBite exercises to treat trismus secondary to head and neck cancer. Support Care Cancer. 2013; 21(4):951–957
[32] Dijkstra PU, Sterken MW, Pater R, Spijkervet FK, Roodenburg JL. Exercise therapy for trismus in head and neck cancer. Oral Oncol. 2007; 43(4): 389–394
[33] Menzel LK. Factors related to the emotional responses of intubated patients to being unable to speak. Heart Lung. 1998; 27(4):245–252
[34] Happ MB. Interpretation of nonvocal behavior and the meaning of voicelessness in critical care. Soc Sci Med. 2000; 50(9):1247–1255
[35] Rodriguez CS, Blischak DM. Communication needs of nonspeaking hospitalized postoperative patients with head and neck cancer. Appl Nurs Res. 2010; 23(2):110–115
[36] Stovsky B, Rudy E, Dragonette P. Comparison of two types of communication methods used after cardiac surgery with patients with endotracheal tubes. Heart Lung. 1988; 17(3):281–289
[37] Costello JM. AAC intervention in the intensive care unit: The Children's Hospital Boston Model. Aug Alternative Comm. 2000; 16(9):137–153
[38] Kraaijenga SA, Oskam IM, van Son RJ, et al. Assessment of voice, speech, and related quality of life in advanced head and neck cancer patients 10-years + after chemoradiotherapy. Oral Oncol. 2016; 55:24–30
[39] McQuestion M, Fitch M, Howell D. The changed meaning of food: physical, social and emotional loss for patients having received radiation treatment for head and neck cancer. Eur J Oncol Nurs. 2011; 15(2):145–151
[40] Martino R, Beaton D, Diamant NE. Perceptions of psychological issues related to dysphagia differ in acute and chronic patients. Dysphagia. 2010; 25(1):26–34
[41] Clavé P, Shaker R. Dysphagia: current reality and scope of the problem. Nat Rev Gastroenterol Hepatol. 2015; 12(5):259–270
[42] Szczesniak MM, Maclean J, Zhang T, Graham PH, Cook IJ. Persistent dysphagia after head and neck radiotherapy: a common and under-reported complication with significant effect on non-cancer-related mortality. Clin Oncol (R Coll Radiol). 2014; 26(11):697–703

45 Posttreatment Dental Considerations

Leah I. Leinbach

Summary
Exposure to cancer therapeutics can cause multiple complications including rapidly progressive dental caries, periodontal diseases, and osteoradionecrosis. These complications are relatively common and can significantly compromise functionality and quality of life. Frequent, consistent follow-up with an oral health provider during the posttreatment period is advised. Recommendations for the prevention and treatment of these common dental complications are reviewed in this chapter.

Keywords: prevention, head and neck radiation, chemotherapy, dental caries, periodontal disease, osteoradionecrosis, salivary dysfunction, self-exams

45.1 Introduction

Frequent, consistent follow-up with an oral health provider is an integral part of both the short- and long-term management of a patient with oral cancer. Salivary dysfunction, dietary changes, immune compromise, direct toxicity to oral structures, and decreased ability to maintain oral hygiene after cancer therapy can lead to the rapid development of dental caries and other odontogenic pathology.[1] These complications can affect overall health as well as seriously compromise quality of life. This chapter will introduce common dental complications of oral cavity cancer, with recommendations for both prevention and treatment. Mucosal complications are explored in Chapter 46, "Oral and Dental Complications of Oral Cancer Treatment."

45.2 Dental Caries

Patients treated for oral cancer are at elevated risk of dental caries, predominantly secondary to salivary dysfunction.[2] Saliva naturally debrides the oral cavity, contains antimicrobial enzymes, and buffers cariogenic acid from foods, beverages, and microorganisms.[3] Although newer treatment techniques, such as parotid transfer and parotid-sparing radiation, are aimed at preserving salivary function, the subjective experience of dry mouth or xerostomia is still commonly reported.[4] Symptoms can be relatively nonspecific: difficulty or painful swallowing, difficulty chewing, pain while eating, taste changes, or a subjective "dry feeling" can all be reported. Patients often describe waking up at night to drink and often present to office visits with a large bottle of water. Clinically, patients can exhibit oral mucosa that is desiccated, cracked, and bleeding. Without a significant serous component, saliva can appear thick and mucus-based. Patients may exhibit rapidly progressive dental caries that are discussed below, and a greater frequency and severity of oral infections such as candidiasis and periodontitis. It is important to note that these sequelae of hyposalivation can be present without the subjective report of xerostomia. Salivary gland dysfunction is mentioned here as it relates to other diseases on topic for this chapter. Treatment recommendations are further discussed in Chapter 46.

Radiation-related hyposalivation and changes in salivary composition favor a shift toward pathogenic bacteria, rapid demineralization of hard tissues, and decreased antimicrobial activity.[5] Salivary flow and composition can be affected by surgical treatment and chemotherapy, but is most compromised after radiation and is worst with concurrent chemoradiation. Decreased salivary function has been reported after exposure to as low as 20 Gy of therapeutic radiation.[5,6] Direct toxicity to odontogenic structures secondary to radiation exposure has also been reported, leading to a decreased repair capacity of hard tissues.[7] Postradiation fibrosis can also make it more difficult to maintain oral hygiene, thereby increasing the risk of dental caries.

45.2.1 Epidemiology

Robust long-term data on the development of caries in postradiation patients are not available. That being said, dental caries after radiation and chemoradiation are common, estimated at 24 and 21%, respectively based on a literature review conducted by Multi-national Association of Supportive Care in Cancer/International Society of Oral Oncology.[8,9] Patients treated with radiation to the head and neck had decayed, missing, and filled teeth scores roughly four times that of healthy controls, indicating an elevated burden of dental caries in this population, with a prevalence that increases with time from treatment.[10,11]

45.2.2 Considerations for Prevention

Prevention is arguably the most important aspect of posttreatment oral care. Oral cancer itself is associated with preexisting poor oral health[12]. Pretreatment dental extractions, infrequent or emergency-only visits to dentist, residence in a community without fluoridated municipal water, a heavily restored dentition, exposed root surfaces, poor oral hygiene, preexisting xerostomia, and a history of gastroesophageal reflux disease/eating disorder are just some factors that may place a patient at additional risk of dental caries. What follows is an outline of daily preventative recommendations that can be reviewed during visits with any member of the treatment team.

45.2.3 Mechanical Debridement

Tooth-brushing two to three times daily is advised with the use of an extra-soft toothbrush. Bristles can be softened in hot water if needed. Oral tissues exposed to chemotherapeutics and radiation tend to be more friable and less resilient than untreated tissues; reducing the likelihood of trauma to these sites is imperative. Harsh-bristled toothbrushes or overbrushing can cause damage to tissues that are already at risk for delayed healing and infection. As such, patients undergoing cancer therapy should be routinely counseled on appropriate oral hygiene techniques. Mechanized toothbrushes are typically recommended, if tolerated. In the case of patients with dexterity limitations, modifications or assistance by a caregiver may be needed. In situations where the use of a bristled toothbrush is not possible, a foam brush dipped in chlorhexidine or saline solution can be utilized. Daily flossing is recommended unless limited by concerns for bleeding or infection. Brushing and flossing methods should be reviewed at each follow-up visit to ensure an atraumatic technique.

45.2.4 Fluoride Therapy

All patients receiving treatment for head and neck cancer should be prescribed 1.1% sodium fluoride toothpaste for use morning and evening, if tolerated. Products with heavy flavoring such as cinnamon and mint as well as whitening agents should be avoided. Fruit-flavored products are a well-tolerated choice that can be specified on the prescription. Regardless of the product prescribed, patients should be advised to brush all surfaces of the teeth for two minutes and then spit but do not rinse. Eating and drinking should be avoided for 30 minutes after application to allow for maximum benefit of the active ingredient. Fabrication of custom fluoride trays for use with fluoride gel may be of additional benefit and can temporarily stimulate salivary flow. In patients who are not able to tolerate toothpaste, especially those with mucositis, a saline solution, chlorhexidine, or water can be used on gauze or a cotton pad to gently debride the teeth and oral cavity. Over-the-counter dentifrices with more natural ingredients, assuming the inclusion of fluoride, may also be less irritating to tissues.

45.2.5 Oral Rinses

Alcohol-containing products can by drying and generally irritating to already sensitive tissues and should be avoided. These include certain over-the-counter oral care products. Chlorhexidine mouth rinses, particularly alcohol-free formulations, are recommended for the treatment and prevention of gingivitis and periodontitis. Chlorhexidine has been shown to decrease burden of pathogenic *Streptococcus mutans* in patients receiving cancer therapy as well as overall plaque deposition.[13,14] Patients should be advised of chlorhexidine's potential to cause taste changes and reversible discoloration of the dentition. Warm saline, baking soda, and other bland rinses can also help with mucosal discomfort and hygiene.

45.2.6 Nutrition Counseling

Many patients will have difficulty maintaining adequate nutrition during and after therapy, increasing the likelihood of consumption of cariogenic foods and beverages. While ensuring adequate nutrition is obviously of primary importance, awareness of the sugar and acid content of what is taken by mouth is necessary as well. Frequent consumption of sugary and/or acidic foods and beverages such as tea, coffee, carbonated beverages, juice, water with lemon or lime, energy drinks, sports drinks, nutritional supplements, and syrup-based medications all increase the risk of dental caries. Patients on a soft diet are more likely to consume high-carbohydrate foods that also have the potential to cause caries. When such foods are consumed, the patient should be advised to, at minimum, rinse the oral cavity with water, or ideally brush the teeth. Professional nutritionists or dieticians included on the care team can provide more specific recommendations. Xylitol products may be recommended as well.

45.2.7 Frequent Follow-up

Oral examinations are advised during radiation therapy if tolerated, 1 month post completion and every 3 to 4 months for at least the first year. Typically professional cleanings are also performed at this frequency. The recall schedule may be adjusted if the patient appears low risk for development of disease after the first year. Diagnostic imaging should be obtained, typically every 6 months for at least the first year. Otherwise, the posttreatment oral evaluation is similar to that outlined in Chapter 10, "Pretreatment Dental Evaluation."

45.2.8 Clinical Presentation

Dental caries related to cancer therapy tend to follow a rapidly progressive pattern, affecting atypical tooth surfaces. Lesions may appear as black or brown, associated with the cervical and incisal aspects of the teeth, as well as any exposed root structure. Patients may also present with generalized erosion of the occlusal aspect of the teeth, which can also appear desiccated and brittle. If untreated, rapid progression of lesions can occur, leading to pulpal involvement and/or crown amputation.[5]

45.2.9 Considerations for Treatment

Diagnosis and evaluation of radiation caries is relatively straightforward given patient history and clinical presentation. Dental imaging should be obtained in order to determine the extent of these lesions. Any lesion extending beyond the dentinoenamel junction requires restoration. Resin composite and amalgam have been shown to have increased longevity compared to glass ionomer materials.[8,15] The fluoride-releasing properties of glass ionomer may be beneficial as temporary restorations or in sites with compromised isolation, but tend to wear more quickly. Lesions extending into the pulp and periradicular sites should be treated endodontically. Dental extractions should be avoided if at all possible. Patients with a known history of radiation-associated caries require more frequent recall. The patient's overall oncologic prognosis and goals for treatment should be considered prior to any proposed treatment, especially in the case of persistent disease.

45.3 Gingivitis and Periodontitis

Hyposalivation, a shift toward pathogenic oral flora, decreased ability to maintain oral hygiene, and compromised bone quality secondary to radiation all place patients at greater risk of periodontal disease. Chemotherapy compromises immune response, decreasing the body's ability to control infection. The chronic inflammatory process characteristic of periodontitis is especially concerning in patients treated for cancer as it increases the risk of Osteoradionecrosis (ORN) and can exacerbate mucositis. Periodontitis is also associated with tooth loss, which can cause issues maintaining nutrition and increases the likelihood of dental extractions.[5]

45.3.1 Epidemiology

Periodontal disease is estimated to affect 47% of the adult population in the United States at any given time.[16] Patients with oral cancer tend to have worse oral health, and periodontal disease tends to worsen after cancer therapy. Furthermore, oral cavity cancer and periodontal disease share some of the same risk factors, such as tobacco use. Chemotherapy and radiation as well as decreased ability to maintain oral hygiene during and after treatment all favor a microbial shift favoring growth of organisms capable of causing periodontitis.[17,18] Additional studies quantifying the burden of periodontal disease in patients with head and neck cancer are required.

45.3.2 Considerations for Prevention

Routine oral hygiene is the best way to prevent and control periodontal disease. Preventive recommendations outlined in the section "Dental Caries" should be reviewed at all recall visits. Patients who have had documented periodontal disease prior to cancer therapy should be treated more aggressively, even if the disease process was addressed. Risk factors that place a patient at elevated risk of periodontitis should also be considered, such as poorly controlled diabetes, certain autoimmune diseases, and continued tobacco use. These higher-risk patients should be seen more frequently to establish patient-specific risk and address any issues at early stages. Cessation counseling can also be provided.

45.3.3 Clinical Presentation

Presentation is similar to that of patients without an oncologic history. Teeth may be mobile with bone loss apparent on routine imaging. Increased probing depths, sulcular purulence, and generalized erythema of the periodontal tissues are all signs of this disease process.

45.3.4 Considerations for Treatment

Conservative management, if at all possible, is favored in cases where periodontitis persists into the posttreatment period. Chlorhexidine oral rinse, except in the case of concurrent mucositis, diligent oral hygiene, antibiotics, scaling, and frequent recall are all advised. Consultation with the patient's radiation oncologist is recommended in cases where surgical intervention is indicated. See section "Osteoradionecrosis" below for additional details. Periodontitis that fails to respond to standard treatment should be further evaluated for possible malignancy.

45.4 Osteoradionecrosis

As described elsewhere in this text, ORN, although relatively uncommon, can be a painful and debilitating complication of cancer therapy. The goal of any posttreatment oral care plan is to avoid the need for any invasive dental procedures and eliminate infection and inflammation. ORN associated with dental trauma, including invasive procedures such as extractions, periodontal surgery, implant placement and some endodontic surgeries, appears to be highest at four years post radiation.[19] Ideally, any dental pathology requiring invasive treatment or resulting in chronic inflammation would have been addressed prior to cancer therapy with the posttreatment phase focused on prevention. In cases where treatment is indicated, the patient's radiation oncologist must be consulted prior to any invasive procedures.

45.4.1 Epidemiology

The estimated incidence of ORN ranges from 2 to 22% based on available data.[20,21] However, recent studies with larger sample sizes reflecting more modern radiation techniques estimate incidence from 2 to 7%.[19,21] Major local risk factors increasing the likelihood of ORN include, but are not limited to, an oral cavity primary site, conventional radiation as opposed to intensity-modulated radiation therapy, extraction of teeth after radiation exposure, and poor oral health, particularly periodontal disease.[19,21] Patient factors include continued use of tobacco and alcohol, poor overall health, increasing age, male sex, immune compromise, and exposure to bisphosphonates.[20–23] Available evidence does not suggest an increased risk with concurrent chemotherapy, however, there is an elevated risk when chemotherapy-associated conditions such as mucositis are present.[21] The association between an oral cavity primary site and ORN likely reflects the increased likelihood that the mandible, a site with higher risk of ORN in and of itself, will be compromised as a consequence of either resection and/or increased radiation dosage. ORN generally becomes a concern in sites receiving at least 50 Gy of radiation, but should be considered a risk in any patient with a history of radiation.[21,22]

45.4.2 Considerations for Prevention

Consultation with the treating radiation oncologist is imperative prior to any planned dental extractions or other invasive dental procedures. The radiation oncologist will typically provide a dose distribution map of the patient's head and neck, outlining the specific radiation dose to specific anatomic locations. While all patients with a history of head and neck cancer should be advised of the elevated risk of ORN, dose maps serve to better estimate the patient's individual risk by anatomic site. Specific treatment recommendations for management of ORN will be detailed elsewhere in this text. What follows is a brief outline of considerations to reduce the likelihood of development.

Dental Extractions

Extractions should be avoided if at all possible in sites exposed to therapeutic radiation. Carious lesions within close proximity to or including the pulp are recommended for endodontic therapy. In situations where extraction is absolutely necessary, removal should be performed as atraumatically as possible. Surrounding bone should be smoothed and any spicules or other potential sites of recurrent trauma should be addressed. There has been some discussion on the use of prophylactic measures such as antibiotics, pentoxifylline/tocopherol and steroids, but additional research is warranted.[21,24]

Hyperbaric Oxygen

Hyperbaric oxygen (HBO) is sometimes recommended prior to invasive dental procedures in patients exposed to therapeutic radiation to the head and neck. It is thought to stimulate circulation and oxygenation of compromised bone thereby decreasing the risk of ORN. That being said, substantial evidence either for or against the use of HBO does not appear to be present.[21] Access to HBO can be limited by geography, insurance coverage, or lack thereof and patient comorbidities. Generally speaking, HBO may be of benefit in a specific population of patients; the decision to recommend its use should come after a discussion of risks and benefits with radiation oncology and the treating provider.

Implant Placement

Previous radiation is not an absolute contraindication for placement but as with any type of treatment, the benefits must outweigh the risk. That being said, limited long-term data regarding implant placement in irradiated bone are available. Available data suggest a roughly similar rate of implant failure in irradiated versus nonirradiated native bone.[25–27] Similarly, available evidence does not seem to suggest a significantly increased risk of ORN in irradiated fibula flaps as compared to native mandible.[26,28] The ideal timing of implant placement is also unclear; it would appear as though earlier placement is best, given the possibility of longer-term improved nutrition and overall functional status. Additional long-term outcomes research with larger cohorts is needed to further guide treatment recommendations.

45.4.3 Clinical Presentation

The presentation of ORN is variable. Depending on grade, ORN can present as anything from a mucosalized site visible only on imaging to a suprainfected, painful area of exposed bone or pathologic fracture. Patients can complain that a prosthesis no longer fits or is painful. Surveillance for ORN should be especially diligent in patients with history of bisphosphonate or angiogenesis inhibitor use as well as those who are taking immunosuppressants. Further recommendations for diagnosis and management of ORN will be detailed elsewhere in this text.

45.5 Tumor Surveillance

Recall visits are an excellent opportunity for disease surveillance. Multiple risk factors may still be present in a patient treated for oral cancer. A head and neck exam should be completed at each visit to potentially identify new primary or recurrent lesions at early stages.

Monthly self-exams are encouraged with routine monitoring of the lips, buccal mucosa, palate, gingival tissue, and dorsal and ventral surfaces of the tongue for any abnormal lesions. Self-evaluation of the submandibular regions and the neck is recommended as well. Patients should be encouraged to become accustomed to what is normal so that any changes can be identified. It is also important to note that after treatment, patients may have a decreased sensory ability to detect pain or become aware of other abnormalities, making self-exams even more important.

Key Points

- Treatment of dental disease is more challenging after exposure to cancer therapeutics. Prevention is paramount.
- Consultation with the patient's radiation oncologist is imperative prior to any planned invasive procedures.
- Overall prognosis and treatment goals should be considered prior to any planned treatment.
- Lifelong follow-up with oral health provider experienced in the treatment of patients with a history of cancer is advised.

References

[1] Cooperstein E, Gilbert J, Epstein JB, et al. Vanderbilt Head and Neck Symptom Survey version 2.0: report of the development and initial testing of a subscale for assessment of oral health. Head Neck. 2012; 34(6):797–804

[2] Buglione M, Cavagnini R, Di Rosario F, et al. Oral toxicity management in head and neck cancer patients treated with chemotherapy and radiation: dental pathologies and osteoradionecrosis (Part 1) literature review and consensus statement. Crit Rev Oncol Hematol. 2016; 97:131–142

[3] Nagy KN, Sonkodi I, Szöke I, Nagy E, Newman HN. The microflora associated with human oral carcinomas. Oral Oncol. 1998; 34(4):304–308

[4] Pfister DG, Spencer S, Brizel DM, et al. National Comprehensive Cancer Network. Head and neck cancers, Version 2.2014. Clinical practice guidelines in oncology. J Natl Compr Canc Netw. 2014; 12(10):1454–1487

[5] Kielbassa AM, Hinkelbein W, Hellwig E, Meyer-Lückel H. Radiation-related damage to dentition. Lancet Oncol. 2006; 7(4):326–335

[6] Gupta N, Pal M, Rawat S, et al. Radiation-induced dental caries, prevention and treatment: a systematic review. Natl J Maxillofac Surg. 2015; 6(2):160–166

[7] Springer IN, Niehoff P, Warnke PH, et al. Radiation caries: radiogenic destruction of dental collagen. Oral Oncol. 2005; 41(7):723–728

[8] Hong CH, Napeñas JJ, Hodgson BD, et al. Dental Disease Section, Oral Care Study Group, Multi-national Association of Supportive Care in Cancer (MASCC)/International Society of Oral Oncology (ISOO). A systematic review of dental disease in patients undergoing cancer therapy. Support Care Cancer. 2010; 18(8):1007–1021

[9] National Cancer Institute, National Institutes of Health. Oral complications of chemotherapy and head/neck radiation (PDQ®). 2014. <http://www.cancer.gov.ezp.welch.jhmi.edu/cancertopics/pdq/supportivecare/oralcomplications/HealthProfessional/page1>. Accessed May 15th, 2018

[10] Deng J, Jackson L, Epstein JB, Migliorati CA, Murphy BA. Dental demineralization and caries in patients with head and neck cancer. Oral Oncol. 2015; 51(9):824–831

[11] Siala W, Mnejja W, Elloumi F, et al. Late toxicities after conventional radiotherapy for nasopharyngeal carcinoma: incidence and risk factors. J Radiother. 2014

[12] Farquhar DR, Divaris K, Mazul AL, Weissler MC, Zevallos JP, Olshan AF. Poor oral health affects survival in head and neck cancer. Oral Oncol. 2017; 73:111–117

[13] Meca LB, Souza FR, Tanimoto HM, Castro AL, Gaetti-Jardim Júnior E. Influence of preventive dental treatment on mutans streptococci counts in patients undergoing head and neck radiotherapy. J Appl Oral Sci. 2009; 17 Suppl:5–12

[14] Pattni R, Walsh LJ, Marshall RI, Cullinan MP, Seymour GJ, Bartold PM. Changes in the periodontal status of patients undergoing bone marrow transplantation. J Periodontol. 2000; 71(3):394–402

[15] De Moor RJ, Stassen IG, van 't Veldt Y, Torbeyns D, Hommez GM. Two-year clinical performance of glass ionomer and resin composite restorations in xerostomic head- and neck-irradiated cancer patients. Clin Oral Investig. 2011; 15(1):31–38

[16] Centers for Disease Control and Prevention. Periodontal disease. <https://www.cdc.gov/oralhealth/periodontal_disease/index.htm>. Accessed May 15th, 2018

[17] Epstein JB, Emerton S, Kolbinson DA, et al. Quality of life and oral function following radiotherapy for head and neck cancer. Head Neck. 1999; 21(1):1–11

[18] Sroussi HY, Epstein JB, Bensadoun RJ, et al. Common oral complications of head and neck cancer radiation therapy: mucositis, infections, saliva change,

fibrosis, sensory dysfunctions, dental caries, periodontal disease, and osteoradionecrosis. Cancer Med. 2017; 6(12):2918–2931

[19] Wang TH, Liu CJ, Chao TF, Chen TJ, Hu YW. Risk factors for and the role of dental extractions in osteoradionecrosis of the jaws: a national-based cohort study. Head Neck. 2017; 39(7):1313–1321

[20] Caparrotti F, Huang SH, Lu L, et al. Osteoradionecrosis of the mandible in patients with oropharyngeal carcinoma treated with intensity-modulated radiotherapy. Cancer. 2017; 123(19):3691–3700

[21] Raggio B, Winters R. Modern management of osteoradionecrosis. Cur Opin Otolaryngol Head Neck Surg. 2018; 26(4):254–259

[22] Owosho AA, Tsai CJ, Lee RS, et al. The prevalence and risk factors associated with osteoradionecrosis of the jaw in oral and oropharyngeal cancer patients treated with intensity-modulated radiation therapy (IMRT): The Memorial Sloan Kettering Cancer Center experience. Oral Oncol. 2017; 64:44–51

[23] Peterson DE, Doerr W, Hovan A, et al. Osteoradionecrosis in cancer patients: the evidence base for treatment-dependent frequency, current management strategies, and future studies. Support Care Cancer. 2010; 18(8):1089–1098

[24] Patel V, Gadiwalla Y, Sassoon I, Sproat C, Kwok J, McGurk M. Prophylactic use of pentoxifylline and tocopherol in patients who require dental extractions after radiotherapy for cancer of the head and neck. Br J Oral Maxillofac Surg. 2016; 54(5):547–550

[25] Colella G, Cannavale R, Pentenero M, Gandolfo S. Oral implants in radiated patients: a systematic review. Int J Oral Maxillofac Implants. 2007; 22(4):616–622

[26] Jackson RS, Price DL, Arce K, Moore EJ. Evaluation of clinical outcomes of osseointegrated dental implantation of fibula free flaps for m0andibular reconstruction. JAMA Facial Plast Surg. 2016; 18(3):201–206

[27] Watzinger F, Ewers R, Henninger A, Sudasch G, Babka A, Woelfl G. Endosteal implants in the irradiated lower jaw. J Craniomaxillofac Surg. 1996; 24(4): 237–244

[28] Salinas TJ, Desa VP, Katsnelson A, Miloro M. Clinical evaluation of implants in radiated fibula flaps. J Oral Maxillofac Surg. 2010; 68(3):524–529

46 Oral and Dental Complications of Oral Cancer Treatment

Arij Kazmi, Amy Cao, and Lauren Levi

Summary
Oral cancer therapy may result in acute and chronic oral/dental consequences which include (but are not limited to) mucositis, hyposalivation/xerostomia, oral infections, neurotoxicity/neuropathy, orofacial pain, taste/smell disorders, and osteoradionecrosis of the jaw. This chapter will discuss in depth on the epidemiology, clinical presentation, diagnosis and evaluation of each dental related complications post oral cancer therapy, as well as treatment considerations to improve patients' quality of life. A collaborative interdisciplinary team is necessary to prepare appropriate treatment plans for patients before the commencement of oncologic therapy.

Keywords: dental oncology, dental care for oral cancer therapy, oral cancer, chemotherapy, head and neck radiation

46.1 Introduction

Oral cancer therapeutic regimens may result in acute and chronic oral and dental sequelae, which indubitably affect a cancer survivor's quality of life. These manifestations may include, but are not limited to, mucositis, hyposalivation and/or xerostomia, osteoradionecrosis (ORN) of the jaw, chemotherapy-induced neuropathy, dysphagia, dysgeusia, an increased risk for developing dental decay, trismus, orofacial pain, mucosal lesions, radiation fibrosis syndrome, and oral infections.[1–60] It is, hence, essential that the patient's oncology team be knowledgeable in the evaluation and management of the oral and dental manifestations associated with head and neck oncologic therapy.

Prior to commencement of therapy, a patient diagnosed with oral cancer should be evaluated by a dental oncologist to help reduce the patient's risk for developing head and neck manifestations associated with his/her proposed oncologic treatment. In addition, clinicians should discuss the patient's proposed cancer treatment with the patient's oncology team and have a detailed discussion with the patient about oral hygiene instruction, the oral and dental sequelae of his/her proposed therapy, and methods to help reduce the patient's risk for developing the associated manifestations. This chapter focuses on the epidemiology, clinical presentation, diagnosis and evaluation of the dental complications of oral cancer therapy as well as treatment considerations and approaches.

46.2 Oral Mucositis

46.2.1 Epidemiology

Oral mucositis is one of the most common complications of head and neck cancer therapy and often reported by patients as the single most debilitating complication of treatment.[24] Sonis et al (2003) reports that chemotherapy and/or radiation therapy (RT) may induce mucosal injury both by direct damage to epithelial cells lining the oral mucosa and also by upregulating an inflammatory response resulting in oral mucositis.[19]

While risk factors may dictate the severity, almost all patients treated with RT for head and neck cancer are expected to develop some degree of oral mucositis.[6,25] Severe oral mucositis has been reported in 29 to 66% of all patients receiving head and neck RT. Increased incidence of mucositis is noted in patients with a primary tumor in the oral cavity, oropharynx, or nasopharynx, those receiving adjunctive chemotherapy, those receiving RT doses ≥ 5,000 cGy, and those receiving altered fractionation RT. Oral mucositis has been reported to occur in approximately 20 to 40% of patients receiving conventional chemotherapy and 80% of patients receiving high-dose chemotherapy.[6,7,25]

46.2.2 Clinical Presentation

Oral mucositis presents as erythematous and ulcerative lesions affecting the oral mucosa.[1,19,25] Signs and symptoms of oral mucositis often vary throughout the progression of head and neck cancer therapy. At the beginning of head and neck RT, cumulative doses as low as 10 Gy may lead to mucosal erythema and superficial tissue sloughing. Patients may complain of discomfort and pain that is similar to a food or chemical burn, although the mucosa at this stage remains intact. As the cumulative doses increase to 20–30 Gy, the mucosa begins to break down resulting in ulcerative mucositis. At this stage, patients may report severe pain and ulcerative lesions present with uneven borders and a pseudomembrane covering, often consisting of bacterial infiltrates and necrotic tissue (▶ Fig. 46.1).

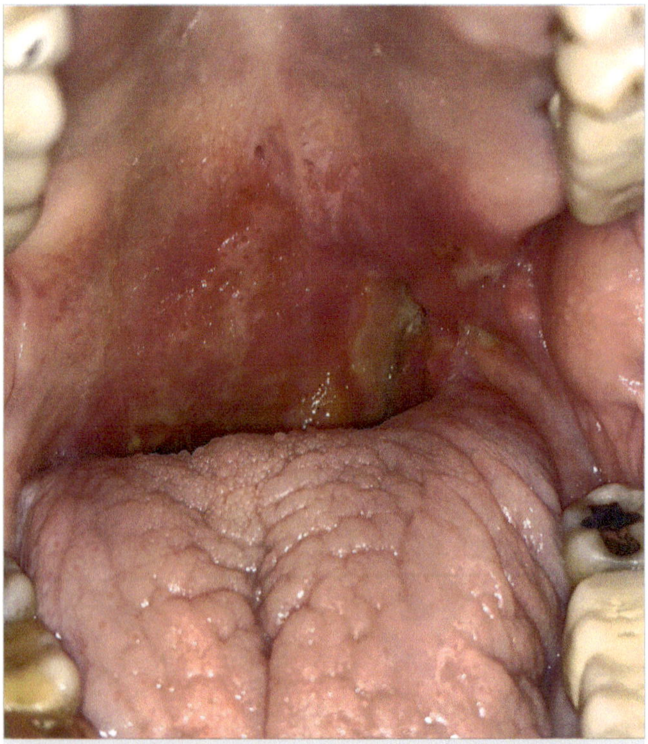

Fig. 46.1 Oral mucositis of the oropharynx in a patient receiving chemoradiation.

This stage of severe pain may persist throughout RT and up to 3 weeks post RT.

Chemotherapy-induced ulcerative mucositis presents at earlier stages of therapy following a more acute course. The initial mucosal changes often present within 5 days of chemotherapy drug infusion and progress to the severely painful ulcerative colitis stage by day seven of therapy. The lesions may persist for 7 to 10 days and commonly heal by 3 weeks post initiation.[25]

46.2.3 Diagnosis and Evaluation

Multiple grading systems attempt to categorize the sequential clinical presentations of oral mucositis (▶ Table 46.1). The World Health Organization (WHO) grading system is based on the clinical presentation and patients' functional status. Other grading systems consider the pathological changes in mucosal tissue.[25,36]

46.2.4 Anatomic Considerations and Approaches

RT and chemotherapy may lead to mucosal injuries that manifest in different locations. RT-induced mucositis is localized to the field of high-dose RT, while chemotherapy-induced mucositis may affect the entire gastrointestinal tract.[1,5,36] Though mucositis may affect the entire oral cavity, it commonly affects the movable mucosa (buccal mucosa, lingual mucosa, floor of the mouth, and soft palate) but rarely presents on keratinized tissue (hard palate, dorsal tongue, and gingiva).[1,25]

46.2.5 Treatment Considerations and Approaches

The Multinational Association of Supportive Care in Cancer (MASCC) recommendations are made only if strong evidence supports effectiveness in the respective treatment settings (▶ Table 46.2). Interventions that are supported with weaker evidence are also listed as suggestions in the detailed review published by MASCC and the Cochrane Group but not included in this chapter.[5,6]

Table 46.1 Classification systems of oral mucositis

World Health Organization (WHO) grading for oral mucositis		National Cancer Institute (NCI) Common Terminology Criteria for Adverse Events (CTCAE) version 3.0	
Grade 0	No oral mucositis	Grade 1	Mucosal erythema
Grade 1	Erythema, oral soreness	Grade 2	Patchy ulcerations or pseudomembranes
Grade 2	Oral erythema, ulcers, solid diet tolerated	Grade 3	Confluent ulcerations or pseudomembranes; bleeding with minor trauma
Grade 3	Oral ulcers, liquid diet only	Grade 4	Tissue necrosis; spontaneous bleeding
Grade 4	Oral ulcers, oral alimentation impossible	Grade 5	Death

46.3 Hyposalivation/Xerostomia

Saliva serves many critical functions that assist in maintaining equilibrium in the oral cavity including playing a vital role in digestion, mastication, deglutition, gustatory sensation, and host defense.[1–4,37,43] Head and neck RT in cumulative doses greater than 25 to 30 Gy may result in salivary tissue damage and temporary or permanent salivary gland dysfunction.[1,37–39,41,43]

46.3.1 Epidemiology

Xerostomia, the subjective sensation of dry mouth, during head and neck RT has a reported prevalence of 93%, which contrasts with the reported prevalence of 6.0% prior to the commencement of RT.[37] Xerostomia is one of the most common late toxicities reported by head and neck cancer patients.

46.3.2 Clinical Presentation

Patients with decreased salivary flow often complain of xerostomia. In addition, they may present with ropey, thick saliva or complain of increased thirst. Reduced salivary flow increases the a patient's risk for developing dental demineralization, dental decay, oral infections, dysgeusia, dysphagia, dysarthria, halitosis, oral soreness and burning, and inability to wear dentures.[1–4,38,39,41,43] The varying symptoms of hyposalivation and/or xerostomia contribute to a reduced quality of life which may affect an individual's psychological and physical health.[1–4,38]

46.3.3 Diagnosis and Evaluation

Damaged salivary glands may lead to altered saliva production resulting in hyposalivation, traditionally defined as resting

Table 46.2 Multinational Association of Supportive Care in Cancer recommendations for management of oral mucositis

Prevention of oral mucositis in patients receiving	**Radiation therapy**	• Benzydamine hydrochloride, nonsteroidal anti-inflammatory agent, *recommended* as mouth rinse for patients with head and neck disease receiving moderate-dose radiation (< 50 Gy) • Antimicrobial lozenges or PTA paste *not recommended* • Iseganan antimicrobial mouthwash *not recommended* • Sucralfate (mucosal coating agent) mouthwash *not recommended*
	Chemotherapy	• Oral cryotherapy, placing ice chips in mouth during chemotherapy delivery, *recommended* in patients receiving bolus dosing of 5-fluorouracil • Sucralfate mouthwash *not recommended*
Treatment of oral mucositis in patients receiving standard-dose chemotherapy		• Chlorhexidine *not recommended*

saliva flow rate of < 0.1 ml/minute and/or stimulated saliva flow rate of < 0.5 ml/minute.[20,21,43] While xerostomia is the subjective measure of dry mouth, hyposalivation serves as an objective measure for assessing salivary flow.[40,43] Xerostomia may be assessed by both patient self-reporting instruments and practitioner-observer assessments; however, patient self-reported assessments are often considered more reliable.[40] Hyposalivation does not always correlate with the subjective symptoms of xerostomia.

46.3.4 Anatomic Considerations and Approaches

The major salivary glands (parotid, submandibular, and sublingual) are commonly included or in close proximity to target radiation fields. Parotid glands are most often irradiated in conventional RT due to their anatomical location.[7,39] In addition, serous glands are often more radiosensitive than mucus glands.[1,2]

46.3.5 Treatment Considerations and Approaches

Reversibility of reduced salivary flow is dose-limited and depends on the field of radiation. Oral health education, prevention, and care are important in maintaining a healthy dentition and preventing further dental complications in oral cancer patients. At the treatment planning stage, patients should be educated on the risks of hyposalivation and loss of protective mechanisms of saliva. Patients should be evaluated by a dentist for dental decay and infections and treated prior to RT. Further dental preventative measures include fluoride-containing mouth rinses, fluoride gels and toothpastes, over-the-counter salivary gland stimulants, sialogogues, and in some cases parasympathomimetics.[38,41–43] Pilocarpine hydrochloride, a parasympathomimetic, has been reported as an effective treatment for radiation-induced xerostomia; however, it may be associated with various side effects due to the parasympathetic stimulation.[38,41,42]

Surgical Options and Approaches

Salivary gland transfer is a surgical procedure that may prevent RT-induced xerostomia and maintain salivary flow rates after RT. Salivary glands that are within the radiation field are surgically transferred to another anatomical space and shielded. For example, submandibular glands may be transferred to the submental space before beginning RT and shielded. The procedure has been reported as highly effective in preventing the incidence of xerostomia in patients receiving RT to treat head and neck cancers. It has also been reported to improve quality of life in these patients.[22,23,39,41]

46.4 Oral Infections

46.4.1 Epidemiology

Oral Candidiasis

Oral candidiasis is extremely common in patients undergoing cancer therapy; however, reports on the incidence, prevalence, and epidemiology are limited.[1,3,4,9,10] A systematic review from 2010 reported that 50% of head and neck cancer patients presented with oral fungal colonization prior to the commencement of RT.[9,10] During RT, 74.5% of the patients presented with oral fungal colonization which remained constant immediately following the completion of RT.[9,10] Of the 74.5% of patients with colonized oral fungi, 37.4% of the patients presented with an oral fungal infection during treatment. After RT, 32.6% presented with oral fungal infection.[9,10] Oral candidiasis may present with pain, dysgeusia, malnutrition, anorexia, and dysphagia.[1,2,4] Patients that are undergoing immunosuppressive therapy, such as chemotherapy, are at an increased risk for the progression of oral candidiasis to oropharyngeal candidiasis and systemic fungemia which can be fatal.[9,10]

Oral Viral Infections

Herpes simplex viral (HSV) recurrence has not been reported in patients after receiving head and neck RT.[1,11,15,16] However, Elad et al (2012) reported that the prevalence of HSV infection is 43.2% in patients treated with chemoradiation.[16]

46.4.2 Clinical Presentation

Bacterial Infections

Bacterial infections in the oral cavity may present as necrotizing ulcerative gingivitis, periodontal infections, odontogenic infections, deep space infections, sialadenitis, or infections secondary to oral mucositis.[3,4,16,17] Oral ulcerations associated with mucositis may provide a nidus for bacterial proliferation and growth.[1,4,14]

Fungal Infections

The most common fungal infections affecting the oral cancer patients may be attributed to oral candidiasis with 90% of candidal infections being associated with *Candida albicans*; nonetheless, other candidal strains have been identified in oral candidiasis including fluconazole-resistant candidal strains.[1,4,9,10] Oral fungal infections may also be attributed to other fungi; yet, these infections are less common than oral candidiasis.[1,4,13] Oral candidiasis may present in various forms including, but not limited to pseudomembranous candidiasis, erythematous candidiasis, mucocutaneous candidiasis, chronic multifocal candidiasis, and angular cheilitis. Erythematous and pseudomembranous candidiasis are most common forms that present in the oncology patient population.[9] Oral candidiasis presentation ranges from intraoral adherent white plaques that may be removed with a gauze to intraoral red lesions in which the tongue may appear red and devoid of filiform papillae. Candidiasis may also present at the commissures of the lips as red, fissured lesions that may be painful.[3,4,13] Occasionally, angular cheilitis may be due to the presence of both *Staphylococcus aureus* and a *Candida* infection, and thus should be treated with both an antibiotic and antifungal ointment.[4]

Viral Infections

Recurrent HSV infections in immunocompromised patients present differently than those in immunocompetent patients.

HSV infections in immunocompromised patients, such as patients undergoing chemotherapy, may present on keratinized and nonkeratinized mucosa which contrasts with typical HSV infections which only affect keratinized mucosa. Moreover, HSV infections in immunocompromised patients may persist longer than 10 to 14 days.[1]

46.4.3 Diagnosis and Evaluation

Bacterial Infections

Culturing oral infection is crucial to diagnosis, evaluation, and management.[3,4] Given the risk of developing a systemic infection in patients undergoing chemotherapy, the oncology team should follow these patients closely for any signs or symptoms of a microbial infection and treat these infections aggressively.[3]

Fungal Infections

Fungal infections are often diagnosed by both clinical appearance and microbial culturing.[2,4,10] Often lesions are diagnosed by clinical presentation alone and response to antifungal medication; however, culture is indicated for lesions that present atypically or resistant to antifungal medications. Lesions that do not respond to antifungal therapy but are suggestive of chronic hyperplastic candidiasis may require biopsy for a definitive diagnosis.[4,13]

Viral Infections

Although often HSV infections may be diagnosed by clinical presentation; atypical presentation may warrant a laboratory culture.[2]

46.4.4 Treatment Considerations and Approaches

Bacterial Infections

Bacterial infections should be treated with broad-spectrum antibiotics. In addition, oral hygiene instruction should be emphasized and reviewed with the patient in order to help eliminate the patient's risk for developing odontogenic infections, periodontal infections, or bacterial infections secondary to mucositis.

Fungal Infections

Antifungal agents are the mainstay of treatment for treating fungal infections with topical medications prescribed as first-line therapy.[1,4] Patients should be encouraged to maintain topical contact time for as long as possible with the mucosa. Patients who do not respond to topical antifungal medication are often prescribed a systemic medication.[4,10] If patients present with a removable dental appliance, they should be prescribed an antifungal suspension to treat the appliance as well.

Viral Infections

HSV infections may be managed with systemic antiviral medications and lesions should be evaluated and followed for resolution. In addition, lesions should be monitored for bacterial or fungal coinfection.

46.5 Neurotoxicity/Neuropathy

46.5.1 Epidemiology

Neuropathic pain affects up to 25 to 40% of cancer patients, and it may result from tumor invasion or cancer treatments.[26,27] Neuropathic pain is associated with increased pain intensity, increased analgesic consumption, decreased quality of life, and negative impacts on sleep and mood.[1,27–29] The most common cause of cancer-induced neuropathy is secondary to tumor neural compression; however, neuropathic pain may also result from oncologic therapy including surgical resection and chemotherapy.[26,30] Chemotherapeutic agents associated with neuropathic pain include vinca alkaloids, taxanes, platinum-derived compounds, suramin, thalidomide, and most recently bortezomib therapy.[26,30]

46.5.2 Clinical Presentation

Cancer-related neuropathic pain is often chronic and commonly presents with pain ranging from dull to sharp in intensity.[29] The pain may be spontaneous and intermittent, and patients may complain of paresthesia and dysesthesia. Touch-evoked allodynia commonly presents, but patients may also complain of thermal-induced allodynia and hyperalgesia.[29]

Chemotherapy-induced peripheral neuropathy is usually a dose-dependent, cumulative side effect with a peripheral distribution.[29] Symptoms include sensory loss, paresthesia, dysesthesia, and pain with muscle weakness. Oxaliplatin-induced neuropathy may result in acute allodynia and pricking dysesthesia affecting the hands and feet, and occasionally, pharyngolaryngeal dysesthesia with sensations of shortness of breath or swallowing difficulties induced by cold drinks.[29,36]

46.5.3 Diagnosis and Evaluation

Diagnosis for neuropathic pain is based on a thorough history and physical examination. Evaluation of a suspected neuropathic condition should include an assessment of pain location, quality, intensity and temporal variation, functional impact on mood, sleep, and other activities of daily living.[27–29]. "Tingling," "burning," and "shooting" are common sensory quality descriptors for neuropathic pain.

Various screening tools for neuropathic pain have been recommended by Neuropathic Pain Special Interest Group of the International Association for the Study of Pain (IASP).[27,31–34] These tools are for screening only and aid in discriminating between neuropathic from nociceptive pain.

46.5.4 Treatment Considerations and Approaches

Pharmacological treatments usually have limited response rates with partial reduction in pain. Treatment for neuropathic pain depends on severity of symptoms, and treatment is aimed at symptom relief. Cancer-related neuropathic pain is often treated with opioids, with more than a 70% response rate.[26]

However, due to nerve sensitization, neuronal suppression with opioids or nonsteroidal anti-inflammatory drugs alone is often insufficient, and thus adjunctive medications are often used. Adjunctive drugs include anticonvulsants, antidepressants, corticosteroids and anesthetics, as well as nutritional supplements such as alpha-lipoic acid, vitamin E, erythropoietin, and acetyl-L-carnitine.[26,29,30] Some evidence for the use of nonpharmacological management strategies (e.g., massage, acupuncture, fitness, and mind-body techniques) to enhance management of neuropathic pain associated with cancer has been found.[35]

46.6 Orofacial Pain

46.6.1 Epidemiology

Orofacial pain is a common prediagnostic complaint in cancer patients that often leads to a cancer diagnosis.[1,26,29] Pain has been reported in 50 to 85% of patients prior to treatment, 81% during chemotherapy or RT, and 70% at the end of the treatment.[1,45–47] Epstein et al (2010) reported that 36% of patients still complained of pain 6 months after therapy, while 33% complained of increased pain after therapy.[47]

Orofacial pain may be attributed to the malignancy or cancer-related therapy. The most common etiology is local tumor invasion through inflammatory and neuropathic mechanisms.[1,26,45,46,48] The severity of pain depends on the size of the mass, presence of pressure, ulceration or inflammation, and stage of invasion. Pain complaints are usually nonspecific, such as a sore throat, pain on swallowing, and pain in the region of tongue, mouth, teeth, and ears.[45,46,48]

Approximately 90% of oral cancers are squamous cell carcinomas (SCC).[48] In oral SCC, pain is observed in 39 to 85% of cases.[46–48] Lymphoma, the second most common neoplasm in the oral region accounting for 3.5% oral malignancies, may induce pain through the periosteum and gingiva.[46] Multiple myeloma also frequently presents with dental pain. Intracranial tumors associated with facial pain have been found to have incidence of 0.8 to 5.9%.[45] Although metastatic neoplasms to the oral cavity only account for 1 to 3% of all oral cancers, pain in metastatic disease to the jaw is reported in 39% and paresthesia in 23% of patients.[47–49]

Pain secondary to cancer therapy depends on treatment modalities.[1,26,45–48] Surgical procedures may lead to myofascial and neuropathic pain syndromes due to local nerve and tissue damage. Resective procedures may result in sensory impairment with 50% experiencing regional hyperalgesia or allodynia.[45,46] Rogers et al (2003) indicated that 88 to 90% patients reported persistent pain at 2 to 5 years post maxillectomy.[45,46] The prevalence of trismus is not well documented with a reported range of 0 to 69%.[2,4,8,52] The wide range may be attributed to the discrepancies in measuring trismus, tumor size, cancer treatment, and the location of the tumor.[2,4,8,52]

46.6.2 Clinical Presentation

Oral SCC may or may not present as a painful lesion. Also, patients with osteosarcoma of the jaws may complain of pain and trigeminal sensory disturbances.[45] Nasopharyngeal cancer is sometimes associated with temporomandibular joint disorder (TMD) signs and symptoms, including headache, earache, and jaw, midface, or neck pain.[45] Intracranial tumors may be associated with trigeminal neuralgia-like symptoms, including burning, dull aching, pressure, or swelling sensations.[45]

Musculoskeletal syndromes, such as TMD associated with muscular fibrosis, scar formation, and trismus, commonly occur after tumor resection. Tissue defects may lead to loss of orofacial function affecting speech, chewing, and swallowing.[1,26,45] In addition, head and neck RT may result in radiation fibrosis syndrome which presents as trismus, fibrotic muscles, cervical dystonia, lymphedema, dysphagia, and orofacial pain impairing a patient's ability to maintain oral hygiene and speak.[2,4]

Dental pain is also common in these patients. Stress and anxiety may cause clenching or bruxism, leading to heavy occlusal stress and discomfort.

46.6.3 Diagnosis and Evaluation

Diagnosing orofacial pain is based on history, clinical examination, and identification of the source of pain. Rating scale techniques are used to assess pain intensity, and appropriate imaging should be used to rule out a suspected pathology.[50] Before undertaking a definitive therapy, clinical diagnosis may also be established through diagnostic analgesic blocking (muscle injections, nerve block injections, intracapsular injections) to differentiate masticatory pain from nonmasticatory myofascial pain.[50] Consultations with other disciplines (medicine, otolaryngology, orthopedics, neurology, rheumatology, or psychology consultation) should be considered for proper identification of the pain disorders. A short period of trial therapy may also aid to confirm the diagnosis.[50]

46.6.4 Treatment Considerations and Approaches

Orofacial pain significantly affects quality of life of cancer patients. Treatment is essential and should be considered through not only palliative care, but also through education and prevention. Basic oral care is essential for prevention and maintenance of oral health.

For patients at risk for developing trismus or radiation fibrosis syndrome, exercises aimed at maintaining vertical dimension of opening may aid in treatment.[8,52] Topical agents may be used for symptomatic relief and may include bland rinses, ice, coating agents, local anesthetics/antihistamine, and topical analgesics.[1,45] A nonpharmacologic approach for pain relief is the use of laser treatments, which may reduce or prevent oral pain.[45] Appropriate referrals to speech pathologists and physical therapists are often indicated.

Opioid analgesics are often prescribed to treat cancer-related facial pain. Systemic medications for pain management can follow the guidelines recommended by WHO Pain Management Ladder (▶ Table 46.3).[1,45,51] Pain management is guided by the severity of pain at the time of presentation, and should be prescribed only as needed. Adjunctive medications include selective serotonin reuptake inhibitors, antihistamines, benzodiazepines, muscle relaxants, antiseizure medications, physiotherapy, cognitive therapy, and acupuncture.[1,45]

Table 46.3 The World Health Organization Pain Management Ladder

Step 1: mild pain Nonopioid with/without adjuvants	Acetaminophen, NSAIDs
Step 2: moderate pain Weak opioid with/without nonopioid/adjuvants	Codeine, hydrocodone, tramadol
Step 3: moderate to severe pain Strong opioid with/without nonopioid/adjuvants	Morphine, oxycodone, hydromorphone, fentanyl, methadone

Modification of the WHO analgesic ladder has been recommended to move from Step 1 to the lowest effective dose of the strong opioids (Step 3), avoiding the weak opioids (Step 2).

46.7 Taste/Smell Disorders

46.7.1 Epidemiology

The prevalence of altered taste and smell perception ranges from 60 to 100% among cancer patients.[1,53,54] Common causes of dysgeusia include oral infection, poor oral hygiene, surgical interventions, medications, and radiation damage to taste buds and salivary glands.[1] Altered taste is reported to be proportional to the cumulative RT dose to the parotid gland.[55] Generally, taste loss is not apparent until a dose of 20 Gy; while at 60 Gy, a relative loss of taste has been reported in 90% of patients.[55] The sense of taste is not only affected by RT but by chemotherapy (platinum-based chemotherapy, cyclophosphamide, doxorubicin, 5-FU and methotrexate) as well.[1,53] RT and chemotherapy-induced xerostomia may also lead to dysgeusia. Chemotherapy may damage olfactory basal cells that may cause patients to become sensitive to odors leading to food aversions and anorexia.[53,54,56]

46.7.2 Clinical Presentation

Patients often report chemosensory changes such as dysgeusia, xerostomia, ageusia, decreased sensitivity to sweet/bitter/salt/sour tastes, and hyperosmia.[53,5454,56] Changes in gustation may also correlate with positive culture of candida in cancer patients, with incidence rate as high of 78%.[56]

46.7.3 Diagnosis and Evaluation

Dysgeusia may be measured and assessed clinically by the recognition threshold values for five basic tastes: sweetness, bitterness, sourness, saltiness, and umami. Tools for quantification include application of filter paper taste strips containing various concentrations of a basic taste or using an electrogustometer for measurement.[55] Olfactory function may be tested with Sniffin' Sticks test® and odors in bottles.[55] Qualitative changes may be reported through patient complaints, interviews, and clinical observations.[1,53–56]

46.7.4 Treatment Considerations and Approaches

Zinc supplementation and acupuncture have been used in management for taste alteration. However, according to a recent systematic review, very low-quality evidence were found to support the use of zinc supplement or acupuncture in comparison to placebo for improvement on taste acuity.[57] Fortunately, chemosensory changes are usually temporary, as new taste and smell receptors are regenerated within 10 to 30 days.[1,53–56] However, it is important to manage taste and smell dysfunctions during RT and chemotherapy to monitor adequate food intake and quality of life of patients. Treatment should focus on patients' subjective sensations and perceived alterations in their chemosensory functions, rather than the objective psychophysical test measurements. Attention should also be placed on the possible causes for taste or smell disturbances, such as a possible candida infection of medication side effect. Caretakers should be sensitive to the increased smell sensations in patients with hyperosmia, as food odors could provoke food aversions and cause nausea.

46.8 Osteoradionecrosis of the Jaw

A late complication of RT, ORN of the jaw presents as an area of exposed bone that fails to heal after receiving high-dose RT.[1–4] Risk factors for ORN include a cumulative radiation dose greater than 60 Gy, trauma and surgery, alcohol abuse, tobacco abuse, and poor oral hygiene. Increased radiation dose greater than 60 Gy presents the highest risk.[60]

46.8.1 Epidemiology

The exact incidence of ORN is unknown, which may be due to the large variation in the clinical parameters used to define ORN. Approximately 5% of patients are affected by ORN.[1] Incidence in the mandible ranges from 2 to 22% and it most commonly affects the body of the mandible.[58,60]

46.8.2 Clinical Presentation

ORN presents as a nonhealing area of exposed bone within an area treated with RT. It often presents after the completion of RT either spontaneously or following invasive dental procedures such as, tooth extractions. Growth of lesions is accelerated in the presence of poor nutrition and poor oral hygiene and may present with secondary infections. Those involving cortical bone may further progress to pathologic fractures and/or formation of sequestra, and/or development of an oroantral or oral-extraoral fistula. While ORN is a rare complication, its clinical presentation may present with severe pain and negatively affect functional prognosis and compromise quality of life.[1–4]

46.8.3 Diagnosis and Evaluation

ORN may present both clinically and radiographically. Clinically, ORN often manifests as mucous membrane ulcers, exposed sequestra, fistulas, paresthesia, or pain (▶ Fig. 46.2). Diagnosis is often made based on clinical presentation and patient's history. Radiographically, ORN may present as decreased bone density, cortical fractures, and/or focal lytic areas[1–4] (▶ Fig. 46.3).

Multiple staging systems for ORN exist in the literature. The varying staging systems are adapted from either the treatments indicated, response to treatment, or according to lesion size

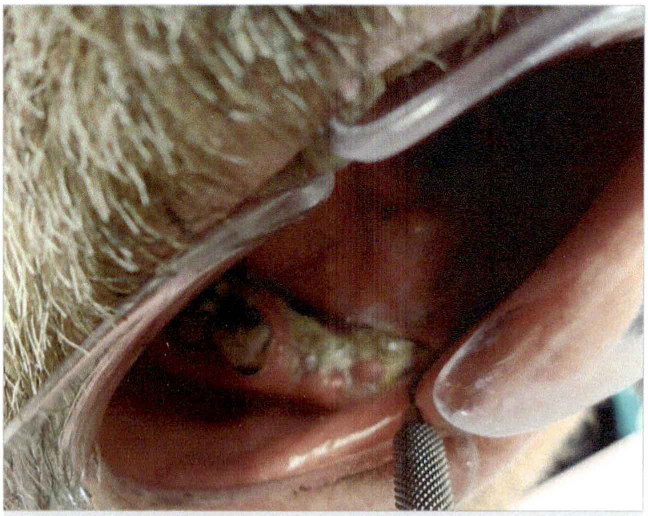

Fig. 46.2 Osteoradionecrosis of the mandible just right of the midline. Note the exposed bone on the alveolar ridge.

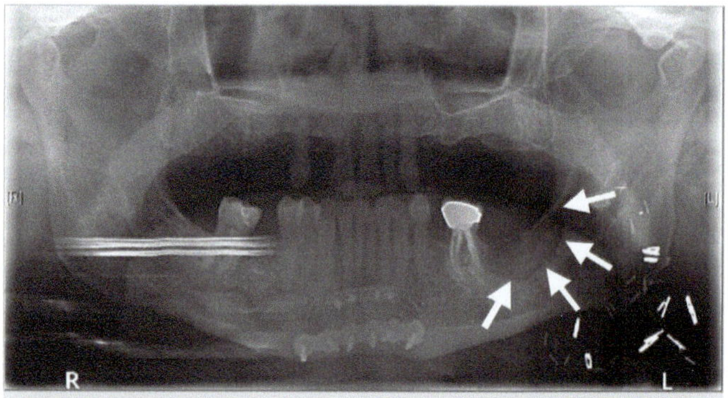

Fig. 46.3 Osteoradionecrosis visualized radiographically on the left side of the mandible. Note the radiolucent lesion on the left mandible infiltrating the inferior alveolar nerve canal.

Table 46.4 Classification of ORN by Notani et al.[60]

I	ORN confined to dentoalveolar bone
II	ORN limited to dentoalveolar bone and/or mandible above the IAN canal
III	ORN involving mandible below the IAN canal, or pathologic fracture, or skin fistula

Abbreviation: IAN, inferior alveolar nerve; ORN, osteoradionecrosis.

and/or symptoms.[59,60] One of the simpler classification systems by Notani et al may be applied to all cases of mandibular ORN (▶ Table 46.4).[60]

46.8.4 Anatomic Considerations and Approaches

ORN presents more commonly in the mandible than in the maxilla and is believed to be due to reduced blood supply. The prognosis of ORN may vary depending on the specific tissues affected. Lesions that are surrounded by keratinized tissue have been reported to have a better prognosis. In addition, lesions that involve the cortical bone present with a greater risk of sequelae including fractures, sequestra formation, and/or fistulas.[1–4]

46.8.5 Treatment Considerations and Approaches

Management of ORN begins with prevention. In the context of RT, a pretreatment comprehensive dental evaluation is extremely important. At this time, a dentist should identify and improve and/or eliminate any risk factors. Patients should be educated on optimal oral hygiene and nutrition. Dental caries and odontogenic sources of infection should either be treated with dental restorations or eliminated by tooth extractions.[1–4] Pretreatment dental care varies with patient motivation and time restrictions limited by the start of RT. All teeth with a questionable prognosis should be extracted, as atraumatically as possible, before beginning RT. Dentists should plan for enough healing time before beginning RT. The suggested healing interval ranges from 10 to 14 days post extraction. However, to reduce the risk a 14 to 21 day healing interval between tooth extraction and initiation of RT is recommended.[4]

Hyperbaric oxygen therapy (HBOT) as an adjunct to surgical interventions is sometimes utilized; however, its efficacy is controversial and questionable. HBOT is associated with adverse effects such as, damage to the ears, sinuses and lungs, increased myopia, claustrophobia, and oxygen poisoning that present controversy.[1,4,59]

Combined pentoxifylline–tocopherol therapy is a recent alternative to existing therapies in treating ORN. Reports suggest that the combined therapy may reduce chronic progressive septic ORN of the mandible.[59] The two drugs may act synergistically as antifibrotic agents.[58]

46.8.6 Surgical Options and Approaches

Early-onset ORN is managed conservatively using systemic antibiotic treatment with limited curettage, debridement, and/or sequestrectomy under local anesthesia. The aim is to remove all devitalized tissue. Advanced or refractive ORN may require more extensive surgical removal of such tissue by extensive sequestrectomy with an additional marginal or complete resection of affected mandibular bone. Such extensive surgical approaches often require a soft-tissue reconstruction to repair the defect.[1,4,58,60]

Key Points

- Clinicians should be aware of the oral and dental sequelae associated with oral cancer therapy and should prepare appropriate treatment plans for patients before the commencement of oncologic therapy.
- Treatment of patients prior to the commencement of therapy may help reduce a patient's risk for developing oral and dental manifestations associated with chemotherapy and head and neck RT.
- Treating cancer is multidisciplinary and requires a collaborative interdisciplinary team.

References

[1] Epstein JB, Thariat J, Bensadoun RJ, et al. Oral complications of cancer and cancer therapy: from cancer treatment to survivorship. CA Cancer J Clin. 2012; 62(6):400–422

[2] Levi LE, Lalla RV. Dental treatment planning for the patient with oral cancer. Dent Clin North Am. 2018; 62(1):121–130

[3] Harrison LB, Sessions RB, Kies MS. Head and Neck Cancer: A Multidisciplinary Approach. Philadelphia: Wolters Kluwer/Lippincott-Raven; 2014

[4] Davies A, Epstein J. Oral Complications of Cancer and its Management. Oxford: Oxford University Press; 2010

[5] Keefe DM, Schubert MM, Elting LS, et al. Mucositis Study Section of the Multinational Association of Supportive Care in Cancer and the International Society for Oral Oncology. Updated clinical practice guidelines for the prevention and treatment of mucositis. Cancer. 2007; 109(5):820–831

[6] Lalla RV, Bowen J, Barasch A, et al. Mucositis Guidelines Leadership Group of the Multinational Association of Supportive Care in Cancer and International Society of Oral Oncology (MASCC/ISOO). MASCC/ISOO clinical practice guidelines for the management of mucositis secondary to cancer therapy. Cancer. 2014; 120(10):1453–1461

[7] Trotti A, Bellm LA, Epstein JB, et al. Mucositis incidence, severity and associated outcomes in patients with head and neck cancer receiving radiotherapy with or without chemotherapy: a systematic literature review. Radiother Oncol. 2003; 66(3):253–262

[8] Dijkstra PU, Kalk WW, Roodenburg JL. Trismus in head and neck oncology: a systematic review. Oral Oncol. 2004; 40(9):879–889

[9] Lalla RV, Latortue MC, Hong CH, et al. Fungal Infections Section, Oral Care Study Group, Multinational Association of Supportive Care in Cancer (MASCC)/International Society of Oral Oncology (ISOO). A systematic review of oral fungal infections in patients receiving cancer therapy. Support Care Cancer. 2010; 18(8):985–992

[10] Bensadoun R-J, Patton LL, Lalla RV, Epstein JB. Oropharyngeal candidiasis in head and neck cancer patients treated with radiation: update 2011. Support Care Cancer. 2011; 19(6):737–744

[11] Epstein JB, Gorsky M, Hancock P, Peters N, Sherlock CH. The prevalence of herpes simplex virus shedding and infection in the oral cavity of seropositive patients undergoing head and neck radiation therapy. Oral Surg Oral Med Oral Pathol Oral Radiol Endod. 2002; 94(6):712–716

[12] Samonis G, Mantadakis E, Maraki S. Orofacial viral infections in the immunocompromised host. Oncol Rep. 2000; 7(6):1389–1394

[13] Neville BW, Damm DD, Allen CM, Chi AC. Oral and Maxillofacial Pathology. St. Louis: Elsevier; 2016

[14] Khan SA, Wingard JR. Infection and mucosal injury in cancer treatment. J Natl Cancer Inst Monogr. 2001; 2001(29):31–36

[15] Villa A, Akintoye SO. Dental management of patients who have undergone oral cancer therapy. Dent Clin North Am. 2018; 62(1):131–142

[16] Elad S, Zadik Y, Hewson I, et al. Viral Infections Section, Oral Care Study Group, Multinational Association of Supportive Care in Cancer (MASCC)/International Society of Oral Oncology (ISOO). A systematic review of viral infections associated with oral involvement in cancer patients: a spotlight on Herpesviridea. Support Care Cancer. 2010; 18(8):993–1006

[17] Raber-Durlacher JE, Epstein JB, Raber J, et al. Periodontal infection in cancer patients treated with high-dose chemotherapy. Support Care Cancer. 2002; 10(6):466–473

[18] Heimdahl A. Prevention and management of oral infections in cancer patients. Support Care Cancer. 1999; 7(4):224–228

[19] Sonis ST. Oral mucositis in cancer therapy. J Support Oncol. 2004; 2(6) Suppl 3:3–8

[20] Cheng SCH, Wu VWC, Kwong DLW, Ying MTC. Assessment of post-radiotherapy salivary glands. Br J Radiol. 2011; 84(1001):393–402

[21] Sreebny LM. Saliva in health and disease: an appraisal and update. Int Dent J. 2000; 50(3):140–161

[22] Liu X-K, Su Y, Jha N, et al. Submandibular salivary gland transfer for the prevention of radiation-induced xerostomia in patients with nasopharyngeal carcinoma: 5-Year outcomes. Head Neck. 2011; 33

[23] Sood AJ, Fox NF, O'Connell BP, et al. Salivary gland transfer to prevent radiation-induced xerostomia: a systematic review and meta-analysis. Oral Oncol. 2014; 50(2):77–83

[24] Bellm LA, Epstein JB, Rose-Ped A, Martin P, Fuchs HJ. Patient reports of complications of bone marrow transplantation. Support Care Cancer. 2000; 8(1): 33–39

[25] Lalla RV, Sonis ST, Peterson DE. Management of oral mucositis in patients who have cancer. Dent Clin North Am. 2008; 52(1):61–77, viii

[26] Clark GT, Ram S. Orofacial pain and neurosensory disorders and dysfunction in cancer patients. Dent Clin North Am. 2008; 52(1):183–202, ix–x

[27] Mulvey MR, Boland EG, Bouhassira D, et al. Neuropathic pain in cancer: systematic review, performance of screening tools and analysis of symptom profiles. Br J Anaesth. 2017; 119(4):765–774

[28] Gilron I, Baron R, Jensen T. Neuropathic pain: principles of diagnosis and treatment. Mayo Clin Proc. 2015; 90(4):532–545

[29] Fallon MT. Neuropathic pain in cancer. Br J Anaesth. 2013; 111(1):105–111

[30] Addington J, Freimer M. Chemotherapy-induced peripheral neuropathy: an update on the current understanding. F1000 Res. 2016; 5:1466

[31] Finnerup NB, Haroutounian S, Kamerman P, et al. Neuropathic pain: an updated grading system for research and clinical practice. Pain. 2016; 157(8): 1599–1606

[32] Bennett M. The LANSS pain scale: the Leeds assessment of neuropathic symptoms and signs. Pain. 2001; 92(1–2):147–157

[33] Bouhassira D, Attal N, Alchaar H, et al. Comparison of pain syndromes associated with nervous or somatic lesions and development of a new neuropathic pain diagnostic questionnaire (DN4). Pain. 2005; 114(1–2):29–36

[34] Freynhagen R, Baron R, Gockel U, Tölle TR. painDETECT: a new screening questionnaire to identify neuropathic components in patients with back pain. Curr Med Res Opin. 2006; 22(10):1911–1920

[35] Cassileth BR, Keefe FJ. Integrative and behavioral approaches to the treatment of cancer-related neuropathic pain. Oncologist. 2010; 15(2) Suppl 2:19–23

[36] Stokman MA, Spijkervet FK, Boezen HM, Schouten JP, Roodenburg JL, de Vries EG. Preventive intervention possibilities in radiotherapy- and chemotherapy-induced oral mucositis: results of meta-analyses. J Dent Res. 2006; 85(8): 690–700

[37] Sasportas LS, Hosford DN, Sodini MA, et al. Cost-effectiveness landscape analysis of treatments addressing xerostomia in patients receiving head and neck radiation therapy. Oral Surg Oral Med Oral Pathol Oral Radiol. 2013; 116(1): e37–e51

[38] Cassolato SF, Turnbull RS. Xerostomia: clinical aspects and treatment. Gerodontology. 2003; 20(2):64–77

[39] Jensen SB, Pedersen AM, Vissink A, et al. Salivary Gland Hypofunction/Xerostomia Section, Oral Care Study Group, Multinational Association of Supportive Care in Cancer (MASCC)/International Society of Oral Oncology (ISOO). A systematic review of salivary gland hypofunction and xerostomia induced by cancer therapies: prevalence, severity and impact on quality of life. Support Care Cancer. 2010; 18(8):1039–1060

[40] Meirovitz A, Murdoch-Kinch CA, Schipper M, Pan C, Eisbruch A. Grading xerostomia by physicians or by patients after intensity-modulated radiotherapy of head-and-neck cancer. Int J Radiat Oncol Biol Phys. 2006; 66(2):445–453

[41] Scrimger R. Salivary gland sparing in the treatment of head and neck cancer. Expert Rev Anticancer Ther. 2011; 11(9):1437–1448

[42] Davies AN, Thompson J. Parasympathomimetic drugs for the treatment of salivary gland dysfunction due to radiotherapy. (review). Cochrane Database Syst Rev. 2015; 10(10):CD003782

[43] Kaae JK, Stenfeldt L, Eriksen JG. Xerostomia after radiotherapy for oral and oropharyngeal cancer: increasing salivary flow with tasteless sugar-free chewing gum. Front Oncol. 2016; 6:111

[44] Brozou V, Vadalouca A, Zis P. Pain in platin-induced neuropathies: a systematic review and meta-analysis. Pain Ther. 2018; 7(1):105–119

[45] Epstein JB, Elad S, Eliav E, Jurevic R, Benoliel R. Orofacial pain in cancer: part II —clinical perspectives and management. J Dent Res. 2007; 86(6):506–518

[46] Fischer DJ, Klasser GD, Epstein JB. Cancer and orofacial pain. Oral Maxillofac Surg Clin North Am. 2008; 20(2):287–301, vii

[47] Epstein JB, Hong C, Logan RM, et al. A systematic review of orofacial pain in patients receiving cancer therapy. Support Care Cancer. 2010; 18(8):1023–1031

[48] Romero-Reyes M, Salvemini D. Cancer and orofacial pain. Med Oral Patol Oral Cir Bucal. 2016; 21(6):e665–e671

[49] Kumar G, Manjunatha B. Metastatic tumors to the jaws and oral cavity. J Oral Maxillofac Pathol. 2013; 17(1):71–75

[50] Gupta R, Mohan V, Mahay V, Yadav PK. Orofacial pain: a review. Dentistry. 2016; 06(03). DOI: 10.4172/2161-1122.1000367

[51] Dios PD, Lestón JS. Oral cancer pain. Oral Oncol. 2010; 46(6):448–451

[52] Bensadoun R-J, Riesenbeck D, Lockhart PB, Elting LS, Spijkervet FKL, Brennan MT, Trismus Section, Oral Care Study Group, Multinational Association for Supportive Care in Cancer (MASCC)/International Society of Oral Oncology

(ISOO). A systematic review of trismus induced by cancer therapies in head and neck cancer patients. Support Care Cancer. 2010; 18(8):1033–1038
[53] Cohen J, Wakefield CE, Laing DG. Smell and taste disorders resulting from cancer and chemotherapy. Curr Pharm Des. 2016; 22(15):2253–2263
[54] Epstein JB, Smutzer G, Doty RL. Understanding the impact of taste changes in oncology care. Support Care Cancer. 2016; 24(4):1917–1931
[55] Hovan AJ, Williams PM, Stevenson-Moore P, et al. Dysgeusia Section, Oral Care Study Group, Multinational Association of Supportive Care in Cancer (MASCC)/International Society of Oral Oncology (ISOO). A systematic review of dysgeusia induced by cancer therapies. Support Care Cancer. 2010; 18(8): 1081–1087
[56] Heckel M, Stiel S, Ostgathe C. Smell and taste in palliative care: a systematic analysis of literature. Eur Arch Otorhinolaryngol. 2015; 272(2):279–288
[57] Kumbargere Nagraj S, George RP, Shetty N, Levenson D, Ferraiolo DM, Shrestha A. Interventions for managing taste disturbances. Cochrane Database Syst Rev. 2017; 12:CD010470
[58] Rivero JA, Shamji O, Kolokythas A. Osteoradionecrosis: a review of pathophysiology, prevention and pharmacologic management using pentoxifylline, α-tocopherol, and clodronate. Oral Surg Oral Med Oral Pathol Oral Radiol. 2017; 124(5):464–471
[59] Fan H, Kim SM, Cho YJ, Eo MY, Lee SK, Woo KM. New approach for the treatment of osteoradionecrosis with pentoxifylline and tocopherol. Biomater Res. 2014; 18(13):13
[60] Nadella KR, Kodali RM, Guttikonda LK, Jonnalagadda A. Osteoradionecrosis of the jaws: clinico-therapeutic management: a literature review and update. J Maxillofac Oral Surg. 2015; 14(4):891–901

47 Trismus in the Head and Neck Cancer Patient

Alexander E. Pazoki and Zachary Saltman

Summary

Trismus in the Head and Neck Cancer Patient provides a comprehensive overview of the condition of "trismus," or the inability or difficulty to open one's mouth, in the head and neck cancer population. The chapter seeks to define this commonly misunderstood clinical finding, as well as review the diagnosis, ramifications, and important anatomical considerations that can lead to this devastating sequela. With emphasis on the etiologic context of head and neck cancer and radiation therapy, best practices and treatment options are explored and considered. The thorough survey of pathogeneses, outcomes, and management are based on the highest quality data available, a combination of both landmark historical studies and novel, ground-breaking investigations. By the end of this chapter, the reader should fully understand and appreciate trismus, the many ways in which it can develop and progress, and the best methods in preventing and addressing it.

Keywords: trismus, masticatory apparatus, radiation fibrosis, intensity-modulated radiation therapy, jaw physiotherapy

47.1 Introduction

The oral cavity is the gateway to health and well-being. A functioning oral cavity is responsible for many things we take for granted on a daily basis. Some of these are directly related to survival, as is the case with mastication, feeding, and nutrition. Others bear an importance that may not affect mortality, but carry an immense psychosocial impact with significant implications on quality of life. Examples of the latter include speech and conversation, eating and taste, as well as intimacy.

While the inability to translate the mandible and adequately separate the jaws does not acutely or invariably lead to death, trismus can have detrimental effects on both the health and well-being of patients, and if not prevented and/or properly treated, it can lead to an irreversible and immeasurable detraction in one's standard of living.

47.2 Definition and Ramifications of Trismus

Determining a precise definition for "trismus" is no easy task. The word itself is derived from the Greek word "trismos," which refers to a grating, grinding, or rasping. Historically, it was first used to describe the inability of tetanus patients to open their mouths, but nowadays it simply refers to an inability to normally open one's mouth for any reason. The metric for mouth opening is known as "maximal inter-incisal opening" (MIO), and this is the measured distance between incisal edges of the maxillary and mandibular incisors, using a ruler or calipers to the nearest millimeter. In an edentulous patient, the measurement would be taken between maxillary and mandibular alveolar crests at the midline. Normal MIO in dentate adults falls within the range of about 35 to 55 mm. The difficulty in defining trismus lays not in the parameters for normal MIO, but in the excess of classification parameters and schemes that have been proposed to diagnose and grade abnormal MIO (▶ Fig. 47.1). Most clinicians and authors agree that a measurement below 35 mm indicates some degree of reduction in mouth opening in a majority of patients, but the threshold at which the function is truly impaired, and furthermore at what point the degree of trismus causes a significant decrease in quality of life or increase in morbidity is difficult to pinpoint. This threshold of 35 mm was advocated as a diagnostic cut-off for trismus by multiple studies. They first based their analysis on criteria of patient's experience of subjective limitation of mouth opening, as well as functional impairment as determined by the Mandibular Function Impairment Questionnaire (MFIQ),[1] which is an assessment based on subjective limitations of 11 mandibular functions (speaking, taking large bites of food, chewing hard food, chewing soft food, work and daily activities, drinking, laughing, chewing resistant food, yawning, and kissing) and of chewing various food consistencies (hard cookie, meat, raw carrot, French bread, nuts, and apple).[2] A more modern study corroborates this cut-off of 35 mm as a point which correlates with both patients' perception of functional disability and decrease in quality of life.[3] Most studies point to the range of 15 to 20 mm as the threshold for "severe" impairment or trismus, and it is speculated that as MIO decreases beyond this level, patients will experience progressive detraction in quality of life.

It is important to note that while a maximum cut-off of 35 mm to identify trismus appears to be appropriate in determining disability and need for intervention in the head and neck cancer population, different values may carry significance in other etiologies of trismus. For example, in the context of head and neck odontogenic infections, an MIO of 30 mm, while less than normal, is more consistent with "guarding" or "splinting" (i.e., limitation or stiffening due to pain) secondary to a less severe infection, such as a vestibular or buccal space abscess. Trismus of 15–20 mm or less in the setting of head and neck infections, however, is almost pathognomonic for infection of the masticator space, a serious condition requiring more urgent intervention.[4]

The ability to normally ingest food begins with mastication and breakdown of incised food, followed by manipulation of chewed food into a bolus largely by the tongue, culminating in complete swallowing of the food bolus and clearance into the esophagus. Lubrication of the bolus and some degree of digestion also occur in the oral cavity by saliva and its components. Normal jaw function and opening determine what can enter the oral cavity and be chewed in the first place, and poor tongue and salivary functions can result in poor bolus organization and food passage respectively, ultimately leading to excess postswallow residue. The ramifications of impairment in this system is not only poor diet and nutrition, but also ineffective airway clearance, increasing the risk of aspiration and thus pneumonias.

It is clear that as the MIO decreases, patients experience severe consequences, beginning with reliance on pureed or

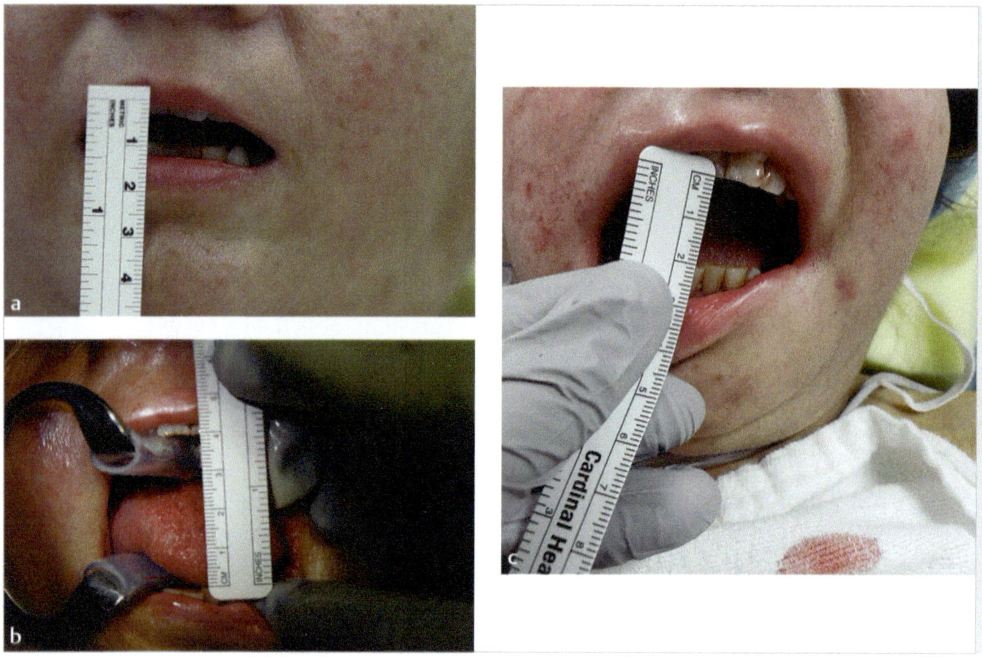

Fig. 47.1 A patient with severe trismus secondary to oral submucous fibrosis, with preoperative MIO of less than 1cm **(a)**, intra-operative opening of 40mm after excision of bilateral fibrotic buccal tissue **(b)**, and then relapse of trismus with MIO of 20mm after soft tissue scarring and contracture at 3 months post-operatively **(c)**. This relapse was attributed to a lapse in home physiotherapy, after which a loss of MIO of approximately 12mm was seen.

liquid diets, and ultimately on enteral tube feeding in the most severe cases. Oral hygiene also becomes increasingly difficult to accomplish, often in a population already at greater risk for dental decay, infection, and oral disease (in the case of those receiving head and neck radiation therapy). So how should MIO be measured and trismus be classified?

Many clinicians employ the finger-breadth technique, with 3 + finger breadths correlating to normal MIO, 2 finger breadths to mildly limited opening, and 1 finger breadth or less to true trismus. This can be effective only as a crude and cursory test, and it is always valuable to obtain precise measurements, especially when following patients over time and monitoring their progress compared to a baseline value. Variation in finger width also renders this technique suboptimal, as what correlates to normal MIO for one clinician may represent limited opening for another. Clinically, the most important consideration is the patients' function and quality of life, as well as ability to monitor their progress with precise values.

47.3 A Brief Review of Anatomy

In order to understand the levels and phases at which masticatory function can break down, one must first know the biomechanics, anatomy, and physiology of jaw opening and closure (▶ Fig. 47.2). The masticatory apparatus is comprised of the bony structures, the **temporomandibular joint (TMJ)** and associated ligaments, and the musculature driving it all.

The bony components of mastication include the maxilla, the mandible, and the glenoid fossa of the temporal bone. The **maxilla** is a nondynamic bone that is fixed to the skull base and discrete from the TMJ, and thus in and of itself contributes minimal variety between individuals vis-à-vis masticatory function. The **mandible** is a U- or V-shaped bone in the dentate segment, with ascending rami that bilaterally give rise to the paired **mandibular condyles** and **coronoid processes**, both of which have major roles in dynamic jaw function. The condyles articulate with the **glenoid** or **mandibular fossa** to form the bony surfaces of the TMJ and are—together with the **meniscus** (or **disk**)—encased in the fibrous, connective tissue **capsule** of the joint. Conversely, the coronoid process is extracapsular, serving primarily as a muscle insertion point for the **temporalis muscle** tendon, working alongside the **medial pterygoid** and **masseter** muscles to drive jaw closure. The fourth primary muscle of mastication, the **lateral pterygoid**, is the predominant muscle involved in jaw opening. Arising from the greater wing of the sphenoid bone and lateral pterygoid plate, it inserts to the pterygoid fovea of the condyle and the meniscus itself, functioning to pull the condyles anteriorly in jaw opening. The complementary, *infra-mandibular* group of accessory muscles also serve as mandibular depressors.

The TMJ itself is a complex structure that encompasses the most intricate and dynamic elements for jaw function and motion. Because of its complexity, it is uniquely classified in several different ways. Anatomically, the TMJ is classified as a *diarthrodial joint*, due to its discontinuous articulation between two bones. Functionally, the TMJ is classified as a *compound joint*, because there are two separate pairs of articulating surfaces: the glenoid fossa with the superior aspect of the disk and the condylar head with the inferior aspect of the disk. This forms two separate joint spaces. The **inferior joint space** allows rotational/hinge (*ginglymoid*) movement of the condyles around a transverse axis drawn in a straight line between the two condylar heads. The **superior joint space** allows anterior translational/sliding (*arthrodial*) movement of the condyles along the articular eminence, in harmony with the overlying disks. In theory, rotational opening can account for about 2.5 cm of interincisal opening, while translation accounts for the remaining 2 cm; however, mandibular function in reality is almost always a synthesis of rotational and translational movements, which gives the TMJ its further classification as a *ginglymoarthrodial* joint.

The TMJ is also a *synovial joint*, referring to the **synovial membrane** or **synovium** that lines the inner surface and

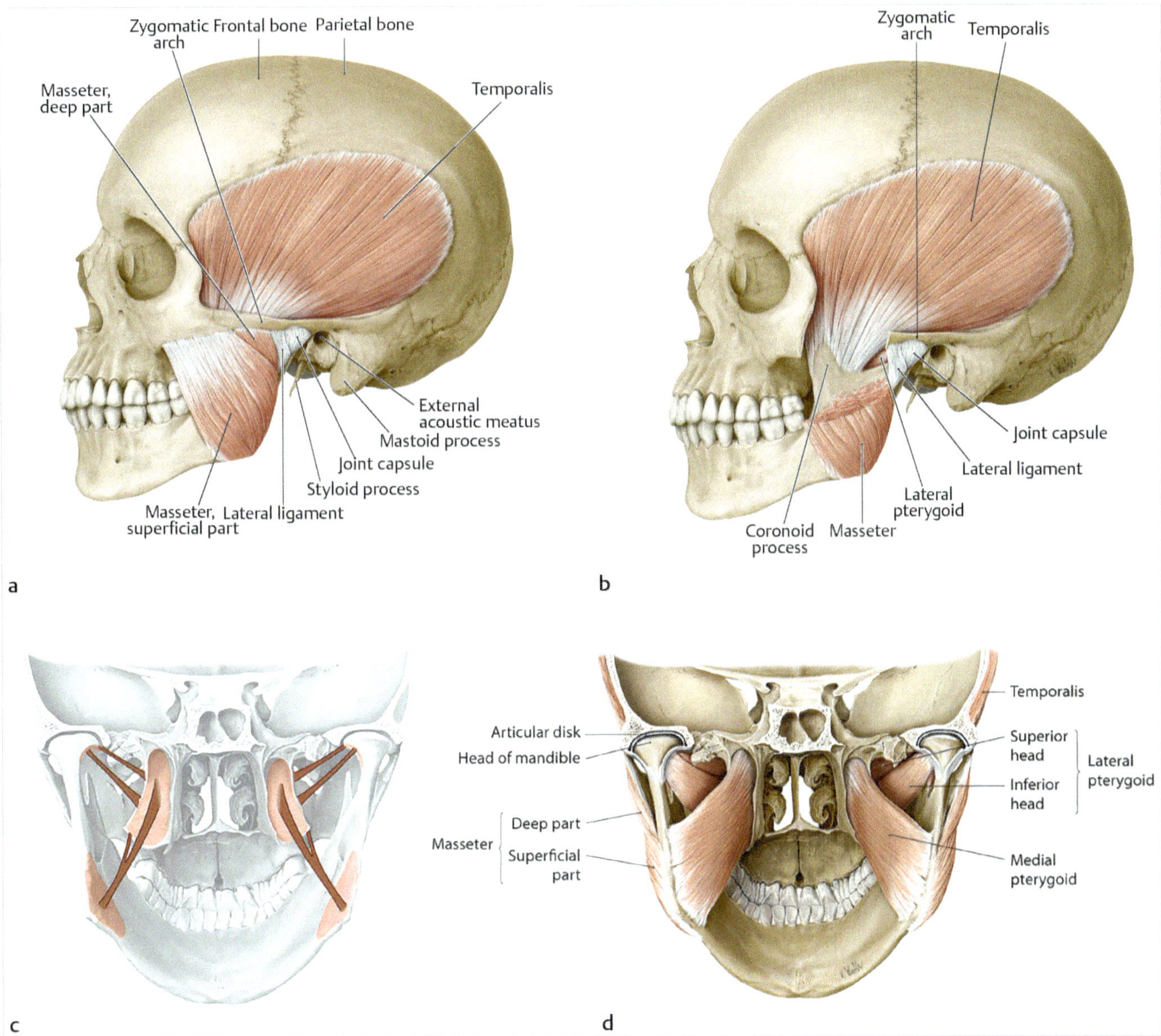

Fig. 47.2 Four masticatory muscles; masseter, temporalis, medial, and lateral pterygoids. **(a)** Masseter with temporalis muscle. **(b)** Temporalis muscle (masseter and zygomatic arch are removed). **(c, d)** Inferior views of the medial and lateral pterygoid muscles. (Source: Schuenke M, Schulte E, Schumacher U. THIEME Atlas of Anatomy: Head and Neuroanatomy. Illustrations by Voll M and Wesker K. 1st Ed. New York:Thieme Medical Publishers; 2010.)

secretes synovial fluid. The functions of this plasma ultrafiltrate include biomechanical lubrication, phagocytosis of intracapsular debris, as well as satisfying the metabolic and nutritional needs of the avascular structures within the TMJ. The synovium itself is able to rapidly regenerate after injury, and is thus a target of much research, along with inflammatory cytokines that are presumed to play a role in the process of TMJ degeneration.

A second type of tissue lining the synovial cavity is the **articular cartilage**, a dense, fibrocartilaginous, connective tissue layer overlying the articular surfaces of the mandibular condyle and temporal bone. This fibrocartilage bears the functional stress of mandibular rotation and translation, reacting to these forces by inducing remodeling and regeneration in its deeper, **proliferative zone** of cells. These cells can differentiate into either cartilaginous or osseous tissue, depending on functional stress.

The meniscus itself is another avascular, noninnervated, densely fibrous connective tissue structure, similarly adapted to resist the stresses of TMJ function. The disk's position is maintained by three functional ligaments and two accessory ligaments. Extending posteriorly, the avascular articular disk crossfades into **retrodiskal tissue**, a continuous but morphologically different tissue, which by contrast has rich vasculature and innervation.

With one U-shaped bone articulating bilaterally against bony fossae of the cranial base via diarthrodial, compound joints, and movements driven by 12 different pairs of muscles and limited by various ligaments, mandibular motion is anything but simple. It comes as no surprise that the TMJ is the most biomechanically complex joint in the human body, and consequently its pathology and the management thereof is a field worthy of many textbooks and resources dedicated to its study alone. The body's ability to adapt to stresses and insults should not be underestimated even in the case of TMJ function, but damage or loss of function at any level or component of mandibular motion can result in dysfunction, pain, and in severe cases trismus.

47.4 Etiology and Pathogenesis of Trismus

Trismus can be acute or chronic and generally arises as a result of a few broad pathologic categories: infection and inflammation, TMJ and myofascial pain dysfunction, trauma, fibrosis, and neoplasia. Every etiology can be distilled down into either causing damage within the TMJ, dysfunction of the muscles driving the TMJ and mandible, anatomical obstruction to mandibular movement, or changes increasing the resistance to stretching of orofacial soft tissues. In many clinical scenarios of trismus, the underlying pathogenesis is multifactorial, involving processes from many of the above categories, but this chapter specifically focuses on trismus in the setting of head and neck cancer.

Trismus can arise in the setting of head and neck neoplasia via three mechanisms: local invasion of a primary or metastatic tumor into structures of mastication (TMJ, musculature, or the innervation thereof), mechanical obstruction of the coronoid or condylar processes of the mandible, or as a result of surgical or radiation therapy of a tumor.

47.4.1 Direct Tumor Involvement and Surgical Changes

Direct tumor extension can cause trismus via invasion into the masticatory muscles, the innervation thereof, the facial skeleton, or in rare cases the TMJ itself. Besides mechanical obstruction of and adhesion to masticatory structures, neurogenic pathways have also been described. Sensory nerve fibers from the TMJ, masticatory muscles, oropharynx, pterygopalatine and infratemporal fossae, pinna, and external auditory canal travel caudally via the glossopharyngeal nerve and branches of the trigeminal nerve, coalescing in the principal sensory trigeminal nucleus in the pons. Stimulation of these nerves may send impulses centrally to the sensory cortex as pain, as well as to the trigeminal motor nucleus, increasing the tone of the muscles of mastication. Given that the mandibular elevators overpower the mandibular depressors by a factor of ten to one, increased tonus alone via this neurogenic pathway may be a contributory factor in head and neck cancer patients presenting with trismus prior to treatment.

Postsurgical trismus is also observed after the excision of lesions leads to scar formation and contracture in areas such as the buccal mucosa, retromolar area, and tonsillar fossa. These known effects of healing and inflammation in such areas can extend to the masseter muscle, pterygoid muscles, or pterygomandibular ligament, for example, functionally shortening these structures and decreasing jaw opening (▶ Fig. 47.3).

In a study by Ichimura and Tanaka of 212 patients with head and neck cancer between 1983 and 1991, overall only 2% presented with trismus at the time of diagnosis, and 1% at the time of recurrence.[5] Other studies, however, have found higher rates specific to certain anatomical sites, such as 56% prevalence of trismus in patients presenting with parapharyngeal malignancy, 72% prevalence in patients with advanced parotid gland tumors, and only 4–9% in patients with nasopharyngeal tumors.[6] It is no surprise that tumor sites in closer proximity to the masticatory apparatus have a higher prevalence of trismus at the time of presentation, and the literature supports this. Of the 212 patients studied by Ichimura and Tanaka, 9 developed trismus via tumor infiltration into muscles of mastication or reflex spasm, and 7 as a result of surgical intervention.

Simple pressure from benign neoplasms on the muscles of mastication have not shown to affect mouth opening.[5] Thus, a benign tumor may only cause trismus in the rare case in which it causes obstruction of the condylar or coronoid processes in translation during jaw opening. Tumors within the TMJ are exceedingly rare, but can arise from bone, cartilage, muscle, or synovium. These can manifest with symptoms similar to internal derangement, sometimes causing delay in diagnosis, which can be extremely dangerous given the proximity to the skull base. The most common benign bone tumors of the TMJ are the **osteoma** and **condylar hypertrophy**, which can impair the enlarged condyle's ability to translate. **Synovial chondromatosis** is the most common benign neoplasm of the synovium. This disease process involves metaplastic calcification of the synovial

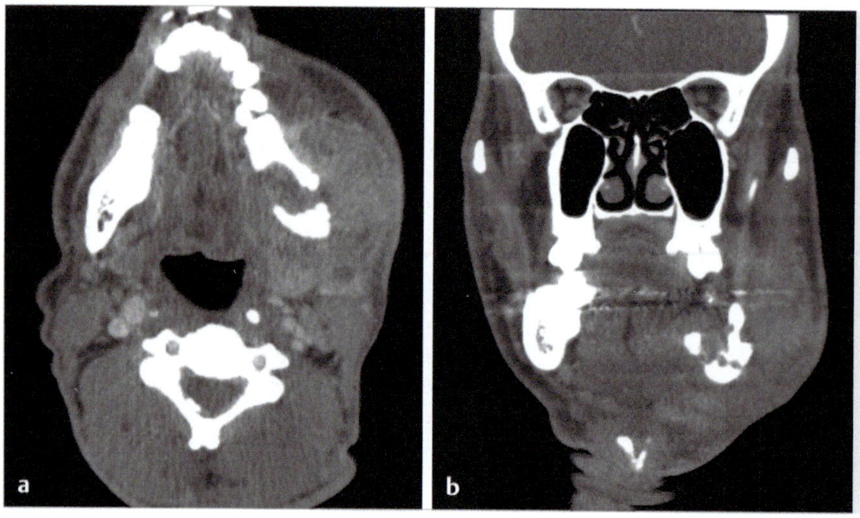

Fig. 47.3 Axial **(a)** and coronal **(b)** CT neck with contrast of an advanced buccal cavity carcinoma. Mandibular destruction is clearly visualized in addition to extensive soft tissue involvement extending through masseter muscle and out to the external skin. (Source: Clinical Cases: In: Genden E., ed. Head and Neck Cancer: Management and Reconstruction. 2nd Edition. Thieme; 2019.)

lining, where the calcified bodies can subsequently detach and suspend in the synovial fluid, develop a perichondrium, and continue to grow. These calcified bodies can often be detected by radiograph, which along with the common initial presentation of preauricular pain and swelling, is helpful in diagnosis. **Ganglionic cysts** are true cystic structures, which have been reported to arise in association with the TMJ capsule or tendon sheaths, sometimes producing TMJD-like symptoms.

Malignancies of the TMJ are very rare and are more likely the result of direct extension of primary lesions from adjacent tissues, rather than metastatic disease, which is more common in the mandibular angle. Adenocarcinomas of the breast, kidney, and lungs are the most common primary lesions to metastasize to the mandibular condyle, and these present with similar early findings as in benign condylar tumors: pain and dysfunction. Early detection is paramount even more so than for benign tumors, due to proximity to skull base.

47.4.2 Head and Neck Radiation Therapy

Trismus is a well-documented complication of radiation therapy for head and neck malignancy, and the prevalence of trismus in this patient population varies wildly from 0 to 100% in the literature, depending on site, extension, radiation dosage, and study design. High incidence of trismus after treatment for head and neck cancer is reported in most studies. For example, a retrospective analysis by Johnson et al found 69 of 246 or 42% of patients with various diagnoses of head and neck cancer developed posttreatment trismus.[7] This incidence was highest specifically with tumors treated in the parotid and nasopharyngeal regions, and both poor baseline function prior to treatment and higher external beam radiation dosages of > 50 Gy were associated with significantly more posttreatment trismus. In a different cohort of 101 head and neck radiation patients, incidence of trismus was found to correlate significantly with anatomic location: 65% in oral/oropharyngeal cancer, 44% in hypopharyngeal cancer, and 31% in laryngeal cancer.[8] Another recent study by Pauli et al showed a postradiation incidence of trismus in head and neck cancer patients to be 28%, with tonsillar tumors most likely to yield posttreatment trismus.[9] A peak incidence of 38% was noted at the 6 months posttreatment mark, with a baseline prevalence of 9% pretreatment.

Radiation therapy is a vastly important treatment modality that has been used for decades in the treatment of head and neck cancer, often in combination with surgery and/or chemotherapy. As discussed throughout this text, the oral complications associated with radiation therapy are extensive and complex, and trismus is among the most debilitating. While the literature exhibits an array of studies and findings, the correlation between radiation to the masticatory apparatus and posttreatment trismus is clear.

The pathophysiology of radiation-induced trismus begins with direct cell damage, combined with compromised regional vascularity and thus perfusion, and activation of fibrosis in soft tissues. These fundamental changes contribute to loss of salivary function, increased susceptibility to caries, soft and hard tissue necrosis, as well as trismus. Fibrosis of damaged muscles of mastication directly impedes function of the masticatory apparatus.[10] The exact biomolecular mechanism is not fully understood, but abnormal fibroblast proliferation has been demonstrated as an important event in this cascade.[11] Scar tissue from radiation therapy and/or surgery can also combine with damage to local innervation for a cumulative deleterious effect. After degeneration of muscles and/or the TMJ has occurred, sustained hypomobility of the mandible leads to further compromise via muscular atrophy and changes within the joint that begin to manifest in as little as three days. These changes can be reversible with return of movement. However, this is a difficult prospect when the cause of hypomobility is structural, as in fibrosis and scarring; hence the importance of physiotherapy in all cases of hypomobility.

The fibrosis and contracture of muscles within the field of radiation arise gradually, often presenting about 9 weeks after completion of treatment, but continuing to progress for months to years. Within the first 9 months following radiation therapy, mouth opening diminishes by an average of 2.4% each month. By the second year postradiation, this drops to about 0.2% decrease in mouth opening each month, and further to 0.1% between 24 and 48 months.[1] Roughly two-thirds of the total loss in mouth opening occurs during the first 9 months of post-radiation therapy. Absolute jaw opening after radiation therapy decreases on average by 18 to 32% compared to pretreatment measurements.[12]

Trismus has been shown to have a dose-dependent relationship with radiation to pertinent components of the masticatory apparatus, and newer radiation-sparing techniques like intensity-modulated radiation therapy (IMRT) seem to lower the degree of trismus of after radiation therapy. Doses as low as 15 Gy result in functional impairment of jaw opening and mastication, while doses in excess of 60 Gy are even more likely to result in trismus.[13] Furthermore, patients undergoing radiation therapy for the second time due to tumor recurrence are at higher risk for trismus than those who are naïve to radiation.[1, 14] Various studies point to specific muscle targets as causative for postradiation trismus, for example, medial pterygoid versus masseter muscles; however, newer IMRT studies indicate that trismus is associated with radiation doses received by both the medial pterygoid and masseter muscles.[15] The fibrotic effects of radiation on either of these muscles limit the range of motion of the mandible in a relatively similar manner, due to their largely parallel anatomy and function.

It is worth noting that most data originated in the treatment era preceding the advent of IMRT and concurrent or concomitant computed tomography (CT). Not only has the addition of CT to IMRT shown to yield no increase in trismus risk compared to conventional radiation therapy,[16] but also IMRT likely decreases the risk of postradiation trismus due to the precision in targeting smaller areas with radiation doses, especially when doses can be minimized in those specific tissues which are known to be susceptible. A recent systematic review found a weighted prevalence of 25.4% in patients after receiving conventional radiation therapy, in contrast to only 5% in patients undergoing IMRT for similar tumors.[17] In a noncontrolled, prospective study by Hsiung and colleagues, 17 patients were treated for nasopharyngeal carcinoma with parotid-sparing IMRT, and the average postradiation mouth opening of the entire cohort was found to be 94% of pretreatment values at 5 months post-IMRT, and 98.1% of pretreatment values at 12 months post-IMRT.[18] This study is limited in power and to only one anatomic site, but one would reasonably hope to see similar benefits of this approach in other head and neck cancer sites. IMRT and concurrent CT appear to be invaluable techniques in reducing the severity and incidence of radiation-induced trismus in many cases, but for those in which tumor proximity to the masticatory apparatus requires curative radiation doses to any of these structures, trismus may still be unavoidable.

47.5 Treatment Approaches and Considerations

Prompt intervention for the treatment of trismus is paramount, as it can minimize or prevent many of the debilitating sequelae of the condition. When a patient presents with postradiation trismus, it is first crucial to discern whether it is a result of treatment, or a harbinger of tumor recurrence. Particularly, if function continues to wane despite physiotherapy or other management, especially if presenting with pain, then a tumor recurrence must be ruled out. Diagnostic imaging such as CT, magnetic resonance imaging (MRI), and positron emission tomography (PET) are effective in surveillance for recurrence in these scenarios (▶ Fig. 47.4). With tumor recurrence ruled out, the clinician should initiate treatment of trismus as soon as possible. As restriction worsens and reversibility becomes less likely, treatment becomes all the more urgent. Pain is a frequent common finding with trismus, with reports of up to 50% of head and neck cancer patients presenting with pain prior to treatment. As previously discussed, if pain prevents an individual from opening his or her mouth, this hypomobility can independently contribute to perpetuation of trismus. Thus, if posttreatment pain persists, analgesia becomes an important consideration during

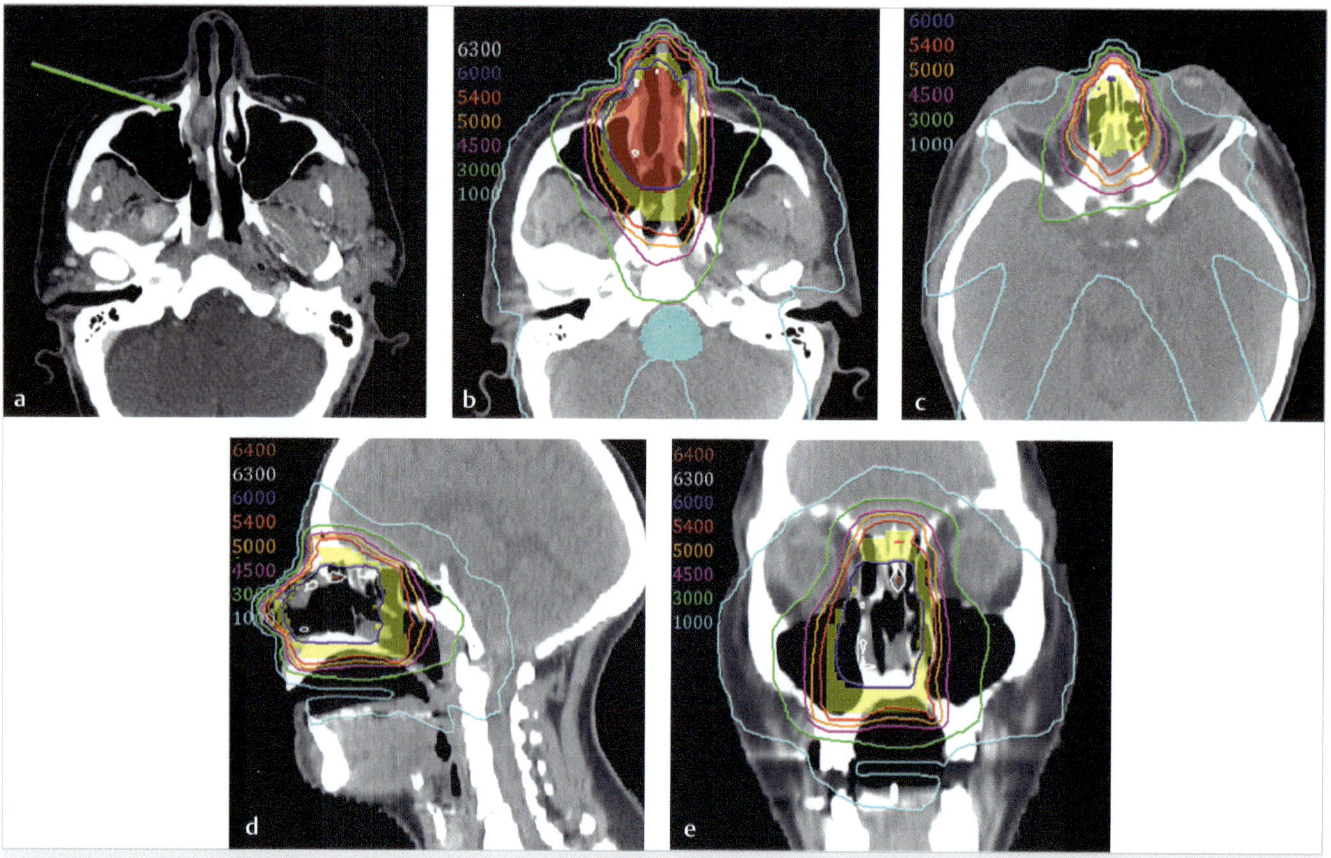

Fig. 47.4 (a–e) A 60-year-old woman presented with nasal obstruction and epistaxis. She was found to have a lesion in the posterior right nasal septum. Biopsy was positive for squamous cell carcinoma; **(a)** shows the tumor (*green arrow*) in an axial slice of diagnostic CT scan. She underwent an endoscopic resection of the tumor. Margins were negative but contained high-grade dysplasia. She was then treated with postoperative IMRT. A mouthopening, tongue-depressing stent was used to minimize dose to the oral structures. As the vCTV was relatively small, it was elected to omit CTV_{ID} but define CTV_{HD} fairly generously to include the septum and right nasal cavity. The remaining left nasal cavity, medial aspect of the right maxillary sinus, hard palate (floor of the nasal cavity), anterior sphenoid sinus, and ethmoid sinuses were defined as CTV_{ED}. CTV_{HD} and CTV_{ED} were prescribed 60 and 54 Gy, respectively, and treatment was delivered in 30 fractions. An axial view of the isodose distribution is shown through the midnose **(b)** along with CTV_{HD} (*red*) and CTV_{ED} (*yellow*). A second axial view **(c)** through the ethmoids and orbits shows only CTV_{ED} at this level. The doses to the optic nerves and lenses were <45 and <10 Gy, respectively. Isodose distributions in sagittal **(d)** and coronal **(e)** views through midplane of the head are also shown. The contour colorwash inside the 60-Gy line is removed so the underlying resected tissues can be appreciated. The mouth-opening stent can also be seen on these views. The patient has done well and is without disease 3 years later. (Source: Tumors of the Nasal Cavity. In: Lund V, Howard D, Wei W, ed. Tumors of the Nose, Sinuses, and Nasopharynx. 1st Edition. Thieme; 2014.)

therapy. Beyond analgesia, the options for management of trismus can be categorized as conservative treatment or surgical.

47.5.1 Conservative/Nonsurgical Management

Conservative management includes both medical and pharmacological interventions, as well as physical therapy, the most effective approach likely involving a combination of the two.

Medical Management

Hyperbaric oxygen (HBO) is a medical intervention that has long been used to stimulate angiogenesis, increasing vascularity and thus perfusion, in tissues with poor vascularity. In this treatment, patients undergo multiple "dives," inhaling 100% oxygen at a minimum of 1.5 atmospheres (150 kPa), in order to dissolve oxygen in the plasma and increase its delivery independent of hemoglobin. While data is limited, HBO is likely ineffective in the treatment of radiation-induced trismus.[19]

Botulinum toxin injection into the muscles of mastication may have some benefits in this patient population, largely via pain reduction due to prevention of painful muscle spasm. Although, unfortunately, its use has not been shown to correlate with measurable improvement in MIO, the ability to control pain caused by radiation fibrosis may justify an adjunctive role for botulinum toxin in the management of trismus.

Pentoxifylline medication and microcurrent electrotherapy have also been employed to increase MIO after head and neck radiation; however, both interventions have shown a very limited effect on trismus.[20,21]

Physiotherapy and Rehabilitation

Physical therapy is the mainstay of trismus management, and while evidence of its efficacy is limited, it should be implemented as soon as possible following surgery and during radiation therapy. Exercises must be carried out as frequently as possible every day and involve both horizontal and vertical range of motion maneuvers. Multiple mechanical implements have been used to facilitate this type of physiotherapy, including stacking tongue depressors, finger-opening spring appliances, acrylic wedges, clothes pegs, and more elaborate appliances from medical manufacturers. While efficacy of such approaches has been widely presented anecdotally, there are known limitations in their use and an absence of adequately sized and controlled studies to prove their value. As with any self-driven treatment protocol, compliance over a long period may be a limiting factor for many patients. There is even some speculation that irradiated patients may regain their masticatory and swallowing function over time without the use of physiotherapy.[22] Despite the limitations and lack of high-powered studies, most authors and clinicians advocate early and aggressive implementation of physical therapy, as the potential for benefit is high, with no associated morbidity or other strong deterrents to treatment. It is key to measure MIO and track progress at baseline and throughout treatment, aiming for a minimum opening of 35 mm. Tracking progress and setting goals are not only helpful for targeted treatment, but also in motivating the patients by providing them with tangible improvements as a direct result of their exercises. Once the goal of 35-mm MIO has been met and sustained, the frequency of exercises may be tapered.[1,23]

Rehabilitative Exercises

Jaw opening exercises (▶ Fig. 47.5) are either active or passive in nature. Active jaw opening exercises involve opening and closing the mouth repeatedly, slow lateral movements of the mandible to the left and right in a slightly open state, and protrusion and retraction of the mandible in a slightly open state. While these are carried out via the patient's head and neck musculature, passive exercises involve opening the mouth either by hand or the use of specific appliances or devices. While the exact therapeutic mechanism is unclear, range of motion and resistance exercises may strengthen the musculature, increase mobility, and improve elasticity within the TMJ. Exercises may even improve local soft-tissue circulation.[22]

Appliances and Devices

Perhaps the oldest and most-used device to facilitate jaw opening exercise is the stacking of wooden tongue depressors. It is inexpensive, effective, and inherently provides patients with incremental benchmarking of progress by the number of tongue depressors that fit between their upper and lower incisors.

Other more sophisticated appliances that are currently and commonly used include the TheraBite Jaw Motion Rehabilitation System and the Dynasplint Trismus System (DTS).[24] The TheraBite relies on passive jaw opening in a vertical dimension to stretch the soft tissues, strengthen musculature, and mobilize joints. Its efficacy has been demonstrated in multiple studies. In one trial of 69 head and neck cancer patients treated with surgery, radiation therapy, chemotherapy, or a combination thereof, TheraBite physiotherapy led to an average increase in MIO of 5.4 mm, with the odds of gaining over 5 mm of opening decreasing as the duration between oncological treatment and initiation of physiotherapy is prolonged.[23] Exercise regimens with the TheraBite were no more effective than those with tongue depressors[25] or simple range of motion exercises,[26] but they were more effective by a mean difference of 5.7 mm than the control group of patients with no structured exercise intervention.[27,28] The Dynasplint or DTS employs prolonged, low-torque stretching to increase MIO, and it similarly has shown to be effective in the literature. A retrospective study of 48 trismus patients following head and neck radiation therapy, dental treatment, oral surgery, and stroke, with the radiation cohort improving MIO by an average of 13.6 mm.[13] Another retrospective study of 26 patients showed a mean MIO increase of 6.2 mm after treatment with DTS, more comparable to the TheraBite.[29]

A different type of physiotherapy is forced mouth opening or manipulation under general anesthesia, which has been shown to improve trismus, but with results that are often transient and accompanied by more potential complications, such as alveolar fracture, soft tissue injury, and reactions to anesthesia.[30]

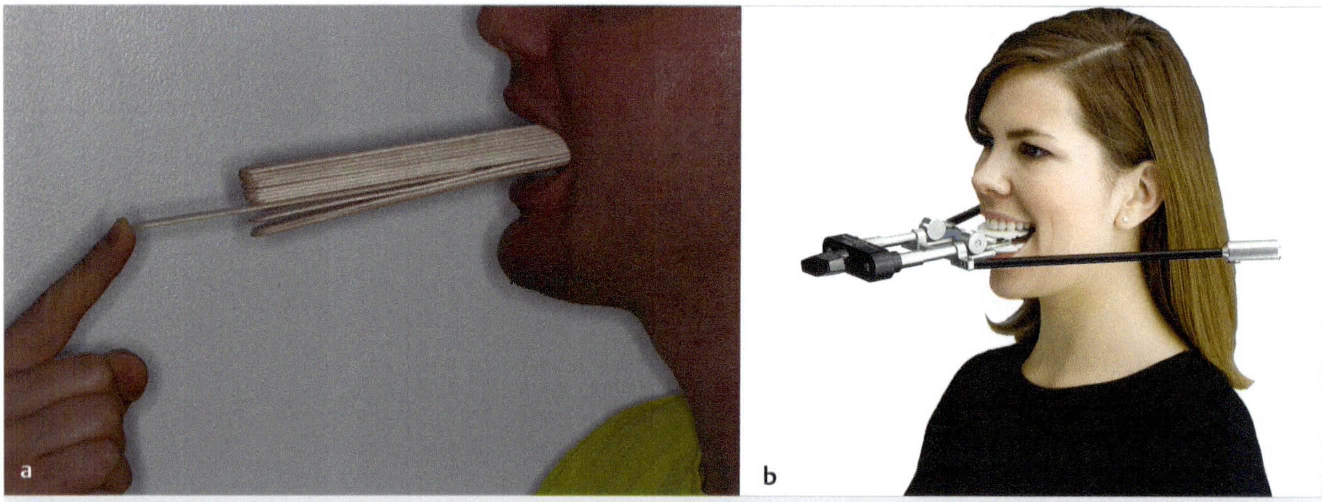

Fig. 47.5 Examples of implements for jaw-opening physiotherapy. **(a)** A demonstration of the tongue-depressor-stacking exercise, which is most economical and widely accessible, and **(b)** the DynaSplint Trismus System, a more advanced medical appliance serving the same purpose (Reproduced with permission of Jaw Dynasplint System and Dynasplint Systems, Inc.)

47.5.2 Surgical Options

Conservative treatment should always be the first-line management of trismus; however, when this fails, coronoidectomy may prove to be effective. Surgical intervention, of course, puts the patients at additional risks when compared to medical and physical therapy, and irradiated patients are particularly susceptible to complications, such as poor wound healing and infection, due to compromised perfusion and existing tissue damage. While coronoidectomy is typically a low-risk procedure, it is an invasive surgery and thus should be carried out judiciously in the head and neck cancer patient population. In tumor patients being treated surgically, whether before or after chemotherapy and/or radiation therapy, and especially in the event of proximity of tumor to the coronoid process, it is recommended to proactively perform coronoidectomies concomitantly to prevent the development of trismus.[13] Available data is limited, but in a noncontrolled study of 18 head and neck cancer patients with trismus refractory to physiotherapy, coronoidectomy proved to drastically improve mouth opening. Patients experienced an immediate increase in MIO of at least 20 mm, with about half of the patients improving by 30 mm. Furthermore, nearly all the patients maintained a normal opening of at least 35 mm for the duration of follow-up. Unfortunately, coronoidectomy is not a panacea in the management of trismus. As the insertion site of the temporalis muscle only, coronoidectomy cannot address radiation fibrosis of other structures, such as the pterygoid or masseter muscles, which are also often involved.[31]

47.6 Prevention

As is the case with many pathologies, attention to prevention is crucial. While some degree of fibrosis and restricted opening is unavoidable in head and neck radiation patients, clinicians must synthesize their knowledge of head and neck anatomy with the known effects seen in irradiated tissues to design treatment plans that minimize damage to structures vital to masticatory function. Similarly, to avoid other negative sequelae, such as ORN, xerostomia, and caries, the dentoalveolar apparatus and salivary glands are ideally kept out of the field of radiation when possible. Tumor eradication is always the priority in head and neck cancer treatment, but newer, dose-sparing radiation techniques like IMRT allow precise targeting of a desired field and thus the ability to spare vital structures from irradiation in many cases. Furthermore, these techniques provide clinicians with an accurate prediction of the structures involved, so that attention can be given to proactively mitigating expected side effects, as well as the ability to give patients proper expectations when going into treatment. Patients absolutely must be warned of the risks of debilitating side effects like trismus before initiating radiation therapy, both to be aware of the consequences as well as the importance of exercises to treat them.

The current dearth of reliable medical treatments for trismus places more importance on proactivity and prevention for clinicians. While more and stronger data is required to assess the extent of the possibilities of proactive techniques like IMRT, the existing evidence is promising. While prophylactic physiotherapy regimens, both during and following radiation therapy, are widely employed to minimize and treat trismus, multiple studies have shown a lack of benefit when compared to care as usual. Given the lack of associated risk with exercise, its use should absolutely continue; however, the current literature may indicate that the greatest potential in reducing the incidence and severity of radiation-induced trismus lies in preventative and proactive efforts.

Key Points

- An MIO of < 35 mm is abnormal and is a threshold below which patients begin to experience diminishing quality of life.
- Damage, obstruction, or dysfunction occurring at any component of the masticatory apparatus can result in acute or chronic trismus, yielding a myriad of etiologies.

- Trismus can be a prognostic indicator and/or guide treatment in some etiologies, such as maxillofacial infections and trauma.
- Trismus can be caused directly by head and neck tumors, as well as by surgical or radiation treatment thereof.
- Trismus is an extremely common and dose-dependent side effect of head and neck radiation due to the resultant fibrosis of soft tissues within the field of radiation.
- Newer radiation modalities such as IMRT likely reduce the incidence of postradiation trismus and also provide accurate expectations based on tissues included in the field.
- Management of trismus should be guided by patient's function and quality of life.
- Physiotherapy is the mainstay of treatment of radiation-induced trismus, and it is similarly effective whether using expensive appliances, cheap implements (i.e., tongue depressors), or fingers.
- When conservative measures fail, coronoidectomy alleviates trismus in many cases; however, it is not a panacea for trismus treatment, as it only addresses the temporalis.

References

[1] Dijkstra PU, Huisman PM, Roodenburg JL. Criteria for trismus in head and neck oncology. Int J Oral Maxillofac Surg. 2006; 35(4):337–342

[2] Stegenga B, de Bont LG, de Leeuw R, Boering G. Assessment of mandibular function impairment associated with temporomandibular joint osteoarthrosis and internal derangement. J Orofac Pain. 1993; 7(2):183–195

[3] Scott B, Butterworth C, Lowe D, Rogers SN. Factors associated with restricted mouth opening and its relationship to health-related quality of life in patients attending a maxillofacial oncology clinic. Oral Oncol. 2008; 44(5):430–438

[4] Flynn TR, Shanti RM, Levi MH, Adamo AK, Kraut RA, Trieger N. Severe odontogenic infections, part 1: prospective report. J Oral Maxillofac Surg. 2006; 64 (7):1093–1103

[5] Ichimura K, Tanaka T. Trismus in patients with malignant tumours in the head and neck. J Laryngol Otol. 1993; 107(11):1017–1020

[6] Rapidis AD, Dijkstra PU, Roodenburg JL, et al. Trismus in patients with head and neck cancer: etiopathogenesis, diagnosis and management. Clin Otolaryngol. 2015; 40(6):516–526

[7] Johnson J, van As-Brooks CJ, Fagerberg-Mohlin B, Finizia C. Trismus in head and neck cancer patients in Sweden: incidence and risk factors. Med Sci Monit. 2010; 16(6):CR278–CR282

[8] Weber C, Dommerich S, Pau HW, Kramp B. Limited mouth opening after primary therapy of head and neck cancer. Oral Maxillofac Surg. 2010; 14(3): 169–173

[9] Pauli N, Johnson J, Finizia C, Andréll P. The incidence of trismus and long-term impact on health-related quality of life in patients with head and neck cancer. Acta Oncol. 2013; 52(6):1137–1145

[10] Wang CJ, Huang EY, Hsu HC, Chen HC, Fang FM, Hsiung CY. The degree and time-course assessment of radiation-induced trismus occurring after radiotherapy for nasopharyngeal cancer. Laryngoscope. 2005; 115(8): 1458–1460

[11] Okunieff P, Augustine E, Hicks JE, et al. Pentoxifylline in the treatment of radiation-induced fibrosis. J Clin Oncol. 2004; 22(11):2207–2213

[12] Goldstein M, Maxymiw WG, Cummings BJ, Wood RE. The effects of antitumor irradiation on mandibular opening and mobility: a prospective study of 58 patients. Oral Surg Oral Med Oral Pathol Oral Radiol Endod. 1999; 88(3):365–373

[13] Stubblefield MD, Manfield L, Riedel ER. A preliminary report on the efficacy of a dynamic jaw opening device (dynasplint trismus system) as part of the multimodal treatment of trismus in patients with head and neck cancer. Arch Phys Med Rehabil. 2010; 91(8):1278–1282

[14] Yeh SA, Tang Y, Lui CC, Huang YJ, Huang EY. Treatment outcomes and late complications of 849 patients with nasopharyngeal carcinoma treated with radiotherapy alone. Int J Radiat Oncol Biol Phys. 2005; 62(3):672–679

[15] van der Molen L, Heemsbergen WD, de Jong R, et al. Dysphagia and trismus after concomitant chemo-intensity-modulated radiation therapy (chemo-IMRT) in advanced head and neck cancer; dose-effect relationships for swallowing and mastication structures. Radiother Oncol. 2013; 106(3): 364–369

[16] Louise Kent M, Brennan MT, Noll JL, et al. Radiation-induced trismus in head and neck cancer patients. Support Care Cancer. 2008; 16(3):305–309

[17] Lee R, Slevin N, Musgrove B, Swindell R, Molassiotis A. Prediction of post-treatment trismus in head and neck cancer patients. Br J Oral Maxillofac Surg. 2012; 50(4):328–332

[18] Hsiung CY, Huang EY, Ting HM, Huang HY. Intensity-modulated radiotherapy for nasopharyngeal carcinoma: the reduction of radiation-induced trismus. Br J Radiol. 2008; 81(970):809–814

[19] King GE, Scheetz J, Jacob RF, Martin JW. Electrotherapy and hyperbaric oxygen: promising treatments for postradiation complications. J Prosthet Dent. 1989; 62(3):331–334

[20] Chua DT, Lo C, Yuen J, Foo YC. A pilot study of pentoxifylline in the treatment of radiation-induced trismus. Am J Clin Oncol. 2001; 24(4):366–369

[21] Lennox AJ, Shafer JP, Hatcher M, Beil J, Funder SJ. Pilot study of impedance-controlled microcurrent therapy for managing radiation-induced fibrosis in head-and-neck cancer patients. Int J Radiat Oncol Biol Phys. 2002; 54(1):23–34

[22] Tang Y, Shen Q, Wang Y, Lu K, Wang Y, Peng Y. A randomized prospective study of rehabilitation therapy in the treatment of radiation-induced dysphagia and trismus. Strahlenther Onkol. 2011; 187(1):39–44

[23] Kamstra JI, Jager-Wittenaar H, Dijkstra PU, et al. Oral symptoms and functional outcome related to oral and oropharyngeal cancer. Support Care Cancer. 2011; 19(9):1327–1333

[24] Bensadoun RJ, Riesenbeck D, Lockhart PB, Elting LS, Spijkervet FK, Brennan MT, Trismus Section, Oral Care Study Group, Multinational Association for Supportive Care in Cancer (MASCC)/International Society of Oral Oncology (ISOO). A systematic review of trismus induced by cancer therapies in head and neck cancer patients. Support Care Cancer. 2010; 18(8):1033–1038

[25] Ren WH, Ao HW, Lin Q, Xu ZG, Zhang B. Efficacy of mouth opening exercises in treating trismus after maxillectomy. Chin Med J (Engl). 2013; 126(14):2666–2669

[26] van der Molen L, van Rossum MA, Rasch CR, Smeele LE, Hilgers FJ. Two-year results of a prospective preventive swallowing rehabilitation trial in patients treated with chemoradiation for advanced head and neck cancer. Eur Arch Otorhinolaryngol. 2014; 271(5):1257–1270

[27] Pauli N, Fagerberg-Mohlin B, Andréll P, Finizia C. Exercise intervention for the treatment of trismus in head and neck cancer. Acta Oncol. 2014; 53(4):502–509

[28] Pauli N, Svensson U, Karlsson T, Finizia C. Exercise intervention for the treatment of trismus in head and neck cancer—a prospective two-year follow-up study. Acta Oncol. 2016; 55(6):686–692

[29] Barañano CF, Rosenthal EL, Morgan BA, McColloch NL, Magnuson JS. Dynasplint for the management of trismus after treatment of upper aerodigestive tract cancer: a retrospective study. Ear Nose Throat J. 2011; 90(12):584–590

[30] Bhrany AD, Izzard M, Wood AJ, Futran ND. Coronoidectomy for the treatment of trismus in head and neck cancer patients. Laryngoscope. 2007; 117(11): 1952–1956

[31] Miloro M, Ghali GE, Larsen PE, Waite PD, eds. Peterson's Principles of Oral and Maxillofacial Surgery. 3rd ed. Shelton, CT: People's Medical Publishing House; 2011

Section IX

Considerations for Recurrent and Metastatic Oral Cavity Cancers

IX

48 Management of Locoregional Recurrent Oral Cavity Cancers

Natasha Cohen, Mark El-Deiry, H. Michael Baddour, and Mihir R. Patel

Summary
Locoregionally recurrent oral cavity cancers occur in up to half of all patients presenting with oral cavity cancers. These tumors are often more aggressive than the index tumor and are associated with poor survival. Various clinical, pathologic, and genetic factors have been associated with increased likelihood of locoregional recurrences. Diagnosis can be challenging since recurrent tumors can mimic side effects of surgical and adjuvant treatments. Current evidence suggests surgical salvage offers the best chance of cure but is associated with significant morbidity.

Keywords: recurrent oral cavity cancer, squamous cell, salvage surgery

48.1 Introduction

Although the incidence of oral cavity cancer (OCC) has been decreasing in North America, it remains one of the most commonly diagnosed cancers worldwide.[1] It is important to understand the pathophysiology of oral cavity carcinoma which predisposes to locoregional recurrence (LRR) in order to optimize the success of primary curative therapy, as well as to undertake successful treatment of LRR. LRR refers to evidence of cancer at the site of primary disease (local) and/or the local draining lymph node basin (regional) after completion of curative treatment. Timely diagnosis of recurrent cancer improves the likelihood of cure; therefore, a high level of clinical suspicion and close follow-up during the high-risk period of follow-up are necessary. This chapter will focus on discussing the epidemiology of recurrent oral cavity cancer (rOCC), risk factors for recurrence, presentation and diagnosis of rOCC, as well as management strategies in this complex disease process.

48.2 Epidemiology: Incidence, Causes, and Clinical Characteristics

The oral cavity is divided into subsites, which include the oral tongue, floor of mouth, hard palate, upper and lower alveolus and gingiva, and buccal mucosa, which is composed of the retromolar trigone, mucosa of the upper and lower lips, cheek mucosa, and the upper and lower buccoalveolar sulci.[2,3] The current standard of care treatment for OCC is comprised of surgical excision with or without adjuvant radiation or chemoradiation.[4,5] Indications for adjuvant radiotherapy include close or positive resection margins, extracapsular nodal extension (ENE), perineural invasion (PNI), N2 or N3 nodal disease, and vascular invasion,[6,7] whereas ENE and positive margins are indications for the addition of chemotherapy to adjuvant treatment.[8,9] Over 80% of patients who present with early stage (T1–T2, N0–N1) OCCs will experience cure with standard therapy. However, nearly half of all patients with OCCs present with locoregionally advanced disease (T3–T4, N2–N3),[10,11] which carries an increased likelihood of developing recurrent disease. In this population, recurrence rates have been reported between 20 and 50%,[12–14] with local recurrences occurring more frequently than regional recurrences (65 vs 25%, respectively).[14]

Although presence of nodal metastases at the time of diagnosis is the most significant prognostic factor for regional recurrence,[15] other factors affecting the propensity for oral cancer to recur include tumor thickness, margin status, histological grade, and extracapsular spread of metastatic nodal disease.[15–18] OCCs have a propensity for bilateral nodal disease, which occurs due to certain OCC subsites having crossover lymphatic drainage, as well as absence of barriers to spread, predisposing to direct invasion to contralateral tissue.[19,20] Therefore, adequate primary treatment of the draining lymph node basin needs to be undertaken at the time of primary treatment to prevent local recurrences. Preservation of the submandibular gland can be considered to improve patients' quality of life by maintaining saliva production which is at risk of decreasing with postoperative radiation treatments. However, careful patient selection is important to avoid an increased risk of LRR. A study by Lanzer et al[21] found that patients with oral cancers originating in the tongue or floor of mouth had higher rates of LRR when the ipsilateral submandibular gland was not resected as part of the neck dissection. Lymph node recurrences were observed in 28.5% of the patients whose submandibular gland was preserved compared with 2.2% where the gland was removed as part of the neck dissection ($p < 0.001$). Elective neck dissections play an important role in the management of OCC with N0 disease, since occult nodal metastases occur in over 20 to 30% of OCC patients.[22,23] The incidence of contralateral occult metastasis has been reported to be around 10% and is statistically significantly predicted by presence of T3 or T4 primary disease, extension of the primary cancer across the midline, presence of positive ipsilateral lymph nodes, poor differentiation on histologic grading, and positive surgical margins.[24,25] A study by Capote-Moreno et al[25] showed that contralateral nodal disease is associated with poor locoregional control and survival outcomes, with 5-year, cause-specific survival rate of 41.2% for those with contralateral nodal metastases compared with 70% in those without contralateral lymph nodes ($p < 0.01$).[25] The study also found that contralateral lymphadenopathy did not occur in primaries originating in the retromolar area and the hard palate, were uncommon in buccal mucosa and gum cancers (3.2 and 5.1%, respectively), and occurred most commonly in cancers of the floor of mouth, followed by tongue cancers (11 and 7.2%, respectively).[25]

There has been a long controversy regarding the pathological features of oral malignancies which should trigger neck dissection in order to prevent regional recurrences, especially in the context of small tumors (T1 or T2). Depth of invasion of the OCC primary has been known to be associated with the development of nodal disease for nearly four decades, with landmark studies published by Spiro et al from Memorial Sloan Kettering as early as 1986.[26,27] These studies identified that tumors with a

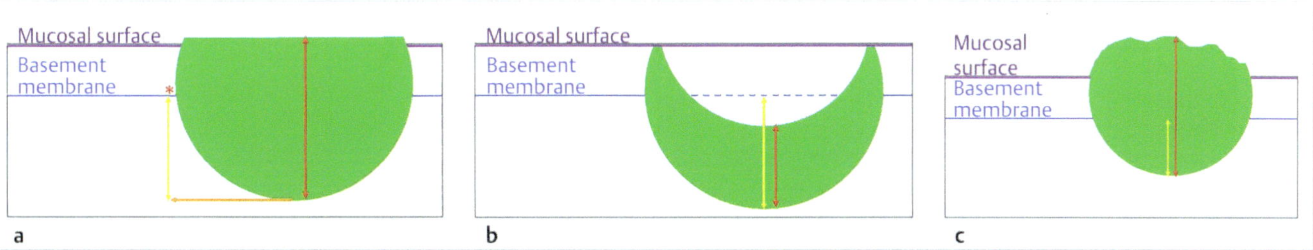

Fig. 48.1 **(a)** Tumor thickness compared with depth of invasion. The graph shows the tumor in green, the depth of invasion in yellow, and tumor thickness in red. The depth of invasion is calculated by measuring the distance between the basement at the adjacent normal mucosa to the level of greatest invasion (*orange line*). Tumor thickness is defined as the distance between the most superficial aspect of the tumor to the level of greatest invasion. **(b)** Tumor thickness in an ulcerative cancer. This image demonstrates that in an ulcerative tumor, tumor thickness will underestimate the depth of invasion. **(c)** Tumor thickness with an exophytic pattern of growth. This image demonstrates an exophytic tumor which overestimates the depth of invasion.

depth greater than 2 mm were associated with a higher rate of treatment failure, and the depth of invasion cutoffs better predicted overall survival than conventional T stage based on tumor size. These studies also emphasized the importance of performing elective neck dissections while nodal metastases remained clinically occult to improve patient outcomes. Subsequent studies continued to show an association between tumor thickness and LRR, but cutoffs for tumor thickness as an indication for elective neck dissections have varied between 2 and 10 mm,[17,26,28–31] and little consensus exists to guide clinical care. This may be due in part to variability in the patterns of tumor growth, as tumor thickness has not reliably reflected the differences between endophytic and exophytic invasion patterns[17] (see ▶ Fig. 48.1a–c). More recently, tumor depth as determined in relation to the basement membrane has been shown to closely and more reliably correlate with disease-free survival. In fact, a recent study by Shim et al[18] found that 5 years disease-free survival in patients with T1 and T2 and N0 or N1 disease was 66% for tumors with 5 mm or greater depth of invasion, compared with 92% for tumors with less than 5 mm depth of invasion ($p = 0.013$). As a result of these findings, the 8th edition of the American Joint Committee on Cancer (AJCC) staging, which has been adopted since January 1, 2018, has now included depth of invasion as a criterion for T staging in order to better reflect prognostic features of cancers into the current staging system.[32]

Tumor resection margin status is also particularly relevant in predicting the likelihood of recurrences. In fact, Loree and Strong[33] first demonstrated this in 1990, showing that a positive margin at the time of surgical excision doubled the rate of recurrence. In this study, patients with negative margins were found to have a recurrence rate of 18% compared with 36% for those with positive margins. Of those with positive margins, patients with in-situ carcinoma at the margins had the highest recurrence rate (44%), followed by microinvasion (36%), margins within 0.5 cm or close margins (35%), and premalignant changes at the margins (33%). They also found that positive margins were more likely to be found in primaries of the buccal mucosa (58%), followed by upper and lower gingiva (42 and 39%, respectively), whereas primaries of the retromolar trigone, tongue, and floor of mouth had the lowest rates of positive margins (24, 27, and 31%, respectively). Moreover, increasing T stage was positively correlated with positive margins and likelihood of recurrence.[33] Since then, studies have confirmed similar findings for reduced overall survival and increased recurrence rate for patients with pathologically positive surgical margins.[34]

Another feature of primary OCC that predicts poor outcomes following primary treatment and higher incidence of recurrence is the subsite of the primary cancer. Although relatively common in Southeast Asia due to use of betel quid,[3] OCCs originating in the buccal mucosa comprises roughly 10% of oral cancers in the Western World; yet they are associated with significantly decreased survival compared to other oral cavity subsites.[35] In fact, the 2- and 5-year disease-specific survival (DSS) were 68.0 and 57.3% compared with 73.4 and 63.8% for other oral cavity subsites, and the overall survival (OS) was 60.49 and 41% for buccal cancers compared with 66.8 and 51.1% for other OCC subsites.[35] Compared to the other oral cancer subsite counterparts, buccal cancers are more likely to present with nodal metastases, and at more advanced local T stage, and affect older patients more than other OCCs.[35–37] In fact, occult metastases occur in 32% of buccal cancers, and 43% of buccal cancers develop nodal metastases.[38] Moreover, nodal metastases occur in over 40% of T1 and T2 disease.[38] It is unclear why buccal cancers present at more advanced stages than OCCs of other subsites, but it is believed that identification of premalignant or early disease may be more challenging than OCCs of other subsites.[35]

Advances in genetic sequencing have allowed us to identify genetic factors that predict aggressive clinicopathologic behavior of oral cavity tumors. For instance, the number of copy number alterations (or CNAs) such as losses or gains of certain chromosomal regions can predict clinical outcomes better, where smaller numbers of CNAs correlate with a more favorable prognosis.[39] This genetic subset of oral cavity malignancies arises from genetic mutations and exhibits a three-gene pattern of an activating mutation of HRAS, an inactivating mutation of CASP8, and a wild-type TP53. These changes are thought to result from chromosome 7 amplifications which include an EGFR locus. Conversely, inactivation or loss of the TGFBR2 gene has also been identified in certain OCC, and is associated with poor prognostic outcomes such as increased risk of metastasis.[40]

48.3 Clinical Presentation

Over 80% of recurrences occur within the first 2 years of treatment.[41–44] After completion of curative treatment of primary oral cavity malignancies, ongoing follow-up is maintained and early identification of recurrences is important to ensure timely salvage treatment if feasible. A thorough history and physical examination are critical for identifying recurrent disease. Signs and symptoms of recurrent locoregional disease can be similar to those of the original presentation of malignancy and can also be confused for side effects of surgical or adjuvant treatment;[45] therefore, maintaining high clinical suspicion for recurrence is essential for identification of recurrent disease. Most patients present with local rather than regional recurrences,[16] with signs and symptoms including new or worsening pain, non-healing oral ulcer, bleeding, dysphagia, odynophagia, trismus, decreased tongue mobility, tooth loss, and numbness of the tongue, oral cavity, lips, and/or face.[44,46] An example of this diagnostic challenge is the difficult to treat sequela of osteoradionecrosis caused by radiotherapy to the mandible, which causes a range of symptoms such as pain, halitosis, pathological fracture of the mandible, and ensuing weight loss. A retrospective case series found that 3% of resected osteoradionecrosis specimens contained unexpected evidence of malignancy.[47]

48.4 Diagnosis and Evaluation

According to the 8th edition of AJCC, recurrent cancer is defined by the presence of cancer after a disease-free period[2,48] following treatment with curative intent, and is not to be mistaken with residual or persistent disease. Although the AJCC does not suggest an explicit cutoff for the duration of a "disease-free period," to prevent confusion between persistent and recurrent disease, experts have suggested 3 to 6 months as the lag time between completion of treatment and designation of cancer as recurrent.[13,14] According to the 2018 National Comprehensive Cancer Network (NCCN) guidelines for treatment of head and neck cancers, follow-up for oral cancers include a complete head and neck examination with fiberoptic or mirror laryngoscopy every 1–3 months for the first year, every 2–6 months for the second year, and then every 4–8 months until 5 years post-treatment.[49] After 5 years, screening is recommended on a yearly basis. Repeat imaging is recommended within 6 months of completion of therapy and subsequently for worrisome signs or symptoms or to evaluate areas that are difficult to examine.[50] The type of imaging used for follow-up assessment should remain consistent with preoperative imaging for ease of comparison, and typically consists of computed tomography (CT) and/or magnetic resonance imaging (MRI), ideally contrast-enhanced.[51] Ultrasonography can also play a role in identifying cervical lymphadenopathy, but contrast-enhanced CT (CECT) imaging remains superior due to its increased diagnostic yield when compared to ultrasound and/or MRI.[52,53] The local effects of surgery and adjuvant radiotherapy and chemotherapy lead to many changes in tissue properties, making it difficult to differentiate the nature of imaging findings, which can be caused by reactive inflammatory processes, scarring, and edema or may represent recurrent disease.[54,55] An imaging modality that can help differentiate posttreatment changes is positron emission tomography (PET)-CT, which has a high sensitivity and specificity for recurrence.[56] Nonetheless, risk stratification for likelihood of LRR based on such imaging has long been challenging and imprecise. In an effort to overcome this challenge, a standardized reporting template[57] was created, similar to those

Table 48.1 Neck Imaging Reporting and Data System (NI-RADS)

NI-RADS Category	Imaging finding	Management
Category 1 No evidence of recurrence	Expected posttreatment change (tissue distortion, scar, radiation change)	Routine surveillance (6 months typically)
Category 2 Low suspicion of recurrence	• Ill-defined abnormality with only mild enhancement and/or 18F-FDG uptake • Subclassification: • 2a: superficial/ mucosal surface • 2b: deep abnormality of < 1 cm • 2c: deep abnormality of > 1 cm	Direct inspection for mucosal findings or short (3-month) follow-up with CECT or PET for deep findings
Category 3 High suspicion of recurrence	Discrete, new, or enlarging lesions with intense enhancement and/or focal FDG uptake	Biopsy
Category 4 Known recurrence	Known recurrence, pathologically proved or definite radiologic or clinical progression	

Abbreviations: CECT, contrast-enhanced computed tomography; FDG, Fluorodeoxyglucose; PET, positron emission tomography.

already existing for malignancies of the breast and prostate. This reporting template for CECT and PET-CT imaging named the Neck Imaging Reporting and Data System (NI-RADS) stratifies patients into four risk categories and proposes management strategies based on NI-RADS Category (see ▸ Table 48.1). The classification system was accurate for identifying primary recurrences, nodal recurrences, and combined sites (area under the curve or AUC, respectively, 0.787, 0.712, and 0.756; $p < 0.001$), and was slightly more accurate for CECT than for PET-CT (AUC 0.779 vs. 0.709).

Ultimately, assessment of rOCC should aim at differentiating and stratifying patients into those amenable to salvage curative therapy and those who are better geared toward palliative therapy. Ability to resect disease is an important factor in making this distinction and is usually defined by encasement of the carotid artery, invasion of prevertebral fascia, and invasion of intracranial structures or mediastinal vessels. Other relevant factors that can affect the decision of pursuing further treatment include the patient's willingness or ability to complete further treatment, performance status, surgeon's comfort with surgical approach, and ability to reconstruct the ensuing defect.[5] Therefore, it is especially important for physicians to set realistic expectations of cure and functional outcomes for patients to make informed care decisions.

48.5 Anatomic Considerations/ Relevant Anatomy

OCC recurrences have poorer prognosis than some of the other common head and neck malignancies such as laryngeal cancer.[20,58] Therefore, careful assessment of the extent of locoregionally recurrent disease should address the structures involved for treatment planning. When possible, salvage surgery has the best oncologic outcomes, whereas additional radiotherapy with or without chemotherapy rarely offers successful long-term cure.[59] When recurrent OCC does not present with unresectable features, it is important to consider other factors that may affect the ability of salvage surgery to achieve cure. Since many OCC patients receive adjuvant radiation therapy with primary treatment, it may be difficult to differentiate posttreatment changes and side effects from tumor invasion. Since adjuvant treatment of recurrent disease is often limited, it is important to be prepared for radical surgery at the time of salvage. In fact, unlike primary resection margins which are considered adequate when measured to be 5 mm,[60–62] margins in the salvage setting may require up to for 1.5 cm peripherally and deep.[63] Since adjacent uninvolved native tissue is typically less resilient and more fibrotic in the recurrent setting, planning for reconstruction is essential and often involves free tissue transfer. Specific reconstructive options will be discussed later in the chapter, but it is important to mention that the resecting surgeon should be mindful to preserve any available arterial and venous branches for vascular anastomoses. Although rotational flaps can be used in the salvage setting, the reconstructive surgeon should be careful and confident that the vascularity of the tissue to be transposed has not been compromised. For example, the submental artery island flap pedicle is often ligated at the time of a level 1 neck dissection, making the vascularity of this flap unreliable in the salvage setting. Another example is the supraclavicular artery island flap which relies on the integrity of the transverse cervical artery and which can be compromised by a level 4 or 5 neck dissection.[64] However, the supraclavicular artery island flap has the advantage of being typically outside of the prior radiation field, making the tissue more desirable for reconstruction than that of previously radiated areas. Confirming the integrity of the blood supply is important in this setting and can be accomplished by preoperative imaging (e.g., computed tomography angiography [CTA] or magnetic resonance angiography [MRA]). Moreover, surgical planning should include options for soft tissue as well as bony reconstruction and should consider the decreased elasticity and resiliency of the neck tissue which will need to accommodate increased volume, which is different from the nonsalvage surgical setting where performing neck dissections leaves ample space to accommodate tissue without risking the vascularity of the reconstruction.

48.6 Surgical Considerations and Approaches

As previously mentioned, salvage surgery for OCCs carries unique challenges due to the biologically aggressive nature of rOCC, as well as due to sequelae from primary treatment. Whereas primary surgical therapy can be geared toward limiting the surgical morbidity of resection without compromising oncologic integrity, salvage surgery can rarely accomplish both due to the adverse healing effects of prior surgery superimposed with the effects of adjuvant radiation/chemoradiation. Therefore, primary closure and rotational flaps with random blood supply should not be considered viable options due to the high likelihood of wound breakdown and adverse outcomes associated with such options. As such, free tissue transfer is essential to improve functional outcomes, achieve reasonable cosmesis, and prevent chronic wound healing issues in these patients. Moreover, in the context of rOCC, especially of the tongue and floor of mouth, total glossectomy may be necessary for adequate oncologic margins (▶ Fig. 48.2). Historically, laryngectomy was performed concurrently with total glossectomy in order to maintain a safe airway and prevent recurrent aspiration pneumonia.[65,66] However, with improvements in reconstruction with free tissue transfer, severe aspiration requiring laryngectomy is rare and there is an increasing body of literature that suggests that laryngeal preservation is safe in the era of free tissue reconstruction.[67]

48.6.1 Defect Analysis and Reconstruction

Analysis of the size and nature of the defect will determine the appropriate reconstructive options. Namely, defects can be qualified as involving skin, mucosa, and bone, and reconstruction should aim to replace components in order to optimize

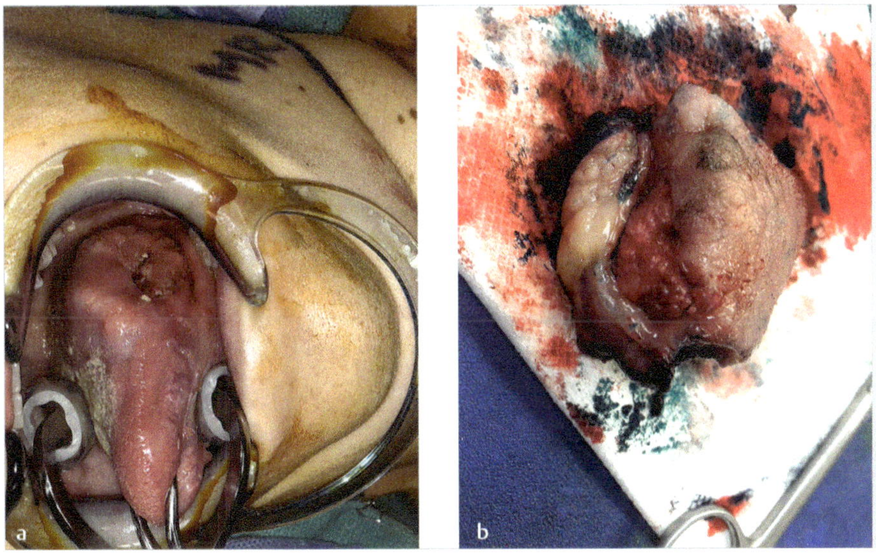

Fig. 48.2 38-year-old female, nonsmoker, with a rT3N0M0 tongue squamous cell carcinoma. **(a)** Intraoral view prior to resection reveals an endophytic tumor involving the left lateral surface. **(b)** Subtotal glossectomy specimen evaluated for margins and depth of invasion.

safety and function of the reconstruction. The introduction of well-vascularized tissue that has not undergone the effects of prior surgery and/or radiation helps minimize the risk of long-term complications.[68]

48.6.2 Radial Forearm Free Flap

The radial forearm free flap is one of the most commonly used free flaps. This fasciocutaneous flap is used for soft tissue reconstruction and has the advantage of having a low flap loss rate, reliable harvest anatomy, and low donor site morbidity.[69] Bulk can be provided by harvest of a proximal fat pad or by including the brachioradialis muscle, and sensation can be restored by anastomosing the lateral antebrachial cutaneous nerve to local nerves such as the lingual, inferior alveolar, or others as indicated by the area of flap inset.[70] An osteocutaneous alternative allows for up to 10 cm of bone available for harvest. The main disadvantage of the radial forearm free flap is the limited amount of tissue available. In the salvage setting, larger flaps may be required, and radial forearm free flap tissue bulk can be variable depending on patient's habitus, limiting its role in certain reconstructions. Some authors have used the beavertail modification to the radial forearm free flap, which allows the inclusion of vascularized fatty tissue to enhance the tissue bulk for an otherwise thin flap.[71,72] Another advantage of this flap is the ability to harvest vascularized tendon that is easily used to restore oral competence in resections involving the lower lip.[73] Donor site morbidity is considered low except in the setting of bone harvest where plating is required to reduce the risk of radial bone stress fractures. The harvest site is closed with a skin graft and the arm is immobilized in a splint for about 7 days.

48.6.3 Anterolateral Thigh Flap

The anterolateral thigh (ALT) flap is commonly used for reconstructing head and neck defects and offers a large tissue surface area with a greater amount of bulk than the radial forearm flap.[74] This free flap is supplied by the descending branch of the lateral circumflex femoral artery and two venae comitantes, which supply septocutaneous or musculocutaneous perforators through the vastus lateralis muscle. Moreover, the lateral femoral cutaneous nerve which is harvested with this flap can be used to innervate the free flap by performing a neurorrhaphy with the lingual nerve, which has been found to generate good swallowing outcomes despite total glossectomy with laryngeal preservation.[75] The ALT flap has the main disadvantage of having a higher flap failure rate than the radial forearm, which is due to the inherent anatomic variability in the origin of the cutaneous perforators providing the blood supply to this flap.[76] Moreover, the pedicle length is shorter than that of the radial forearm free flap, ranging between 8 and 16 cm,[77] which can pose a challenge in the salvage setting where availability of vascular donor vessels can be limited. Although tissue bulk is considered a desirable feature of the ALT flap, it can also be a limitation of this flap, but can be managed by performing a suprafascial harvest and thinning to tailor its use to the head and neck.[77,78] Donor site morbidity is minimal since the primary site can almost always be closed primarily despite large amounts of tissue being harvested.[79]

48.6.4 Fibula Free Flap

The fibula free flap is the workhorse for bony reconstructions of the head and neck. It provides up to 30 cm of good quality bone with reliable cortical thickness, which is important for dental rehabilitation (▶ Fig. 48.3). It can be harvested as an osteocutaneous flap to provide tissue for mucosal or skin reconstructions. Its blood supply is the peroneal artery and two venae comitantes that are frequently good size matches for vessels in the neck, and its pedicle is long (up to 15 cm), allowing for greater flexibility in the salvage setting which may be vessel-depleted. However, vascular insufficiency and unfavorable anatomy can pose a challenge when harvesting the fibular free flap; therefore, vascular mapping must be performed preoperatively (e.g., angiography).[80] In cases where the fibular skin paddle is insufficient to reconstruct the defect, a double flap can be used to achieve successful functional and cosmetic outcomes.[81]

48.6.5 Scapular and Parascapular Free Flap

The scapular free flap is a good alternative for defects requiring both bony as well as large soft tissue reconstructions. Supplied

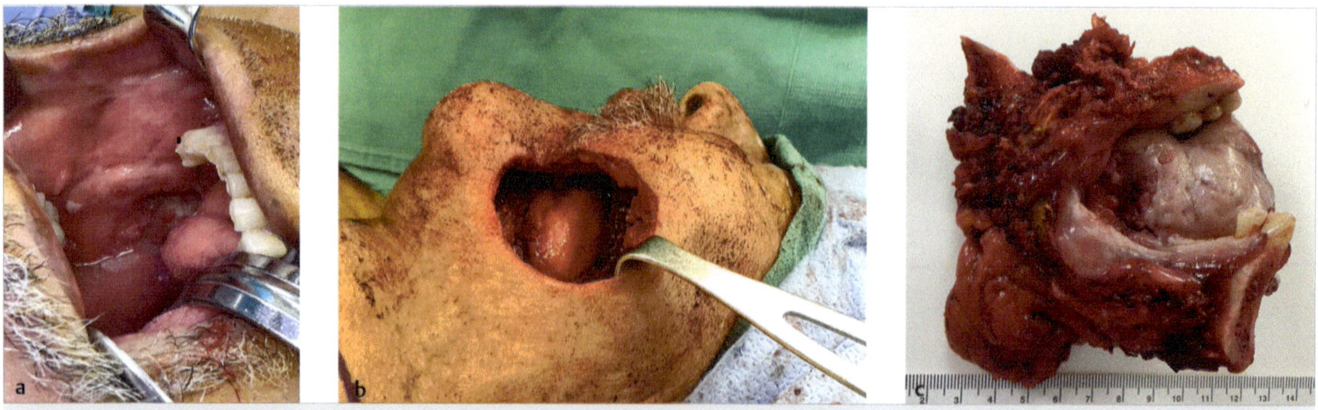

Fig. 48.3 77-year-old male, former smoker, with rT4bN0M0 buccal cavity squamous cell carcinoma. **(a)** Intraoral view of tumor demonstrates deceptively small appearing tumor. **(b)** Radical resection of tumor and surgical defect that was reconstructed with a scapula free flap. **(c)** En bloc resection of the mandible and maxilla, with level Ib given invasion of masticator space, achieved with negative margins.

by the circumflex scapular artery, harvest of the lateral border of the scapula allows for harvest of up to 14 cm of bone with a pedicle length ranging between 11 and 14 cm.[82] Very large skin paddle can be harvested, and the muscle supplied by branches of the circumflex scapular artery such as the latissimus dorsi, teres major, or serratus muscles can be used to provide additional tissue to close large defects.

48.7 Surgical Sequelae (Short- and Long-term)

Despite offering the best chance of cure, salvage surgery for rOCC carries significant morbidity and offer poor survival outcomes. Even in carefully selected patients, recurrent squamous cell carcinoma of the oral cavity has a 30 to 50% 5-year survival following salvage surgery,[43,58,63,83,84] whereas nonsurgical treatments lead to overall survival between 9 and 17%.[20] Time to recurrence is one of the most important factors in predicting curability, with short times to recurrence predicting poorer outcomes.[43] A study by Liao et al[63] looked at specific time-to-recurrence cutoffs that predict survival outcomes, and showed that in patients with negative primary surgical margins who had early relapses within the first 10 months following primary definitive treatment, only 13% of patients remained alive at the completion of follow-up, compared with 50.5% of those with late relapses presenting 10 or more months after treatment. Five-year DSS was found to be 53.5% for late recurrences compared with 13.8% for early recurrences. Fifty percent of patients with early relapse underwent salvage treatment of which 78% had surgery with or without adjuvant radiation or chemoradiation. Of those with late recurrences, 72.6% underwent salvage treatment and of those 84% underwent salvage surgery with or without adjuvant radiation or chemoradiation.[63] The 5-year DSS and 5-year OS for patients with early recurrences who underwent salvage treatment were 38.4 and 35.8% compared with 0% for those who selected for palliative therapy. Conversely, the 5-year DSS and 5-year OS for patients with late recurrences who underwent salvage treatment were 80 and 79.2% compared with 9.3 and 12.4% for those who did not undergo salvage treatment. Multivariate analysis identified that tumor depth of 10 mm or more of the primary, distant metastases, and absence of salvage therapy significantly decreased 5-year DSS and 5-year OS in early recurrences, whereas distant metastases, neck recurrence, and absence of salvage therapy worsened the same survival outcomes in late recurrences.[63] Moreover, patients who are initially treated with surgery and radiation have a 1.3-fold increased risk of death from disease compared with those treated with surgery alone.[43] Other factors predicting poor outcomes for salvage treatment of recurrent disease include advanced primary disease, regional rather than local recurrence, and failure of initial surgery plus adjuvant chemoradiation therapy.[43] Factors that indicate good prognosis are regional recurrence in the absence of previous neck dissection, local recurrence in previously positive tumor margin resections, delayed, interrupted, or inadequately dosed radiotherapy, and recurrence outside the radiotherapy field.[43,46]

Salvage therapy for OCC also carries increased risk of infection and salivary fistula.[65] However, free flap reconstruction has been shown to lower the incidence of these complications in the salvage setting,[85] making this a critical component of salvage surgery as previously discussed. A study by Kostrzewa et al[86] found that the rates of infection and fistula were 36%, incidence of flap failure and severe hemorrhage were 11%, and over 58% of patients remained gastrostomy tube dependent for their nutritional needs. In this study, fistulas were salvaged by use of a pedicled pectoralis major flap, which is standard practice at our center as well. Moreover, few patients return to satisfactory diets (25% for oral cavity recurrence, 18% for neck recurrences) and other functional outcomes such as speech, public eating, and performance status are also significantly negatively impacted by salvage surgery.[83] Moreover, these outcomes are all negatively impacted by presalvage advanced stage.

Despite the narrow therapeutic ratio in the head and neck, re-irradiation following salvage surgery has been undertaken with some success. However, toxicity is significant, with a study from the Dana Farber Institute describing 91% of re-irradiated patients developed at least 1 grade 3 acute toxicity and 46% developed late grade 3 toxicity. Moreover, 11% of their cohort died of salvage treatment side effects with no evidence of disease, with causes of death including aspiration, oropharyngeal hemorrhage, and infection.[87] Nonetheless, a systematic review of studies addressing re-irradiation concluded that re-irradiation conferred a 10–30% survival benefit and should be offered in high-risk cases following salvage surgery.[68] Evidence suggests that microvascular reconstruction helps to prevent major complications such as carotid rupture and tissue necrosis.[88] Brachytherapy has been described as a reasonable alternative to re-irradiation with external beam radiation therapy to minimize morbidity when exceeding normal tissue tolerance to radiation (see Chapter 34). In fact, when used in the adjuvant setting alongside external beam therapy, it has been shown to improve local tumor control rates by up to 60%, and 43% when used alone following salvage surgery.[89] However, severe local side effects are common, and include wound healing issues, tissue breakdown, infection, and osteonecrosis.[89]

48.8 Conclusion

Recurrent oral cavity cancer is a complex entity within head and neck malignancies and requires a multidisciplinary approach. In fact, members of the team such speech language pathologists, nutritionists, occupational therapists, physiotherapists, and other allied health care providers are invaluable for assessing, maintaining, and rehabilitating patients with rOCC. However, it is important to be realistic when discussing either surgical or nonsurgical outcomes, as well as identifying those who are best suited for a palliative approach. Counseling the patient for smoking and drinking cessation as well as cessation of other carcinogenic exposures is necessary for improving the patient's oncologic and overall healing outcomes.

Key Points

- Locoregionally recurrent OCCs occur in up to half of all patients presenting with OCCs.
- These tumors are often more aggressive than the index tumor and are associated with poor survival.
- Various clinical, pathologic, and genetic factors have been associated with increased likelihood of LRRs.

- Diagnosis can be challenging since recurrent tumors can mimic side effects of surgical and adjuvant treatments.
- Surgical salvage offers the best chance of cure but is associated with significant morbidity.

References

[1] Chaturvedi AK, Anderson WF, Lortet-Tieulent J, et al. Worldwide trends in incidence rates for oral cavity and oropharyngeal cancers. J Clin Oncol. 2013; 31(36):4550–4559

[2] Brierley J, Gospodarowicz MK, Wittekind C. TNM Classification of Malignant Tumours. 8th ed. ed. Chichester, West Sussex, UK; Hoboken, NJ: John Wiley & Sons, Inc.; 2017

[3] Chi TH, Yuan CH, Chen RF. Screening for oral cavity cancer: a 1-year experience of a regional hospital in Taiwan. JNMA J Nepal Med Assoc. 2014; 52 (195):902–906

[4] da Silva SD, Hier M, Mlynarek A, Kowalski LP, Alaoui-Jamali MA. Recurrent oral cancer: current and emerging therapeutic approaches. Front Pharmacol. 2012; 3:149

[5] Kerawala C, Roques T, Jeannon JP, Bisase B. Oral cavity and lip cancer: United Kingdom National Multidisciplinary Guidelines. J Laryngol Otol. 2016; 130 S2:S83–S89

[6] Bernier J, Cooper JS, Pajak TF, et al. Defining risk levels in locally advanced head and neck cancers: a comparative analysis of concurrent postoperative radiation plus chemotherapy trials of the EORTC (#22931) and RTOG (# 9501). Head Neck. 2005; 27(10):843–850

[7] Liao CT, Chang JT, Wang HM, et al. Analysis of risk factors of predictive local tumor control in oral cavity cancer. Ann Surg Oncol. 2008; 15(3):915–922

[8] Cooper JS, Zhang Q, Pajak TF, et al. Long-term follow-up of the RTOG 9501/ intergroup phase III trial: postoperative concurrent radiation therapy and chemotherapy in high-risk squamous cell carcinoma of the head and neck. Int J Radiat Oncol Biol Phys. 2012; 84(5):1198–1205

[9] Lin CY, Lee LY, Huang SF, et al. Treatment outcome of combined modalities for buccal cancers: unilateral or bilateral neck radiation? Int J Radiat Oncol Biol Phys. 2008; 70(5):1373–1381

[10] Olsen MH, Bøje CR, Kjær TK, et al. Socioeconomic position and stage at diagnosis of head and neck cancer—a nationwide study from DAHANCA. Acta Oncol. 2015; 54(5):759–766

[11] Funk GF, Karnell LH, Robinson RA, Zhen WK, Trask DK, Hoffman HT. Presentation, treatment, and outcome of oral cavity cancer: a National Cancer Data Base report. Head Neck. 2002; 24(2):165–180

[12] Mücke T, Mitchell DA, Ritschl LM, et al. Influence of tumor volume on survival in patients with oral squamous cell carcinoma. J Cancer Res Clin Oncol. 2015; 141(6):1007–1011

[13] Liu SA, Wong YK, Lin JC, et al. Impact of recurrence interval on survival of oral cavity squamous cell carcinoma patients after local relapse. Otolaryngol Head Neck Surg. 2007; 136(1):112–8

[14] Mücke T, Wagenpfeil S, Kesting MR, Hölzle F, Wolff KD. Recurrence interval affects survival after local relapse of oral cancer. Oral Oncol. 2009; 45(8):687–691

[15] Denis F, Garaud P, Manceau A, et al. [Prognostic value of the number of involved nodes after neck dissection in oropharyngeal and oral cavity carcinoma]. Cancer Radiother. 2001; 5(1):12–22

[16] Woolgar JA, Rogers SN, Lowe D, Brown JS, Vaughan ED. Cervical lymph node metastasis in oral cancer: the importance of even microscopic extracapsular spread. Oral Oncol. 2003; 39(2):130–137

[17] Kirita T, Okabe S, Izumo T, Sugimura M. Risk factors for the postoperative local recurrence of tongue carcinoma. J Oral Maxillofac Surg. 1994; 52(2): 149–154

[18] Shim SJ, Cha J, Koom WS, et al. Clinical outcomes for T1-2N0-1 oral tongue cancer patients underwent surgery with and without postoperative radiotherapy. Radiat Oncol. 2010; 5:43

[19] Fan S, Tang QL, Lin YJ, et al. A review of clinical and histological parameters associated with contralateral neck metastases in oral squamous cell carcinoma. Int J Oral Sci. 2011; 3(4):180–191

[20] Ho AS, Kraus DH, Ganly I, Lee NY, Shah JP, Morris LG. Decision making in the management of recurrent head and neck cancer. Head Neck. 2014; 36(1): 144–151

[21] Lanzer M, Gander T, Lübbers HT, Metzler P, Bredell M, Reinisch S. Preservation of ipsilateral submandibular gland is ill advised in cancer of the floor of the mouth or tongue. Laryngoscope. 2014; 124(9):2070–2074

[22] Wensing BM, Merkx MA, Krabbe PF, Marres HA, Van den Hoogen FJ. Oral squamous cell carcinoma and a clinically negative neck: the value of follow-up. Head Neck. 2011; 33(10):1400–1405

[23] O'Brien CJ, Traynor SJ, McNeil E, McMahon JD, Chaplin JM. The use of clinical criteria alone in the management of the clinically negative neck among patients with squamous cell carcinoma of the oral cavity and oropharynx. Arch Otolaryngol Head Neck Surg. 2000; 126(3):360–365

[24] Koo BS, Lim YC, Lee JS, Choi EC. Management of contralateral N0 neck in oral cavity squamous cell carcinoma. Head Neck. 2006; 28(10):896–901

[25] Capote-Moreno A, Naval L, Muñoz-Guerra MF, Sastre J, Rodríguez-Campo FJ. Prognostic factors influencing contralateral neck lymph node metastases in oral and oropharyngeal carcinoma. J Oral Maxillofac Surg. 2010; 68(2):268–275

[26] Spiro RH, Huvos AG, Wong GY, Spiro JD, Gnecco CA, Strong EW. Predictive value of tumor thickness in squamous carcinoma confined to the tongue and floor of the mouth. Am J Surg. 1986; 152(4):345–350

[27] Spiro RH, Spiro JD, Strong EW. Surgical approach to squamous carcinoma confined to the tongue and the floor of the mouth. Head Neck Surg. 1986; 9 (1):27–31

[28] Pinto FR, de Matos LL, Palermo FC, et al. Tumor thickness as an independent risk factor of early recurrence in oral cavity squamous cell carcinoma. Eur Arch Otorhinolaryngol. 2014; 271(6):1747–1754

[29] Balasubramanian D, Ebrahimi A, Gupta R, et al. Tumour thickness as a predictor of nodal metastases in oral cancer: comparison between tongue and floor of mouth subsites. Oral Oncol. 2014; 50(12):1165–1168

[30] O'Brien CJ, Lauer CS, Fredricks S, et al. Tumor thickness influences prognosis of T1 and T2 oral cavity cancer—but what thickness? Head Neck. 2003; 25 (11):937–945

[31] Matos LL, Manfro G, Santos RV, et al. Tumor thickness as a predictive factor of lymph node metastasis and disease recurrence in T1N0 and T2N0 squamous cell carcinoma of the oral tongue. Oral Surg Oral Med Oral Pathol Oral Radiol. 2014; 118(2):209–217

[32] Lydiatt WM, Patel SG, O'Sullivan B, et al. Head and neck cancers—major changes in the American Joint Committee on Cancer eighth edition cancer staging manual. CA Cancer J Clin. 2017; 67(2):122–137

[33] Loree TR, Strong EW. Significance of positive margins in oral cavity squamous carcinoma. Am J Surg. 1990; 160(4):410–414

[34] Jan JC, Hsu WH, Liu SA, et al. Prognostic factors in patients with buccal squamous cell carcinoma: 10-year experience. J Oral Maxillofac Surg. 2011; 69(2): 396–404

[35] Camilon PR, Stokes WA, Fuller CW, Nguyen SA, Lentsch EJ. Does buccal cancer have worse prognosis than other oral cavity cancers? Laryngoscope. 2014; 124(6):1386–1391

[36] Diaz EM, Jr, Holsinger FC, Zuniga ER, Roberts DB, Sorensen DM. Squamous cell carcinoma of the buccal mucosa: one institution's experience with 119 previously untreated patients. Head Neck. 2003; 25(4):267–273

[37] DeConde A, Miller ME, Palla B, et al. Squamous cell carcinoma of buccal mucosa: a 40-year review. Am J Otolaryngol. 2012; 33(6):673–677

[38] Lubek JE, Dyalram D, Perera EH, Liu X, Ord RA. A retrospective analysis of squamous carcinoma of the buccal mucosa: an aggressive subsite within the oral cavity. J Oral Maxillofac Surg. 2013; 71(6):1126–1131

[39] Cancer Genome Atlas N, Cancer Genome Atlas Network. Comprehensive genomic characterization of head and neck squamous cell carcinomas. Nature. 2015; 517(7536):576–582

[40] Lu SL, Herrington H, Reh D, et al. Loss of transforming growth factor-beta type II receptor promotes metastatic head-and-neck squamous cell carcinoma. Genes Dev. 2006; 20(10):1331–1342

[41] Eckardt A, Barth EL, Kokemueller H, Wegener G. Recurrent carcinoma of the head and neck: treatment strategies and survival analysis in a 20-year period. Oral Oncol. 2004; 40(4):427–432

[42] Wong LY, Wei WI, Lam LK, Yuen AP. Salvage of recurrent head and neck squamous cell carcinoma after primary curative surgery. Head Neck. 2003; 25 (11):953–959

[43] Kernohan MD, Clark JR, Gao K, Ebrahimi A, Milross CG. Predicting the prognosis of oral squamous cell carcinoma after first recurrence. Arch Otolaryngol Head Neck Surg. 2010; 136(12):1235–1239

[44] Kissun D, Magennis P, Lowe D, Brown JS, Vaughan ED, Rogers SN. Timing and presentation of recurrent oral and oropharyngeal squamous cell carcinoma and awareness in the outpatient clinic. Br J Oral Maxillofac Surg. 2006; 44(5): 371–376

[45] Halczy-Kowalik L, Wiktor A, Rzewuska A, Kowalczyk R, Wysocki R, Posio V. Compensatory mechanisms in patients after a partial or total glossectomy due to oral cancer. Dysphagia. 2015; 30(6):738–750

[46] Sharma P, Shah SV, Taneja C, Patel AM, Patel MD. A prospective study of prognostic factors for recurrence in early oral tongue cancer. J Clin Diagn Res. 2013; 7(11):2559–2562
[47] Marwan H, Green JM, III, Tursun R, Marx RE. Recurrent malignancy in osteoradionecrosis specimen. J Oral Maxillofac Surg. 2016; 74(11):2312–2316
[48] AJCC Cancer Staging Manual. New York, NY: Springer Science + Business Media; 2016
[49] Adelstein D, Gillison ML, Pfister DG, et al. NCCN guidelines insights: head and neck cancers, version 2.2017. J Natl Compr Canc Netw. 2017; 15(6):761–770
[50] Pfister DG, Spencer S, Adelstein D, et al. NCCN Clinical Practice Guidelines in Oncology - Head and Neck Cancers. 2018; February 15, 2018: https://www.nccn.org/professionals/physician_gls/pdf/head-and-neck.pdf, 1.2018
[51] Liu G, Dierks EJ, Bell RB, Bui TG, Potter BE. Post-therapeutic surveillance schedule for oral cancer: is there agreement? Oral Maxillofac Surg. 2012; 16 (4):327–340
[52] Atula TS, Varpula MJ, Kurki TJ, Klemi PJ, Grénman R. Assessment of cervical lymph node status in head and neck cancer patients: palpation, computed tomography and low field magnetic resonance imaging compared with ultrasound-guided fine-needle aspiration cytology. Eur J Radiol. 1997; 25(2):152–161
[53] Rottey S, Petrovic M, Bauters W, et al. Evaluation of metastatic lymph nodes in head and neck cancer: a comparative study between palpation, ultrasonography, ultrasound-guided fine needle aspiration cytology and computed tomography. Acta Clin Belg. 2006; 61(5):236–241
[54] Lell M, Baum U, Greess H, et al. Head and neck tumors: imaging recurrent tumor and post-therapeutic changes with CT and MRI. Eur J Radiol. 2000; 33 (3):239–247
[55] Kunkel M, Förster GJ, Reichert TE, et al. Detection of recurrent oral squamous cell carcinoma by [18F]-2-fluorodeoxyglucose-positron emission tomography: implications for prognosis and patient management. Cancer. 2003; 98 (10):2257–2265
[56] Abgral R, Querellou S, Potard G, et al. Does 18F-FDG PET/CT improve the detection of posttreatment recurrence of head and neck squamous cell carcinoma in patients negative for disease on clinical follow-up? J Nucl Med. 2009; 50(1):24–29
[57] Aiken AH, Farley A, Baugnon KL, et al. Implementation of a novel surveillance template for head and neck cancer: Neck Imaging Reporting and Data System (NI-RADS). J Am Coll Radiol. 2016; 13(6):743–746.e1
[58] Arnold DJ, Goodwin WJ, Weed DT, Civantos FJ. Treatment of recurrent and advanced stage squamous cell carcinoma of the head and neck. Semin Radiat Oncol. 2004; 14(2):190–195
[59] Koo BS, Lim YC, Lee JS, Choi EC. Recurrence and salvage treatment of squamous cell carcinoma of the oral cavity. Oral Oncol. 2006; 42(8):789–794
[60] Pandey M, Bindu R, Soumithran CS. Results of primary versus salvage surgery in carcinoma of the buccal mucosa. Eur J Surg Oncol. 2009; 35(4):362–367
[61] Varvares MA, Poti S, Kenyon B, Christopher K, Walker RJ. Surgical margins and primary site resection in achieving local control in oral cancer resections. Laryngoscope. 2015; 125(10):2298–2307
[62] Dillon JK, Brown CB, McDonald TM, et al. How does the close surgical margin impact recurrence and survival when treating oral squamous cell carcinoma? J Oral Maxillofac Surg. 2015; 73(6):1182–1188
[63] Liao CT, Chang JT, Wang HM, et al. Salvage therapy in relapsed squamous cell carcinoma of the oral cavity: how and when? Cancer. 2008; 112(1):94–103
[64] Atallah S, Guth A, Chabolle F, Bach CA. Supraclavicular artery island flap in head and neck reconstruction. Eur Ann Otorhinolaryngol Head Neck Dis. 2015; 132(5):291–294
[65] Magrin J, Kowalski LP, Sabóia M, Sabóia RP. Major glossectomy: end results of 106 cases. Eur J Cancer B Oral Oncol. 1996; 32B(6):407–412
[66] Weber RS, Ohlms L, Bowman J, Jacob R, Goepfert H. Functional results after total or near total glossectomy with laryngeal preservation. Arch Otolaryngol Head Neck Surg. 1991; 117(5):512–515
[67] Dziegielewski PT, Ho ML, Rieger J, et al. Total glossectomy with laryngeal preservation and free flap reconstruction: objective functional outcomes and systematic review of the literature. Laryngoscope. 2013; 123(1):140–145
[68] Strojan P, Corry J, Eisbruch A, et al. Recurrent and second primary squamous cell carcinoma of the head and neck: when and how to reirradiate. Head Neck. 2015; 37(1):134–150
[69] Orlik JR, Horwich P, Bartlett C, Trites J, Hart R, Taylor SM. Long-term functional donor site morbidity of the free radial forearm flap in head and neck cancer survivors. J Otolaryngol Head Neck Surg. 2014; 43:1
[70] Baas M, Duraku LS, Corten EM, Mureau MA. A systematic review on the sensory reinnervation of free flaps for tongue reconstruction: does improved sensibility imply functional benefits? J Plast Reconstr Aesthet Surg. 2015; 68 (8):1025–1035
[71] Henry A, McCaul JA. Osseocutaneous radial forearm flap with beavertail modification; a case report of a novel, single, reconstructive free flap for the tongue, floor of mouth and mandible. Int J Surg Case Rep. 2016; 28:270–273
[72] Seikaly H, Rieger J, O'Connell D, Ansari K, Alqahtani K, Harris J. Beavertail modification of the radial forearm free flap in base of tongue reconstruction: technique and functional outcomes. Head Neck. 2009; 31(2):213–219
[73] Jeremić JV, Nikolić ZS. Versatility of radial forearm free flap for intraoral reconstruction. Srp Arh Celok Lek. 2015; 143(5–6):256–260
[74] Song YG, Chen GZ, Song YL. The free thigh flap: a new free flap concept based on the septocutaneous artery. Br J Plast Surg. 1984; 37(2):149–159
[75] Tuhar ZD, Zamfirescu D, Gheorghiță C, Slăvescu D, Frunză A, Lascăr I. Ablation of advanced tongue cancer and mobile tongue reconstruction by using a sensitive anterolateral thigh and vastus lateralis muscle free flap. J Med Life. 2015; 8(1):64–67
[76] Kimata Y, Uchiyama K, Ebihara S, Nakatsuka T, Harii K. Anatomic variations and technical problems of the anterolateral thigh flap: a report of 74 cases. Plast Reconstr Surg. 1998; 102(5):1517–1523
[77] Wei FC, Jain V, Celik N, Chen HC, Chuang DC, Lin CH. Have we found an ideal soft-tissue flap? An experience with 672 anterolateral thigh flaps. Plast Reconstr Surg. 2002; 109(7):2219–2226, discussion 2227–2230
[78] Lu M, Sun G, Hu Q, Tang E, Wang Y. Functional assessment: free thin anterolateral thigh flap versus free radial forearm reconstruction for hemiglossectomy defects. Med Oral Patol Oral Cir Bucal. 2015; 20(6): e757–e762
[79] Kimata Y, Uchiyama K, Ebihara S, et al. Anterolateral thigh flap donor-site complications and morbidity. Plast Reconstr Surg. 2000; 106(3):584–589
[80] Disa JJ, Cordeiro PG. The current role of preoperative arteriography in free fibula flaps. Plast Reconstr Surg. 1998; 102(4):1083–1088
[81] Kuzon WM, Jr, Jejurikar S, Wilkins EG, Swartz WM. Double free-flap reconstruction of massive defects involving the lip, chin, and mandible. Microsurgery. 1998; 18(6):372–378
[82] Cannon TY, Strub GM, Yawn RJ, Day TA. Oromandibular reconstruction. Clin Anat. 2012; 25(1):108–119
[83] Goodwin WJ, Jr. Salvage surgery for patients with recurrent squamous cell carcinoma of the upper aerodigestive tract: when do the ends justify the means? Laryngoscope. 2000; 110(3 Pt 2) Suppl 93:1–18
[84] Zafereo M. Surgical salvage of recurrent cancer of the head and neck. Curr Oncol Rep. 2014; 16(5):386
[85] Withrow KP, Rosenthal EL, Gourin CG, et al. Free tissue transfer to manage salvage laryngectomy defects after organ preservation failure. Laryngoscope. 2007; 117(5):781–784
[86] Kostrzewa JP, Lancaster WP, Iseli TA, Desmond RA, Carroll WR, Rosenthal EL. Outcomes of salvage surgery with free flap reconstruction for recurrent oral and oropharyngeal cancer. Laryngoscope. 2010; 120(2):267–272
[87] Sher DJ, Haddad RI, Norris CM, Jr, et al. Efficacy and toxicity of reirradiation using intensity-modulated radiotherapy for recurrent or second primary head and neck cancer. Cancer. 2010; 116(20):4761–4768
[88] Suh JD, Kim BP, Abemayor E, et al. Reirradiation after salvage surgery and microvascular free flap reconstruction for recurrent head and neck carcinoma. Otolaryngol Head Neck Surg. 2008; 139(6):781–786
[89] Grabenbauer GG, Rödel C, Brunner T, et al. Interstitial brachytherapy with Ir-192 low-dose-rate in the treatment of primary and recurrent cancer of the oral cavity and oropharynx: review of 318 patients treated between 1985 and 1997. Strahlenther Onkol. 2001; 177(7):338–344

49 Management of Metastatic Oral Cavity Cancers

Won Jin Ho and Hyunseok Kang

Summary

Oral cavity cancers rarely present with metastatic disease, but development of metastatic disease is not uncommon and is associated with poor outcome. Current standard therapies include first-line platinum-based systemic therapy in combination with fluorouracil and cetuximab, an anti-epidermal growth factor receptor (anti-EGFR) antibody, and second-line immune check point inhibitor therapy with anti-PD-1 antibodies such as pembrolizumab and nivolumb. Appropriate selection of therapy entails assessment of the patient's pretreatment performance status, evaluation of other comorbidities, and judicious consideration of metastasectomy or stereotactic body radiotherapy. Patients with suboptimal performance status may instead be treated with upfront doublet chemotherapy or even single-agent therapy involving platinum-based agents, taxanes, cetuximab, or methotrexate. Ongoing research efforts to improve the treatment of metastatic disease include identifying predictive biomarkers based on genomics and immune phenotypes; investigating the utility of novel molecularly targeted agents; and formulating innovative approaches to incorporate biologics and immune therapy agents into the treatment paradigm.

Keywords: distant metastasis, oligometastatic disease, systemic therapy, combination chemotherapy, immunotherapy, metastasectomy

49.1 Introduction and Epidemiology

Approximately 20% of all oral cavity and pharyngeal cancers are diagnosed with distant metastatic disease.[1] Among oral cavity cancers only, at least 5–8% of patients present with distant metastatic disease at the time of diagnosis.[2] Furthermore, a retrospective review of 889 patients with oral cavity cancer who underwent curative intent radical surgery revealed that about 10% of patients develop distant metastasis in 5 years.[3] While the overall 5-year survival rate of all oral cavity and pharyngeal cancers is roughly 65%,[1] the median survival of patients with distant metastatic head and neck squamous cell cancers (HNSCC) remains dismal at approximately 7–10 months.[4–6] The central focus of management in patients with metastatic oral cavity cancers has been limited to palliative treatments, especially given the often poor performance status of such patients. However, empowered by better understanding of the underlying cancer biology, there have been remarkable advancements in the development of systemic therapy options in the past decade, providing for new therapeutic approaches with significant benefits (▶ Table 49.1).

49.2 Current Management

49.2.1 Biological Overview

Head and neck cancers have long been linked to exposure to tobacco carcinogens in association with accumulation of key genomic changes along the course of cancer development.[19] Within the past decade, human papillomavirus (HPV) has emerged as a major prognostic factor in oropharyngeal squamous cell carcinoma (OPSCC).[20] However, the presence of HPV is less common—approximately 25%—in oral cavity squamous cell carcinoma (OCSCC), and the role of HPV in the development of OCSCC still remains largely unclear.[21,22] There is no significant association between HPV status and prognosis in OCSCC,[23] which could be a reflection of low transcriptional activity of viral oncoproteins E6 and E7 in OCSCC.[24]

Both HPV-positive and HPV-negative HNSCCs manifest dysregulated cell cycles from inactivation of the p53 and Rb pathways.[25] Recent genomic landscape analysis of HNSCC confirmed frequent loss-of-function alterations in *TP53* as well as loss of *CDKN2A* (leading to inactivation of $p16^{INK4A}$) in HPV-negative HNSCC; and helical domain mutations in *PIK3CA* as the most common genomic alteration in HPV-positive HNSCC.[26] The scarcity of mutations in cell cycle regulating proteins among HPV-positive HNSCC is not suprising given that HPV-positive tumors already harbor disrupted p53 and Rb pathways through the actions of viral oncoproteins E6 and E7.[27] Heightened proliferative activity due to dysregulated cell cycle has been the basis of traditional chemotherapeutic agents such as anti-metabolites, platinum-based drugs, and taxanes. Further insights from genomics research will continue to provide the grounds for development of novel therapies.

Table 49.1 Standard systemic therapies for metastatic oral cavity cancers

Treatment	Ref	Study design
First-line options		
Preferred triplet therapy for patients with robust PS		
• Cisplatin, 5FU, cetuximab (EXTREME regimen)	6	Phase III RCT
Doublet chemotherapy regimens		
• Cisplatin, 5FU (CF)	7	Phase III RCT
• Cisplatin, paclitaxel (CP)	5	Phase III RCT
• Cisplatin, cetuximab	4	Phase III RCT
• Paclitaxel, cetuximab	8	Phase II SAT
• Docetaxel, cetuximab	9	Retrospective
Second-line options for platinum-refractory disease		
Immunotherapeutic agents		
• Nivolumab	10	Phase III RCT
• Pembrolizumab	11	Phase III RCT
Doublet chemotherapy regimen		
• Gemcitabine, pemetrexed	12	Phase II SAT
Other agents with evidence of monotherapy activity		
Carboplatin	13	
Capecitabine	14	Phase II SAT
Docetaxel	15	Phase II SAT
Paclitaxel	16	Phase II SAT
Afatinib	17	Phase III RCT
Methotrexate	18	

Abbreviations: PS, performance status; RCT, randomized control trial; SAT, single arm trial.

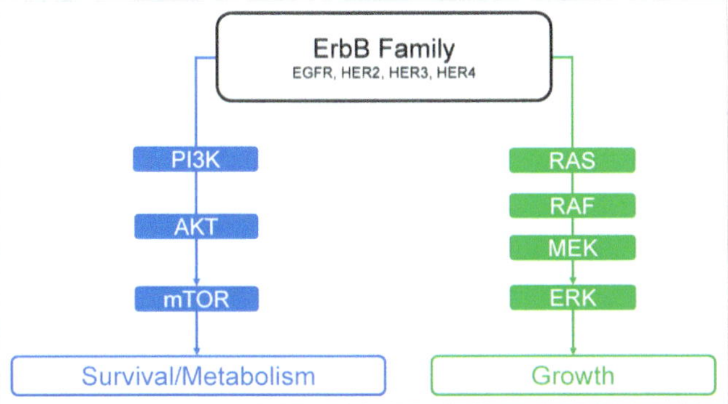

Fig. 49.1 Oncogenic signaling pathways in head and neck cancers. Epidermal growth factor receptor (EGFR), one of ErbB family receptors, is overexpressed in many head and neck cancers. Both PI3K-AKT-mTOR and RAS-RAF-MEK-ERK pathways are downstream of ErbB family receptors; head and neck carcinogenesis may depend on increased activation of either of these pathways. Gain-of-function alterations in PI3K and RAS are established as significant oncogenic events in head and neck cancers.

Early studies utilizing immunohistochemistry techniques have shown that overexpression of epidermal growth factor receptor (EGFR) is frequent in HNSCC in association with worse outcomes.[28–30] Subsequently confirmed by molecular techniques, EGFR amplification has been reported in up to 31% of OCSCCs[31] and 15% of all HPV negative HNSCCs.[26] EGFR activation can trigger downstream oncogenic pathways such as PI3K-AKT-mTOR and RAS-MEK-ERK (▶ Fig. 49.1). The Cancer Genome Atlas (TCGA) analysis also demonstrated activating alterations of these downstream pathways, such as mutations in the *PIK3CA* and *HRAS*, reinforcing the critical role of these pathways in the oncogenesis of HNSCC.[26] This has led to successful therapeutic strategies incorporating anti-EGFR agents and insight into resistance mechanisms to such therapies.[4,6,32,33]

Also in recent decades, landmark studies in cancer research renewed cognizance for the tumorigenic role of immune escape or immune editing by the tumor against immune surveillance mechanisms.[34,35] Key cellular components of an immune-suppressive tumor microenvironment such as myeloid-derived suppressor cells,[36] regulatory T cells,[37] and tumor-associated macrophages[38] have now been well-characterized. Dysregulation of inflammatory cytokines such as TGFβ,[37,39] IL-6,[38] IL-10,[37,38] and PGE2[40] has been shown to play a role in suppressing activation of dentritic cells, NK cells, and/or T cells. Furthermore, tumor cells are able to evade T cell-mediated immune recognition via mutations in HLA expression and antigen processing machinery.[41] In HNSCC, these concepts were not only recapitulated in large-scale genomic characterization of tumors revealing alterations in genes responsible for proper antigen presentation,[26] but also in specific studies utilizing oral cavity cancer samples exploring specific ligand–receptor co-signaling interactions, e.g., PD-1/PD-L1, responsible for dampening T cell-mediated immune responses.[42,43] When comparing across many different cancer types, HNSCC is among those with the highest levels of overall immune cell infiltration, immunoregulatory presence as measured by regulatory T cell infiltration, and cytotoxic antitumor NK cells.[44] These observations suggest that the HNSCC immune microenvironment may in fact be poised to respond to immune-modulating treatment approaches. Thus, much of the recent efforts on improving the treatment of HNSCCs have focused on establishing and expanding the role of immunotherapy in the overarching treatment paradigms.

49.2.2 Clinical Considerations

When treating patients with metastatic oral cavity cancers, major clinical factors to consider include the performance status and presence of other comorbidities. Performance status is useful for predicting how well the patient will tolerate intensive chemotherapy regimens. Developed by the Eastern Cooperative Oncology Group (ECOG) in 1982,[45] the ECOG numeric scale is a common way to define a patient's performance status, i.e., daily living abilities: Grade 0 represents patients who are fully active without restrictions; Grade 1 represents patients who are ambulatory and able to undergo limited exertion such as light house work or office work; Grade 2 is for patients who are capable of self-care but not work activities, with less than 50% of waking hours spent sitting down or lying down; Grade 3 defines patients who spend more than 50% of waking hours confined to bed or chair; Grade 4 represents complete disability without any self-care capabilities; and Grade 5 signifies death. Studies in the 1980s have shown that chemotherapy in patients with poor performance status does not lead to much benefit but rather high toxicities and short survival.[46] Thus, both American Society of Clinical Oncology (ASCO) expert panel and National Comprehensive Cancer Network (NCCN) guidelines have generally advised against administering chemotherapy to patients with ECOG performance status of 3 or more.[47,48] For patients with ECOG performance status of 2, single-agent chemotherapy may be favored over multi-agent chemotherapy.

Patients' comorbidities also play a critical role in determining the type of chemotherapy agent to be administered. Key platinum-based drugs used to treat metastatic oral cavity cancers include cisplatin and carboplatin. Cisplatin is notorious for nephrotoxicity and is thus avoided altogether in patients with compromised renal function or used cautiously with appropriate renal dosing and aggressive hydration protocols. Since this parameter serves as a critical limiting factor for the use of cisplatin, carboplatin is often used in place of cisplatin due to its lower toxicity profile. Both agents, however, are associated with development of peripheral neuropathy and should be used judiciously in patients who have history of diabetes or alcoholism. Along with platinum-based drugs, taxane-based chemotherapeutic agents, e.g., docetaxel and paclitaxel, are also used with caution in patients with increased risk of neurotoxicity.

49.2.3 Considerations for Oligometastatic Disease

In line with the "cascade" theory of metastatic spread as described by Viadana et al in the late 1970s,[49] lung is thought to be a disseminating site for further metastatic spread of head and neck cancers. This has provided the rationale for studies involving surgical resection of pulmonary metastases of head and neck primary cancers. Collective evidence demonstrates that pulmonary metastasectomy in patients with oligometastatic relapse of head and neck squamous cell carcinomas without extrapulmonary metastasis may achieve 5-year survival in as much as 30% of patients.[50–52] Favorable features associated with survival advantage in prior studies include longer disease-free interval prior to metastatic relapse,[53–55] younger patients with age less than 50 or 60 years,[50,55–57] and complete resection.[50,51,53] Interestingly, however, several subset analyses have shown that, compared to other metastatic head and neck squamous cell carcinomas, oral cavity primary site is a predictor of poor outcome, i.e., no survival advantage was seen with pulmonary metastasectomy in patients with oral cavity primary.[53,57–59] Thus, while metastasectomy may be considered for select patients who exhibit positive prognostic characteristics as well as sufficient performance status and pulmonary function to undergo surgery, its utility remains unclear in patients with metastatic oral cavity cancers.

Development of stereotactic body radiation (SBRT) has enabled delivery of ablative doses of radiation to oligometastatic sites. SBRT has been adopted for palliative treatment and has been evaluated in many nonrandomized studies involving patients with various cancers; results from these studies suggest that SBRT is safe and effective,[60] but data on the use of SBRT in oligometastatic HNSCC are limited. Likewise, there is no currently available data to support adjuvant chemotherapy after metastasis-directed local therapies (surgery or SBRT) for oligometastatic disease.

49.2.4 Current Standard of Care

First-line Treatment for Recurrent/Metastatic HNSCC

The current standard of care for first-line treatment in recurrent/metastatic HNSCC is triplet therapy combining platinum, fluorouracil, and cetuximab based on the results of the EXTREME trial.[6] In this landmark phase III trial, adding cetuximab significantly prolonged the median overall survival to 10.1 months from 7.4 months when using doublet chemotherapy. This observed benefit was accompanied by increased risk for adverse effects including grade 3 skin toxicity, hypomagnesemia, and sepsis. Cetuximab is a chimeric mouse-human IgG1 monoclonal antibody, which can cause hypersensitivity reactions through the presecence of specific preformed IgE antibodies more prevalent in the Southeastern United States.[61] A fully humanized anti-EGFR monoclonal antibody, panitumumab, was investigated in a phase III study in a design similar to the EXTREME trial but failed to improve overall survival compared to platinum and 5FU alone.[62] Combination of platinum, docetaxel, and cetuximab has demonstrated overall response rate (ORR) of 44% and overall survival of up to 14 months in a single-arm phase II study[63] and is currently being evaluated in a randomized study (NCT02268695). Importantly, all of these trials restricted the enrollment to exclude patients who developed recurrent or metastatic disease within 6 months of systemic platinum-based chemotherapy, typically given with concurrent radiation. Such patients are considered to have platinum-refractory disease and probably would not benefit from platinum-based chemotherapy. There is, however, some variation in what is defined as platinum-refractory disease; for example, an ECOG study evaluating the role of bevacizumab defined platinum refractoriness as disease progression within 4 months from the last dose of platinum-based chemotherapy.[64] Thus, an interval of 4 to 6 months is generally used to determine platinum refractoriness. For platinum-refractory patients, continued treatment with nonplatinum subsequent line therapies are more appropriate.

For patients who do not have the appropriate performance status for standard triplet combination therapy, doublet chemotherapy can be an effective alternative. A phase III study has demonstrated that both overall survival and response rates were similar between cisplatin with fluorouracil (CF) and cisplatin with paclitaxel (CP).[5] Subsequent studies have shown that platinum-based doublet regmens such as CF, CP, and cisplatin/carboplatin with cetuximab are active alternatives and historically have yielded median overall survival of roughly 6–8 months.[4,5,7] Alternatively, combination of taxanes and cetuximab have also been explored in the first-line setting for patients who are not candidates for platinum-based chemotherapy. Weekly paclitaxel and cetuximab showed 54% response rate and overall survival of 8.4 months with acceptable toxicity in a single arm phase II study.[8] A small retrospective analysis investigated biweekly docetaxel and cetuximab in a similar population and showed comparable overall survival (8.3 months).[9] Finally, patients who are not candidates for combination therapies may also be treated with single-agent therapies involving any of the agents above including even methotrexate, an early anti-metabolite drug studied in head and neck cancers dating back to the 1960s.[65]

Second-line and Subsequent Line Treatment for Recurrent/Metastatic HNSCC

For patients who have progressed on first-line platinum-based regimens including patients who have progressed within 6 months of completing platinum-based chemoradiation, options have been very limited. Fortunately, recent research advancements have led to new subsequent line therapies that have demonstrated to be significant for such patients. Development of anti-PD-1/PD-L1 antibodies has led to pivotal trials studying the efficacy of immunotherapy strategies in treating platinum-refractory metastatic head and neck cancers. Notably, CheckMate 141, a phase III trial, demonstrated that patients with platinum-refractory recurrent/metastatic HNSCC treated with nivolumab have median overall survival of 7.5 months versus 5.1 months when treated with a standard single-agent therapy (methotrexate, docetaxel, or cetuximab).[10] The FDA has approved the use of nivolumab and pembrolizumab in metastatic head and neck cancer patients, with approval of pembrolizumab based on early phase trials showing meaningful clinical activity of the drug.[66] Although a follow-up phase III study (KEYNOTE-040) did not demonstrate significant improvement in overall survival with pembrolizumab compared to standard single-agent therapy, pembrolizumab did exhibit a favorable toxicity profile and led to significantly improved overall survival in patients with positive PD-L1 expression.[11] These findings have thus established nivolumab and pembrolizumab as standard second-line therapies for patients with metastatic oral cavity cancers.

Combination chemotherapy can still be used as subsequent line therapy for select patients with good performance status. For example, the combination of pemetrexed and gemcitabine was investigated in a small phase II study in patients who have progressed through at least one chemotherapy-based regimen, showing an ORR of 16%.[12] However, single-agent chemotherapy, such as methotrexate, typically exhibits poor ORR, i.e., less than 10%.[17,67] As for targeted therapeutics, exploration of single-agent cetuximab in the second-line setting has demonstrated a rather disappointing best ORR of 13%.[33] Afatinib, an irreversible pan-ErbB2 inhibitor which targets EGFR, HER2, and HER4, was evaluated in a randomized phase III trial, demonstrating significant improvement in progression-free survival when compared to methotrexate (median 2.6 months vs. 1.7 months) but not in the primary endpoint of overall survival.[17]

49.3 Future Directions

49.3.1 Precision Medicine: Molecularly Driven Treatment Approaches

Advances in cancer genomics have opened the door to precision medicine; major efforts stemming from aggregate gene/protein expression data are underway to exploit the individual patient's molecular profile for drug targeting beyond EGFR. In addition to frequent *TP53* alterations, the TCGA revealed frequent mutations in *PIK3CA*, a gene coding for a subunit of the enzyme phosphatidyl-inositol 3-kinase (PI3K) involved in downstream signaling pathways important for cell proliferation and survival, in up to 21% of HNSCC cases.[26] It is the only mutated oncogene with statistical significance in HNSCC, and more than one-third of HPV-negative and the majority of HPV-positive HNSCC cases have gain-of-function alterations in *PIK3CA*.[26] Indeed, almost one-third of HPV-negative HNSCCs harbor mutations in genes involved in the PI3K pathway including *PIK3CA*, *AKT1/2/3*, *mTOR*, *PTEN*, *TSC1/2*, *RICTOR*, and *RPTOR*.[68] Primarily characterized to activate the PI3K-AKT-mTOR pathway which is dysregulated in many other cancer types, PI3K serves as a targetable biomarker prompting the development of specific inhibitors.[69] There have been several clinical trials using PI3K inhibitors such as buparlisib in patients with metastatic HNSCC, which have shown mixed results, possibly due to heterogeneous genetic makeup of the tumors with regards to their *PIK3CA* mutational status.[70] More PI3K inhibitors are under clinical development including the p110α selective inhibitor alpelisib, which is expected to engender antitumor activity without affecting other isoforms of PI3K.[71] Inhibitors of other components of the PI3K pathway such as AKT and mTOR are also actively being investigated in recurrent/metastatic HNSCC.[72]

Another frequently mutated oncogene in HNSCC is *HRAS*, a member of the RAS gene family, which is observed in approximately 5% of HPV-negative HNSCCs.[26] It is downstream of ErbB family and activates RAF1 and BRAF or PI3K signaling, along RAF/MEK/ERK or PI3K/AKT/mTOR cascade.[73] *HRAS* is the only isoform of RAS that is completely dependent on farnesyltransferase for its membrane localization and has been demonstrated to be susceptible to inhibition by tipifarnib, a highly selective farnesyltransferase inhibitor.[74] Notably, preliminary results from an ongoing phase II study examining the efficacy of tipifarnib in patients with HNSCC resistant to prior chemotherapy, cetuximab, and immunotherapy revealed an ORR of 67% which is very encouraging, although the results are based on a cohort of only six patients.[75]

Another highly altered gene from the TCGA is the tumor suppressor *CDKN2A*; exclusively found among HPV-negative HNSCCs, loss-of-function alterations in *CDKN2A* were present in 58% of the cases analyzed ($n = 243$).[26] *CDKN2A* can be inactivated by epigenetic silencing through promoter methylation[76] or loss of expression.[77] *CDKN2A* encodes for $p16^{INK4a}$, which functions as an inhibitor of cyclin dependent kinases 4 and 6 (CDK4/6) and regulates Rb function. *CDKN2A* also encodes for $p14^{arf}$ which mediates proper p53 function via regulation of Mdm2. Thus, inactivation of *CDKN2A* can lead to loss of cell cycle regulation and uncontrolled cell growth.[78] Indeed, CDK4/6 inhibitors such as palbociclib, ribociclib, and abemaciclib are already approved for breast cancer[79,80] and have shown promising activity in non-small cell lung cancers with *KRAS* mutation.[81] To explore the use of targeting this specific pathway, multiple phase I/II trials are in progress to assess the safety and efficacy of treating metastatic HNSCC patients with a combination of CDK4/6 inhibitors and cetuximab (NCT02429089, NCT02499120).

Despite many active areas of investigation into biomarker-targeted therapies supported by sound scientific rationale, much of the efforts in the past have not been successful. For example, while *EGFR* is one of the more commonly mutated or amplified genes, several trials capitalizing on anti-EGFR drugs other than cetuximab such as panitumumab, zalutumumab, and afatinib all have failed to demonstrate substantial clinical efficacy in patients with metastatic HNSCC.[17,62,82] One potential underlying reason for the minimal benefit observed may be due to the lack of biomarker specifications within such trials or understanding of resistance mechanisms. For example, it has previously been shown that high levels of ErbB2 (HER2) and ErbB3 (HER3) are associated with anti-EGFR resistance and that combined targeting of EGFR with HER2[83] or HER3[84] is more efficacious than EGFR targeting alone. Such observations indicate the critical importance as well as the challenge of pursuing more molecularly defined trials in the future.[85]

49.3.2 Immunotherapy: Beyond Anti-PD-1/PD-L1 Blockade

Encouraged by the successes of immune checkpoint inhibitors in the second-line setting, there is enormous interest in improving the use of immunotherapeutic agents in treating metastatic head and neck cancer patients. Key strategies include: (a) identifying predictive biomarkers for response or resistance, (b) exploring optimal combination approaches, and (c) adopting immune therapy into first-line setting.

PD-L1 expression has been associated with positive response in many cancers including head and neck cancers (KEYNOTE-040) and has been adopted as an integral biomarker for specific indications such as first-line treatment for non-small cell lung cancers.[86] It is, however, notable that treatment responses are often observed in even PD-L1 negative/low HNSCC patients in the second-line setting.[10] Another biomarker under intense investigation is the tumor mutational burden (TMB). Higher TMB correlates with higher response rates to immune checkpoint inhibitors, and HNSCC is among the cancers with relatively higher TMB.[87]

Although single-agent anti-PD-1 antibodies have been approved and established as part of the standard of care, majority of patients experience progression of disease on this treatment. Thus, combination approaches have been explored to improve the efficacy of immune checkpoint inhibitors. For example, agents targeting indoleamine 2,3-dioxygenase (IDO), an enzyme that catalyzes degradation of tryptophan to kynurenine leading to T cells suppression, have shown promising activity in combination with anti-PD-1 antibodies in head and neck cancers.[88] Augmentation of NK cell activity by blocking inhibitory signals through killer-cell immunoglobulin-like receptors (KIRs) also has shown encouraging results in a small number of head and neck cancer patients.[89] Combinations with other immune checkpoint inhibitors such as anti-CTLA4 antibody and anti-LAG3 antibody are being actively explored in head and neck cancer.

Another major focus of research efforts has been to bring immunotherapy to front-line therapy. For example, CheckMate 651 has been comparing the use of nivolumab in combination with ipilimumab, an anti-CTLA4 antibody, to the EXTREME regimen (NCT02741570). Similarly, the KESTREL trial has also been studying the combination of an anti-PD-L1 antibody, durvalumab, and an anti-CTLA-4 antibody, tremelimumab, in comparison to the EXTREME regimen (NCT02551159).[90] Also, KEYNOTE-048 has been exploring the use of pembrolizumab with chemotherapy versus pembrolizumab alone vis-à-vis the EXTREME regimen (NCT02358031). The results of these studies have the potential to impact the field significantly and are highly anticipated.

Key Points

- The prognosis for metastatic oral cavity cancers remains very poor.
- Assessing the patients' performance status and other existing comorbidities is critical for determining the most appropriate treatment regimen.
- Current first-line standard treatment for patients with metastatic OCSCC is the EXTREME regimen, which combines cisplatin/carboplatin, fluorouracil, and cetuximab.
- Standard subsequent line therapy for platinum-refractory disease is anti-PD-1 immunotherapy with nivolumab or pembrolizumab. Other agents that could be considered are methotrexate, cetuximab, or taxane-based monotherapy.
- Precision oncology approaches based on genomics and immunologic biomarkers are expected to improve outcomes with less toxicity for patients with metastatic oral cancer. Several clinical trials on molecularly targeted therapies and immunotherapies are underway.

References

[1] Siegel RL, Miller KD, Jemal A. Cancer Statistics, 2017. CA Cancer J Clin. 2017; 67(1):7–30

[2] Carvalho AL, Nishimoto IN, Califano JA, Kowalski LP. Trends in incidence and prognosis for head and neck cancer in the United States: a site-specific analysis of the SEER database. Int J Cancer. 2005; 114(5):806–816

[3] Liao CT, Wang HM, Chang JT, et al. Analysis of risk factors for distant metastases in squamous cell carcinoma of the oral cavity. Cancer. 2007; 110(7):1501–1508

[4] Burtness B, Goldwasser MA, Flood W, Mattar B, Forastiere AA, Eastern Cooperative Oncology Group. Phase III randomized trial of cisplatin plus placebo compared with cisplatin plus cetuximab in metastatic/recurrent head and neck cancer: an Eastern Cooperative Oncology Group study. J Clin Oncol. 2005; 23(34):8646–8654

[5] Gibson MK, Li Y, Murphy B, et al. Eastern Cooperative Oncology Group. Randomized phase III evaluation of cisplatin plus fluorouracil versus cisplatin plus paclitaxel in advanced head and neck cancer (E1395): an intergroup trial of the Eastern Cooperative Oncology Group. J Clin Oncol. 2005; 23(15):3562–3567

[6] Vermorken JB, Mesia R, Rivera F, et al. Platinum-based chemotherapy plus cetuximab in head and neck cancer. N Engl J Med. 2008; 359(11):1116–1127

[7] Forastiere AA, Metch B, Schuller DE, et al. Randomized comparison of cisplatin plus fluorouracil and carboplatin plus fluorouracil versus methotrexate in advanced squamous-cell carcinoma of the head and neck: a Southwest Oncology Group study. J Clin Oncol. 1992; 10(8):1245–1251

[8] Hitt R, Irigoyen A, Cortes-Funes H, Grau JJ, García-Sáenz JA, Cruz-Hernandez JJ, Spanish Head and Neck Cancer Cooperative Group (TTCC). Phase II study of the combination of cetuximab and weekly paclitaxel in the first-line treatment of patients with recurrent and/or metastatic squamous cell carcinoma of head and neck. Ann Oncol. 2012; 23(4):1016–1022

[9] Posch D, Fuchs H, Kornek G, et al. Docetaxel plus cetuximab biweekly is an active regimen for the first-line treatment of patients with recurrent/metastatic head and neck cancer. Sci Rep. 2016; 6:32946

[10] Ferris RL, Blumenschein G, Jr, Fayette J, et al. Nivolumab for recurrent squamous-cell carcinoma of the head and neck. N Engl J Med. 2016; 375(19): 1856–1867

[11] Cohen EE, Harrington KJ, Le Tourneau C, et al. LBA45_PRPembrolizumab (pembro) vs standard of care (SOC) for recurrent or metastatic head and neck squamous cell carcinoma (R/M HNSCC): Phase 3 KEYNOTE-040 trial. Annals of Oncology. 2017; 28(suppl_5). DOI: https://doi.org/10.1093/annonc/mdx44 0.040

[12] Fury MG, Haque S, Stambuk H, Shen R, Carlson D, Pfister D. A phase 2 study of pemetrexed plus gemcitabine every 2 weeks for patients with recurrent or metastatic head and neck squamous cell cancer. Cancer. 2011; 117(4):795–801

[13] Al-Sarraf M, Metch B, Kish J, et al. Platinum analogs in recurrent and advanced head and neck cancer: a Southwest Oncology Group and Wayne State University Study. Cancer Treat Rep. 1987; 71(7–8):723–726

[14] Martinez-Trufero J, Isla D, Adansa JC, et al. Phase II study of capecitabine as palliative treatment for patients with recurrent and metastatic squamous head and neck cancer after previous platinum-based treatment. Br J Cancer. 2010; 102(12):1687–1691

[15] Catimel G, Verweij J, Mattijssen V, et al. EORTC Early Clinical Trials Group. Docetaxel (Taxotere): an active drug for the treatment of patients with advanced squamous cell carcinoma of the head and neck. Ann Oncol. 1994; 5 (6):533–537

[16] Grau JJ, Caballero M, Verger E, Monzó M, Blanch JL. Weekly paclitaxel for platin-resistant stage IV head and neck cancer patients. Acta Otolaryngol. 2009; 129(11):1294–1299

[17] Machiels JP, Haddad RI, Fayette J, et al. LUX-H&N 1 investigators. Afatinib versus methotrexate as second-line treatment in patients with recurrent or metastatic squamous-cell carcinoma of the head and neck progressing on or after platinum-based therapy (LUX-Head & Neck 1): an open-label, randomised phase 3 trial. Lancet Oncol. 2015; 16(5):583–594

[18] Woods RL, Fox RM, Tattersall MH. Methotrexate treatment of squamous-cell head and neck cancers: dose-response evaluation. Br Med J (Clin Res Ed). 1981; 282(6264):600–602

[19] Haddad RI, Shin DM. Recent advances in head and neck cancer. N Engl J Med. 2008; 359(11):1143–1154

[20] Ang KK, Harris J, Wheeler R, et al. Human papillomavirus and survival of patients with oropharyngeal cancer. N Engl J Med. 2010; 363(1):24–35

[21] Annertz K, Rosenquist K, Andersson G, Jacobsson H, Hansson BG, Wennerberg J. High-risk HPV and survival in patients with oral and oropharyngeal squamous cell carcinoma—5-year follow up of a population-based study. Acta Otolaryngol. 2014; 134(8):843–851

[22] Reuschenbach M, Kansy K, Garbe K, et al. Lack of evidence of human papillomavirus-induced squamous cell carcinomas of the oral cavity in southern Germany. Oral Oncol. 2013; 49(9):937–942

[23] Isayeva T, Li Y, Maswahu D, Brandwein-Gensler M. Human papillomavirus in non-oropharyngeal head and neck cancers: a systematic literature review. Head Neck Pathol. 2012; 6 Suppl 1:S104–S120

[24] Lingen MW, Xiao W, Schmitt A, et al. Low etiologic fraction for high-risk human papillomavirus in oral cavity squamous cell carcinomas. Oral Oncol. 2013; 49(1):1–8

[25] Leemans CR, Braakhuis BJ, Brakenhoff RH. The molecular biology of head and neck cancer. Nat Rev Cancer. 2011; 11(1):9–22

[26] Cancer Genome Atlas N, Cancer Genome Atlas Network. Comprehensive genomic characterization of head and neck squamous cell carcinomas. Nature. 2015; 517(7536):576–582

[27] Chung CH, Gillison ML. Human papillomavirus in head and neck cancer: its role in pathogenesis and clinical implications. Clin Cancer Res. 2009; 15(22): 6758–6762

[28] Dassonville O, Formento JL, Francoual M, et al. Expression of epidermal growth factor receptor and survival in upper aerodigestive tract cancer. J Clin Oncol. 1993; 11(10):1873–1878

[29] Maiorano E, Favia G, Maisonneuve P, Viale G. Prognostic implications of epidermal growth factor receptor immunoreactivity in squamous cell carcinoma of the oral mucosa. J Pathol. 1998; 185(2):167–174

[30] Rubin Grandis J, Melhem MF, Gooding WE, et al. Levels of TGF-alpha and EGFR protein in head and neck squamous cell carcinoma and patient survival. J Natl Cancer Inst. 1998; 90(11):824–832

[31] Sheu JJ, Hua CH, Wan L, et al. Functional genomic analysis identified epidermal growth factor receptor activation as the most common genetic event in oral squamous cell carcinoma. Cancer Res. 2009; 69(6):2568–2576

[32] Bonner JA, Harari PM, Giralt J, et al. Radiotherapy plus cetuximab for squamous-cell carcinoma of the head and neck. N Engl J Med. 2006; 354(6):567–578

[33] Vermorken JB, Trigo J, Hitt R, et al. Open-label, uncontrolled, multicenter phase II study to evaluate the efficacy and toxicity of cetuximab as a single agent in patients with recurrent and/or metastatic squamous cell carcinoma of the head and neck who failed to respond to platinum-based therapy. J Clin Oncol. 2007; 25(16):2171–2177

[34] Dong H, Zhu G, Tamada K, Chen L. B7-H1, a third member of the B7 family, co-stimulates T-cell proliferation and interleukin-10 secretion. Nat Med. 1999; 5(12):1365–1369

[35] Leach DR, Krummel MF, Allison JP. Enhancement of antitumor immunity by CTLA-4 blockade. Science. 1996; 271(5256):1734–1736

[36] Ostrand-Rosenberg S, Sinha P. Myeloid-derived suppressor cells: linking inflammation and cancer. J Immunol. 2009; 182(8):4499–4506

[37] Alhamarneh O, Amarnath SM, Stafford ND, Greenman J. Regulatory T cells: what role do they play in antitumor immunity in patients with head and neck cancer? Head Neck. 2008; 30(2):251–261

[38] Komohara Y, Jinushi M, Takeya M. Clinical significance of macrophage heterogeneity in human malignant tumors. Cancer Sci. 2014; 105(1):1–8

[39] Moutsopoulos NM, Wen J, Wahl SM. TGF-beta and tumors—an ill-fated alliance. Curr Opin Immunol. 2008; 20(2):234–240

[40] Harris SG, Padilla J, Koumas L, Ray D, Phipps RP. Prostaglandins as modulators of immunity. Trends Immunol. 2002; 23(3):144–150

[41] Ogino T, Shigyo H, Ishii H, et al. HLA class I antigen down-regulation in primary laryngeal squamous cell carcinoma lesions as a poor prognostic marker. Cancer Res. 2006; 66(18):9281–9289

[42] Malaspina TS, Gasparoto TH, Costa MR, et al. Enhanced programmed death 1 (PD-1) and PD-1 ligand (PD-L1) expression in patients with actinic cheilitis and oral squamous cell carcinoma. Cancer Immunol Immunother. 2011; 60 (7):965–974

[43] Tsushima F, Tanaka K, Otsuki N, et al. Predominant expression of B7-H1 and its immunoregulatory roles in oral squamous cell carcinoma. Oral Oncol. 2006; 42(3):268–274

[44] Mandal R, Şenbabaoğlu Y, Desrichard A, et al. The head and neck cancer immune landscape and its immunotherapeutic implications. JCI Insight. 2016; 1(17):e89829

[45] Oken MM, Creech RH, Tormey DC, et al. Toxicity and response criteria of the Eastern Cooperative Oncology Group. Am J Clin Oncol. 1982; 5(6):649–655

[46] Pater JL, Loeb M. Nonanatomic prognostic factors in carcinoma of the lung: a multivariate analysis. Cancer. 1982; 50(2):326–331

[47] Schnipper LE, Smith TJ, Raghavan D, et al. American Society of Clinical Oncology identifies five key opportunities to improve care and reduce costs: the top five list for oncology. J Clin Oncol. 2012; 30(14):1715–1724

[48] Network NCC. Head and Neck Cancer (Version 2.2017). 2017; https://www.nccn.org/professionals/physician_gls/pdf/head-and-neck.pdf. Accessed December 26, 2017

[49] Viadana E, Bross I, Pickern J. Cascade Spread of Blood-Borne Metastases in Solid and Nonsolid Cancers in Humans. Boston: G.K. Hall; 1978

[50] Liu D, Labow DM, Dang N, et al. Pulmonary metastasectomy for head and neck cancers. Ann Surg Oncol. 1999; 6(6):572–578

[51] Winter H, Meimarakis G, Hoffmann G, et al. Does surgical resection of pulmonary metastases of head and neck cancer improve survival? Ann Surg Oncol. 2008; 15(10):2915–2926

[52] Young ER, Diakos E, Khalid-Raja M, Mehanna H. Resection of subsequent pulmonary metastases from treated head and neck squamous cell carcinoma: systematic review and meta-analysis. Clin Otolaryngol. 2015; 40(3):208–218

[53] Shiono S, Kawamura M, Sato T, et al. Metastatic Lung Tumor Study Group of Japan. Pulmonary metastasectomy for pulmonary metastases of head and neck squamous cell carcinomas. Ann Thorac Surg. 2009; 88(3):856–860

[54] Finley RK, III, Verazin GT, Driscoll DL, et al. Results of surgical resection of pulmonary metastases of squamous cell carcinoma of the head and neck. Am J Surg. 1992; 164(6):594–598

[55] Nibu K, Nakagawa K, Kamata S, et al. Surgical treatment for pulmonary metastases of squamous cell carcinoma of the head and neck. Am J Otolaryngol. 1997; 18(6):391–395

[56] Yotsukura M, Kinoshita T, Kohno M, et al. Survival predictors after resection of lung metastases of head or neck cancers. Thorac Cancer. 2015; 6(5):579–583

[57] Haro A, Yano T, Yoshida T, et al. Results of a surgical resection of pulmonary metastasis from malignant head and neck tumor. Interact Cardiovasc Thorac Surg. 2010; 10(5):700–703

[58] Mochizuki T, Okumura S, Ishii G, et al. Surgical resection for oral tongue cancer pulmonary metastases. Interact Cardiovasc Thorac Surg. 2010; 11(1):56–59

[59] Mazer TM, Robbins KT, McMurtrey MJ, Byers RM. Resection of pulmonary metastases from squamous carcinoma of the head and neck. Am J Surg. 1988; 156(4):238–242

[60] Tree AC, Khoo VS, Eeles RA, et al. Stereotactic body radiotherapy for oligometastases. Lancet Oncol. 2013; 14(1):e28–e37

[61] Chung CH, Mirakhur B, Chan E, et al. Cetuximab-induced anaphylaxis and IgE specific for galactose-alpha-1,3-galactose. N Engl J Med. 2008; 358(11): 1109–1117

[62] Vermorken JB, Stöhlmacher-Williams J, Davidenko I, et al. SPECTRUM investigators. Cisplatin and fluorouracil with or without panitumumab in patients with recurrent or metastatic squamous-cell carcinoma of the head and neck (SPECTRUM): an open-label phase 3 randomised trial. Lancet Oncol. 2013; 14 (8):697–710

[63] Guigay J, Fayette J, Dillies AF, et al. Cetuximab, docetaxel, and cisplatin as first-line treatment in patients with recurrent or metastatic head and neck squamous cell carcinoma: a multicenter, phase II GORTEC study. Ann Oncol. 2015; 26(9):1941–1947

[64] Argiris A, Li S, Savvides P, et al. Phase III randomized trial of chemotherapy with or without bevacizumab (B) in patients (pts) with recurrent or metastatic squamous cell carcinoma of the head and neck (R/M SCCHN): Survival analysis of E1305, an ECOG-ACRIN Cancer Research Group trial. Journal of Clinical Oncology. 2017; 35(15_suppl):6000

[65] Lane M, Moore JE, III, Levin H, Smith FE. Methotrexate therapy for squamous cell carcinomas of the head and neck: intermittent intravenous dose program. JAMA. 1968; 204(7):561–564

[66] Seiwert TY, Burtness B, Mehra R, et al. Safety and clinical activity of pembrolizumab for treatment of recurrent or metastatic squamous cell carcinoma of the head and neck (KEYNOTE-012): an open-label, multicentre, phase 1b trial. Lancet Oncol. 2016; 17(7):956–965

[67] Kushwaha VS, Gupta S, Husain N, et al. Gefitinib, Methotrexate and Methotrexate plus 5-Fluorouracil as palliative treatment in recurrent head and neck squamous cell carcinoma. Cancer Biol Ther. 2015; 16(2):346–351

[68] Lui VW, Hedberg ML, Li H, et al. Frequent mutation of the PI3K pathway in head and neck cancer defines predictive biomarkers. Cancer Discov. 2013; 3(7):761–769

[69] Dienstmann R, Rodon J, Serra V, Tabernero J. Picking the point of inhibition: a comparative review of PI3K/AKT/mTOR pathway inhibitors. Mol Cancer Ther. 2014; 13(5):1021–1031

[70] De Felice F, Guerrero Urbano T. New drug development in head and neck squamous cell carcinoma: the PI3-K inhibitors. Oral Oncol. 2017; 67:119–123

[71] Massacesi C, Di Tomaso E, Urban P, et al. PI3K inhibitors as new cancer therapeutics: implications for clinical trial design. OncoTargets Ther. 2016; 9:203–210

[72] Pons-Tostivint E, Thibault B, Guillermet-Guibert J. Targeting PI3K signaling in combination cancer therapy. Trends Cancer. 2017; 3(6):454–469

[73] Keeton AB, Salter EA, Piazza GA. The RAS-effector interaction as a drug target. Cancer Res. 2017; 77(2):221–226

[74] Chen X, Makarewicz JM, Knauf JA, Johnson LK, Fagin JA. Transformation by Hras(G12V) is consistently associated with mutant allele copy gains and is

reversed by farnesyl transferase inhibition. Oncogene. 2014; 33(47):5442–5449

[75] Ho A, Chau N, Wong DJ, et al. Abstract LB-A10: Preliminary results from a phase 2 proof of concept trial of tipifarnib in tumors with HRAS mutations. Mol Cancer Ther. 2018; 17(1 Supplement):LB-A10:-LB-A10. DOI: 10.1158/1535-7163.TARG-17-LB-A10. https://mct.aacrjournals.org/content/17/1_Supplement/LB-A10

[76] Guerrero-Preston R, Michailidi C, Marchionni L, et al. Key tumor suppressor genes inactivated by "greater promoter" methylation and somatic mutations in head and neck cancer. Epigenetics. 2014; 9(7):1031–1046

[77] Lim AM, Do H, Young RJ, et al. Differential mechanisms of CDKN2A (p16) alteration in oral tongue squamous cell carcinomas and correlation with patient outcome. Int J Cancer. 2014; 135(4):887–895

[78] Liggett WH, Jr, Sidransky D. Role of the p16 tumor suppressor gene in cancer. J Clin Oncol. 1998; 16(3):1197–1206

[79] Hortobagyi GN, Stemmer SM, Burris HA, et al. Ribociclib as first-line therapy for HR-positive, advanced breast cancer. N Engl J Med. 2016; 375(18):1738–1748

[80] Turner NC, Ro J, André F, et al. PALOMA3 Study Group. Palbociclib in hormone-receptor-positive advanced breast cancer. N Engl J Med. 2015; 373(3):209–219

[81] Patnaik A, Rosen LS, Tolaney SM, et al. Efficacy and safety of Abemaciclib, an inhibitor of CDK4 and CDK6, for patients with breast cancer, non-small cell lung cancer, and other solid tumors. Cancer Discov. 2016; 6(7):740–753

[82] Machiels JP, Subramanian S, Ruzsa A, et al. Zalutumumab plus best supportive care versus best supportive care alone in patients with recurrent or metastatic squamous-cell carcinoma of the head and neck after failure of platinum-based chemotherapy: an open-label, randomised phase 3 trial. Lancet Oncol. 2011; 12(4):333–343

[83] Erjala K, Sundvall M, Junttila TT, et al. Signaling via ErbB2 and ErbB3 associates with resistance and epidermal growth factor receptor (EGFR) amplification with sensitivity to EGFR inhibitor gefitinib in head and neck squamous cell carcinoma cells. Clin Cancer Res. 2006; 12(13):4103–4111

[84] Wang D, Qian G, Zhang H, et al. HER3 targeting sensitizes HNSCC to cetuximab by reducing HER3 activity and HER2/HER3 dimerization: evidence from cell line and patient-derived xenograft models. Clin Cancer Res. 2017; 23(3):677–686

[85] Szturz P, Seiwert TY, Vermorken JB. How standard is second-line cetuximab in recurrent or metastatic head and neck cancer in 2017? J Clin Oncol. 2017; 35(20):2229–2231

[86] Reck M, Rodríguez-Abreu D, Robinson AG, et al. KEYNOTE-024 Investigators. Pembrolizumab versus chemotherapy for PD-L1-positive non-small-cell lung cancer. N Engl J Med. 2016; 375(19):1823–1833

[87] Yarchoan M, Hopkins A, Jaffee EM. Tumor mutational burden and response rate to PD-1 inhibition. N Engl J Med. 2017; 377(25):2500–2501

[88] Hamid O, Bauer TM, Spira AI, et al. Epacadostat plus pembrolizumab in patients with SCCHN: preliminary phase I/II results from ECHO-202/KEYNOTE-037. 2017; 35(15_suppl):6010

[89] Althammer S, Steele K, Rebelatto M, et al. 31st Annual Meeting and Associated Programs of the Society for Immunotherapy of Cancer (SITC 2016): late breaking abstracts. J Immunother Cancer. 2017; 4(2):91

[90] Jacobs C, Lyman G, Velez-García E, et al. A phase III randomized study comparing cisplatin and fluorouracil as single agents and in combination for advanced squamous cell carcinoma of the head and neck. J Clin Oncol. 1992; 10(2):257–263

50 Immunotherapy

Ruth J. Davis and Rajarsi Mandal

Summary

The paradigm shift from conventional chemotherapy and targeted therapy to immunotherapy represents an exciting frontier in the medical management of human cancer. Head and neck cancers are ideal candidates for these immune-based approaches due to their high degree of immune cell infiltration. Two PD-1 inhibitors (pembrolizumab and nivolumab) were recently FDA approved for the treatment of head and neck cancer. Ongoing studies are investigating the role of checkpoint inhibition in the neoadjuvant setting and in combination with other novel immune modulating agents to maximize patient responses.

Keywords: immunotherapy, immune checkpoint blockade (ICB), PD-1, tumor infiltrating lymphocyte (TIL), head and neck squamous cell carcinoma (HNSCC)

50.1 Introduction

Immunotherapy represents an exciting frontier in the development of nonsurgical treatments for human cancers. Oral cavity cancer is one of the most promising avenues for the field. General approaches to triggering immune eradication of cancers have included tumor vaccines, adoptive cell transfer (ACT), and immune checkpoint blockade (ICB). The unprecedented successes of checkpoint inhibitors in a variety of cancer types have led to their approval by the FDA for the treatment of melanoma, non-small cell lung, renal cell, head and neck, and bladder cancers. These are the first agents since conventional chemotherapy to be applied successfully across a variety of tumor types, and are the subject of a rapidly developing body of research to expand responses and refine treatment regimens.

Immunotherapeutic strategies are distinct from conventional chemotherapy or targeted therapy, and represent a paradigm shift toward harnessing the body's own immune system to attack a tumor. The nonspecific destruction of rapidly dividing cells achieved with conventional chemotherapy is associated with significant morbidity and toxicity. Targeted therapies have shown promise in subsets of tumors with specific mutations; however, the whirlwind of growth and mutational evolution that define most cancers can also lead to rapid development of resistance. Immunotherapy, on the other hand, seeks to harness the power of the body's immune system against invading tumor cells to generate a widespread and durable response.

Responses to chemoradiation in the oral cavity cancer population have historically been modest, and surgery is increasingly preferred as the primary treatment modality when feasible.[1] Oral cavity cancer is an area with unmet need for improved nonsurgical alternatives, and these patients are poised to benefit greatly from advances in immunotherapy research. This chapter will explore our baseline understanding of immune infiltration in head and neck cancer, particularly in oral cavity cancer, and highlight the successes and failures of recent immunotherapy clinical trials for head and neck cancer. Additionally, this chapter will address clinical biomarkers for response, resistance mechanisms, and ongoing clinical trials and research efforts to improve immunotherapy for head and neck cancer.

50.2 Immune Infiltration in Head and Neck Cancer

Cancer types that are susceptible to checkpoint inhibition tend to be immunologically active at baseline with a high level of immune cell infiltration in the tumor microenvironment. These tumors generally have a high mutational load, creating neoantigens that are displayed on the surface of antigen-presenting cells (APCs), and lead to activation of the T lymphocytes and natural killer (NK) cells that destroy tumor cells. The development of a clinically relevant cancer requires evasion of this immune response. Immunotherapeutic approaches such as ICB aim to reverse this immune escape, restoring the body's ability to reject invading tumor cells.

Head and neck squamous cell carcinoma (HNSCC) lies at the high end of the spectrum of immune-infiltrated cancers, making it a particularly appealing candidate for the use of immunotherapy. Human papillomavirus (HPV) + HNSCC is the third most immune-infiltrated human cancer, and HPV– HNSCC ranks seventh.[2] The degree of tumor-infiltrating lymphocytes (TILs) in HNSCCs varies both by HPV status and by anatomic subsite, with HPV + oropharyngeal squamous cell carcinoma (OPSCC) at the top.[3] The fact that oral cavity cancer has lower immune infiltration than some other subtypes provides a rationale for therapeutic approaches aimed at enhancing immune infiltration (i.e., Toll-like receptor [TLR], Stimulator of Interferon Genes [STING]) in addition to reversing immune suppression (i.e., ICB).

A variety of studies have demonstrated a correlation between tumor-infiltrating immune cells and positive outcomes. Infiltration of T cells into HNSCCs has been associated with increased locoregional control and survival, regardless of treatment modality.[4–6] Not only is the number of lymphocytes in the tumor microenvironment an independent prognostic factor,[7] but lymphocyte functionality is also associated with prognosis.[8] The prognostic value of immune cell infiltration extends far beyond HNSCC in the landscape of human cancers, and has also been demonstrated reproducibly in melanoma,[9] ovarian,[10] and colorectal cancers.[11]

The inflamed microenvironment of HNSCC sets the stage for reversal of immune exhaustion. A variety of co-stimulatory and co-inhibitory immune checkpoint receptors modulate T-lymphocyte activation by APCs at the immune synapse (▶ Fig. 50.1). The use of monoclonal antibodies to block co-inhibitory immune checkpoints (i.e., programmed death-1 [PD-1], CTLA-4), or activate co-stimulatory checkpoints (i.e., CD40, OX40, 4–1BB, CD28) can alter the balance in favor of antitumor immunity.

PD-1 is of particular interest due to FDA approval of antibodies targeting this checkpoint. PD-1 is expressed on the surface of activated T cells and NK cells, and limits an overactive immune response, preventing autoimmune destruction. However, long-term antigen exposure in the setting of tumor

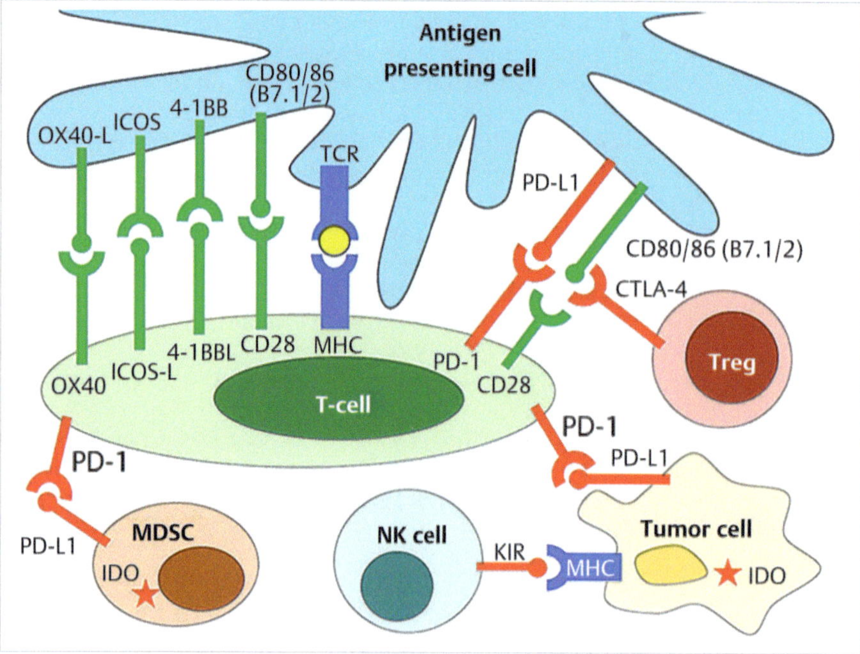

Fig. 50.1 The immune synapse: Immune stimulatory (green) and inhibitory (red) signals between tumor cells and host immune cells that are therapeutic targets for immunotherapy.

development may lead to overexpression of PD-1 and T lymphocyte exhaustion. When engaged by its ligands, PD-L1 or PD-L2 (on tumor cells), PD-1 inhibits immune activation and allows tumor growth to proceed. Reversal of this immunologic suppression can lead to profound changes in immune response and patient prognosis.

50.3 Immunotherapy for Head and Neck Cancer

50.3.1 Previous Attempts

Prior to the advent of ICB, cetuximab was the first new agent to be approved by the FDA for HNSCC in many years. Cetuximab is a monoclonal antibody (mAb) that targets the epidermal growth factor receptor (EGFR) on the surface of HNSCC cells, and is approved by the FDA for the treatment of advanced HNSCC in combination with radiation, as monotherapy, or in combination with chemotherapy for recurrent/metastatic HNSCC. Cetuximab functions as an immunotherapeutic agent through activation of antibody-dependent cellular cytotoxicity (ADCC). The cetuximab antibody serves as a bridge that at one end (Fab region) binds EGFR on the surface of tumor cells and at the other end (Fc region) binds CD16/FcRIII on the surface of NK cells. This binding activates NK cells to release perforin and granzyme B, which lyse the tumor cell. Although 80% of HNSCCs overexpress EGFR, only 10–20% of patients respond to cetuximab, spurring efforts to combine it with additional agents to circumvent this resistence.[12]

Additional approaches that have been evaluated with limited success in early phase HNSCC trials include vaccination and ACT. Antitumor vaccines aim to augment immune recognition of tumor cells through increased presentation of antigen by dendritic cells, and induce immunologic memory to prevent recurrence. Vaccination approaches involve injection of tumor-associated antigens[13] or injection of autologous dendritic cells loaded with p53 antigen *ex vivo*.[14] However, compared to other cancer types with well-defined tumor antigens (i.e., prostate cancer, for which the Sipuleucel-T vaccine is FDA approved), identification of a highly immunogenic peptide for broad use in HNSCC remains a challenge.

ACT is another approach that has shown promising results in melanoma,[15,16] and was recently approved by the FDA for treatment of acute lymphoblastic leukemia. Traditionally, ACT involves purification of autologous TILs from a surgical specimen, *ex vivo* stimulation, expansion, and re-injection of TILs that are active against the patient's tumor.[15,16] These autologous T lymphocytes may also be engineered to express T-cell receptors (TCRs) or chimeric antigen receptors (CARs) with high specificity for particular tumor-associated antigens, thereby increasing the potency and specificity of the antitumor response. In HNSCC, a clinical trial evaluating CARs specific for HPV-16 E6 has recently been completed (NCT02280811).

50.3.2 Current State

Currently, the use of checkpoint inhibitors targeting PD-1 is the only immunotherapeutic strategy that has demonstrated clear clinical benefit in the treatment of HNSCC. Data from recent trials evaluating the PD-1 inhibitors pembrolizumab and nivolumab resulted in FDA approval in 2016 of both agents for the treatment of recurrent or metastatic HNSCC that progressed either during or after treatment with platinum-based chemotherapy.

The phase Ib KEYNOTE-012 trial of pembrolizumab in recurrent or metastatic HNSCC demonstrated an 18% overall response rate with median progression-free survival of 2 months and overall survival of 13 months, and a 17% rate of grades 3–4 adverse events.[17] The phase III CheckMate 141 trial compared nivolumab to standard therapy in patients with recurrent or metastatic, platinum-refractory HNSCC.[18] The identification of a significant survival benefit led to early conclusion of the trial: nivolumab reduced the risk of death by 30% compared to standard treatment with median overall survival extending from 5.1 to 7.5 months. With an overall response rate of 13.3% compared to 5.8% with standard therapy, nivolumab also more than doubled 1-year survival from 16.6 to 36%. Additionally, nivolumab was better tolerated, with only 13.1% experiencing grades 3–4 adverse events compared to 35.1% in the standard therapy group.

The KEYNOTE-040 phase III trial compared pembrolizumab to standard therapy in patients with recurrent or metastatic platinum-refractory HNSCC.[19] This study failed to meet its primary endpoint: a 19% improvement in overall survival achieved with pembrolizumab did reach the pre-specified criteria for statistical significance. Median survival with pembrolizumab was only marginally improved to 8.4 months compared to 7.1 months with standard therapy. However, the use of salvage immunotherapy in the standard arm may confound these results, and could contribute to 2 months longer median survival in the standard arm of KEYNOTE-040 compared to CheckMate 141. Similar to the results of CheckMate 141, only 13.4% experienced grades 3–5 adverse events with pembrolizumab compared to 36.3% with standard therapy.

The KEYNOTE-055 phase II trial also evaluated pembrolizumab in HNSCC that was refractory to both platinum and cetuximab.[20] In this population, an overall response rate of 16% was identified, with responses lasting for a median of 8 months. Although the response rates to ICB in these studies remain modest, the durability of benefit and translation into improved clinical outcomes in these heavily pre-treated populations provide the foundation for current and future work aimed at expanding responses and identifying patients likely to benefit.

50.4 Ongoing and New Trials

50.4.1 Ongoing Monotherapy Trials

The KEYNOTE-048 (NCT02358031) phase III trial is currently evaluating pembrolizumab as first-line treatment compared to standard of care in patients with recurrent/metastatic HNSCC. In addition, phase II trials are evaluating adjuvant pembrolizumab vs. placebo, in patients at high risk for recurrence (PATHWay, NCT02841748) or after salvage surgery in patients with relapsed, locally recurrent HNSCC (NCT02769520). A randomized phase II trial comparing pembrolizumab to methotrexate in frail or cisplatin-ineligible HNSCC patients has not yet begun recruitment (ELDORANDO, NCT03193931). Pembrolizumab is also under evaluation for patients with residual disease following definitive radiation (XRT) (NCT02892201).

50.4.2 Neoadjuvant Trials

When feasible, surgical resection or radiation remains the primary treatment for oral cavity cancer, with chemoradiation typically reserved for the adjuvant setting in patients with high risk features, or as upfront treatment for patients with unresectable disease. However, with the addition of checkpoint inhibitors to the armamentarium, interest has been renewed in the use of neoadjuvant therapy for HNSCC at large.[21] Theoretical advantages of immunotherapy in the neoadjuvant setting include intact lymphatics allowing for improved infiltration of immune cells to the tumor, reversal of lymphocyte exhaustion at an early stage, and presence of significant intact antigen to prime immune memory and keep postsurgical recurrence at bay. The successful use of neoadjuvant therapy may lead to early identification of responsive tumors, and the possibility of decreasing tumor burden to minimize the degree of resection or downstage unresectable to resectable disease.[21]

A phase II trial evaluating neoadjuvant pembrolizumab in surgically resectable stage III/IV HNSCC is currently underway (NCT02296684).[22] Preliminary analysis identified pathologic response to a single dose of neoadjuvant pembrolizumab in 43% of patients at the time of surgery, and 48% of patients experienced clinical-to-pathologic downstaging.[22] The CheckMate-358 phase I/II study is an ongoing international multicenter study evaluating nivolumab in virus-associated cancers. A cohort of 29 patients with HPV+and HPV– resectable HNSCC were treated with two doses of nivolumab prior to surgery, and 48% experienced reduction in tumor size by the time of surgery.[23]

50.4.3 Rationale Surrounding Combination Studies

Although clinical response rates to ICB have been low in the heavily pretreated recurrent/metastatic HNSCC population (13.3–18%), the clinical improvements seen in responders are impressive.[17,18] Tumors may downregulate co-stimulatory receptors or increase signaling through alternative immune checkpoints at the immune synapse (▶ Fig. 50.1) to maintain immunosuppression in the face of ICB. Efforts have turned to the development of combination therapy regimens to broaden responses through the simultaneous targeting of multiple immune mechanisms. For example, 4–1BB (CD137) is a co-stimulatory receptor that is the target of two mAbs (utomilumab and urelumab) in clinical development. Of additional interest are studies combining PD-1 inhibition with the CTLA-4 inhibitor ipilimumab, which was the first checkpoint inhibitor to achieve FDA approval in 2011. CTLA-4 is expressed on the surface of regulatory T lymphocytes (Tregs), and binds CD80/86 on the surface of APCs to competitively inhibit T-cell activation (▶ Fig. 50.1).[24] A phase III clinical trial comparing a combination of nivolumab (PD-1) and ipilimumab (CTLA-4) to the EXTREME regimen (cetuximab, cisplatin/carboplatin, and fluorouracil) is currently recruiting (NCT02741570).

Combinations of ICB with conventional chemotherapy and radiation are also of interest due to the tremendous release of antigen achieved with these cytotoxic therapies. Several studies are evaluating the timing of ICB administration, either concurrent with conventional therapy or as an adjuvant treatment. See ▶ Table 50.1 and ▶ Table 50.2 for a summary of active clinical trials evaluating nivolumab or pembrolizumab in combination therapy regimens.

50.4.4 Innate Immune Activation

Strategies to activate the innate immune system represent alternatives or complementary approaches to the stimulation of adaptive immune cell function through ICB or activation of co-stimulatory pathways. Not all tumors have a high degree of lymphocyte infiltration, and these immunologically "cold"

Table 50.1 Clinical trials evaluating combinations including nivolumab

Targets	Treatments	Phase	Clinical trial ID	HNSCC patient eligibility	Status
CTLA-4	+ Ipilimumab	II	NCT02919683	Oral cavity SCC Stage T2 + and/or N1 +	Recruiting
CTLA-4	+ Ipilimumab + XRT	I	NCT03162731	HPV– HNSCC Stage IVA-B	Recruiting
CTLA-4	+ Ipilimumab	II	NCT02823574	Recurrent/metastatic HNSCC	Recruiting
PI3K-γ	+ IPI-549	I	NCT02637531	HNSCC refractory to PD-1 alone	Recruiting
CSF1R	+ FPA008	I	NCT02526017	Recurrent/progressive HNSCC	Recruiting
EGFR TLR8	+ Cetuximab + Motolimod	Ib	NCT02124850	Untreated HNSCC Stages II–IVA (neoadjuvant)	Recruiting
Oncolytic virus	+ Enadenotucirev	I	NCT02636036	Advanced/metastatic HNSCC	Recruiting
Spleen tyrosine kinase (SYK)	+ TAK-659	I	NCT02834247	Recurrent/metastatic HNSCC	Recruiting
CD27	+ Varlilumab	I/II	NCT02335918	Platinum-refractory HNSCC Stage III/IV	Recruiting
LAG3	Relatlimab + /– Nivolumab	I/II	NCT01968109	Immunotherapy-naïve HNSCC	Recruiting
EGFR	+ Cisplatin or Cetuximab or IMRT	I	NCT02764593	Intermediate & high-risk locoregionally advanced HNSCC	Recruiting
PDE-5	+ Tadalafil	I	NCT03238365	Surgically resectable HNSCC	Recruiting
KIR	+ Lirilumab	II	NCT03341936	Locoregionally recurrent HNSCC	Not yet recruiting
PD-1 + CTLA-4 vs. EXTREME	Nivolumab + Ipilimumab vs. Cetuximab + Cisplatin/ Carboplatin + 5-Fluorouracil	III	NCT02741570	Recurrent/metastatic HNSCC	Recruiting
PD-1 + IDO + Platinum vs. EXTREME	Nivolumab + Epacadostat + Platinum + 5-Fluorouracil vs. Cetuximab + Platinum + 5-Fluorouracil	III	NCT03342352	Recurrent/metastatic HNSCC	Not yet recruiting
	SBRT + /– Nivolumab	II	NCT02684253	Metastatic HNSCC	Recruiting
	+ XRT	II	NCT03313804	Metastatic HNSCC	Recruiting
	+ XRT	I/II	NCT03247712	Surgically resectable HNSCC (neoadjuvant)	Not yet recruiting
	+ Carboplatin + Paclitaxel	II	NCT03342911	Stages III–IV resectable HNSCC	Not yet recruiting

Abbreviations: EGFR, epidermal growth factor receptor; HNSCC, head and neck squamous cell carcinoma; IDO, indoleamine 2,3-dioxygenase; KIR, killer cell immunoglobulin-like receptor; SCC, squamous cell carcinoma, SYK; XRT.

tumors may benefit from stimulation of innate immunity and the production of Th1-polarizing cytokines that induce infiltration and activation of lymphocytes.

TLRs are transmembrane receptors that recognize molecular patterns associated with microbial invasion, and mediate responses through activation of innate immunity. In 2010 the FDA approved a topical TLR7/8 agonist, imiquimod, for the treatment of actinic keratosis, basal cell carcinoma, and warts. More recently, a selective TLR8 agonist, motolimod (VTX-2337), has been shown to induce elevated levels of immune-activating cytokines in a phase I trial,[25] and a phase Ib trial of motolimod + cetuximab identified a 54% disease control rate in 13 patients with recurrent/metastatic HNSCC (NCT01334177).[26] Most recently, the Active8 randomized phase II trial (NCT01836029) failed to demonstrate improved progression-free or overall survival with the addition of motolimod to the EXTREME regimen in recurrent/metastatic HNSCC.[27] However, a subgroup of patients who experienced an immune-related injection site reaction did obtain significant benefit. This data indicates that further refinement in treatment approach will be required before motolimod advances to further phases of study. Currently, a phase Ib study of nivolumab, cetuximab, and motolimod in the neoadjuvant setting is recruiting (NCT02124850). In addition, the TLR-9 agonist, SD101, is also under study in combination with pembrolizumab in recurrent/metastatic HNSCC (NCT02521870).

Another immune activating approach that has reached phase I clinical trials in HNSCC (NCT02675439, NCT03172936) is agonism of the STING receptor. The STING receptor represents a TLR-independent pathway of innate immune activation, through which microbial (or tumor) associated cytosolic DNA stimulates production of type I interferon and activation of innate immunity. In preclinical studies, synthetic cyclic dinucleotides have been shown to activate the STING receptor and reduce growth of T-cell inflamed head and neck cancers, and combine with PD-1 pathway blockade to induce tumor rejection.[28]

Table 50.2 Clinical trials evaluating combinations including pembrolizumab

Targets	Treatments	Phase	Clinical trial ID	HNSCC patient eligibility	Status
Platelets	+ /– (clopidogrel + ASA)	I	NCT03245489	Recurrent/metastatic HNSCC	Recruiting
TLR9	+ SD-101	Ib/2	NCT02521870	Recurrent/metastatic HNSCC	Recruiting
Galectin	+ GR-MD-02	I	NCT02575404	HNSCC progressive after 1 + platinum-containing regimens	Recruiting
EGFR	+ Cetuximab	II	NCT03082534	Recurrent/metastatic HNSCC	Recruiting
Angiogenesis	+ EphB4-HSA	II	NCT03049618	HNSCC progressive after 1 + platinum-containing regimens	Recruiting
Nitric oxide synthetase	+ L-NMMA	Ib	NCT03236935	HNSCC recurrent/refractory to platinum-based regimen	Not yet recruiting
Oncolytic virus	+ Talimogene Laherparepvec	Ib/3	NCT02626000	Recurrent/metastatic HNSCC	Recruiting
Bruton tyrosine kinase	+ /– Acalabrutinib	II	NCT02454179	Recurrent/metastatic HNSCC	Ongoing, not recruiting
CSF-1R	+ PLX3397	I/II	NCT02452424	Recurrent/metastatic solid tumors	Ongoing, not recruiting
CD40	SEA-CD40 + /– pembrolizumab	I	NCT02376699	Recurrent/metastatic solid tumors	Recruiting
B7-H3	+ Enoblituzumab	I	NCT02475213	B7-H3 + unresectable/locally advanced/ metastatic solid tumors	Recruiting
IDO	+ Epacadostat	II	NCT03238638	Advanced HNSCC, failed PD-1/PD-L1 therapy	Not yet recruiting
IDO	+ Epacadostat (neoadjuvant) → surgery	II	NCT03325465	Surgically resectable HNSCC	Not yet recruiting
Histone deacetylase	+ Vorinostat	I/II	NCT02538510	Recurrent/metastatic/inoperable HNSCC or salivary gland cancer	Active not recruiting
	+ XRT	I	NCT02318771	Recurrent/metastatic HNSCC	Recruiting
	+ XRT	II	NCT03313804	Metastatic HNSCC	Recruiting
	+ XRT	II	NCT02609503	Stages III–IV (nonmetastatic) HNSCC, not eligible for cisplatin	Recruiting
	+ XRT	II	NCT03085719	Metastatic HNSCC unresponsive to PD-1	Recruiting
	+ Reirradiation	II	NCT02289209	Locoregional inoperable recurrent or second primary HNSCC	Recruiting
	SOC (surgery, XRT + /– cisplatin) + adjuvant pembrolizumab	II	NCT02641093	Advanced, resectable HNSCC	Recruiting
	+ SOC (chemoradiation)	I/II	NCT02759575	Locally advanced laryngeal SCC	Recruiting
	+ cisplatin-IMRT vs. after cisplatin-IMRT	II	NCT02777385	Intermediate or high risk nonmetastatic HNSCC	Recruiting
	+ chemoradiation (CRT)	I	NCT02586207	Stages III–IVB HNSCC	Recruiting
	CRT + pembrolizumab vs. CRT	III	NCT03040999	Locally advanced HNSCC	Recruiting

Abbreviations: CRT; EGFR, epidermal growth factor receptor; HNSCC, head and neck squamous cell carcinoma; IDO, indoleamine 2,3-dioxygenase; XRT.

50.5 Improving Patient Selection Using Genetic and Immunologic Criteria

50.5.1 Current Biomarkers

Responses to ICB are highly variable across patients and cancer types, with HNSCC response rates remaining below 20%. Expression of PD-L1 in the tumor microenvironment initially emerged as a logical biomarker of response to anti-PD1 therapy, with 36% response observed in patients with PD-L1 positive tumors compared to 0% response in those lacking PD-L1 expression.[29] Further studies have confirmed this tendency for higher response rates in PD-L1 positive patients, and PD-L1 expression is currently the most widely used biomarker; however, it has been found to be highly imperfect as a predictor of response. Across cancers, the majority of PD-L1 positive patients still do not respond to PD-1 inhibition, whereas a small but significant proportion of PD-L1 negative patients do respond.[30] In HNSCC, the KEYNOTE-012 phase Ib trial observed a 22% response to pembrolizumab in PD-L1 positive patients compared to 4% in those lacking PD-L1 expression.[31] In the phase III CheckMate 141 trial the trend toward improved

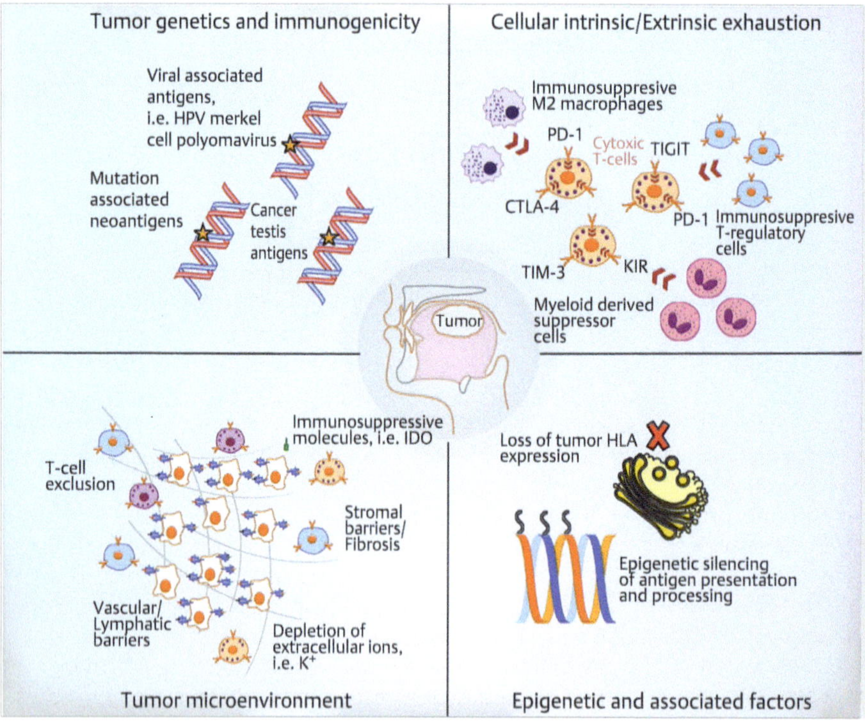

Fig. 50.2 Determinants of response/resistance to oral cavity immunotherapy.

responses to nivolumab in PD-L1 positive tumors did not reach statistical significance.[18]

The genetic and immunological basis of immunotherapeutic resistance in head and neck cancer is multifactorial and involves components of inherent tumor immunogenicity, T-cell exhaustion, unfavorable tumor microenvironments, and epigenetic factors (▶ Fig. 50.2). Predicting response to PD-1 inhibitors is clearly more complex than simply identifying expression of PD-L1. Possible confounding factors include the potential role of an additional PD-1 ligand, PD-L2, in responders who lack PD-L1 expression, poor T-cell infiltration in poorly responsive PD-L1 positive tumors, and alternative mechanisms of immune evasion in PD-L1 positive patients that are not reversed through ICB alone.[32] A recent study has demonstrated the utility of a T-cell inflamed gene expression profile for predicting responses to pembrolizumab.[33] This 18-gene profile was validated using HNSCC data from the KEYNOTE-012 trial, with the area under the receiver operating characteristic (ROC) curve of 0.75, compared to 0.65 for PD-L1 expression (however this unplanned comparison did not reach statistical significance). A clinical assay based on this gene expression profile is currently under study in clinical trials of pembrolizumab.

50.5.2 Tumor Genetics

The genetic landscape of a specific tumor also plays a vital role in the initiation of antitumor immunity and responsiveness to ICB. Tumors with more nonsynonymous mutations can generate greater numbers of neoantigens that can be recognized as non-self, becoming targets of immune destruction. Higher mutational load has been associated with clinical benefit both in non-small cell lung cancer patients treated with pembrolizumab[34] and melanoma patients treated with a CLTA4-targeting agent.[35] However, the role of nonsynonymous mutations in predicting responses to ICB appears to be more complicated than the number of mutations. Not all patients with high mutational load are responsive to ICB, and some patients with low mutational load still benefit.[30] Specific neoantigen signatures have been identified in responders to ICB, suggesting that certain neoantigens (i.e., those with homology to microbe-associated antigens) may be more powerful than others in igniting antitumor immunity in the context of checkpoint inhibition.[35]

One class of mutations that appear to be particularly relevant are mutations in mismatch repair (MMR) genes. These mutations can play a role in tumorigenesis by allowing for inaccurate DNA replication and generation of oncogenes or loss of tumor-suppressor genes. In addition, MMR dysfunction leads to inaccurate DNA replication, and subsequent generation of more neoantigens.[30] Recent studies have correlated efficacy of pembrolizumab with MMR mutations in patients with non-small cell lung cancer;[34] however, further research to evaluate its utility in HNSCC is necessary.

50.5.3 Immunosuppressive Characteristics

A T-cell inflamed phenotype appears to be necessary but insufficient for clinical response to ICB,[33] suggesting that additional mechanisms of immune evasion are at work in these immunologically "hot" tumors.[24] Analysis of the most immune-infiltrated human cancer types revealed HNSCC to have the highest median Treg/CD8 + T-cell ratio and the highest level of NK cell infiltration.[2] This data highlights the importance of Tregs in maintaining the immunosuppressive microenvironment of HNSCC. Tregs release immunosuppressive cytokines that inhibit T cell and NK cell recruitment and function. Through surface expression of CTLA-4, Tregs also limit T-cell activation.[24]

Blockade of CTLA-4 with the monoclonal antibody ipilimumab enhances antitumor immunity and survival in melanoma. However, clinical trials evaluating CTLA-4 inhibition in HNSCC are underway. In addition to CTLA-4, therapies targeting Treg surface receptors such as inducible T cell costimulator (ICOS), CCR4, CD25, OX40, and GITR are the subject of ongoing research. NK cells also express a variety of stimulatory and inhibitory surface receptors that represent interesting targets given the high degree of NK cell infiltration in HNSCC.[2] The killer cell immunoglobulin-like receptor (KIR) on the surface of NK cells is the target of the mAb lirilumab, which is under study in combination with nivolumab in relapsed, resectable HNSCC (NCT03341936).

In addition to Tregs, myeloid-derived suppressor cells (MDSCs) are another immunosuppressive cell type deployed by tumors to evade host immunity. These immature myeloid cells inhibit antitumor immunity through secretion of immunosuppressive cytokines, production of reactive oxygen and nitrogen species, depletion of arginine and tryptophan from the tumor microenvironment, and expression of PD-L1.[24] MDSCs have been associated with recurrence and metastasis in HNSCC patients after definitive treatment, and have been the target of a variety of inhibitory strategies.[24] In preclinical studies of oral cavity cancer, responses to ICB have been enhanced by functional inhibition of MDSCs with a selective PI3Kδ/γ inhibitor, and by depletion of MDSCs from the tumor microenvironment.[36,37] Inhibition of phosphodiesterase-5 with tadalafil has been shown to inhibit MDSCs functionally, and enhance markers of antitumor immunity in HNSCC in the neoadjuvant setting.[38] MDSCs and tumor cells express an enzyme indoleamine 2,3-dioxygenase (IDO), which mediates immunosuppression by decreasing tryptophan in the tumor microenvironment and activating Tregs. IDO inhibitors such as epacadostat may target both MDSC function and Treg activation, and are currently under study in combination with ICB in a variety of solid tumors.[2,24]

50.5.4 HPV Status

Although most HPV + OPSCCs are highly infiltrated with T lymphocytes and have an excellent prognosis, a subset of these tumors with low TIL levels carry a poor prognosis no better than that of HPV- HNSCC.[39] The significance of HPV positivity in non-OPSCC has been a subject of debate. However, recent work by Chakravarthy et al demonstrated a causal role of HPV in 4.1% of non-OPSCCs.[3] In this study, HPV-driven non-OPSCC lacked the positive prognosis classically associated with HPV + OPSCC and had lower levels of T-cell infiltration. These data suggest that the positive prognosis associated with HPV + OPSCC may be in part attributed to the strong antitumor immune response generated by the HPV virus. However, a recent analysis of T cells of two patients who experienced complete regression of metastatic HPV + cervical cancer in response to adoptive transfer of TILs selected for HPV-E6/E7 oncoprotein reactivity revealed predominant reactivities against tumor-related antigens rather than the viral antigens. This suggests that even in the setting of HPV + disease, nonviral antigens still represent excellent targets.[40] Further work is needed to fully understand the role of HPV infection in development and targeting of antitumor immunity.

50.6 Conclusion

The future of immunotherapy for HNSCC is very promising. Given the high degree of T cell and NK cell infiltration into human HNSCCs, there is great potential for reversing tumor-mediated immune suppression through the use of FDA-approved checkpoint inhibitors and development of novel immunotherapeutic regimens. Oral cavity cancer has a unique advantage due to the accessibility of the tumor for serial biopsies, making it an ideal candidate for further study of immunotherapeutic approaches. In addition, the development of new technologies allowing for precise characterization of the genetic and immunologic landscape of these tumors will inevitably lead to the development of improved immune-based treatment approaches for patients with oral cavity cancer.

Key Points/Pearls

- Immunotherapy represents a paradigm shift from targeted therapy or conventional chemotherapy to harness the body's immune system to attack a tumor.
- HNSCCs are highly infiltrated with immune cells, making them an ideal candidate for immunotherapeutic approaches.
- Pembrolizumab and nivolumab are two PD-1 inhibitors approved by FDA for the treatment of recurrent or metastatic HNSCC that has progressed either during or after treatment with platinum-based chemotherapy.
- Ongoing studies suggest a possible role for PD-1 inhibitors in the neoadjuvant setting.
- Immune agonists (i.e., TLR or STING agonists) may be useful in combination with checkpoint inhibitors.
- PD-L1 expression is an imperfect biomarker of response to ICB, and tumor genetics may prove to be a more reliable alternative.
- Reversing additional mechanisms of tumor-mediated immunosuppression may expand responses to ICB.

References

[1] Fujiwara RJT, Burtness B, Husain ZA, et al. Treatment guidelines and patterns of care in oral cavity squamous cell carcinoma: primary surgical resection vs. nonsurgical treatment. Oral Oncol. 2017; 71:129–137

[2] Mandal R, Şenbabaoğlu Y, Desrichard A, et al. The head and neck cancer immune landscape and its immunotherapeutic implications. JCI Insight. 2016; 1(17):e89829

[3] Chakravarthy A, Henderson S, Thirdborough SM, et al. Human papillomavirus drives tumor development throughout the head and neck: improved prognosis is associated with an immune response largely restricted to the oropharynx. J Clin Oncol. 2016; 34(34):4132–4141

[4] Badoual C, Hans S, Rodriguez J, et al. Prognostic value of tumor-infiltrating CD4 + T-cell subpopulations in head and neck cancers. Clin Cancer Res. 2006; 12(2):465–472

[5] Balermpas P, Michel Y, Wagenblast J, et al. Tumour-infiltrating lymphocytes predict response to definitive chemoradiotherapy in head and neck cancer. Br J Cancer. 2014; 110(2):501–509

[6] Xu Q, Wang C, Yuan X, Feng Z, Han Z. Prognostic value of tumor-infiltrating lymphocytes for patients with head and neck squamous cell carcinoma. Transl Oncol. 2017; 10(1):10–16

[7] Nguyen N, Bellile E, Thomas D, et al. Head and Neck SPORE Program Investigators. Tumor infiltrating lymphocytes and survival in patients with head and neck squamous cell carcinoma. Head Neck. 2016; 38(7):1074–1084

[8] Shibuya TY, Nugyen N, McLaren CE, et al. Clinical significance of poor CD3 response in head and neck cancer. Clin Cancer Res. 2002; 8(3):745–751. Accessed September 4, 2017

[9] Clemente CG, Mihm MC, Jr, Bufalino R, Zurrida S, Collini P, Cascinelli N. Prognostic value of tumor infiltrating lymphocytes in the vertical growth phase of primary cutaneous melanoma. Cancer. 1996; 77(7):1303–1310
[10] Sato E, Olson SH, Ahn J, et al. Intraepithelial CD8+tumor-infiltrating lymphocytes and a high CD8+/regulatory T cell ratio are associated with favorable prognosis in ovarian cancer. Proc Natl Acad Sci U S A. 2005; 102(51): 18538–18543
[11] Pagès F, Berger A, Camus M, et al. Effector memory T cells, early metastasis, and survival in colorectal cancer. N Engl J Med. 2005; 353(25):2654–2666
[12] Srivastava RM, Lee SC, Andrade Filho PA, et al. Cetuximab-activated natural killer and dendritic cells collaborate to trigger tumor antigen-specific T-cell immunity in head and neck cancer patients. Clin Cancer Res. 2013; 19(7): 1858–1872
[13] Yoshitake Y, Fukuma D, Yuno A, et al. Phase II clinical trial of multiple peptide vaccination for advanced head and neck cancer patients revealed induction of immune responses and improved OS. Clin Cancer Res. 2015; 21(2):312–321
[14] Schuler PJ, Harasymczuk M, Visus C, et al. Phase I dendritic cell p53 peptide vaccine for head and neck cancer. Clin Cancer Res. 2014; 20(9): 2433–2444
[15] Rosenberg SA, Yang JC, Sherry RM, et al. Durable complete responses in heavily pretreated patients with metastatic melanoma using T-cell transfer immunotherapy. Clin Cancer Res. 2011; 17(13):4550–4557
[16] Besser MJ, Shapira-Frommer R, Itzhaki O, et al. Adoptive transfer of tumor-infiltrating lymphocytes in patients with metastatic melanoma: intent-to-treat analysis and efficacy after failure to prior immunotherapies. Clin Cancer Res. 2013; 19(17):4792–4800
[17] Seiwert TY, Burtness B, Mehra R, et al. Safety and clinical activity of pembrolizumab for treatment of recurrent or metastatic squamous cell carcinoma of the head and neck (KEYNOTE-012): an open-label, multicentre, phase 1b trial. Lancet Oncol. 2016; 17(7):956–965
[18] Ferris RL, Blumenschein G, Jr, Fayette J, et al. Nivolumab for recurrent squamous-cell carcinoma of the head and neck. N Engl J Med. 2016; 375(19): 1856–1867
[19] Cohen EE, Harrington KJ, Le Tourneau C, et al. Pembrolizumab (pembro) vs standard of care (SOC) for recurrent or metastatic head and neck squamous cell carcinoma (R/M HNSCC): Phase 3 KEYNOTE-040 trial. Ann Oncol. ESMO 2017; 28:v605–v649
[20] Bauml J, Seiwert TY, Pfister DG, et al. Pembrolizumab for platinum- and cetuximab-refractory head and neck cancer: results from a single-arm, phase II study. J Clin Oncol. 2017; 35(14):1542–1549
[21] Hanna GJ, Adkins DR, Zolkind P, Uppaluri R. Rationale for neoadjuvant immunotherapy in head and neck squamous cell carcinoma. Oral Oncol. 2017; 73: 65–69
[22] Uppaluri R, Zolkind P, Lin T, et al. Neoadjuvant pembrolizumab in surgically resectable, locally advanced HPV negative head and neck squamous cell carcinoma (HNSCC). J Clin Oncol. 2017; 35(15_suppl):6012–6012
[23] Ferris RL, Gonçalves A, Baxi SS, et al. An open-label, multicohort, phase 1/2 study in patients with virus-associated cancers (CheckMate 358): safety and efficacy of neoadjuvant nivolumab in squamous cell carcinoma of the head and neck (SCCHN). Ann Oncol. 2017; 28(suppl_)(5):605–649
[24] Davis RJ, Van Waes C, Allen CT. Overcoming barriers to effective immunotherapy: MDSCs, TAMs, and Tregs as mediators of the immunosuppressive microenvironment in head and neck cancer. Oral Oncol. 2016; 58:59–70
[25] Northfelt DW, Ramanathan RK, Cohen PA, et al. A phase I dose-finding study of the novel Toll-like receptor 8 agonist VTX-2337 in adult subjects with advanced solid tumors or lymphoma. Clin Cancer Res. 2014; 20(14): 3683–3691
[26] Chow LQM, Morishima C, Eaton KD, et al. Phase Ib trial of the Toll-like receptor 8 agonist, motolimod (VTX-2337), combined with cetuximab in patients with recurrent or metastatic SCCHN. Clin Cancer Res. 2017; 23(10):2442–2450
[27] Cohen E, Saba NF, Gitlitz B, et al. Immunotherapy of cancer Active8: a randomized, double-blind, placebo-controlled study of chemotherapy plus cetuximab in combination with motolimod immunotherapy in patients with recurrent or metastatic squamous cell carcinoma of the head and neck. Ann Oncol. 2016; 27(Suppl_)(6)
[28] Moore E, Clavijo PE, Davis R, et al. Established T cell-inflamed tumors rejected after adaptive resistance was reversed by combination STING activation and PD-1 pathway blockade. Cancer Immunol Res. 2016; 4(12):1061–1071
[29] Topalian SL, Hodi FS, Brahmer JR, et al. Safety, activity, and immune correlates of anti-PD-1 antibody in cancer. N Engl J Med. 2012; 366(26):2443–2454
[30] Mandal R, Chan TA. Personalized oncology meets immunology: the path toward precision immunotherapy. Cancer Discov. 2016; 6(7):703–713
[31] Chow LQM, Haddad R, Gupta S, et al. Antitumor activity of pembrolizumab in biomarker-unselected patients with recurrent and/or metastatic head and neck squamous cell carcinoma: results from the phase Ib KEYNOTE-012 expansion cohort. J Clin Oncol. 2016; 34(32):3838–3845
[32] De Meulenaere A, Vermassen T, Aspeslagh S, et al. Turning the tide: clinical utility of PD-L1 expression in squamous cell carcinoma of the head and neck. Oral Oncol. 2017; 70:34–42
[33] Ayers M, Lunceford J, Nebozhyn M, et al. IFN-γ-related mRNA profile predicts clinical response to PD-1 blockade. J Clin Invest. 2017; 127(8):2930–2940
[34] Rizvi NA, Hellmann MD, Snyder A, et al. Cancer immunology: mutational landscape determines sensitivity to PD-1 blockade in non-small cell lung cancer. Science. 2015; 348(6230):124–128
[35] Snyder A, Makarov V, Merghoub T, et al. Genetic basis for clinical response to CTLA-4 blockade in melanoma. N Engl J Med. 2014; 371(23):2189–2199
[36] Davis RJ, Moore EC, Clavijo PE, et al. Anti-PD-L1 efficacy can be enhanced by inhibition of myeloid-derived suppressor cells with a selective inhibitor of PI3Kδ/γ. Cancer Res. 2017; 77(10):2607–2619
[37] Clavijo PE, Moore EC, Chen J, et al. Resistance to CTLA-4 checkpoint inhibition reversed through selective elimination of granulocytic myeloid cells. Oncotarget. 2017; 8(34):55804–55820
[38] Califano JA, Khan Z, Noonan KA, et al. Tadalafil augments tumor specific immunity in patients with head and neck squamous cell carcinoma. Clin Cancer Res. 2015; 21(1):30–38
[39] Ward MJ, Thirdborough SM, Mellows T, et al. Tumour-infiltrating lymphocytes predict for outcome in HPV-positive oropharyngeal cancer. Br J Cancer. 2014; 110(2):489–500
[40] Stevanović S, Pasetto A, Helman SR, et al. Landscape of immunogenic tumor antigens in successful immunotherapy of virally induced epithelial cancer. Science. 2017; 356(6334):200–205

51 Palliative Care/Considerations for Metastatic Oral Cavity Cancers

Kershena Liao and Andrew G. Sikora

Summary
Head and neck cancer patients face unique challenges in symptom management and maximization of quality of life throughout their course of treatment. Multidisciplinary engagement in delivery of palliative care, as well as addressing palliative concerns earlier in the course of treatment, can enhance patient's quality of life, and potentially lead to improvement of other clinical outcomes. Much of what is known about palliative care and best practices for its delivery stems from studies in other cancers, providing numerous opportunities for meaningful research into symptom- and quality of life-related issues and delivery of palliative care in head and neck cancer.

Keywords: palliative care, end-of-life considerations, pain management in oral cancer

51.1 Introduction

Palliative care is an approach to delivery of health care interventions that focus on improving quality of life and minimizing pain as well as other distressing symptoms, whether they be physical or psychosocial.[1] Palliation may be provided early on in the course of a chronic illness such as oral cancer, in conjunction with treatment with curative intent, and may take on a more prominent role later in a patient's treatment trajectory.[1–3] As such, it is a misconception to view palliation as synonymous with hospice care, which attends to needs exclusively during the end-of-life period.[1] With regards to the care of the oncologic patient, studies have shown unmet palliative needs exist throughout a patient's cancer treatment trajectory, not just in the end-of-life phase.[3–5] In this chapter, we aim to provide an overview of the most common palliative needs of oral cancer patients, as well as demonstrate the need for early integration of palliative care services in the multidisciplinary health care team for these patients. Finally, we consider some ethical quandaries relevant to palliative care for oral cancer patients.

51.2 Surgeons as Frontline Providers of Palliation in Oral Cancer

Head and neck cancer surgeons typically serve as primary coordinators of care for their cancer patients amongst multidisciplinary team members. As such, oral cancer surgeons are charged with the task of identifying and addressing symptomatic concerns for their patients, requiring a basic knowledge of palliative concerns of oral cancer patients.[2] Widespread implementation of communication aids such as standardized surveys enquiring about patients' feelings about treatment and prognosis, quality of life, and end-of-life concerns may prove useful in identifying palliative needs and may itself help to address patients' anxiety.[6] A considerable amount of research delves into the unique symptomatology of oral cancer, including the specific challenges of oral cancer pain, as well as quality of life concerns such as the ability to breathe without distress, to chew and/or swallow or otherwise maintain adequate nutrition, to communicate, and to manage sequelae of treatments such as xerostomia and trismus.[7,8]

51.3 Challenges in Pain Control for Oral Cancer Patients

Pain is one of the top concerns for patients with advanced cancer of the oral cavity and is distinct from other types of oncologic pain in its severity and intrusiveness. Pain has been found to be a primary concern for roughly 80% of terminally ill head and neck cancer patients.[7,9–11] In a meta-analysis investigating prevalence of pain among cancer patients, head and neck cancer pain was more widely prevalent than gynecologic, gastrointestinal, lung, and breast cancers.[12] These patients' cancer pain is experienced with a unique keenness due to the anatomy and functional demands of the oral cavity. Specifically, in contrast to the visceral pain derived from solid tumors in the abdomen, for example, the pain experienced by patients with advanced cancer in the oral cavity can be sharply localized due to trigeminal nerve innervation.[9] Additionally, the oral cavity is responsible for numerous specialized functions, including mastication, swallowing, and speech; these mechanical requirements further stimulate function-related pain.[9,13] Furthermore, the molecular biology of oral cavity squamous cell carcinoma (SCC) directly contributes to the pain experienced by patients: nociceptive mediators such as endothelin-1 (ET-1), proteases and protease-activated receptors (PAR_1 to PAR_4), and nerve growth factor (NGF) are secreted by oral SCC cells, leading to sensitization and stimulation of nociceptors in the tumor microenvironment.[9,14]

51.3.1 Airway Management

A report showed 43% of head and neck cancer patients have respiratory difficulties in the end-of-life period.[15] In one study by Timon and Reilly, one-fifth to one-sixth of patients were deemed to need tracheostomy tube placement for airway concerns.[7] As discussed by Shuman et al, airway concerns are an integral part of head and neck cancers, particularly as a patient's disease progresses and evolves.[16] Preparation for the possibility and in some cases eventuality of airway obstruction in head and neck cancer patients is of utmost importance; health care providers must ensure adequate patient education and discussion of preferences for urgent/emergent airway interventions should the need arise.[16] Alternatives to emergency airway management include supportive care and medications that help to mitigate air hunger and dyspnea as well as the anxiety associated with breathing symptoms.[16]

Functional Impairments in Mastication, Swallowing, and Speech

In addition to the pain elicited during mastication and swallowing mentioned previously, functional limitations in these actions pose significant challenges to maintaining adequate nutrition.[17] Alternative feeding routes often must be sought to prevent or treat malnutrition and cachexia, with 25% patients requiring percutaneous gastrostomy placement in one study of head and neck cancer patients in general.[7] Furthermore, mastication and swallowing dysfunction narrows the range of therapeutic options to treat patients' pain, necessitating delivery through alternative feeding routes (if any have been established) or devising alternate pain regimens.

Patients benefit from multidisciplinary team coordination of adjunctive therapy with speech therapy and nutrition services.[18] Additionally, communication barriers that often result from treatment should prompt health care providers to initiate early discussions of patient's wishes regarding his/her care in order to achieve a more thorough and nuanced understanding, particularly regarding end-of-life/resuscitative preferences.[19]

51.3.2 Gustatory Alterations

Xerostomia, altered taste sensation, and trismus are common side effects of radiotherapy that can have a significant impact on patients' quality of life.[8] Oral mucositis, experienced by more than 80% of head and neck cancer patients, often limits their ability to endure full planned courses of radiotherapy as a result of the oral pain, bleeding, dysphagia, and resultant decreased nutritional intake, infections, and hospitalizations.[11,20] Interventions to prevent or decrease severity of oral mucositis include proper oral care and hygiene, regular assessment by care providers using one of several validated scales (from the National Cancer Institute [NCI], Radiation Therapy Oncology Group [RTOG], European Organization for Research and Treatment of Cancer [EORTC]), limiting alcohol/tobacco use, and employing radiotherapeutic precautions when possible.[20]

Additionally, osteoradionecrosis is a major complication resulting from radiation treatments which may require preemptive full dental extraction.[8] Therefore, because pretreatment evaluation by dental team may help prevent posttreatment complications (such as osteoradionecrosis) and symptom management (such as avoidance of dental infections by removing diseased dentition), involvement of dentist at an early stage is advisable for improved symptom control in the long term.[8,21]

51.3.3 Psychosocial Distress

Oral cavity cancers and their treatment may cause distressing psychological symptoms because of their unique location and functional impact. Compared to treatments for other types of cancers, e.g., pneumonectomy, prostatectomy, and bowel resection, interventions for head and neck cancer are easily visible to others, altering patients' appearance and interactions with others in an especially debilitating way, particularly in the context of intimate relationships with loved ones.[22,23] Disfigurement of the face resulting from treatments or the malignancy itself may feel socially isolating and can provoke a sense of losing one's identity at the very moment of grappling with one's existence.[22,23]

Evidence suggests that patients with advanced oral cancers experience greater emotional and psychological distress than patients with other malignancies including other head and neck cancers.[17,24,25] Studies estimate that overall 30–40% of head and neck cancer patients experience significant depression and anxiety, which also amplifies the perception of pain.[24–26] In fact, in a study by Misono et al, patients with cancers of the oral cavity and pharynx were found to have the third highest suicide rate when ranked by anatomic location of patients' cancers, and a rate three to four times higher than that of the general US population.[27] It is difficult to determine whether this elevated risk of depression and suicide is due to the nature of head and neck cancer itself or common comorbidities such as tobacco and alcohol abuse, but the resultant psychosocial distress requires management nonetheless.[16,27]

Strategies to address these psychosocial symptoms include support network, education, emotional support, and psychotherapy (e.g., cognitive behavioral therapy), as well as providing patients with a sense of control.[17,24,25] Additionally, a collaborative care approach involving multidisciplinary teams of specialists, primary care providers, and care management in conjunction with psychopharmacology is a systems-based strategy that decreases cancer patients' depression, which in turn can affect length of hospital stay and treatment compliance in addition to quality of life.[28]

51.4 Deficits in Palliation of Oral Cancer

Despite the severity and specificity of oral cancer pain and symptomatology, several indications exist that palliative care interventions and services remain underutilized in the care of oral cancer patients. For example, treatment of metastatic oral cancer pain largely entails opiates; however, head and neck cancers have displayed a higher Opioid Escalation Index (a measure of the amount of increase in opioid requirement for pain control over time) than other cancers, indicating that tolerance rapidly develops, and that pain coverage is often insufficient and limited in oral cancer patients.[13,29] Novel strategies to harness endogenous opioid systems such as endothelin and cannabinoid receptors for relief of nociception are being investigated.[9]

Particularly in the end-of-life period, an assessment of key indicators of quality of life (including adequate symptom control for patient's comfort and dignity, desired place of death, presence of relatives, absence of futile interventions, and minimization of time in the hospital) reflects areas with room for improvement.[30] Traditionally, most terminally ill patients report a preference for dying at home rather than in the hospital; however, studies have found that up to 86% of head and neck cancer patients died in the hospital rather than at home.[7,15] Also one study estimated that only 22% had family members present at the time of death.[30] Emergency hospital admission was identified in about half of head and neck cancer patients in the end-of-life period; the most common reason was for bleeding.[30] These data suggest that more remains to be done to improve oral cancer patients' quality of life particularly in the terminal phase of illness.

51.5 Benefit of Improved Palliative Care Integration

Bakitas et al in Project ENABLE (Educate, Nurture, Advise, Before Life Ends) found that a psychoeducational intervention aimed at assessing and advising patients on anticipated symptoms of their cancer led to a significantly greater quality of life as well as a trend toward mitigation of symptom intensity.[31] In another paradigm-changing study by Temel et al, patients with non-small cell lung cancer were randomized into two groups: early palliative care intervention alongside standard oncologic therapy versus standard oncologic treatment alone. Results of this study showed that patients randomized to the early palliative intervention group displayed improved quality of life, lower rates of depression, and also longer median survival time.[5] Those patients receiving earlier palliative care also received less aggressive or futile treatment in the end of life, and more commonly had resuscitation preferences documented.[5] Greer et al posit that the improved outcomes in these studies were not a result of pharmacologic interventions or referrals to mental health professionals but rather improved symptom management through enhanced attention and support, counseling, and coordination of care.[2] Though these studies were performed in patients with non-head and neck cancers, it may reasonably be extrapolated that early and better integration of palliative care services would similarly benefit patients with advanced oral cavity cancer—and might perhaps be of even greater import given the unique pain and symptomatology of oral cancer. Indeed, one study by Shuman et al seems to support this conclusion, as they found that palliative care team involvement in a variety of health care settings (inpatient, hospice, outpatient) was associated with improved symptom control and care in the end-of-life period.[32]

Of note, family and other caregivers for these patients undertake a significant workload managing the myriad, complex symptoms associated with this disease, which may ultimately limit feasibility of any interventions or proposed palliative measures.[33] Early inclusion of palliative care services in the care of lung and gastrointestinal cancer patients aided caregivers' psychological well-being, as measured by decreased symptoms of psychological distress and depression.[34] Further studies are needed to confirm how the benefits of earlier integration of palliative care translate to the oral cancer patient and caregiver populations, as well as to identify the key elements of palliative care interventions that yield improved outcomes.[2]

51.6 Ethical Considerations in the Palliation of Oral Cancer Patients

51.6.1 Challenges in Decision-making

As mentioned earlier in the chapter, barriers to communication often encountered by oral cancer patients particularly in late stages of their disease impede facile discourse; therefore, earlier initiation of discussions about possible palliative interventions should be undertaken in order to maximize patient's decision-making autonomy. In one study in the Netherlands, 13% of close relatives felt that patients received care that was incongruent with their wishes, underlining the need for improved communication that facilitates end-of-life decision-making.[35] However, physicians should note that patients desire varying levels of autonomy and decision-making independence, and acknowledge the need to include family members in the decision-making process.[33] Understandably, whether the final decision-making role is taken on by the patient, family member, and/or physician/other health care provider varies according to psychosocial dynamics specific to each patient and his or her support network.[33,36,37]

Additionally, physicians should assess their own subconscious biases, as they have the potential to influence their recommendations to patients: physician demographics such as age, specialization, and practice setting have been associated with increased willingness to withdraw life-sustaining treatments.[38–42] Interestingly, health care providers at a regional head and neck cancer center in the United Kingdom tended to overestimate the impact that deficits in speech, saliva, and swallowing had on head and neck cancer patients' health care-related quality of life (HRQoL).[43] This discrepancy between provider- and patient-reported assessments of those parameters is important to note because underestimating patient's quality of life may skew providers' assessments when considering transitioning to palliative therapy.[19] Finally, in order to achieve informed consent for treatment, physicians should endeavor to relay accurate representations of treatment alternatives, stressing that while palliative surgery, radiation, and chemotherapy may help relieve cancer pain to some degree, these interventions do not reliably lead to improved survival outcomes and may likely lead to new symptomatic concerns.[9,26]

51.6.2 Resource Utilization

The US lags behind many other countries in life expectancy gains and other health outcomes despite per capita health care expenditures that are among the highest in the world.[44] As a result, curtailment of health care costs and judicious resource utilization have become an increasingly important part of the conversation. Patro et al discussed the ethical conflict in treating head and neck cancer patients who continue to smoke during treatment.[45] On the one hand, the ethical principles of beneficence and nonmaleficence and the virtue of compassion would argue for prompt surgery in spite of active smoking, particularly since decreased likelihood of cessation tends to correlate more with certain demographic groups that are victims of health care disparities (inconsistent with the ethical principle of justice). On the other hand, actively smoking patients tend to experience greater postoperative complications, entailing increased days of hospitalization, surgeon and operating room time, and resources to manage complex wounds. The head and neck cancer surgeon has an ethical imperative to balance these competing interests when offering palliative surgery or other interventions for these patients.

Along with the impetus for palliative care involvement for improved patient outcomes, a mounting body of evidence suggests that palliative care involvement may also result in cost savings for hospitals and more cost-efficient, higher quality health care.[2] How to restructure payment and reimbursement systems to appropriately incentivize palliative interventions and palliative care team involvement remains to be determined.[2]

Key Points

- Oral cancer surgeons, as frontline providers and coordinators of care for their cancer patients, must be fluent in identifying palliative concerns unique to oral cancer patients, including pain control, airway symptoms, functional impairments in mastication, swallowing, speech, and taste, and psychosocial distress.
- Oral cancer care providers must also consider the unique challenges of assessing palliative care needs of patients with oral cancer, who often have significant barriers to communication that increase the difficulty of articulating their needs and concerns and engaging in shared decision-making with their providers.
- Despite the severity and specificity of the symptomatology of oral cancer patients, palliative care interventions are underutilized, as evidenced by inadequate pain control and deteriorating quality of life, particularly toward the end-of-life period. However, studies of other oncologic anatomic sites suggest that improved palliative care interventions and integration may offer not only improved symptom control, but also higher quality care and prolonged survival outcomes.

References

[1] World Palliative Care Alliance. Global atlas of palliative care at the end of life. http://www.who.int/cancer/publications/palliative-care-atlas/en/. Published 2014. Accessed January 14, 2015

[2] Greer JA, Jackson VA, Meier DE, Temel JS. Early integration of palliative care services with standard oncology care for patients with advanced cancer. CA Cancer J Clin. 2013; 63(5):349–363

[3] Beernaert K, Pardon K, Van den Block L, et al. Palliative care needs at different phases in the illness trajectory: a survey study in patients with cancer. Eur J Cancer Care (Engl). 2016; 25(4):534–543

[4] Jacox A, Carr DB, Payne R. New clinical-practice guidelines for the management of pain in patients with cancer. N Engl J Med. 1994; 330(9):651–655

[5] Temel JS, Greer JA, Muzikansky A, et al. Early palliative care for patients with metastatic non-small-cell lung cancer. N Engl J Med. 2010; 363(8):733–742

[6] Yeh JC, Cheng MJ, Chung CH, Smith TJ. Using a question prompt list as a communication aid in advanced cancer care. J Oncol Pract. 2014; 10(3):e137–e141

[7] Timon C, Reilly K. Head and neck mucosal squamous cell carcinoma: results of palliative management. J Laryngol Otol. 2006; 120(5):389–392

[8] Rogers SN. Quality of life perspectives in patients with oral cancer. Oral Oncol. 2010; 46(6):445–447

[9] Viet CT, Schmidt BL. Biologic mechanisms of oral cancer pain and implications for clinical therapy. J Dent Res. 2012; 91(5):447–453

[10] Wotherspoon RJ, Kanatas AN, Rogers SN. Review of HaNDLE-on-QoL: a database of published papers that use questionnaires to report quality of life in patients with cancer of the head and neck. Br J Oral Maxillofac Surg. 2018; 56 (2):e5–e9

[11] Bossi P, Cossu Rocca M, Corvò R, et al. The vicious circle of treatment-induced toxicities in locally advanced head and neck cancer and the impact on treatment intensity. Crit Rev Oncol Hematol. 2017; 116:82–88

[12] van den Beuken-van Everdingen MH, de Rijke JM, Kessels AG, Schouten HC, van Kleef M, Patijn J. Prevalence of pain in patients with cancer: a systematic review of the past 40 years. Ann Oncol. 2007; 18(9):1437–1449

[13] Connelly ST, Schmidt BL. Evaluation of pain in patients with oral squamous cell carcinoma. J Pain. 2004; 5(9):505–510

[14] Schmidt BL, Hamamoto DT, Simone DA, Wilcox GL. Mechanism of cancer pain. Mol Interv. 2010; 10(3):164–178

[15] Shedd DP, Carl A, Shedd C. Problems of terminal head and neck cancer patients. Head Neck Surg. 1980; 2(6):476–482–. Accessed May19, 2018

[16] Shuman AG, Fins JJ, Prince ME. Improving end-of-life care for head and neck cancer patients. Expert Rev Anticancer Ther. 2012; 12(3):335–343

[17] Farris C, Petitte DM. Head, neck, and oral cancer update. Home Healthc Nurse. 2013; 31(6):322–328, quiz 328–330

[18] Yamauchi T, Edahiro A, Watanabe Y, et al. Risk factors for postoperative dysphagia in oral cancer. Bull Tokyo Dent Coll. 2012; 53(2):67–74

[19] Liao K, Blumenthal-Barby J, Sikora AG. Factors influencing head and neck surgical oncologists' transition from curative to palliative treatment goals. Otolaryngol Head Neck Surg. 2017; 156(1):46–51

[20] De Sanctis V, Bossi P, Sanguineti G, et al. Mucositis in head and neck cancer patients treated with radiotherapy and systemic therapies: literature review and consensus statements. Crit Rev Oncol Hematol. 2016; 100:147–166

[21] Thanvi J, Bumb D. Impact of dental considerations on the quality of life of oral cancer patients. Indian J Med Paediatr Oncol. 2014; 35(1):66–70

[22] Schenck DP. Ethical considerations in the treatment of head and neck cancer. Cancer Contr. 2002; 9(5):410–419

[23] Frank HA, Davidson TM. Ethical dilemmas in head and neck cancer. Head Neck Surg. 1989; 11(1):22–26.

[24] Katz MR, Irish JC, Devins GM. Development and pilot testing of a psychoeducational intervention for oral cancer patients. Psychooncology. 2004; 13(9): 642–653

[25] Semple CJ, Sullivan K, Dunwoody L, Kernohan WG. Psychosocial interventions for patients with head and neck cancer: past, present, and future. Cancer Nurs. 2004; 27(6):434–441

[26] Narayanan RS, Nair MK, Padmanabhan TK. Palliation of pain in advanced oral cancer. Headache. 1988; 28(4):258–259

[27] Misono S, Weiss NS, Fann JR, Redman M, Yueh B. Incidence of suicide in persons with cancer. J Clin Oncol. 2008; 26(29):4731–4738

[28] Li M, Kennedy EB, Byrne N, et al. Systematic review and meta-analysis of collaborative care interventions for depression in patients with cancer. Psychooncology. 2017; 26(5):573–587

[29] Mercadante S, Dardanoni G, Salvaggio L, Armata MG, Agnello A. Monitoring of opioid therapy in advanced cancer pain patients. J Pain Symptom Manage. 1997; 13(4):204–212

[30] Ethunandan M, Rennie A, Hoffman G, Morey PJ, Brennan PA. Quality of dying in head and neck cancer patients: a retrospective analysis of potential indicators of care. Oral Surg Oral Med Oral Pathol Oral Radiol Endod. 2005; 100(2):147–152

[31] Bakitas M, Lyons KD, Hegel MT, et al. Effects of a palliative care intervention on clinical outcomes in patients with advanced cancer: the Project ENABLE II randomized controlled trial. JAMA. 2009; 302(7):741–749

[32] Shuman A, Yang Y, Taylor JMG, Prince ME. End-of-life care among head and neck cancer patients. Otolaryngol Head Neck Surg. 2011; 144. DOI: 10.1177/0194599810397603.End

[33] O'Sullivan EM, Higginson IJ. "I'll continue as long as I can, and die when I can't help it": a qualitative exploration of the views of end-of-life care by those affected by head and neck cancer (HNC). BMJ Support Palliat Care. 2016; 6(1): 43–51

[34] El-Jawahri A, Greer JA, Pirl WF, et al. Effects of early integrated palliative care on caregivers of patients with lung and gastrointestinal cancer: a randomized clinical trial. Oncologist. 2017; 22:1528–1534

[35] Offerman MP, Pruyn JF, de Boer MF, et al. Experience of palliative care for patients with head and neck cancer through the eyes of next of kin: impact of an expert center. Head Neck. 2014; 36(10):1459–1466

[36] Chen H, Haley WE, Robinson BE, Schonwetter RS. Decisions for hospice care in patients with advanced cancer. J Am Geriatr Soc. 2003; 51(6):789–797

[37] Weissman DE. Decision making at a time of crisis near the end of life. JAMA. 2004; 292(14):1738–1743

[38] Marmo S. Recommendations for hospice care to terminally ill cancer patients: a phenomenological study of oncologists' experiences. J Soc Work End Life Palliat Care. 2014; 10(2):149–169

[39] Silverman HJ. How decisive are physician values in end-of-life decision-making? Crit Care Med. 1996; 24(6):909–911

[40] Sohoni A. Physician decision making: an observation. Am J Hosp Palliat Care. 2009; 26(4):320–322

[41] Christakis NA, Asch DA. Physician characteristics associated with decisions to withdraw life support. Am J Public Health. 1995; 85(3):367–372

[42] Cassell J, Buchman TG, Streat S, Stewart RM. Surgeons, intensivists, and the covenant of care: administrative models and values affecting care at the end of life—updated. Crit Care Med. 2003; 31(5):1551–1557, discussion 1557–1559

[43] Parhar S, Rogers SN, Lowe D. Perspectives of the multidisciplinary team on the quality of life of patients with cancer of the head and neck at 2 years. Br J Oral Maxillofac Surg. 2015; 53(9):858–863

[44] Health at a Glance 2017: Indicators OECD. www.oecd.org/health/health-at-a-glance.htm. Accessed May 20, 2018

[45] Patro A, Guerrini CJ, Huang AT, Sikora AG. The patient who continues to smoke on-treatment: an ethical dilemma. Otolaryngol Head Neck Surg. 2018; 158(3):469–472

Section X

Future Directions

52 Cancer Prevention and Oral Preneoplasia

Ashok Jethwa, Gerard J. Ondrey, and Frank Ondrey

Summary

Currently, the efforts to reduce and treat oral leukoplakia have not resulted in any cancer prevention treatments for dysplastic leukoplakia or field carcinogenesis. A large number of National Institutes of Health funded research projects and clinical trials has not resulted in a "tamoxifen equivalent" for head and neck preneoplasia or tobacco-induce field carcinogenesis. There are currently 24 clinical trials listed for "oral leukoplakia" in the U.S National Library of Medicine (clinicaltrials.gov). As precision medicine develops, the authors have a strong hope that studies of the tumor milieu in the pathophysiology of leukoplakia (genomics, etc.) will reveal dysregulated metabolic pathways and biomarkers in precancerous squamous cells and milieu cells that become intervention targets.

Keywords: oral leukoplakia, chemoprevention, preneoplasia, tobacco abuse, type II agents, retinoidsa

52.1 Oral Preneoplasia Background

Oral leukoplakias and related lesions occur in approximately 1% of the adult population worldwide. This translates into approximately 2.8 million patients in the United States who harbor these lesions. Oral leukoplakia was originally described in 1877 by Schwimmer, who described and illustrated a lesion on the tongue of an individual.[1] However, there is a wide range of oral lesions and conditions that are associated with the subsequent development of cancer. Oral leukoplakias can anatomically occur anywhere in the mouth, including the inner aspect of the lip contiguous with the buccal mucosa, the lateral aspect of the tongue and the floor of the mouth, the tongue dorsum, and the soft and hard palates. They can occur in the endolarynx as well, but are infrequently observed in the pharynx or hypopharynx.

Oral lesions vary in terms of their likelihood to develop into cancer based on their anatomic site, but the tongue and the floor of the mouth are considered especially high risk sites. Certain lesions, such as those that occur in a socket from a tooth extraction or where the upper and lower teeth meet in the buccal mucosa, pose no significant risk of developing into oral cancer. Dentures and related prosthetic devices can commonly rest at aspects of the upper and lower gingiva and are associated with hyperkeratosis at sites of contact. As a category, these areas are called friction ridges, and the associated lesion is called a friction ridge keratosis. Linea alba is the term commonly used to describe a friction ridge in the buccal mucosa that occurs at the junction of the upper and lower teeth. In aggregate, these types of keratoses are almost always benign. However, these regions can harbor dysplasia if they are associated with chewing tobacco placement or direct inhalational contact of tobacco, so it is not safe to assume these locations are benign until a careful history is obtained.

There are several options to consider for a patient that presents with oral cavity leukoplakia. If the anatomic region and the lesion have been under professional observation for a long period of time, one can immediately perform an incisional biopsy of the lesion, which is a gold standard for diagnosis. There are no biomarkers or special stains that one would normally need to request outside of standard histopathology. However, if a lesion is discovered at the time of a visit or documentation of prior presence of a lesion is unclear, one would recommend reducing or eliminating potential risk factors with re-examination of the oral cavity again in 6 weeks. This a standard recommendation for such patients. When biopsies are performed, they are preserved in formalin and sent for routine histopathology. At our institution, we orient biopsied lesion tissue by laying them flat, mucosal side up, on chromatography filter paper for a few moments. The filter paper with the lesion is then placed in 10% formalin. We do this for all incisional biopsies, many of which are taken with 3–6 mm Baker punches to avoid any crush or tissue folding artifact. This allows high fidelity biopsies for pathologic evaluation for diagnosis, clinical trials, and tissue procurement purposes.

52.2 Risk Factors

The most important risk factors for head and neck squamous cell carcinoma (HNSCC) are smoking and alcohol consumption.[2] These factors are associated with 75% of head and neck cancers and their effects are synergistic.[2] Both combustible and smokeless forms of tobacco have been linked to head and neck cancer, and their use is variable based on geographic location. Cigarettes and cigars are the most commonly used combustible tobacco products, while chewing tobacco, betel quid, and snuff are the most commonly used smokeless tobacco products.

The odds ratio (OR) of developing HNSCC in tobacco users compared to those who have never used tobacco is approximately 2.13.[3] While cessation does lower the risk, it is unclear whether the risk returns to that of a person who has never used tobacco.[4] Some data suggest that the risk returns to that of a person who has never used tobacco after about 20 years of cessation.[5]

Hashibe et al have extensively studied the association between carcinogenesis in the head and neck, and tobacco and alcohol use in humans.[3] At least 75% of HNSCC in Europe, the United States, and other industrialized nations are attributable to the combinations of alcohol and tobacco.[3] However, the respective contributions of each risk factor can be difficult to understand as they are strongly associated with each other. In this study, Hashibe et al attempted to understand the independent associations of tobacco and alcohol with HNSCC.[3] They performed a pooled analysis to investigate the extent to which head and neck cancer was associated with cigarette smoking in never drinkers and with alcohol consumption among never smokers. Data was pooled from 15 case control studies to include 10,244 head and neck cancer case subjects and 15,227 control subjects. 1,072 case subjects and 5,775 control subjects had never smoked tobacco, while 1,598 case subjects and 4,051 control subjects had never consumed alcohol. Among never drinkers, cigarette smoking was associated with an increased risk of HNSCC (OR for ever smoking versus never smoking was = 2.13, 95% CI = 1.52 to 2.98).[3] In addition, they demonstrated a clear dose–response relationship for the frequency, duration, and number of pack-years of cigarette smoking.[3] Approximately 24% (95% CI = 16 to 31) of head and neck cancer cases among nondrinkers in this study would have been prevented if these individuals had never smoked cigarettes.[3]

Recently, Wyss et al studied the association between cancer and several tobacco products.[6] For combustible products, they found increased risks of HNSCC for cigarettes (OR = 3.46, 95% CI = 3.24–3.70), cigars (OR = 2.54, 1.93–3.34), and pipes (OR = 2.08, 1.55–2.81).[6] In regards to smokeless tobacco, the use of snuff was shown to be associated with HNSCC (OR = 1.71, 1.08–2.70), particularly for oral cavity cancers (OR = 3.01, 1.63–5.55).[7] Chewing tobacco was weakly associated with HNSCC among patients who had never smoked (OR = 1.20, 0.81–1.77).[7] However, when restricted to oral cavity cancers, chewing tobacco had a stronger association (OR = 1.81, 1.04–3.17).[7] Furthermore, while human papillomavirus (HPV)-induced HNSCC is rising in incidence, a 2013 analysis of over 100,000 subjects showed 66% of HNSCC diagnoses were tobacco and alcohol related.[8] Thus, tobacco remains a prominent cause of HNSCC.

Alcohol was first recognized as a convincing risk factor for head and neck cancer by the International Agency for Research on Cancer in 1988. Since then, many studies have been published that support this statement. A recent meta-analysis investigated 572 studies, including 486,538 cancer cases.[9] This study indicated that the relative risks for heavy drinkers compared with nondrinkers and occasional drinkers were 5.13 (95% CI, 4.31–6.10) for oral and pharyngeal cancer and 2.65 (95% CI, 2.19–3.19) for laryngeal cancer.[9] A dose–risk relationship was observed between light, moderate, and heavy drinking among the cancer subsites.

The synergistic effect of tobacco and alcohol is supported by analysis of pooled data from 17 European and American studies.[10] The population attributable risk was 72%, which included 4% for alcohol alone, 33% for tobacco alone, and 35% for both alcohol and tobacco. The ORs of developing HNSCC are 2.37 (1.66–3.39) for tobacco users who are nondrinkers, 1.06 (0.88–1.28) for alcohol users who have never used tobacco, and 5.73 (3.62–9.06) for those who use both.[10] This effect was more than multiplicative. Similar steep rises in the risk of HNSCC among alcohol and tobacco users, especially those using high amounts of each product, have been demonstrated by Dal Maso et al.[11]

52.3 Pathogenesis

To date, over 70 known carcinogens have been described in cigarette smoke.[12] Of the many toxic and carcinogenic substances resulting from tobacco exposure, tobacco-specific nitrosamines (TSNAs) and polycyclic aromatic hydrocarbons (PAHs) have been most heavily studied with regard to exposure and carcinogenicity. TSNAs are found in tobacco and tobacco smoke and are formed during the curing and processing of tobacco. They exist in both combustible and smokeless forms of tobacco. Of the TSNAs, N'-nitrosonornicotine (NNN) carries the highest risk for development of head and neck cancer. In rats, NNN reproducibly induces head and neck tumors. Subcutaneous or gavage administration of NNN to rats produces nasal tumors predominantly.[13] However, when administered in drinking water or a liquid diet, NNN exposure results in oral, esophageal, and nasal tumors.[13] PAHs represent a diverse group of carcinogenic compounds that share a similar structure of multiple benzene rings. Several PAHs have also demonstrated carcinogenicity in animal models.[14] The most well-studied constituents in this group include benzo[*a*]pyrene (BaP) and 1-hydroxypyrene (1-HOP).[4] When given orally, PAHs result in tongue and esophageal cancers and tumors of the upper respiratory tract, including in the nose, larynx, and trachea. When given by inhalation, tumors are found in the upper digestive tract including the pharynx, esophagus, and forestomach.[4]

While the above animal studies clearly implicate tobacco and alcohol in the carcinogenicity of HNSCC, not all people who use tobacco products will develop HNSCC. There are complex mechanisms of genetic predisposition, carcinogen metabolism and excretion, immunologic competency, and genetic alterations that put some tobacco users on the path to developing cancer. However, others are able to exit this pathway by excreting the carcinogens or repairing DNA damage, for example.[15]

The exact mechanisms for alcohol-related carcinogenesis are not fully understood. However, several carcinogenic effects of ethanol and its major metabolite, acetaldehyde, have been identified.[16] Acetaldehyde disrupts DNA synthesis and repair.[16] Additionally, ethanol is oxidized to acetaldehyde in the oral cavity by microbes. Thus, the concentration of acetaldehyde in saliva is 10- to 100-fold higher than in the blood, increasing the level of carcinogen contact to the oral mucosa.[16] Ethanol is associated with aberrations in several tumor suppressor and oncogene pathways.[16] Ethanol also acts as a solvent for several other carcinogens introduced by tobacco smoking, diet, and chemicals into cells. This is one mechanism by which alcohol and tobacco are thought to act synergistically in head and neck cancer carcinogenesis.

52.4 Other Etiologic Risk Factors for Oral Cavity Carcinoma

It is well established that oral lichen planus has an associated risk of conversion to oral cavity carcinoma about 4% of the time. This 4% risk is realized more frequently in patients who have persistent lesions or who have more severe lesions with dysplasia coexisting in their lesions.[17] In our practice, we regularly screen for and vigorously treat oral lichen planus. Erosive oral lichen planus is the more severe form of the disease. We generally employ various topical agents, including steroid containing mouthwashes, steroid containing creams, antihistamines, and at times, the transplant rejection drug tacrolimus.

Proliferative verrucous leukoplakia is a condition that occurs along the gingiva of the teeth. This is a rare condition of the mouth and frequently converts to gingival malignancies. Affected patients are treated aggressively with topical steroids. Once these lesions convert to malignancy, patients must undergo surgical resections, including cortical mandibulectomy. Despite surgical resection, these lesions can aggressively recur.[18]

Submucous fibrosis is another precancerous condition; it seems to be more common in East Asia as a consequence of betel nut chewing. There is often an associated difficulty with trismus that may require surgical intervention for oral rehabilitation.[19]

52.5 Diagnostic Aids

52.5.1 Optical Coherence Tomography

Optical coherence tomography (OCT) uses infrared light waves to create a high-resolution image.[20] OCT images are generated by measuring the intensity of back scattered light after the tissue is probed with a low-power, near-infrared light source (wavelengths ranging from 750 to 1300 um).[21] The signal is converted from a luminous signal to a digital signal, which is sent to a computer for graphical processing.[22] In healthy mucosa, OCT can distinguish among the squamous epithelium, the underlying lamina propria, and the transition to the basement membrane. Structures such as minor salivary glands and filiform papillae can be identified. In buccal mucosa, healthy mucosa, epithelial hyperplasia, moderate dysplasia, and oral cavity squamous cell carcinoma (SCC) can be distinguished from each other by OCT. In abnormal oral mucosa samples, as the standard deviation of the scan's signal profile increases, the spatial-frequency spectrum exponential decay constant becomes smaller, and the epithelium becomes thicker. This feature can be useful in disease monitoring.[22] Limitations of OCT include operator and technology dependence.

52.6 Management of Oral Cavity Leukoplakia

Currently there are no effective permanent treatments for oral cavity leukoplakia. Cochrane Reviews have been performed several times over a number of years with similar conclusions. These reviews demonstrate that lesions can be completely excised but they frequently return.[23] However, treatment of these lesions must occur and there are a number of strategies for treatment despite their frequent recurrence after treatment.

52.6.1 Excision

Once the diagnosis of a premalignant lesion has been made, and more importantly, invasive carcinoma has been ruled out, there are several methods for treatment. These include medical and surgical treatments. Surgical excision can be performed with scalpel and laser techniques. Ablation or vaporization of the lesion can also be performed with laser techniques. Several laser wavelengths can be used; however, the CO_2 laser is most commonly used.[24] Surgical excision is performed to remove areas at high risk to harbor foci of early carcinoma and attempts at complete removal of all premalignant lesions are impractical in most situations.[20]

Due to the widespread field effect of oral carcinogens in the oral cavity, premalignant changes are often found over wide areas of the oral cavity. Recurrence rates of 10–34% after excision of leukoplakia have been reported.[20] Additionally, complete excision of premalignant lesions does not have a significant impact on the development of oral carcinoma.[20] Arnaoutakis et al[25] performed a retrospective study and compared wide excision or ablation of oral premalignant lesions to observation. They demonstrated that excision/ablation is more effective than observation in preventing recurrence of premalignancy and progression to malignancy.[25]

52.6.2 Photodynamic Therapy

Photodynamic therapy (PDT) is another form of ablative therapy. A photosensitizing agent, such as 5-aminolevulinic acid (5-ALA), is applied topically or given intravenously. The tissue to be targeted is then exposed to a specific wavelength of light that matches the absorption characteristics of the photosensitizer, which activates the photosensitizer, causing it to transfer energy to molecular oxygen generating reactive oxygen species and causing tissue damage.[20]

The main drawback to PDT is photosensitivity after treatment. Additionally, the depth of penetration is dependent upon the photosensitizer and light conditions required to activate it. For example, 5-ALA is activated by 635 nm of light and penetrates only about 2 mm.[26] Some larger solid tumors cannot be effectively treated with PDT.

52.7 Chemoprevention Efforts

There is a long rich history of trying to prevent oral cavity leukoplakia lesions from progressing to oral cavity carcinoma. There is also a high level of interest in treating field carcinogenesis with cancer prevention agents to lower the incidence of conversion to oral cavity carcinoma. In the realm of preventive oncology, there are several operational definitions.

Primary prevention of oral cavity carcinoma (or any malignancy) consists of eliminating agents that are considered risk factors, or preventing their use in the first place. Tobacco and alcohol use and addiction start in adolescents and young adults and may culminate in oral cavity leukoplakias and cancer several decades later. Primary prevention currently consists of tobacco and smoking cessation counseling for patients who are current smokers. Counseling about oral cancer should also be considered with moderate or greater alcohol users, particularly when they are encountered as preneoplasia patients in your practice.

Primary prevention needs to be distinguished from **chemoprevention**. There is both **primary chemoprevention** and **secondary chemoprevention. Primary chemoprevention** is defined as prescribing a pharmaceutical agent or natural product in order to prevent patients who are at high risk for oral cavity carcinoma from their preneoplastic state from progressing to oral cavity carcinoma. In **secondary chemoprevention**, the agent would be taken after successful treatment for oral carcinoma to prevent recurrence or second malignancies in the mouth or elsewhere. After oral cancer treatment, field carcinogenesis remains and the patients are at risk for second primary malignancies at a rate of 3–7% per year. These second primaries may occur in any organ at risk—primarily in the oral cavity, but also in the lung, esophagus, and bladder. A common example of current secondary chemoprevention would be the use of tamoxifen or raloxifene in females who have had a history of breast cancer. In this case, the estrogen antagonist is taken for a period of 5 years or more. With effective agents, secondary chemoprevention would be practical in the post head and neck cancer treatment scenario, as we generally follow up our patients with frequent examinations and endoscopies for a period of 5 years. One may assume that the highest risk of cancer returning as a second primary malignancy would occur in the first 5 years, but we commonly see patients in our clinics with new cancers after 10, 15, and even 20 years after their primary malignancy.

52.8 Aerodigestive Chemoprevention Agents

If one examines the agents that have been utilized and the themes that have been addressed for chemoprevention, they generally fall into discrete categories. Principal mechanisms for currently postulated chemoprevention drugs include forced differentiation and anti-inflammatory agents. With regard to agents that are hypothesized to force maturation, vitamin A and derivatives have been the most commonly used agents over the past 30 years. It was originally noted that vitamin A is necessary for the maintenance of normal health and maturation of mucosal tissues, particularly tissues in the oral cavity and the oropharynx.[27] As a consequence of this observation, the earliest cancer prevention efforts in oral cavity carcinoma involved the use of naturally occurring or synthetic retinoids for periods of time ranging from 3 months to several years, depending on the type of clinical trial that was conducted. The initial landmark randomized controlled trial study for oral cancer prevention involved the use of 13-cis-retinoic acid.[28] The outcome of the study demonstrated that oral cavity leukoplakia lesions were reduced significantly in size after 6 months of retinoid treatment. The clinical reductions in size of leukoplakia lesions were quite common but histologic improvement from high-grade to low-grade dysplasia or from low-grade dysplasia to normal were not nearly as common. From the earliest 13-cis-retinoic acid study, a number of studies were co-opted by MD Anderson and related institutions. These involved a variety of retinoids including fenretinide (4HPR), and there was additional success.[29]

Ultimately, a Phase III randomized secondary primary prevention trial with low dose 13-cis-retinoic acid (30 mg/day isotretinoin) in oral carcinoma failed to show utility in a large randomized clinical trial.[30] Over the course of a number of trials, dose reductions were needed secondary to toxicity. Particularly, skin toxicities and hypertriglyceridemia were dose limiting toxicities. Over the years, doses were reduced to a point where they were no longer clinically effective. It is important to note that currently there is ongoing research to find safe retinoids that do not have dose limiting side effects. Dozens of retinoids have been synthesized, and a couple of compounds have made their way to early phase clinical trials. Specifically, a drug called UAB 30 has been used in early phase clinical trials for breast cancer prevention, and it appears to be a safe agent with achievable serum levels to be effective.[31] This drug might represent a nontoxic retinoid suitable for aerodigestive cancer prevention. There has also been considerable interest in using retinoids as topical agents to avoid systemic toxicity. A number of publications point to the use of mucoadhesive patches with retinoids to treat oral leukoplakia.[32,33]

It is established that the degree of inflammation escalates as the level of dysplasia increases in oral preneoplastic lesions. Our group and others have shown considerable pro-inflammatory cytokine production in the milieu of oral cavity carcinoma, preneoplastic lesions, and from cell lines and animals. In addition to producing inflammatory cascades in the milieu, these substances can act as paracrine factors for tumorigenesis, and may even be contributed to by the microbiome in the vicinity. Therefore, there is considerable rationale for applying anti-inflammatory strategies in the oral cavity cancer prevention setting. Both topical and systemic anti-inflammatory strategies have been applied to oral leukoplakia clinical trials. In an initial study by Mulshine and colleagues, the cyclooxygenase inhibitor and anti-inflammatory drug ketorolac (toradol) was dissolved in a mouthwash preparation, and this mouthwash was used twice daily by patients with oral precancerous lesions for a period of 3 months. The response rate was similar for ketorolac and the placebo arm without changes in histology.[34] A second large randomized study utilized the cyclooxygenase-2 inhibitor celecoxib. Forty-nine patients were studied after twice daily celecoxib for 3 months, and again no statistically significant differences were found between the placebo and agent arms. Celecoxib was generally well tolerated. Patients with higher baseline celecoxib-2 mRNA levels had an increased risk of disease progression.[35]

Another strategy has been to target invasion with protease inhibitors. The agent most studied in this category has been the Bowman-Birk inhibitor, which was featured in studies that were advanced to the randomized Phase II setting by Meyskens. Again, this agent was not successful, with similar placebo and agent response rates.[36]

More recent studies have focused on Type II diabetes agents, which actually can fulfill both the forced differentiation and anti-inflammatory targeting strategies of aerodigestive cancer prevention. There have been multiple studies performed with anti-diabetic agents, including both biguanides and thiazolidinediones. It has been observed in large patient cohorts that cancers can be reduced in patients taking either class of drugs for a period of time. With regard to thiazolidinedione drugs, the principal agent under consideration is pioglitazone. Pioglitazone is a peroxisome proliferator-activated receptor γ (PPARγ) activator involved in pro-differentiation features of adipocytes and other lineages. In vitro studies support the use of PPARγ ligands in the treatment and prevention of aerodigestive cancers. Chang and Szabo examined the expression of PPARγ in normal lung and non-small cell lung cancer (NSCLC) cell lines and the effects of PPARγ ligands on NSCLC growth and differentiation status.[37] In head and neck cancer, pioglitazone suppressed tongue carcinoma development in a transgenic animal model of oral SCC.[38] In a study of male diabetics followed in Veterans Administration (VA) hospitals, Govindarajan et al demonstrated a 33% reduction in lung cancer risk among thiazolidinedione users compared with nonusers.[39] Using the same VA database, the authors also reported a 41–55% reduction in head and neck cancer in diabetics using thiazolidinediones in combination with other agents or alone. An open-label phase 2a trial conducted by Ondrey and colleagues at University of Minnesota treated subjects with high-risk oral premalignant lesions with pioglitazone (45 mg/day) for 3 months (NCT00099021). There was a significant partial clinical response rate in over 70% of patients after 3 months. A phase IIB randomized trial has also been performed and is currently undergoing final write-up for publication.

With regard to biguanides, metformin, a first-line drug commonly used to treat diabetes mellitus, also directly inhibits cell growth. Vitale-Cross et al showed that metformin prevented the development of oral SCCs in a murine model of HNSCC.[40]

Further evidence in support of metformin's cancer chemopreventive efficacy has come from epidemiologic studies. Population studies and several meta-analyses have revealed that treatment with metformin is significantly associated with reduced cancer risk, suggesting that metformin might have chemoprevention efficacy in humans.[41,42] The magnitude of the risk reduction varies across studies, ranging from 10 to 30% decrease in overall cancer risk. Several studies have focused on metformin's potential as a cancer prevention drug in common obesity-associated cancer, such as in the breast, prostate, pancreas, and colon.[41–46]

Dietary compounds and natural products are also an area of interest in oral cancer prevention and leukoplakia treatment. There is significant interest in the use of raspberry derivatives with some successful human studies performed with demonstrated efficacy for topical preparations.[47,48] The use of curcumin is also of significant interest as this spice will function in an anti-inflammatory fashion that may decrease preneoplastic lesions as well.[49–51]

Key Points

- Oral cavity surveillance indicates a significant issue, in that patients with oral cavity leukoplakia are not kept under the same type of surveillance that patients with high PSA levels are kept.
- In oral cavity leukoplakia, we have very minimal ways to examine and stratify risks within the entire population of oral cavity leukoplakia patients.
- High-grade oral cavity leukoplakia (moderate, severe dysplasia, and carcinoma in situ) has a much higher chance of progressing to invasive cancer than hyperplasia or low grade dysplasia.

References

[1] Bánóczy J. The therapy of oral leukoplakia. In: Oral Leukoplakia; Hague, The Netherlands: Martinus Nijhoff Publishers; 1982:182–189

[2] Argiris A, Karamouzis MV, Raben D, Ferris RL. Head and neck cancer. Lancet. 2008; 371(9625):1695–1709

[3] Hashibe M, Brennan P, Benhamou S, et al. Alcohol drinking in never users of tobacco, cigarette smoking in never drinkers, and the risk of head and neck cancer: pooled analysis in the International Head and Neck Cancer Epidemiology Consortium. J Natl Cancer Inst. 2007; 99(10):777–789

[4] Khariwala SS, Carmella SG, Stepanov I, et al. Elevated levels of 1-hydroxypyrene and N′-nitrosonornicotine in smokers with head and neck cancer: a matched control study. Head Neck. 2013; 35(8):1096–1100

[5] Winn DM, Lee YC, Hashibe M, Boffetta P, INHANCEcconsortium. The INHANCE Consortium: toward a better understanding of the causes and mechanisms of head and neck cancer. Oral Dis. 2015; 21(6):685–693

[6] Wyss A, Hashibe M, Chuang SC, et al. Cigarette, cigar, and pipe smoking and the risk of head and neck cancers: pooled analysis in the International Head and Neck Cancer Epidemiology Consortium. Am J Epidemiol. 2013; 178(5): 679–690

[7] Wyss AB, Hashibe M, Lee YA, et al. Smokeless tobacco use and the risk of head and neck cancer: pooled analysis of US studies in the INHANCE Consortium. Am J Epidemiol. 2016; 184(10):703–716

[8] Hashibe M, Hunt J, Wei M, Buys S, Gren L, Lee YC. Tobacco, alcohol, body mass index, physical activity, and the risk of head and neck cancer in the prostate, lung, colorectal, and ovarian (PLCO) cohort. Head Neck. 2013; 35(7):914–922

[9] Bagnardi V, Rota M, Botteri E, et al. Alcohol consumption and site-specific cancer risk: a comprehensive dose-response meta-analysis. Br J Cancer. 2015; 112(3):580–593

[10] Hashibe M, Brennan P, Chuang SC, et al. Interaction between tobacco and alcohol use and the risk of head and neck cancer: pooled analysis in the International Head and Neck Cancer Epidemiology Consortium. Cancer Epidemiol Biomarkers Prev. 2009; 18(2):541–550

[11] Dal Maso L, Torelli N, Biancotto E, et al. Combined effect of tobacco smoking and alcohol drinking in the risk of head and neck cancers: a re-analysis of case-control studies using bi-dimensional spline models. Eur J Epidemiol. 2016; 31(4):385–393

[12] Khariwala SS, Hatsukami D, Hecht SS. Tobacco carcinogen metabolites and DNA adducts as biomarkers in head and neck cancer: potential screening tools and prognostic indicators. Head Neck. 2012; 34(3):441–447

[13] Hecht SS. Biochemistry, biology, and carcinogenicity of tobacco-specific N-nitrosamines. Chem Res Toxicol. 1998; 11(6):559–603

[14] IARC Working Group on the Evaluation of Carcinogenic Risks to Humans. Tobacco smoke and involuntary smoking. IARC Monogr Eval Carcinog Risks Hum. 2004; 83:1–1438

[15] Hecht SS. Tobacco carcinogens, their biomarkers and tobacco-induced cancer. Nat Rev Cancer. 2003; 3(10):733–744

[16] Kawakita D, Matsuo K. Alcohol and head and neck cancer. Cancer Metastasis Rev. 2017; 36(3):425–434

[17] Fitzpatrick SG, Hirsch SA, Gordon SC. The malignant transformation of oral lichen planus and oral lichenoid lesions: a systematic review. J Am Dent Assoc. 2014; 145(1):45–56

[18] Muddana K, Thadudari D, Maloth AK, Pupala G, SRK Nanadan. Proliferative verrucous leukoplakia—a clinico pathological entity: an update. Indian J Dent Adv. 2016; 8(3):183–186

[19] Pillai R, Balaram P, Reddiar KS. Pathogenesis of oral submucous fibrosis: relationship to risk factors associated with oral cancer. Cancer. 1992; 69(8): 2011–2020

[20] Gillenwater A, Papadimitrakopoulou V, Richards-Kortum R. Oral premalignancy: new methods of detection and treatment. Curr Oncol Rep. 2006; 8 (2):146–154

[21] Steele TO, Meyers A. Early detection of premalignant lesions and oral cancer. Otolaryngol Clin North Am. 2011; 44(1):221–229, vii

[22] Gentile E, Maio C, Romano A, Laino L, Lucchese A. The potential role of in vivo optical coherence tomography for evaluating oral soft tissue: a systematic review. J Oral Pathol Med. 2017; 46(10):864–876

[23] Lodi G, Franchini R, Warnakulasuriya S, et al. Interventions for treating oral leukoplakia to prevent oral cancer. Cochrane Database Syst Rev. 2016; 7: CD001829

[24] Novakovic D, Rickert S, Blitzer A. Office-based laser treatment of oral premalignant lesions. Operative Techniques in Otolaryngology.. 2011; 22:159–164

[25] Arnaoutakis D, Bishop J, Westra W, Califano JA. Recurrence patterns and management of oral cavity premalignant lesions. Oral Oncol. 2013; 49(8):814–817

[26] Biel MA. Photodynamic therapy in head and neck cancer. Curr Oncol Rep. 2002; 4(1):87–96

[27] Johnson JE, Ringsdorf WM, Jr, Cheraskin E. Relationship of vitamin A and oral leukoplakia. Arch Dermatol. 1963; 88(5):607–612

[28] Hong WK, Endicott J, Itri LM, et al. 13-cis-retinoic acid in the treatment of oral leukoplakia. N Engl J Med. 1986; 315(24):1501–1505

[29] William WN, Jr, Lee JJ, Lippman SM, et al. High-dose fenretinide in oral leukoplakia. Cancer Prev Res (Phila). 2009; 2(1):22–26

[30] Khuri FR, Lee JJ, Lippman SM, et al. Randomized phase III trial of low-dose isotretinoin for prevention of second primary tumors in stage I and II head and neck cancer patients. J Natl Cancer Inst. 2006; 98(7):441–450

[31] Kolesar JM, Hoel R, Pomplun M, et al. A pilot, first-in-human, pharmacokinetic study of 9cUAB30 in healthy volunteers. Cancer Prev Res (Phila). 2010; 3(12):1565–1570

[32] Wu X, Desai K-GH, Mallery SR, Holpuch AS, Phelps MP, Schwendeman SP. Mucoadhesive fenretinide patches for site-specific chemoprevention of oral cancer: enhancement of oral mucosal permeation of fenretinide by coincorporation of propylene glycol and menthol. Mol Pharm. 2012; 9(4):937–945

[33] Desai K-GH, Mallery SR, Holpuch AS, Schwendeman SP. Development and in vitro-in vivo evaluation of fenretinide-loaded oral mucoadhesive patches for site-specific chemoprevention of oral cancer. Pharm Res. 2011; 28(10):2599–2609

[34] Mulshine JL, Atkinson JC, Greer RO, et al. Randomized, double-blind, placebo-controlled phase IIb trial of the cyclooxygenase inhibitor ketorolac as an oral rinse in oropharyngeal leukoplakia. Clin Cancer Res. 2004; 10(5):1565–1573

[35] Papadimitrakopoulou VA, William WN, Jr, Dannenberg AJ, et al. Pilot randomized phase II study of celecoxib in oral premalignant lesions. Clin Cancer Res. 2008; 14(7):2095–2101

[36] Armstrong WB, Taylor TH, Kennedy AR, et al. Bowman Birk inhibitor concentrate and oral leukoplakia: a randomized phase IIb trial. Cancer Prev Res (Phila). 2013; 6(5):410–418

[37] Chang TH, Szabo E. Induction of differentiation and apoptosis by ligands of peroxisome proliferator-activated receptor gamma in non-small cell lung cancer. Cancer Res. 2000; 60(4):1129–1138

[38] Yoshida K, Hirose Y, Tanaka T, et al. Inhibitory effects of troglitazone, a peroxisome proliferator-activated receptor gamma ligand, in rat tongue carcinogenesis initiated with 4-nitroquinoline 1-oxide. Cancer Sci. 2003; 94(4):365–371

[39] Govindarajan R, Ratnasinghe L, Simmons DL, et al. Thiazolidinediones and the risk of lung, prostate, and colon cancer in patients with diabetes. J Clin Oncol. 2007; 25(12):1476–1481

[40] Vitale-Cross L, Molinolo AA, Martin D, et al. Metformin prevents the development of oral squamous cell carcinomas from carcinogen-induced premalignant lesions. Cancer Prev Res (Phila). 2012; 5(4):562–573

[41] Evans JMM, Donnelly LA, Emslie-Smith AM, Alessi DR, Morris AD. Metformin and reduced risk of cancer in diabetic patients. BMJ. 2005; 330(7503):1304–1305

[42] Gandini S, Puntoni M, Heckman-Stoddard BM, et al. Metformin and cancer risk and mortality: a systematic review and meta-analysis taking into account biases and confounders. Cancer Prev Res (Phila). 2014; 7(9):867–885

[43] Landman GWD, Kleefstra N, van Hateren KJ, Groenier KH, Gans RO, Bilo HJ. Metformin associated with lower cancer mortality in type 2 diabetes: ZODIAC-16. Diabetes Care. 2010; 33(2):322–326

[44] Hirsch HA, Iliopoulos D, Struhl K. Metformin inhibits the inflammatory response associated with cellular transformation and cancer stem cell growth. Proc Natl Acad Sci U S A. 2013; 110(3):972–977

[45] Zakikhani M, Dowling R, Fantus IG, Sonenberg N, Pollak M. Metformin is an AMP kinase-dependent growth inhibitor for breast cancer cells. Cancer Res. 2006; 66(21):10269–10273

[46] Li D, Yeung S-CJ, Hassan MM, Konopleva M, Abbruzzese JL. Antidiabetic therapies affect risk of pancreatic cancer. Gastroenterology. 2009; 137(2): 482–488

[47] Mallery SR, Tong M, Shumway BS, et al. Topical application of a mucoadhesive freeze-dried black raspberry gel induces clinical and histologic regression and reduces loss of heterozygosity events in premalignant oral intraepithelial lesions: results from a multicentered, placebo-controlled clinical trial. Clin Cancer Res. 2014; 20(7):1910–1924

[48] Mallery SR, Zwick JC, Pei P, et al. Topical application of a bioadhesive black raspberry gel modulates gene expression and reduces cyclooxygenase 2 protein in human premalignant oral lesions. Cancer Res. 2008; 68(12):4945–4957

[49] Ardito F, Perrone D, Giuliani M, Testa NF, Muzio LL. Effects of curcumin on squamous cell carcinoma of tongue: an in vitro study. Curr Top Med Chem. 2018; 18(3):233–243

[50] Kuriakose MA, Ramdas K, Dey B, et al. A randomized double-blind placebo-controlled phase IIB trial of curcumin in oral leukoplakia. Cancer Prev Res (Phila). 2016; 9(8):683–691

[51] Cheng AL, Hsu CH, Lin JK, et al. Phase I clinical trial of curcumin, a chemopreventive agent, in patients with high-risk or pre-malignant lesions. Anticancer Res. 2001; 21 4B:2895–2900

Index

Note: Page numbers set **bold** or *italic* indicate headings or figures, respectively.

D

E

M

N

O

S

T

U

V

W

X

Z